Fundamentals of
ORTHOPEDICS

Fundamentals of
ORHTOPEDICS

Second Edition

Mukul Mohindra MS (Orthopaedics) DNB MNAMS
Dip SICOT (Belgium) FNB (Arthroscopy and Sports Medicine)
Specialist
CGHS Specialist Wing and Central Institute of Orthopaedics
Vardhman Mahavir Medical College and Safdarjung Hospital
New Delhi, India

Jitesh Kumar Jain MS (Orthopaedics)
FNB (Arthroscopy and Sports Medicine)
Registrar
Institute of Orthopaedics and Traumatology
Sawai Man Singh Medical College
Jaipur, Rajasthan, India

Words of Wisdom

Deepak Chaudhary

Forewords

Ramesh Kumar
RC Meena
Himanshu Kataria

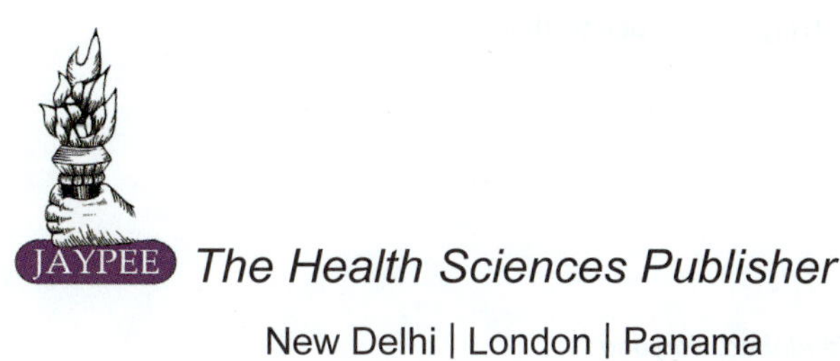

JAYPEE *The Health Sciences Publisher*

New Delhi | London | Panama

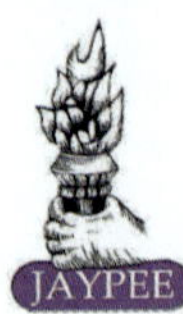 **Jaypee Brothers Medical Publishers (P) Ltd.**

Headquarters

Jaypee Brothers Medical Publishers (P) Ltd.
4838/24, Ansari Road, Daryaganj
New Delhi 110 002, India
Phone: +91-11-43574357
Fax: +91-11-43574314
E-mail: jaypee@jaypeebrothers.com

Overseas Offices

J.P. Medical Ltd.
83, Victoria Street, London
SW1H 0HW (UK)
Phone: +44 20 3170 8910
Fax: +44(0) 20 3008 6180
E-mail: info@jpmedpub.com

Jaypee Brothers Medical Publishers (P) Ltd.
17/1-B, Babar Road, Block-B, Shaymali
Mohammadpur, Dhaka-1207
Bangladesh
Mobile: +08801912003485
E-mail: jaypeedhaka@gmail.com

Jaypee Highlights Medical Publishers Inc.
City of Knowledge, Building 235, 2nd Floor
Clayton, Panama City, Panama
Phone: +1 507-301-0496
Fax: +1 507-301-0499
E-mail: cservice@jphmedical.com

Jaypee Brothers Medical Publishers (P) Ltd.
Bhotahity, Kathmandu, Nepal
Phone: +977-9741283608
E-mail: kathmandu@jaypeebrothers.com

Website: www.jaypeebrothers.com
Website: www.jaypeedigital.com

Fundamentals of Orthopedics

First Edition: 2016

Second Edition: **2018**

ISBN: 978-93-5270-132-2

Printed at Ajanta Offset & Packagings Ltd., Faridabad, Haryana.

Dedicated to

My mom and dad, for their blessings;
my wife Bhumika, for her unconditional love; and
my family, for always being there to my support.

—Mukul Mohindra

My parents, whose nurturing gave me
courage to dream; my wife Zeepee, who strengthened me
to realize my dreams; and, my brother Manish, who has
always been there, whenever I needed support.

—Jitesh Kumar Jain

Contributors

Ammar Aslam MS (Orthopaedics)
Assistant Professor
Department of Orthopaedics
Hamdard Institute of Medical Sciences
and Research
Jamia Hamdard University
New Delhi, India
(*Spondyloarthropathies*)

Ankit Thora MS (Orthopaedics) DNB
Consultant Orthopaedics and
Joint Replacement Specialist
Shalby Hospital
Indore, Madhya Pradesh, India
(*Electrodiagnostic Studies, Compression Neuropathies*)

Ankur Wadera MD (Radiodiagnosis) DNB
Consultant Radiologist
Deepak Hospital
New Delhi, India
(*Imaging in Orthopedics*)

Anurag Tiwari MS (Orthopaedics) DNB
Assistant Professor
Department of Orthopaedics
All India Institute of Medical Sciences
Bhopal, Madhya Pradesh, India
(*Osteomyelitis and Septic Arthritis and Skeletal Tuberculosis*)

Ashish Rana Dip Orthopaedics DNB (Ortho)
Consultant Orthopaedics and
Joint Replacement Specialist
NIMS University
Jaipur, Rajasthan, India
(*Rickets and Osteomalacia*)

Balaji Sambandam MS (Orthopaedics) DNB
Assistant Professor
Department of Orthopaedics
Sri Manakula Vinayagar Medical College
and Hospital, Puducherry, India
(*Injuries around Ankle, Orthopedic Instruments and Implants*)

Milind Tanwar MS (Orthopaedics)
Senior Resident
Sports Injury Centre
Vardhman Mahavir Medical College and
Safdarjung Hospital, New Delhi, India
(*Amputations, Orthotics and Prosthotics Splints and Tractions*)

Paritosh Gogna MS (Orthopaedics) DNB
Dip SICOT (Belgium)
Consultant Orthopaedics
Artemis Hospitals
Gurugram, Haryana, India
(*Ligament Injuries of Knee,
Latest Trends in Orthopedic Surgery*)

RC Meena MS (Orthopaedics)
Head of the Department
Institute of Orthopaedics and Traumatology
Sawai Man Singh Medical College
Jaipur, Rajasthan, India
(*Management of Polytrauma Patients*)

RL Dayma MS (Orthopaedics)
Professor
Institute of Orthopaedics and Traumatology
Sawai Man Singh Medical College
Jaipur, Rajasthan, India
(*Upper Limb Traumatology*)

Ruchi Dudeja MD (Paediatrics)
Consultant Paediatrician and Neonatologist
Krishna Medicare Centre
Gurugram, Haryana, India
(*Skeletal Dysplasias*)

Sahil Batra MS (Orthopaedics) DNB FNB (Spine)
Consultant Spine Surgeon
Caremax Superspeciality Hospital
Jalandhar, Punjab, India
(*Spinal Injuries*)

Sahil Gaba MS (Orthopaedics)
Senior Resident
Department of Orthopaedics
All India Institute of Medical Sciences
New Delhi, India
(*Pediatric Orthopedics*)

Saurabh Agarwal MS (Orthopaedics)
Consultant Orthopaedics
Indraprastha Apollo Hospital
New Delhi, India
(*Anatomy and Composition of Bone
and Bone Growth*)

Shivali Arya MBBS
Maulana Azad Medical College
New Delhi, India
(*Sketches*)

Simran Kaur MBBS
Pandit Bhagwat Dayal Sharma University
of Health Sciences
Rohtak, Haryana, India
(*Multiple Myeloma and Soft Tissue Sarcomas,
Osteoporosis*)

Words of Wisdom

'Hard work beats talent when talent fails to work hard, is a universal truth. The master key to success is determination, to do that extra bit and to go that extra mile. But effort should always be well disciplined. Discipline means persistence and perseverance—the ability to continue through bad times, obstacles and problems in a competent manner. This book is a diligent effort by a team of people to share the knowledge and experience they gained over the sleepless nights of hard work to give you the best. So, get set to reach your goals with a mentor to guide, and steer yourself through till you reach what you deserve.

Always remember the **6Ps** that demarcate the bridge between mediocrity and excellence.

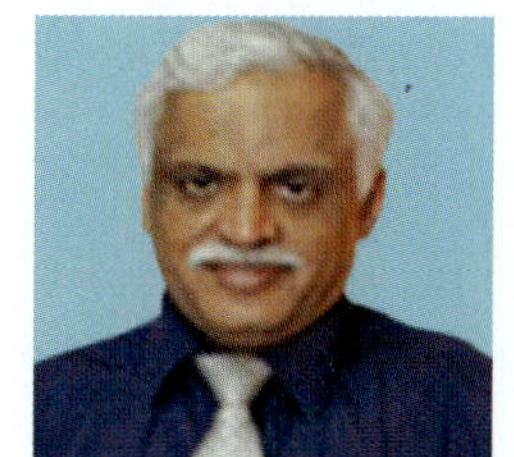

Proper

Prior

Planning

Prevents

Poor

Performance

Deepak Chaudhary
Director
Sports Injury Centre
Vardhman Mahavir Medical College
and Safdarjung Hospital
New Delhi, India

Foreword

In today's world, where each of us wants to contribute his/her share towards having a healthy and better life, this book does complete justice. It has covered all the basic and advanced topics in the minutest of details, while maintaining the length to an extent as not to lose interest of the reader. The pictorial insets are the catchpoints to explain the synonyms used, in the best possible manner making the related topic not only interesting but also enhancing the visual memory.

The simplicity of the words is a complete feast for the reader. It is a must read not only for undergraduates but also for those pursuing higher studies. The entire effort makes the subject simplified, interesting, reproducible and applicable, getting the best out of you, for you and your patients. I congratulate the authors and offer my best wishes!

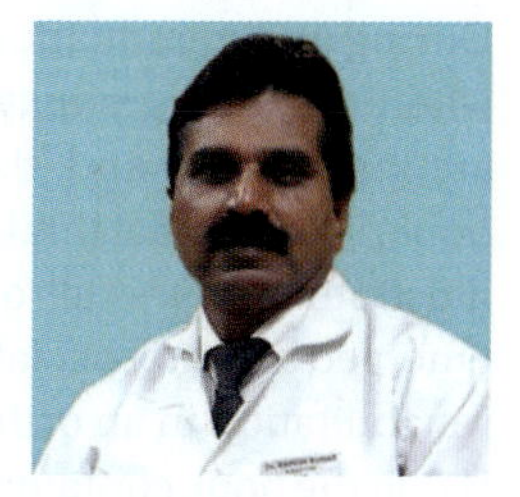

Ramesh Kumar
Director
Central Institute of Orthopaedics
Vardhman Mahavir Medical College
and Safdarjung Hospital
New Delhi, India

Foreword

During undergraduation, orthopedics is one among the least read subjects and this is such a specialty in India, where the undergraduates and postgraduates read different books as most of the books meant for undergraduates are insufficient; and, those for postgraduates, are indigestible for undergraduates. After going through this book, I believe that this is a fine balance between undergraduate and postgraduate teachings. It is an extensively illustrated book—full of diagrams, X-rays, flow charts and high-yield points. Of late, sports medicine has emerged as a subspecialty of orthopedics, and I am happy to see a separate chapter on sports injuries and their rehabilitation in an orthopedic textbook for undergraduates. What makes it desirable for all medical students is that the book contains so much updated information, and covers all important and rare topics of orthopedics that the students will not require any other book for preparation of their postgraduate entrance examination. I wish all the best to the authors!

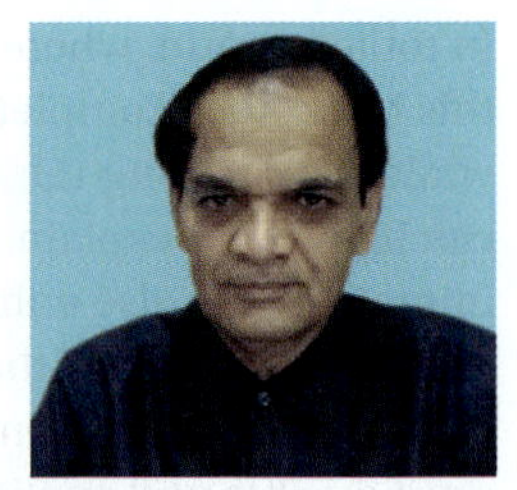

RC Meena
Head of the Department
Institute of Orthopaedics and Traumatology
Sawai Man Singh Medical College
Jaipur, Rajasthan, India

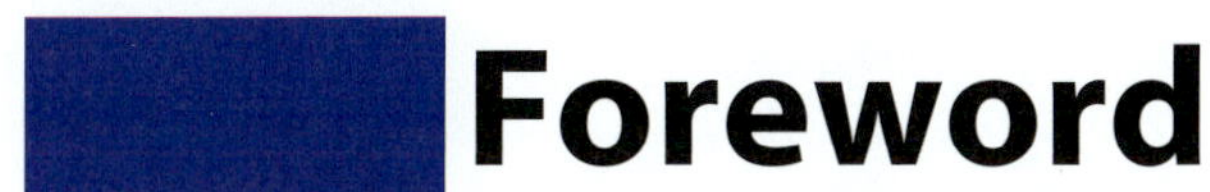

Foreword

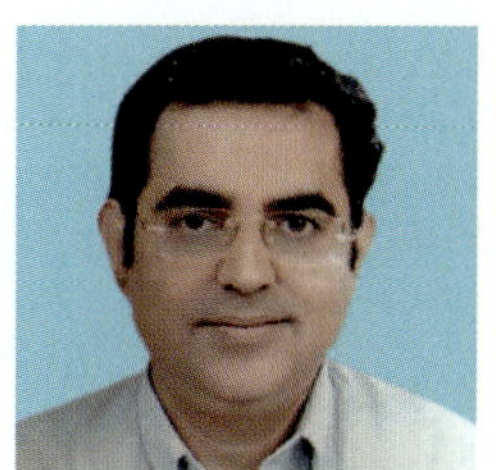

Teaching methodology and orthopedics course curriculum have undergone plethora of changes in the past decade. The quantum jump in orthopedic technology witnessed in diagnosis and management of various orthopedic pathologies and procedures calls for a compact reading material, which keeps pace with the change.

Fundamentals of Orthopedics by Drs Mukul Mohindra and Jitesh Kumar Jain has narratively and comprehensively explained the basic concepts, diagnosis and management of key orthopedic conditions, which the undergraduates must know as a part of their MBBS curriculum. The inclusion of excellent X-rays, clinical photographs and box depictions, besides elaborating high-yield points after each relevant pathology or concept, are highly informative, with an eye on postgraduate entrance examination.

Having gone through a few chapters, I am fully convinced that this book with its lucidity and in-depth elaboration of orthopedic pathologies, will be an asset to every undergraduate student.

Drs Mukul Mohindra and Jitesh Kumar Jain have worked with me at the Sports Injury Centre, Vardhman Mahavir Medical College and Safdarjung Hospital, New Delhi, India, and have an amazing clarity of clinical foundations of orthopedics. I strongly feel that the book is a must on the shelf of every undergraduate student of medicine. I am sure that the authors will further justify every subsequent edition, keeping in mind the fast-changing orthopedic technology.

I wish the book and the authors all success in furthering the knowledge of orthopedics among the undergraduate students.

Himanshu Kataria
Professor
Sports Injury Centre
Vardhman Mahavir Medical College
and Safdarjung Hospital
New Delhi, India

Preface

'When the going gets tough, the tough gets going'. This perspective well holds its worth in today's era where the examination system has undergone a paradigm shift. To keep pace with the growing expectations of the varied examiners, what is required from a medical student, today, is extreme versatility. Not only it is important to acquire sound principles to attempt the subjective papers and pass the clinical examinations, but it is also equally mandatory to build an elaborative knowledge bank that is accurate and up-to-date with the current trends to score well in the objective examinations. This book is just a perfect answer to this tough task that time has posed to a medical aspirant.

The book has been written to offer an all-in-one package to conquer every version of the examination system. The information given in the book is elaborate yet it is concise and to the point. Latest trends in the field have well been addressed by addition of units such as Sports Injuries and their Rehabilitation. A number of contributors have shared their knowledge and concepts to ensure the material delivered is highly accurate. Considering the paucity of time that lies with an aspirant, the contributors have especially worked hard to ensure complete delivery of the material in topics such as polytrauma management, arthritis, metabolic bone diseases, spinal injuries, etc. that lie sandwiched between orthopedics and other branches.

Since we have been actively involved in teaching for many years, we were well versed with the changing recent trends. All topics have an incredible touch of simplicity yet they are comprehensive. An amazing feature of the book is the vast collection of images. Almost every clinical sign, clinical test, radiological sign, an instrument or an implant has been depicted in the form of a well-labeled figure. Similes have been drawn to enable clear and easier understanding of all fancy signs in the subject—an idea that is first of its kind. We remember well our times as undergraduates when looking at them we would ponder as what to look for. We are hopeful that this addition will not only enhance the practical skills of the readers but also help them steer through the increasing image-based puzzles being put up to them in the online versions. The book features the first-ever introduced image-based quiz section to help to understand the matter.

Keeping in mind the objective entrance pattern, well-sorted statements have been added at the end of all topics as 'High-yield Points' to facilitate answering the multiple choice questions. We have not only ensured that nothing is missed but also confirmed that information is highly accurate, for we understand well enough the worth every single correct answer holds in shaping your future.

When we sit back and share memories of times we used to prepare, we would often smile together at some common moments—that around 20 different subjects and all to be mastered for just one exam. It is indeed a herculean task for which we have jotted an excellent and well-organized Synopsis of Orthopedics with efforts that spanned over sleepless nights. This chapter has all that you need to brush up a day before the examination when the adrenaline rush is high but the brain glucose is low.

'All is well that ends well', a quote that needs no description. So to ensure the end is just not dump, rather just perfect, a smartly prepared MCQs collection comprising both controversial and non-controversial questions from all recent examinations have been sorted and jotted to rightly make this edition an "All-in-One" book. These MCQs are just the perfect feast for the hungry PG aspirants.

And, to sum up, we will share with you a quote well said, "You seldom improve when you have no role models but yourself to copy." This book has been written to give you just a perfect mentor that will teach you sound principles and practices of orthopedics, make you versatile to an extent the trend demands, and simply make you the best what you really deserve to be, for you have proven you are different from the lot by choosing a profession that is one of the most noble ones.

Mukul Mohindra
Jitesh Kumar Jain

Acknowledgments

"Where there is will, there is a way and to steer you through that way, there are always these hands disguised as teachers, colleagues, juniors and friends." To accomplish the herculean task of concisely and comprehensively compiling the knowledge yet keeping it simple to understand and memorize, there were so many brains and hands working day and night selflessly behind the stage. This book was a dream project started and thought by us but a long list of people got involved along, in one way or the other. It is our pleasure to acknowledge them, though their support and our gratitude cannot be justified by these words, and it is not a single word of exaggeration to say that this project would have not reached its final destination, had these people not been the silent and the strongest pillars.

Our journey kickstarted in Sports Injury Centre, Vardhman Mahavir Medical College and Safdarjung Hospital, New Delhi, India, where the thought of this venture first striked. It was the vision of our Director, Dr Deepak Chaudhary, who motivated us to step forward. Problems unfolded as we traveled the path but the guidance and blessings by our teachers Dr Himanshu Kataria, Dr Deepak Joshi and Dr Vineet Jain helped us pave our way through. Drs Ankit Goyal, Nitin Mehta, Pallav Mishra, Himanshu Gupta, Ajay Lal, Vivek Shankar and Ashutosh Jha were all a source of motivation whenever we got into any dilemma. Our co-fellows, Drs Mohd Shafi Bhat, Navdeep, Naveen MG, Lalit Bafna, and our colleagues Drs Darsh Goyal, Rahul, Manoj Arya, Shiv Chouksey, Parth Chaudhary, Sanjay Ramavat, Rakesh Daripa, Himanshu Bhargava, Brahma Prakash, Pawan Sharma, Utkarsh, Atul Mahajan, Pankaj, Sunny, Rajat, Prashant, Sunil, Mukul Mittal, Sushmita, Rafat, and Shikha, all deserve special thanks for sharing our load of responsibilities and taking over the work so that we could give our best.

I, Dr Mukul Mohindra, would take this pleasure to thank my teachers whom I owe what I am today. Orthopedics for me started with Dr Mohammed Yamin, Head, Department of Orthopaedics, Dayanand Medical College and Hospital, Ludhiana, Punjab, India, and other mentors from the institute, to name a few, Drs Rajoo Singh Chhina, Sandeep Puri, Hemlata Badyal, Sunil Juneja, Harpal Singh Selhi, Rajneesh Garg, Poonam Singh, Lily Walia, Jagjiv Sharma, Alka Dogra, Bajwa, Hitant Vohra, Deepinder Chhina, Sarit Sharma, and Harpreet Puri, who made me worth to a level that I could make it my choice. The Department of Orthopaedics, Pandit Bhagwat Dayal Sharma Post Graduate Institute of Medical Sciences, Rohtak, Haryana, India, carved a stone which had no meaning into a well-shaped, knowledgeable youth well deserved to serve. I am short of words to thank Dr SS Sangwan (Professor) (former Vice-Chancellor, University of Health Sciences, Rohtak) who was not just my guide but my mentor and Senior Dr RC Siwach (Professor) and Dr NK Magu (Professor) for they have always been my role models. I also offer my thanks to Drs ZS Kundu, A Devgun, Roop Singh, R Gupta, R Rohilla, Pradeep Kamboj, Amit Batra, Vineet Verma, Sanjay Arora, and Gaurav Saini for getting the right concepts and the right surgical skills into me. I would be failing in my duty if I do not thank my teachers at Maulana Azad Medical College, New Delhi, Drs VK Gautam (Professor), AK Dhal, AK Gupta, Lalit Maini, Vinod Kumar, Manoj, Sumit Sural, and Dhananjay Sabat, who gave me the space to grow and allowed my skills to flourish. I am also thankful for the constant support provided by Dr Ramesh Kumar, Director, Central Institute of Orthopaedics and also the faculty and seniors at Vardhman Mahavir Medical College and Safdurjung Hospital from various specialties, Drs R Wadhwa, SP Singh, Shayama Gupta, BP Sharma, LG Krishna, RK Chopra, Vikas Gupta, R Beniwal, Hitesh Lal, Ashish Jainum, Sandeep Shaina, Anurag Jain, SK Pandey, and Ankit Ruhella. Equally supportive were my colleagues and junior Drs Sahu, Heemendra, Amit, Ashwani, Ratish, and Pankaj. No point of missing Dr George Macheras and his team who provided me the golden opportunity to train at KAT Hospital, Athens, Greece, and sharpen my concepts on joint replacement surgeries. I would also extend my thanks to my motivators Dr Mukesh Bhatia and Dr Sumer Sethi. Last but not least, my friends for being physical, emotional and professional pillars to hold on to whenever I needed them, Drs Kamal Bali, Rishav Gupta, Dickey Richard, Ashwani Singh, Chandan Jasrotia, Vikas Kataria, Kulbhushan Kamboj, Rohit Singla, Milind Tanwar, Vivek Bansal, Anish Aggarwalla, Tushar Mehta, and Pritish Singh. Thank you is a very petite word to express my heartfelt gratitude for that every moment you invested in me and trusted me and my decisions.

Prima facie, I, Dr Jitesh Kumar Jain, would be grateful to Lord Mahavira and Shiva for catering me good mental and physical health that made timely completion of this book possible. I owe my success to Department of Orthopaedics, Jawaharlal Nehru Medical College, Aligarh, Uttar Pradesh, India, for sculpturing me into an orthopedic surgeon and shaping me into what I'm today. I would extend my gratitude to my teachers, Drs RC Meena (Professor), Mahesh Bansal (Professor), RL Dayma (Professor), SL Sharma (Professor), Anurag Dhakad (Professor), Ravinder Lamoria, Prashant Modi, Umesh Meena, Arun Sharma, Rajkumar (all from Swai Man Singh Medical College, Jaipur, Rajasthan, India), Professor M Zahid, MKA Sherwani (Professor), Mazhar Abbas (Professor), Naiyer Asif (Professor), AQ Khan, Lateef Z Jeelani, S Ahmad, Owais A Qureshi, Yasir S Siddqui, Zulfqar, Hatif, and Matloob Rehman (all from Jawaharlal Nehru Medical College and Hospital, Aligarh) for seeding in me the aptitude and the ethics of this field. I owe my practicing skills to my mentor Dr JVS Vidyasagar, Head of Department, Global Hospital, Hyderabad, Telangana, India, and Dr Rajeev K Sharma, Senior Consultant,

Indraprastha Apollo Hospital, New Delhi, India. I also thank my close inmates, Drs Sachin Khurana, Kushesh Gupta, Himanshu Gupta, and Varun Mittal for always being a backing to fall on. I would like to include a special note of thanks to my friend Nitesh Patni and Dr Praveen Sharma in encouraging me to start, endure and finally publish this book. I fail in my duty if I do not thank Drs Rahul Upadhyay, Vijay Yadav, Vaibhav Agarwal, Gaurav Deshwar, Divyansh, Mahaveer Mali, Rahul Temani, Rohit Kavishwer, Ashwini Kumar, Sheshkant, Amit Jain, Deepak Beniwal, Chandan, Jalaj, Jaskaran, Gaurav Gupta, Faizan, Ravish Chabra, Nitin Agarwal, Deepak Raghav, Sachin Ingole, Hiren Patel, and Matad Lokeshwaraiah Chetan for their valuable help and critical comments.

The contributors of this book deserve special thanks for their immense patience, hard work, time and energy they have put in. Despite their busy schedules, they stood by us to write the chapters comprehensively at a single call. Guys this project would never have been accomplished without your efforts. We also thank *Radiopedia.org. Learning Radiology.com*, The Radiology Assistant and Dr Charlie Goldburg (UCSD, California, US) for providing the image banks that has made this book different and unique.

Last but not least, we extend our thanks to our little artist Dr Shivali Arya, for her amazing sketches that gave real shapes to our weird ideas and words and to Ms Ritu, Ms Preeti and the staff at Sports Injury Centre, who helped us even beyond the working hours. We sincerely thank M/s Jaypee Brothers Medical Publishers (P) Ltd, New Delhi, India, and their wonderful team for accepting our work and making sincere efforts to let our work come down to reality.

Contents

Introduction to Orthopedics

ORTHOPEDICS—HISTORY AND EVOLUTION

INTRODUCTION

It will be interesting to know that orthopedics was born as a specialty for correcting deformities in children. In 1741 Nicolas Andry **(Fig. 1.1)** coined the word "orthopaedics", which was derived from Greek words for "correct" or "straight" (orthos) and "child" (paidion). Both "orthopaedics" and "orthopedics" are accepted spellings and in vogue worldwide. Until the end of 18th century, orthopedics was limited to correction of deformities in children and fracture treatment was largely restricted to traction, splints and bandages.

In 19th century, three landmark discoveries in this surgical field made surgeries safe, painless and enthusiastic. These were development of principles of antisepsis by Sir Joseph Lister **(Fig. 1.2)**, the discovery of ether anesthesia in 1846 by William Morton (1819–1868) and the invention of X-rays by Wilhelm Conrad Roentgen (1845–1923). Discovery of X-rays revolutionized the way of making a diagnosis in orthopedic cases. Another vital contribution which modernized the management of fractures was the invention of plaster of Paris (POP) bandage by Antonius Mathijsen in 1851. Thereafter, in 20th century the World Wars I and II contributed a lot to the development of core orthopedics by producing countless number of patients requiring amputation, debridement, fracture management, tendon surgeries, etc. In fact many great orthopedic surgeons were military surgeons like Sir Robert Jones, Gerhard Küntscher, and Antonius Mathijsen. Today, the scope of orthopedics has extended way beyond fracture fixation and deformity correction and many subspecialty branches have emerged like spine surgery, orthopedic oncology, pediatric orthopedics, sports medicine, reconstructive orthopedics (joint replacement), etc.

SOME ORTHOPEDIC LEGENDS AND THEIR CONTRIBUTION

Galen (129–199 BC): Father of Sports Medicine. He is also credited with describing for the first time the use of longitudinal traction for reduction of overlapping bone fragments.

Nicolas Andry (1658–1742) (Fig. 1.1): He published the first book in orthopedics "L'Orthopedie" in 1741, which conferred him the title of "Father of Orthopedics". For correction of deformity of tibia he suggested bandaging the limb to an iron plate. His famous engraving **(Fig 1.3)** of the "crooked tree" published by him in his book soon became the symbol of orthopedics worldwide.

Percival Pott (1714–1788): Pott's fracture. Pott's paraplegia. In 1756, this great English surgeon sustained a broken leg after fall from his horse. It was assumed that he had sustained a bimalleolar fracture so it began to be called Pott's fracture but in reality he had sustained a much serious open fracture of tibia.

Jean-André Venel (1740–1791): He is considered by some as "Father of Orthopedics". He established the first orthopedics institute in the world in Switzerland.

Hugh Owen Thomas (1834–1891): He devised the popular Thomas splint and Thomas test for flexion deformity of the hip. He is also known as "Father of British Orthopedics".

James Paget (1814–1899): He was the great English surgeon-cum-pathologist who is best known for his contributions, viz. Paget's disease of bone and Paget's disease of nipple. He popularized the term "Fracture disease" to refer to stiffness that occurs following conservative treatment of fractures. He was also

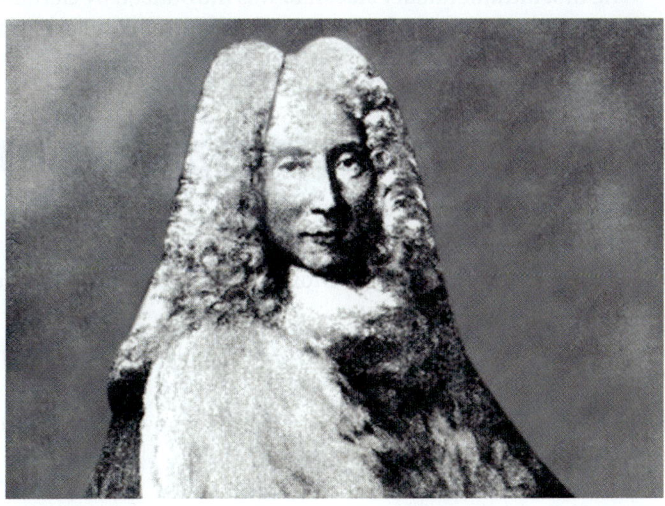

Fig. 1.1: Nicolas Andry (1658–1742)

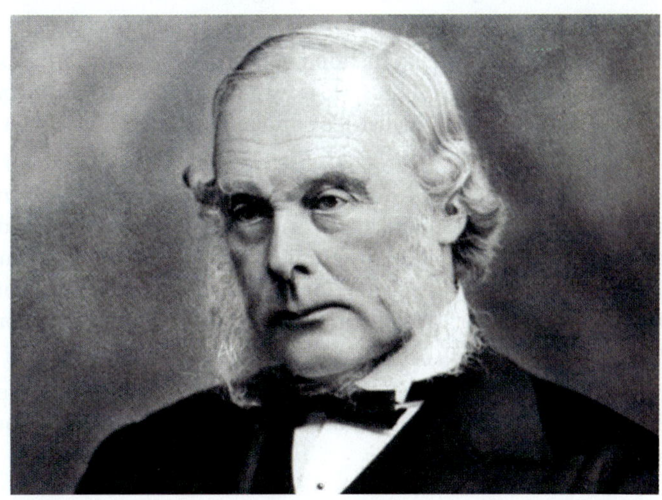

Fig. 1.2: Sir Joseph Lister (1827–1912)

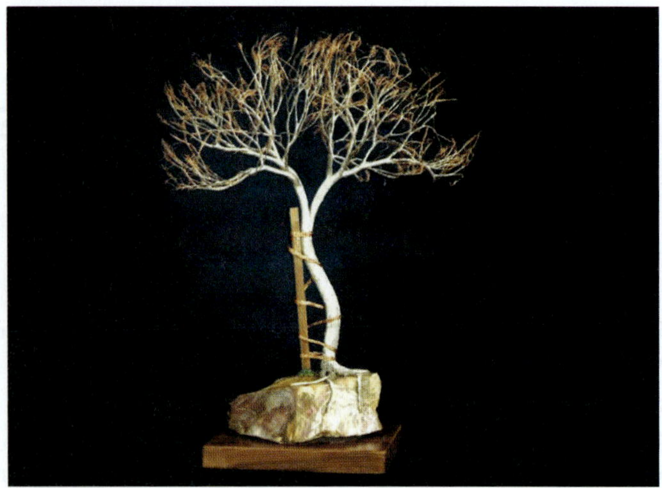

Fig. 1.3: Famous engraving of "Crooked tree" from the book of Nicolas Andry

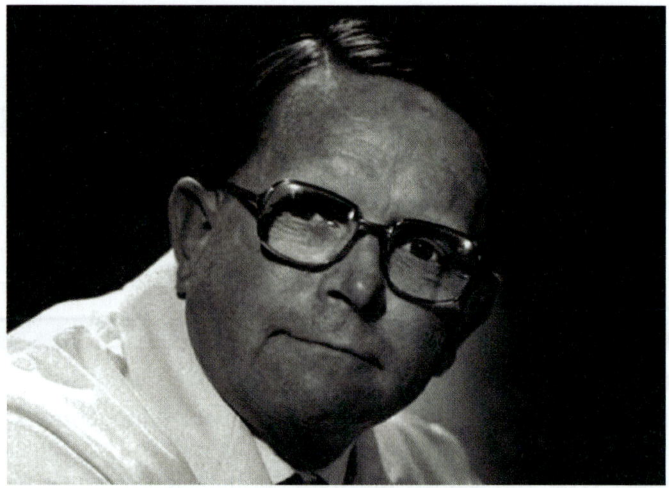

Fig. 1.4: Sir John Charnley (1911–1982)

the first to describe "Carpal Tunnel Syndrome" in 1854 although the term was coined by Moersch later in 1938.

Robert Jones (1857–1933): He was the nephew of great Hugh Owen Thomas. He is known as "Father of Modern Orthopedics". He described the Jones fracture and the Robert Jones bandage. He published first report of use of X-rays in orthopedics.

Albin Lambotte (1866–1955): Belgian surgeon, coined the term "osteosynthesis" meaning internal fixation and is regarded as the "Father of Modern Internal Fixation". He also devised the first modern external fixator and was first to describe the use of biodegradable implants.

Martin Kirschner (1879–1942): He contributed the very simple but the very useful "K wire" to orthopedics.

Lorenz Böhler (1885–1973): Father of Trauma Surgery.

Austin Moore (1899–1963): He performed the first metallic hip replacement. He designed the Austin-Moore prosthesis, which is still in use.

Gerhard Küntscher (1900–1972): His biggest contribution to orthopedics was the intramedullary nail which revolutionized the treatment of diaphyseal fractures of long bones.

Reginald Watson-Jones (1902–1972): He devised the Watson-Jones approach (anterolateral approach) to the hip joint. He was the student of Sir Robert Jones. He was the first editor of *Journal of Bone and Joint Surgery* (British), a popular journal on the subject.

Maurice E. Müller (1918–2009): He was a Swedish surgeon who was instrumental in the development of internal fixation techniques (fixation of fractures with metal implants placed inside the skin). In 1958 he co-founded "Arbeitsgemeinschaft fur Osteosynthesefragen" (German for "Association for the Study of Internal Fixation", or "AO", a popular organization that works for improving the standard of patient care in orthopedics.

Paul Randall Harrington (1911–1980): Harrington invented the Harrington rod, a device that is used during corrective surgery for scoliosis.

John Charnley (1911–1982) (Fig. 1.4): Father of Total Hip Arthroplasty. He was the great innovator of the modern total hip replacement and popularized the use of bone cement in total hip replacement.

Gavriil Abramovich Ilizarov (1921–1992): He gave the famous Ilizarov theory that bone would grow if gradually distracted. His work pioneered a new way of treating some of the most difficult cases in orthopedics, viz. infected nonunion, deformity correction and limb lengthening.

Kenji Takagi (1888–1963): Father of Arthroscopy. Takagi, a Japanese surgeon carried out the first successful arthroscopy of a joint (knee).

Masaki Watanabe (1911–1995): Father of Modern Arthroscopy. He performed the first arthroscopic partial meniscectomy.

William Enneking (1926–2014): Father of Orthopedic Oncology. He gave a classification system for bone tumors.

HIGH-YIELD POINTS

- Nicolas Andry is also called as the Father of Parasitology.
- The first intramedullary steel nail was introduced by Gerhard Küntscher. However, first interlocking intramedullary nail was performed by Modney and Bambara in 1953.
- First reamed intramedullary nailing was done by Fischer.

ORTHOPEDIC TERMINOLOGY

Abduction (Figs 1.5A to C):* Movement of limb away from the mid-sagittal plane of the body.

Adduction (Figs 1.5A to C):* Movement of limb toward the mid-sagittal plane of the body.

Ankylosis (Fig. 1.6A): Fusion of a joint due to a disease that causes abnormal adhesions between two joint surfaces.

Arthrocentesis: Joint aspiration (withdrawing synovial fluid/blood from the joint).

---

*Abduction and adduction movements occur in coronal plane of the body.

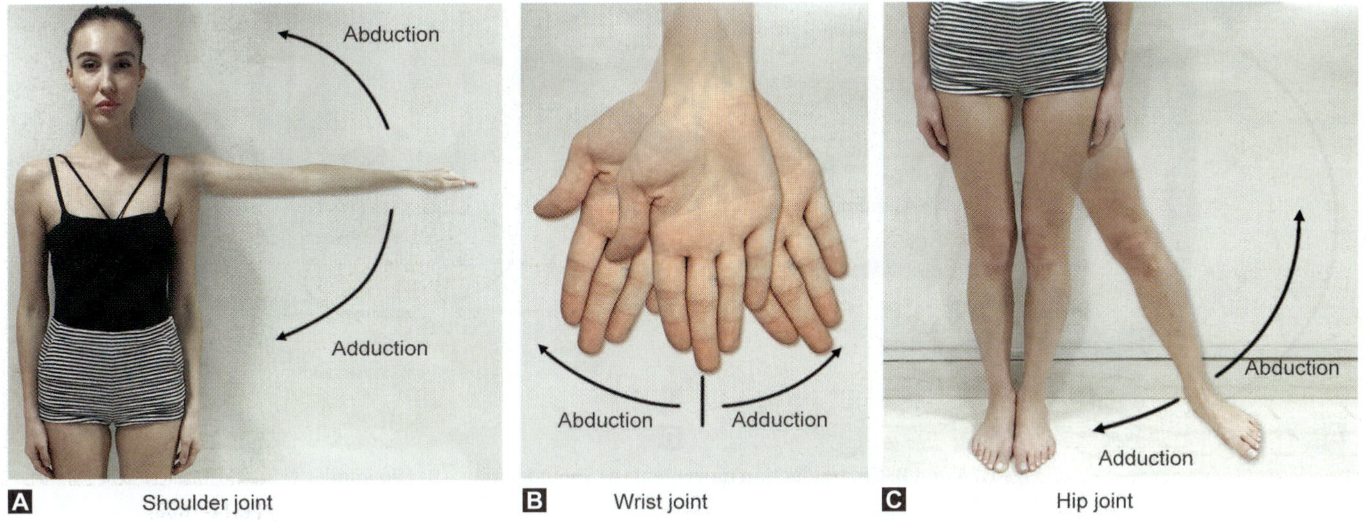

Figs 1.5A to C: Abduction and adduction movements

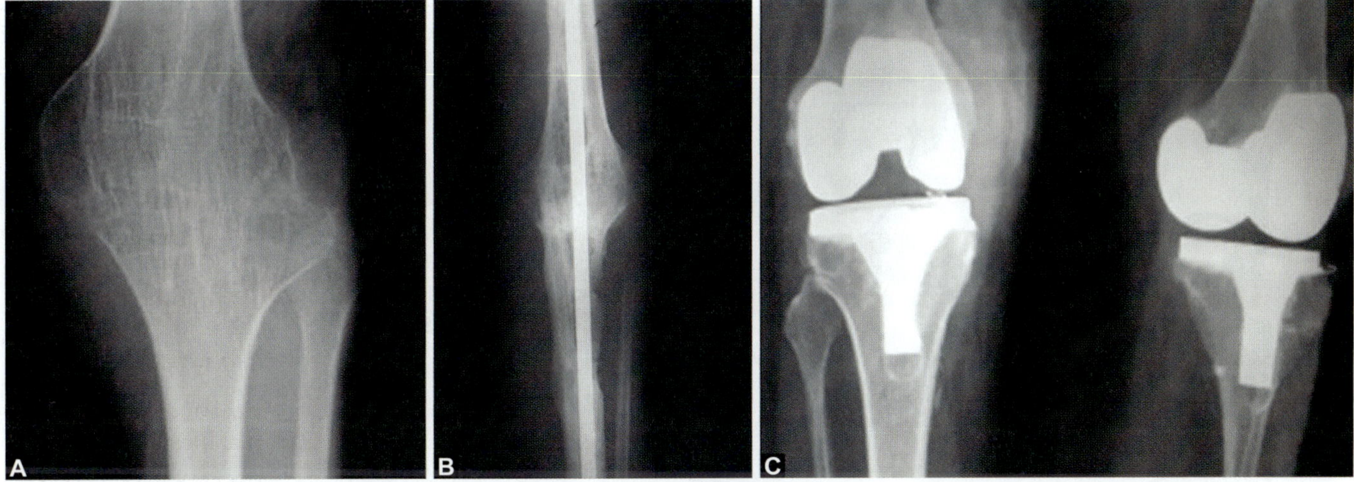

Figs 1.6A to C: X-rays of the knee showing (A) Ankylosis; (B) Arthrodesis; and (C) Arthroplasty (knee replacement)

Arthrodesis (Fig. 1.6B): Surgically-induced fusion of two joint surfaces.

Arthroeresis: It refers to an operation carried on a joint to restrict an undue mobility.

Arthrography: X-ray examination of joint after injecting contrast material (now largely been replaced by MRI).

Arthropathy: A disease of a joint.

Arthroplasty (Fig. 1.6C): Replacement of a joint with a prosthesis.

Arthrosis: Degenerative wear and tear of cartilage of the joint (osteoarthritis).

Arthrotomy: A procedure where surgeons cut into the joint (usually to drain pus from the joint).

Calcaneus: Deformity of ankle joint with the foot fixed in dorsiflexion.

Calcification: Deposition of amorphous (powdered/noncrystalline) calcium phosphate.

Cavus: Exaggeration of medial longitudinal arch of the foot.

Clonus: Successive, rhythmic and involuntary muscular contraction and relaxation (pathological hyperreflexia of normal deep tendon reflex). More than 5 beats are significant.

Chemonucleolysis: Injection of chymopapain (a proteolytic enzyme) into disc space to dissolve the disc (as a treatment of prolapsed disc).

Circumduction (Figs 1.7A and B): It is a combination of flexion, extension, abduction and adduction. In this movement, distal end of a limb makes a conical movement and the apex of the cone is at the proximal end of the limb.

Corticotomy: A surgery that involves cutting only the cotex of bone, leaving the meduallary vessels and periosteum intact. The bone may or may not be split into two pieces.

Coxa: Pertaining to the hip.

Cubitus: Pertaining to the elbow.

Dorsum: Upper/back surface of an animal/human (dorsal surface of the hand is the surface opposite the palm).

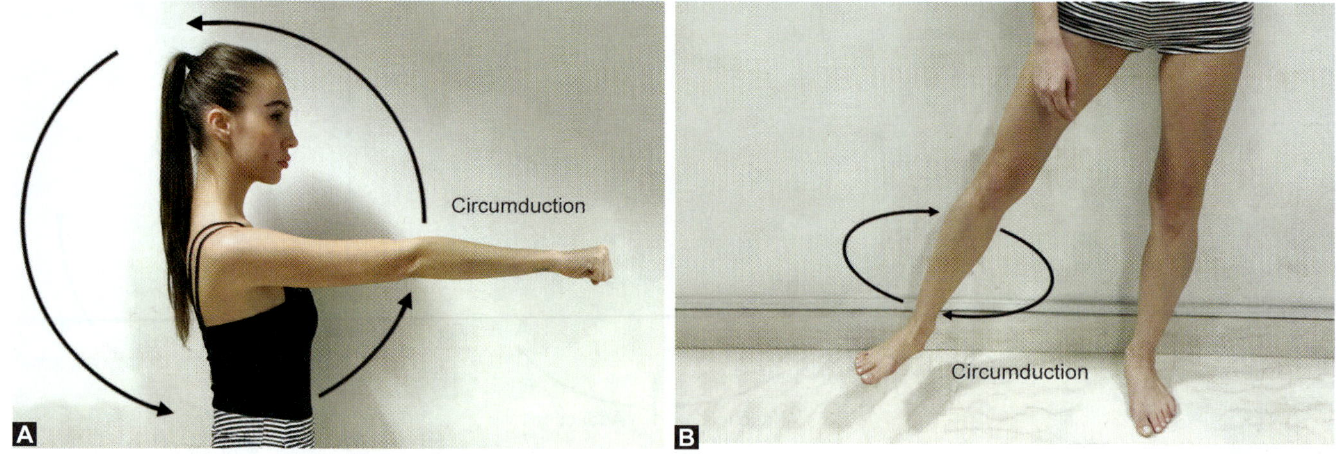

Figs 1.7A and B: Circumduction movement (A) Shoulder joint; (B) Hip joint

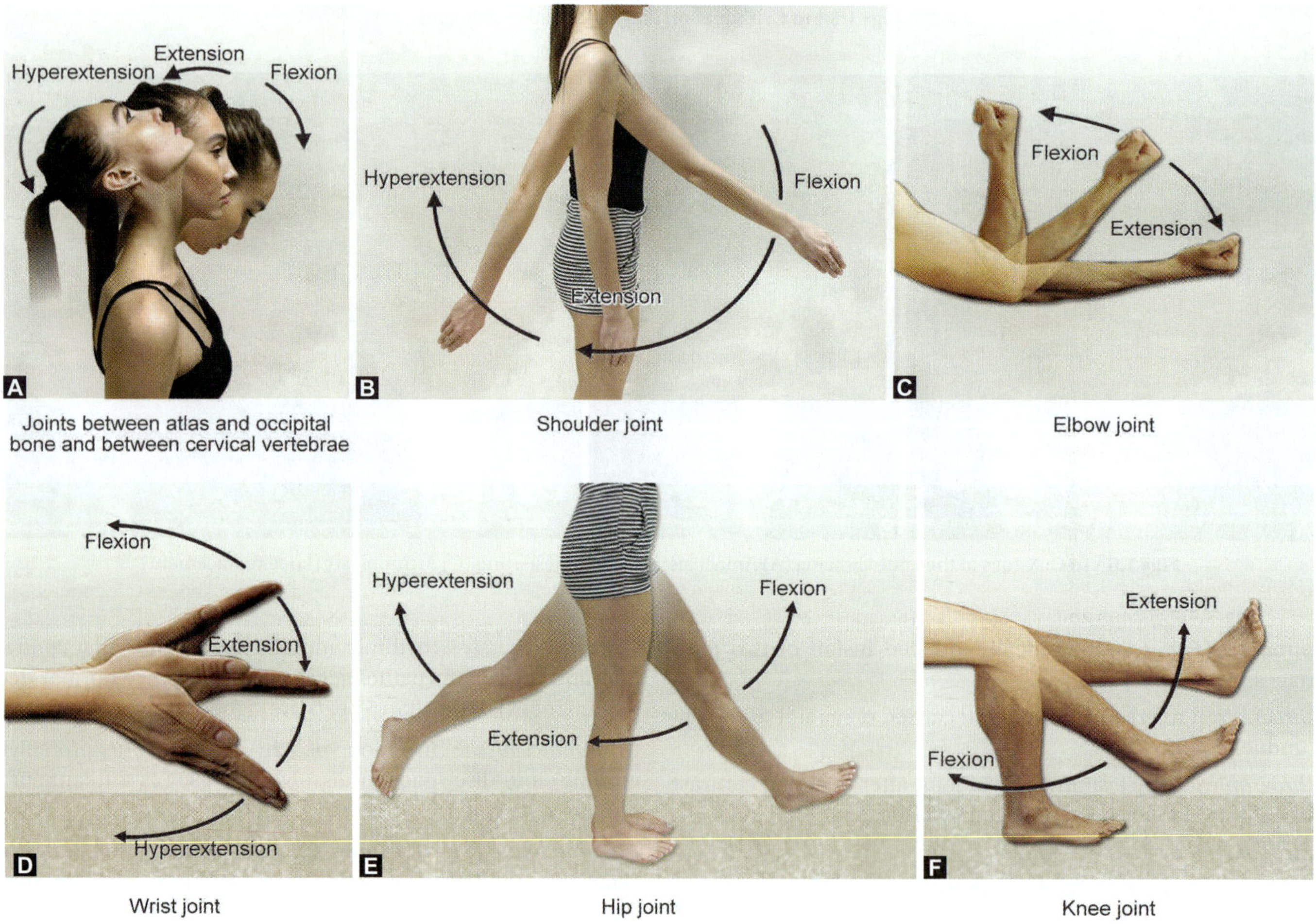

Figs 1.8A to F: Extension and flexion movements

Dislocation: Two joint surfaces loosing total contact with each other.

Epiphyseal plate/growth plate or physis: Hyaline cartilage present above the proximal metaphysis and below the distal metaphysis separating metaphysis from epiphysis.

Epiphysiodesis: Surgically-induced fusion of the epiphyseal plate or physis to metaphysis and/or epiphysis.

Equinus: Deformity of ankle joint with foot fixed in plantar flexion.

Extension (Figs 1.8A to F): Movement in sagittal plane, which increases the angle between two body parts.

Eversion (Fig. 1.9): Plantar surface (sole) of foot rotates away from mid-sagittal plane (can be called valgus).

Flexion (Figs 1.8A to F): Movement in sagittal plane, which decreases the angle between two body parts.

Genu: Pertaining to knee.

Hemarthrosis: Bleeding into the joint space.

Impacted fracture: When fracture fragments are driven into each other.

Interosseous membrane: A fibrous sheath that separates two bones (between two forearm bones or two leg bones).

Inversion **(Fig. 1.9):** Plantar surface of the foot (sole) rotates toward the mid-sagittal plane (can be called as varus).

Kyphosis: Normal backward convex curvature of spine in thoracic and sacral region.

Laminectomy: Removal of spinal lamina (usually to decompress the spinal cord or nerves).

Lordosis: Normal backward concave curvature of spine in cervical and lumbar region.

Laminotomy: Removal of a part of lamina.

Manus: Pertaining to the wrist.

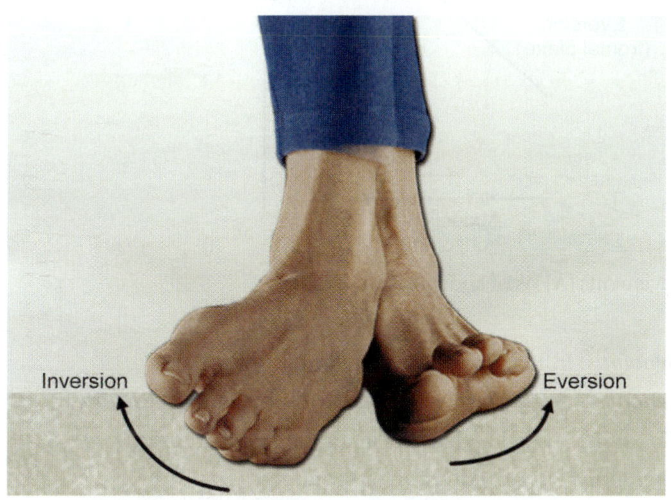

Fig. 1.9: Eversion and inversion movements of the foot

Myositis: Inflammation of the muscles.

Neurolysis: Interruption of the transmission of nerve signal (usually for pain relief) by application of physical agents (heat or freezing) or chemicals (such as phenol or alcohol) to a nerve.

Neurorraphy: Surgical suturing of a divided nerve.

Open reduction: Reduction of fracture fragments by surgical exposure and under direct vision. In open reduction fracture hematoma is drained.

Opposition (apposition) of thumb **(Fig. 1.10):** A movement unique to thumb in which thumb rotates around its long- axis and its palmar surface comes in contact with the palmar surface of little finger.

Orthotic: Orthotic is a device that aids/supports a body part and enhances the structural and functional characteristics of the skeletal system.

Ossification: Deposition of crystalline calcium phosphate to form new bone.

Osteoclasis: Surgically-induced fracture of the bone (to correct a bone deformity).

Osteogenesis: Bone formation.

Osteometric devices: Theses are used to measure bone length.

Osteonecrosis: Death of bone tissue.

Osteosynthesis: Stabilization and internal fixation of fracture.

Osteotomy: A surgical procedure in which bone is cut in order to correct deformity.

Plantar surface: Inferior surface of the foot, which comes in contact with the ground.

Plantaris: Equinus that occurs at the forefoot is called plantaris (forefoot fixed in plantarflexion).

Planus: Flattened medial longitudinal arch.

Pronation **(Figs 1.11A and B):** Rotation of the forearm and hand so that the palm faces downward. Pronation of foot is a combination of eversion, abduction and dorsiflexion.

Prosthesis: An artificial device that replaces a body part.

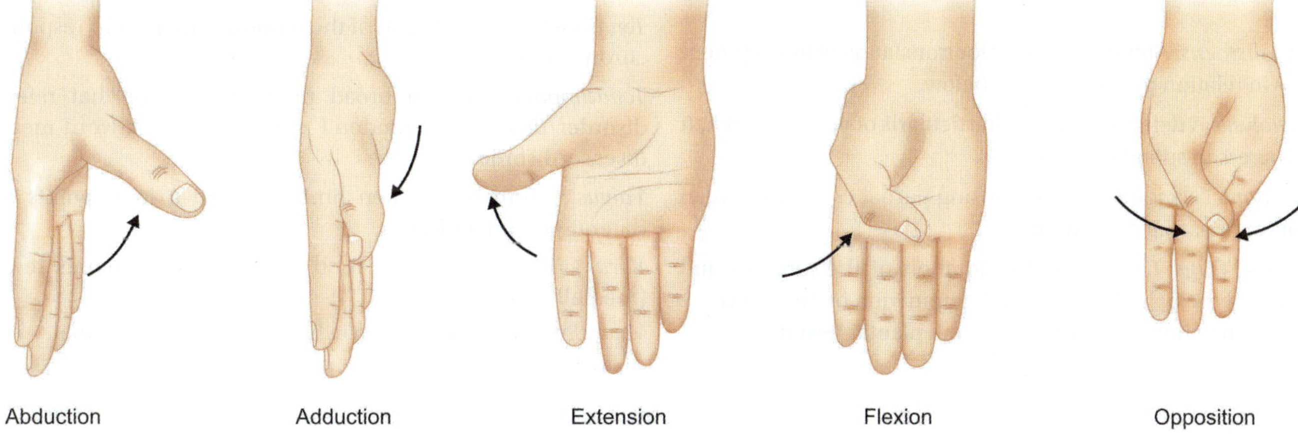

Fig. 1.10: Thumb movements

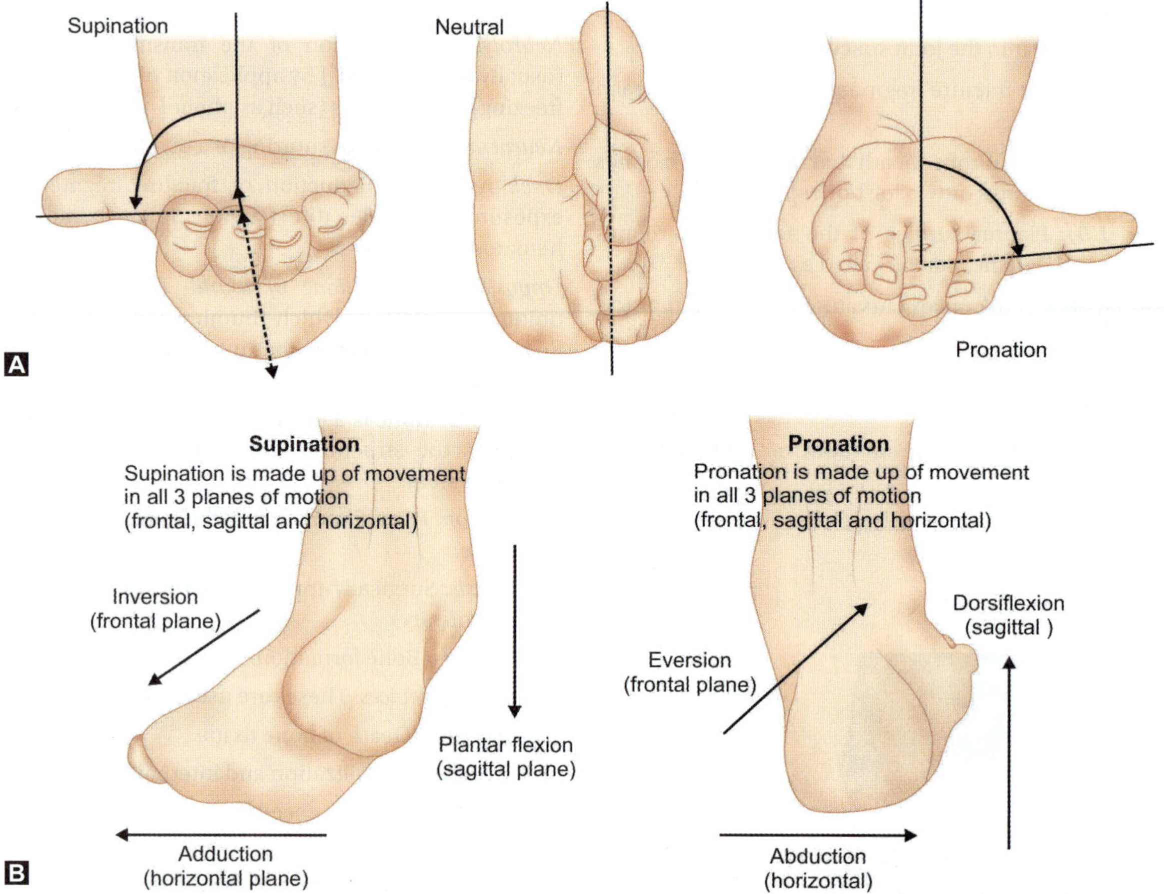

Figs 1.11A and B: Supination and pronation movements (A) Wrist and forearm; (B) Foot

Recurvatum: Excessive extension deformity of a joint (Genu Recurvatum is hyperextension deformity of knee joint, i.e. knee bends backwards). It is opposite to flexion deformity.

SLAP lesion: Tear of superior labrum in shoulder, from anterior to posterior aspect.

Spondylitis: Inflammation of vertebrae.

Spondylosis: An umbrella term that refers to degenerative changes in the spine, viz. bone spurs, degenerated intervertebral discs, etc.

Spondylolisthesis: Anterior or posterior translation of one segment of spine in relation to the vertebrae below.

Spondylolysis: A defect in pars-interarticularis of vertebral arch. It may progress to spondylolisthesis.

Subluxation: Two joint surfaces loosing partial contact between each other (a partial dislocation).

Supination (Figs 1.11A and B): Rotation of the forearm and hand so that the palm faces upward. Supination of the foot is the combination of inversion, adduction and plantar flexion.

Synovitis: Inflammation of synovium.

Tenodesis: Surgical suturing/anchoring of tendon to bone.

Tenolysis: Surgical release of a tendon from adhesions.

Tenotomy: Surgical division of a tendon.

Tenosynovitis (syn. tenovaginitis): Inflammation of a tendon and its surrounding sheath.

Tendonitis (syn. tendinitis): Inflammation of the tendon (an acute condition usually).

Tendinosis: Degeneration of the tendon's collagen in response to chronic overuse.

Tendinopathy: It is a broad nonspecific term that refers to disorder/disease of a tendon ("pathy" is a greek word meaning disease/disorder).

Valgus:* Term used when limb distal to a joint points away (laterally) from mid-line.

Varus:* Term used when limb distal to a joint points towards (medially) mid-line.

Volar: Pertaining to the palm in hand or the sole in the foot.

---

*Varus and valgus movements/deformities occur in coronal plane of the body and the terms can be used in context to any joint in the body. For example, if the limb distal to elbow points laterally, it is called cubitus valgus.

General Orthopedics

INTRODUCTION

The human skeleton is composed of 206 bones. It is divided into axial (80 bones) and appendicular (126 bones) parts. *Axial skeleton* consists of the skull, vertebral column and thoracic cage. *Appendicular skeleton* consists of shoulder girdle and upper limbs, pelvic girdle and lower limbs. While clavicle, scapulae and pelvis belong to appendicular skeleton; ossicles of the middle ear and the hyoid bone are categorized under the axial skeleton.

FUNCTIONS OF SKELETON SYSTEM

- Skeleton framework gives shape to the body and in coordination with muscles, it allows for the body movements.
- It protects vital organs. For example, rib cage provides protection for the lungs and skull provides protection to the brain.
- Bone is a storehouse of minerals, especially calcium and phosphorus and plays a vital role in the calcium metabolism (mineral homeostasis) in the body.
- In adults, flat bones such as pelvis, sternum, cranium, ribs, vertebra and scapulae contain the red bone marrow and are an important site of blood production.

STRUCTURE OF BONE

The basic unit of the skeletal system of the body is "bone". Bones along with ligaments and cartilage provide a strong yet flexible framework on which muscles attach through tendons to generate coordinated movements of the body.

Bones are made up of:
- Bone cells (osteoblast, osteoclast and osteocytes); and
- Intercellular matrix.

Bone Cells

There are three types of bone cells: (1) osteoblast (2) osteoclast and (3) osteocytes.

Osteoblasts

These are bone forming cells derived from mesenchymal precursors in the bone marrow. These are mononuclear cells, which have a well-developed rough endoplasmic reticulum and a large Golgi complex. They lay down new matrix which is known as osteoid (uncalcified matrix). These are rich in alkaline phosphatase and produce type I collagen and other noncollagenous bone proteins. Osteoblasts are activated by parathyroid hormone and they control osteoclastic activity (*see* Page 412, **Fig. 15.8**).

Osteocytes

These are terminally differentiated stage of osteoblasts. When osteoblasts become trapped in the matrix they secrete, they become osteocytes. Osteocytes are linked to each other via long cytoplasmic extensions called canaliculi, which are used for exchange of nutrients through gap junctions. Although osteocytes have reduced synthetic activity and (like osteoblasts) are not capable of mitotic division, they are actively involved in the routine turnover of bony matrix, through various mechanisms. They can also destroy bone through a rapid, transient mechanism (different from osteoclasts) called osteocytic osteolysis.

Osteoclasts

These are bone reabsorbing multinucleated giant cells derived from mononuclear precursors of macrophage lineage (specifically monocytes) in the marrow. These cells are activated by osteoblasts only upon appropriate signals (parathormone). Their main function is to resorb bone and are thus involved in bone remodeling. Active osteoclasts are present in excavations in bone formed by them after erosion of the matrix, the excavations being called as "Howship's lacunae" (lacunae means "pit").

Intercellular Matrix

Matrix consists of organic (biological) and inorganic (mineral) components. Organic component includes collagen fibers (mostly type I collagen). Inorganic matter is composed mainly of calcium and phosphorus in a crystalline form called "hydroxyapatite". Bone also contains other minerals in small amount, i.e. magnesium, potassium, strontium and ferrous salts, etc. Organic matter gives the bone its flexibility and elasticity while inorganic matter gives strength and hardness to the bone. Bones are densest tissue in the body due to deposition of minerals in the intercellular matrix.

Exact chemical composition of bone is given in **Box 2.1**.

TYPES OF BONES

Bones can be classified based on their macroscopic (anatomical) or microscopic structure or their maturity (**Table 2.1**).

Box 2.1: Chemical composition of bone (based on dry weight)

- *Bone cells:* Make up approximately 5%
- Intercellular matrix (95%)
    - *Inorganic matrix:* 65% (mainly calcium and phosphorus)
    - *Organic matrix:* 30% [80% of which is type I collagen with rest being noncollagenous proteins (osteocalcin/bone Gla protein, osteopontin, osteonectin and alkaline phosphatase)]

Table 2.1: Classification of bones

Based on anatomy	*Long*: Have length more than width, e.g. tubular bones of upper and lower limbs
	Short: Have width more than length, e.g. short bones of foot and hand (tarsals and carpals)
	Flat: These are bones expanded into flat plates, e.g. bones of the skull, pelvis, sternum, etc.
	Irregular: These have nonuniform shape and hence do not fall into any above category. These include facial bones, vertebrae and sacrum
	Sesamoid: Which is present within a tendon or a muscle, e.g. patella in quadriceps tendon and pisiform in flexor carpi ulnaris tendon
	Accessory bones: These are extra bones which have failed to fuse during development, e.g. accessary navicular
Based on microscopic structure	Cortical (compact) and cancellous (trabecular) bones
Based on maturity	Woven and lamellar bone

Classification based on Macroscopic Structure

Classification based on anatomy/macroscopic shape is a very commonly used mode of categorization. Based on macroscopic structure, bones can be long, short, flat, irregular, sesamoid and accessory. Long bone in a growing child can be divided into epiphysis, physis (growth plate/epiphyseal plate), metaphysis and diaphysis **(Fig. 2.1)**. In mature bone epiphysis fuses with metaphysis and growth plate gets replaced by bone (visible on X-ray as epiphyseal line). Few important facts about each of these parts are provided below.

Parts of a growing long bone:

- *Epiphysis*: Epiphysis is present on either ends of a long bone except the metacarpals, metatarsals and phalanges where it is present only at one end. It primarily consists of cancellous bone covered by a thin layer of compact bone. On its ends,

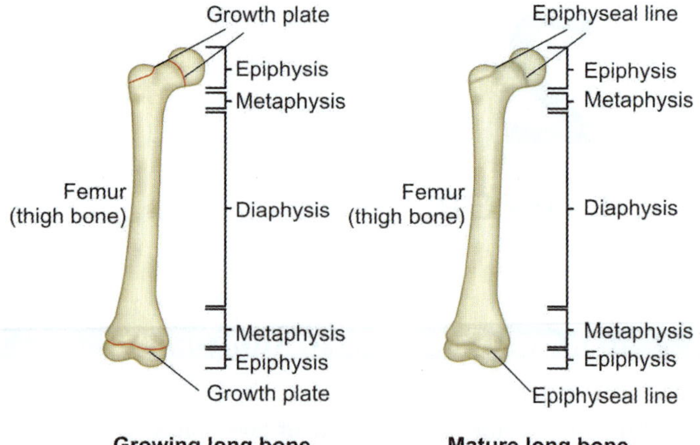

Fig. 2.1: Parts of growing and mature bone

it is covered by articular cartilage where it forms the joint. However, epiphyses at different sites in body can be grouped into different categories depending on primary function they perform as outlined below:

- *Pressure epiphysis*: They take part in joint formation and hence weight transmission, e.g. lower end of femur.
- *Traction epiphysis*: Their primarily provide attachments to muscles, e.g. tuberosities (humerus) and trochanters (femur).
- *Atavistic epiphysis*: These are phylogenetically independent but become fused in man., e.g. coracoid process of scapula.
- *Aberrant epiphysis*: These are epiphyses that are not always present, e.g. epiphysis at head of 1st metacarpal.
- *Physis*: Physis (growth plate/epiphyseal plate) is a thin region of actively growing bone cells between the epiphysis and the metaphysis in a growing bone. This is present on both the ends of the long bones and is responsible for the longitudinal growth of the bones (interstitial growth).

It consists of four zones **(Fig. 2.2)**:

- Germinal zone/Resting zone
- Proliferative zone

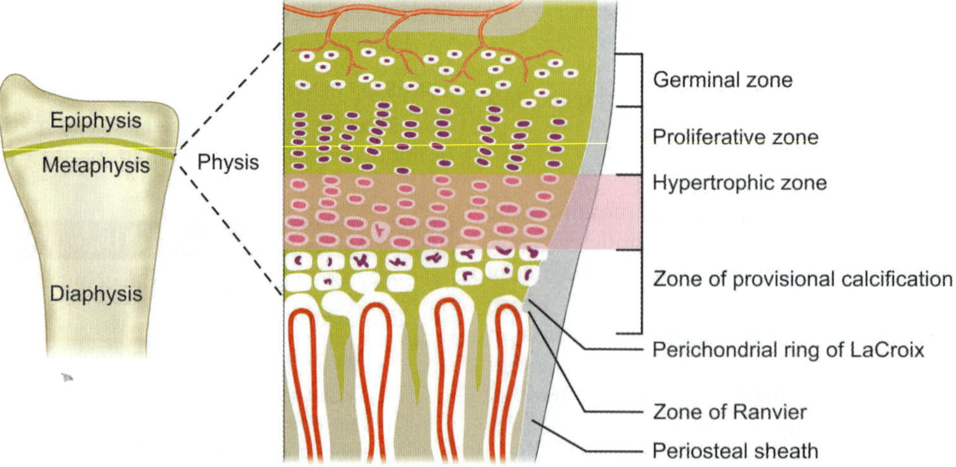

Fig. 2.2: Structure of physis (growth plate)

– Hypertrophic zone (maturation zone)
– Zone of provisional calcification (endochondral ossification).

Germinal zone provides the developing chondrocytes. These chondrocytes divide and get organized into columns in proliferative zone. In hypertrophic zone chondrocytes stop mitoses and undergo hypertrophy (increase in size). In the zone of provisional calcification apoptosis of chondrocytes and calcification of the cartilaginous matrix occurs. Since the hypertrophic zone has large sized cells lying loosely in scanty intercellular tissue, it is the weakest zone of physis. Hence, most physeal injuries occur through this plane. In Rickets, due to lack of calcification, cells accumulate in hypertrophic zone, resulting in weakened growth plates that eventually deform under body weight.

Physis is connected to the epiphysis and metaphysis by the zone of Ranvier and the perichondral ring of LaCroix. The zone of Ranvier contains germinal cells, which are responsible for the circumferential growth of the physis (appositional growth). Ring of LaCroix is a fibrous structure that connects the zone of Ranvier with the periosteum of the metaphysis thereby strengthening the metaphyseal-physeal interphase.

- *Metaphysis*: It is the part of the bone between the wide growth plate above and the narrow diaphysis below. It has abundant cancellous bone and hence fractures in this area exhibit excellent union properties owing to massive surface area and abundant vascularity of the cancellous bone.
- *Diaphysis*: It is the narrow region between the two metaphyses. It consists of compact cortical bone that provides strength needed for weight bearing and movement. It has a hollow medullary canal or cavity which harbors bone marrow and is surrounded all around by cortex. Cortex is lined on outside by a layer of dense connective tissue called as periosteum which is anchored to cortex by special fibers called as Sharpey's fibers. Periosteum is further comprised of two layers: (1) an outer fibrous layer that has abundant blood vessels and (2) an inner cambium layer that harbors osteogenic cells and has bone forming capabilities. During bone growth, the width of the bone increases (appositional growth) as osteoblasts in cambium layer lay new bone tissue at the periosteum. The inside of compact bone is lined by cancellous (spongy) bone that has an inside lining called endosteum, a cellular layer rich in osteogenic cells and osteoblasts. Bone formation is more than bone resorption on the periosteal surface and bone resorption is more than bone formation on the endosteal surface, so with aging bones normally increase in diameter and marrow spaces expand.

Classification based on Microscopic Structure

Based on microscopic structure bones can be classified into cortical (compact) or cancellous (spongy) types with the adult human skeleton having almost 80% cortical and 20% cancellous bone.

Cortical bone are the long bones of the body like the femur or humerus and the small bones of the hand and foot like metacarpals and metatarsals. Cortical bone **(Fig. 2.3)** consists of a number of columns of cells called "osteon". Each osteon has layers of bone cells (osteoblasts, osteocytes and osteoclasts arranged in a lamellar pattern) around a central canal called "Haversian canal". The outer border of an osteon is lined by a cement line which is a region of collagen-poor bone matrix. The Haversian canal surrounds the blood vessels and nerve cells throughout the bone and communicates with the osteocytes in the lacunae through canaliculi. "Volkmann's canals" run perpendicular to the "Haversian canals". They interconnect the Haversian canal with each other and with the periosteum and allow for the transfer of nutrients. Sharpey's fibers are type I collagen fibers that connect periosteum to bone and also help attaching muscles to bone.

Cancellous bone (trabecular or spongy bone) is dominant in small bones of the wrist, the bones of the hand and mid-foot like calcaneum and talus. The epiphyseal and metaphyseal areas of long bones, flat bones (pelvis, ribs, skull, etc.), and vertebrae are also cancellous bones. Cancellous bones are more porous, more vascular and have a much larger surface area than compact bone. They contain sheets (lamellae) of bone called "trabeculae" which interconnect to form open spaces giving a honeycomb appearance **(Fig. 2.4)**. Spaces between these trabeculae contain red or yellow marrow depending on person's age and which bone is it. Hence, spongy bone is important for production of blood cells.

Classification based on Maturity

Based on the development stage or maturity bone can be categorized into woven and lamellar types. Lamellar bone pattern is one that is present in normal adult compact as well as cancellous bones. Lamellar bone is stress oriented with a parallel arrangement of collagen fibers into sheets called lamellae **(Fig. 2.4)**. Woven bone is characterized by random organization of collagen fibers (as the name "woven" suggests) and is relatively a weak structure in comparison to lamellar bone that is mechanically stronger. It is immature bone which is not stress oriented. Woven bone pattern is present in all fetal bones and in the initial stages of fracture healing (later it gets replaced by lamellar bone). Woven bone is quickly produced and it has a high rate of turnover compared to lamellar bone.

BLOOD SUPPLY OF BONE

The skeleton receives approximately 5–10% of the cardiac output. A typical long bone derives its blood supply from nutrient artery, periosteal vessels and epiphyseal-metaphyseal vessels **(Fig. 2.5)**. Epiphyseal-metaphyseal regions are supplied by epiphyseal and metaphyseal vessels which are direct branches of periarticular blood vessels. The dominant supply comes from nutrient artery that enters the medullary canal, branches up and down and supplies the inner two-thirds of the cortices of the diaphysis and metaphysis. The periosteal vessels (present in the outer fibrous layer of the periosteum) mainly supply blood to the outer one-third of the cortex. If the nutrient artery is damaged (as in nailing a bone), periosteal vessels are usually sufficient to nourish the bone and when the periosteal vessels are damaged (as in plating a bone), the nutrient artery takes over.

HIGH-YIELD POINTS

- The largest internal organ in the body is skeletal muscles (639-840 muscles).
- Osteocytes are the most abundant (90%) and most long lived cells in the bone tissue.
- Osteocalcin is a protein that is exclusively produced by osteoblasts and hence a marker the detection of which is sufficient to label a structure as bone. Its concentration in the blood is a direct measure of osteoblastic activity.

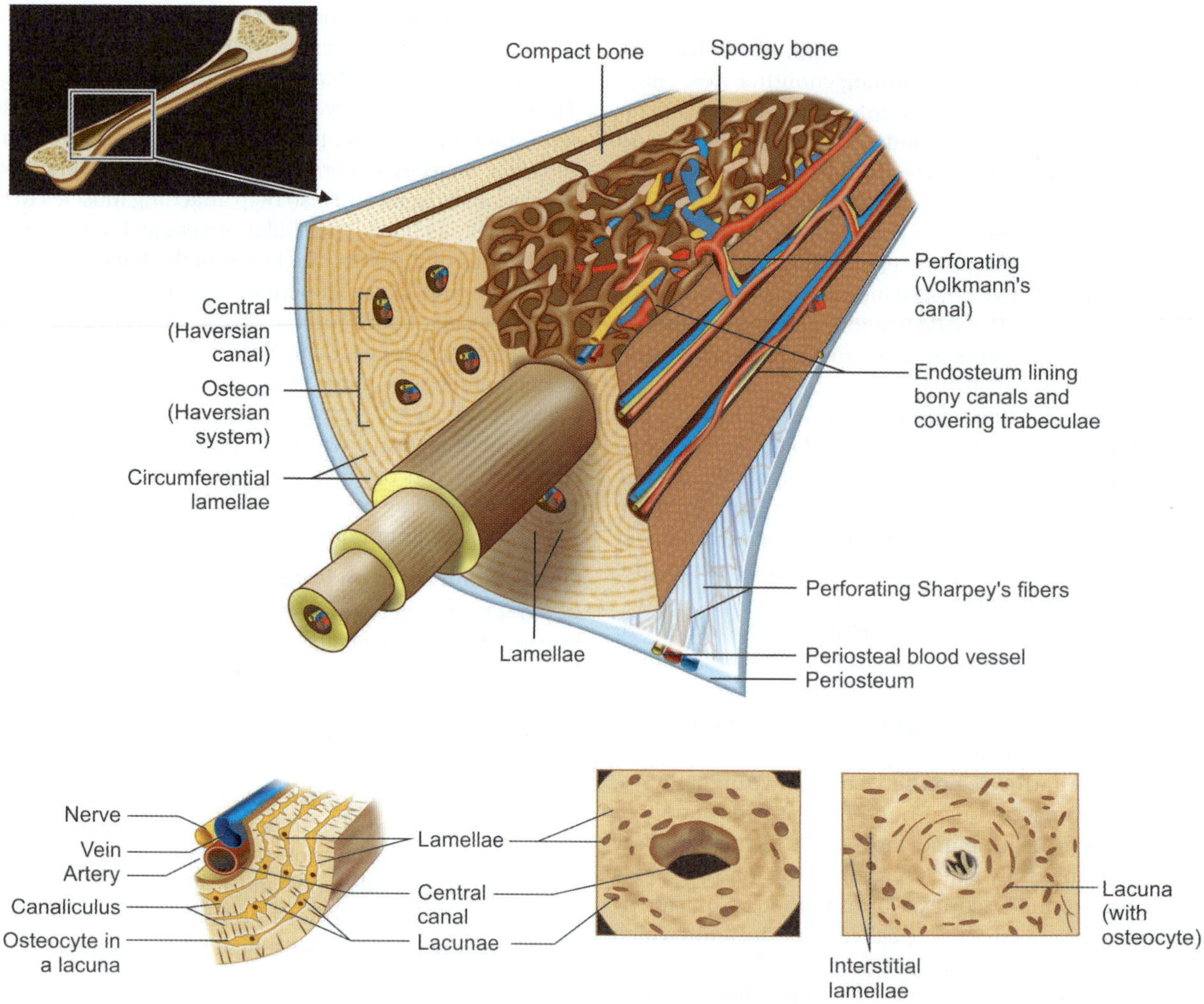

Fig. 2.3: Microscopic structure of cortical bone

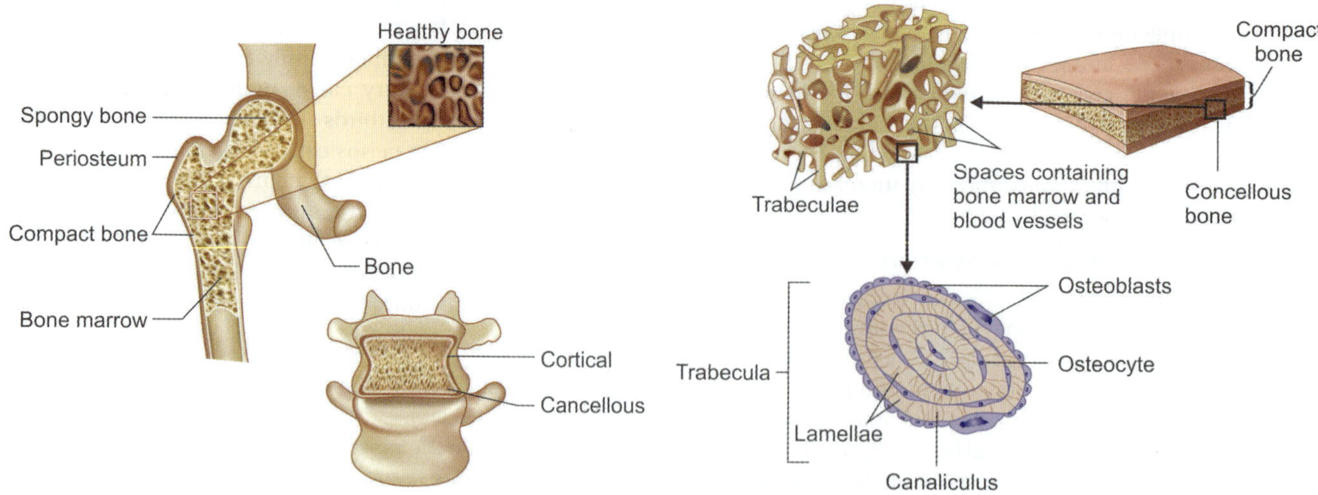

Fig. 2.4: Microscopic structure of cancellous bone

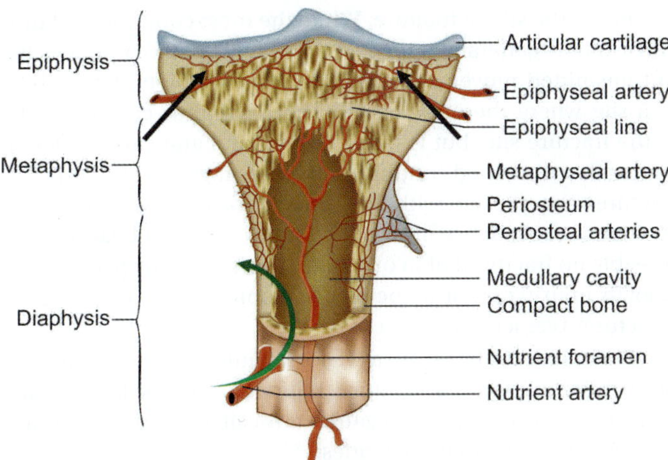

Fig. 2.5: Blood supply of bone

- A long bone is defined as one which has length more than width. By this definition, phalanx followed by metacarpal/metatarsal is the shortest long bone in the body.
- Although clavicle is classified as a long bone, it has no medullary (bone marrow) cavity.
- Porosity of cortical bones mostly falls in the range of 5– 10%, while that of cancellous bones ranges between 75% and 95%. Hence, cancellous bones are highly porous.
- Vertebrae have maximum ratio of cancellous bone compared to any other bone in the body (their cancellous to cortical bone ratio is 75:25).
- Like lamellar bone, matrix in trabecular (cancellous) bone is also deposited in the form of lamellae only. So, the trabecular bone is also lamellar bone, but it does not contain Haversian systems.
- Physis or growth plate can be considered a temporary primary cartilaginous joint. It is a hyaline cartilage plate conventionally taken to be a part of metaphysis.
- *Hueter Volkmann law*: As per this rule, compression forces across the physes inhibit growth while tensile forces across the physes stimulate growth.
- Bones in the body are in a continuous state of formation and resorption (remodeling) and the process is maximum at the endosteal surface. Hence, endosteum can be considered as the most metabolically active part of a bone.

GROWTH OF BONE

The process of formation of bone is called "ossification". During the fetal stage bone formation occurs either by "intramembranous ossification" or by "endochondral ossification".

Endochondral ossification: Endochondral ossification is seen in the long bones of the body. It involves formation of a cartilage model and its subsequent replacement by calcium hydroxyapatite deposition to form bone. During endochondral ossification, some mesenchymal cells develop into chondrocytes. These chondrocytes proliferate and secrete extracellular matrix which is mineralized to form the cartilage model. Now cartilage cells start dying and few cells surrounding these dead cartilage cells become osteoblast and form what is called an "ossification

center". These osteoblasts now secrete bony matrix into the degrading surrounding cartilage. In this way, the whole cartilage gets replaced by bone.

The ossification centers are of two types. Primary ossification centers appear in the cartilage during the fetal development. These are responsible for the formation of the diaphysis of the bones. By rule there is generally one primary center that appears before birth for every diaphysis except in clavicle that has two primary centers for its diaphysis. Primary center ossifies diaphysis, metaphysis and growth plate cartilage. Secondary ossification centers mostly appear after birth and are responsible for the formation of the epiphysis of the long bones and the extremities of flat and irregular bones.

Intramembranous ossification: It occurs in flat bones and in the clavicle. Here calcium hydroxyapatite is directly deposited into a preexisting membrane (derived from primitive connective tissue) without any intervening cartilage model stage. During intramembranous ossification, mesenchymal cells, derived from neural crest enter the bone formation site and proliferate. Some of these cells now differentiate into osteoblasts forming the ossification center. The osteoblasts in the ossification center secrete collagen and proteoglycans to form an extra cellular matrix. Calcification occurs in this collagen matrix. During this process of calcification, bony (calcified) spicules are formed. A layer of mesenchymal cells that surround the calcified spicule forms the periosteum.

Appositional (Increase in Width) and Interstitial Growth (Increase in Length)

In fetal life, each long bone is represented by a rod of hyaline cartilage surrounded by perichondrium. Interstitial growth in this cartilage model occurs when chondrocytes within the cartilage divide and secrete new matrix and increase the length of cartilage model. Appositional growth occurs when chondroblasts in the perichondrium produce new matrix at the periphery and increase the width of cartilage model.

In contrast to cartilage in fetus, adults have mature bone. Mature bone grows only by appositional growth. Inner layer of periosteum (cambium layer) contains osteoprogenitor cells, which develop into osteoblasts. These osteoblast secret new bone matrix and increase the thickness of bone. Longitudinal growth, which occurs before maturity is primarily due to cartilage proliferation at the growth plate or physis, which subsequently undergoes mineralization to form bone.

HIGH-YIELD POINTS

- *Ossification centers*: Ossification centers for the distal femur, calcaneum, talus and sometimes cuboid are present at term birth. Ossification centers for proximal tibia are either present at birth or appears within 2 months.
- The first bone to start ossifying in the human skeleton is the clavicle. It is only long bone to ossify by intramembranous ossification. It starts ossifying at fifth week of intrauterine life and that is when the human skeleton starts forming. The clavicle is also the last bone to complete ossification when its medial end fuses with the shaft. The mandible is the second bone to ossify after clavicle by intramembranous ossification.

- *Law of ossification:* As per this law, the secondary center that appears first fuses last. The bone that does not obey this law is "fibula".
- In first metacarpal, secondary center of ossification is present at its base, but the same is present in the heads in all other metacarpals.
- *Ossification of carpals:* Carpal bones ossify by rule from one center only. Capitate is the first carpal bone to ossify (at 2 months) and before 3 years of age, only capitate and hamate ossify in a child's hand.

FRACTURE: TYPES AND CLASSIFICATIONS

INTRODUCTION

A fracture is a break in the continuity of bone (even a single cortex) with or without displacement. **Box 2.2** gives list of some common fractures encountered in orthopedics in different situations.

While the term fracture is used in context of an injury to bone, injury to joints leads to a dislocation or subluxation. Dislocation refers to two joint surfaces loosing total contact with each other and subluxation (a partial dislocation) term is used when the two joint surfaces retain some contact with each other **(Fig. 2.6)**. Most common dislocation encountered in orthopedics is shoulder > elbow. Since shoulder dislocation is rarely seen in children, elbow is the most common dislocation in pediatric age group.

Signs and symptoms: Pain/tenderness, swelling, loss of transmitted movements and abnormal mobility are classical signs present at the site of fracture. While the most common and most consistent is generally tenderness, the most pathognomic is loss of transmitted movements and abnormal mobility (i.e. mobility at a site where there is normally not). Crepitus can be elicited at the fracture site, but is often very painful and can be there in some other unrelated conditions like gas gangrene, etc. Displaced fractures may present with deformity at fracture site. The patient is often not able to use his fracture limb, i.e. weight bearing is not possible on fractured tibia or femur. Any fracture (especially high velocity injury) may be associated with injury to surrounding vital structures (vessels and nerves).

Fractures are almost always accompanied by varying amounts of surrounding soft tissue injury. Injury to a muscle is referred to as a "strain" while injury to ligaments is called as "sprain". Sprains can be classified into three grades:

- *Grade I:* Tear of less than one-third fibers of a ligament
- *Grade II:* Tear of more than one-third ligament fibers (but not a complete tear)
- *Grade III:* Complete tear of a ligament.

Classification Systems for a Fracture

Why is a classification system needed for fractures?

- It guides the treatment—a common treatment approach is usually followed for same injuries, e.g. interlocking nailing for diaphyseal fracture of femur or tibia.
- It explains prognosis—open fractures are more likely to carry a poorer prognosis than close fractures, high chance of avascular necrosis in some fracture, e.g. fracture proximal pole of scaphoid and basal fracture neck of femur.
- It makes easy to describe a fracture, i.e. to give details of fracture to other surgeons.

There are many ways to classify fractures **(Table 2.2)**. Classification systems have evolved from a description of the clinical appearance of fracture (before the invention of X-rays, e.g. Colle's fracture) to X-ray based fracture's descriptions. A fair idea of the mechanism of injury can be inferred from X-ray appearance of a fracture and hence fractures can also be classified based on mechanism of injury **(Table 2.3)**.

AO Classification of Fractures (Muller's AO/OTA Classification)

This is a unique and comprehensive classification **(Figs 2.7 and 2.8)** published initially by AO foundation in 1987, which can be applied to fracture of all bones. It is an alphanumerical classification, i.e. numbers and alphabets are used to classify a fracture which allows fracture patterns to be given a digital platform. Recently a pediatric version has also been published.

In AO classification, a unique and uniform pattern **(Box 2.3)** is followed to classify every fracture.

- Each major bone is given a number **(Fig. 2.8A)** like humerus, forearm bones, femur and leg bones have been assigned 1, 2, 3 and 4, respectively.
- Further in long bone fractures, each long bone is divided into three segments; (1) proximal segment, (2) diaphysis and (3) distal segment, which are assigned 1, 2 and 3 numbers, respectively **(Fig. 2.8B)**.
- Fracture sustained by concerned segment is further given an alphabetic categorization from A to C depending upon the fracture pattern **(Fig. 2.8C)**.

Box 2.2: Most common fractures

Most common fractures overall—clavicle > distal end radius

Age wise:

- Most common fracture at birth—clavicle > humerus
- Most common fracture in children—greenstick fracture of forearm bones
- Most common fractures in elderly—vertebral fracture > distal end radius fractures

In a patient presenting with history of the fall on an outstretched hand:

- Most common fracture if the patient is a child (especially less than 10 years)—supracondylar humerus
- Most common fracture if the patient is a young adolescent—scaphoid fracture
- Most common fracture in adult (especially postmenopausal osteoporotic female)—distal end radius

---

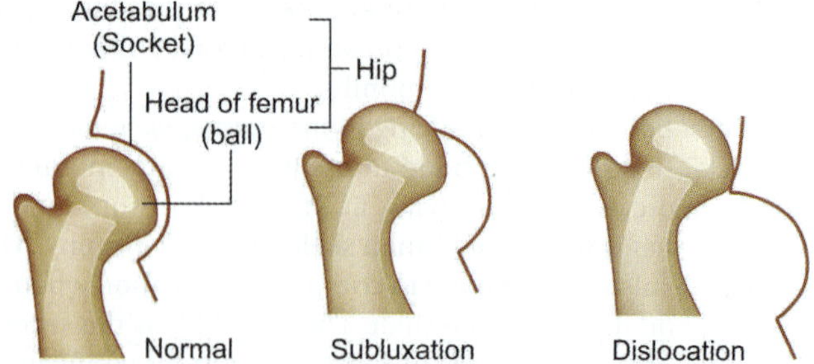

Fig. 2.6: Diagrammatic representation of subluxation and dislocation

Table 2.2: Various classification systems of fractures

Based on displacement

- *Undisplaced fractures*: Bone only breaks but fracture fragments do not displace
- *Displaced fractures*: Minimally to completely displaced fractures
- *Impacted fracture*: When fracture fragments are pushed into each other. It is usually seen in distal radius and proximal femur fracture

Based on communication with environment

- *Close*: No contact with external environment
- *Open fractures*: Where fracture communicates with environment. In open fractures, fracture hematoma is drained out of wound

Based on completeness

- *Complete fracture*: Complete loss of bone continuity
- Incomplete fractures (only one cortex is broken), e.g. greenstick fracture
- *Traumatic fracture*: Which is sustained due to injury

Based on etiology

- *Pathological fracture*: Which occurs in diseased bone due to trivial trauma or no injury
- *Stress/Fatigue fracture*: Which occurs in normal bone due to excessive stress overload
- *Fragility/Insufficiency fracture*: A type of pathological fracture which occurs due to osteoporosis

Based on radiology

- *X-ray features based*: Most currently used classifications are X-ray based, i.e. Garden classification of fracture neck femur
- *CT scan based*: Sanders classification of calcaneus fracture

Based on fracture pattern

- Transverse, oblique, spiral, comminuted and segmental

Based on location

- *Intra-articular fractures*: Which involve the articular surface
- *Extra-articular fractures*: Diaphyseal and metaphyseal fractures

Other types

- *Avulsion fracture*: A small chunk of bone is torn away from the bone due to pull of ligament or tendon
- *Periprosthetic fractures*: Fractures around joint replacement prostheses

Table 2.3: Mechanism of injury and fracture patterns		
Type of force	*Geometry of fracture*	
1. Bending	*Transverse or oblique:* In transverse fracture, fracture line runs transversely to the long axis of bone	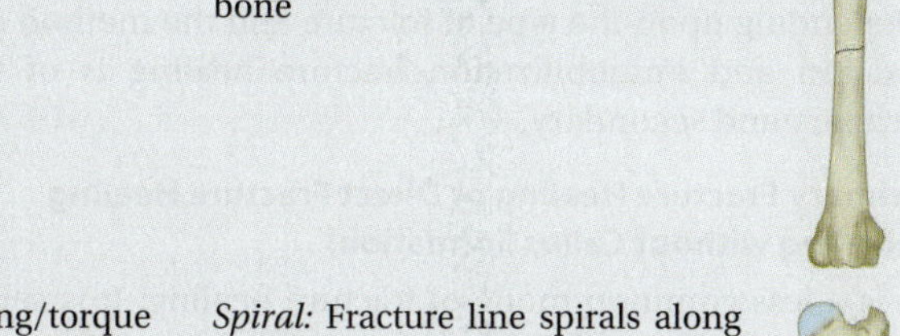
2. Twisting/torque	*Spiral:* Fracture line spirals along the long axis of bone in more than one plane	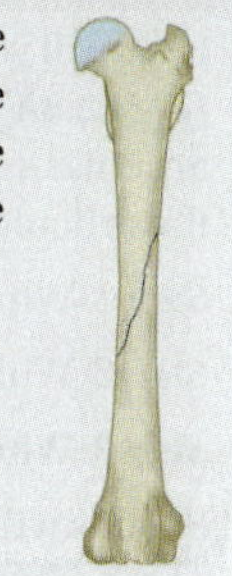
3. Axial compression combined with bending and torsion	*Oblique:* Fracture line runs oblique to the long axis of the bone (angle with horizontal is >30°) and the two cortices of each fragment are in the same plane	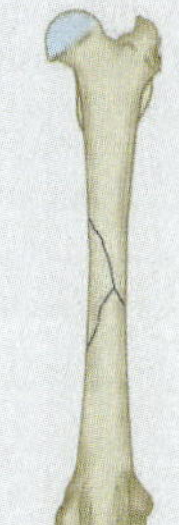
4. High energy direct impact	*Comminuted fracture:* More than three fracture fragments	

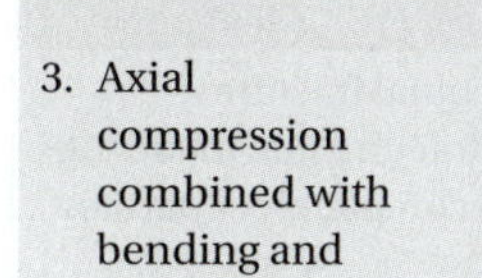

- A further division into groups and subgroups can also be made, which differs from bone to bone.

HIGH-YIELD POINT

- "Occult fracture" is a general term applied to those subtle fractures where clinical examination points to a fracture, but the fracture is not visible on an X-ray. Fatigue and insufficiency fractures, many a times present as occult fractures. The investigation of choice for occult fractures is MRI (better than CT). Occult fractures are seen on X-rays after 2–4 weeks when there is evidence of new bone formation.

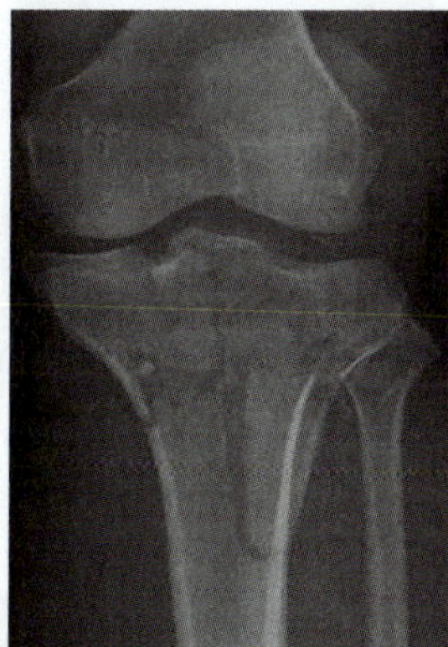

Fig. 2.7: Proximal tibial metaphyseal fracture with articular involvement with metaphyseal-diaphyseal separation (41-C by AO classification, see **Box 2.3**)

BIOLOGY OF FRACTURE HEALING AND NONUNION

FRACTURE HEALING

Fracture healing is a remarkable process that aims at the restoration of exact anatomy of bone. Although it is a continuous process, but divided into five phases which overlap each other. Depending upon the type of fracture and the method of fracture fixation and immobilization fracture healing is of two types primary and secondary.

Primary Fracture Healing or Direct Fracture Healing (Healing without Callus Formation)

It is a less common mode of fracture healing. It is seen in rigid internal fixation of fractures (compression plating) and in unicortical fractures (Greenstick fractures). It is a direct attempt of bone to restore its continuity without forming fracture callus. It is of two types: (1) gap healing and (2) contact healing.

Gap healing occurs when there is a minimal gap in between rigidly fixed fracture ends. Woven bone (immature bone having

---

Box 2.3: Example of AO classification **(Fig. 2.7)**

How will you classify a proximal metaphyseal tibial fracture **(Figs 2.8A to C)** which is comminuted with a fracture line involving articular surface and metaphysis and fracture completely separates the articular surface from diaphysis?

Step 1: Which bone—humerus (4)

Step 2: Which segment—proximal segment (1)

Step 3: Which type— complete articular (C)

So, this will be classified as fracture 41-C*

---

*A digital number is designating the fracture morphology, serving the purpose of AO classification.

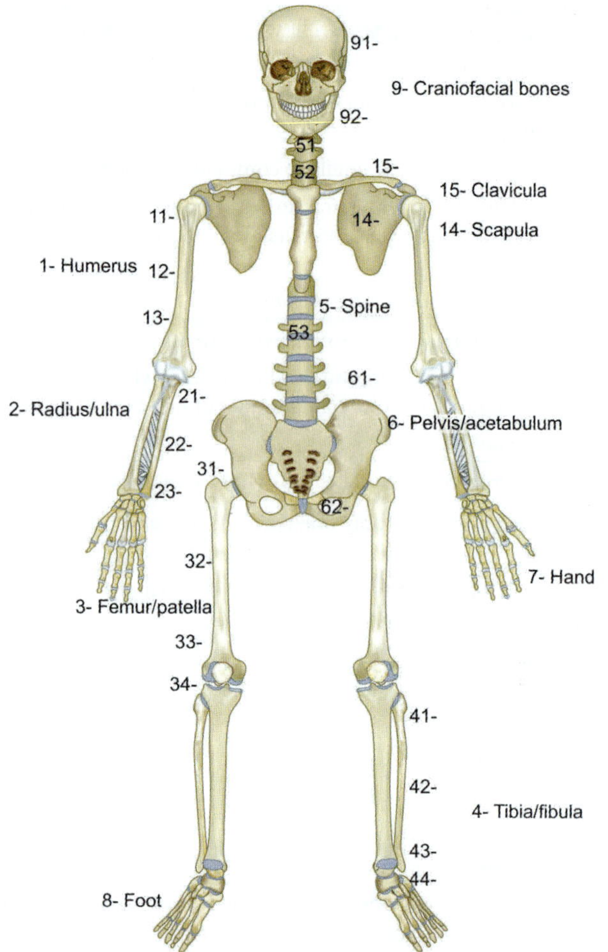

Fig. 2.8A: AO classification: Each major bone is assigned a number (1–9)

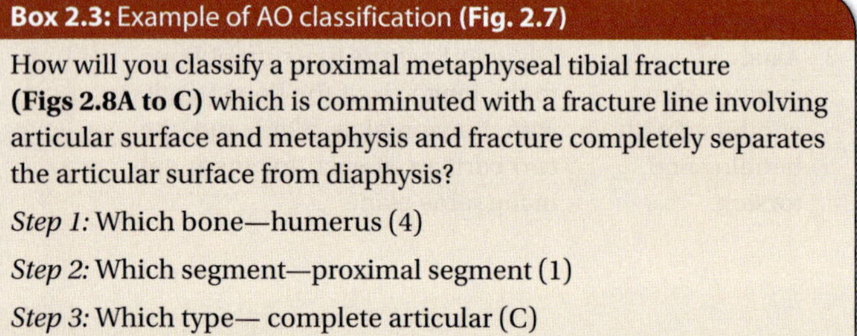

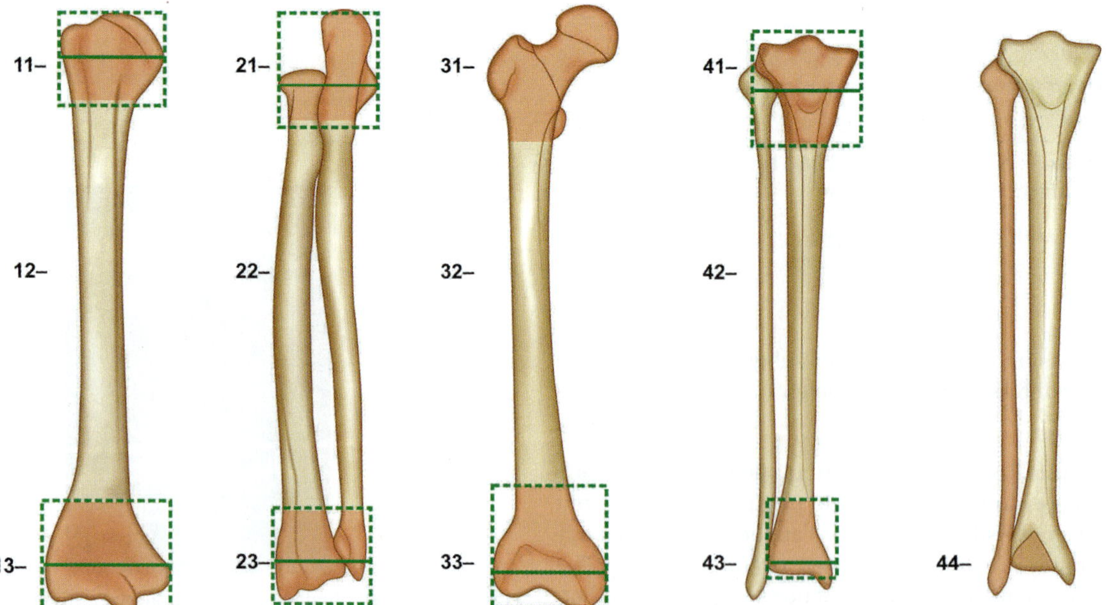

Fig. 2.8B: AO classification: Assigning number for the segment of long bone involved (c.f. malleoli in tibia and fibula are considered separately under segment categorization and assigned number 4)

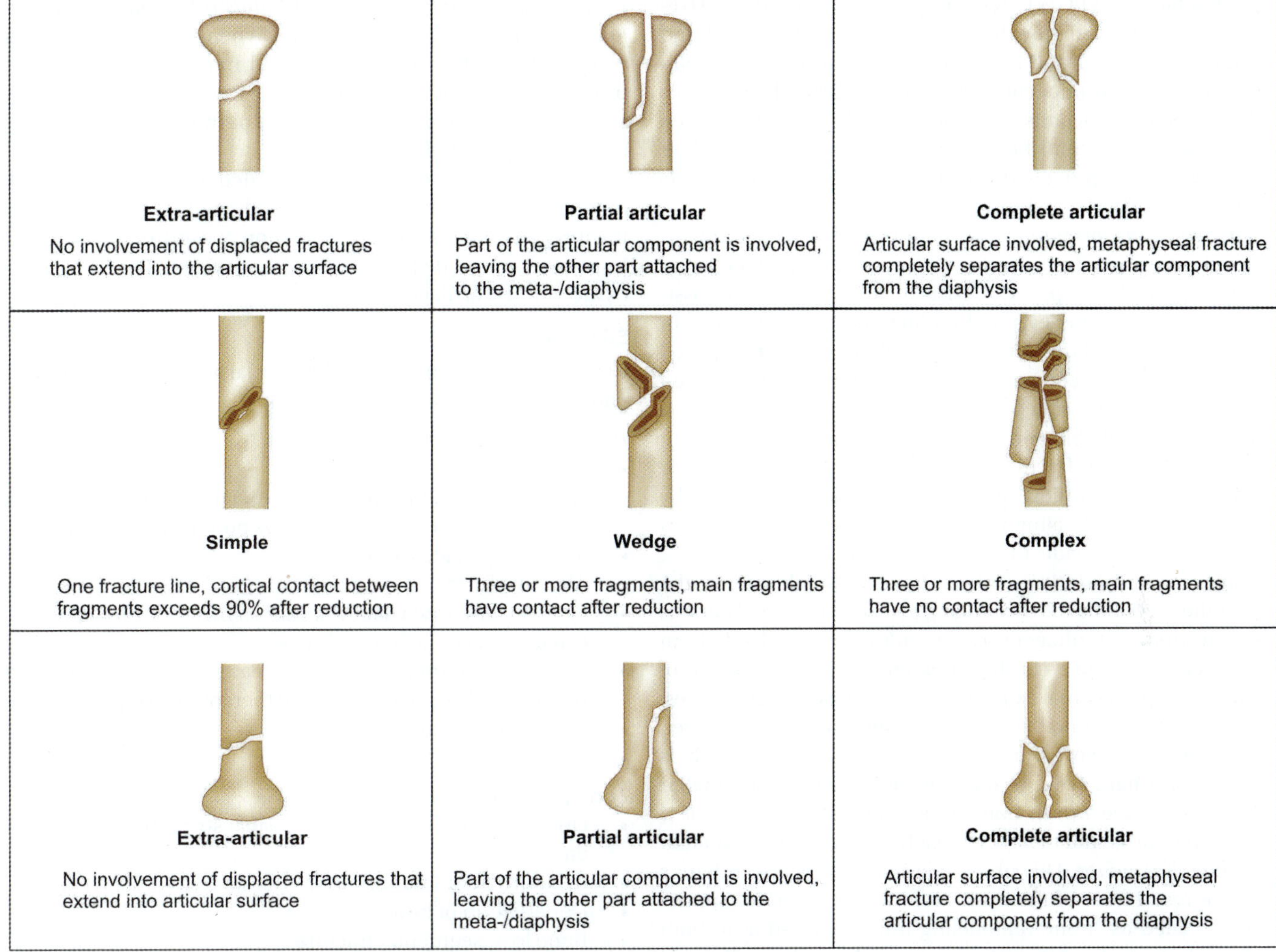

Fig. 2.8C: AO classification: Assigning alphabet to fracture pattern of the involved segment

a random arrangement of collagen fibers) is initially formed in transverse orientation between fracture gaps which is later replaced by lamellar bone (regular parallel alignment of collagen into sheets/lamellae).

Contact healing is seen when fracture ends are closely approximated to each other without any gap. Osteoclasts at one end of fracture cause bone resorption to form so called "cutting cones" such that the fracture gap widens initially. In these cones, osteoblasts lay down new bone.

Secondary Fracture Healing or Indirect Fracture Healing (Healing by Callus Formation)

This is the more common method of fracture healing. It is seen in the absence of rigid fixation (e.g. in cast immobilization, intramedullary nailing and bridge plating for comminuted metaphyseal fractures). It is divided into five phases **(Box 2.4)**:

1. *Stage of hematoma formation*: Hematoma formation starts within a few hours of a fracture. Periosteal and intramedullary vessel disruption produces the hematoma at the fracture site.
2. *Stage of granulation tissue (inflammatory phase)*: Hematoma accumulates beneath the periosteum and between fracture

> **Box 2.4:** Approximate timing of various stages of fracture healing
>
> - Hematoma is fully organized by 2–3 days
> - Granulation tissue is fully formed by 2–3 weeks
> - Provisional (soft) callus is seen first around 3 weeks (First radiological sign of union) but callus is nicely formed by 3 months
> - Woven bone/hard callus is formed by 3 months (First clinical sign of union) but bone attains its natural strength (consolidation) by 2–3 years. Implants used for fracture fixation can be removed by this time
> - Remodeling continues to occur after 2–3 years and is an ever-going process

ends and acts as a source of growth factors and cytokines that initiate cellular events of healing. Inflammatory response peaks at 24 hours with accumulation of neutrophil, platelets, lymphocytes, macrophages, endothelial cells and fibroblasts. These cells produce a number of growth factors and cytokines like fibroblast growth factors (FGFs), vascular endothelial growth factors (VEGFs), transforming growth factor-β (TGF-β), platelet-derived growth factor (PDGF), interleukin-1 and interleukin-6 (IL-1 and IL-6), tumor necrosis factor-α (TNF-α) and bone morphogenetic proteins (BMPs). These factors act as chemoattractants for mesenchymal stem cells derived from periosteum and bone marrow and also induce their differentiation into chondroblasts, osteoblasts, fibroblasts and angioblasts.

3. *Stage of callus formation*: The stem cells that have differentiated into osteoblasts synthesize new bone to affect repair (repair phase). This phase consists of intramembranous ossification, chondrogenesis and endochondral ossification. In the initial stage of this phase, the healing tissue is composed of mixed fibrous connective tissue, cartilage, some woven bone and osteoid, called as provisional callus or soft callus. This callus is pliable and weak but good enough to prevent shortening at the fracture site, although not angulation or rotation. Callus earliest becomes visible on radiographs by 3 weeks. As this healing progresses, pH gradually becomes alkaline from an acidic pH of inflammatory phase.

4. *Stage of consolidation (woven bone)*: Osteoblasts at the periphery of callus start producing bone by intramembranous ossification. Simultaneously chondrocytes derived from stem cells lay down cartilaginous matrix. Mineralization of this cartilaginous matrix takes place by these chondrocytes. Ultimately at the end of this phase whole callus is composed of hard callus/woven bone (mineralized callus) which is strong and hard (as it is mineralized) but lacks a lamellar structure. Since woven bone is rigid and strong, when it is formed bone is said to have clinically united or consolidated.

5. *Remodeling phase*: This phase continues for years and aims at the restoration of the exact architecture of bone. Special units called as "bone remodeling units" consisting of both osteoclasts and osteoblasts are formed on the surface of the bone. The osteoclasts reabsorb the woven bone and osteoblasts deposit more and more osteoid. In this way, the whole woven bone is eventually replaced by lamellar bone. Thicker lamellar bone is laid in the area of high stresses (these are compression sites having more of osteoblastic activity) while in areas with no stress (these are tension sites having more of osteoclastic activity) unwanted bony buttresses are carved away to make the bone attain anatomical shape (Wolf's law—bone formation occurs only along the lines of stress). While remodeling phase classically refers to this normalization of the lamellar (internal) structure of bone, some biologists use the phrase "modeling phase" to refer to the normalization of the normal anatomical (external) shape of bone that ensues with the above changes.

Some authors divide the process of fracture healing into three phases: (1) Inflammatory (hematoma formation and granulation tissue formation), (2) reparative (soft and hard callus formation) and (3) remodeling/modeling phase.

DELAYED UNION AND NONUNION

There is no universal definition of fracture nonunion, which is applicable to all fractures. Arbitrarily nonunion fracture is one that has not united and is neither expected to unite without intervention.

United States Food and Drug Administration panel has given following definition of nonunion: "When union does not take place in 9 months after fracture and fracture shows no visible progressive signs of healing at least for 3 months". Most orthopedic surgeons do not consider nonunion of fracture of shaft of long bones to happen before 6 months.

Delayed union of fracture is defined as when fracture takes more than usual time to unite depending on the type and site of fracture, but shows some progression toward union over time. In nonunion and delayed union, fracture gap is filled by fibrous tissue or fibrocartilage.

Etiology

Causes of nonunion are multifactorial and may be related to patient, injury, fracture or treatment.

Patient- or host-related factors:
- *Age*: Old age
- *Malnutrition*: Albumin less than 3.5 mg/dL and lymphocytes less than 1,500 cells/mL indicates poor healing potential.
- Smoking/tobacco abuse
- Alcohol abuse
- *Systemic diseases*: Diabetes, cancer, metabolic bone diseases, osteomalacia, Cushing's disease.
- *Drugs*: Nonsteroidal anti-inflammatory drugs (NSAIDs), antineoplastic drugs, corticosteroid therapy and bisphosphonates
- Radiation therapy
- Infection.

Local factors related to injury:
- Open fractures (excessive periosteal stripping and soft tissue damage)
- Intra-articular fracture
- Denervation of bone
- Bone loss, segmental fracture
- High velocity injury/severely comminuted fracture
- Intact fellow bone (intact fibula may prevent apposition of fracture fragments in case of fracture tibia)
- Soft tissue interposition

Fracture-specific factors:
- *Vicarious blood supply*: Some fractures are prone to nonunion due to the vicarious blood supply of the bone **(Box 2.5)**.
- Pathological fractures have poor healing potential.
- Neuropathic fractures

Factors related to treatment:
- Inadequate reduction **(Fig. 2.9)**
- *Inadequate internal fixation*: Implant too short, construct too stiff.

Box 2.5: Some fractures commonly prone to nonunion

- Fracture neck of femur
- Fracture proximal pole and waist of scaphoid
- Fracture body of talus
- Fracture lateral condyle in children
- Fracture base of fifth metatarsal
- Fracture distal one-third of tibia and distal one-third of the ulna

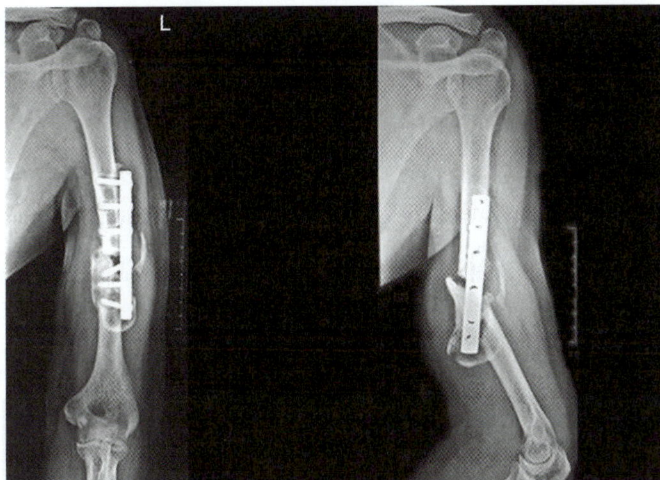

Fig. 2.9: X-ray humerus (AP and lateral views) showing nonunion following inadequate reduction

- *Inadequate immobilization*: Excessive motion at the fracture site leads to disruption of early bridging callus
- *Wrong surgical technique*: Excessive periosteal stripping.

Clinical Features

The most common nonunion that presents to an orthopedic surgeon is fracture of the distal one-third of tibia and most common cause of nonunion overall is inadequate immobilization. A patient who has been waiting for union of a fracture for a long time, presents with functional disability (inability to use a limb or bear weight). Persistent pain and tenderness may be present at the fracture site especially in initial stages. Nonunion, however, at times may be painless especially when a false joint (pseudoarthrosis) forms. Instability (abnormal mobility, crepitus) is generally frank in such cases. The patients especially with painful nonunion must always be evaluated for signs of infection like swelling, increased local temperature, discharge, etc. Some blood and urine markers are also available that can help evaluate the process of bone formation or resorption **(Box 2.6)**.

Radiology

Defining union on X-rays needs two orthogonal views (AP and lateral) showing healing of three out of four cortices without appreciable mobility or pain clinically. X-ray of fracture nonunion may show following signs **(Fig. 2.10)**: Persistent fracture line, paucity of callus, sclerotic and rounded fracture ends with obliteration of the medullary canal and osteopenia in the surrounding bone. A CT scan may show persistent fracture line in doubtful cases. Scintigraphy helps to distinguish between biologically active (rich blood supply) and unresponsive nonunion (poor blood supply).

Types

Fracture nonunion is classified based on the blood supply of fracture ends into atrophic and hypertrophic varieties. Both types are further divided into various subtypes **(Table 2.4)**. Hypertrophic nonunion is usually seen where immobilization is not adequate and abundant callus formation occurs in an attempt to attain stability.

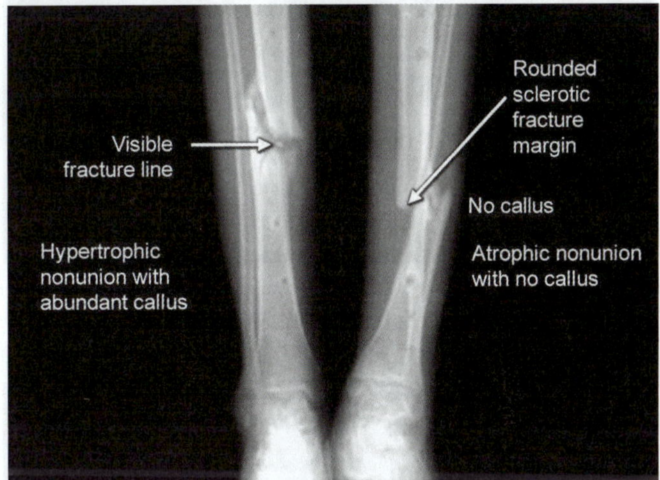

Fig. 2.10: X-ray bilateral legs (AP views) showing classical radiographic signs of hypertrophic (right leg) and atrophic nonunion (left leg) in a patient

A special type is "pseudoarthrosis" which is characterized by fluid-filled cavity (clear fluid) which is lined by a membrane (synovial like cells), between fracture ends. Bone scan shows vascularized bone ends. It occurs due to insecure fixation where excessive motion leads to false joint formation **(Fig. 2.11)**.

Treatment

In hypertrophic nonunion, just a stable internal fixation may promote union, but treatment of oligotrophic and atrophic noninfected nonunion requires open reduction, debridement of sclerotic fracture ends followed by stable internal fixation along with bone grafting (pivotal step). Nonunion with bone loss, shortening and deformity are difficult cases and require distraction osteogenesis using ring fixator based on the Ilizarov's principles (*see* Page 30). Nonunion may also occur following surgery due to infection. Treatment of infection takes priority over treatment of nonunion. First step is to control infection by implant

Table 2.4: Types of nonunion **(Figs 2.11 to 2.13)**

Hypertrophic nonunion **(Figs 2.10 and 2.11)**	They are characterized by vascularized bone ends. Callus formation is generally seen and may be abundant, but this callus is nonbridging in nature	• *Elephant's foot:* Rich in callus—it results from insecure fixation and early weight bearing in a reduced fracture • *Horse's hoof:* Less abundant callus—it is seen in moderately unstable fracture fixation • *Oligotrophic:* Minimal or no callus but vascularized bone ends. It is seen in distracted/displaced bone ends
Atrophic nonunion **(Figs 2.10 and 2.12)**	Characterized by absence of callus. Bone scan shows avascular fracture ends. Fracture ends become atrophic and osteoporotic	• *Torsion wedge*: Characterized by an avascular intermediate fragment between fracture ends, which has united to one main fracture end • *Comminuted*: Characterized by presence of one or more avascular fragments between fracture ends • *Defect (gap) nonunion* **(Fig. 2.13)**: Characterized by loss of bone between fracture ends

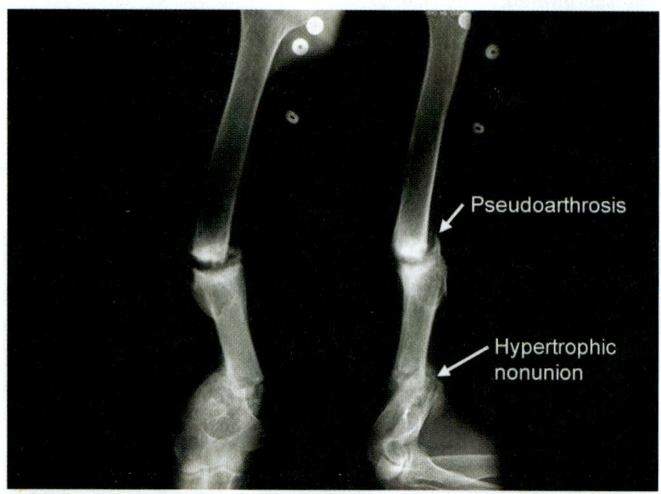

Fig. 2.11: X-ray of humerus (AP and lateral views) showing hypertrophic nonunion with abundant callus formation (lower label) and pseudoarthrosis (upper label)

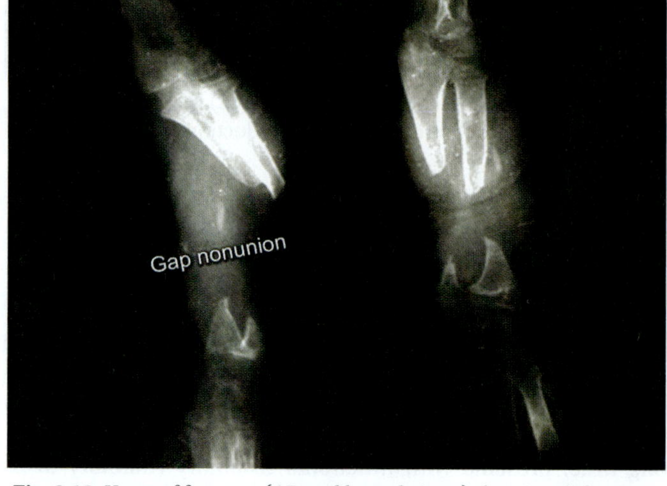

Fig. 2.13: X-ray of forearm (AP and lateral views) showing defect/gap nonunion—a type of atrophic nonunion

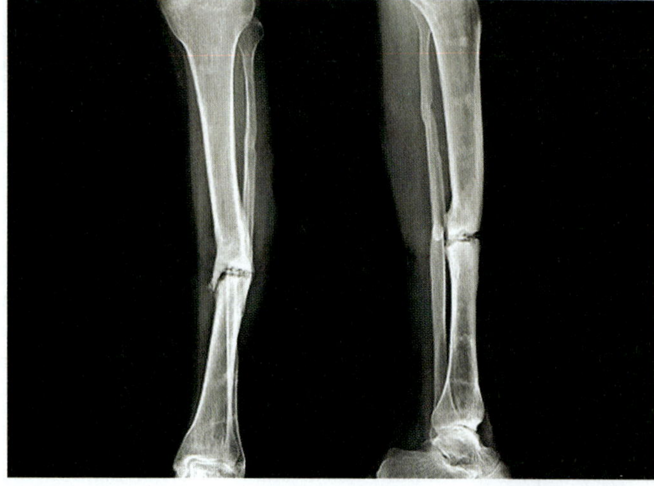

Fig. 2.12: X-ray of leg (AP and lateral views) showing sclerosed fracture ends and scanty callus with obliterated marrow cavity—typical of atrophic nonunion

removal, adequate debridement and use of antibiotic cement beads. Once infection is controlled nonunion can be managed on above stated principles. **Figure 2.14** shows radiological progress to union following use of bone graft after nonunion of fracture shaft of humerus.

Apart from surgical methods some biophysical methods **(Box 2.7)** have also been used in the treatment of delayed and nonunion with varying success.

BONE GRAFTING (FIG. 2.14)

A pivotal step in treatment of any nonunion is to graft the fracture site. A bone graft is a transplanted bone. Its use is indicated to stimulate bone union, to replace lost bone or to assist in revascularization of avascular segments.

Types

- Autogenous (autologous) bone graft is a graft transplanted from one site of skeleton (donor site) to another site (recipient site) within the same individual. It is considered the gold standard and most commonly used. Autogenous cancellous grafts are usually harvested from the iliac crest (most common site), the fibula, proximal tibia, the distal radius, the olecranon, the greater trochanter and distal femoral condyles.
- Allografts are harvested from one individual and transplanted into a different individual of the same species. Allografts are preserved by various techniques (lyophilization/freeze-drying, deep-frozen/fresh-frozen, cryopreservation, etc.) and treated (ethylene oxide treatment or gamma irradiation) before transplantation to reduce graft rejection.

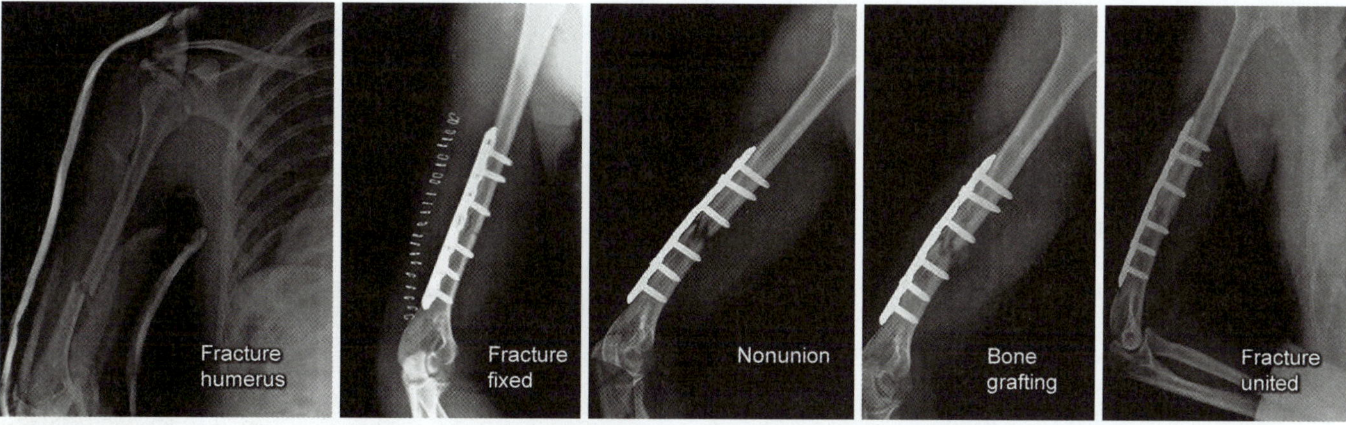

Fig. 2.14: Fracture shaft humerus as it unites in a 24-year-old male

Box 2.7: Biophysical methods for treating fracture nonunion

- Low intensity pulsed ultrasound (intensity < 0.1 W/cm^2)
- Electrical stimulation
- High-energy extracorporeal shock wave therapy

- Xenografts are transplanted from one species to a member of a different species.
- Isograft is transplanted from one monozygotic twin to the other.

Additionally, the graft may be described as cortical, cancellous, corticocancellous and osteochondral (having both bone and cartilage piece). Cancellous bone graft serves the purpose of osteoinduction and osteoconduction and also provides for osteoprogenitor cells. Cortical grafts are poor in osteoinduction and do not provide for osteoprogenitor cells. Iliac crest (the most common bone graft harvest site) is a source of tricortical graft (cancellous bone surrounded by cortex on three sides). Cortical grafts are mostly harvested from fibula and ribs while the best site for harvesting a cancellous bone graft is considered to be postero-superior iliac spine (part of iliac crest).

A division into vascularized and nonvascularized grafts can also be made. Vascularized grafts carry their own blood supply while nonvascularized grafts do not and they are simple free grafts. The vascularized bone grafts can be harvested in two ways. One is to take a bone (usually fibula) and keep its blood vessel intact (free vascularized bone graft) and anastomose the same to a vessel at the recipient site. The other is to take a bone along with an attached pedicle of muscle such that the vessel of the muscle is kept intact (muscle pedicle bone graft). This bone can be transplanted to a nearby site and the muscle's vessel continues to supply the bone.

Properties of a Bone Graft

Osteoinduction: Process of inducing pluripotent/primitive mesenchymal cells to differentiate into bone forming cells osteoblasts.

Osteoconduction: Graft acts as a scaffold for the growth of new bone on its surface and deep down its pores, when placed in contact with native bone.

Osteogenesis: Graft itself provides bone forming cells osteoblasts.

Table 2.5: Bone graft substitutes

Type	Example	Properties
Ceramic based	Calcium phosphate and its collagen composites, hydroxyapatite, tricalcium phosphate, bioactive glass, etc.	Osteoconductive
Polymer based	Biodegradable polymers	Osteoconductive
Growth factors based	Bone morphogenetic proteins and platelet rich plasma (PRP)	Osteoinductive
Cell based	Bone marrow aspirate	Osteogenic potential

BONE GRAFT SUBSTITUTES

Limited availability of autologous bone graft and associated donor site morbidity limits the use of autogenous bone graft. Allogenic bone grafts have limited potential of osteoinduction and inferior mechanical strength as compared to autologous bone graft due to storage and sterilization techniques employed. They also carry a small risk of disease transmission. These shortcomings led to developments of bone graft substitutes. **Table 2.5** summarizes the different bone graft substitutes used in orthopedics.

HIGH-YIELD POINTS

- During fracture healing, cells from the cambium layer of periosteum are the earliest to produce bone.
- Excessive motion and very rigid fixation (no motion) both may lead to nonunion whereas micromotion at fracture ends promotes callus formation and is a desirable factor.
- Bone is continuously in a remodeling state. In adult skeleton (after skeletal growth has ended) for bone deposition to occur a raw surface would be needed. This is prepared by osteoclasts (bone resorbing cells that are derivatives of monocytes). These cells resorb cortical bones by forming cones, but they resorb cancellous bone by forming lacunae/pits (Howship's lacunae).
- Bone apposition/formation is best seen in Howship's lacunae followed by cutting cones prepared by osteoclasts in a normal adult bone. However, in a fractured bone (bone resorption

is not needed) so the apposition would be best seen in the subperiosteal cambium layer.

- The first radiological stage of union is callus (provisional callus/soft callus) that may be visible earliest by 3 weeks but the first clinical stage of union is woven bone (hard callus) formation.
- Indium-111-labeled leukocyte imaging is very sensitive and specific in diagnosing infected nonunion.
- Tetracycline labeling is a special method used to estimate the rate of mineralization in newly laid osteoid or in other words it estimates the rate of bone turnover. It is used in diagnostic situations in cases like osteomalacia, bone tumors, etc.
- Better fracture remodeling is seen in younger patients, fracture nearer to the growth plate and when deformity/angulation is in plane of joint movement.
- The cancellous bone graft is slowly replaced by new bone by a complex process known as "creeping substitution".
- A number of growth factors have been identified that are produced by osteoblasts that regulate cell development and differentiation in bone. BMP 2 and 7 are one of them that have recently received a bit of attention. They have been synthesized in purified form from demineralized bone matrix (DBM) and are commercially available for therapeutic use to enhance osteogenesis. Marshal Urist (1964) is credited with this invention.
- *Demineralized bone matrix:* It is an allogeneic bone graft prepared by acid extraction of cortical bone. It is rich in collagen I, noncollagenous proteins and has some BMPs. BMPs convey osteoinductive property to DBM.
- *Induced membrane technique (Masquelet):* This is a relatively new technique introduced to deal with gap nonunion with large bone defect. A cement (polymethylmethacrylate) spacer is introduced into the gap after radical debridement of fibrous tissue. A membrane forms over the spacer in 6–8 weeks. Now the spacer is removed and cancellous bone graft is packed inside the membrane. The biological chamber created by the membrane harbors growth factors, prevents graft resorption and enhances union of the fracture site.
- Fractures which are prone to malunion are:
  - Supracondylar humerus fracture in children
  - Intertrochanteric fracture of femur
  - Colles' fracture.

All these are metaphyseal fractures occurring in cancellous that rapidly unites but often malunites. Nonunion is generally more common with diaphyseal fractures involving compact or cortical bone.

SPLINTS AND TRACTIONS

SPLINTS

Any "rigid" device "used to immobilize" the injured part of the body is called a splint. Almost any rigid material can be used to splint the injured limb in emergency **(Fig. 2.15)**. The primary purpose of splinting is preventing further trauma and reducing pain, until a diagnosis is made and primary management is done. Splints may also be used in postoperative period for support, rest

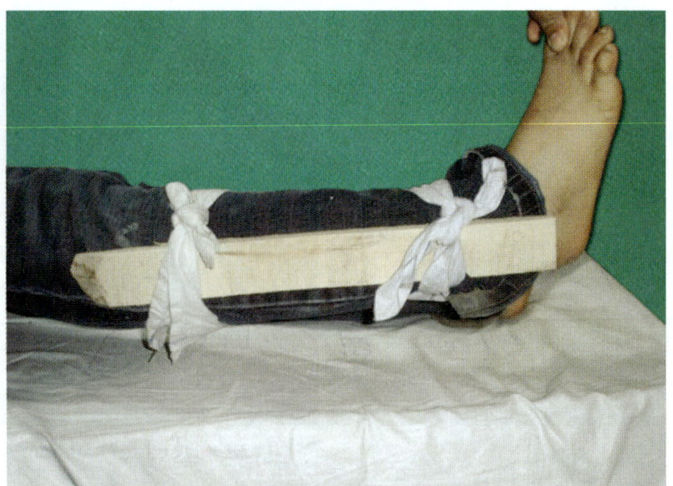

Fig. 2.15: Use of wooden plank as an emergency splint

or even as a definitive measure to treat an orthopedic injury/deformity in the form of a plaster of Paris (POP) back slab/cast. There are a wide variety of methods to splint an injured limb depending on the site of trauma. Few commonly used splints/braces are mentioned in **Table 2.6**.

Plaster of Paris Splint (Fig. 2.16)

It is a commonly used splint which can be used to support any fracture. It can be molded according to shape of the limb. When one molds it to cover only three-fourths of the circumference of a limb, this splint is called a POP slab; if it covers the entire circumference, it is called a cast. It is often used to support the fractured limb for transportation of the patient while the patient is awaiting definitive treatment.

Thomas Splint (Figs 2.17A and B)

It was designed by HO Thomas for tuberculosis of the knee. It has one outer bar, one inner bar and one ring. The ring is at an angle of 120° to the inside bar and the outer bar has a curve to accommodate the greater trochanter.

Size and preparation of Thomas splint: Appropriate length of the Thomas splint should be chosen for proper splinting. Ring size is chosen by adding 2 inches to the thigh circumference at the highest point of groin. Length is measured by adding 6 inches to the length from the highest point on the medial side of groin to heel. After having chosen the appropriate size, Thomas splint is prepared by padding on it by cotton bandages and cotton. The ring should also be padded well to avoid impingement on the skin.

Use: It is used for immobilization of the lower limb in hip and thigh injuries. It is efficient and easy to use tool for transportation of patients with lower limb injuries. Fixed and sliding traction can also be given on Thomas splint.

Cramer Wire Splint (Figs 2.18A and B)

It is made up of two thick and parallel wires with many interlacing wires (ladder splint). It is a flexible splint which can be bent into different shapes to accommodate different body parts. It is used

Table 2.6: Commonly used splints and braces

Name	Use
Aeroplane splint	Brachial plexus injury
Aluminum splint	Fracture of phalanges
Anterior spinal hyperextension (ASHE) brace	Dorsolumbar spinal injury
Ankle support	Ankle sprain, ankle fractures
Bohler-Braun splint	Lower limb fractures—tibia and femur
Buddy strapping	Phalangeal fracture
Cramer wire splint	Fractures of arm, forearm, and leg
Cock up splint	Radial nerve palsy
Denis Brown splint	CTEV
Figure of eight brace	Clavicle fracture
Four post collar, SOMI brace, Philadelphia collar	Cervical spine injury
Forearm sugar tong splint	Distal forearm and wrist fracture
Knuckle bender splint	Ulnar nerve palsy
Lumbo-Sacral corset	Lumbar strain
Mallet finger splint/Stack splint	Mallet finger
Milwaukee/Boston brace/Lyon brace/Providence brace/Charleston brace/Wilmington brace/SpineCor brace	Scoliosis
Radial gutter splint	Fracture of radial-sided metacarpals
Sling and swathe	Shoulder and humeral injuries
Taylors brace	Dorsolumbar spinal injury
Thomas splint	Lower limb fractures
Toe raising splint/AFO brace	Foot drop
Tripoint splint	Boutonniere deformity, swan-neck deformity
Ulnar gutter splint	Fracture of ulnar-sided metacarpals, Boxer's fracture
Volkmann's splint and Turn buckle splint	Volkmann's ischemic contracture
Von Rosen's splint, Pavlik Harness, Frejka pillow	Congenital dislocation of hip

Abbreviations: SOMI, sterno-occipital mandibular immobilizer; CTEV, congenital talipes equinovarus; AFO, ankle foot orthosis.

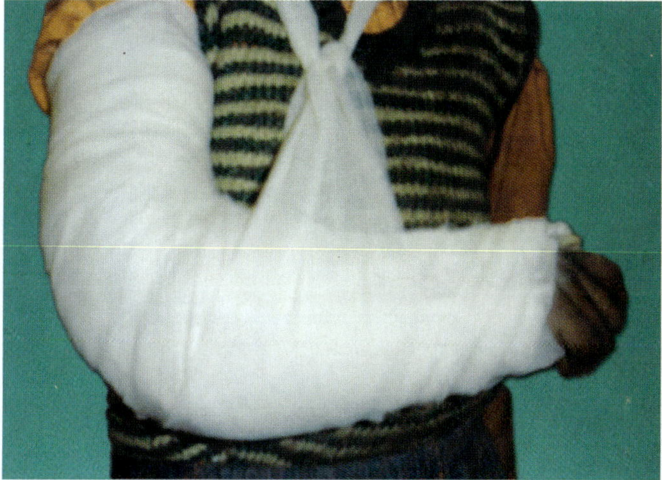

Fig. 2.16: Plaster of Paris (POP) splint

for temporary splinting of fractures of both upper and lower limbs during transportation.

Bohler-Braun Splint (Figs 2.19A and B)

Bohler modified the Braun's splint which had only one pulley for tibial traction. Bohler-Braun (BB) splint has three pulleys for simultaneous tibial and femoral tractions and to change the angle of traction. Commercially available BB splint has three or four pulleys. It is used for both tibial and femoral fractures.

Functions of Pulleys

- *Pulley A:* Calcaneal/tibial traction
- *Pulley B:* Femoral traction
- *Pulley C:* It is used to change the line/angle of traction. It is also used to prevent equinus deformity of the ankle or foot drop.

One disadvantage of BB splint is that ambulation of patients is difficult with it.

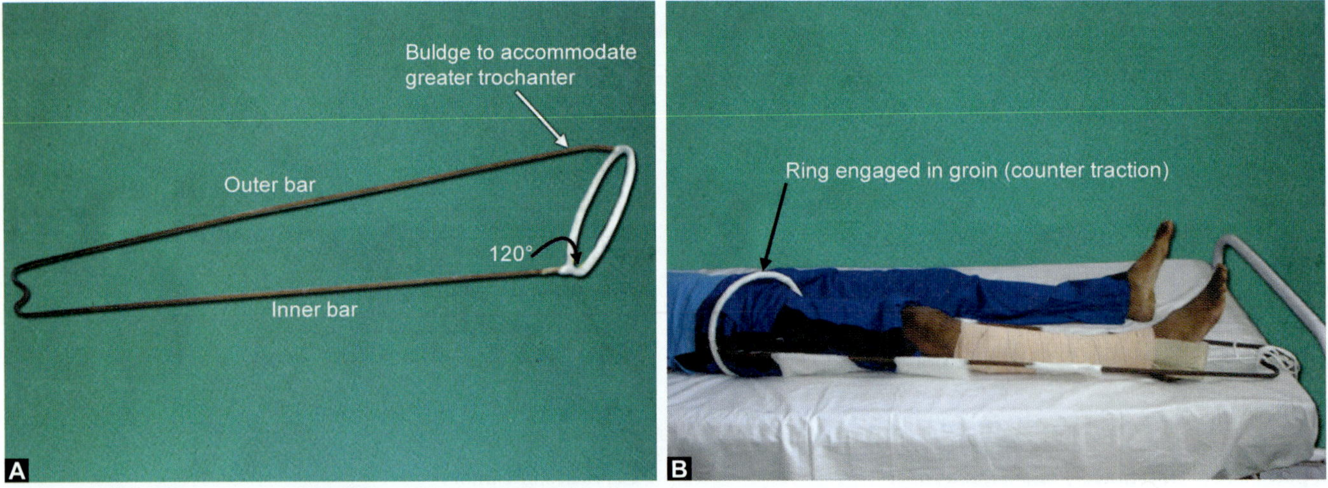

Figs 2.17A and B: (A) Thomas splint and (B) Fixed traction on Thomas splint

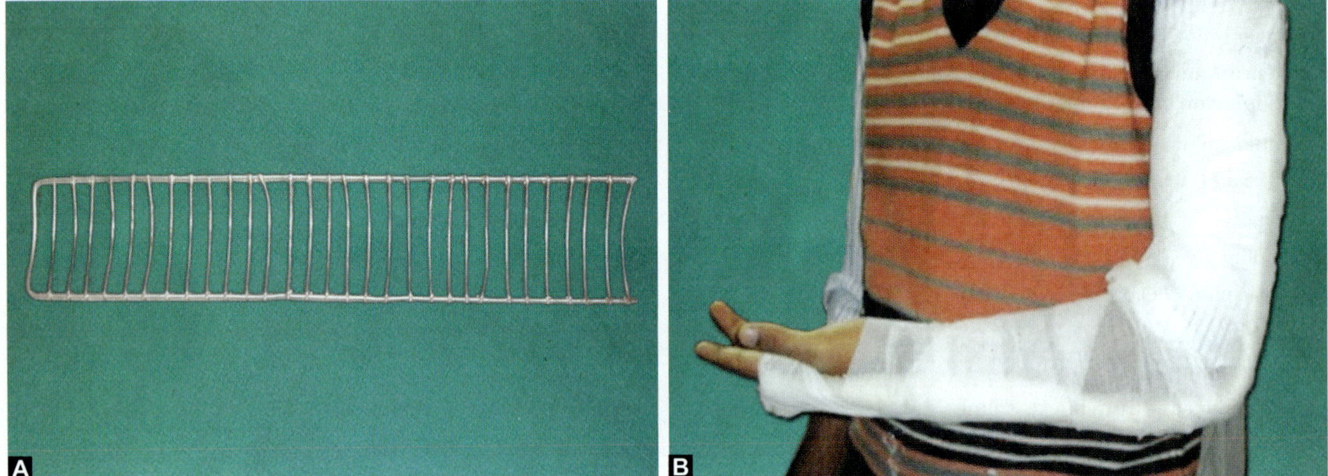

Figs 2.18A and B: (A) Cramer wire splint and (B) It can be easily bent to support fractures of limbs

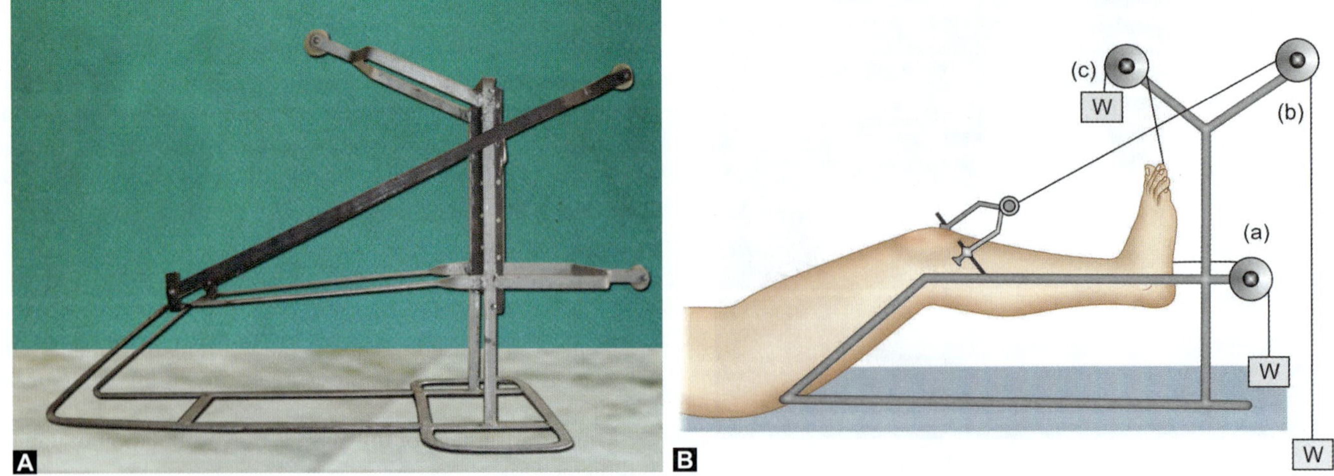

Figs 2.19A and B: (A) Bohler-Braun (BB) splint and (B) Traction on BB splint

HIGH-YIELD POINTS

- Two great surgeons are associated with BB splint. (1) Lorenz Böhler, the "Father of Traumatology", and (2) Heinrich Braun, the "Father of Local Anesthesia".
- *Tobruk splint*: Fixes traction of lower limb on a Thomas splint. Mostly used in treatment of pediatric femur shaft fractures.
- *Fisk splint*: Modified Thomas splint to which a knee flexion piece is attached.

Indications of Splinting

Splints are indicated in initial management of acute musculo-skeletal injuries. They are used for short-term before the definitive treatment is done. Splints are noncircumferential immobilizers and can accommodate swelling so they are best indicated for injuries where swelling is anticipated.

Indications for use of a splint are as follows:
- *Used for transportation*: Splinting of the injured limb provides and makes the transportation of the patient easy and less painful before the definitive treatment. Thomas splint and Cramer wire splint are particularly used for this purpose.
- *Used for traction*: Some splints are used for preoperative traction of the fractured limb. This helps in reducing the pain and spasm, correcting deformity and maintaining limb alignment, e.g. BB splint and fixed traction on Thomas splint.
- *Therapeutic use*: Splints are also used to maintain deformity correction [e.g. Dennis-Brown splint in congenital talipes equinovarus (CTEV)] and to prevent deformity (Cock-up splint in radial nerve palsy). A valgus knee splint is used in medial compartment osteoarthritis for pain relief.
- To provide rest for acutely inflamed joints as a knee brace in TB knee and ankle brace in an ankle sprain.

- They are also used in the postoperative period in the form of immobilizers (especially at the shoulder and the knee) for helping in early cautioned mobilization of patients.

Precautions and Care

- Always splint the joint above and below the site of trauma.
- Use appropriate amount and type of "padding to avoid pressure sores". Properly pad bony prominences and high-pressure areas before application of a splint.
- Properly position the extremity before, during, and after application of splints/casts.
- Always assess the skin condition and dress the wound before splinting. Keep the limb elevated and document the neurovascular status of the affected limb before splinting.
- Always have an eye on the presence/development of compartment syndrome in an injured limb. Diagnosis is made on clinical suspicion of tense swelling and pain on passive stretching of digits. Always keep the distal extremity uncovered for serial assessment of neurovascular status.
- Encourage active toe/finger movements to reduce swelling and advise cryotherapy for pain relief.

TRACTION

Traction is defined as the application of a continuous, well-sustained pulling force on a limb or muscle group in order to achieve a normal anatomical orientation and correction of bony deformity which occurred due to the fracture or dislocation. Traction relieves pain by counteracting the muscle spasm and allows limb to rest in functional position. Commonly used traction systems in orthopedics are listed in **Table 2.7**.

For traction to be effective countertraction is needed. Countertraction is the pull acting to offset or oppose primary

Table 2.7: Commonly used traction systems in orthopedics	
Traction	*Use*
Agnes hunt traction	Hip flexion deformity correction
Bryant's traction, Gallows traction, 90-90 traction, Fisk traction	Fracture shaft femur
Buck's traction/skin traction	Preoperatively in femoral fractures, to give rest to the infected joint of the lower limb, undisplaced/minimally displaced fracture of acetabulum, after reduction of dislocated hip joint
Calcaneal traction	Preoperatively used in tibial fracture
Crutchfield tongs, head halter traction, Gardner well tongs, halo-pelvic traction	Cervical spine injury
Dunlop traction, smith traction	Supracondylar fracture humerus
Halo-pelvic traction	Spinal deformities (scoliosis)
Head Halter traction	Neck pain
Lower tibial traction	Tibial fracture
Metacarpal traction	Comminuted forearm fractures
Olecranon traction	Supracondylar humeral fracture or comminuted distal humeral fracture
Perkin's traction	Tibial and femoral fractures
Pelvic belt traction (Intermittent lumbar traction)	Low back ache (given on OPD basis)
Russel Hamilton traction	Trochanteric fracture, femoral shaft fracture
Supracondylar femoral traction	Proximal femoral and shaft fracture
Upper tibial traction	Femoral fracture
Well leg traction	Correction of adduction or abduction deformities of hip joint

traction force used for the reduction and to maintain the reduction. Depending on the force providing countertraction, the tractions may be grouped as:

- *Fixed (Fig. 2.17B):* When the countertraction is produced by the traction system itself. A part of traction system gets purchase on a part of the patient's body. For example, in the Thomas splint, ring takes purchase around the groin and produces countertraction. Fixed traction cannot obtain reduction, but can maintain it.
- *Sliding/balanced (Fig. 2.20):* Where the countertraction is applied by the horizontal component of body weight. The body is kept at an angle by raising the foot end of the bed and gravity/weight of the patient provides the countertraction. Roughly 1 inch elevation is required for each pound of traction weight.
- *Combined traction:* Uses both fixed and sliding tractions. Tractions can also be grouped depending on the methods of application of traction. The two methods are:
  1. *Skin traction/Buck's traction (Fig. 2.21):* It is a noninvasive method which can sustain no more than 10 lbs or 6 kg force. It is commonly used in children as their muscle mass and hence spasm is less. It should not be used to obtain or maintain the reduction. It can be applied by two methods, adhesive skin traction and nonadhesive skin traction (vent-foam skin traction).

     Contraindications to skin traction: It cannot be used where skin condition is poor (wound, allergy, dermatitis, impairment of circulation, venous ulcers, impending gangrene) or in cases of marked shortening/overriding of bony fragments.

     Complications: Excoriation of skin from slipping of the adhesive strapping, pressure sores around the bony prominences and rarely common peroneal nerve palsy are a few complications.
  2. *Skeletal traction (Figs 2.22 and 2.23):* It is a more definitive form of traction. It is applied by a metal pin (Steinmann or Denham pin) passed through bone and a Bohler stirrup attached to it. It is used for reducing as well as maintaining the reduction of a fracture.

     Usual sites of skeletal traction are the upper third tibia, distal third tibia, supracondylar femur and the calcaneum in fractures of the lower limb. Olecranon, 2nd and 3rd metacarpals are usual sites in upper limb for passage of pins for skeletal traction.

     Complications: Pin site infections, distraction at the fracture site, skin necrosis at the entry site, damage to the epiphyseal plate in children and rarely osteomyelitis are a few complications of skeletal traction.

Indications of Traction

- To regain "anatomical alignment" and relation in cases of fractures and dislocations when surgery is delayed or not possible due to medical reasons.
- To "reduce muscle spasm", deformities and relieve pain, e.g. poliotic/spastic limb, TB hip, psoas abscess.
- For "decompression of nerve root impingement" (sciatica, spondylolisthesis, compression fractures of spine).

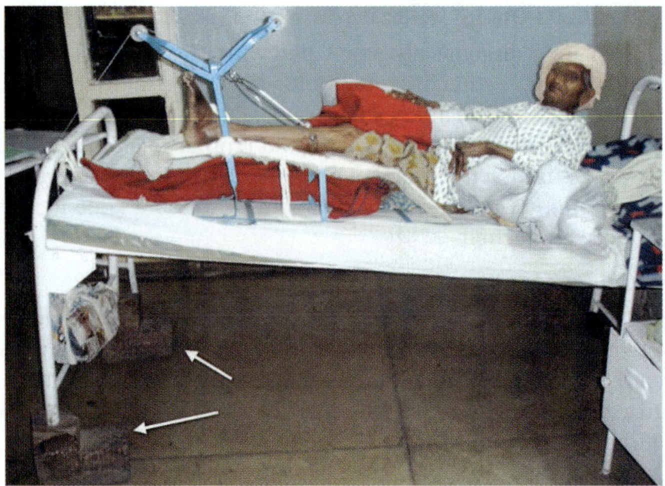

Fig. 2.20: Sliding traction on Bohler-Braun (BB) splint where the foot end of the bed is elevated (arrows) to give countertraction by virtue of gravity

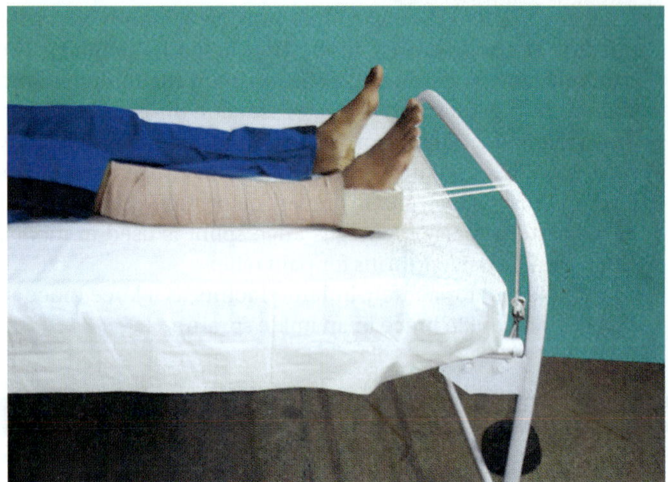

Fig. 2.21: Nonadhesive skin traction

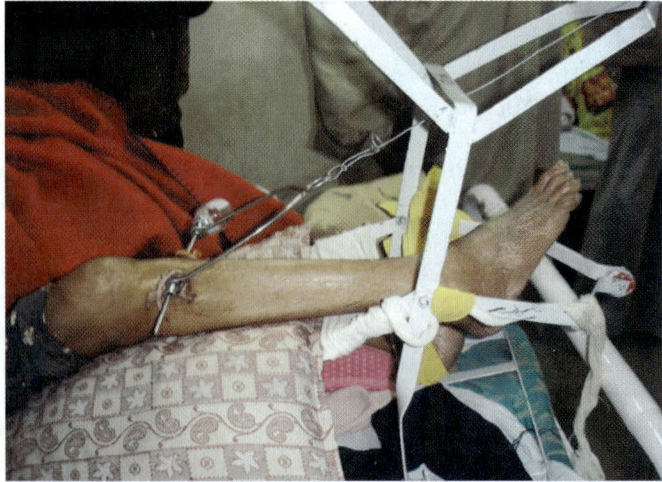

Fig. 2.22: Upper tibial skeletal traction on Bohler-Braun (BB) splint

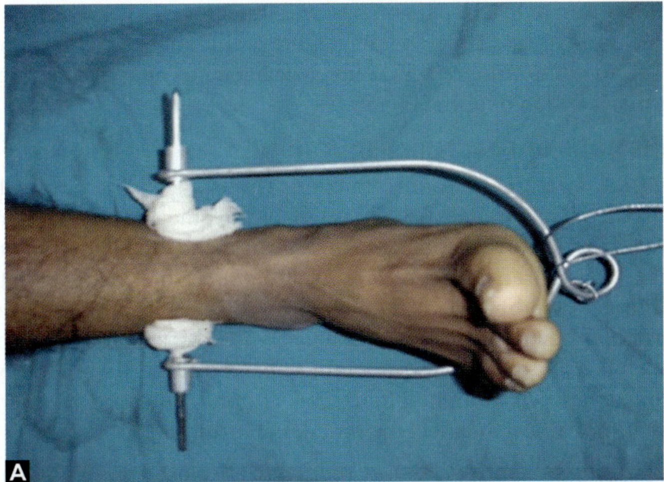

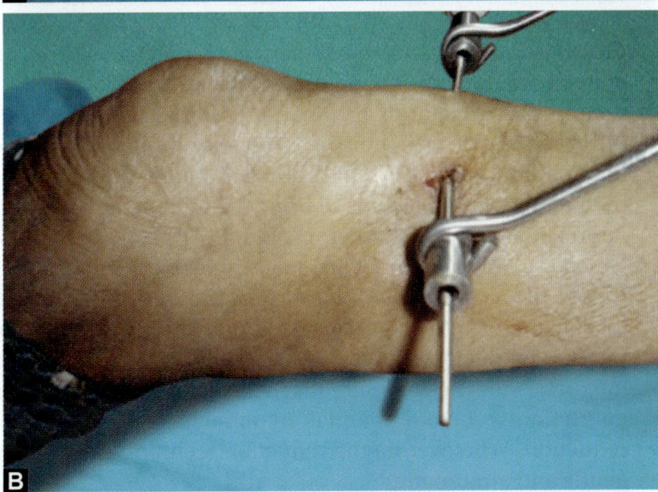

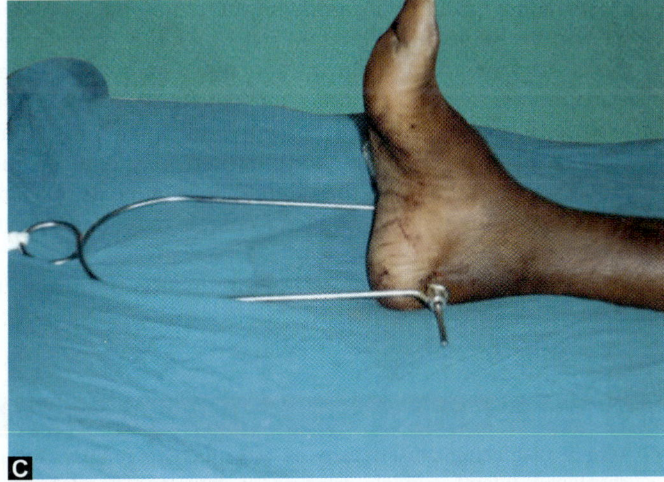

Figs 2.23A to C: Common orthopedic tractions: (A) Lower tibial traction;
(B) Upper tibial traction and (C) Calcaneal traction

Contraindications

- "Active" stage of inflammatory (rheumatoid) or infective arthritis
- Spinal instability
- Signs of "vascular disease", i.e. ischemia

- Increased pain or worsening of symptoms with traction
- Fractures with metastatic bone disease
- Pregnancy.

Precaution and Care

- The limb should be "comfortably placed" and "adequate weight" should be applied depending on the site of fracture/deformity and the built of the patient. Up to 20 kg weight can be put on skeletal traction.
- The "weight" should "never touch the ground" and counter should always be in place if the traction is sliding. The ropes should be on the pulley only.
- Proper "pin site care" and daily cleaning and dressing is must to minimize chances of pin site infection.
- Good nursing care is very important to avoid complications of recumbency, i.e. frequent turning over in bed to avoid pressure sores, active and passive physiotherapy to avoid joint stiffness and muscle wasting.
- Frequent documentation of neurovascular status is very important. Swelling of the toes may indicate tight skin traction. Any tingling/paresthesia may indicate towards excessive traction causing traction palsy of nerve.
- Regular X-ray of the limb should be done to see the reduction of fracture.

BEDS AND FRAMES

Ideal orthopedic bed for patients with multiple injuries is one with adjustable height, i.e. Bradford frame. It allows for change of bed pan and linen without moving the patient.

Balkan beam frame (Florschutz frame) **(Fig. 2.24)** is still used in orthopedic wards where Bradford frame is not available. It is an overhead frame attached to the patient's bed consisting of overhead bars with pulleys attached to them which allow patient to lift up pelvis, turn postures easily preventing bed sores and hence improves self-care.

HIGH-YIELD POINTS

- The first use of traction for correcting overriding of bone fragments was described by Galen.
- *Perkins' traction*: Its a skeletal traction without use of any splint.

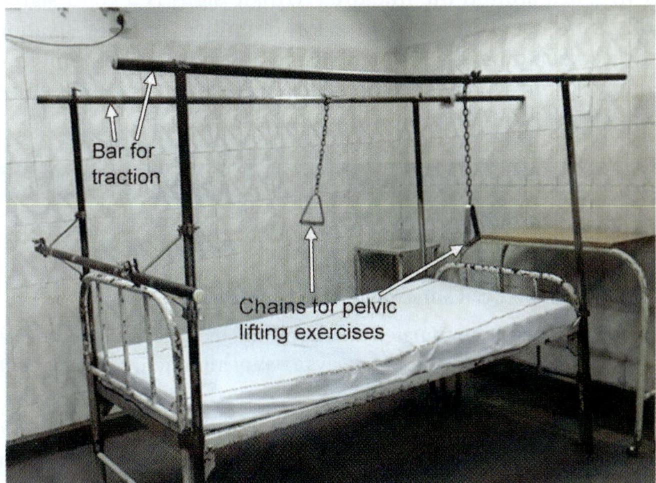

Fig. 2.24: Balkan's beam frame

GENERAL PRINCIPLES OF FRACTURE FIXATION

PRINCIPLES OF FRACTURE MANAGEMENT

Management of a fractured bone should aim not only at restoration of bony anatomy, but functional rehabilitation of the limb also. Diagnosis of a fracture with modern diagnostic modalities is usually straightforward. Management of a fracture can be summarized in the following headings:

- *Resuscitation and patient stabilization:* Based on advanced trauma life support (ATLS) guidelines
- Management of soft-tissue injury
- Fracture reduction
- *Maintenance of reduction by fracture immobilization:* Cast immobilization, internal fixation or external fixation
- Rehabilitation.

RESUSCITATION AND PATIENT STABILIZATION

Orthopedic trauma patients are often victims of high-velocity road traffic accidents and may sustain multiple injuries. Some injuries may be life-threatening and need immediate intervention before the definitive treatment of fracture is begun (save life, then save the limb, then save joint, then save function). ATLS guidelines provide comprehensive and speedy management of such injuries (*see* Chapter 3 for details).

MANAGEMENT OF SOFT-TISSUE INJURY

Traumatic fracture of the bone is almost always associated with injury to its soft-tissue cover.

Tscherne graded the soft-tissue injury associated with closed fracture in four grades **(Table 2.8)**.

The soft-tissue injury does not mean injury to only skin and muscles. Look also for blood vessels injury (signs of ischemia), nerve injury (paresthesia, sensory loss, motor weakness), ligament injury (joint instability), etc.

In Grade 0 or I injuries, the focus is on treatment of fracture only. However, in Grade II or III injuries, outcome of fracture management depends upon the timely and effective dealing with soft-tissue injury. The limb should be splinted to provide rest to injured tissues and put on traction to keep the fracture aligned. Elevation of the limb helps in subsidence of swelling. Appearance of wrinkles around the fracture (Wrinkle sign) is a good sign of soft-tissue recovery and time for definitive fracture fixation. Always keep an eye with high suspicion on the development of compartment syndrome in both closed and open fractures. Out of

proportion pain and pain on passive stretching of muscles are the earliest features. Timely management is the only key to save the limb in compartment syndrome. Management of open fractures is discussed in detail in Chapter 3.

METHODS OF FRACTURE REDUCTION

Not all fractures require reduction. Undisplaced or minimally displaced fractures are usually amenable to direct immobilization. The criteria for acceptable reduction depend on many factors like site of fracture, age, etc. As a general rule, acceptability criteria are more generous for children than adults and for extra-articular fractures than intra-articular fractures. In some fractures like clavicle fracture and fractured neck of humerus in elderly, conservative treatment often gives a good outcome as slight malunion does not affect the functional result.

Two main methods of fracture reduction are closed reduction and open reduction.

1. *Closed reduction:* In closed reduction, fracture site is not opened so fracture hematoma is retained. Reduction is done under general or regional anesthesia, but sometimes intravenous (IV) sedation or local anesthesia may suffice. Manual traction is given to disimpact the fracture ends and then manipulation is done to bring the fracture ends in close approximation in both anteroposterior (AP) and lateral views which is confirmed under an image intensifier.

   Closed reduction by mechanical traction: In some fractures, displacing force of muscles is too much to reduce the fracture manually, e.g. in a fractured shaft of femur, cervical fractures, etc. These require mechanical traction (via special instruments) before manual manipulation for achieving reduction. Whatever be the reduction technique, it must be gentle and atraumatic.

2. *Open reduction:* In open reduction, fracture site is opened so fracture hematoma is drained. Reduction is done under direct vision with the help of reduction forceps and other instruments. Heroic efforts for anatomical reduction (excessive use of reduction forceps and other tools) may cause excessive periosteal stripping and may damage the blood supply to bone. So they should be avoided as they are actually detrimental to healing. Acceptable reduction should be aimed.

Fractures that mostly require open reduction are listed in **Box 2.8**.

Table 2.8: Tscherne's classification of soft-tissue injury in closed fracture	
Grade	*Classification*
0	No or minor soft-tissue injury
I	Superficial abrasion or skin contusion
II	Deep contaminated abrasions and localized skin or muscle contusions. There is always a risk of imminent compartment syndrome in this group
III	Extensive skin contusion, destruction of muscle or subcutaneous tissue avulsion (closed degloving). High chances of compartment syndrome and vascular injuries compared to other grades

Box 2.8: Fractures requiring open reduction

- Where displacing muscle force is too much to reduce close; displaced lateral condyle fracture of humerus in children, displaced fracture patella
- Where restoration of anatomy is of utmost importance; displaced intra-articular fracture, displaced type III and IV epiphyseal injury in children
- Atrophic nonunion requiring bone grafting
- Fractures with vascular injury
- Where closed reduction fails

IMMOBILIZATION METHODS

There are four methods of fracture immobilization and maintaining the reduction achieved.

- *Cast immobilization*: Mostly used for fractures that have been reduced closed.
- *Continuous traction*: Used in cases where one cannot apply cast or fix a fracture with an implant.
- *External fixation*: Primarily a method of immobilization for open fractures.
- *Internal fixation (osteosynthesis)*: It is a rule for fixing fractures that have been reduced by open incisions. Implants put inside the skin are used to fix fractures reduced in a closed manner (*see* below).

Cast Immobilization

Plaster of Paris cast immobilization is still the standard method of immobilization for most fractures that have been reduced closed. In acute fractures, casts are applied as slabs (plaster that covers three-fourth circumference of a limb) and not as full circumference plasters due to risk of swelling and development of compartment syndrome. When the swelling subsides, usually after a week, the slab is converted into a full cast.

Fiber cast is now available, which is light weight, radiolucent and impervious to water but costlier than POP cast. In acute displaced fractures, the plaster cast is preferred because molding of plaster cast according to body contours is easier than fiber cast.

Some common fractures where cast is usually a preferred method of immobilization are given in **Box 2.9.** Commonly used cast methods are tabulated in **Table 2.9.**

Wedging of a cast (Figs 2.25A and B): This is a reduction technique used in long bone diaphyseal fractures with angular malalignment. In this technique, a window is cut in the cast at fracture level, leaving a hinge intact on the apex of the deformity. For example, in valgus deformity (distal fragment going laterally) window is cut on lateral side leaving a hinge on medial side and varus force is applied distal to the fracture. Once the correction is obtained, more cast material is applied to fix the achieved reduction.

Precautions and Care of Cast

- Adequate padding of cotton or stockinette and synthetic wool should be done before applying cast.
- The plaster cast is a circumferential splint and well-fitted cast does not accommodate swelling. If swelling appears after casting it can hamper arterial blood flow. Keep a careful watch for signs and symptoms of compromised circulation. Excessive swellings of digits and out of proportion pain are alarming signs and if present, plaster should be cut and limb should be assessed for development of compartment syndrome.
- The limb should be kept elevated to prevent development of swelling.
- There should not be any indentations on the cast as it may impinge upon underlying soft tissues. Similarly edges of the cast should not impinge upon the skin.

Table 2.9: Common cast and slabs

Cast and slab	Joints and fractures
Burkhalter cast	Metacarpals and phalangeal fractures
Colles' cast	Colles' fracture
Cylindrical cast	Undisplaced patellar fracture, ligament injuries around knee
Hanging cast	Fractured shaft of humerus
Hip spica	Fractured shaft of femur in children
James slab	Metacarpals and phalangeal fractures
Minerva cast	Cervical spine injury
Patellar tendon bearing (PTB) cast	Fractured shaft of tibia
Risser's cast	Scoliosis
Scaphoid cast	Scaphoid fracture
Thumb spica	Fractures involving the base of thumb
Turn buckle cast	Scoliosis
U slab	Fractured shaft of humerus

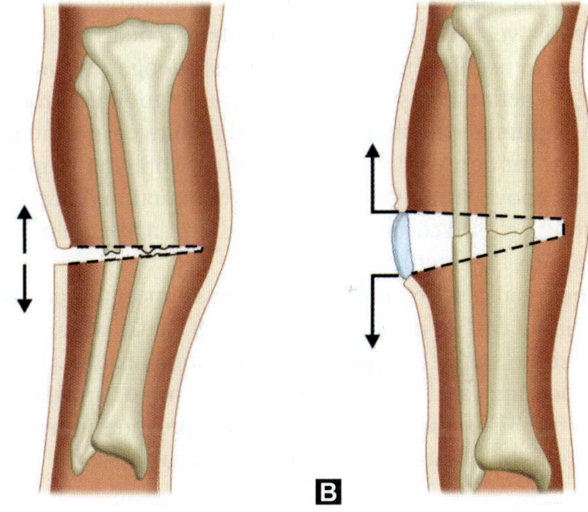

Figs 2.25A and B: Wedging of a cast

Box 2.9: Fractures where cast immobilization is commonly used

- Most pediatric fractures (as remodeling is very good)
- Adult fractures:
  - Metacarpal and metatarsal fractures
  - Colles' fracture
  - Fracture of surgical neck of humerus in elderly
  - Stress fractures
  - Undisplaced fractures of the carpal and tarsal bones
  - Undisplaced/minimally displaced ankle fractures

HIGH-YIELD POINTS

- *The "Rule of Two" for cast application*: A cast for any fracture should always immobilize one joint above and one joint below the fracture site.
- Charnley popularized the concepts of fracture reduction and cast immobilization for many fractures.

- *Cast syndrome (superior mesenteric artery syndrome)*: It is a rare complication of body casts or hip spicas that is characterized by gastric dilatation due to partial or complete obstruction of the duodenum. Obstruction occurs as there is compression of the first part of duodenum between the superior mesenteric artery anteriorly and the aorta and spinal column posteriorly. It is treated by removal of cast and nasogastric decompression, fluid replacement, proper positioning and hyperalimentation. Surgery is rarely needed.
- *Fracture disease (a term popularized by James Paget)*: It is the name given to the constellation of symptoms which occur following immobilization in a cast. It is characterized by pain, swelling, stiffness, muscle atrophy, etc. Early physiotherapy should be encouraged to prevent it. As per some workers, this term is a part of reflex sympathetic dystrophy syndrome (*see* Page 97).

Functional Cast Bracing *(Fig. 2.26)*

Functional cast bracing concept was popularized in the late 1960s by Sarmiento. Initially it was done for tibial fractures, but later on for femur and upper limb fractures also. The technique of functional cast bracing consists of applying a splint (called brace) to the fractured limb that while supporting the fracture allows early weight bearing and movement of nearby joints. Early mobilization in this manner encourages osteogenesis and tissue healing. Functional cast brace is accurately molded around the limb in segments which are connected by hinges around joint to allow joint motion while conventional cast bracing immobilizes the joints above and below the fracture. Functional brace works by creating a closed compartment simulating a hydraulic cylinder that supports the fracture.

Functional cast bracing provides less support to fracture than conventional cast so it is applied after 2–3 weeks when fractured ends become sticky and pain and swelling subsides. The early weight bearing is allowed with painless minor movement on fracture site. Thus, functional cast bracing prevents joint stiffness, speeds-up rehabilitation and promotes osteogenesis.

Continuous Traction

Role of traction for immobilization in modern orthopedic practice is very limited. Only valid indication for which continuous traction is still widely practiced is cervical fractures and dislocations. In some fractures like fractured shaft of femur, proximal femoral fractures, acetabular fractures, comminuted Pilon fracture and fracture dislocation of the hip joint, if surgery is delayed or postponed due to medical or other reasons, patient is put on continuous skeletal traction to maintain the limb alignment and achieve union in acceptable position. Cast immobilization is not appropriate to hold the fragments in the proper position in these fractures.

Immobilization by External Fixation

In this method, fractured fragments are anchored to an external bar with the help of pins inserted into proximal and distal fragments of bone. Two or three pins are inserted into each fragment and connected to a rod or bar with the help of clamps **(Fig. 2.27)**. This method is mainly applied in cases of open and infected fractures where internal fixation carries a high risk of infection or its exacerbation. An external fixator in this situation provides a stabilizing assembly that simultaneously allows dressing of the wound, and since most of its assembly is outside the skin, there are least chances of infection. Commonly used external fixator frames are one plane (monolateral) frame, two planes (bilateral) frame and ring fixator.

Ilizarov Ring Fixator

Russian surgeon, Gavriil Ilizarov pioneered the revolutionary technique of bone and soft-tissue regeneration based on distraction osteogenesis in the 1960s.

Principle: It is based on the principle of "distraction histogenesis" which states that gradual distraction of bone at the rate of 1 mm/day, regenerates new bone at the distraction site. At the site of distraction, fibroblast-like cells become metabolically active and secrete collagen. Dormant mesenchymal cells at the site get converted into osteoblasts and secrete osteoid. Growth

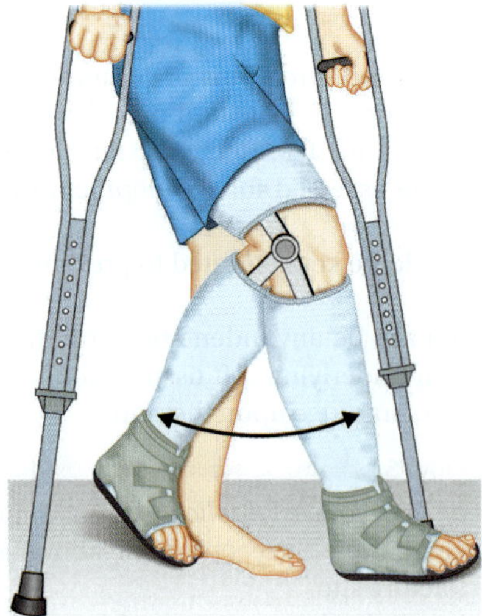

Fig. 2.26: Functional bracing for tibial diaphyseal fracture

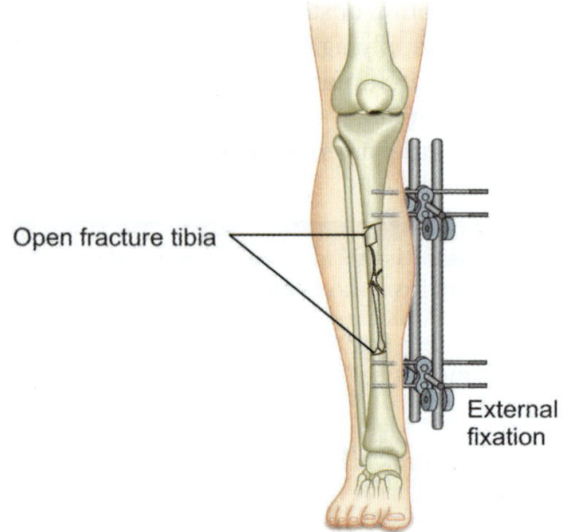

Fig. 2.27: External fixator assembly being used in treating open fracture of the tibia

changes are also seen in soft tissues with cellular hypertrophy and hyperplasia in myocytes, capillary formation and development of nerves in the direction of tension vector, so all tissues including bone are lengthened.

*Assembly and technique (**Figs 2.28A and B**):* The Ilizarov external fixator is a special modified external fixator that has a complex assembly of metal rings, threaded rods and Kirschner wires. Wires are passed through skin and soft tissue and drilled through both bony cortices. Wires are attached under tension to half and full metal rings encircling the bone. Assembly is completed by connecting the rings to threaded rods. Assembly can be angulated using hinges if deformity correction is planned. After fixation of the assembly, corticotomy (cutting the cortices of bone while leaving a posterior hinge of periosteum intact for vascular supply) is done in the bone to be lengthened. Corticotomy is usually done at the metaphysis because of high potential for osteogenesis in metaphyseal cancellous bone. Gradual distraction is started after a few days of corticotomy. Few days are given as a latency period for hematoma to form and organize at site of corticotomy. Rate of distraction is kept slow at 1 mm/day at a rhythm of 0.25 mm every 6 hours. New bone is formed by gradual distraction at the corticotomy site. Additionally, corticotomy increases blood flow to the involved extremity and since thin tensioned wires are used for fixation, the construct has a "trampoline-like effect" allowing micromotion at fracture that further encourages union **(Fig. 2.28B)**. Uses of Ilizarov method are given in **Box 2.10**.

HIGH-YIELD POINTS

- Taylor spatial frame **(Fig. 2.28C)** and Limb Reconstruction System (LRS, **Fig. 2.28D**) also called as Rail road fixator are other external fixator modifications used for limb lengthening, in the treatment of nonunion and deformity correction. They are easier to apply than Ilizarov fixator, but costlier.
- Intramedullary devices are also available for limb lengthening, but not for deformity correction.
- Even up to 10 cm of bone has been reported to be lengthened by the use of Ilizarov.

Complications: Ilizarov technique is a complex procedure and should be done by experts only. Complications related to the procedure are muscle contracture, neurovascular insult, pin site infection, premature or delayed consolidation at corticotomy site and problems regarding patient compliance. Since Ilizarov frame needs to be kept for a long time (~1 cm of bone is formed per month), this often leads to social isolation of the patient and also it is cumbersome to carry the heavy frame.

Managing complications: Pin site infection is the most common complication. Daily pin care with saline cleaning and Betadine dressing of the pin tract should be done. In severe infection, the pin is removed and new pin is inserted elsewhere. Thorough knowledge of neurovascular anatomy is necessary to avoid neurovascular injury during pin insertion. During the distraction if sensory symptoms appear, rate of distraction is slowed or even stopped until symptoms disappear. Proper splinting and physiotherapy is necessary to prevent soft-tissue contractures. Regular radiological examination of the whole limb should be done to judge the consolidation at corticotomy site and also for earliest detection of subluxation or dislocation of adjacent joints.

Internal Fixation (Osteosynthesis)

In modern orthopedic practice, the trend has been changed in favor of internal fixation (fixing a fracture with implants applied inside the skin) of most fractures. Benefits of internal fixation are early mobilization preventing joint stiffness and more anatomical fracture alignment.

Internal fixation is the rule for all fractures that are treated by open reduction where the complete treatment is called as open reduction and internal fixation (ORIF).

However, in some special situations, internal fixation can also be done in some fractures that have been reduced closed, e.g. while nailing a long bone **(Figs 2.29A to C)**. Here the treatment is called as close reduction and internal fixation (CRIF) as skin incision (e.g. at greater trochanter in femur nailing) being away from fracture site does not drain the hematoma (so closed reduction) while the fracture is fixed with an implant that lies inside the skin (internal fixation).

Classical examples of closed reduction (hematoma not drained) and internal fixation (implant inside the skin) include:
- Nailing of a long bone
- Fixing of a neck femur fracture with multiple screws*
- Pinning (putting K wires) in supracondylar humerus fractures*

Various methods of internal fixation available include:
- *Screws*: They are inserted either directly across the fracture (lag screw) to compress it or put through the plates to fix a fracture. Common types of screws are cortical, cancellous and locking screws (*see* Pages 491 and 493).
- *Kirschner wires (K-wires)*: These are stainless steel wires which are available in 1–3 mm diameters. These are used mainly in pediatric fractures or in fractures of the small bones of hands and feet.
- *Plates*: These are available in different designs and contour for different fractures. Five basic principles on which plates work are listed in **Table 2.10** and **Figures 2.30 and 2.31**.
- *Intramedullary nails*: These have drastically evolved over time from k-nail of 1940s to present-day interlocking nails (*see* below)

Box 2.10: Use of Ilizarov method

- In the treatment of infected nonunion and gap nonunion
- In deformity correction, malunion and burn contracture
- To gain length of limb
- In joint arthrodesis
- Proximal focal femoral deficiency
- Chronic osteomyelitis
- Chronic dislocations
- *Neglected clubfoot:* For distracting posteromedial side of the foot

---

*In the latter two situations, the skin incisions are minimal such that the hematoma is not drained so closed reduction, but since an implant has been put within the body (inside the skin cover) to fix the fracture, it is an internal fixation.

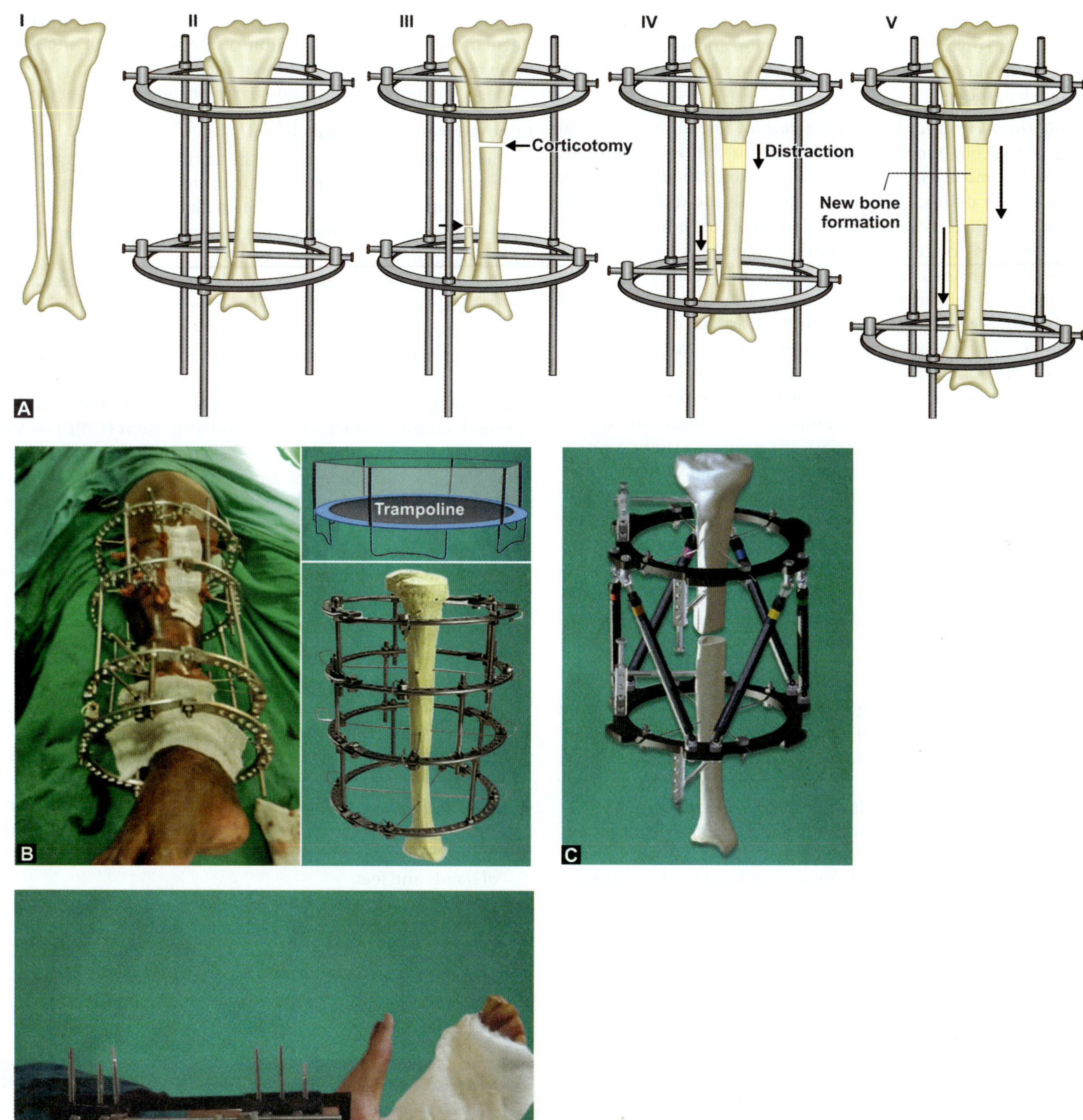

Figs 2.28A to D: (A) Limb lengthening by Ilizarov ring fixator (I to V); (B) Ilizarov ring fixator depicting "trampoline effect"; (C) Taylor spatial frame; (D) LRS fixator

Some Special Implants for Internal Fixation

Dynamic compression plate (DCP): In DCP, tightening of eccentrically placed screws in screw holes of plate causes axial compression of fracture. First centrally placed screws are used to compress the plate against bone in one fragment. Now in opposite fragment screws are placed eccentrically in a hole that

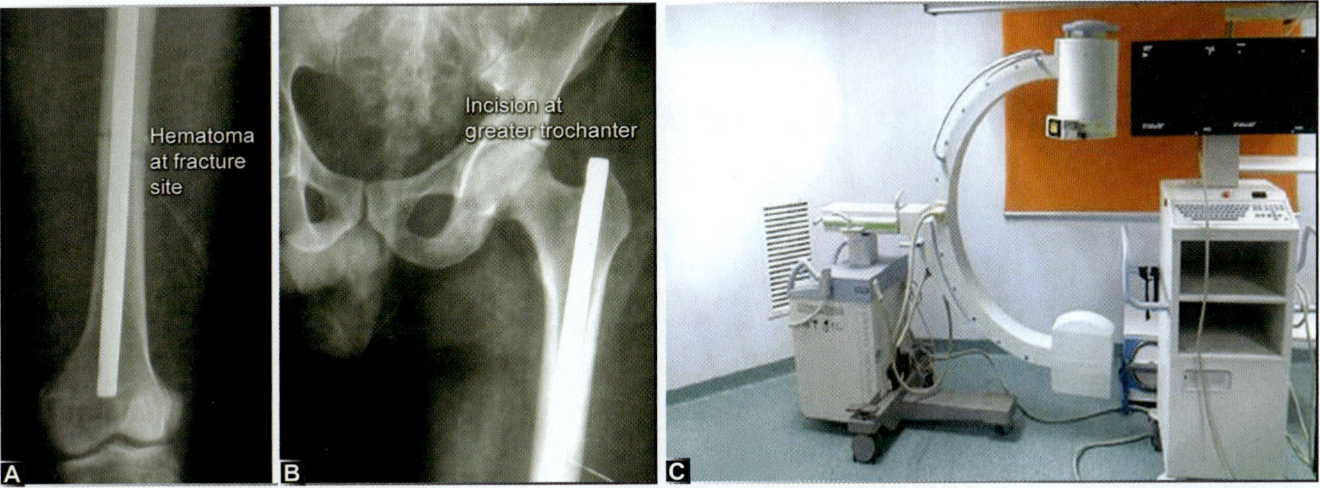

Figs 2.29A to C: A shaft femur fracture fixed by close reduction and internal fixation (CRIF) using intramedullary nail (Figs A and B). Fracture reduction is achieved closed under X-ray guidance thorough use of image intensifier (Fig. C)

Table 2.10: Principles of plate fixation **(Figs 2.30 and 2.31)**

Parameters	Principles	Example
Compression	This plate produces compression across the fracture when it is fixed plate across the fracture with screws (*read dynamic compression plate*)	Transverse or oblique forearm fractures
Neutralization plate	Its main function is to link the bones above and below the fracture without producing any compression across the fracture. It is used to protect the lag screw which is used to compress the fracture	Butterfly fracture (fracture with a separated wedge-shaped chip of bone) of metaphysis or diaphysis
Bridge plate	It is used to bridge "a comminution" in metaphyseal and diaphyseal fractures. It is a less rigid fixation than compression plating	Comminuted metaphyseal or diaphyseal fractures
Buttress plate	It is a plate with a broad surface area that is used to prevent displacement of a large fracture fragment, mostly of an articular surface	Tibial plateau or distal femur or distal radius fractures
Tension band plate (TBP)	Tension band principle (*read below*) can be exploited, if a plate can be fixed on convex side of a curved bone. Axial load causes concave bone surface to collapse, generating tensile (distraction) stresses on opposite side in plate. By Newton's III Law, reaction occurs in form of compression at fracture site	Plating convex surfaces in femur, radius, tibial fractures (when fracture geometry permits)

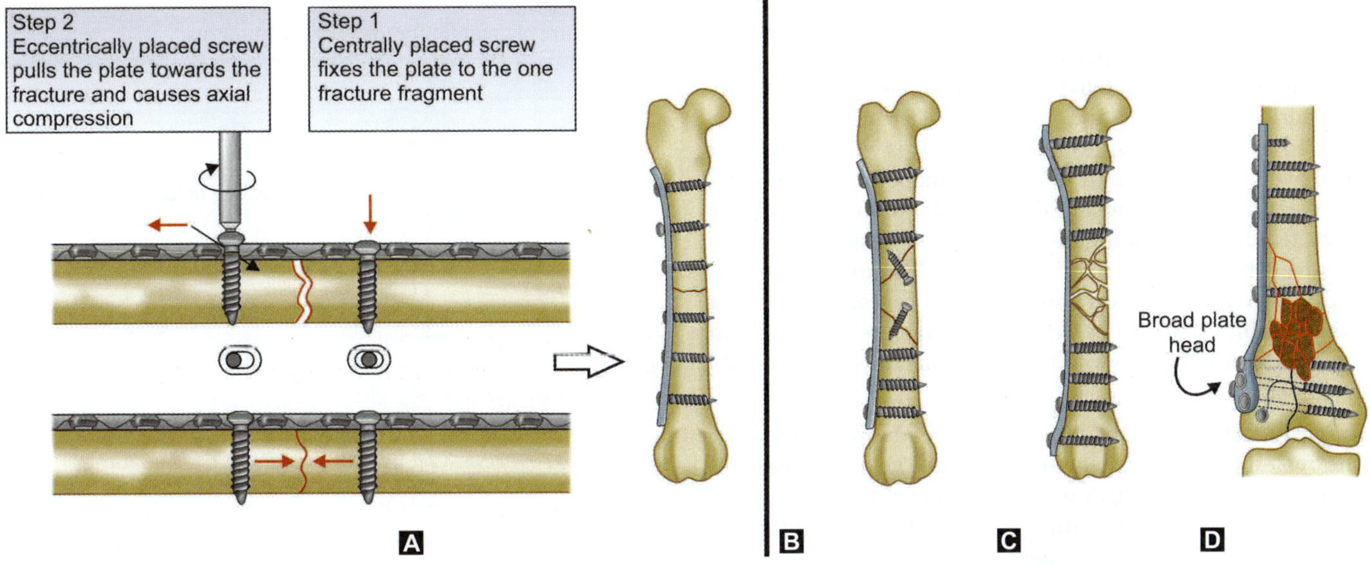

Figs 2.30A to D: (A) Compression plating; (B) Neutralization plate; (C) Bridge plate; (D) Buttress plate

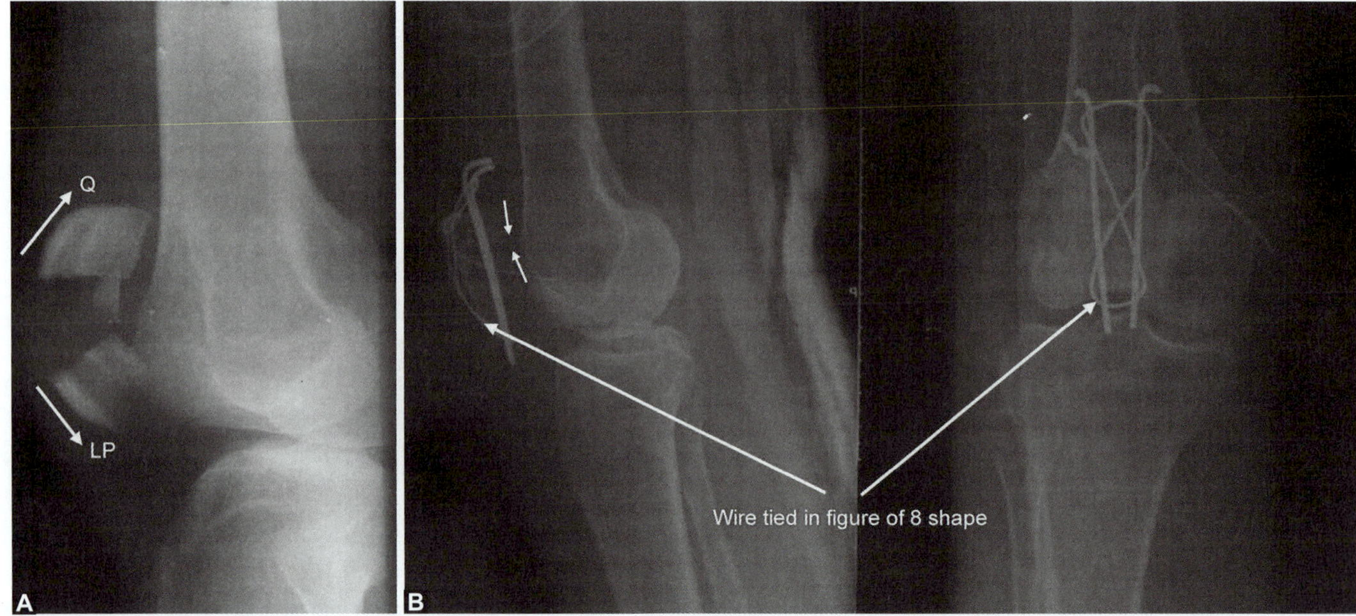

Figs 2.31A and B: Tension band wiring of patella fracture (Q, pull by quadriceps; LP, pull by ligamentum patellae)

has a sloping surface. When this eccentric screw is tightened, the plate (along with bone to which it is fixed) is pushed axially causing compression at fracture site **(Fig. 2.30A)**.

Locking plate: In this plate, screw heads have threads which get locked into plate holes and provide a very good stability even in osteoporotic bone (*see* Page 472). Locking is possible at different angles (almost up to 40°) which enables plate to provide good angular stability as well. Locking plates are used mainly for comminuted metaphyseal fractures, osteoporotic fractures and periprosthetic fractures where the screw hold in the bone may not be good.

Tension band principle: Here tensile/distractive forces of convex surface are converted into compressive forces on concave surface by applying the device (either plate or tension band wire) on convex surface (tension surface) of a fractured bone. A classical example is a transverse patellar fracture as shown in **Figures 2.31A and B**. Here the patellar fragments are being distracted by the quadriceps pull above and ligament patellae below. A wire has been tied on the convex side of the patella. This will get stretched due to patellar distraction by quadriceps and just like a stretched rubber band it will reciprocally exert compression pull upon this stretch to compress the fracture (Newton's III law of motion). Fractures where tension band principle is commonly used are listed in **Box 2.11**. Tension band principle can also be used in plating **(Table 2.10)** to achieve better fracture compression, if fracture geometry allows to fix a plate on convex surface of a curved bone.

Intramedullary nail: First successful intramedullary nailing was done by Gerhard Küntscher in the year 1939. The nail he used was a V-shaped steel nail which was later changed to hollow clover leaf model. This nail relied on a frictional fit between the nail and the bone (*see* Page 470). Since then intramedullary nailing has seen many changes in design as well as in the technique. In

1942, Fischer introduced the use of intramedullary reamers to increase the contact area between the nail and host bone, thus increasing the stability of the fracture. Later Modney invented the interlock nails that get locked into the bones to provide additional rotational stability in case of comminuted fractures **(Fig. 2.32)**. Then in the 1960s, the development of image intensifiers allowed surgeons to do intramedullary nailing with better confidence and with closed reduction (as explained in **Figs 2.29A and B**).

Box 2.11: Fractures commonly fixed by tension band principle

- Transverse fracture of the patella
- Fracture of the olecranon
- Fracture of greater trochanter of the femur
- Fracture of the medial malleolus
- Fracture of greater tuberosity of the humerus

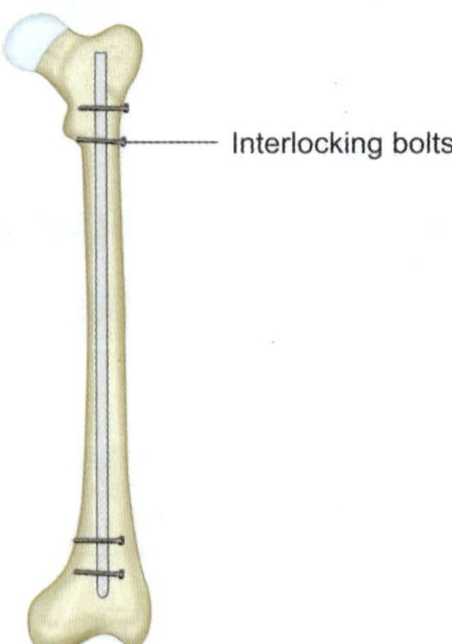

Fig. 2.32: Interlocking nail

Flow chart 2.1: A general algorithm for deciding treatment for any fracture

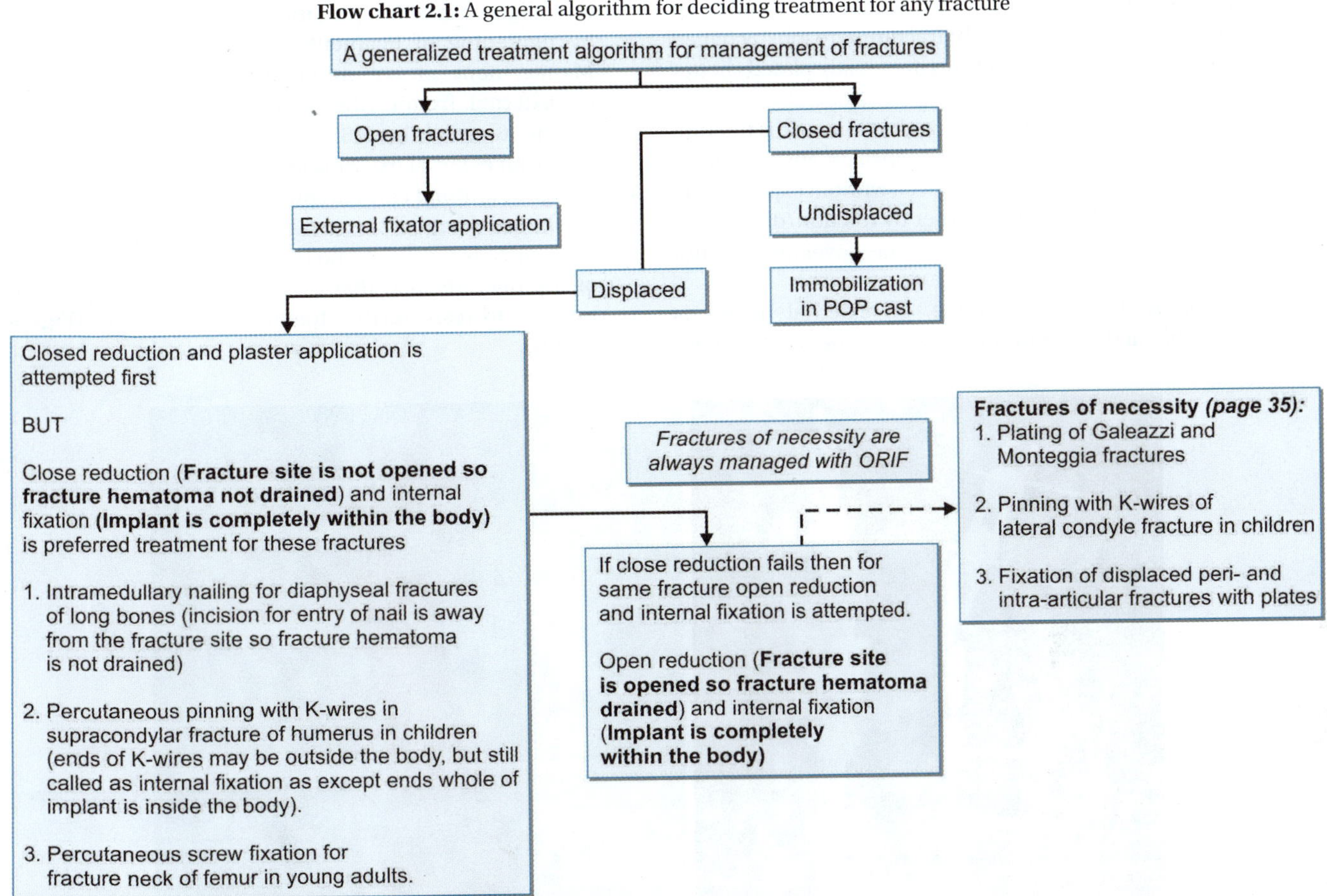

Abbreviations: POP, plaster of Paris; ORIF, open reduction and internal fixation.

Principle of intramedullary nailing: Fracture is reduced under image intensifier and after reaming of medullary cavity, nail is inserted into it which acts as an internal splint to resist bending. Interlocking nails are provided with slots for locking bolts which prevent rotation and shortening.

Advantages of intramedullary nailing: It is an ideal implant for long bone diaphyseal fractures. It can be implanted by minimally invasive technique without exposing the fracture hematoma. Thus, it is a biological method of fracture fixation.

A treatment algorithm for management of any fracture is given in **Flow chart 2.1**.

Biodegradable implants: Derived from materials like polyglycolic acid and polylactic acid, these are inert implants that undergo gradual degradation by biological processes and are absorbed by the body over time. Sice the need for fixation is temporary until the bone unites, considerable interest has come up off to explore their use. Atleast they have a theoretical advantage of avoidance of a second surgery of implant removal. However, high cost and allergic reactions have kept their use limited. They are mostly used in form of bioabsorbable screws and anchors (a device that is designed to fix soft tissues to bone) in arthroscopic surgeries.

HIGH-YIELD POINTS

- First use of "splinting" was described by Hippocrates.
- First use of internal fixation in form of cerclage (circumferential) wiring can be traced back to 1775 in French literature but formally Jean-Francois Malgaigne is credited with describing the first internal fixator as well as the first external fixator devices around 1840s. For internal fixation he used a wire loop and for external fixation he drove a spike into the tibia that was held by straps. First plating was done by Hansmann in Germany in 1886. However, the credit for pioneering the modern external and internal fixation devices is given to Albin Lambotte from Belgium, who in early 1900s coined the term "Osteosynthesis" (in Greek "osteo" means bone and "synthesis" means joining fragments of bone with metal) to refer to internal fixation, which earned him the title of "Father of Modern Internal Fixation". He is also considered to be the first to describe the use of biodegradable implants in orthopedics.
- A plate is considered to be a load-bearing device. It bears all the weight if loaded before a fracture unites and hence cracks. A nail is a load-sharing device. It allows vertical translation of bone ends and shares the load with the bone. So even if the

fracture is not united, it does not fail under load. Hence, in weight bearing bones (lower limb) fractures are mostly nailed while in upper limb bones, fractures are mostly plated (better stability).

- *Direct and indirect reduction*: Direct reduction means fracture fragments are manipulated directly by instruments or hands. In indirect reduction, fracture is reduced without exposing the fracture. Reduction is achieved either by traction/distraction or by applying forceps on the soft-tissue envelope and not directly on the bone.
- *Ligamentotaxis*: In this technique, an external fixator is applied in distraction around the fracture site. Here, length and alignment of fracture fragments are achieved indirectly by tightening of ligaments surrounding the fracture site. Management of comminuted distal radius fractures by an external fixator (distractor) is based on principles of ligamentotaxis **(Figs 2.33A and B)**. This is one of the places where an external fixator is used in a closed fracture.
- *Antiglide plating*: This is a special type of buttress plating used in oblique fracture patterns that are prone to displacement. Here plate is fixed to bone by inserting screws near the apex of the fracture such that the other part of the plate acts as buttress to resist further fracture displacement **(Figs 2.34A and B)**.

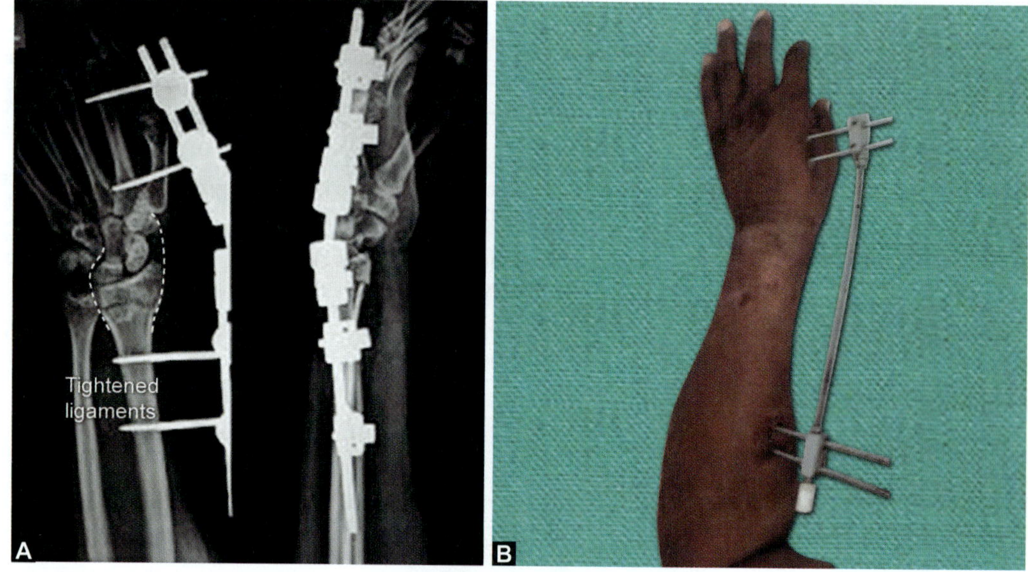

Figs 2.33A and B: (A) X-ray of wrist joint anteroposterior (AP) and lateral views showing fixation of distal radius fracture by external fixator (tightened ligaments are shown by broken white lines) and (B) The clinical picture of distractor used for distal end radius fracture

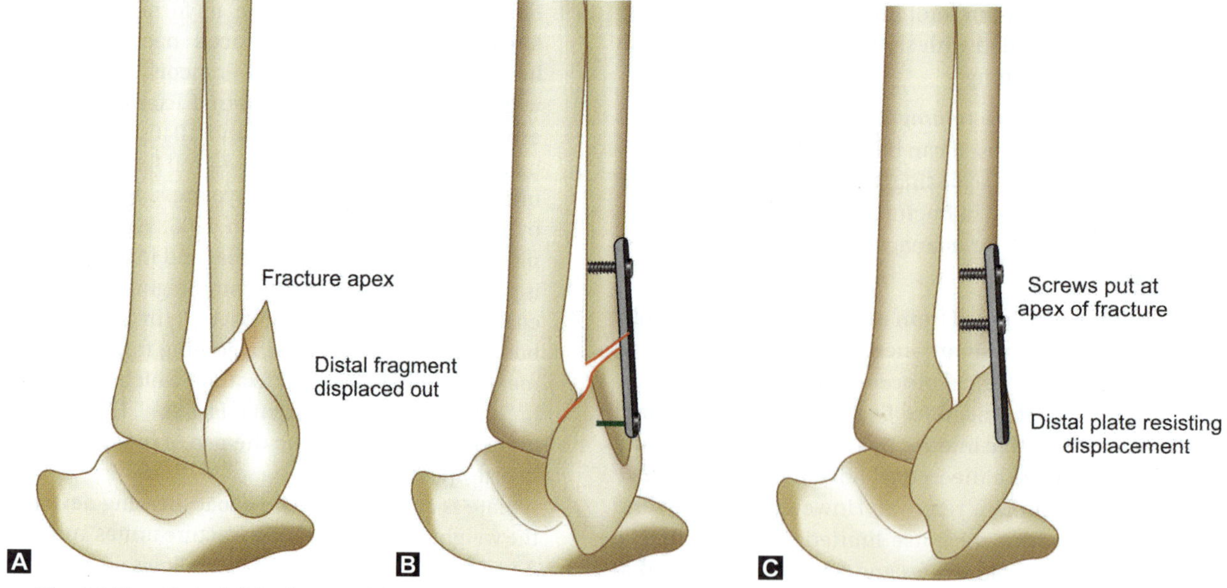

Figs 2.34A to C: Antiglide plating: Oblique fracture is prone to displacement if fixed in routine fashion (A, B) and in antiglide plating screws are put near apex of fracture (C) so that distal part of plate opposes fracture displacement

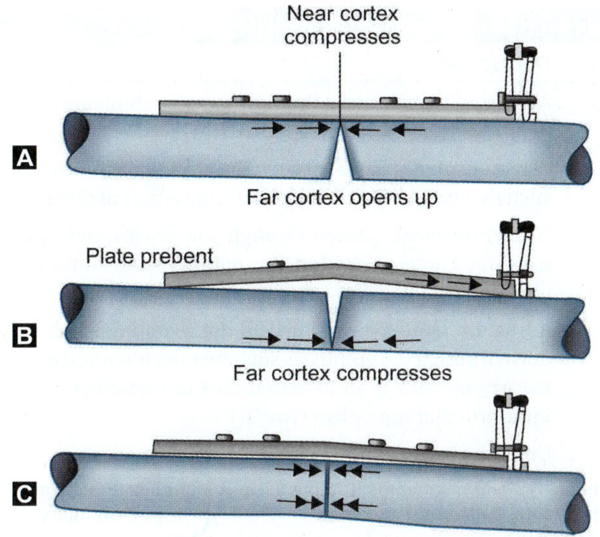

Figs 2.35A to C: Schematic diagram to explain prebending of a plate

- *Prebending of a plate*: Bending a plate little bit before application is a usual practice by most surgeons. When a plate is applied to a bone in compression mode, near cortex compresses but far cortex opens up **(Fig. 2.35A)**. Prebending of a plate before application **(Fig. 2.35B)** causes far cortex to compress and allows uniform compression at fracture site eventually **(Fig. 2.35C)**. It is not to be confused with tension band plate (TBP) **(Figs 2.31A and B)** as in prebending straight plate is fixed to a straight bone, unlike TBP where a straight plate is fixed on curved side of bone.
- *Fractures of necessity*: These are the fractures which essentially require ORIF for their management as a primary step.
  - Galeazzi fracture, Monteggia fracture
  - Lateral condyle humerus fracture in children
  - All displaced intra-articular fractures (displaced intra-articular fractures need absolute anatomical reduction to prevent joint arthritis so they are always reduced open and fixed).

FRACTURE CONSIDERATIONS IN CHILDREN AND PHYSEAL INJURIES

A pediatric bone is anatomically and biomechanically different from an adult bone. It behaves differently from an adult bone to injury and also during healing.

UNIQUE FEATURES OF PEDIATRIC BONE

- Periosteum is much thicker and stronger than adult bone. The thicker periosteum requires much greater energy to disrupt than in adults. Hence one finds the characteristic greenstick fracture pattern in children (*see* below). Also, the periosteum is lot more vascular which allows rapid healing of fractures and confers a lot better remodeling capacity.
- Pediatric bone has low bending strength and low modulus of elasticity compared to adult bone (more flexible); hence, it absorbs much greater energy before failure which makes plastic deformation and greenstick fracture patterns common. Also, since pediatric bone is more porous than adult bone peripheral extension of the main fracture line does not occur, so comminuted fractures are rarely seen in children.
- The bone mineral density of pediatric bone is also low in comparison to adult bone.
- *Open physis* presents a scenario unique to children. Physis/growth plate is the weakest part of child's bone and hence physeal injuries in this age group are not uncommon. Most common consequence of such injury is a partial or complete closure of the growth plate resulting in growth disturbances (angular deformity and shortening).

CHARACTERISTIC FRACTURE PATTERNS OF PEDIATRIC BONE

- *Greenstick fracture*: Flexible bones bend in response to injuring force causing one cortex to break. However, thicker periosteum resists the deforming forces more than in adult, and prevents the other cortex from cracking. This causes characteristic greenstick fracture pattern in children where one cortex breaks and other cortex remains intact or only deforms **(Fig. 2.36A)**. Greenstick fracture is the most common fracture pattern seen in a child and most commonly involves the forearm bones.
  Treatment of greenstick fracture: CR and POP application is the standard treatment. Traction is given to align the bone and reduction force is applied directly at the fracture. Overcorrection is often done, this may complete the fracture. After alignment fracture is immobilized in a cast.
- *Torus/Buckle fracture*: These fractures classically occur at the junction of the metaphysis and diaphysis. Distal radius is the most common site. The fracture pattern comprises an incomplete and stable injury with buckling (compared to buckle of a bag pressed inside to lock it) of a single cortex of bone **(Fig. 2.36B)**. The mechanism involved is axial loading with bending causing compression of trabeculae of single cortex. Fracture line is usually not visible and sometimes angulation is the only clue to the fracture. Splinting is usually all that is required for treatment as children display excellent remodeling capacity.

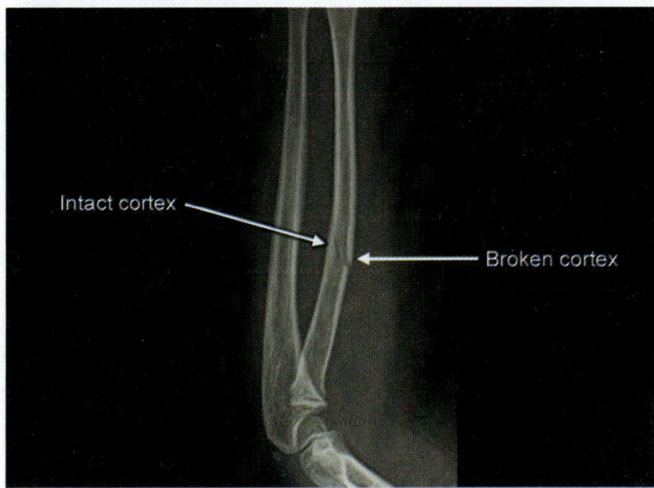

Fig. 2.36A: X-ray forearm lateral view showing greenstick fracture of the radius

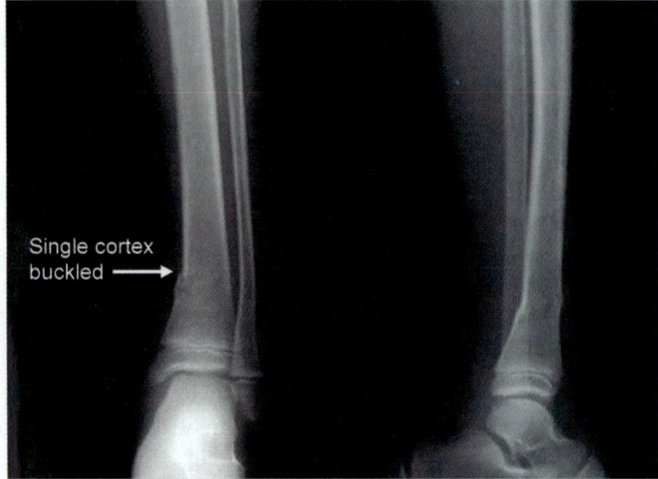

Fig. 2.36B: X-ray leg AP and lateral views showing torus fracture of the distal tibial metaphysis

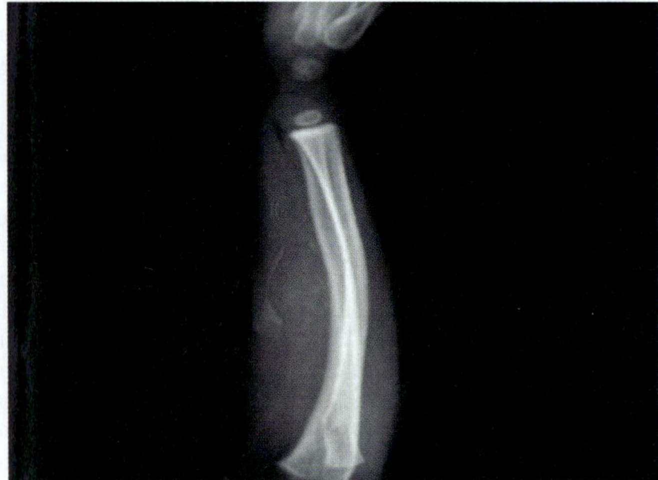

Fig. 2.37: Plastic deformity—see the angulation without any break

Source: Reproduced from Chee Y (2009). Plastic deformity. EURORAD. DOI:10.1594/EURORAD/CASE.2791.

- *Plastic deformation*: Bones in children are more flexible than in adults. When force is not sufficient to break the bone it may inflate or bend the bone permanently (beyond the elastic limit). Plastic deformation **(Fig. 2.37)** is most common in forearm bones, especially in ulna. Severe deformity (angulation more than 20° in older children) requires reduction and splintage.

PHYSEAL INJURIES

Physis is the weakest part of pediatric bone with hypertrophic zone being the weak link. Open physes are susceptible to injury in children. These are common injuries in children especially in adolescent age group (12–14 years) nearer to the growth spurts. The most common site of physeal injury is phalanx followed by distal radius.

Classification: There are many classification systems for physeal injuries viz. Ogden classification, Poland classification, Peterson classification, etc. It is the Salter–Harris classification **(Table 2.11)**

Type	Description
I	A fracture plane passes through the growth plate separating epiphysis from metaphysis
II	A fracture plane passes through the physis and the metaphysis such that epiphysis separates carrying a part of metaphysis*
III	A fracture plane passes through the physis and epiphysis (causing a fracture within the epiphysis; an intra-articular injury)
IV	A fracture plane passes through the metaphysis, physis and down through the epiphysis such that the fractured epiphysis is carrying with it an attached part of metaphysis (also an intra-articular injury like type III)
V	Crushing injury of the physis

Table 2.11: Salter–Harris classification **(Fig. 2.38)**

*Thurston–Holland fragment is a triangular piece of metaphysis that remains attached to the epiphysis. It is characteristic of type II physeal injury (but also seen in type IV).

that is most commonly used system across the globe to classify physeal injuries in children. It is based on the extent of fracture line whether the epiphysis, physis or metaphysis is involved **(Fig. 2.38)**. The most common type encounterd in clinical practice is type II while the rarest is type V. The classification is useful in predicting the outcome/prognosis, with type I having the best and type V having the worst prognosis. Infact, type V involves physeal crushing and is mostly a retrospective diagnosis made after years when the child presents with a deformity. Mnemonic SALTER is useful in remembering this classification **(Table 2.12)**.

Diagnosis of physeal injuries: Physeal injury should be suspected in every child who presents with pain and swelling around the joint. Diagnosis can be ascertained and type defined on routine X-rays **(Figs 2.39A and B)**. Some rare varieties also exist beyond the standard five types that the treating doctor must know **(Box 2.12)**. Whenever in doubt about the diagnosis, comparison with X ray views of the normal side or obtaining an MRI are very useful measures.

Treatment: In children, fractures heal at a faster rate so timely reduction of physeal injuries is of paramount importance. Attempt of reduction in cases presenting late can further damage the growth plate. In type I and II fracture reduction should not be attempted after 7–10 days, however type III and type IV fractures must be reduced open as they involve the joint. Once reduced, reduction can be secured with pins or/and cast. Type V needs special mention. Here diagnosis first hand is very difficult and deformity is inevitable as growth plate is crushed. Treatment in these cases involves treatment of deformity by measures like osteotomy, limb lengthening with Ilizarov or chondrodiastasis (*see* Page 378).

HIGH-YIELD POINTS

- *Growing pains*: These are muscular (nonarticular) pains complained by children particularly of age group 3–12 years during evening or night hours in the region of anterior thigh, calf, or behind the knee. They are thought to be due to growth spurts although scientific evidence for same is lacking.

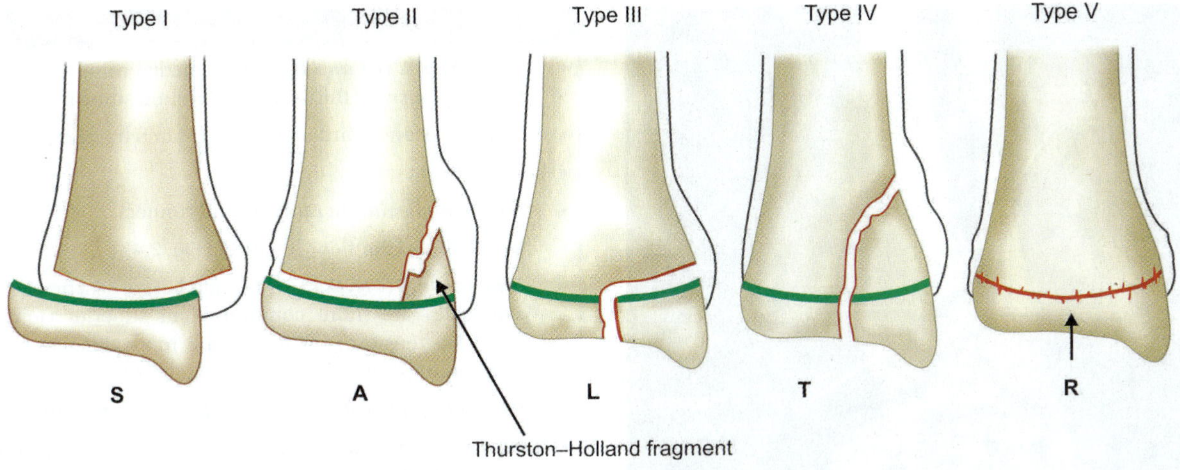

Fig. 2.38: Salter–Harris classification

Table 2.12: Mnemonic for Salter–Harris classification—"SALTR"				
Type I	*Type II*	*Type III*	*Type IV*	*Type V*
Slipped (slippage of epiphysis)	Above (fracture passes up in the metaphysis)	Lower or below (fracture passes below in epiphysis)	Through (fracture passes through the all; epiphysis, physis and metaphysis)	Rammed or crushed physis

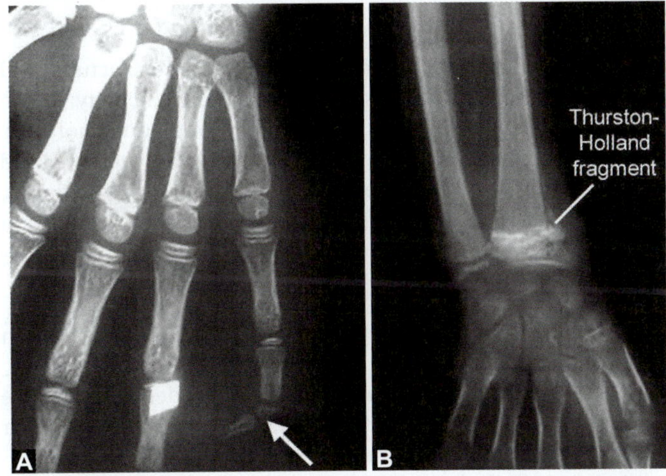

Figs 2.39A and B: (A) X-ray of hand showing type I physeal injury of distal phalanx of little finger (arrow); (B) X-ray of wrist showing type II physeal injury of distal radius with Thurston-Holland fragment (labeled)

Box 2.12: Rare types of physeal injuries (beyond Salter–Harris type V)

- *Type VI*: Injury to the peripheral portion of the physis and a resultant bony bridge formation which may produce an angular deformity (added in 1969 by Mercer Rang)
- *Type VII*: Isolated injury to the epiphyseal plate (VII–IX added in 1982 by JA Ogden)
- *Type VIII*: Isolated injury to the metaphysis, with a potential injury related to endochondral ossification
- *Type IX*: Injury to the periosteum that may interfere with membranous growth

However, they are self-limiting phenomena which means children grown out of them.

- *Growing fractures*: These are skull fractures seen mainly in infancy and early childhood characterized by progressive diastatic enlargement of the fracture line. A complication can be a cystic mass filled with cerebrospinal fluid, called as a "leptomeningeal cyst".
- *Toddler's fracture (see Page 147)*: It is undisplaced or minimally displaced spiral fracture of shaft of tibia, usually seen in small children. Treatment is long leg cast immobilization for 2–3 weeks.
- *Triplane fractures* **(Fig. 2.40)**: These are a variety of Salter-Harris type IV injuries seen classically in adolescents. The fracture line characteristically runs in all three planes: vertically across epiphysis, horizontally in physis and obliquely across metaphysis. These fractures are classically seen around distal tibia (as the physeal closure first occurs medially, the lateral physis that remains open till late sustains this fracture) and occasionally around distal radius or proximal tibia.
- Pediatric bone has more remodeling capacity than adult bone. Deformity in plane of motion remodels to greater extent than deformity in other plane. Rotational deformity remodels less than angular deformity.
- The weakest part of a child's bone is growth plate while the strongest are the periosteum and the adjacent ligaments and joint capsule.
- The weakest zone of growth plate that is ruptured in most physeal injuries is the hypertrophic zone.
- The largest and the fastest growing of all growth plates is the distal femoral physis (contributes 70% to femur length and 37% to leg length). It is the first physis in the body to ossify. Also, it is the most common physis to be injured around the

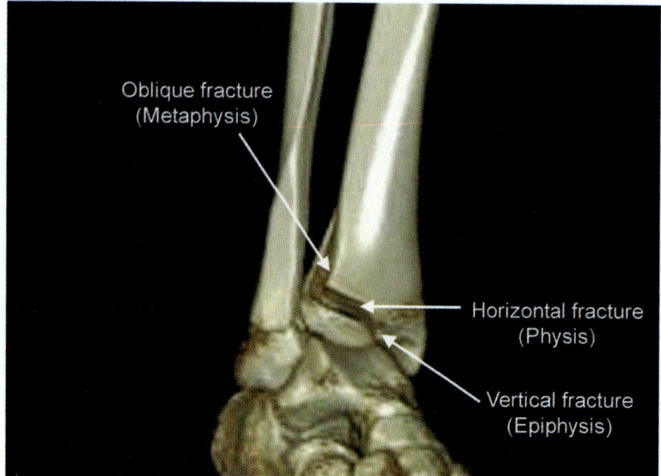

Fig. 2.40: Diagrammatic representation of a Triplane fracture involving distal tibia

knee. Injury can occur during birth in a breech delivery leading to Salter–Harris type I lesion. More commonly it is injured in a child by knee hyperextension (distal fragment displaced anteriorly) or when there is a valgus force to the knee (distal fragment goes laterally). The former mostly causes a type II lesion and a risk to popliteal artery rupture while the latter mechanism is more commonly associated with a type III or a type II Salter–Harris lesion. In either type characteristically multiple layers of the growth plate are injured (not just the hypertrophic zone).

SPECIAL FRACTURE GROUPS

STRESS FRACTURES

The term "Stress fracture" refers to a partial or complete fracture that results from inability of bone to bear stress applied in a rhythmical, repeated, sub-threshold, non-violent manner. Stress fractures are further divided into two categories:

1. *Fatigue fractures*: Here a bone with normal elastic resistance is subjected to abnormal compressive or tensile stresses (neither of which alone are capable of producing the fracture), leading to mechanical failure over time.
2. *Insufficiency fractures*: Here normal physiological stress is applied to a bone with abnormal elastic resistance (deficient mineralization), e.g. in osteoporosis, osteomalacia, hyperparathyroidism or renal osteodystrophy.

Fatigue stress fractures are the most common in weight-bearing bones of lower limb especially in dancers, runners, jumpers, gymnast and military recruits. The most common sites include distal third tibia followed by metatarsals (second and third) and fibula. In foot, the metatarsals (March fracture, *see* Page 161) are the most common site while among the tarsal bones of the foot, the calcaneum and navicular mostly sustain stress injuries. Stress fractures of non-weight bearing bones (upper limbs and torso) may also occur following repetitive stress. The most common non-weight bearing sites involved are the ribs (most commonly first rib) followed by ulna and olecranon. While stress fractures of ribs are mostly found in rowers, stress fractures

---

Box 2.13: Common sites of fatigue stress fractures

- *Tibia* **(Figs 2.41A and B)**: Posteromedial compression injuries in distal or proximal thirds (most common stress fractures)
- Shaft of second/third metatarsal (March fracture)
- Other metatarsals
- *Medial malleolus*: In jumpers and runners
- Distal fibula (Runner's fracture) **(Fig. 2.42)**
- *Femoral neck* **(Fig. 2.43)**: Inferomedial cortical breaks (compression side) are more common than superior (tension side). However, tension side breaks are more dangerous and often progress to complete fracture without fixation
- *Femoral shaft*: Posteromedial or medial cortical breaks
- *Navicular*: In central third of bone in runners/sprinters, ballet dancers, football players
- *Calcaneus*: Tuberosity fractures in military recruits and in runners
- *Ribs*: Fractures of middle ribs (4th–9th) common in rowers due to traction by serratus anterior
- Pubic rami stress fractures in female long distance runners

of olecranon are particularly common in baseball players. **Box 2.13** shows common sites of fatigue stress fractures.

Pathophysiology

Repetitive cyclical loading alters bone's microstructure and leads to increase in osteoblastic and osteoclastic activity. When repetitive loading occurs at a rate at which body does not have time to recover, bone formation (osteoblastic activity) lags behind bone resorption (osteoclastic activity). If this stress continues, fatigued bone may develop microfractures that eventually end in full cortical breaks.

Risk Factors for Stress Fracture

- *Alteration in the training program*: Sudden increase in duration/intensity/frequency of training.
- *Alteration in biomechanics*: Stiff ankle (decreased ankle dorsiflexion), increased hip external rotation and hyper pronation at subtalar joint.
- Limb length discrepancy.

Clinical Features

After a period of stressful activity (athletic training, unaccustomed activity), patient presents with complaints of gradual development of pain at the site of stress fracture. Patient describes it as activity-related pain and that he gets relief with rest. On examination, the involved area displays focal bony tenderness. Mild swelling over the affected region may be present.

Radiology

It takes 2–3 weeks for the stress fracture to become visible on X-ray. Low-density cortical area (gray cortex) is the earliest sign. Later a radiolucent line extending across the cortex appears at the site of fracture. Endosteal thickening with solid thick periosteal new bone formation **(Figs 2.41 and 2.42)** guides the diagnosis in early stages while a frank fracture line with cortical break is usually a late feature (appear 2–3 months after the stress fracture).

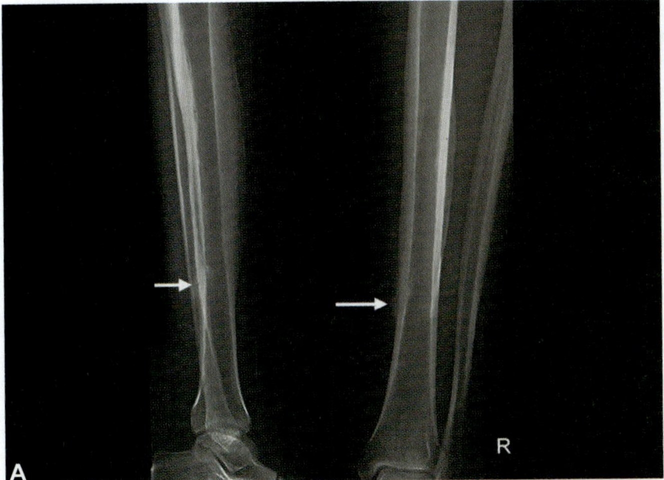

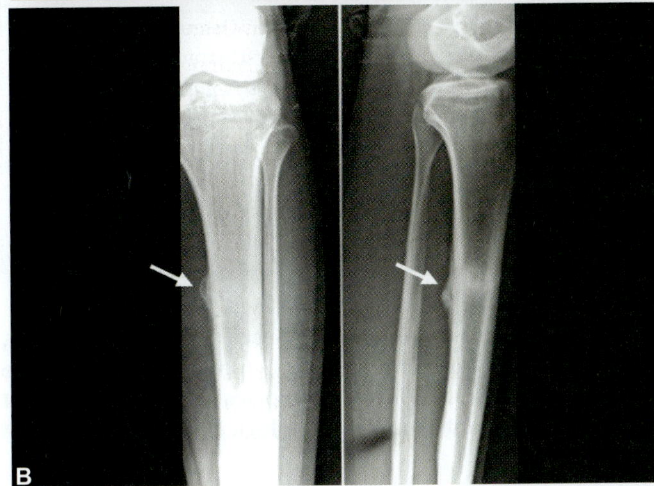

Figs 2.41A and B: X-ray of leg, AP and lateral views, showing stress fracture of distal tibia (A) and proximal tibia (B) (arrow marks are pointing to characteristic periosteal reaction, seen due to healing of stress fracture)

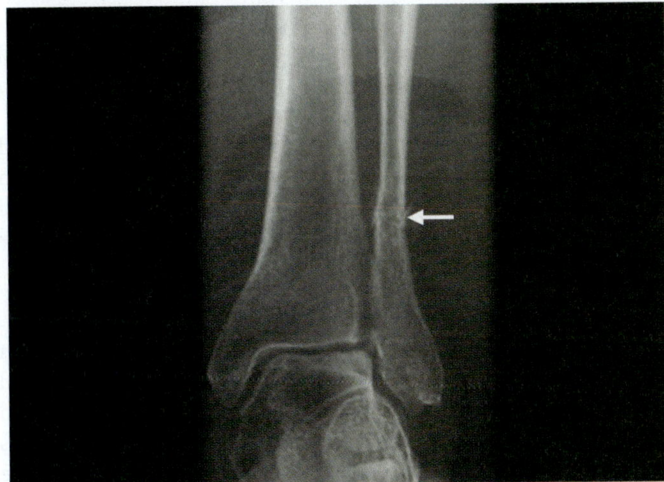

Fig. 2.42: X-ray of distal leg showing stress fracture of distal fibula (runner's fracture) (arrow)

Bone scan [technetium-99m (Tc 99m) methylene diphosphonate] shows increased osteoblastic activity and can be useful in early

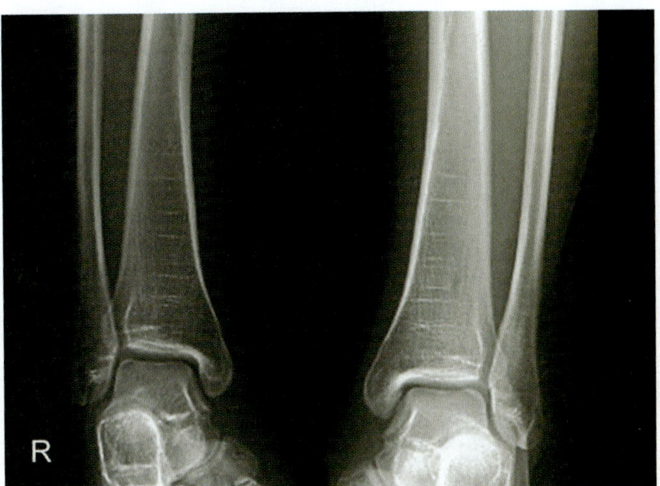

Fig. 2.43: Growth arrest lines (should not be confused with stress fracture)

stages; however, magnetic resonance imaging (MRI) is the investigation of choice (IOC) for detection of stress fractures and provides the earliest diagnosis.

Stress fractures must be differentiated from Harris lines/ Park lines/growth arrest lines **(Fig. 2.43)** which are bilateral symmetrical dense trabecular metaphyseal lines mostly seen in rapidly growing bone ends.

Treatment

Activity modification is enough for management of most of the stress fractures. However, for lower limb stress fractures (metatarsals, navicular, etc.), a non-weight bearing below knee cast immobilization for 4–6 weeks is considered the treatment of choice. High-grade (MRI showing wide or transcortical increased signal intensity) tension-side (superior) femoral neck stress fractures require prophylactic internal fixation with cancellous screws.

HIGH-YIELD POINTS

- *Stress fractures are categorized into two types*: (1) High risk and (2) low risk. The high-risk stress fractures are those that generally need surgery (e.g. neck of femur, **Fig. 2.44**) while the low-risk group is mostly managed with cast immobilization (e.g. metatarsals).
- Use of running shoes, shock absorber inserts in shoes and modification of running mechanics (increase in cadence and decrease in stride length) are simple measures to prevent lower limb stress fractures in high risk groups.
- Low intensity pulsed ultrasound (LIPUS) at intensity < 0.1 W/cm² (normally ultrasound is used at 0.1–3 W/cm²) can also be used to enhance fracture healing in stress fractures.
- Magnetic resonance imaging has equal sensitivity rather more specificity than bone scan and it is the IOC in detecting stress fractures, providing the earliest diagnosis. However, at times stress fractures may be bilateral and MRI may not prove cost effective. Although there are no strict recommendations in literature, the authors prefer a bone scan in cases suspected of having bilateral stress injuries, as a single investigation can guide a bilateral diagnosis.

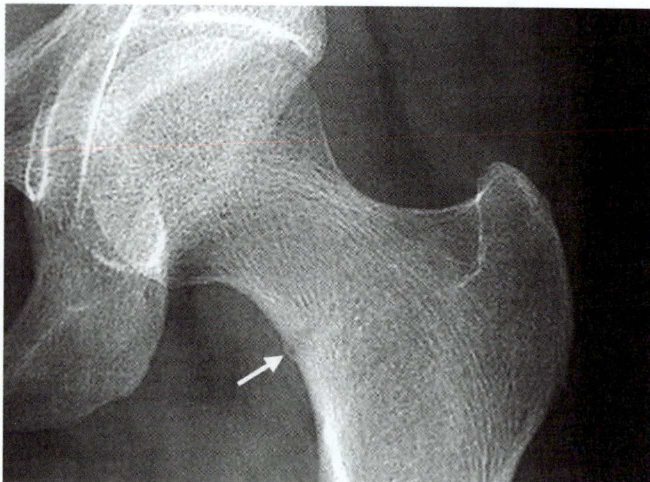

Fig. 2.44: Compression side femoral neck stress fracture (arrow mark)

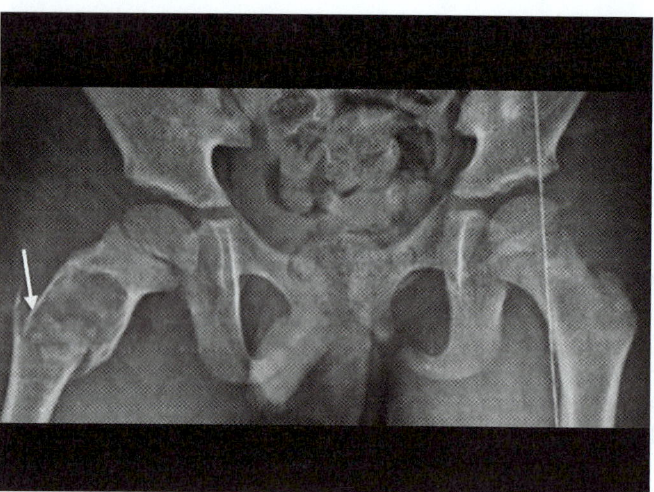

Fig. 2.45: X-ray pelvis (AP view) shows a pathological fracture of the proximal femur (arrow) due to a simple bone cyst

PATHOLOGICAL FRACTURES

Pathological fractures **(Fig. 2.45)** occur in bones which have been abnormally weakened either by a systemic affection (e.g. osteoporosis) or by a localized disease process (malignant or nonmalignant in nature). Trivial trauma/stress which would have left the normal bone intact causes a pathological fracture in a weak bone. Although the term can be used in the setting of a generalized metabolic bone disease like osteoporosis, it is usually reserved for fractures caused through a focal abnormality like a bone tumor or infection or for fractures occurring due to an inherited bone disorder. **Table 2.13** summarizes the association of bone quality and load applied in causing various types of fractures.

The most common site of affection varies with the age of presentation. In people under the age of 60 years, pathological fractures mostly occur in neck of femur secondary to malignancy (metastasis). In elderly, over the age of 60 years, osteoporosis is the most common implicating factor, with most fractures being

Table 2.13: The relation between bone quality and bone load in producing various types of fractures

Type	Bone quality	Load
Traumatic	Normal	Single large
Fatigue (stress)	Normal	Repetitive
Insufficiency (stress)	Abnormal (metabolic)	Minimal
Pathological	Abnormal (tumor)	Minimal

Box 2.14: Causes of pathological fractures

- *Reduced bone mass*: Osteoporosis
- *Neoplastic*: Primary bone tumor (benign and malignant), metastatic bone lesions
- *Tumor-like lesions*: Simple bone cyst, aneurysmal bone cyst, fibrous dysplasia, nonossifying fibroma
- *Metabolic and hormonal imbalance*: Osteomalacia, Rickets, Scurvy, Cushing's syndrome, hyperparathyroidism
- *Developmental disorders and bony dysplasias*: Osteogenesis imperfecta, osteopetrosis, achondroplasia, diaphyseal aclasis (multiple exostosis), Ollier's disease
- *Defect of bone remodeling*: Paget's disease, osteopetrosis
- *Infections*: Osteomyelitis, hydatid disease of bone
- *Marrow cell disorders*: Histiocytosis, Gaucher's disease

compression fractures of vertebral bodies of dorsal spine. Overall, osteoporotic vertebral compression fractures in elderly are the most common presentation of pathological fractures. **Box 2.14** shows some important causes of pathological fractures.

Diagnosis

Pathological fracture should be suspected when a fracture occurs:
- In an elderly who is a known patient of cancer
- Spontaneously or after trivial trauma
- In a patient with history of irradiation
- With the complaint of pain or limp preceding the fracture
- With unusual fracture pattern, for example, a horizontal fracture line in subtrochanteric femur **(Fig. 2.46)** is often pathological.

A detailed workup **(Box 2.15)** of the patient with a suspected pathological fracture should be done including the search for occult primary. If investigations fail to reveal the cause of pathological fracture, biopsy should be done to establish the diagnosis.

Management

Management of pathological fracture should focus on pain relief, management of cause of the pathological fracture and fracture stabilization. Often a combination of NSAIDs and narcotics is required for adequate pain relief. Bisphosphonates and radiotherapy are also used for pain relief and to halt the progression of bone destruction in metastatic bone cancer. Radionuclide therapy is the recent addition in the treatment for palliative pain relief from metastatic bone disease. Commonly used agents are phosphorus-32 orthophosphate and strontium-89 chloride.

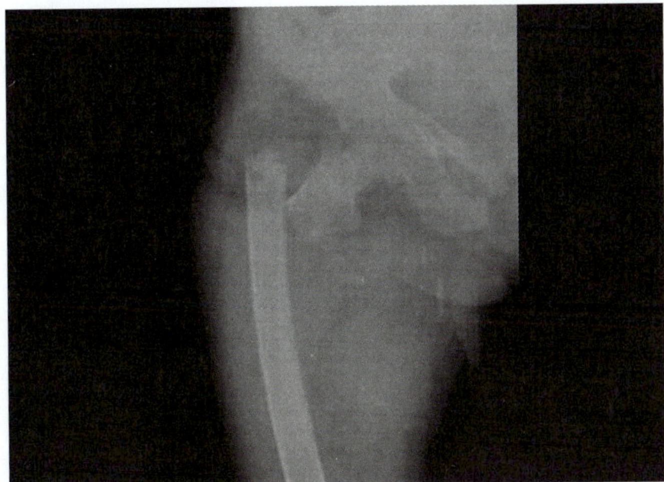

Fig. 2.46: X-ray of proximal femur (AP view) demonstrating a horizontal/transverse subtrochanteric fracture in a 30-year-old epileptic female due to osteomalacia. Such patterns must be evaluated for a pathological background

---

Box 2.15: Workup of a patient with suspected pathological fracture

- *Blood investigations*: CBC, ESR, CRP, renal function tests, liver function tests, thyroid function tests
- Bone densitometry (DEXA)
- *Metabolic profile*: Serum calcium, serum phosphorus, serum alkaline phosphatase, PTH
- *Search for occult primary*: Tumor markers, plasma protein electrophoresis, immunoelectrophoresis, clinical examination of breast, thyroid and prostate, mammography, etc.
- *Radiology*: X-ray of involved bone, CT scan of the chest, pelvis and abdomen, MRI to know the local spread, PET scan, bone scan for the occult metastasis

Abbreviations: CBC, complete blood count; ESR, erythrocyte sedimentation rate; CRP, C-reactive protein; DEXA, dual-energy X-ray absorptiometry; PTH, parathyroid hormone; PET, positron emission tomography.

Fracture fixation: Conventional methods [cast immobilization or ORIF (open reduction and internal fixation)] are usually enough for pathological fractures secondary to cystic lesions of bone, benign neoplasm and due to generalized systemic diseases (osteoporosis, Paget's disease, osteogenesis imperfecta, etc.). Metastatic pathological fractures often fail to unite with casting and require internal fixation with intramedullary rod or long plate with addition of bone cement to fill the defect or replacement of affected bone with prosthesis. Joint arthroplasty is a favorable option for lesions near the joint. For the involvement of large area of bone often replacement of whole bone with a tumor prosthesis (megaprosthesis) is required (*see* Page 481). Fracture in case of osteomyelitis requires primary management of infection with temporary stabilization of fracture followed by definite treatment of fracture, once infection is controlled.

Impending Pathological Fracture

At times a patient may present with a large lytic lesion of bone, highly likely to fracture but not fractured yet. Prophylactic internal fixation of bone is warranted in such cases, if the risk of fracture is high. Mirel's criteria **(Table 2.14)** are used to quantify the risk of impending fracture in such cases and thereby plan prophylactic fixation in high-risk fractures.

HIGH-YIELD POINTS

- Most common presentation of pathological fracture is the fracture itself.
- The term "fragility fracture" is used for pathological fractures occurring in osteoporotic bone with low energy trauma (e.g. fall in an elderly). Vertebral fractures (most common), proximal femoral fractures and wrist fracture (Colles' fracture) are the three most common fragility fractures.
- Bisphosphonates inhibit the osteoclast-mediated bone resorption by inducing osteoclast apoptosis, inhibiting osteoclast maturation and decreasing their activity. They hold important place in medicinal treatment of pathological fractures secondary to bony metastasis or osteoporosis. However, no role of bisphosphonates has been proven yet in managing stress fractures.
- Although bisphosphonates are mainstay of treatment of osteoporosis but long-term treatment (>5 years) can cause subtrochanteric fractures in femur (*see* Page 402) due to severe suppression of bone turnover and inhibition of bone remodeling.

IMAGING IN ORTHOPEDICS

Radiology plays a pivotal role in management of orthopedic patients. X-rays, ultrasonography (USG), CT scan, MRI and nuclear imaging, all have specific roles in different orthopedic pathologies.

X-RAYS

Discovered by Wilhelm Conrad Roentgen in 1895, X-rays are basically electromagnetic waves in the wavelength of 0.01–10 nm. These electromagnetic radiations are produced when high-energy electrons strike the tungsten target in a special X-ray tube (cathode ray tube). These radiations when sent by X-ray machine

---

Table 2.14: Mirel's criteria for prophylactic fixation of impending pathological fractures

Score	1	2	3
Site	Upper limb	Lower limb	Peritrochanteric
Pain	Mild	Moderate	Severe
Lesion	Blastic	Mixed	Lytic
Size	<1st/3rd diameter of bone	1st/3rd to 2nd/3rd diameter of bone	>2nd/3rd diameter of bone

Mirel's score > 8 warrants prophylactic fixation

Box 2.16: Uses of X-rays in orthopedics

- Use in trauma:
  - Usually the first investigation in trauma
  - To see the location and type of fracture
  - Glass pieces can be seen on X-ray due to the presence of lead within them
  - Also used after fracture reduction by plaster fixation/nailing to confirm proper fixation of fracture fragments
- Use in infection (osteomyelitis):
  - Loss of soft-tissue planes is the first change in pyogenic osteomyelitis (24–48 hours)
  - Periosteal reaction is the first bone change (7–10 days)
  - Chronic osteomyelitis shows sclerosed dead bone (sequestrum) with thick onion peel type of periosteal reaction (differential diagnosis—Ewing's sarcoma)
  - Air pockets may be seen in soft tissues in spread of infection to soft tissues—necrotizing fasciitis
- Use in bone tumors:
  - *Tumor location:* Epiphyseal, metaphyseal or diaphyseal
  - *Tumor matrix:* Cartilaginous tumors have characteristic rings and arcs pattern of calcification, bone-forming tumors like osteosarcoma show osteoid tumor matrix
  - Periosteal reaction, adjacent soft-tissue involvement
- Use in degenerative arthritis:
  - Reduced joint space in involved joint (indicates cartilage damage as cartilage is not visualized on X-ray and forms the joint space)
  - Osteophytes, subchondral cysts, subchondral sclerosis — seen in osteoarthritis

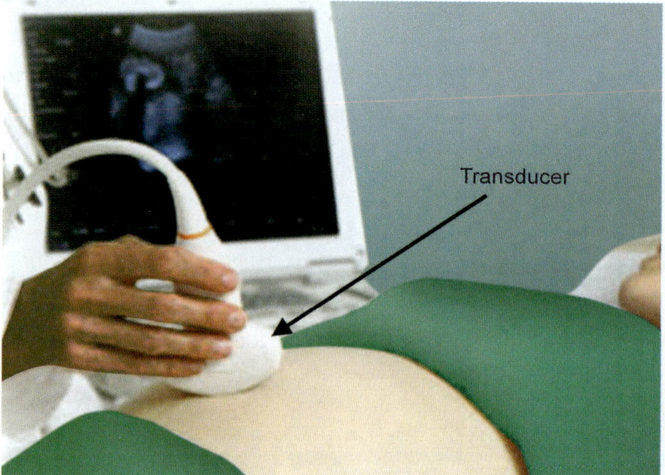

Fig. 2.47: Ultrasound machine in use

Box 2.17: Uses of ultrasound in orthopedics

- Infection or inflammatory arthritis
  - Useful for evaluation of soft-tissue infections, any abscesses, muscle edema and status of draining lymph nodes
  - Joint effusion can be noted—best for visualization of septations or internal echoes within the joint fluid that are often seen in septic arthritis
  - USG-guided aspiration of joint fluid to make a diagnosis
  - Thickened synovium with increased vascularity (pannus formation) is seen in rheumatoid arthritis
- Trauma
  - *Mainly used for evaluation of vessels by using color Doppler:* Vascular injury with a localized hematoma can be well appreciated in short time
  - *Traumatic tendon tears:* Acute or chronic tendon tears can be seen on USG, facilitated by dynamic evaluation
- Degenerative conditions
  - Tendon tears (e.g. Rotator cuff tears), muscle atrophy
- Nerve compression
  - Useful in evaluation of carpal tunnel syndrome
  - USG of both hip joints is a useful screening test for hip dysplasia in newborns

through various tissues of body are differentially absorbed, giving their images on X-ray films. Since these rays can pass well thorough the soft tissues and organs, the same are not visible on the film while the bones get photographed distinctly, making them the first line radiographic investigation in most orthopedic cases. Uses of X-rays in orthopedics are given in **Box 2.16.**

- *Advantages:* Cheap, easily available even in peripheral centers.
- *Drawbacks:* Radiation risk (avoid in pregnant women), image obtained is uniplanar, less sensitivity as compared to CT/MRI, minimal details about cartilage/soft tissues.

ULTRASOUND (SONOGRAM)

Word "ultrasound" in physics refers to sound that humans cannot hear. Ultrasound waves are high-frequency sound waves (2–18 MHz) generated by a special effect called "piezoelectric effect". An electric current is passed through a piezoelectric crystal (made of lead zirconate titanate), which makes it change its shape and generate these high-frequency sound waves. The ultrasound machine possesses a "transducer" **(Fig. 2.47)**, which houses this piezoelectric crystal that generates these waves and then transmits them through tissues before receiving them back as "echoes". There is differential passage of these waves through various tissues, hence giving their images on the machine's monitor (hyper or hypoechoeic). The main benefit is that the information is relayed in real time.

High-frequency, high-resolution "linear" transducer is characteristically used (8–13 MHz) for musculoskeletal ultrasound. These linear transducers have better resolution (but lesser penetration) as compared to the conventional convex transducers.

A special mode called "Doppler mode" can identify vascular flow in channels and also measure the direction and speed of flow. It can be used to mark an artery, distinguish it from a vein and pin point site of stenosis/block to flow. Uses of ultrasound in orthopedics are given in **Box 2.17.**

- *Advantages*: No radiation risk, easily available, high sensitivity for soft tissues, very good to detect presence of fluid in any plane, information relayed is in real time so useful for dynamic examination (patient can be asked to move a limb to see the status of specific muscles/tendons), useful in evaluating patients with metallic implants which limits the evaluation by CT and MRI.
- *Drawbacks*: Status of bone not well seen (as bones completely reflect the waves allowing no passage), operator-dependent investigation, limited field of view.

COMPUTED TOMOGRAPHY SCAN

The credit for discovery of computed tomography (CT) scan is given to Godfrey Hounsfield. The machine consists of a rotating X-ray tube and a series of detectors placed directly 180° opposite to the tube in a "gantry" (**Fig. 2.48**), with a table that moves in and out of the gantry as required. The rotation of the X-ray tube in the gantry enables generation of cross-sectional images of the scanned portion of the body. Uses of CT scan in orthopedics are given in **Box 2.18**.

- *Advantages*: Takes less time than MRI, high sensitivity for bone pathologies (but not for marrow), multiplanar reconstruction is possible as X-ray tube rotates 360° in the gantry (coronal, sagittal, axial and oblique), three-dimensional (3D) reconstruction of data sets is possible (useful in planning surgeries). CT angiography (CT imaging done after vascular introduction of a contrast agent) is useful in showing status of vessels in relation to the pathology (tumor/trauma).

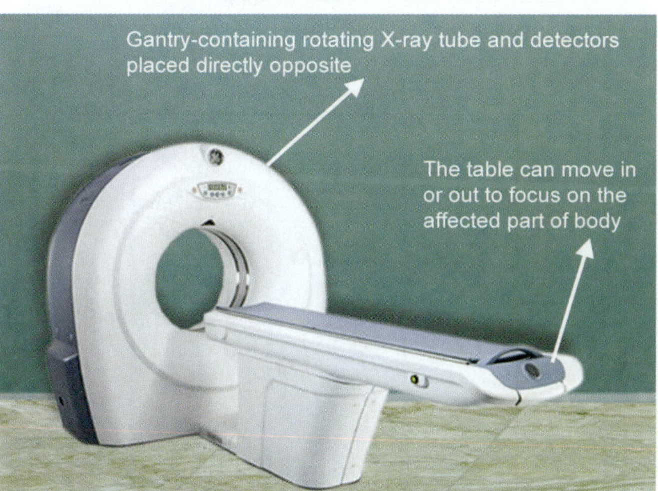

Fig. 2.48: CT scan machine (gantry and the table)

- *Drawbacks*: High radiation exposure, expensive, poor image quality and artifacts in metallic implants (due to beam hardening), poor resolution for soft tissues.

MAGNETIC RESONANCE IMAGING

This is a highly advanced imaging mode that generates images of the body structures with the use of powerful magnets that can create a strong magnetic field and produce radiofrequency (RF) pulses (radio waves are electromagnetic waves). Images can be acquired in all three planes: (1) axial, (2) coronal and (3) sagittal, enabling a 3D reconstruction.

Principle of Magnetic Resonance Imaging

The machine as shown in **Figure 2.49** has a gantry that hoists a powerful electromagnet (bore magnet) and special coils called "gradient coils". A "part specific conductive field coil" is attached to the body part of the patient to be imaged.

Principle: An atom has in its center a nucleus, containing protons (positively charged particles) and neutrons (neutral particles) in a specific arrangement, with electrons (negatively charged particles) revolving around them in their orbits. MRI makes use of the magnetic properties of those atomic nuclei that contain "free protons". An example is the hydrogen atom nucleus (has a single free proton) present in water molecules, and therefore in all body tissues.

The basic concept of MRI needs understanding of two important principles of nuclear magnetic resonance (NMR). First, nuclei with odd number of protons will have a spin. And second, a moving/spinning electric charge (moving charge is electric current) produces a magnetic field. Since hydrogen nucleus has a free proton, it will have a spin and hence possess a magnetic field.

Now, these nuclei are randomly aligned in the absence of a strong magnetic field (**Fig. 2.50A**). When a strong magnetic field is applied (by bore magnet in the MRI gantry), the hydrogen nuclei (containing charged free protons) align themselves along the direction of the magnetic field. The external magnetic field is directed along the Z axis, which is also the longitudinal axis of the patient. The forces of the aligned protons add up together to form a net magnetic vector along the Z axis (**Fig. 2.50B**), and is called longitudinal magnetization (LM). At this stage a RF signal (excitation pulse) is sent in the XY plane (90 to LM) and some of the protons pick some energy from this RF pulse and go to higher energy levels. The new magnetic vector is now formed in XY plane (**Fig. 2.50C**) and is called transverse magnetization (TM). The motion in TM vector produces electric current, which is received as a signal in the part specific conductive field coil attached on imaged body part of patient and then processed into MR image by the computers.

A typical spin-echo sequence consists of a 90° pulse followed by a 180° pulse, at the end of which signal (also called as "echo") is received. The parameters detected in part specific coils are:

Time to repeat (TR): It is the time interval between start of one RF pulse and the start of next RF pulse, i.e. duration between the beginnings of the two 90° pulses.

Time to echo (TE): It is the time interval between the start of RF pulse and reception of the echo (signal).

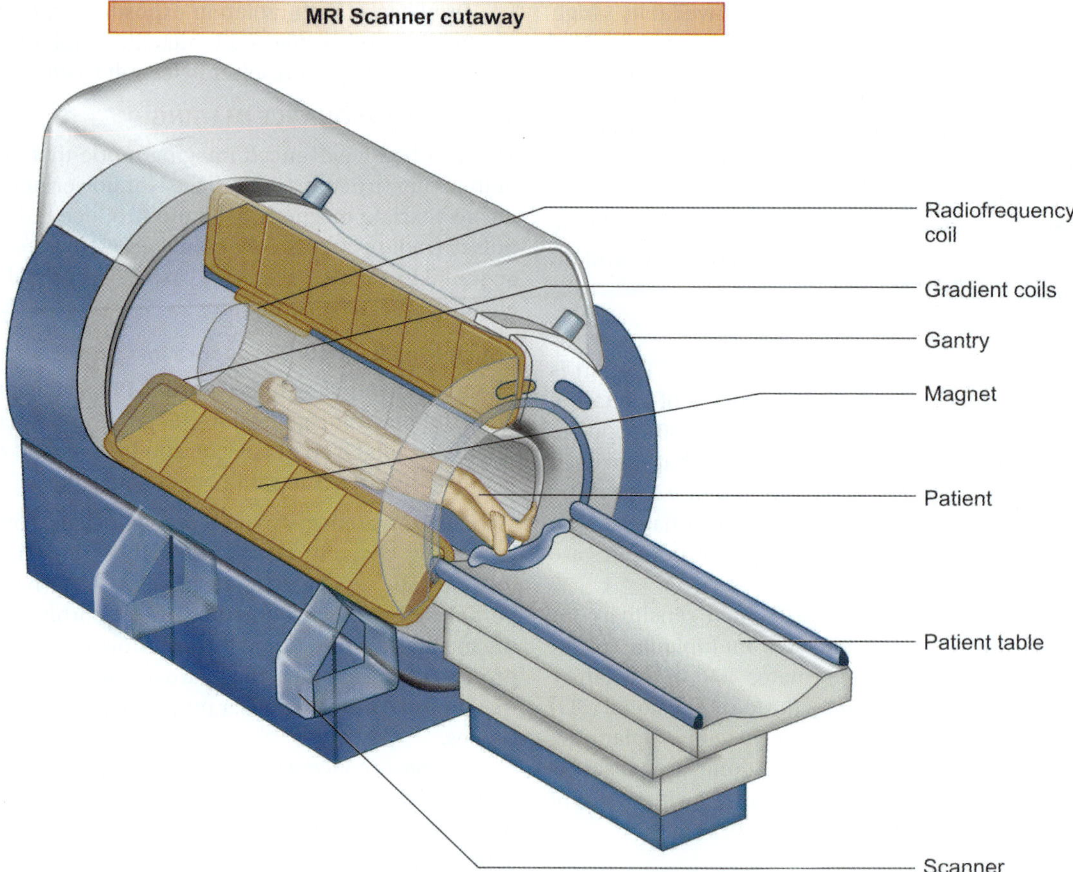

Fig. 2.49: Diagram showing parts of an MRI machine

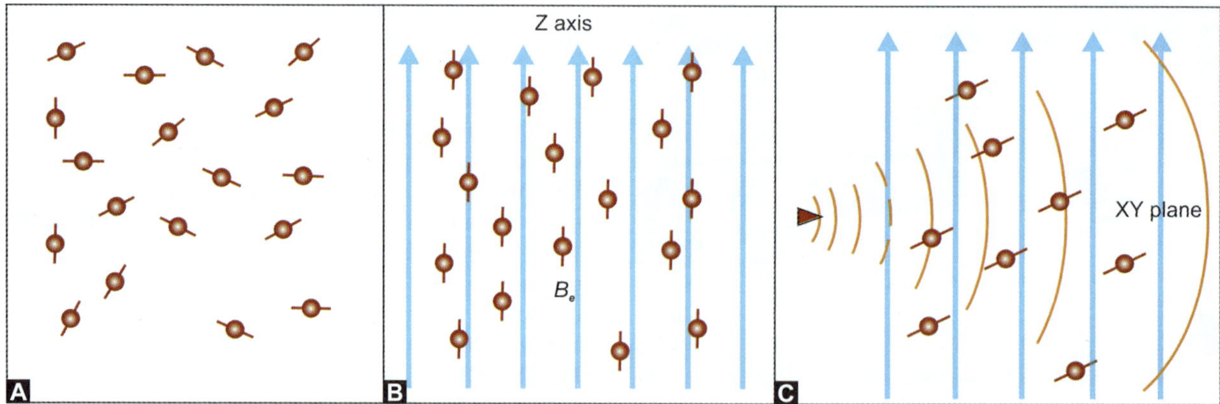

Figs 2.50A to C: Diagram explaining basic principle of MRI. (A) Hydrogen nuclei randomly arranged in absence of a strong magnetic field; (B) The nuclei "being charged" particles aligning along the applied external magnetic field (Z axis) resulting in longitudinal magnetization; (C) An RF excitation signal (90° pulse) being applied perpendicular to LM state magnetic moment causing transverse magnetization (in XY plane) and hence generation of an electric signal

Abbreviations: RF, radiofrequency; LM, longitudinal magnetization.

The signal thus obtained and contrast produced in the images will depend upon two factors:

1. The density of mobile free protons in the imaged organ. Tissue with high proton density will emit stronger signals.

2. The intensity and frequency of the RF excitation signal applied. By altering the characteristics of the RF excitation signal, variations in TR and TE times can be achieved, thereby producing several different pulse sequences, each

of which can be specific to highlight a different tissue or pathology.

Basic Magnetic Resonance Imaging Pulse Sequences

Variations in TR and TE* can be used in procuring a variety of image patterns. For example, a short TR and short TE gives T1-weighted images while a long TR and long TE gives T2-weighted images. A long TR and short TE gives proton density images. In addition to the main bore magnet, there are three more "gradient specific coils" in the gantry, which further modify the magnetic field and help in increasing the types of image sequences/patterns that can be attained.

Important MRI pulse sequences and their characteristics are as follows:

- *T1-weighted*: Useful for obtaining anatomic detail, detecting fat and hemorrhage. Fat and hemorrhage are hyperintense (bright) on T1-W images.
- *T2-weighted*: Useful for detecting pathology. Since water is hyperintense on T2-W images (pneumonic: World War 2—WW2, water is white on T2), sites of inflammation shine out.
- *Proton density (PD) images*: Useful for meniscal pathology and anatomic details.
- *Gradient echo-T2 images (produced by using signals from gradient coils in gantry)*: Calcified areas and hemorrhage (appear hypointense/dark) are better identified, in fact, said to "bloom" out. This characteristic can be useful in detecting loose bodies and pathologies like PVNS (*see* Page 332). Fibrocartilage, i.e. meniscus in the knee and labrum in the shoulder, can be visualized very nicely. 3D reconstruction of the images can be done.
- *STIR (short tau inversion recovery/FAT-SAT images)*: Fat is suppressed easing marrow and soft-tissue pathology identification.
- *FLAIR (fluid attenuation inversion recovery) images*: Used for imaging brain (as CSF is suppressed).
- *Diffusion weighted images*: Highlight sites of decreased proton movement, so useful to identify brain infarcts or cerebral abscess (which appear bright).

Role of Contrast

Both CT scan and MRI employ use of contrast medium to further enhance the pathology and make its identification easier. While CT scans use iodine or barium compounds as contrast, Gadolinium compounds are commonly employed as contrast material in MRI as they have seven unpaired electrons and create significant local magnetic field disturbances to alter the signal.

For visualizing joint pathologies, contrast materials can either be given by intravenous injection (indirect arthrography) or can be directly injected into the joint (direct arthrography).

Indirect arthrography: Here the contrast material is injected via the intravenous (IV) route. Enhancement by IV route relies on the fact that the *sites of inflammation or active tumor tissue* will have increased vascular supply and leaky cell membranes, causing contrast to leak into the lesion or joint, providing the enhancement at the site of affection.

> **Box 2.19:** Uses of MRI in orthopedics
>
> - Trauma
>   - Not routinely used
>   - IOC for unilateral stress fractures (bone scan can be preferred for bilateral stress fractures) and occult fractures
>   - Bone contusions can be seen, even when the cortex is intact
>   - Traumatic tendon ruptures, hematomas
> - Infection/inflammation
>   - MRI is IOC in acute, subacute and chronic osteomyelitis as it shows the status of marrow of involved bone as well as adjacent soft tissues
>   - Also, the preferred modality in septic arthritis and soft-tissue infections like pyomyositis, necrotizing fasciitis
> - Tumors
>   - Useful in assessing intramedullary spread, skip lesions, soft-tissue extent, status of adjacent neurovascular bundles

Direct arthrography: Here the joints are directly punctured (under USG guidance) and contrast is injected. It distends the joint capsule, thereby separating many of the closely applied soft tissue structures, making their identification easier on the image.

Uses of MRI in orthopedics are given in **Box 2.19**.

- *Advantages*: Excellent soft-tissue details, marrow details, no radiation exposure. MRI is the investigation of choice (IOC) in soft tissue (marrow, brain, spine, muscles, tendons, ligaments, cartilage, nerves) pathology detection. It is also the IOC for diagnosis of occult fractures and stress fractures (as it can detect marrow edema which appears prior to a frank cortical break).
- *Drawbacks*: Expensive, time consuming, high chances of motion artifacts when metal implants (casing magnetic disturbances) are in situ.
- *Contraindications*: Permanent pacemaker, metallic implants (presently MRI compatible titanium implants are being used in most places), neurostimulators, metallic auditory implants, claustrophobic patients (open MRI is available for claustrophobic patients).

POSITRON EMISSION TOMOGRAPHY-COMPUTED TOMOGRAPHY SCAN

It is a combination of two modalities—positron emission tomography (PET) and CT scan. A substrate molecule is infused and its uptake by sites of high metabolism (sites of pathology) is detected by CT imaging. Unlike bone scan that is indicative of only osteoblastic activity, PET-CT detects any tumor cell activity. 18-FDG (fluorodeoxyglucose) is the most commonly used agent to study metabolism while 13-N ammonia is most commonly used agent to study perfusion.

In orthopedics, PET-CT is mainly used for finding occult primary in suspected patients with bone tumors, in follow up of oncologic imaging to assess treatment response and for assessing distant/widespread metastasis.

---

* Typically, long TR is greater than 1,500 ms (millisecond) and short TR is less than 500 ms. Long TE is above 70–75 ms and short TE is around 15–20 ms. TR is always higher than TE.

BONE SCAN

Bone scan is a nuclear medicine test, i.e. it makes use of a small amount of radioactive substance (Tc 99m-labeled methylene diphosphonate) called as tracer, to scan body tissues, especially bones. The tracer is injected into a vein and as it perfuses various tissues, the activity (radiations emitted by various tissues with uptake) is detected by using a gamma camera.

Activity in bone scan is recorded in three phases:

1. *Early perfusion/Flow phase (image taken 2–5 seconds after injection)*: Here the isotope is still in the blood, so perfusion to a lesion can be evaluated. Areas of cellulitis show up in this phase.
2. *Middle blood pooling phase (image taken 5 minutes after injection)*: Areas that have moderate to severe soft tissue infection have dilated capillaries. So, blood pools up in these areas showing them up on the scan, better than phase I.
3. *Delayed bone phase (image taken 2–4 hours after injection)*: After 2–4 hours, most of isotope in blood is metabolized while the rest is taken up by the bone, so this phase is positive (in addition to above two phases) when a bone pathology is present. Areas with increased bone turnover/osteoblastic activity appear as areas of increased uptake (hot spots) on the scan and vice versa.

Uses of bone scan are given in **Box 2.20**. Since specificity of bone scan is very low, it is mainly used as a screening tool. Also it has limited ability to determine intraosseous extent of bone lesions or to demonstrate extra osseous soft tissue extensions where MRI serves a much better tool.

HIGH-YIELD POINTS

- *The rule of two in imaging:* Always obtain an X-ray of one joint above and one joint below the site of injury, in any suspected fracture.

Box 2.20: Uses of bone scan*

- *Hot spots (increased tracer uptake)*: Metastasis, trauma, neoplasm, infection
- *Cold spots (decreased tracer uptake)*: Multiple myeloma, histiocytosis X, metastasis from renal cell carcinoma/thyroid carcinoma (due to the replacement of normal bone or marrow)
- *Superscan (generalized/diffuse increased uptake)*: Hyperparathyroidism, renal osteodystrophy, widespread Paget's disease, diffuse metastasis

**Bone marrow agents:* Tc 99m-labeled sulfur colloid and Tc 99m minimicroaggregated albumin colloid are used for evaluating hematopoietically active marrow and marrow infiltrative diseases (e.g. glycogen storage disease).

- *Order of investigations in inflammatory joint swelling (e.g. septic arthritis)*: X-ray → USG-guided aspiration of joint fluid → MRI.
- Edward Purcell and Felix Bloch received Nobel Prize in 1954 for discovery of NMR phenomena but credit for developing MRI is given to Peter Mansfield and Paul Lauterbur who designed it's clinical application in the form of MRI imaging.
- In general, fat has a high signal (bright) on T1-weighted MRI images and fluid has a high signal on T2-weighted MRI images. Structures with little water or fat, such as cortical bone, tendons, and ligaments are hypointense (dark) in all types of sequences **(Table 2.15)**.
- Multiacquisition variable-resonance image combination and slice-encoding for metal artifact correction are specialized MRI sequences designed to minimize metallic artifacts around implants and prosthesis.
- Magnetic resonance imaging gives the earliest diagnosis and is the IOC for occult (hidden) fractures and unilateral stress

---

Table 2.15: Table depicting character shown by different structures on T1-W vs. T2-W MRI images

Tissue/fluids	T1 image	T2 image
Fat in marrow or cancellous bone or degenerated areas	White	Greyish-white
Muscles	Gray	Gray
CSF or clear fluid or water in tissues	Black	White
White matter brain/spine	Dark gray	Gray
Gray matter brain/spine	Blackish	Whitish gray
Granulation tissue	Gray	Whitish gray
Air	Black irregular	Black irregular
Bone	Black	Black
Flowing blood	Black	Black
Ligament or capsule (mature fibrous tissue)	Black line/band	Black line/band
Cord contusion or edema (myelitis)	dark gray	Whitish
Prevertebral hematoma	White (subacute stage)	Whitish
Ischemic/necrosed/sequestrated bone	Gray dead bone surrounded by black zone	Gray dead bone surrounded by white zone
Syrinx	Black cavity in cord	White cavity in cord
Myelomalacia	Dark	White
Nucleus pulposus hydated	Black/gray	White
Nucleus pulposus desiccated	Black	Black

Adapted from Tuberculosis of the skeletal system (by Dr SM Tuli).

fractures (authors prefer bone scan in suspected bilateral stress fractures).

- For osteomyelitis, MRI gives the earliest diagnosis (within 24 hours) and is the IOC. Bone scan is next in preference to MRI, and can establish the diagnosis within 48–72 hours (the area of infection has increased uptake due to osteoblastic activity). The gold standard is aspiration of pus and isolation of organism (i.e. culture and sensitivity testing).
- Magnetic resonance imaging is also the IOC for evaluating marrow extent, micrometastasis, skip lesions and soft-tissue involvement in cases of bone tumors. However, for confirming diagnoses of any tumor, biopsy is the gold standard.
- Although USG is considered the IOC for diagnosing developmental dysplasia of hip, the best investigation is MRI as it allows evaluation of complete disease spectrum.
- In heterotopic ossification, the earliest detection can be done by a bone scan. However, the screening investigation for the purpose is alkaline phosphatase levels and prostaglandin E2 level in 24-hour urine sample. A sudden increase in 24-hour urinary excretion of PGE2 is an indication for bone scan.
- When patient has problems around a prosthetic joint, bone scan can be used to differentiate between infection and aseptic (noninfective) loosening of the prosthesis.
- A bone scan is highly sensitive for osteoblastic (sclerotic) lesions while FDG-PET CT is more sensitive for osteolytic lesions and marrow involvement. Hence, IOC for osteoblastic or sclerotic metastasis is bone scan while for osteolytic metastasis it is FDG-PET CT.

TOURNIQUET IN ORTHOPEDICS

INTRODUCTION

Tourniquets (French "tourner" meaning "to turn") are commonly used in orthopedic surgeries to achieve bloodless clean surgical field. They are applied proximally on the limb to get bloodless clean field distally, thus, they are used for surgeries around the elbow, forearm and hand in upper limb and around the knee, leg and foot in the lower limb.

HISTORY

- First documented use of tourniquet dates back to 1674 by French army surgeon Etienne J Morel. In 1874, Joseph Lister described the first use of tourniquet in elective civilian practice.
- Friedrich von Esmarch developed a flat rubber bandage (Esmarch bandage) for exsanguination.
- The modern pneumatic tourniquet was first introduced by Harvey Cushing in 1904.

TYPES

- *Pneumatic tourniquets:* These are operated by air/gas under pressure (cuff is inflated by air/oxygen/nitrogen).
- *Nonpneumatic tourniquets:* Petit (belt) tourniquet and Esmarch (elastic) tourniquet.
  In modern orthopedic surgeries, pneumatic tourniquets have replaced nonpneumatic tourniquets.

HOW TO USE (FIGS 2.51A TO C)

Proximal part of the limb is wrapped with several (atleast two) layers of cast padding (usually of cotton wool) and then tourniquet is applied over the padding (minimum 5 cm proximal to planned surgical site). The limb is first exsanguinated by elevation and applying Esmarch bandage from distally to proximally. After exsanguination of the limb, tourniquet is inflated. Inflated tourniquet prevents blood flow distal to tourniquet and provides blood free clean surgical field.

PRINCIPLES OF TOURNIQUETS USE

- Tourniquets are available in several sizes. Mostly used is 10 cm wide cuff for arm and 15 cm or wider for thigh. Wide tourniquets are more effective at lower inflation pressures than narrow cuff tourniquets, so widest possible cuff size should be used.
- Solutions used in limb cleaning and painting (Savlon, Betadine, etc.) should not be allowed to seep underneath the tourniquet. It may cause chemical burns. So occlude tourniquet edges to prevent soakage of wool.
- *Safe time and pressure:* 2 hours are usually considered as the safe upper limit for tourniquet application. A general practice is to keep the pressure 100 mm Hg plus the systolic blood pressure for the upper arm and 100–150 mm Hg plus the systolic blood pressure for the thigh tourniquet. If more than 2 hours are required, then tourniquet should be deflated for 10 minutes and then again inflated.
- *Limb occlusion pressure (LOP):* Ideally LOP should be used to calculate the tourniquet inflation pressure. LOP is the pressure at which the distal arterial blood flow as evidenced by the Doppler probe, stops. Tourniquet should be inflated to a pressure higher than the LOP to cover the intraoperative fluctuations in arterial pressure. If LOP is less than 130 mm Hg, the safety margin is 40 mm Hg; for LOP 131–190 mm Hg, the margin is 60 mm Hg; and if LOP is more than 190 mm Hg, the margin is 80 mm Hg.

CONTRAINDICATIONS

Peripheral vascular disease, deep vein thrombosis (due to few reports citing increased thromboembolic phenomena), severe infection of the limb and compromised cardiac status are relative contraindications to use of tourniquets. Exsanguination prior to tourniquet application should preferably be avoided in cases of infection and malignancy to prevent dissemination.

COMPLICATIONS

- Nerve injury is the most common complication of tourniquet application. Nerve injuries are more common in upper limb tourniquets and radial nerve is the most common nerve to be involved. Excessive pressure and insufficient pressure (causing venous congestion) both may cause nerve palsy. Direct pressure by cuff on the nerves is the most common cause followed by ischemia, so nerve injury is related more to cuff pressure than duration.
- *Post-tourniquet syndrome:* It is mainly related to ischemia. It presents with postoperative edema, redness, pain dysesthesia and stiffness. It is caused by muscle injury due to high mechanical pressure.

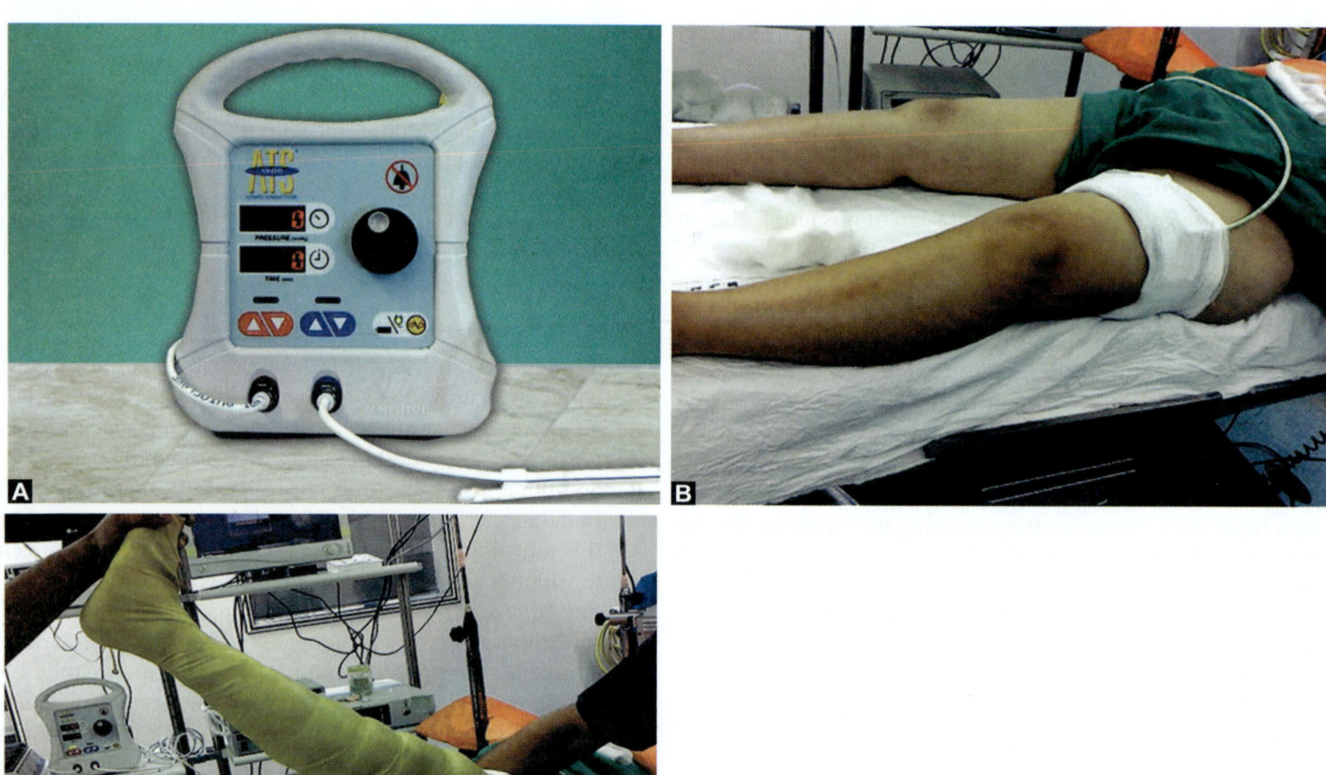

Figs 2.51A to C: (A) Modern pneumatic tourniquet; (B) Application of tourniquet; (C) Application of Esmarch before tourniquet inflation

- *Chemical burns*: It may occur due to see page of antimicrobial solutions used for skin preparation underneath the tourniquet cuff.

- Compartment syndrome is rare but most devastating complication.

3

CHAPTER

Management of Polytrauma Patients and Open Fractures

INTRODUCTION

Traumatology (trauma; greek; injury or wound) refers to study of injuries or wounds caused by accident or violence to a person. With cases on rise as if an epidemic, this domain now forms the backbone of Orthopedics. Over past century, world has witnessed many mass traumatic events like terrorist bombings, war disasters, rail accidents, fires, etc. and not uncommon for a surgeon is to encounter polytrauma patients in mass number.

Polytrauma patients are those patients who have sustained two or more severe injuries which endanger life [injury severity score (ISS) >18, *see* later]. The leading cause of polytrauma and death are road traffic accidents and mostly involved are the young and active population of society. Care of these polytrauma patients begins right from the scene of the accident. Highly coordinated team efforts are required to manage the victims effectively. Often these patients are a part of mass casualty and hence the immediate step that comes into operation is triage.

TRIAGE

In case of mass casualties the injured persons often outnumber the helping medical experts. The immediate step in such situation is to sort the patients based on their need for treatment and the resources available, this process is called *triage*. Simply this is a system deciding which patient should be treated first, depending on how severe they are injured. Patients are sorted into four color-coded groups of priority based on their need for evacuation and immediate treatment as outlined below:

1. *Priority 1 (Red)—(Immediate care needed):* These patients cannot survive without immediate treatment, but have a chance of survival with immediate intervention.
2. *Priority 2 (Yellow)—(Urgent care needed):* These patients are stable for the moment but require observation in a hospital. These patients have injuries that are less severe than red categories, but may be life or limb threatening if treatment is delayed beyond several hours. These patients may require a retriage.
3. *Priority 3 (Green)—(Delayed care needed):* These patients have only minor injuries and are tagged as walking wounded. These are segregated from more seriously injured patients of the above two categories and treated after the red and yellow category patients have been treated.
4. *Priority 4 (Black)—(Dead):* These are patients without obvious vital signs.

Priority 1 patients are those who are likely to deteriorate without medical help (requiring immediate intervention to save lives) are attended first while injured, but walking in patients with stable vitals, classified into delayed (Priority 3) category, are attended later as the situation permits.

GUIDELINES FOR CARE OF SERIOUSLY INJURED

Once the priority order is decided, the doctor in emergency starts attending the priority 1 patient. The first step is to ensure that the patient in question does not have a cardiac arrest. The recommendation [by American Heart Association (AHA)] is to check the carotid pulse for atleast 10 seconds while simultaneously assessing the breathing pattern of the patient. Three situations may arise (**Flow chart 3.1**):

1. *Pulse detectable and patient breathing normally:* In this situation, the polytrauma patient is subjected to the Advanced Trauma Life Support protocol (ATLS, read later) described by the American College of Surgeons to prevent an impending cardiac arrest and hence collapse.
2. *Pulse detectable but breathing not normal:* The situation is characteristic of patients having respiratory depression secondary to causes like opioid poisoning. They should be managed according to suspected cause.
3. *Pulse absent and no normal breathing (e.g. gasping respiration):* These are the patients in cardiac arrest that need immediate cardiopulmonary resuscitation (CPR) and are subjected to the AHA's Basic Life Support (BLS) protocol (if resuscitation is performed without use of special equipment, drugs or invasive skills, as in collapsed patients lying roadside) or Advanced Life Support (ALS) protocol (if there is availability of equipment like cardiac monitors, endotracheal tubes, drugs, etc. as in an ambulance or hospital setting).

BASIC LIFE SUPPORT

This is a protocol for CPR that includes a series of steps that are instituted on an emergency basis in any collapsed patient suspected to have a cardiac arrest. The protocol is designed to be performed not just by a doctor, but a medical technician, a paramedic or even a qualified bystander who identifies such a patient. Since the care of the patient has to start from the accident scene, the protocol steps are designed barring the use of any special equipment, drugs or invasive skills (except a defibrillator that is available at most locations and is simple to use as automated equipment are largely installed in most locations).

Before the protocol is formally instituted, the performer is advised to brush through three quick steps to ensure personal as well as patient's safety. These are designated by mnemonic "DRS" viz. "Danger" (remove the patient from the site of danger like from middle of the road to a safe place), "Response" (command patient to assess his response to get a quick idea

Flow chart 3.1: Emergency guidelines for the care of a seriously injured polytrauma patient (modified from American Heart Association's 2015 guidelines)

Verify scene safety

Victim is unresponsive
Shout for nearby help
Activate emergency response system
via mobile device (If appropriate)
Get AED and emergency equipment
(or send someone to do so)

Normal breathing, has pulse → Follow th ATLS protocol for polytrauma patient to prevent an impending cardiac arrest that could be life threatening

Look for no breathing or only gasping and check pulse (simultaneously). Is pulse **definitely** felt within 10 seconds?

No normal breathing, has pulse → Provide rescue breathing: 1 breath every 5–6 seconds, or about 10–12 breaths/min.
• Activate emergency response system (if not already done) after 2 minutes
• Continue rescue breathing: Check pulse about every 2 minutes. If no pulse, begin CPR (go to "CPR" box)
• If possible opioid overdose, administer naloxone if available per protocol

No breathing or only gasping, no pulse

Cardiac arrest

Basic life support

CPR
Begin cycles of
30 compressions and 2 breaths
Use AED as soon as it is available

AED arrives

Check rhythm. Shockable rhythm?

Yes, shockable → Give 1 shock. Resume CPR immediately for about 2 minutes (until prompted by AED to allow rhythm check). Continue until ALS providers take over or victim starts to move

No, nonshockable → Resume CPR immediately for about 2 mintues (until prompted by AED to allow rhythm check). Continue until ALS providers take over or victim starts to move

Abbreviations: ALTS, advanced trauma life support; AED, automated external defibrillator; CPR, cardiopulmonary resuscitation.

of the seriousness of the injury) and "Send for help" (alert the nearby persons of the situation and ask send them to seek immediate help or call an ambulance). Immediately thereafter the steps to be endorsed are best remembered by the mnemonic "CABD" viz. starting immediate "Chest compressions", managing "Airway", providing rescue "Breathing" and ensuring early "Defibrillation". The important details of each step are outlined here.

Chest Compressions

Chest compressions, take precedence even over airway assessment in patients with cardiac arrest. It is postulated that when a person enters into a cardiac arrest, the blood still has some oxygen that can be harnessed by the tissues in the body (as metabolic acidosis shifts the oxygen-hemoglobin dissociation curve). Immediate chest compressions ensure that the blood gets delivered to the dying tissues, buying them some additional time for survival. Compressions are given by placing both hands one on top of another, with "heel part" centered over the chest around two fingers above xiphoid (i.e. the lower tip of the sternum), while body weight is being used to administer compressions **(Figs 3.1A and B)**. 100–120 compressions are given per minute for all age groups and chest is allowed to recoil fully in between. For adults, children and infants, chest is pushed up to 5, 4 and 3 cm, respectively.

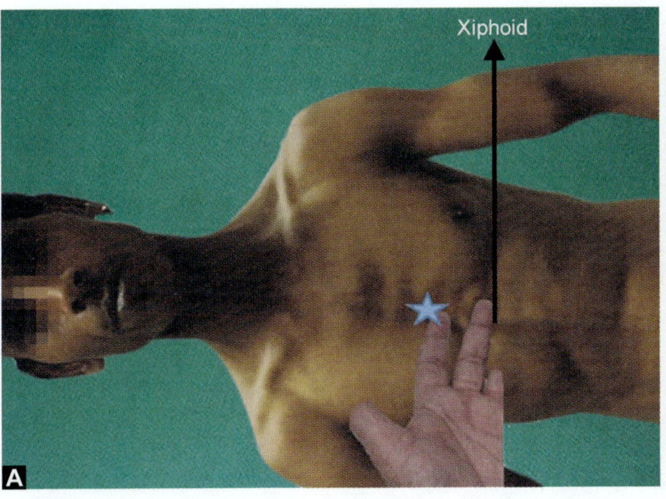

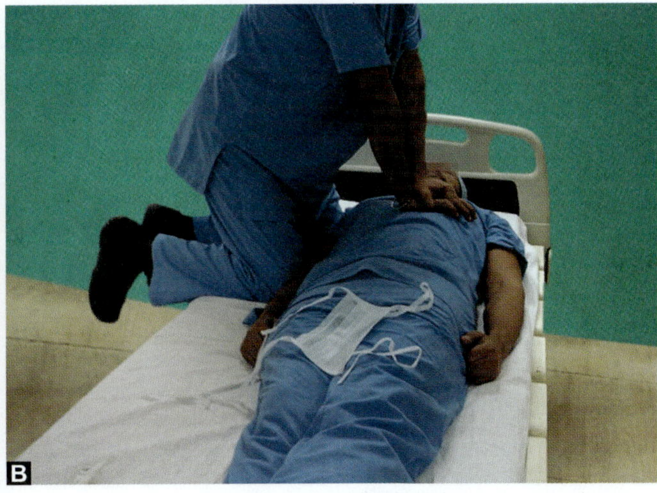

Figs 3.1A and B: (A) Site of chest compression (marked with a star) is two finger breadths above the xiphoid in the middle of the chest; (B) Doctor in action during a cardiopulmonary resuscitation (CPR). Note the hands one on top of another, elbows straight and the doctor up on bed to utilize his body weight to administer compressions via "heel" of his palm

Airway Management

Next step is to assess airway patency. Chin lift or jaw thrust (more effective) is the recommended maneuvers **(Figs 3.2A and B)** to establish the patency of a nonpatent airway. Blind finger sweeps should rather be avoided, as they may push foreign objects deeper into the airway. Once patent, the rescuer can try possible insertion of oral (oropharyngeal airway) or nasal (nasopharyngeal airway) adjuncts of proper size **(Figs 3.3A to C)** to maintain airway patency.

Breathing

Once the patency of the airway is secured, rescue breathing is to be provided. After every 30 chest compressions, give two rescue breaths in both adult and child victims, verifying that the chest rises and falls. Attempt the two artificial ventilations either using the mouth-to-mouth technique, or preferably a bag-valve-mask (BVM) apparatus **(Fig. 3.4)**, if available. The mouth-to-mouth technique is not recommended, unless a face shield is present. Continue for five cycles (or 2 minutes) of "CAB" before reassessing pulse.

Defibrillation

While the rescuer is performing the CPR as described earlier, the helper is asked to arrange an automated external defibrillator (AED). The AED is to be used as soon as it is available **(Fig. 3.5)**. The device is attached to the patient's chest. It assesses the cardiac rhythm and guides the performer whether the rhythm is shockable or not. Give the shock if the AED prompts, else continue with CPR for another 2 minutes, after which the rhythm is to be rechecked by the AED. The BLS protocol continues until— (1) the patient regains a pulse, (2) the rescuer is relieved by another rescuer of higher training (i.e. an ALS team arrives, *see* later), (3) the rescuer is too physically tired to continue CPR, or (4) the patient is pronounced dead by a medical doctor.

ADVANCED LIFE SUPPORT AND ADVANCED CARDIOVASCULAR LIFE SUPPORT

Advanced Life Support is a treatment consensus for CPR in patients with cardiac arrest and related medical problems (e.g.

stroke), as agreed in Europe by the European Resuscitation Council, most recently in 2010. The Americans use a parallel protocol called Advanced Cardiovascular Life Support (ACLS), endorsed from the AHA, latest updated in 2015. These protocols are a continuum of the BLS protocol as the ambulance team arrives at the scene or patient reaches the hospital where there are certified practitioners (trained emergency medicine technicians or medics), having training and skills in the use of special equipment and invasive techniques (e.g. endotracheal intubation) and drugs (e.g. adrenaline, oxygen). The basic steps are the same as outlined earlier, however, the appropriate equipment is taken to use wherever needed, e.g. the laryngeal masks **(Fig. 3.6A)** or endotracheal tubes **(Fig. 3.6B)** to secure and maintain the airway, and drugs for managing cardiac arrest **(Table 3.1)**.

The most important point to highlight in the ALS system is the use of cardiac monitors to analyze the patient's heart rhythm. In contrast to an AED in BLS, where the machine decides when

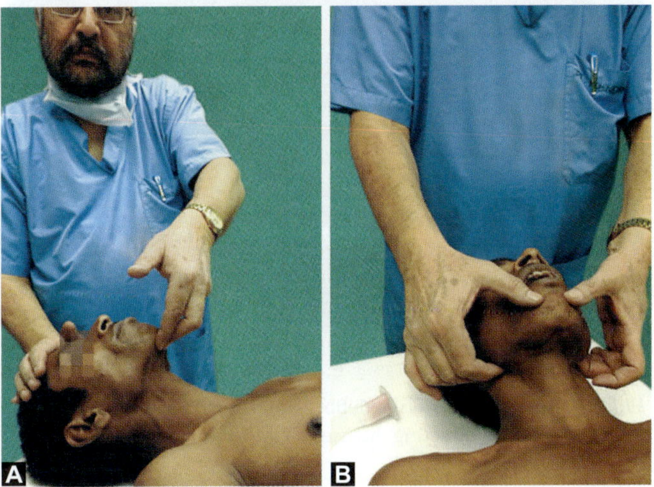

Figs 3.2A and B: (A) Demonstrating chin lift technique; (B) Jaw thrust technique for achieving airway patency. The latter is preferred

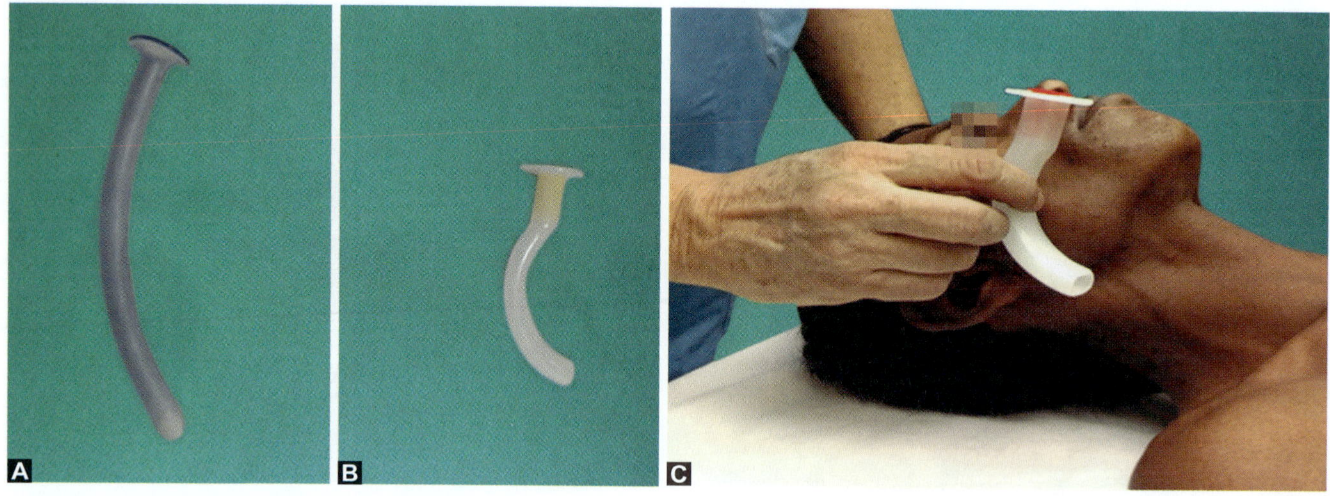

Figs 3.3A to C: (A) Nasopharyngeal airway; (B and C) Oropharyngeal airway, with the latter being sized from the incisors to the angle of the jaw

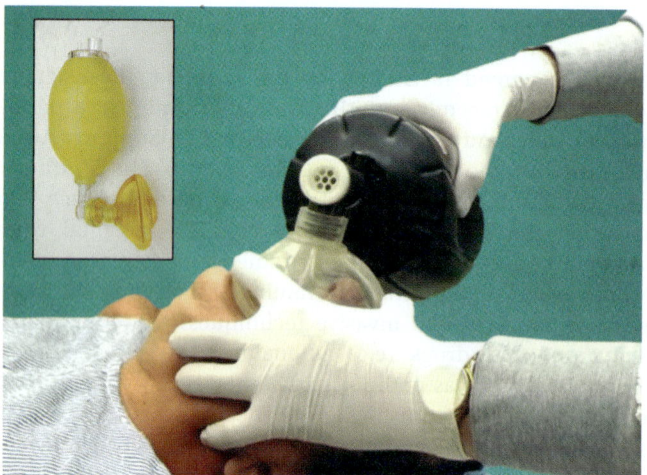

Fig. 3.4: Bag valve mask (inset) ventilation

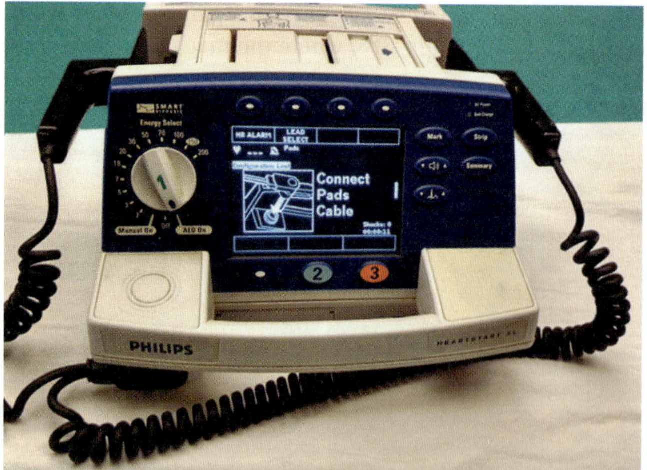

Fig. 3.5: Automated external defibrillator (note the command on the screen directing the user for appropriate steps)

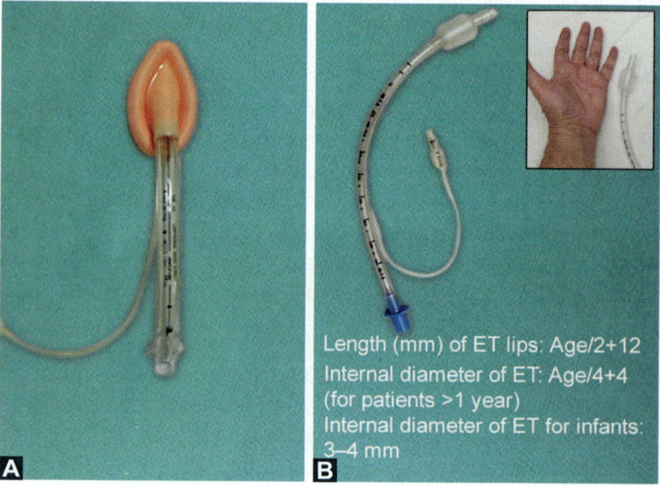

Figs 3.6A and B: (A) Laryngeal mask airway; (B) Endotracheal tube. The internal diameter of the tube generally chosen is matchable to the diameter of patient's little finger. However, correct ways to determine diameter and size are as shown in the **Figure 3.6B**

signs. Further steps in ACLS involve insertion of intravenous (IV) lines and placement of various airway devices and use of emergency drugs, such as epinephrine and amiodarone. An essential step in the ALS system is to quickly search for possible reversible causes of cardiac arrest (i.e. the Hs and Ts, **Table 3.2**). Based on their diagnosis, more specific treatments are administered. These treatments may be medical such as IV injection of an antidote for drug overdose, or surgical such as insertion of a chest tube (or performing needle thoracocentesis) for those with tension pneumothorax. The legitimate factor in the decision to terminate resuscitation is an end-tidal CO_2 production ($EtCO_2$) of less than 10 mm Hg, measured on waveform capnography, after at least 20 minutes of resuscitation.

ADVANCED TRAUMA LIFE SUPPORT

Advanced trauma life support is a periodically updated, evidence-based training course (by the American College of Surgeons) for physicians and surgeons who are involved in the care of trauma

and how to shock a patient, the ACLS team leader makes those decisions based on rhythms on the monitor and patient's vital

Table 3.1: Drugs used in Advanced Life Support (ALS) protocol for cardiopulmonary resuscitation (CPR)

Rhythm	Drugs*
Shockable	Adrenaline 1 mg after second shock and then every second cycle Amiodarone 300 mg after third shock
Nonshockable	Adrenaline 1 mg immediately and then every second cycle

Caution: Routine atropine use is no longer recommended unless there is a high risk for bradycardia.

Table 3.2: The Hs and Ts—reversible causes of cardiac arrest

The "Hs"	The "Ts"
• Hypoxia	• Tension pneumothorax
• Hypovolemia	• Tamponade cardiac
• Hypokalemia/Hyperkalemia	• Toxins (medicinal poisonings)
• Hypothermia/Hyperthermia	• Thromboembolism
• Hydrogen ions (acidosis)	
• Hypoglycemia	

patients. Concept behind ATLS is that save the life (i.e. prevent an impending cardiac arrest) by addressing the most dangerous threat to life first. "Correct sequence" for assessment and management of a polytraumatized patient (not in cardiac arrest or revived from arrest) is triage; primary survey; adjuncts to primary survey; patient transfer if needed; secondary survey; adjuncts to secondary survey; re-evaluation and definitive care.

Primary Survey

This part involves identifying and managing life-threatening injuries. A catastrophic exsanguinating external hemorrhage, if seen, should be immediately managed with a tamponade. Patients are rapidly assessed on the basis of "ABCDE" resuscitation protocol:

- **A**irway control with stabilization of the cervical spine.
- **B**reathing assessment—management of respiratory distress.
- **C**irculation—assessment of shock and management.
- **D**isability or neurological status—management of head injury.
- **E**xposure or undressing of the patient.

Airway Management with Cervical Spine Protection

Management of the airway is the first and foremost priority. A patient lying prone should be log rolled to supine position for airway assessment. Start with assessing the patency of the airway by suctioning and cleaning and look for any foreign body and facial fractures that may obstruct the airway. Management of foreign body obstruction has been summarized in **Flow chart 3.2**. However, more commonly than a foreign body, it is the tongue that falls back and obstructs the airway in the unconscious patient. Chin lift and jaw thrust **(Figs 3.2A and B)** maneuvers as outlined earlier can be performed if required to establish patency. Oropharyngeal or nasopharyngeal airways **(Figs 3.3A and B)** can be inserted if these maneuvers are not successful. Indications for definite airway management, i.e. tracheal intubation/ cricothyroidotomy **(Figs 3.7A and B)** include the inability to

Flow chart 3.2: Protocol for the management of foreign body obstruction

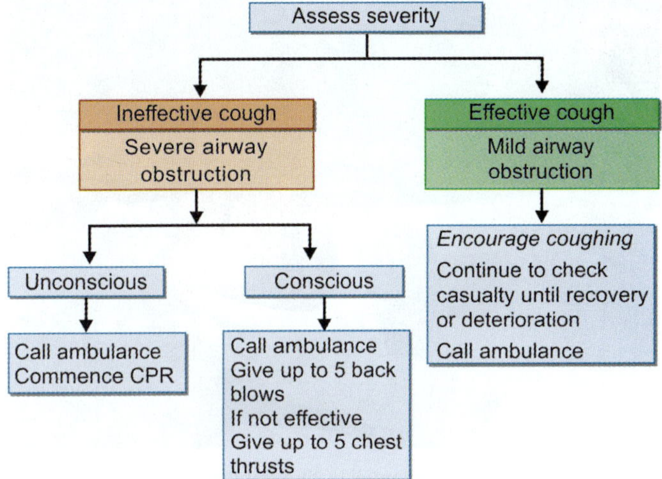

Abbreviation: CPR, cardiopulmonary resuscitation.

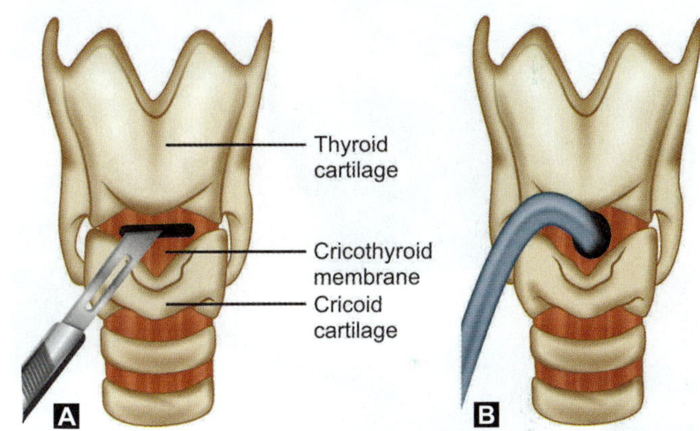

Figs 3.7A and B: Cricothyroidotomy

maintain an adequate airway by abovementioned measures, the risk of aspiration or score less than 8 on Glasgow Coma Scale (GCS). Cervical spine should be manually protected all the time while managing the airway by manual in-line stabilization **(Fig. 3.8)** and neck should not be hyperflexed, hyperextended or rotated. Once the definite airway management has been done, a proper sized cervical collar is applied **(Figs 3.9A and B)**.

Breathing and Ventilation

Adequate breathing and ventilation require proper functioning of chest wall, diaphragm and lung. Chest wall should be exposed to look for the position of the trachea, symmetrical chest movements, rate and depth of respiration. Auscultate the chest for breath sounds. The most serious injuries that can compromise breathing in a polytrauma patient include tension pneumothorax, massive hemothorax and flail chest (defined as three or more contiguous rib fractures, each in two places). Oxygen is administered by high flow non-rebreathing mask. If breathing is inadequate, then BVM ventilation is started **(Fig. 3.4)**. Tension pneumothorax and massive hemothorax require immediate chest decompression **(Fig. 3.10)**.

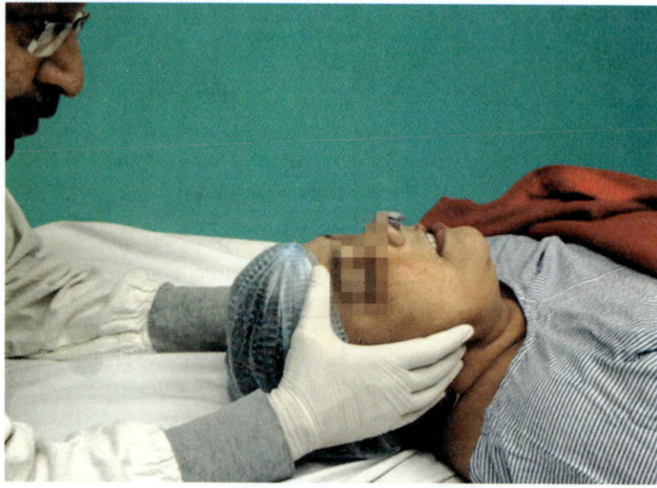

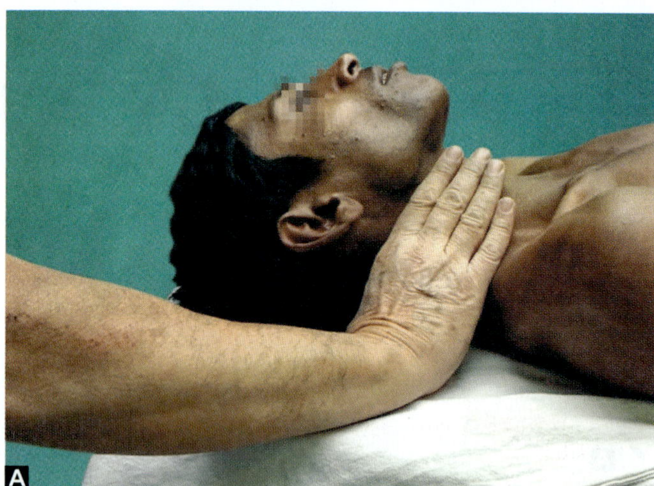

A

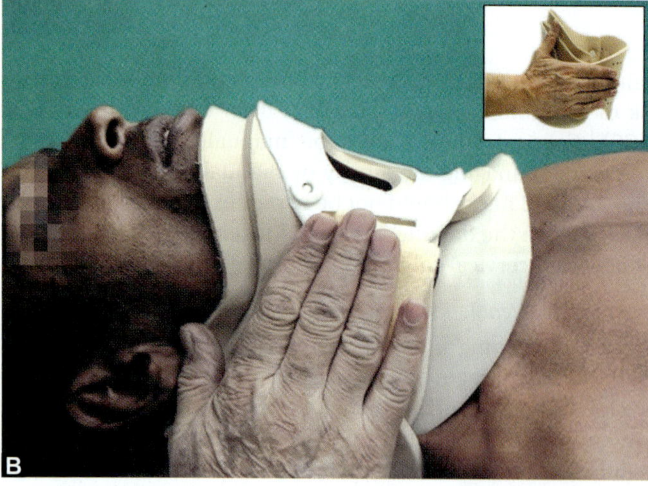

B

Figs 3.9A and B: Sizing and application of cervical collar

Fig. 3.8: Manual in-line stabilization

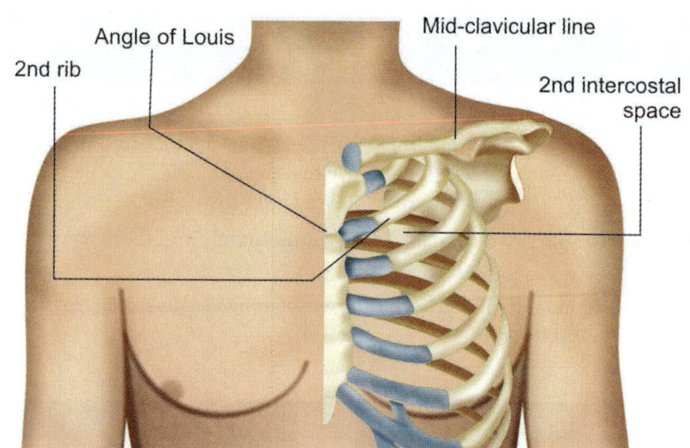

Fig. 3.10: Landmarks for needle thoracocentesis in cases of tension pneumothorax. A large bore needle is inserted in the 2nd intercostal space in mid-clavicular line to decompress the pleural space

Circulation

Control of internal and external hemorrhage is the most important preventable cause of death. Any external hemorrhage is controlled by direct pressure, wound packing or by use of a tourniquet. Internal hemorrhage may occur in the pelvis, abdomen, chest, retroperitoneum and from a fractured bone. Bleeding site is identified by clinical examination and imaging (X-ray, USG, etc.). Management depends on the site of the bleeding like pelvic binder for the hemorrhage in the pelvis and use of a splint for a fracture of a long bone and surgical packing for suspected internal bleeding. IV access is established using two wide bore cannulas placed in the antecubital fossa or groin. The patient is assessed for signs and symptoms of the shock **(Box 3.1)**. IV fluid therapy is started with crystalloid fluids, preferably 1 L (20 mL/kg) of warm (39°C) Ringer lactate (RL), titrated to patient's pulse and blood pressure response.

Disability and Neurological Examination

Level of consciousness is conventionally assessed by GCS **(Table 3.3)**. A practical approach of rapid assessment is simply asking the name or details of the accident and rating the patient as per the AVPU Scale. In AVPU scale **(Box 3.2)** after assessment, patient is assigned a letter score (A, V, P, U) based on the alertness, voice response, pain response and unresponsiveness. Patients with score below "A" level must be carefully assessed for pupillary size and reaction, signs of raised intracranial pressure and lateralizing signs and a formal GCS must be calculated. GCS less than 8 indicates a severe reduction in consciousness and such patients require urgent intubation and mechanical ventilation. Indications for neurological referral include deterioration in GCS, GCS less than 8, seizures, focal neurological signs and CSF leak. Cervical X-rays may be ordered to look for cervical spine injury while CT scan is the investigation of choice in suspected head injury cases. The criteria for imaging are given in **Table 3.4**.

Exposure and Environment Control

Undress the patient and examine the abdomen, flanks and back for any suspected injury, limb deformities and suspected fractures and dislocations. Examination of back requires "log rolling" the patient, a technique that is very critical and requires at least five team members as shown in **Figure 3.11**.

Box 3.1: Classification of hemorrhage

- Class I: Less than 15% loss of circulating blood volume
  - *Diagnosis:* No change in blood pressure, pulse, or capillary refill
  - *Treatment:* Crystalloid
- Class II: 15–30% loss of circulating blood volume
  - *Diagnosis:* Tachycardia with normal blood pressure
  - *Treatment:* Crystalloid
- Class III: 30–40% loss of circulating blood volume
  - *Diagnosis:* Tachycardia, tachypnea, and hypotension
  - *Treatment:* Rapid crystalloid replacement, then blood
- Class IV: More than 40% loss of circulating blood volume
  - *Diagnosis:* Marked tachycardia and hypotension
  - *Treatment:* Immediate crystalloid and urgent most blood replacement

Box 3.2: AVPU Scale

A	Awake and alert patient, eyes open spontaneously
V	Patient does not open eyes spontaneously, but opens to verbal stimulation
P	Patient only responds to painful stimuli
U	Unresponsive patient

Table 3.3: Glasgow Coma Scale

	Score
Best eye opening	
Spontaneous	4
To voice	3
To pain	2
None	1
Best verbal response	
Orientated	5
Confused/disorientated	4
Inappropriate words	3
Incomprehensible sounds	2
None	1
Best motor response	
Obeys commands	6
Localizes to pain	5
Withdraws to pain	4
Abnormal flexion to pain	3
Extension to pain	2
None	1

Adjuncts to Primary Survey

These are the diagnostic and monitoring investigations which support the diagnosis of primary survey. These include: ECG, arterial blood gas analysis, pulse oximetry, insert urinary and gastric catheters, monitoring of exhaled CO_2, chest and pelvis X-rays, etc.

Table 3.4: Criteria for cervical spine imaging and CT head in polytrauma

NEXUS criteria for cervical spine imaging	*Canadian CT head rule*
No posterior mid-line tenderness	GCS < 15, 2 hours postinjury
No focal neurological deficit	Suspected depressed or open skull fracture
Normal alertness with no evidence of intoxication	Any signs of basal skull fracture (raccoon eyes, battle sign, CSF rhinorrhea, etc.)
No clinically apparent painful distracting injury	>1 episode of vomiting Age > 64 years Dangerous mechanism of injury (e.g. fall > 1 m height)
No need of cervical spine X-rays if all above conditions are met	Undertake a CT head study if any of the above condition is met

Abbreviations: NEXUS, National Emergency X-Radiography Utilization Study; GCS, Glasgow Coma Scale; CSF, cerebrospinal fluid.

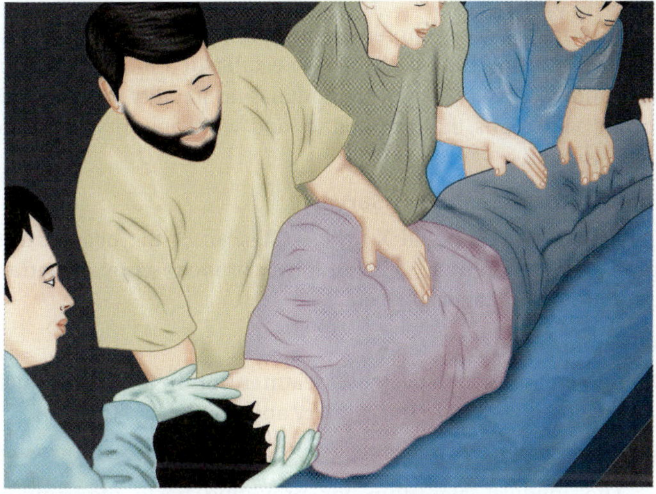

- The team leader takes control of the head and cervical spine and is responsible for coordinating the roll.
- Three members of the team are positioned on the side to which the face is to be turned controlling the chest, hips and knees respectively.
- The fifth member stations on the posterior side and inspects the back as the patient is log rolled.

Fig. 3.11: Log rolling technique

Patient Transfer

Once the primary survey is done and life-threatening injuries have been identified and managed, patient transfer may be needed to a higher center or other facility in the same set-up in order to undertake appropriate investigations, to provide missing treatment or simply to provide a safer environment. It is mandatory that all such transfers, strictly be made after fixing the patient on a spine board, the same being readily available in every emergency facility **(Fig. 3.12)**.

Secondary Survey

This part involves identifying and managing non-life threatening minor injuries, which can be missed during the primary survey. Secondary survey involves taking an "AMPLE" history (Allergies,

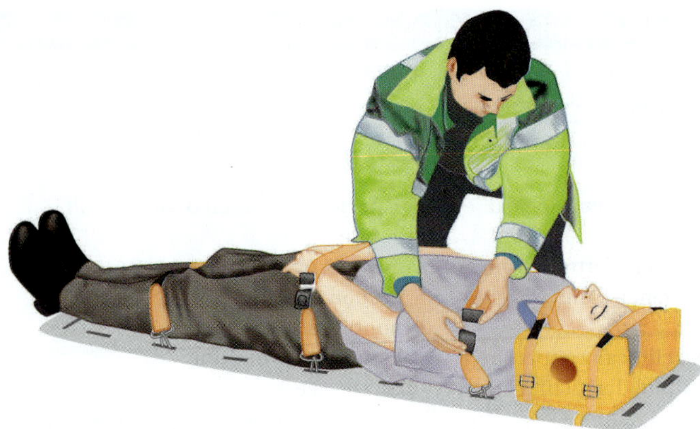

Fig. 3.12: Polytrauma patient being fixed to a spine board for transport

Medications currently used, Past illness/Pregnancy, Last meal, Events/Environment related to the injury), performing a detailed examination from head to toe and from front to back and reassessment of vital signs.

Secondary survey should begin only after primary survey is completed, resuscitation efforts are established and the patient is hemodynamically stable. Hemodynamic stability is defined as normal vital signs that are maintained with only maintenance fluid volumes.

Adjuncts to the Secondary Survey

These include additional X-rays, a CT scan of the head, chest, spine and abdomen, angiography, bronchoscopy, contrast urography, esophagoscopy, etc.

Definitive Care

Definitive care is the specialist treatment of the injuries, which have been diagnosed in the primary and secondary surveys.

HIGH-YIELD POINTS

- The medical algorithm for providing basic life support to adults in the USA was published in 2005 in journal "Circulation" by the AHA.
- The AHA 2015 ACLS update has advised on the use of mobile phones to notify emergency medical services (EMS) or nearby rescuers of the serious situation. The update also encourages lay persons to perform continuous "hands-only CPR" at a minimum, until the EMS arrives.
- Targeted temperature goal range of 32–36°C is advised to be maintained by AHA, during cardiac resuscitation.
- A common complication occurring during CPR is rib fractures, seen in up to one-third of the patients undergoing resuscitation. Vast majority of these fractures are bilateral and most commonly involved are anterior segments of 3rd–5th ribs. Despite fractured ribs, the doctor is supposed to continue with the CPR.
- In managing a polytrauma patient in shock, although RL, normal saline (NS) and hypertonic saline (HS), all are used world over, debate exists in context of crystalloid of choice. RL is mostly preferred, owing to the theoretical advantages it offers. RL is converted in the liver to pyruvate which is further broken down to CO_2 and H_2O. The two interact in

aqueous solution to release the bicarbonate ions ($H_2CO_3 \leftrightarrow H^+ + HCO_3^-$), which act as a buffer in the setting of metabolic acidosis secondary to shock. NS on the other hand is a hyperchloremic solution (chloride ion rich fluid) that does not produce any ion that can be metabolized into HCO_3^- and hence, worsens acidosis (referred to as dilution acidosis) apart from lowering fibrinogen levels thereby increasing chances of coagulopathy. The concern using RL is the lower sodium content it has in comparison to the extracellular fluid. There is a risk of hyponatremic encephalopathy although very rare. HS on the other hand also has no proven benefit over these standard crystalloids.

- *Focused assessment with sonography for trauma (FAST):* An adjunct to surveys, this is basically a rapid bedside USG evaluation done in patients with suspected blunt trauma to the torso in order to find sites of unrecognized hemorrhage. The examination is a kind of a screening test (90% sensitivity) meant to replace historical methods like diagnostic peritoneal lavage, in searching for evidence of traumatic free fluid suggestive of bleeding into the peritoneal, pericardial or pleural cavities. The procedure involves examination of four quadrants around the abdomen (Morrison and splenorenal pouch, and around the pericardium) and the pelvis in a supine patient using 3.5–5 MHz convex USG transducers. An extended examination may also be used to evaluate the lungs for possibility of the presence of a pneumothorax (extended FAST).

MANAGEMENT OF OPEN FRACTURES

INTRODUCTION

An open fracture (old term—compound fracture) is one that communicates with external environment or in other words where the hematoma is draining out from the wound **(Fig. 3.13)**. Open fractures are orthopedic emergencies. They carry increased morbidity due to severe soft tissue injury and risk for fracture contamination. Open fractures of the tibia are the most common open long bone fractures.

CLASSIFICATION

Gustilo-Anderson classification is the most commonly used classification system for open fractures **(Table 3.5)**. Gustilo-Anderson grading must be done after debridement of the wound as the grading can change after debridement.

MANAGEMENT

Open fractures are usually high velocity injuries and patient may require resuscitation in the emergency room. Start IV antibiotics and give tetanus prophylaxis once resuscitation is complete. Active bleeding may require compression bandaging. Give IV analgesics or regional block for pain relief and remove the gross contamination. Splint the fracture, place sterile saline dressing on the wound and shift the patient to the operation theater urgently. Thorough surgical wound debridement (removal of devitalized tissue, foreign objects and any visible contamination) should be done as soon as possible (ideally within 6 hours). Vitality of muscles is assessed by *4 Cs*—color (pink), consistency (firm), contractility (should respond to pinch or electrocautery) and capillary circulation (actively bleeding). Patients often require serial debridements and low pressure saline lavage is the most effective way of reducing bacterial load of the wound **(Table 3.6)**. IV antibiotics should be continued for 24 hours after wound closure in Gustilo type I and type II and for 3 days in Gustilo type III fractures.

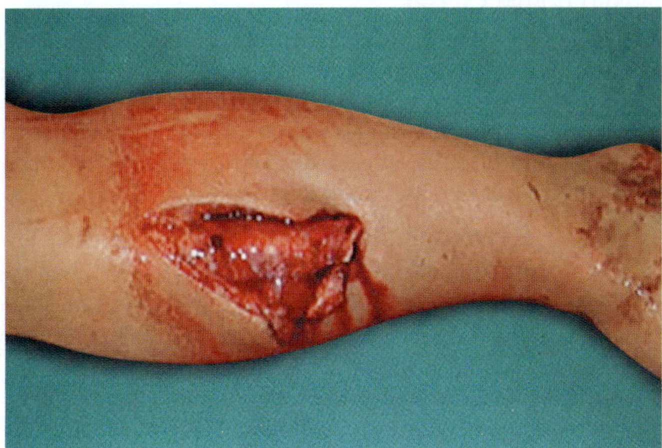

Fig. 3.13: Open or compound fracture

Table 3.5: Gustilo-Anderson classification of compound fractures*

Type/Grade	Features
I	Fracture wound < 1 cm with minimal soft tissue injury and fracture comminution. Usually, it is low energy trauma with clean wound
II	Fracture wound > 1 cm without extensive soft tissue damage and fracture comminution. There is mild-to-moderate soft tissue injury and mild-to-moderate wound contamination
IIIA	Fracture wound > 10 cm with extensive soft tissue injury and wound contamination, but with adequate soft tissue coverage (at least periosteum over bone is intact)
IIIB	Fracture wound > 10 cm with extensive soft tissue damage and contamination. Soft tissue coverage is inadequate (periosteal stripping occurs and bone may be exposed) and require skin or flap grafting
IIIC	Any size of open wound with major vascular injury requiring repair

*Gunshot wounds with fractures and open segmental fractures are classified as type IIIA Gustilo-Anderson injuries.

Fracture Fixation and Wound Closure

Primary definitive internal fixation of Gustilo type I fracture can be done if the soft tissue condition permits, but Gustilo type II or beyond categories, mostly need temporary external fixation (for wound management) while internal fixation is opted once infection settles and wound heals. Wound healing can be hastened by a primary closure when the soft tissue damage is limited, however, in few cases of Gustilo type II and III fractures, primary closure may not be possible and decision of closure is taken after second relook debridement. These patients often require skin grafting or coverage with muscle flaps for wound healing.

CRUSH SYNDROME (TRAUMATIC RHABDOMYOLYSIS)

INTRODUCTION

It is the systemic manifestation of extensive muscle injury due to severe crushing of muscles and subsequent release of cellular components of muscle cells into circulation. It is most commonly seen in victims of road traffic accidents with prolonged extrication.

PATHOPHYSIOLOGY

Severe crushing causes lysis of muscle cells, leading to significant metabolic derangements and eventual organ failure. The process starts with crushing and compression, opening stretch activated channels and shutting down Na/K channels at the cellular level. This leads to increased intracellular calcium, which in turn stimulates protease activity in cell leading to cellular lysis. After extrication (i.e. removal from entangled situation) restoration of blood flow to injured muscles, causes reperfusion injury. The limb may swell up rapidly leading to compartment syndrome (*see* Page 79).

Metabolic derangements include hyperkalemia, hypocalcemia and hyponatremia. With shifting of intravascular fluid into the cells, the patient frequently develops shock. Renal symptoms are the most serious complications. Myoglobin is released from damaged myocytes into circulation and precipitates into proximal tubules causing renal injury. Patients with crush syndrome are also likely to develop acute respiratory distress syndrome (ARDS) due to deregulated inflammatory mediators.

TREATMENT

It is largely supportive. Restoration of circulating blood volume to re-establish urine output and normalization of metabolic derangements are the main goals of treatment. Up to one-third

Table 3.6: Open fracture management recommendations

Type of fracture	Infection risk	Prophylactic antibiotics	Recommended saline irrigation	Wound closure
G-A type I	Increased (0–2%)	1st generation cephalosporin	With 3 liters	Usually, immediately after surgical intervention
G-A type II	Much increased (2–10%)	1st generation cephalosporin plus aminoglycoside	With 6 liters	Immediate or early (within 24–72 hours)
G-A type III	Maximum (10–50%)	1st generation cephalosporin plus aminoglycoside	With 9 liters	Immediate or early or delayed (after 72 hours)

Abbreviation: G-A, Gustilo-Anderson classification.

of patients develop acute renal failure and require dialysis. The impending compartment syndrome may necessitate fasciotomy.

DAMAGE CONTROL ORTHOPEDICS

This relatively new concept aims at reducing mortality by advocating a temporary management of the fractures and soft tissue injury initially in a multiply injured patient till the patient is stable enough to tolerate a definitive procedure. The concept advocates that a multiply injured patient has already sustained a "hit" in the form of high energy impact during trauma. Subjecting him to "second hit" in the form of a major surgery (for definitive fracture management) when he is not too stable to bear with it may not be a rational option. Surgery itself is a kind of trauma and this second hit in an already polytraumatized patient may worsen his condition. Hence, management in multiply injured patients should be split up into emergent and definitive procedures.

The external fixator is one of the most important weapons of damage control orthopedics (DCO), in armamentarium of an orthopedic surgeon, in the care of polytrauma patients **(Figs 3.14A and B)**. It provides for rapid temporary stabilization of fractures during the early phase, reduces further tissue damage and helps in patient ambulation. Once the patient's condition is optimized (5–7 days later), definitive fixation of fractures can be undertaken.

TRAUMA SCORING SYSTEMS

INTRODUCTION

Several scoring systems are in use to classify trauma patients and to predict the outcome of multiply injured patients. These are broadly classified into anatomical, physiological and combination scores. Examples of commonly used physiological scores are revised trauma score (RTS) and acute physiology and chronic health evaluation (APACHE) score. Commonly used anatomical scores are abbreviated injury score (AIS) and injury severity score (ISS).

Following are some commonly used scores in orthopedic practice for severely injured patients:

REVISED TRAUMA SCORE

Revised trauma score is calculated from the sum of patient's respiratory rate, systolic blood pressure and GCS (GB Road*) and is used to decide which patients should be sent to a higher level trauma center. The score ranges from 0 to 12. In triage, a patient with RTS score of 12 is labeled delayed (green), 11 as urgent (yellow) and 3–10 (red) as immediate.

INJURY SEVERITY SCORE

It is an anatomical score and provides an overall score for patients with multiple injuries, helping in predicting the chances of survival. Its value is directly proportional to mortality, morbidity and hospital stay. Each injury is assigned an AIS and six body regions (head, face, chest, abdomen, extremities, including pelvis and external) are taken into consideration. Only the highest AIS score in each body region is used. The ISS score is the sum of squares of scores of three most severely injured regions. An AIS takes values between 1 and 6, and 6 is graded as unsurvivable, so the highest ISS score can be 25 + 25 + 25 = 75. If an injury is assigned an AIS of 6 (unsurvivable injury), the ISS score is automatically assigned to 75.

MANGLED EXTREMITY SEVERITY SCORE**

This score is used to predict the chances of amputation after severe extremity trauma. In cases of massive crushing of the limb, this score helps to predict whether to go for limb salvage or to

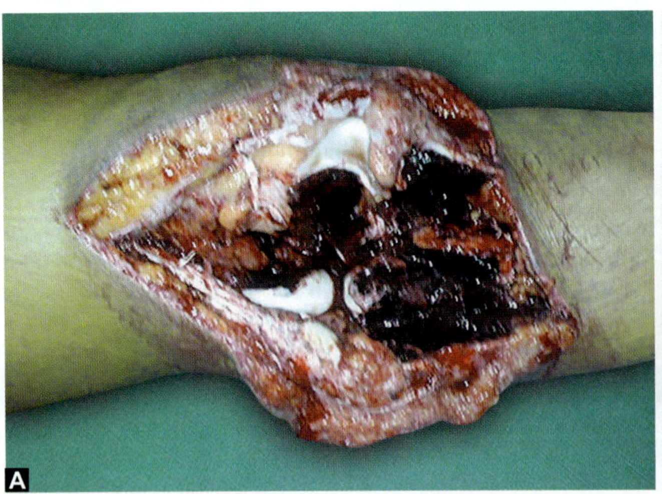
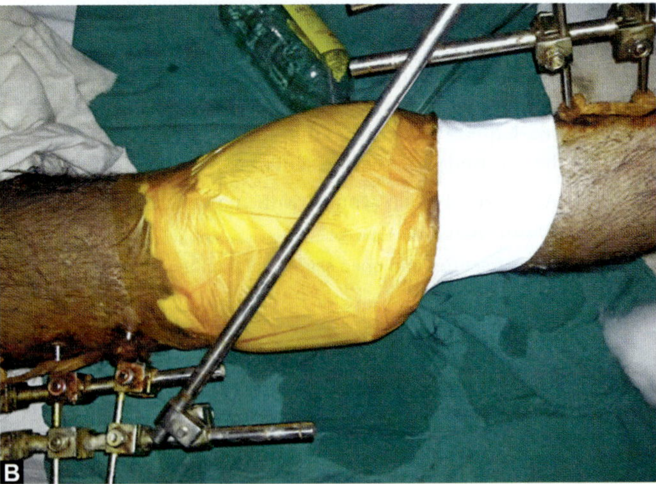

Figs 3.14A and B: External fixator being used for the initial management of multiply injured patient with open fracture (Damage Control Orthopedics) providing temporary stabilization while facilitating wound dressings

Courtesy: Dr Pradyumna Krishna M, Assistant Professor, Ortho Department, PGIMS, Rohtak.

Mnemonic GB Road: Glasgow coma scale, Blood pressure, Respiratory rate
**Mnemonic LISA: Limb ischemia, Injury severity, Shock, Age of patient*

empirically amputate the limb to save the life of the patient. It consists of the four variables and the final score is the sum of all four variables:

1. Skeletal and soft tissue injury (graded 1–4)
2. Ischemia of limb (graded 1–3, score is doubled for ischemia of more than 6 hours)
3. Shock (graded 0–2)
4. Age (graded 0–2).

A score of 7 or more is highly predictive of amputation. It is highly specific but less sensitive score in predicting the fate of the injured limb.

HANNOVER FRACTURE SCALE (1983, UPDATED IN 1998)

Having evolved from the Tscherne's classification, the scale provides a reliable measure of limb salvage (better predictability than MES score). The scale considers every detail of the injury (extent of fracture bone loss, skin injury as a percent of limb circumference, muscle injury as a percent of limb circumference, wound contamination, deperiostation, local circulation, systolic blood pressure, neurologic findings) to the involved extremity and provides a score ranging between 0 and 22. A score more than or equal to 11 indicates significant trauma, with amputation recommended.

GANGA HOSPITAL OPEN INJURY SEVERITY SCORE (Rajasekaran, Ganga Hospital, India)

Open fractures are conventionally classified by Gustilo-Anderson classification. Gustilo classification is mainly based on the size and nature of the wound and not on the extent of the injury to the different components of the limb. Severity of the injury to different components of the limb (skin, muscles, bone, etc.) may not be related to the size of the wound. Type IIIB injuries in Gustilo classification actually include a very wide spectrum, making treatment planning rather difficult. Ganga Hospital Score was devised to ensure more uniform decision making amongst surgeons on deciding soft tissue reconstruction in such injuries. The score **(Table 3.7)** accesses three areas—skin and fascia (i.e. the covering soft tissues), the musculotendinous units (i.e. functional units) and bone (i.e. skeletal support), with the severity scale in each category ranging from 1 to 5. Further points are added if the patient has certain comorbidities. Depending on the Ganga score (calculated post-debridement) patients of type IIIB injury are grouped in 4 groups:

Group I: Score of five or less
Group II: Score between six and ten
Group III: Score of 11 to 15 and
Group IV: Score of more than 15.

Table 3.7: Ganga Hospital Open Injury Severity Score

Components	Description		Scores
Covering structures: Skin and fascia	Wound not over the bone	Without skin loss	1
		With skin loss	2
	Wound over the bone	Wounds exposing the skeleton but without skin loss and bone can be covered during debridement	3
		Wounds exposing bone due to skin loss or which require extensive debridement of the skin	4
	Wounds involving skin loss over the entire circumference of the limb exposing bone circumferentially		5
Functional tissues: Musculotendinous and nerve units	Exposed musculotendinous (MT) units without injury		1
	Injury to MT units which can be primarily repaired		2
	Crushing with loss/Irreparable injury to MT units (often involved tendon transfer) Repairable nerve injuries		3
	Extensive damage of one entire compartment MT units Irreparable nerve injuries		4
	Loss of two or more compartments/Subtotal amputation		5
Skeletal structures: Bone and joints	Transverse/Oblique fracture with periosteal stripping		1
	Unicortical comminution, presence of a large butterfly fragment involving more than 50% of the circumference or segmental fractures without bone loss		2
	Periarticular comminution with joint disorganization		3
	Circumferential comminution of bone with or without bone loss of <4 cm		4
	Comminuted/Segmental fracture with bone loss >4 cm		5
Comorbid conditions: Add 2 points for each condition present	1. Open injury >12 hours. 2. Sewage or organic contamination/farmyard injuries 3. Age >65 years 4. Debilitating diseases (DM, COPD, IHD, etc.) 5. Fat embolism 6. Associated systemic injuries 7. Another major injury to the same limb/Compartment syndrome		

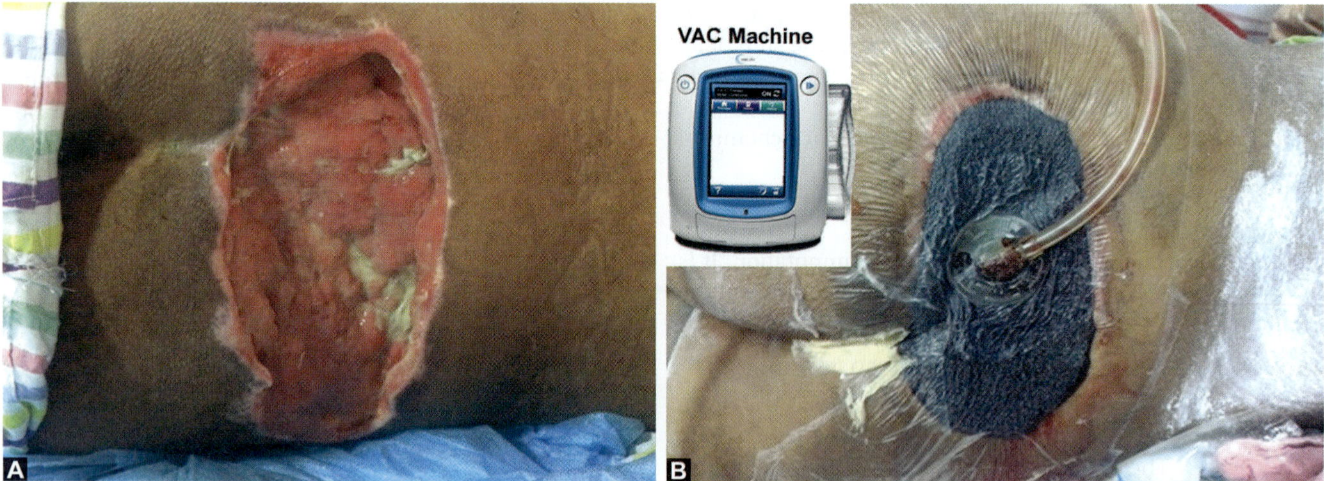

Figs 3.15A and B: (A) A nonhealing bed sore; (B) This bed sore has been debrided, dressed and sealed with a special drape. A tube from the wound has been connected to a VAC apparatus to generate negative pressure inside the wound

Courtesy: Mr. Nijo.

Score more than three in any component entails the need for plastic surgeon. Salvage is challenging and functional outcome is often guarded for a limb which gets a score of more than three in two or more components. Chances of amputation increase with increasing scores and almost all patients with a score of five in more than one component and all Group IV patients eventually require amputation.

HIGH-YIELD POINTS

- The greatest priority step in treatment of contaminated open fractures is debridement followed by external fixation. The Gustilo-Anderson classification category is also to be assigned to an open fracture, post wound debridement only.
- In grossly contaminated wounds, local antibiotic delivery may also be considered. Bead pouch technique with the use of antibiotic mixed bone cement (polymethylmethacrylate) is the commonly used method. Antibiotic impregnated cement beads are left in the wound and removed once infection settles and wound heals.
- Vacuum-assisted closure (VAC) or negative pressure wound therapy (NPWT) is a useful adjunct to wound management when primary closure is not possible. This is a sealed, negative pressure dressing applied over the wound that helps draw the wound edges together, removes infectious material by suction effect, increases local blood flow and actively promotes granulation tissue formation **(Figs 3.15A and B)**.
- *EUSOL (University of Edinburgh solution):* It is a solution made up of chlorinated lime (12.5 g) and boric acid (12.5 g) mixed in 1 L of distilled water. It is used for wound dressing as it is capable of "chemical debridement".

CHAPTER 4

Traumatology: Injuries of Upper Limb, Skull and Face

INJURIES AROUND THE SHOULDER GIRDLE AND FRACTURE SHAFT OF HUMERUS

CLAVICLE FRACTURE

The clavicle is the most common fractured bone during childbirth and overall. Clavicle fractures account for about 4–10% of skeletal trauma presenting to orthopedic emergency. A direct blow on the shoulder or direct fall onto the shoulder is the most common mechanism of injury.

Relevant Anatomy

The clavicle is a horizontally placed S-shaped subcutaneous long bone, which is convex forward in the medial two-thirds and convex backward in the lateral one-third. At its distal end it is connected to coracoid process and acromion by coracoclavicular (CC) ligaments (inner conoid and outer trapezoid) and acromioclavicular (AC) ligaments **(Fig. 4.1)**.

More than 80% of the fractures of the bone are located in the middle third of the clavicle (specifically at the junction of the medial two-thirds and lateral one-third) followed by acromial and sternal part (least common).

The reasons for this location are:
- *Peculiar anatomy*: This is a junction point of two curvatures
- There is a defect in this area of bone as the nutrient artery has to enter at this point.

After fracture the medial fragment is elevated by unopposed pulling of sternoclenoid muscle and distal fragment is displaced inferiorly and medially by the pull of the deltoid and pectoralis major muscles **(Figs 4.2A and B)**, assisted by the weight of the extremity.

Diagnosis

Patients present with a history of trauma followed by swelling, tenderness and crepitus at the site of fracture. Bone can be easily palpated for deformity, hematoma and crepitus. The patient must be examined for neurovascular deficit due to vicinity of vital structures to the fracture site. Diagnosis is confirmed on an anteroposterior (AP) **(Fig. 4.2B)** and Zanca X-ray view (10–15° cephalic tilt AP view of the shoulder).

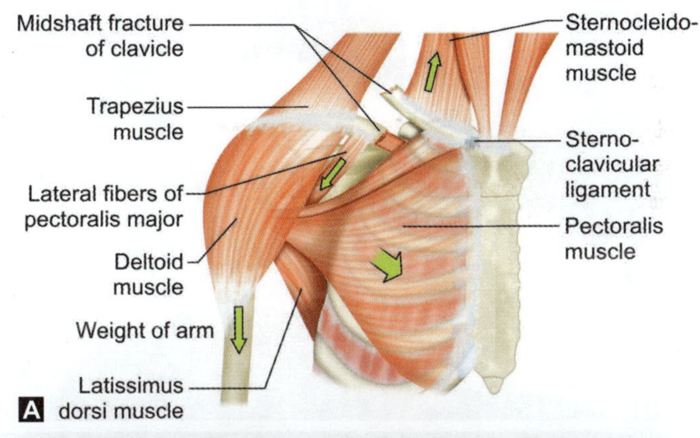

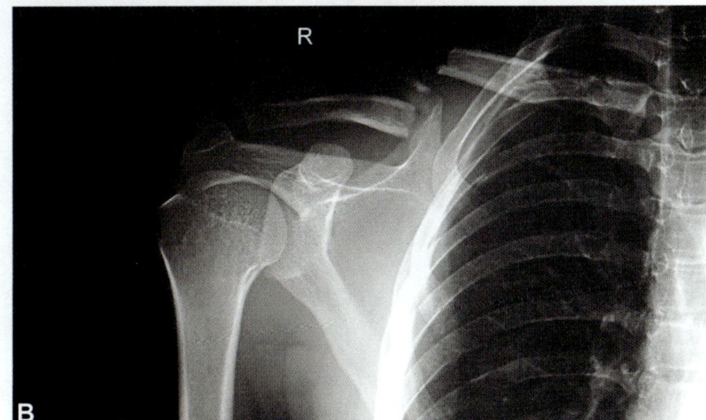

Figs 4.2A and B: (A) Schematic representation of displacements in clavicular fracture; (B) X-ray anteroposterior view of shoulder showing the classic displacements in clavicle fracture

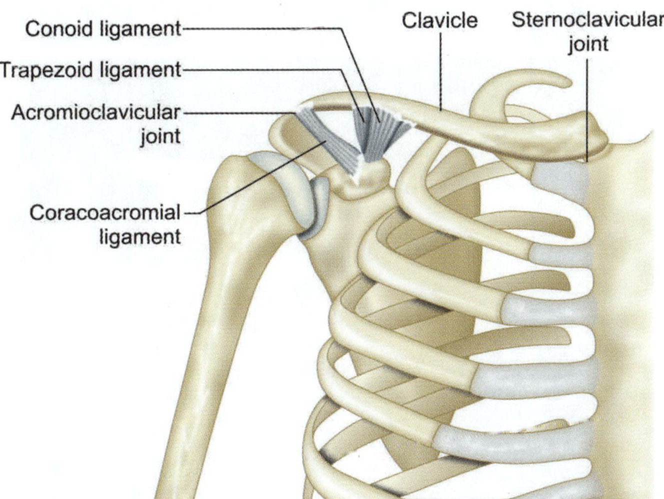

Fig. 4.1: Diagram showing the ligaments around the clavicle

Management

Management is nonoperative in most of the cases as this bone almost always unites. Most surgeons prefer using ready-made clavicular braces **(Figs 4.3A to C)** to provide some support. A figure-of-eight bandage is outdated, but may be used for infants. Immobilization with a simple sling **(Fig. 4.3A)** produces the same result with less pain compared to the traditional figure-of-eight bandage or a clavicular brace. It is especially preferred in undisplaced lateral end clavicle fractures. The active shoulder physiotherapy should be started as early as pain allows. Full range of shoulder motion can be expected in 6–8 weeks.

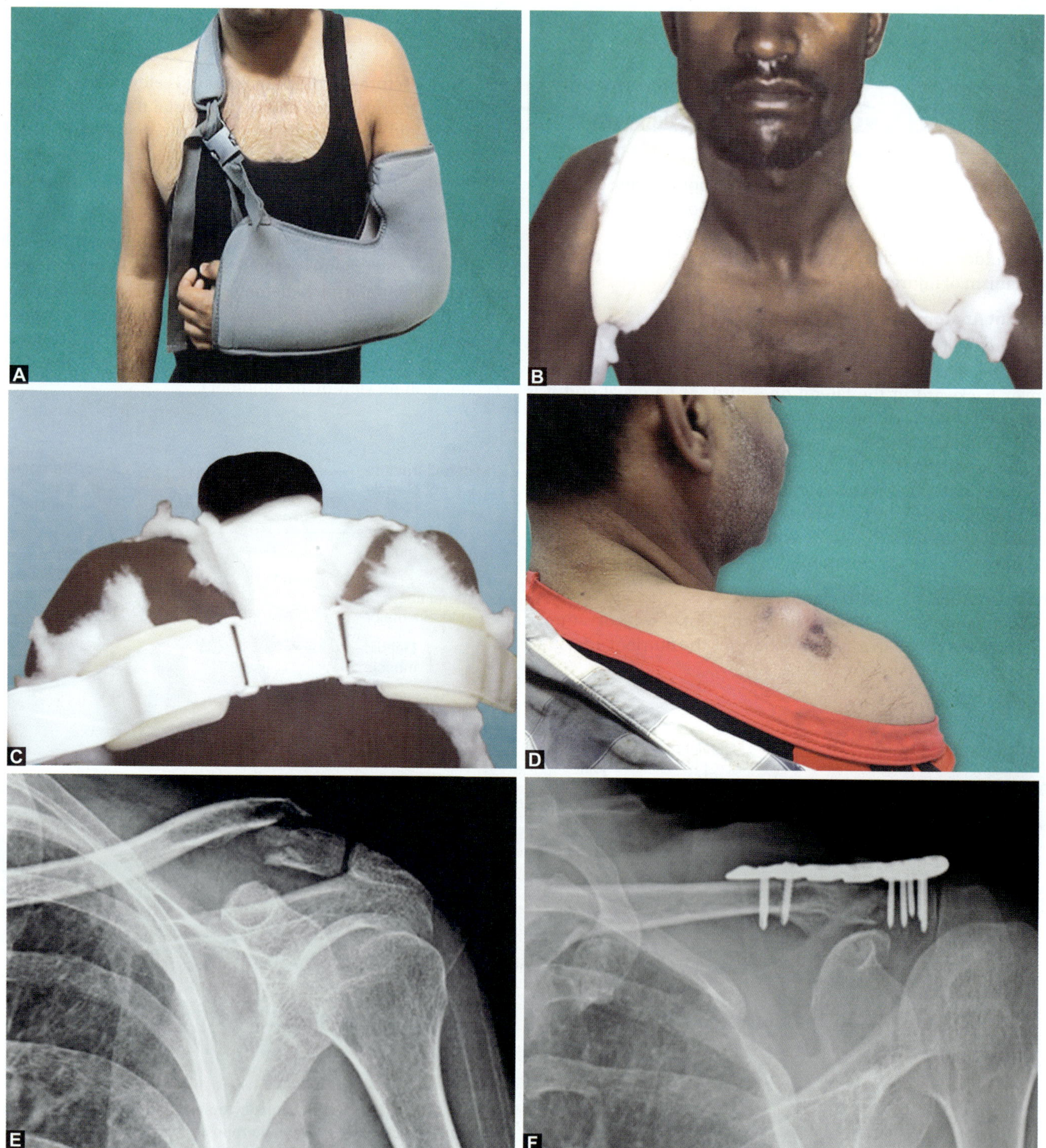

Figs 4.3A to F: Immobilization in a (A) simple sling or in (B and C) clavicular brace is enough for most of the cases of clavicle fractures. (D) Fracture lateral end of clavicle that was tenting the skin is shown in (E) anteroposterior X-ray of the shoulder. (F) The fracture was fixed with a clavicular plate

Indication for operative fixation (with a plate or intramedullary pinning): Open fractures, associated neurovascular deficit, polytrauma patient, floating shoulder (*see* **Figs 4.5A and B**), displacement and shortening greater than 2 cm, tenting of the skin by elevated fragment and displaced fracture of lateral end clavicle **(Figs 4.3D to F)** are the indications for operative fixation.

Complications

Malunion is the most common complication and may result in the formation of an undue prominence that is a relative indication for surgery in patients having problem with cosmesis. However, surgery leads to the formation of an unacceptable scar so the patient has to be explained that. Other complications are neurovascular injury, mostly in the lower trunk of brachial plexus (acute as well as delayed due to encroachment of thoracic outlet by malunited or nonunited displaced fractures), nonunion and infection (following operative fixation and open fracture). The rate of nonunion is less than 1% and requires open reduction internal fixation (ORIF) with bone grafting. Supraclavicular nerve (superficial to clavicle) and subclavian vessels are at risk during operative repair. The brachial plexus is closest to clavicle at its mid portion and must be protected in operative fixations involving the area.

HIGH-YIELD POINTS

- The clavicle is the first bone to start ossification (at the 5th week of gestation), however, medial (sternal end) clavicular epiphysis is generally the last long bone epiphysis to fuse, at 22–25 years of age.
- Although conventionally categorized as a long bone (as it has length greater than breadth), the clavicle is a long bone of exceptions. It is the only long bone to lie horizontally in the body. It ossifies by intramembranous ossification (while other long bones ossify by endochondral ossification) and has two primary centers of ossification for its shaft (as opposed to one in other long bones). And to add more, it is a long bone with no medullary cavity.

FRACTURE OF SCAPULA

Blunt trauma in road traffic accidents is the most common cause of this relatively infrequent fracture. A majority of the fractures are undisplaced or minimally displaced and successfully managed with conservative treatment. Associated injuries are more important from a clinical point of view. Rib fracture is the most common-associated injury followed by head and chest injury (pneumothorax and pulmonary contusions).

Diagnosis

Patients present with a history of trauma followed by swelling, local tenderness, crepitus and ecchymosis. Diagnosis can be made on X-rays **(Figs 4.4A and B)**—anteroposterior, lateral and axillary views. **Figure 4.4A** shows the description of an AP view of the shoulder joint.

Classification

These fractures are generally classified based on the anatomy. Body and spine fractures are the most common, followed by scapular neck and glenoid cavity. Fracture of the acromion and coracoid are less common.

Treatment

Nonoperative treatment is sufficient for the majority of the fractures. Scapula being surrounded all around by muscles has a very good vascularity and hence rapidly unites. Shoulder immobilization is required until pain alleviates. Early physiotherapy in form of pendulum and active range of motion exercises is started early. ORIF is required for significantly displaced fractures and fracture of the coracoid with AC joint dislocation.

HIGH-YIELD POINTS

- Os acrominale is a separate ossification center, which fails to unite with the main body of the acromion. It should not be mistaken for a fracture. However, it can be a cause of impingement in the shoulder (**Fig. 17.10B**, *see* Page 455).
- *Floating shoulder (**Figs 4.5A and B**)*: It is defined as ipsilateral scapular (glenoid) neck fractures with mid shaft clavicle

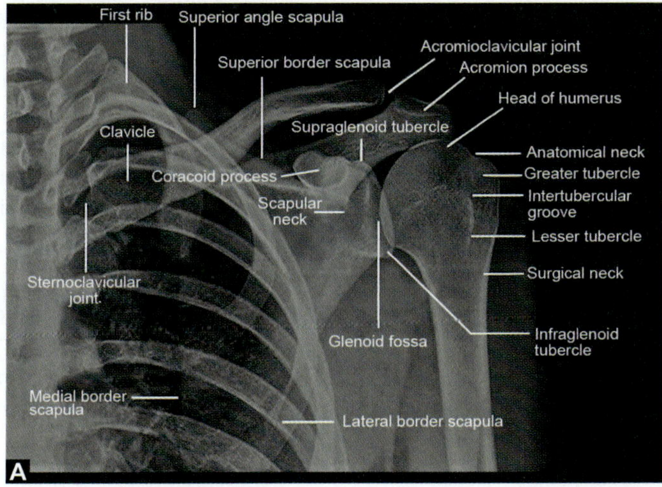

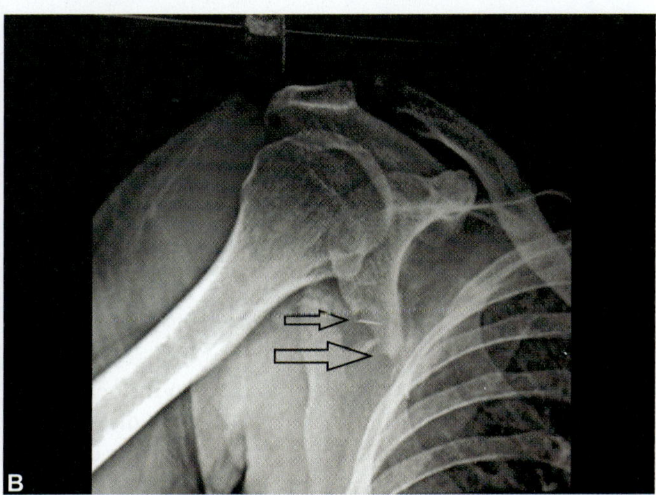

Figs 4.4A and B: (A) Descriptive X-ray of shoulder joint anteroposterior (AP) view; (B) X-ray shoulder AP view showing scapular fracture at infraglenoid tubercle (arrows)

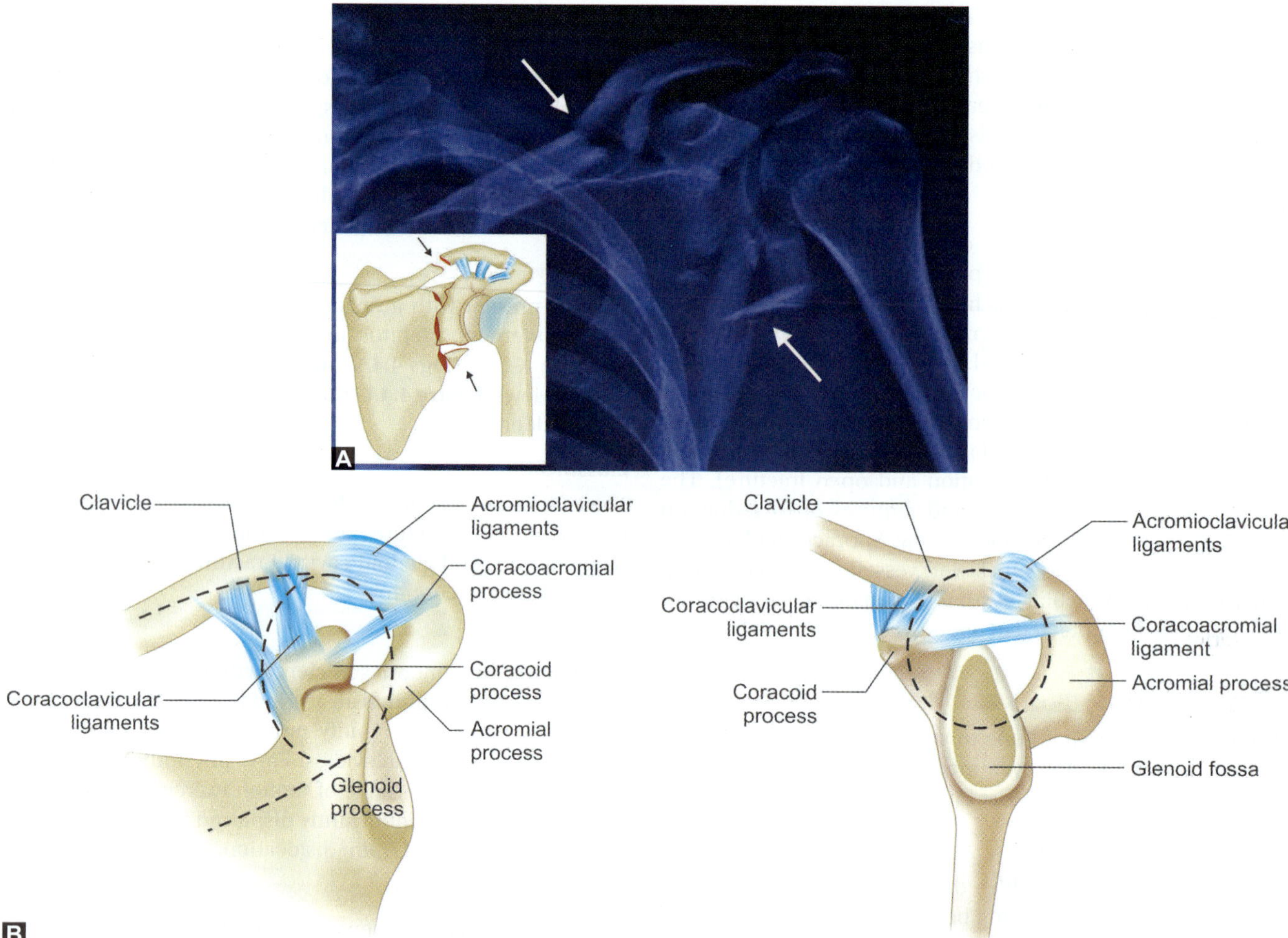

Figs 4.5A and B: (A) Floating shoulder in X-ray anteroposterior view. Note fractures in clavicle (arrow) and scapular neck (arrow); (B) The superior suspensory shoulder complex (Goss)

fracture. Goss has better defined it technically as a double disruption of so called "superior suspensory shoulder complex (SSSc)". SSSc is a bone and soft-tissue ring securing the upper limb to the trunk by superior and inferior struts **(Fig. 4.5B)**.

- *Scapulothoracic dissociation*: This is a limb-threatening injury where the upper limb is separated from the thorax with fractures in clavicle, scapula and first rib. There may be traction injury to the plexus leading to paralysis in the whole limb or at times intimal injury in the subclavian vessels leading to thrombosis and gangrenous changes in upper limb.

SHOULDER DISLOCATION

Dislocation of the shoulder is the most common dislocation in orthopedic practice comprising of almost 50% of all dislocations that present to an orthopedic clinic. Uncommon in children (where proximal humeral physis rather gives way), it most commonly affects young, active males below 30 years of age.

Relevant Anatomy

The structure of the shoulder joint can be imagined to be like a golf ball and a tee **(Fig. 4.6)**. At any time only one-fourth of a humeral head articulates with the glenoid. Hence, the bony articulation is inherently unstable and the prime restraint to dislocation is provided by the soft tissue cover around the joint.

Important structures that stabilize the shoulder joint include the primary or static restraints and the secondary or dynamic restraints (dynamic because these can be built-up with exercises to improve joint stability).

Important static restraints are:

- *Joint capsule*: A strong capsule encloses the joint all around to keep it located.
- *Glenohumeral ligaments (**Fig. 4.7A**)*: These are a group of ligaments (superior, middle and inferior) that run across the anterior and inferior aspects of the shoulder from the glenoid margin to the neck of the humerus. They reinforce the anterior capsule, adding to the anterior stability. Inferior

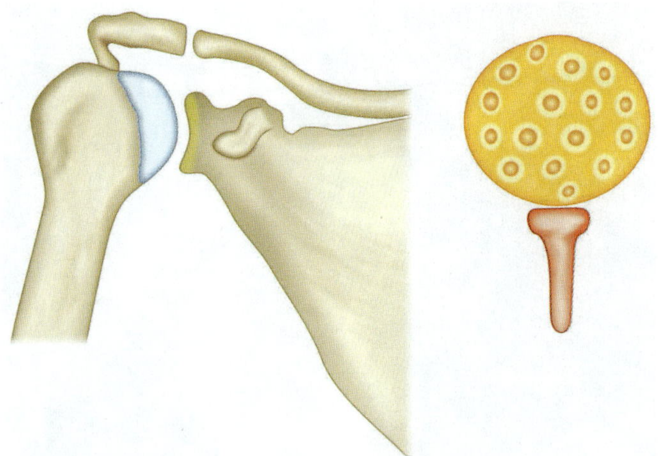

Fig. 4.6: Schematic representation of the shoulder joint showing the similarity to golf ball and a tee

glenohumeral ligament (IGHL) has anterior and posterior bands that create a "hammock" inferiorly especially adding to inferior stability where the capsule is the weakest.

- *Glenoid labrum (Fig. 4.7B):* This is a fibrocartilaginous rim around the glenoid. Glenoid is deepened to almost 50% by the presence of labrum around it.
- *Negative intra-articular pressure*: The joint has a minimal amount of synovial fluid such that there is a cohesive force between the opposing surfaces.
- *Bony articulating surfaces*: Their contribution as explained above is limited.

Important dynamic restraints **(Figs 4.8A and B)** include:

- *Rotator cuff*: This is a group of four muscles, viz. subscapularis, supraspinatus, infraspinatus and teres minor that encircle and surround the shoulder joint in front and back. The subscapularis originates from the coastal surface of scapula and extends anteriorly across the shoulder to insert into the lesser tuberosity of humerus. The other three muscles attach to the greater tuberosity of humerus and strengthen the anterosuperior and posterior aspects as shown in **Figure 4.8A**.

- *Deltoid and biceps*: The anterior aspect of the shoulder is well covered by the deltoid and if the muscle is strong it would not allow the joint to dislocate. Similarly, the tendon of long head of biceps **(Fig. 4.8B)** originates from the supraglenoid tubercle and travels in front of the humeral head to enter into the bicipital sulcus, reinforcing the anterior aspect of the joint thereby acting as another dynamic restraint.

Now from the knowledge of anatomy one can now well imagine that since this is a joint primarily stabilized by soft tissues, it would dislocate with minimal force and hence it is the most common dislocation in orthopedic practice. Also, most of the times the doctor reduces the joint, but the soft tissues fail to heal up. In all such cases when an important restraint is nonfunctioning the patients land up with the well-recognized complication of shoulder dislocation, i.e. recurrent dislocations.

Classification

Dislocation of shoulder can be anterior, posterior or inferior (depending upon where the humeral head goes in relation to the glenoid). A superior dislocation is not seen as superiorly the presence of a strong coracoacromial arch prevents the head from riding up **(Fig. 4.8B)**.

Anterior Dislocation

This is the most common type (90–95%). Dislocated head lies anteroinferiorly in relation to the glenoid **(Fig. 4.9A)**.

Anterior dislocation is further subdivided into following subtypes **(Fig. 4.9B)**:

- Subcoracoid—it is the most common subtype. The head lies inferior to the coracoid process.
- Subglenoid—next common subtype. The head lies anterior and below the glenoid.
- Subclavicular—the head lies below the clavicle.
- Intrathoracic—it is very rare.

Posterior Dislocation

This accounts for less than 5% of shoulder dislocation cases. There are three subtypes: subacromial, subglenoid and subspinous. The subacromial type in which the head lies posterior to glenoid and inferior to acromion is the most common subtype.

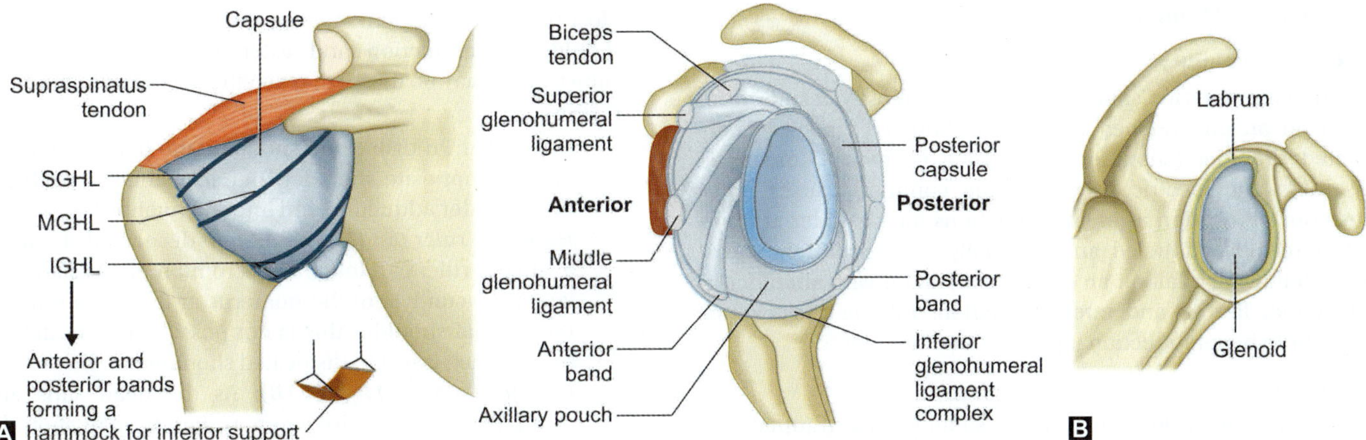

Figs 4.7A and B: (A) The superior (SGHL), middle (MGHL) and inferior (IGHL) glenohumeral ligaments (GHL); (B) Diagrammatic representation of the glenoid labrum

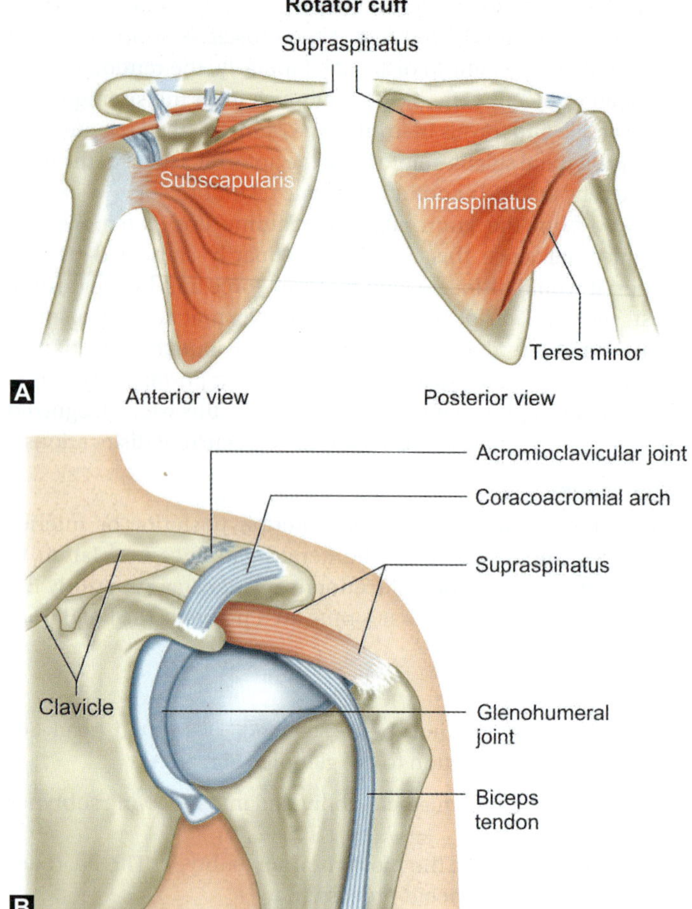

Figs 4.8A and B: (A) The rotator cuff muscles; (B) Diagram depicting biceps as a dynamic restraint *(subscapularis that overlaps anterior aspect has been omitted)*

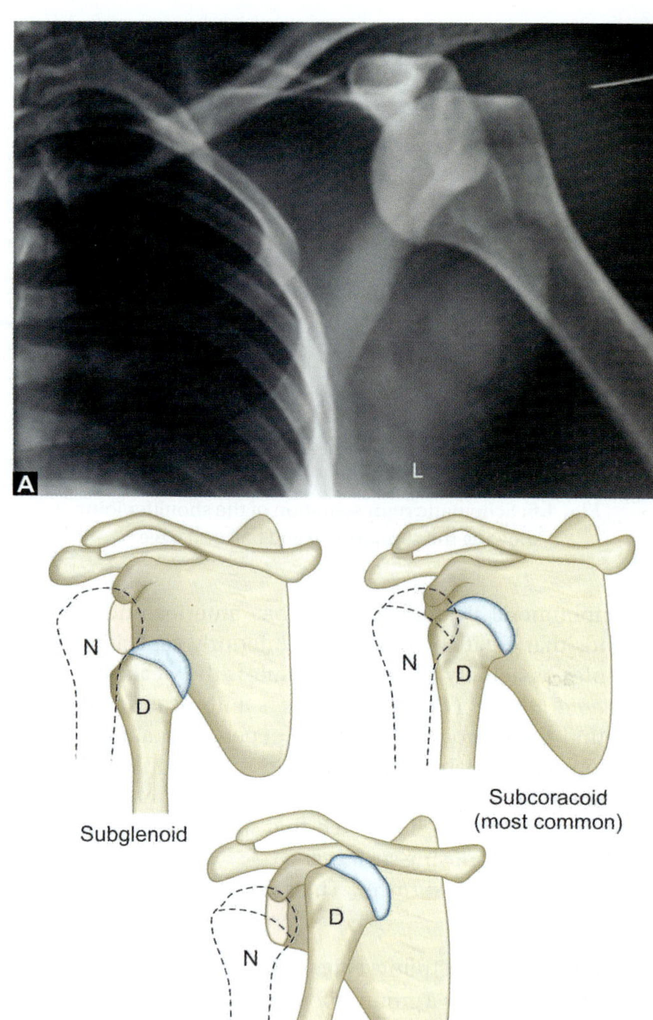

Figs 4.9A and B: (A) Anteroposterior X-ray of shoulder showing anterior shoulder dislocation; (B) Diagrammatic representation of subtypes of anterior dislocation of shoulder

Abbreviations: N, normal; D, dislocated.

Inferior Dislocation or Luxatio Erecta

This is the rarest type in which the humeral head lies inferior to glenoid rim with a hyperabducted humerus (the arm locked in full abduction). The patient typically comes in emergency with abducted and locked shoulder supported by other hand over his head **(Figs 4.10A and B)**.

Mechanism of Injury

A traumatic anterior shoulder dislocation mostly results from a fall on an outstretched hand with abducted and externally rotated shoulder (shoulder in throwing position). Convulsive disorders and electric shock are the common causes for a posterior dislocation as in such situations the shoulder at times gets forcefully adducted and internally rotated. Rarely can it occur following a fall on an outstretched hand with shoulder in adduction, flexion and internal rotation. Inferior dislocations result from hyperabduction injuries of the shoulder.

Diagnosis

Most first-time dislocations of the shoulder are traumatic in nature. Patients present with a history of trauma and severe pain in the shoulder with inability to use the limb.

- Most patients sustain an anterior dislocation and keep their shoulder in abduction and external rotation. Following clinical tests may be useful to reach the diagnosis in doubtful cases:
    - *Duga's test*: In dislocated shoulder, the hand cannot be taken to opposite shoulder (due to inability to achieve full shoulder adduction and internal rotation).
    - *Hamilton ruler test* **(Fig. 4.11A)**: In dislocated shoulder, a straight ruler can touch the acromion process and the lateral epicondyle of the humerus at the same time. In the normal shoulder this is not possible due to deltoid bulge which is lost in dislocated shoulder.
    - *Callaway's test* **(Fig. 4.11B)**: As the head slips and occupies the axilla, girth from axillary base to shoulder top (i.e. the vertical circumference of axilla) increases as compared to the opposite shoulder.

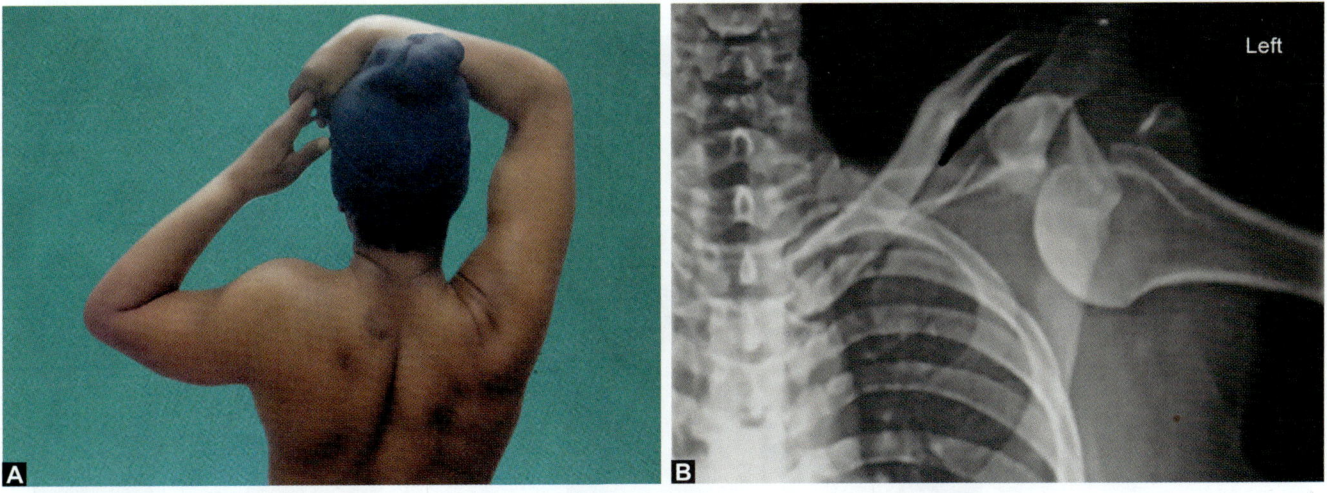

Figs 4.10A and B: (A) Typical posture of a patient of Luxatio Erecta (salute posture); and (B) X-ray of shoulder anteroposterior view showing inferior dislocation of the shoulder

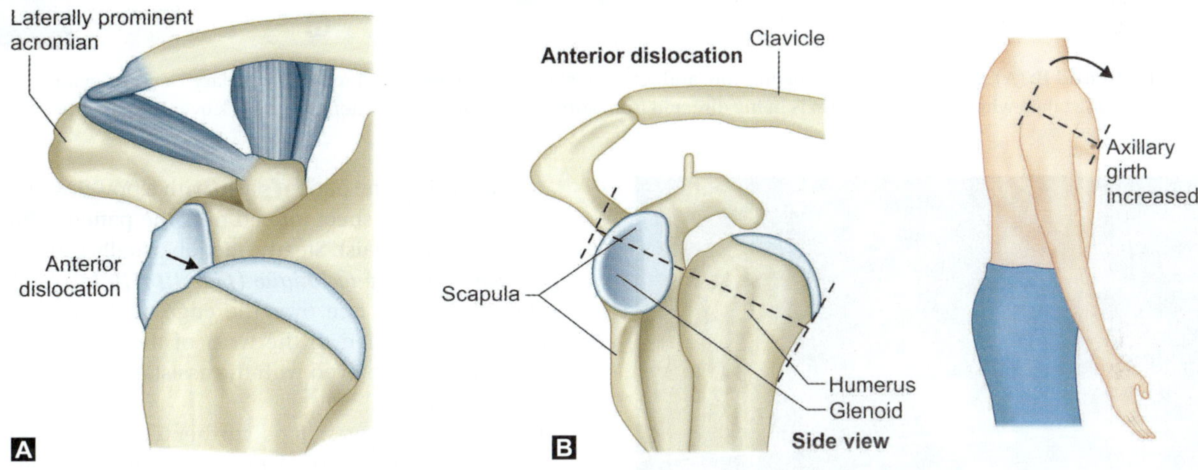

Figs 4.11A and B: (A) Hamilton ruler test; and (B) Callaway's test

- The patients who sustain posterior dislocation keep their shoulder in adduction and internal rotation. External rotation is limited. Coracoid process may be more prominent and humeral head may be palpable posteriorly. In routine anteroposterior X-ray, posterior dislocation often is missed initially as the humeral head appears to be almost normally aligned with the glenoid. A lateral view (axillary view) would show the head to be posterior, but needs shoulder abduction, which is not possible in patients with a dislocated shoulder. However, a modified axillary view (Velpeau axillary view) can rather be opted **(Figs 4.12A and B)**. Else, some important radiological signs may be sought to suggest the diagnosis in doubtful cases **(Fig. 4.13)**. In posterior dislocation of the shoulder the humeral head remains in internal rotation and looks like a light bulb (light bulb sign). Anterior glenoid fossa looks empty as head dislocates posteriorly (vacant glenoid sign). Trough sign indicates an impression fracture that may develop on the anterior humeral head as it strikes against the posterior rim of the glenoid. And if on anteroposterior view, space between anterior rim of glenoid and humeral head is more than 6 mm (rim sign positive), it is highly suggestive of a posterior dislocation.

- Inferior dislocation is the rarest but the classical attitude is generally diagnostic **(Fig. 4.10A)**.

Treatment

Acute shoulder dislocation is reduced on urgent basis under sedation or general anesthesia and then arm is kept in a sling or a chest-arm bandage for 3 weeks (to allow the soft tissues to heal up). Gentle physiotherapy is started as soon as the pain subsides.

Techniques of closed reduction of shoulder dislocation are as follows:

- *Traction counter-traction techniques*: It is further categorized into Hippocratic technique and Metsen's technique.

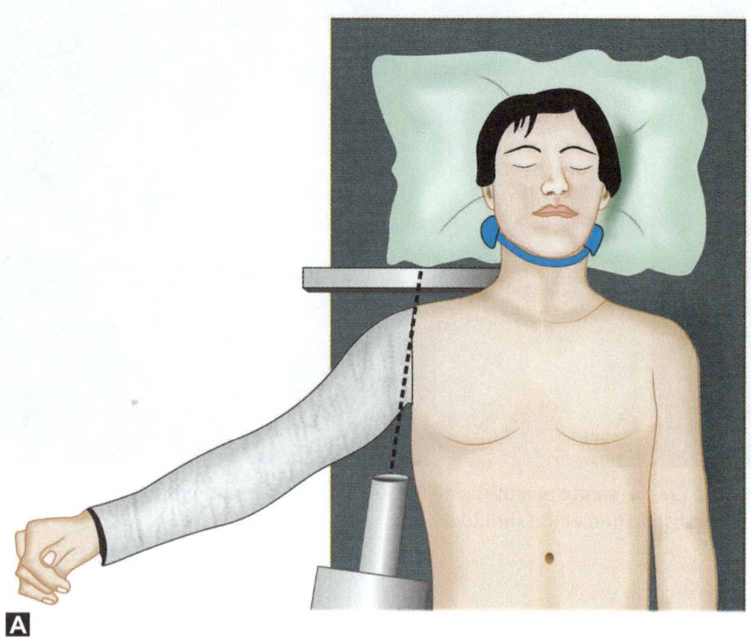

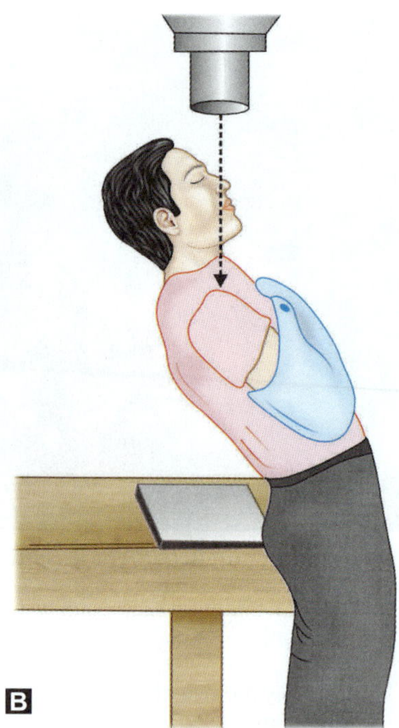

Figs 4.12A and B: (A) Axillary view being taken. Note abduction at shoulder needed; (B) A modified axillary view (Velpeau view) is being taken where the X-ray beam is being directed from superior to inferior as patient leans back over the cassette

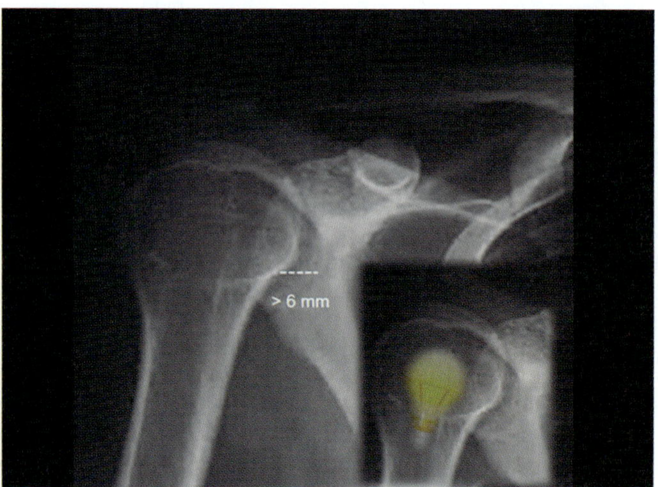

Fig. 4.13: Light bulb sign and rim sign in posterior dislocation of shoulder (note the head is appearing in reduced position even though it is dislocated posteriorly)

- *Hippocratic technique (Fig. 4.14A):* In supine position, surgeon holds the patient hand with arm in 30–40° abduction and gives sustained traction for about 1 minute. Counter traction is given by putting the surgeon's heel into the patient's axilla. This acts as a fulcrum and arm is gradually adducted. Internal and external rotation of the shoulder may aid in reduction. This is less favored nowadays as it is more painful method and brachial plexus and vessels are at risk during the maneuver.
- *Metsen's technique (Fig. 4.14B):* Patient lies supine with a sheet around the chest and also looped over the assistant's waist for counter traction. Steady traction along the axis of the patient's arm with elbow flexed to 90° given by another sheet looped over the patient's forearm and surgeon's waist. Steady traction usually causes reduction.

- *Stimson's gravity technique (Fig. 4.14C):* In prone position, shoulder hangs free over the edge of the table and about 3-kg weight is tied to the wrist of the dislocated shoulder. Reduction is achieved with the assistance of gravity in about 20–30 minutes.
- *Leverage techniques*: It is further classified into Kocher's technique (conventional method widely practiced), Spaso technique and Milch technique.
  - *Kocher's technique (Figs 4.15A to D)*: In supine position, arm is kept by the side of the body and the elbow is flexed to 90°. Now slowly externally rotate the shoulder by grasping the wrist and supporting the elbow until resistance is felt (70–80°). Now lift the externally rotated upper arm in the sagittal plane as far as possible. Now internally rotate the shoulder (bring the patient's hand towards the opposite shoulder). The humeral head slips back into the glenoid with a palpable and audible click.
  - *Spaso technique (Fig. 4.16)*: In supine position, the affected arm is grasped around the wrist and gently lifted vertically, applying gentle traction. While maintaining vertical traction, the shoulder is rotated externally. A clunk is heard and/or felt when the reduction is completed.
- *Scapular manipulation*: In prone position, patient's arm is kept in forward flexion and external rotation (suspended at the edge of the table) and 3–7 kg weight or manual traction is applied to the wrist. Now the tip of scapula is pushed medially with thumb while physician externally rotates the superior and medial aspects of the scapula. This method is claimed to be fast and relatively painless.

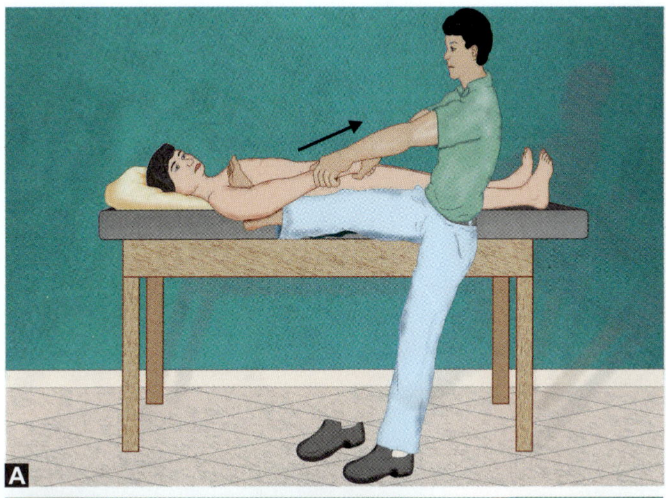

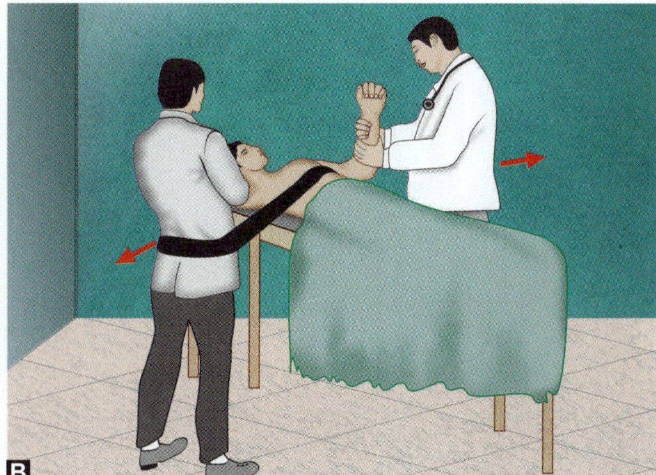

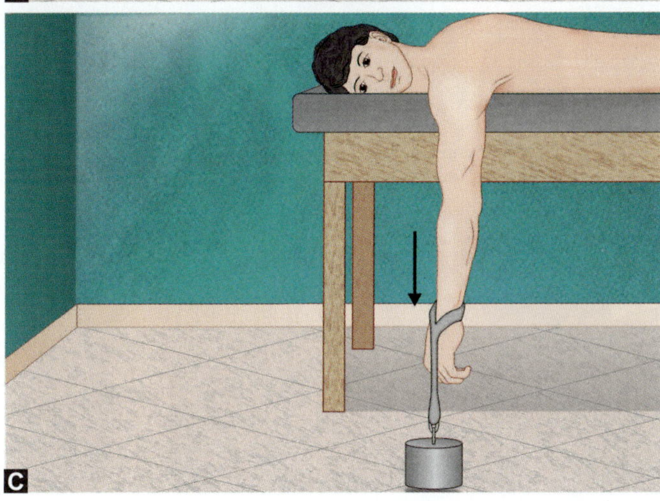

Figs 4.14A to C: (A) Schematic depiction of Hippocratic technique; (B) Metsen's traction-counter traction technique; (C) Stimson's gravity technique (reduction is achieved with the assistance of gravity)

- *Cunningham technique*: This is a newer method and claimed to be effective, painless and fast. Shoulder dislocation produces spasm of surrounding muscles which pull the dislocated humeral head and prevents its reduction. The Cunningham technique involves massaging the trapezius, deltoid and biceps sequentially, thus relieving the spasm and allowing for reduction. In sitting position, support the arm and keep it adducted and with elbow flexed to 90° or more. Now massage the trapezius and deltoid for 1–2 minutes, gently and ask the patient to shrug his shoulder. Now massage the biceps at a mid humerus level and keep the patient relax. As the patient relaxes and spasm relieves head of humerus slips back into the glenoid.

In most cases, the doctor is able to achieve a reduction by either of the methods mentioned above. If in case one is unable to reduce closed reduction (due to any intervening soft tissue structure), then without wasting any time the patient should be planned up for an urgent open reduction under anesthesia.

Complications

The complications post-shoulder reduction show a bimodal age distribution. In patients aged 40 years and above most common complication is rotator cuff tear and shoulder stiffness. In young patients, recurrent dislocation is the most common complication after first episode of dislocation. In fact, recurrent dislocation is overall the most common (long-term) complication, and has been discussed in detail in Chapter 6. Osteoarthritis of glenohumeral joint can be another long-term sequel of shoulder dislocation. Neurovascular injury is not uncommon so all patients should be thoroughly examined. Axillary nerve injury (circumflex branch) is the most common acute complication and can be present in almost 7–10% of cases (although transient in most cases). It can be detected by absent deltoid contraction or better by loss of sensation over the skin of a small part of the lateral upper arm (regimental badge sign, *see* Page 267 for details). After axillary nerve the other nerve that is injured (frequency wise) is the suprascapular nerve.

ACROMIOCLAVICULAR JOINT INJURY

Acromioclavicular joint disruption accounts for 3–5% of all shoulder injuries. It can especially be common among sports person involved in contact sports, occurring when they sustain a direct blow on acromion with the arm in adducted position.

Relevant Anatomy

The AC joint is a diarthrodial joint between the clavicle and the acromion. Stability to this joint is given by the capsule and AC ligaments (anteroposterior stability) and CC ligaments (superoinferior stability) **(Fig. 4.1)**. The medial CC ligament is conical-shaped conoid ligament which runs from the conoid

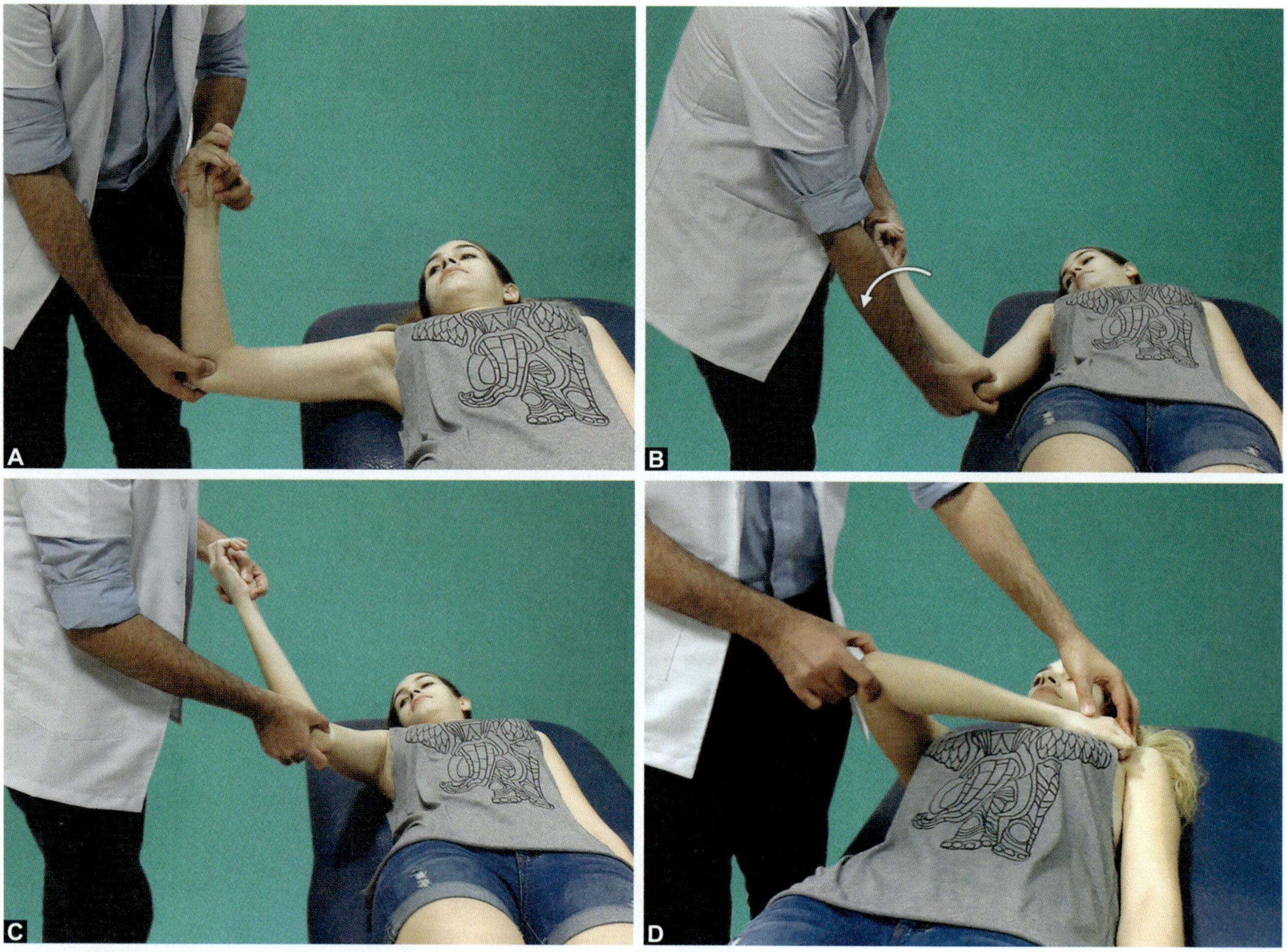

Figs 4.15A to D: Kocher's technique of reduction of anterior dislocation of the shoulder. (A) Patient comes with abducted shoulder; (B) Gently adduct the shoulder and then externally rotate the arm; (C) Elevate the externally rotated arm; and (D) Internally rotate the shoulder

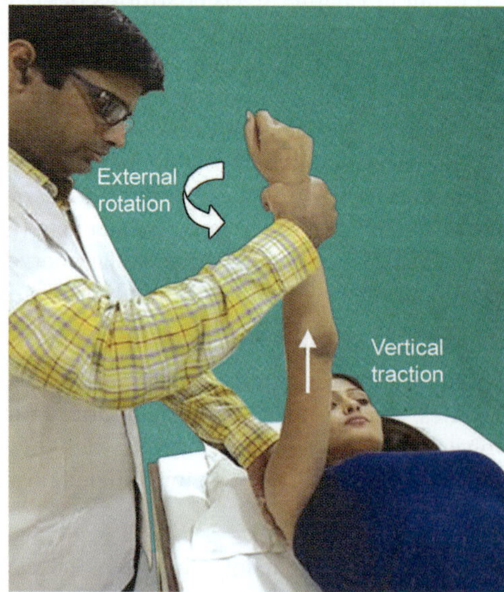

Fig. 4.16: Spaso technique

tubercle of the clavicle to the base of the coracoid process and provides resistance to superior translation and joint rotation. The lateral CC ligament is the trapezoid ligament which lies anterior and lateral to the conoid tubercle and inserts more laterally on the base of the coracoid and provides resistance to joint compression.

Classification

Rockwood (RW) classification **(Table 4.1 and Fig. 4.17)** is most commonly used to classify AC joint injuries.

Diagnosis

The patient presents with pain, swelling and deformity of AC joint following history of injury. Diagnosis can be confirmed by X-ray of the shoulder—anteroposterior **(Fig. 4.18A)**, axillary lateral view and Zanca view (10–15° cephalic tilt anteroposterior view of shoulder).

Management

Rockwood types I and II are managed conservatively by rest in a sling and analgesic. Treatment of RW type III is controversial and should be individualized (surgical for athletes and high-demanding young and conservative for older, less active). Surgical treatment may be considered if the patient does not get relief with conservative trial. RW types IV through VI should be managed by surgical reconstruction. Weaver Dunn **(Fig. 4.18B)** is the conventional surgical procedure performed, although modern techniques involving arthroscopic fixation are evolving very fast.

Table 4.1: Rockwood classification of acromioclavicular (AC) joint disruption

Type I	Sprain of the AC ligament, no significant instability is present
Type II	A complete tear of the AC ligaments, but the coracoclavicular (CC) ligaments remain intact. There may be slight vertical displacement (<30%) of the AC joint
Type III	Both sets of ligaments (AC and CC) are disrupted. A type III occurs when the distal clavicle is completely displaced. Up to 100% translation of clavicle relative to the acromion occurs
Type IV	Both sets of ligaments (AC and CC) are disrupted with posterior displacement of the clavicle through the trapezius muscle
Type V	Both sets of ligaments (AC and CC) are disrupted with gross displacement (often between 100% and 300%) of the clavicle
Type VI	Both sets of ligaments (AC and CC) are disrupted and the distal clavicle displaces inferiorly into a subacromial or subcoracoid position

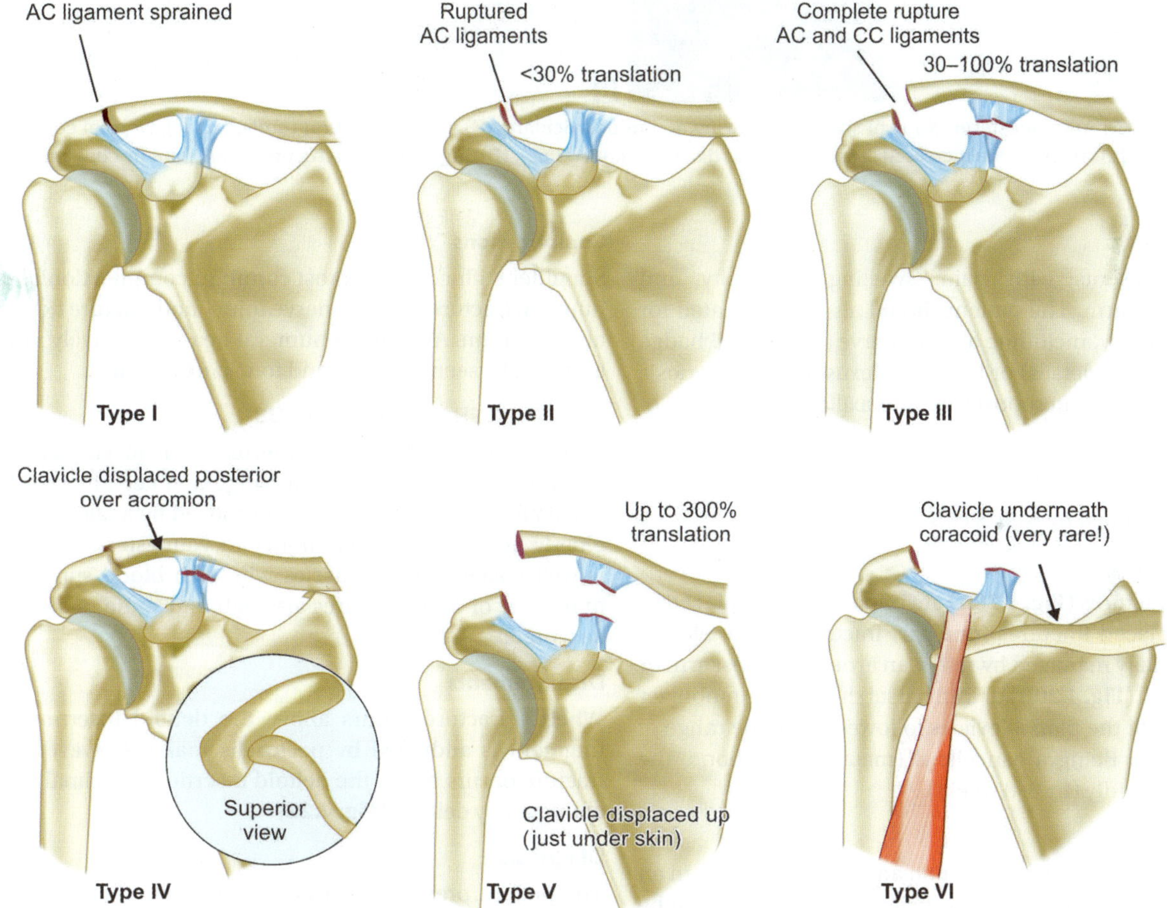

Fig. 4.17: Diagrammatic depiction of Rockwood classification
Abbreviations: AC, acromioclavicular; CC, coracoclavicular.

STERNOCLAVICULAR JOINT DISLOCATION

These are rare injuries. A posterior dislocation of the clavicle is a dangerous injury as the vital structures in the chest can get injured. However, an anterior subluxation or dislocation (medial end of clavicle is displaced anteriorly or anterosuperiorly to the anterior margin of the sternum) is far more common than posterior (medial end of clavicle is displaced posteriorly or posterosuperiorly to posterior margin of the sternum).

Most of sternoclavicular (SC) joint injuries can be managed conservatively (observation/close reduction and rest in figure-of-eight straps). Only irreducible posterior dislocation and chronic posterior dislocation may require surgery.

HIGH-YIELD POINT

- Serendipity view and Hobbs views are special views for SC joint injuries.

FRACTURE OF PROXIMAL HUMERUS

These are common in elderly patients and most of them are osteoporotic fractures in postmenopausal women. Most commonly these are caused by low-energy domestic fall on an outstretched arm.

Classification

Neer's classification **(Table 4.2 and Fig. 4.19)** is most commonly used to classify these fractures, which is based on the number of displaced fragments.

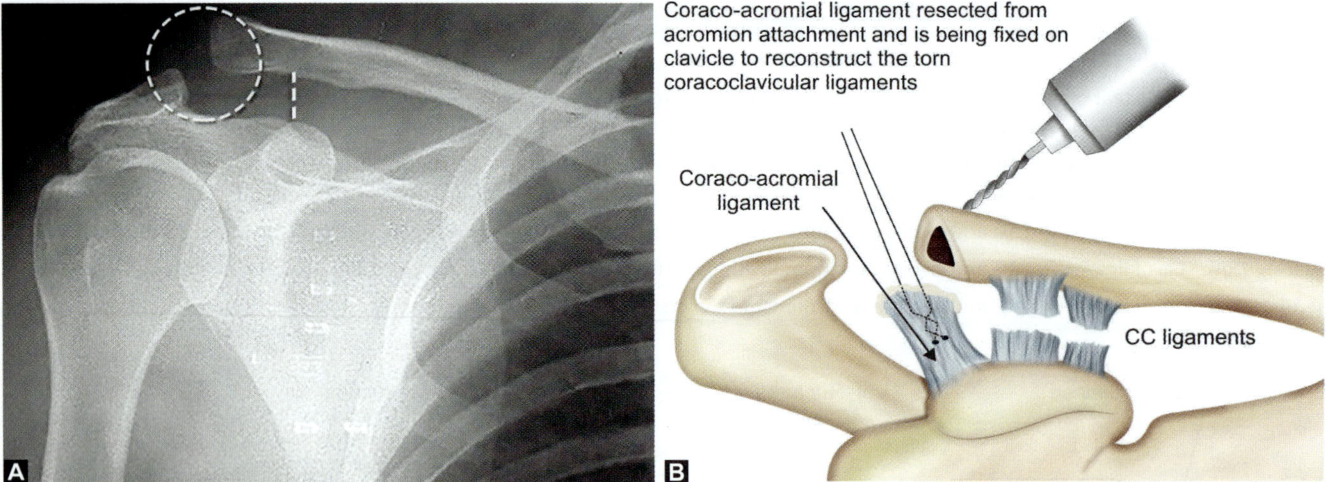

Figs 4.18A and B: (A) Anteroposterior X-ray of shoulder showing acromioclavicular (AC) joint dislocation (*dotted circle*). Normal coracoclavicular (CC) distance is 1.1–1.3 cm. Note the increased coracoclavicular distance (*dotted line*); (B) Surgical reconstruction of AC joint by conventional Weaver Dunn technique

Clinical Features

The patient presents with pain, swelling, deformity and bruising of upper arm. The patient should also be evaluated for neurovascular injury, including axillary nerve (regimental badge sign, *see* Page 267 for details) or brachial plexus injury. Diagnosis can be confirmed by anteroposterior and axillary X-ray views of the shoulder joint.

Management

Management is guided by Neer's classification.

One-part Fractures

Most of these fractures **(Fig. 4.20A)** are impacted, undisplaced or minimally displaced fractures (one-part fracture). In an elderly patient, it is usually managed by rest in an arm sling, chest arm or Velpeau bandage **(Fig. 4.20B)** or a universal shoulder immobilizer **(Fig. 4.20C)**, until the pain alleviates followed by gentle range of motion exercises. Being a cancellous (metaphyseal) bone, the fractures unite rapidly (by 6–8 weeks).

Two-part Fractures

Surgical neck fractures: Close reduction and immobilization in an arm sling for 3 weeks are usually sufficient. If fracture cannot be reduced close satisfactorily, then fixation with percutaneous pins, intramedullary nail or with a locked compression plate (LCP) is required.

Greater tuberosity fracture: This is usually associated with anterior dislocation of the shoulder. Greater tuberosity usually comes to its place when shoulder joint is reduced. If it does not reduce (displacement remains >1 cm or angulation >45°), then fixation with intraosseous sutures or cancellous screws is required.

Three- and Four-part Fractures

These are difficult to reduce closed and require operative fixation with intramedullary nailing or plating **(Fig. 4.21)**. In highly comminuted fractures chances of avascular necrosis (AVN) of humeral head are high and replacement arthroplasty may be required.

Complications

Shoulder stiffness is the most common complication of proximal humeral fracture. Axillary nerve injury and fracture nonunion are also common. AVN of the humeral head is relatively uncommon and usually seen in three- and four-part fractures.

FRACTURE SHAFT OF HUMERUS

This is a fracture of the humerus distal to surgical neck but proximal to the supracondylar ridge and accounts for less than 1% of all fractures. This is usually caused by a fall on the hand in elderly and motor vehicle injury in youngsters. Since humerus is well enveloped by muscles with rich blood supply, chances of healing of shaft fractures are high and some malunion is well accepted.

Displacements

When a fracture occurs above the deltoid insertion proximal fragment is adducted by pectoralis major. However, when the fracture occurs below the deltoid insertion, proximal fragment is abducted by deltoid **(Fig. 4.22)**.

Diagnosis

The patient presents with pain and swelling of arms. The arm is usually bruised and tender. Injury to radial nerve is the most common complication and patient should be assessed for radial nerve injury [wrist drop and loss of active extension of metacarpophalangeal (MCP) joints]. Diagnosis can be confirmed on X-ray of the arm.

Management

Nonoperative treatment **(Figs 4.23A to C)** of humeral shaft fracture enjoys high healing and success rate. Anatomical reduction is not necessary and angular and rotational malunion are easily masked by a good range of motion at the shoulder and elbow joints. Hanging cast (applied from an inch proximal to fracture site to wrist with elbow flexed to 90°, such that weight of plaster distracts and reduces fracture) and plaster of Paris U-slab (extending from base of neck, over the shoulder, lateral aspect of the arm, under the elbow to the medial side of the arm) are popular methods for the

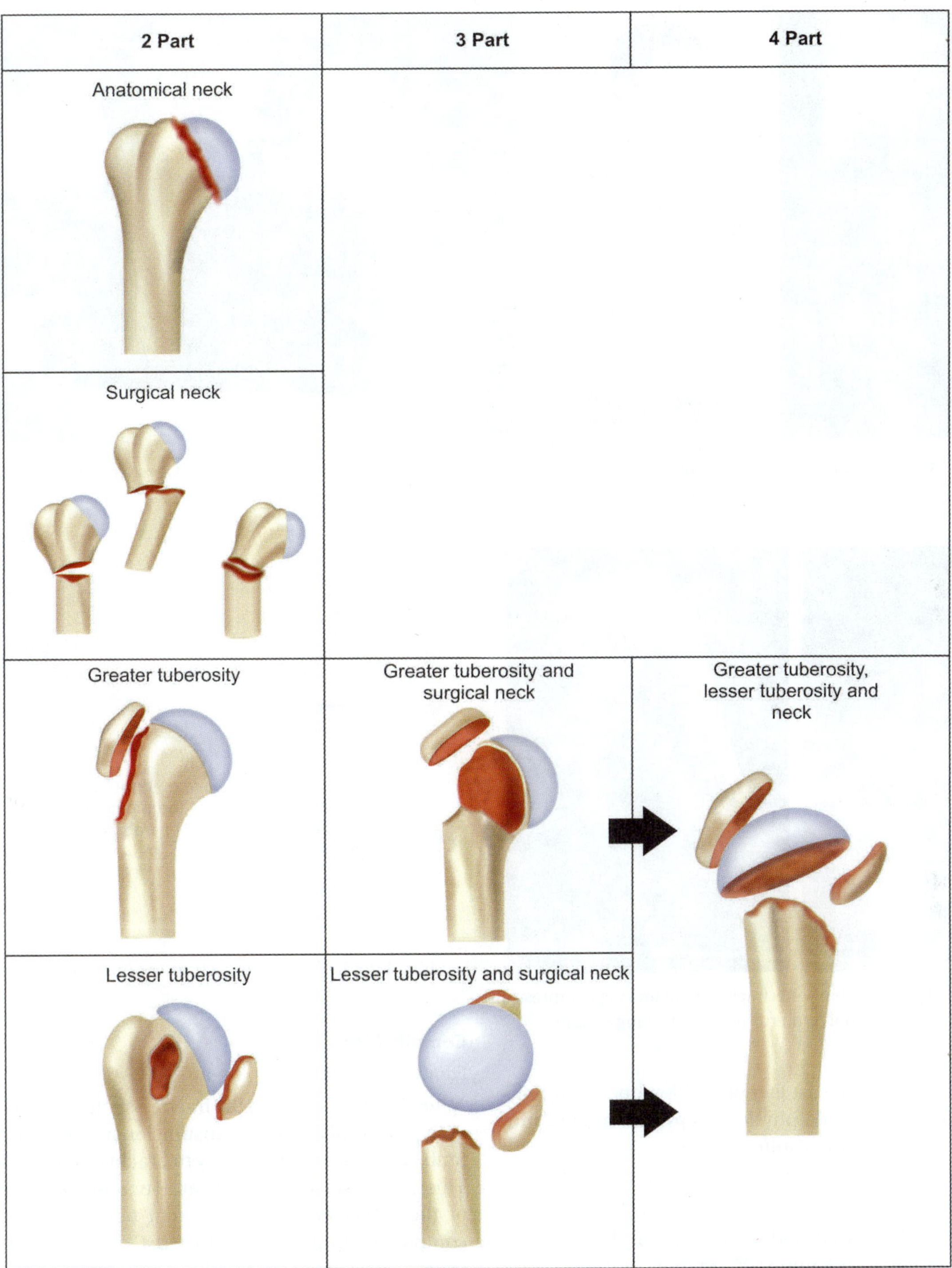

Fig. 4.19: Neer's classification of proximal humerus fractures

Table 4.2: Neer's classification of fracture of proximal humerus

One-part fracture	The fragments are undisplaced **(Fig. 4.20A)**
Two-part fracture	One segment is displaced from other (surgical neck fracture, anatomical neck fracture, greater tuberosity fracture, lesser tuberosity fracture, etc.)
Three-part fracture	Two segments are displaced
Four-part fracture	All the major parts (head, shaft, greater and lesser tuberosity) are displaced

Note: Displacement is defined as the separation between fragments is more than 1 cm or an angulation is more than 45°.

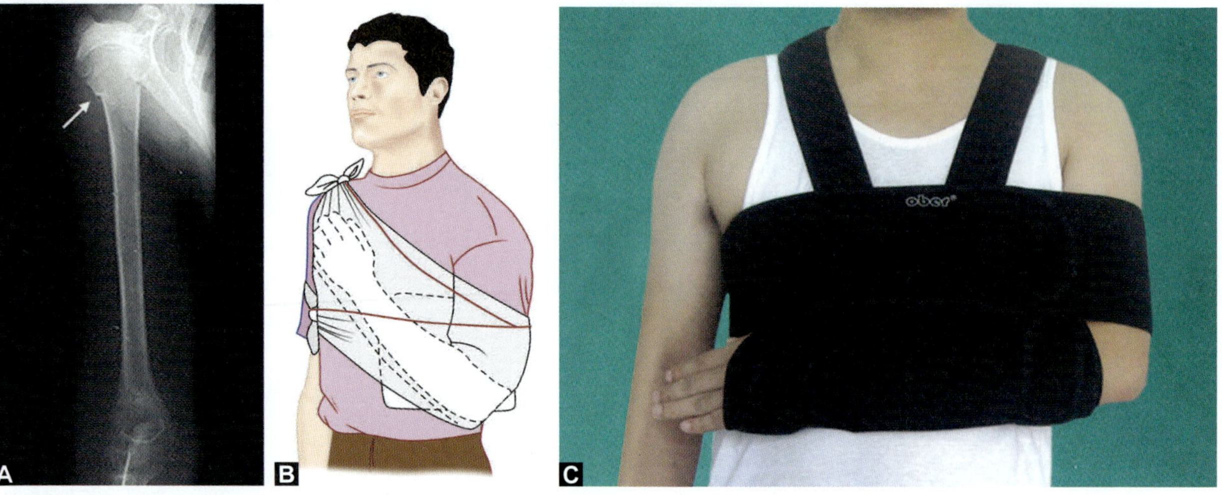

Figs 4.20A to C: (A) X-ray showing one-part fracture of the proximal humerus (arrow); (B) Chest arm bandage (Velpeau bandage*); (C) Universal shoulder immobilizer

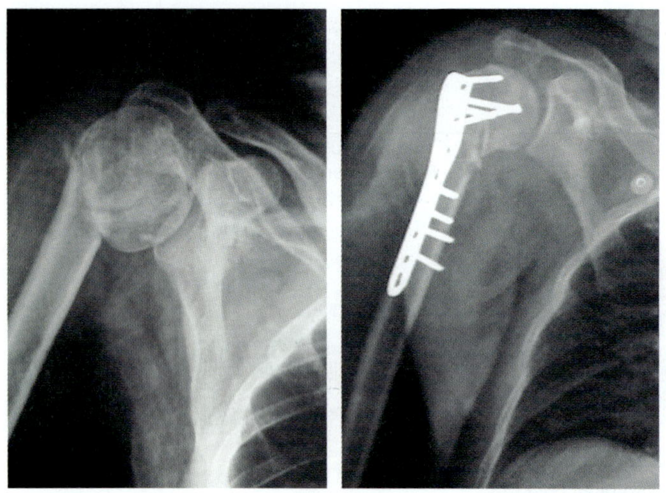

Fig. 4.21: Fixation of proximal humerus fracture with locking compression plate (PHILOS—proximal humerus internal locking system)

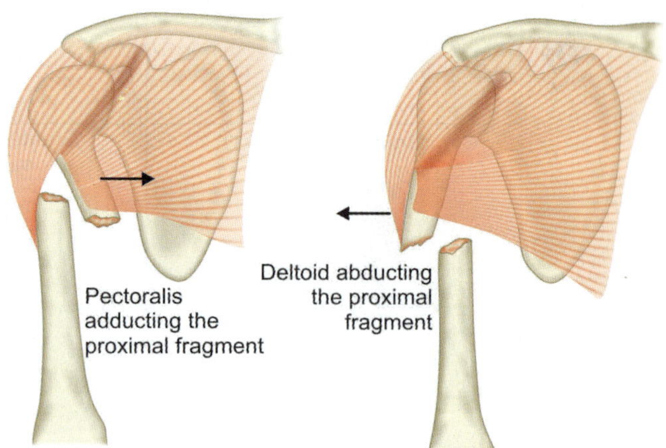

Fig. 4.22: Deforming muscle forces in a fracture shaft of humerus

conservative treatment. The cast is replaced by functional brace after about 2 weeks and gentle physiotherapy and mobilization are started early to prevent joint stiffness.

Operative Indications

- When acceptable closed reduction cannot be obtained (shortening >3 cm, angulation >20°, rotation >30°)
- Open wound, associated neurovascular injuries
- Polytrauma patient, ipsilateral forearm, shoulder or elbow fracture
- Pathological fractures and segmental fracture
- Operative fixation can be achieved with close reduction and intramedullary nailing, open reduction and plating **(Figs 4.24A and B)**. The external fixator is applied in case of an open fracture.

Complications

Early Complications

Neurovascular injury: If the fracture shaft of humerus is associated with signs of vascular insufficiency (decreased pulse, cold limb, paresthesia, etc.) injury to brachial artery must be excluded. This needs an emergency and urgent exploration and repair of the artery is required. Radial nerve injury (most common complication) presents with wrist drop and loss of MCP joint extension. This is particularly common with open fractures, polytrauma, vascular injury and multiple ipsilateral fractures. Mostly this is a stretching injury to the nerve in the spiral groove (neurapraxia) and usually recovers. Exploration of the radial nerve is usually not required except in cases of the open wound. Passive range of motion physiotherapy must be instituted and cock-up wrist splint should be given until nerve recovers to prevent joint stiffness. The nerve should be explored if there is no sign of recovery by 3 months.

---

*Velpeau bandage was originally devised for sternoclavicular dislocations, but it is also used in acromioclavicular joint dislocations, fractures of clavicle, scapula and neck of humerus and immobilizing dislocated shoulder after reduction.

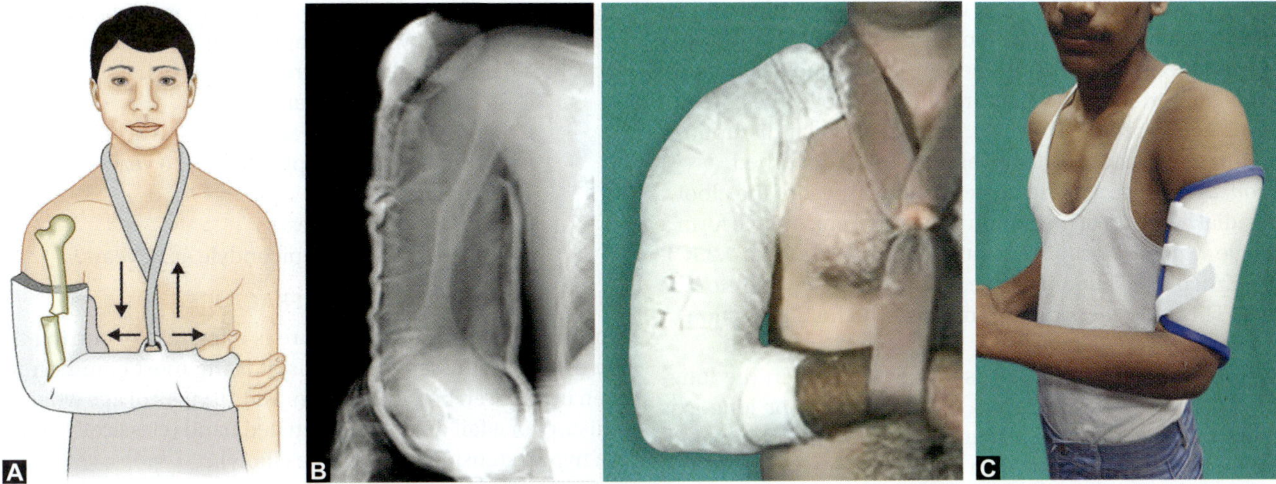

Figs 4.23A to C: Conservative treatment methods for fracture shaft humerus. (A) Schematic depiction of hanging cast; (B) Fracture shaft humerus reduced and held in a U-slab; (C) Functional brace applied for fracture shaft humerus

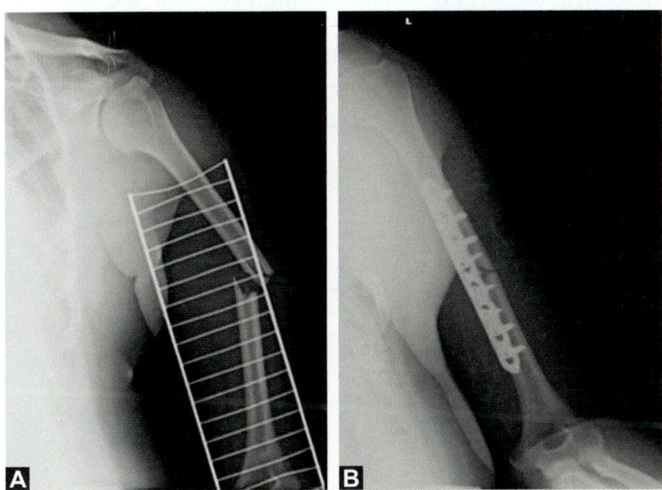

Figs 4.24A and B: (A) X-ray arm anteroposterior view showing fracture mid shaft of humerus; and (B) After fixation with plate

Late Complications

Delayed union and nonunion: This can occur following closed and operative treatment. Common causes are technical error (inadequate plate size, inadequate reduction before fixation and inadequate screw purchase), mechanical failure due to osteoporotic bone in which screws fail to hold the bone, fracture site distraction (most common cause) due to heavy hanging cast, fracture geometry (transverse fracture) and fracture type (segmental and open fracture). If there are signs of callus formation wait for expected union. Treatment of established nonunion in cancellous bone grafting and operative fixation.

Joint stiffness: It is common and can be prevented simply by early range of motion physiotherapy.

HIGH-YIELD POINTS

- Holstein Lewis fracture is a special variant of humerus fractures that occurs at the junction of upper two-thirds and lower one-third. In this region, the radial nerve is adherent to

the lateral intermuscular septum as the nerve crosses from posterior to lateral compartment. Hence, this fracture gets very commonly complicated by radial nerve palsy, the nerve being relatively fixed structure gets stretched due to fracture movements. Fortunately, the palsy is mostly transient.

- Although the most common complication of fracture shaft humerus is radial nerve palsy, in most cases it is mostly a stretch of nerve and spontaneous recovery occurs. Hence, no exploration and repair are needed acutely. However, if a palsy develops during manipulation and casting of fracture, the nerve is likely trapped at the fracture site and urgent exploration and repair should be sought.

INJURIES AROUND THE ELBOW

RELEVANT ANATOMY AROUND THE ELBOW

Relevant anatomy around the elbow is discussed as follows:

- Elbow joint is a synovial hinge joint having the ulnohumeral and radiohumeral components **(Fig. 4.25A)**. The ulnohumeral joint acts as a hinge where spool-shaped trochlea of the articular surface of the humerus articulates with the trochlear notch of ulna. The radiohumeral joint is formed between the spheroidal capitulum of the humerus and the head of the radius. In the upper radioulnar joint circumference of the head of the radius articulates with the radial notch of the ulna. Flexion and extension take place at the ulnohumeral joint (mainly) and radiocapitellar joint whereas pronation and supination take place mainly at the proximal radioulnar joint.
- Stability of the elbow joint depends on the congruency of articulating surfaces and surrounding capsule, medial collateral ligament (MCL) and lateral collateral ligament (LCL). MCL (particularly anterior band) is the primary restraint to valgus force. The lateral ulnar collateral ligament (part of LCL complex) is the primary stabilizer against varus and posterolateral instability.
- *Three-point bony relationship (**Fig. 4.25B**)*: Medial epicondyle, lateral epicondyle and the tip of olecranon form

a straight horizontal line when the elbow is extended and an isosceles triangle when the elbow is flexed to 90°. This three-point relationship is maintained in supracondylar fracture of the humerus as the fracture line is above the level of interepicondylar line. However, in intra-articular disruptions (fractures or dislocation), the relationship is disturbed.

- *Anconeus triangle*: On the posterolateral aspect of the elbow, the radial head, tip of olecranon and lateral epicondyle form a triangle which is occupied by anconeus muscle **(Fig. 4.25C)**. Intra-articular injections in the elbow can be given into this space. This space becomes prominent with fluid collection in the joint.
- *Carrying angle* **(Fig. 4.26)**: It is an angle between the long-axis of humerus and long-axis of the forearm (or long-axis of ulna) with elbow fully extended and forearm supinated. In extended position forearm and arm are not perfectly aligned and forearm is slightly deviated outside, forming an angle with the long-axis of the arm. This is known as carrying angle. Mean value in male is 11° and in females is 14°. This allows forearms to swing freely without hitting the hips.
- *Ossification around elbow* **(Fig. 4.27)**: Evaluation of elbow fractures may pose difficulty in children due to the changing anatomy of growing elbow. There are six ossification centers around the elbow, which appear in a predictable sequence. CRITOE is a simple way to remember this.
  - C—Capitellum at 2 years
  - R—Radial head at 4 years
  - I—Internal (medial) epicondyle at 6 years
  - T—Trochlea at 8 years
  - O—Olecranon at 10 years
  - E—External (lateral) epicondyle at 12 years.

SUPRACONDYLAR HUMERUS FRACTURE

Supracondylar humerus fracture is a fracture occurring through the olecranon fossa of humerus. It is the most common fracture seen in children between 3 years and 10 years of age when there is a history of a fall on the outstretched hand (classically when there is a hyperextension injury to the elbow).

Following factors account for the same:
(i) Thin shell of bone in the area (as there is coronoid fossa anteriorly and olecranon fossa posteriorly)
(ii) In hyperextension olecranon impinges into the fossa and breaks it
(iii) Lax soft tissues in children allow hyperextension very easily
(iv) Bone is growing and actively remodeling at this age

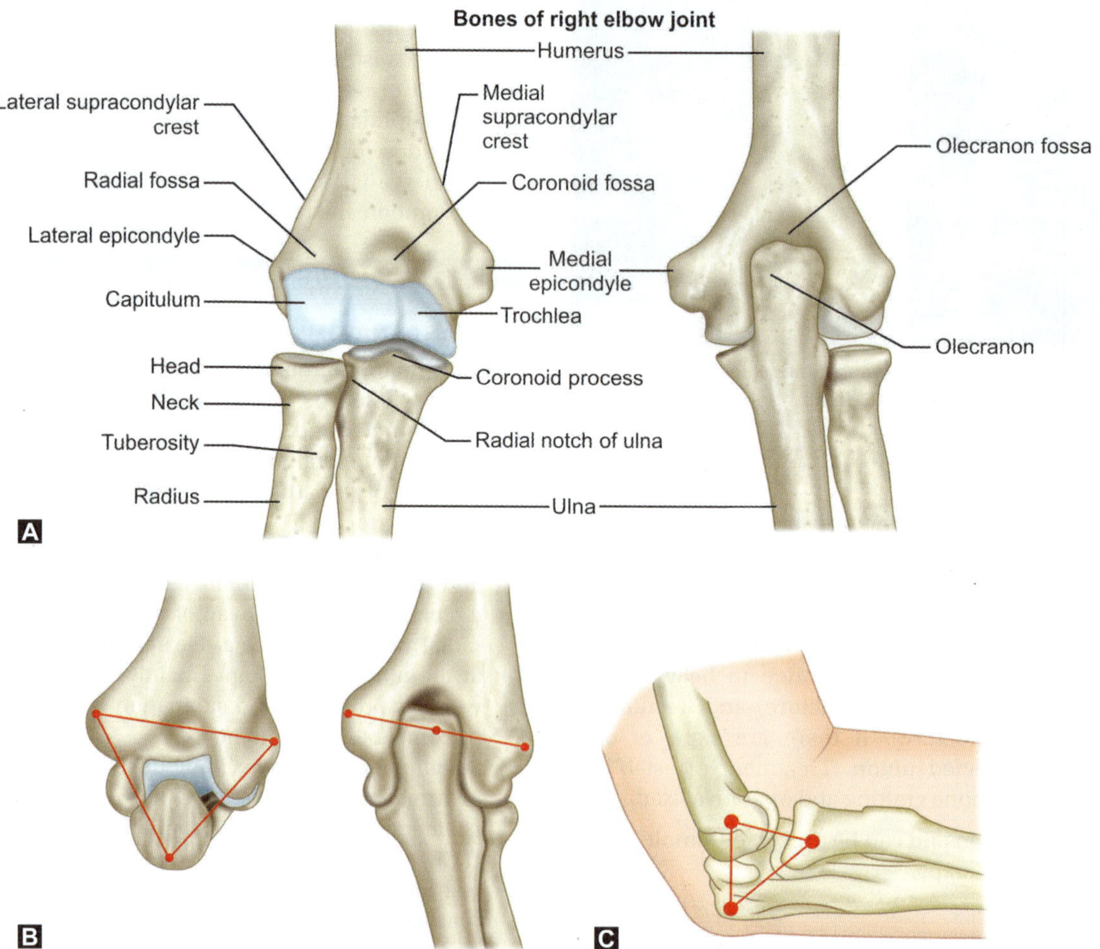

Figs 4.25A to C: (A) Anatomy of elbow joint; (B) Three-point bony relationship of elbow; (C) Anconeus triangle

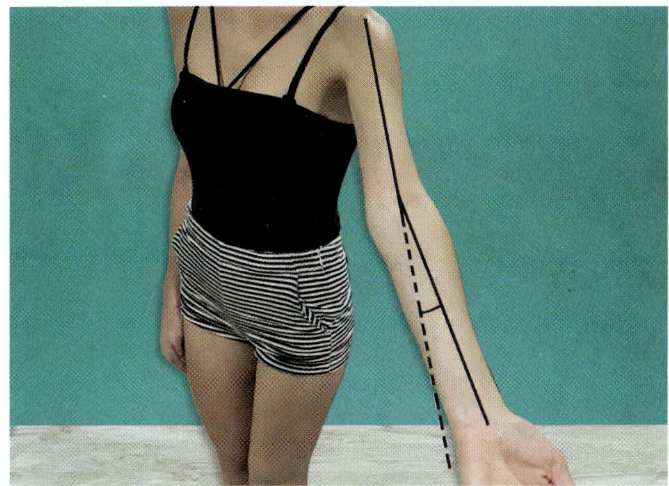

Fig. 4.26: Carrying angle

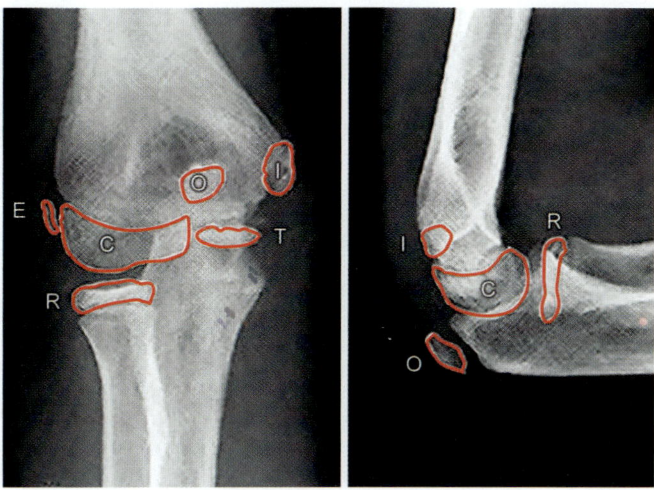

Fig. 4.27: Ossification around elbow

(v) A tight anterior capsule allows the olecranon tip to hinge against the fossa.

Displacements and Types of Fracture

The distal fragment in supracondylar humerus fracture can have a proximal shift, medial/lateral tilt or shift, anterior/posterior tilt or shift and/or can be in internal rotation. Based on mechanism of injury and displacements* (of distal fragment), the fracture can be of two types:

- *Extension type supracondylar fracture*: Most common type. Here the distal fragment is pulled posteriorly by the triceps as shown in **Figure 4.28**. It is caused by falling on an outstretched hand with the elbow in extension.
- *Flexion type supracondylar fracture*: This accounts for less than 5% cases. It is caused by a direct blow on the posterior aspect of flexed elbow. Distal fragment is displaced anteriorly.

Gartland Classification

As per the Gartland classification fractures are categorized into:

- *Type I*: Nondisplaced or minimally displaced fracture.
- *Type II*: One cortex (or at least periosteum) is intact such that there is only angulation but no displacement. Posterior angulation occurs with intact posterior cortex in extension type injury. Anterior angulation occurs with intact anterior cortex in flexion type injury.
- *Type III*: Completely displaced fracture with disruption of both cortices. Posteriorly displaced type III fractures may further be grouped into posteromedially displaced (occur when forearm is pronated at fall) or posterolaterally displaced (occur when forearm is supinated at fall). Since the former situation is more common and since an oblique fracture line causing the collapse of the medial column is the commoner result, most fractures tend to be displaced posteromedially.

Diagnosis

The patient presents with pain, elbow swelling and tenderness at supracondylar ridges. In completely displaced fracture there may be "S" shaped angulation deformity at the elbow. Dimpling

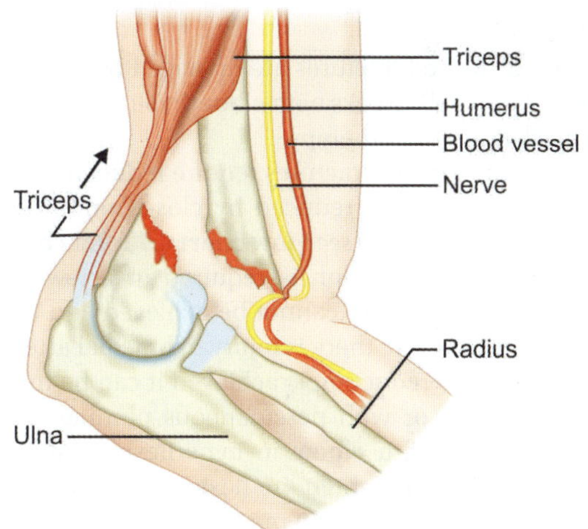

Fig. 4.28: Schematic representation of supracondylar fracture showing the distal fragment being displaced posteriorly by the triceps muscle

of the skin may be visible anteriorly secondary to penetration of the proximal fragment into the brachialis muscle (pucker sign). Nondisplaced or minimally displaced fractures may have only subtle clinical features with no swelling of the elbow. Radiography (*see* fat pad sign) is the mainstay of diagnosis in such cases. A thorough neurovascular examination must be done as this fracture is notorious to end up with dreadful complications.

Radiological Examination

Diagnosis can be confirmed on anteroposterior and lateral views of the elbow. In minimally displaced fracture fat pad sign (radiolucency anterior or posterior to distal humeral diaphysis, **Fig. 4.29**) may be seen on the lateral X-ray view. As the fracture hematoma fills up the coronoid and olecranon fossa, the fat in these fossae is displaced, that gives rise to this lucency on radiographs. Since missing this fracture can have grave consequences a thorough evaluation of the normal radiographic elbow parameters and indices is essential before ruling out a fracture **(Figs 4.30A and B)**.

---

*Displacements in orthopedics by convention always refer to position of the distal fragment.

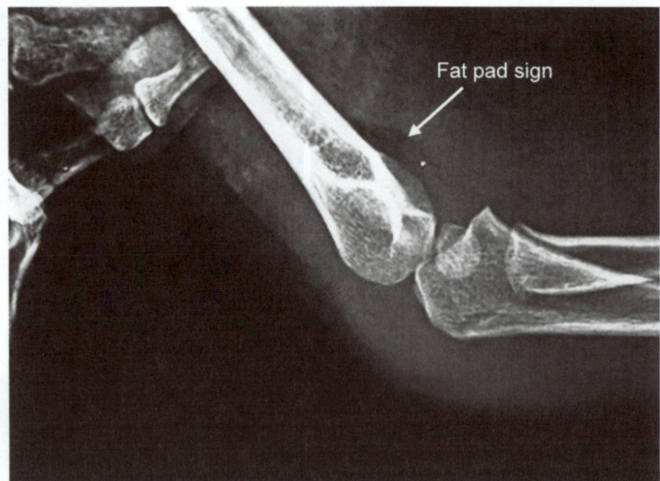

Fig. 4.29: Fat pad sign in undisplaced supracondylar humerus fracture

Management

Type I nondisplaced fractures are managed by above elbow cast immobilization for 3 weeks with elbow in 90° flexion, followed by range of motion physiotherapy.

Type II and type III fractures require reduction. The majority of the fractures can be reduced by close manipulation under C-arm image intensifier (*see* **Flow chart 4.1** for method of closed reduction). Open reduction is required in a few cases where adequate close reduction cannot be achieved and in cases with open wounds or where there is injury to brachial artery requiring a repair. Once the reduction is achieved it can be maintained in above elbow cast or with percutaneous pinning. Since plaster splinting is done with elbow in hyperflexion (intact posterior capsule and triceps tighten in flexion and form a posterior support) and excessive flexion may risk neurovascular structures, pinning is mostly the preferred method **(Figs 4.31A and B)**. However, at times one is unable to take up these patients for reduction attempt due to anesthetic problems or other issues. In such situations, the fracture can be temporary splinted by applying a Dunlop (skin traction, **Fig. 4.31C**) or a Smith's traction (skeletal traction).

Assessment of Reduction

Common missed displacements are varus tilt, posterior displacement and internal rotation of distal fragment. Following parameter may be useful in assessing adequacy of reduction:

(i) *Varus tilt:* This can be predicted from a Baumann's angle in AP view or Crescent sign in lateral view. In the latter, a crescent-shaped shadow may be seen in the small radiolucent gap of elbow joint **(Fig. 4.32A)** due to overlap of capitulum over the olecranon tip. Baumann's angle **(Fig. 4.32B)** is drawn between a line drawn perpendicular to the long-axis of the humeral shaft and physeal line of lateral condyle of humerus in AP view (normal 8–28°). A small angle may result in fracture malunion leading to a cubitus varus deformity at elbow.

(ii) *Abnormal horizontal rotation:* Internal rotation is common and it's presence manifests as Fish tail sign **(Fig. 4.31A)**. Due to internal rotation of distal fragment, the anterior margin of proximal fragment appears as a sharp spike.

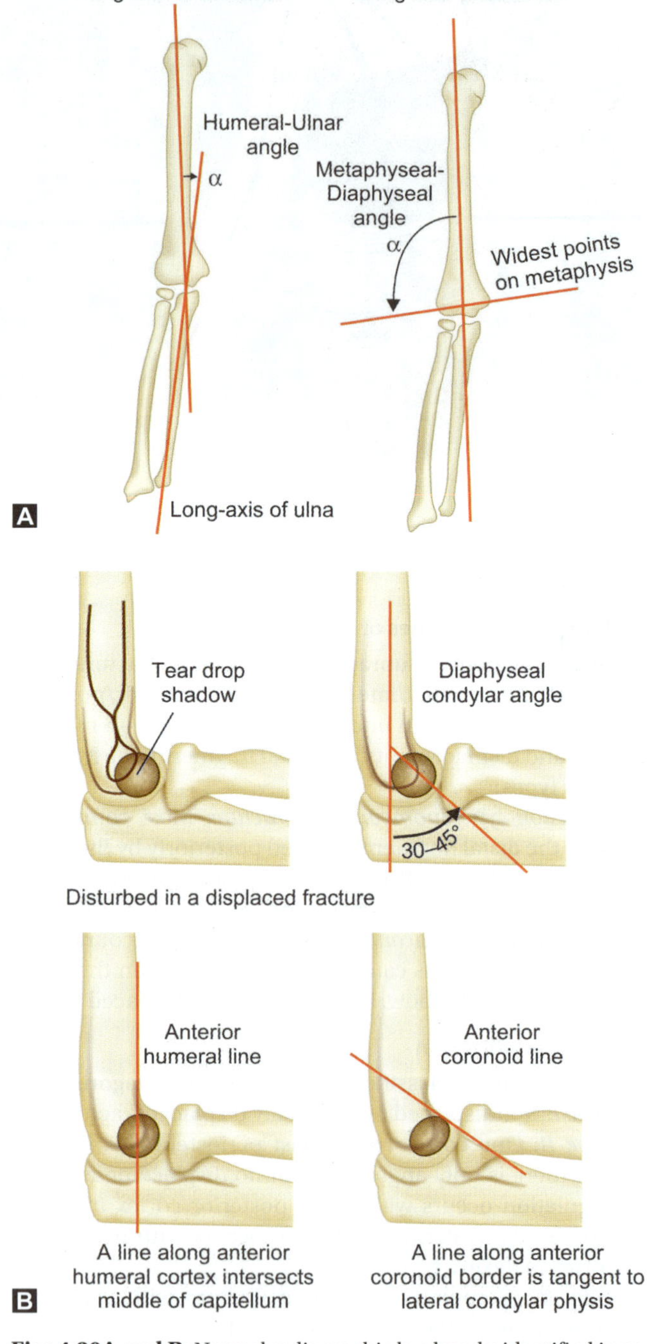

Figs 4.30A and B: Normal radiographic landmarks identified in an X-ray of pediatric elbow in AP (A) and lateral (B) projections

(iii) *Posterior displacement:* Disruption of tear drop, anterior humeral line and anterior coronoid line **(Fig. 4.30B)** may give a clue.

Once reduction is confirmed to be acceptable, the fracture may be splinted. Since splinting is done with the elbow in hyperflexion and pronation, routine X-rays views are difficult to obtain in plaster. A special X-ray view called Jones view (hyperflexion shoot through elbow; **Fig. 4.33**) may be used to assess the fracture, post-reduction.

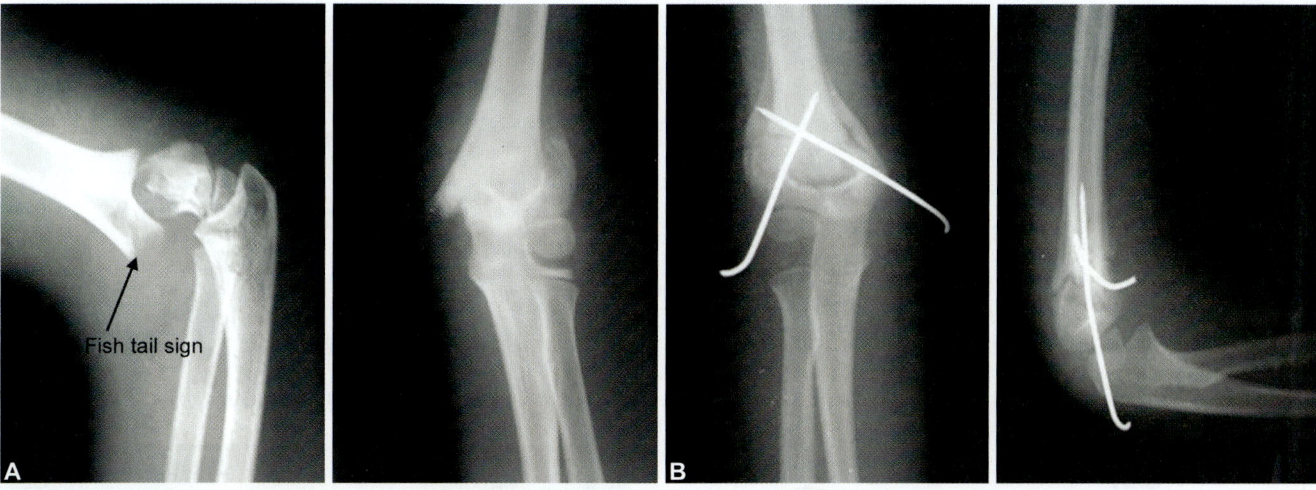

Figs 4.31A and B: (A) Anteroposterior and lateral X-rays of elbow showing supracondylar fracture of humerus; and (B) Close reduction and percutaneous pinning of supracondylar fracture of humerus

Flow chart 4.1: Method of closed reduction for extension type supracondylar humerus fracture

Steady continuous traction with elbow in full extension (surgeon holds the forearm and assistant grasps the arm)

↓

While traction is maintained valgus/varus deformity is corrected by direct pressure with thumb on the distal fragment

↓

Now, surgeon pushes the distal fragment anteriorly with thumb and proximal fragment posteriorly with fingers of dominant hand (traction is maintained with nondominant hand)

↓

Reduction is maintained with dominant hand and nondominant hand flexes the elbow and pronates the forearm for posteromedially displaced fracture and supinates the forearm for posterolaterally displaced fracture

↓

Reduction is checked in image intensifier (Anteroposterior and lateral views)

In flexion type fracture same steps are followed but instead of anteriorly directed force, distal fragment is reduced by posteriorly directed force

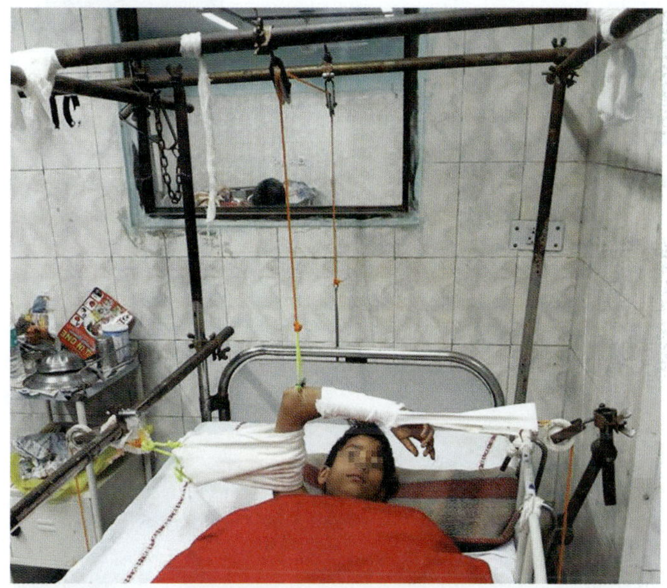

Fig. 4.31C: A modified Dunlop traction for supracondylar fracture management in a child

capillary refill, absent radial pulses and absent or decreased pulse oximeter saturation), angiography may be done and exploration of brachial artery may be warranted. However, if the radial pulse disappears after fracture reduction (and elbow is not acutely flexed for plaster), it indicates that artery is entrapped between fracture fragments and this requires immediate surgical exploration.

Complications

Early Complications

Vascular Injury

Brachial artery may be compressed by fracture fragment or get entrapped between two fracture fragments **(Fig. 4.28)**. Whenever a patient with supracondylar humerus fracture presents with an absent radial pulse, immediate reduction should be attempted as reduction relieves compression and frequently restores circulation. If even after reduction, limb remains ischemic (absent/decreased

Compartment Syndrome **(Fig. 4.34)**

Supracondylar fracture humerus is the most common cause of compartment syndrome in children. Compartment syndrome results when pressure rises within the closed compartment of forearm, causing a vascular compromise, the insult occurring secondary to the supracondylar humerus fracture at the elbow **(Flow chart 4.2)**. Muscle hypoxia as a result of ischemia causes increased capillary permeability and intramuscular edema which further causes a rise in compartmental pressure. Decreased

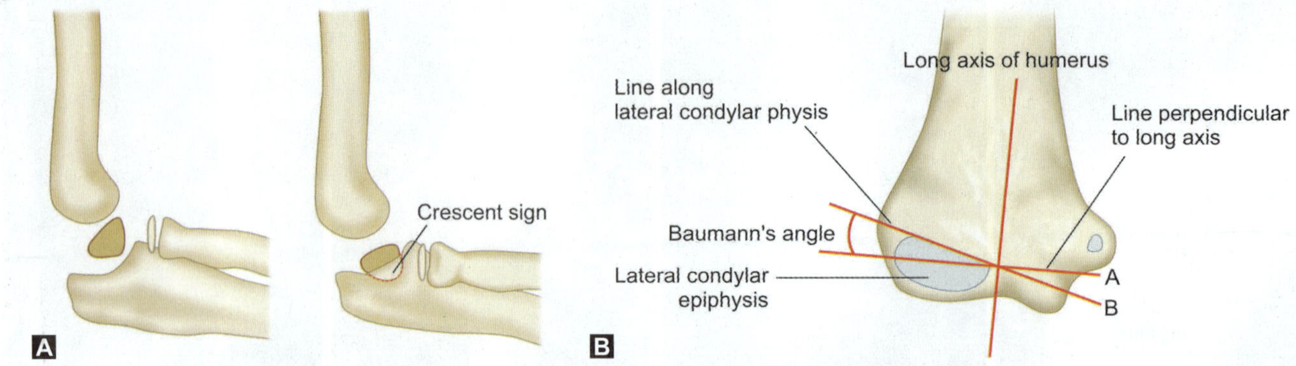

Figs 4.32A and B: (A) Schematic representation of crescent sign in lateral elbow X-ray; (B) Baumann's angle

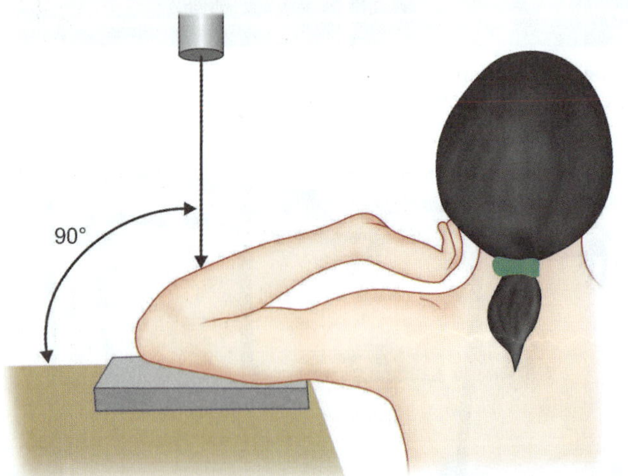

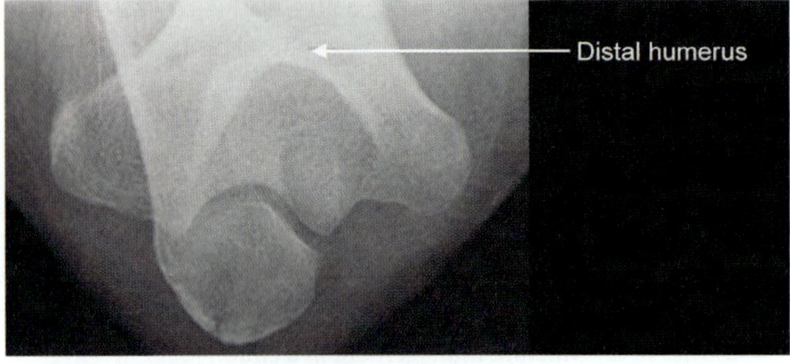

Fig. 4.33: Jones view of elbow (an axial view of elbow)

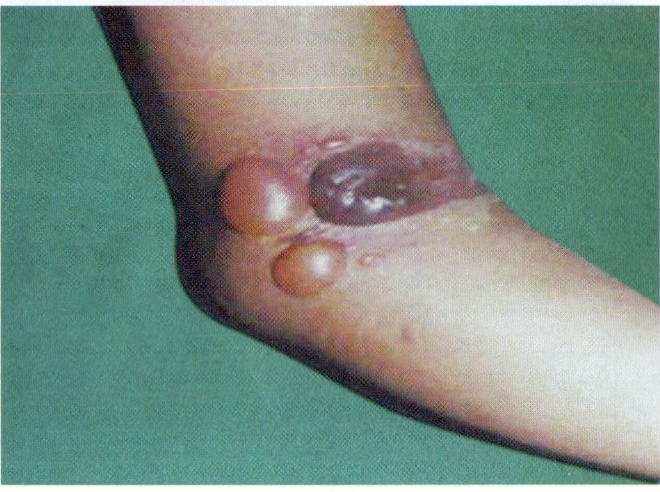

Fig. 4.34: Compartment syndrome following supracondylar fracture of humerus—see massive swelling and blebs

Flow chart 4.2: Events in development of compartment syndrome

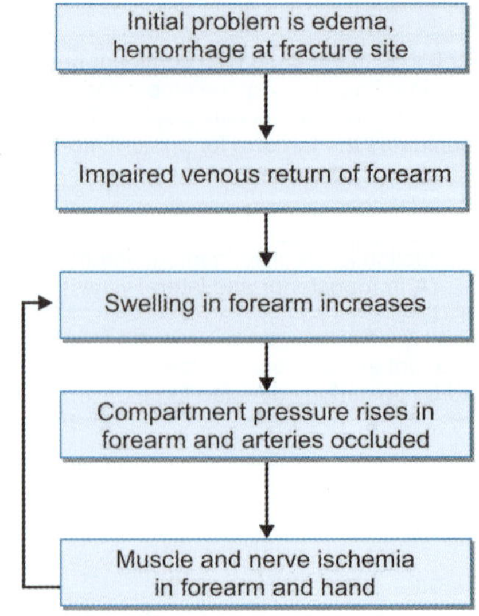

venous return also contributes to raise compartment pressure. Thus, a vicious cycle is set which can only be stopped with the immediate surgical release of involved compartment by fasciotomy (there is no benefit of fasciotomy after 72 hours).

Diagnosis: Diagnosis should be made on clinical ground by looking for the six "P"s—puffiness (swelling), pain on passive stretch of the fingers (passive stretch test), pallor, pulselessness, paresthesias and paralysis. The earliest and most reliable sign is the passive stretch test. Pulse is an unreliable sign and distal pulses may be present or absent. Development of paresthesia and paralysis are late features. Wick or slit catheter technique or an arterial line pressure monitor can measure the compartment pressure accurately. Pressure more than 30 mm Hg (normal compartment pressure is less than 10 mm Hg) usually indicates the need for surgical intervention, although threshold pressure is different with different measurement techniques and decision of surgical release of compartment (fasciotomy) should be taken on clinical ground.

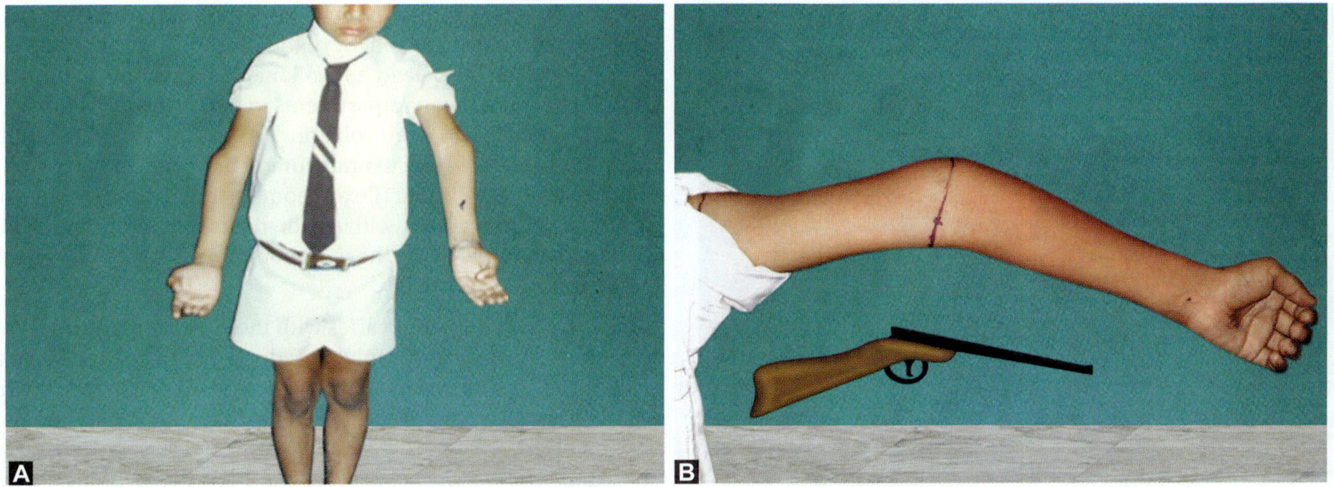

Figs 4.35A and B: (A) Cubitus varus deformity following malunited supracondylar fracture of humerus; and (B) The typical appearance of gunstock deformity

Prevention and treatment: Best treatment for compartment syndrome is vigilant avoidance. Injured limb should be kept elevated to decrease soft tissue swelling and edema. However, in impending compartment syndrome limb should be kept at heart level because limb elevation also reduces arterial blood flow and thus oxygen delivery to tissues. Tight circumferential dressing should be removed. Treatment of impending or established compartment syndrome is essentially fasciotomy of the involved compartment. A fracture can be stabilized after surgical decompression of the compartment.

Nerve Injury

Anterior interosseous nerve injury is the most common nerve injury followed by median and then radial nerve injury in extension type of supracondylar humerus fracture. In flexion type fractures and in postoperative cases it is the ulnar nerve that is most commonly involved. The adequate neurological examination is although difficult to do with an injured child and so initially diagnosis may be missed. Fortunately, almost all nerve injuries are neurapraxia only (approximately 11% patients have neuropraxias) and improve with time. Watchful expectancy is all that is required. If recovery does not happen in 12 weeks than nerve conduction studies and electromyographic studies should be done. If a nerve is found transected then either nerve grafting or tendon transfer should be considered.

Late Complications

Malunion

This is the most common complication of supracondylar fracture. Cubitus varus deformity (gunstock deformity, **Figs 4.35A and B**) is more common than cubitus valgus deformity because postero-medially displaced fractures which tend to develop varus angula-tion, are more common than posterolaterally displaced fractures. These problems which occur months after fracture heals, cause more cosmetic problem and less functional problem. However, lateral condylar fracture, elbow and shoulder instability and distal humeral epiphyseal separation all have been reported as complications following cubitus varus deformity.

Cubitus varus deformity is actually a three-dimensional deformity with rotational malalignment along with a coronal plane deformity that occurs due to an uncorrected medial tilt and internal rotation of the distal fragment. Rotational component is largely compensated by shoulder movement so only coronal plane deformity correction is all that is necessary.

For mild degree of deformity nothing is required except reassurance. In severe cases, corrective osteotomy is required to improve cosmetic appearance and functional deficit. Lateral closing wedge osteotomy (French or modified French) with single plane (coronal) correction and fixation with K-wires, screws or a plate is the most commonly done procedure.

Elbow Stiffness

This can be a problematic complication in cases with prolonged immobilization. Early range of motion physiotherapy at 3 weeks should be commenced to prevent elbow stiffness. A rare cause of elbow stiffness is myositis ossificans that needs special attention.

Myositis Ossificans (Aka Hematoma Ossificans)

It is a benign pathological bone formation (heterotopic ossifica-tion) in muscles and other soft tissues **(Fig. 4.36)**. Trauma is the most common inciting event, but may occur without trauma in paraplegics, Guillain-Barré (GB) syndrome, acquired immuno-deficiency syndrome (AIDS) encephalopathy, closed head injury, following extensive burns and in a comatose patient. One-third cases are idiopathic.

Most commonly affected muscles are quadriceps, glutei and brachialis. However, the elbow joint is most commonly involved joint by myositis ossificans. After injury, massage to the elbow and vigorous passive physiotherapy may provoke the development of myositis ossificans.

Pathology: It is a calcium hydroxyapatite deposition (ossifi-cation*) in soft tissues being composed of a benign matrix rich in fibroblasts and osteoclast like giant cells. Ackerman

---

*Ossification is the deposition of crystalline calcium phosphate (i.e. calcium hydroxyapatite) while calcification is the deposition of amorphous (powdered) calcium phosphate in soft tissues.

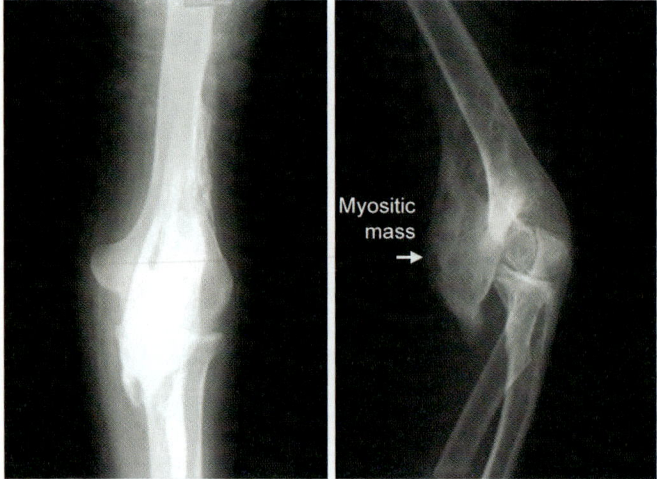

Fig. 4.36: Myositis ossificans of elbow joint
Courtesy: Dr Sachin Ingole.

zonal phenomenon is a characteristic feature. In the center actively proliferating fibroblast with numerous mitotic figures, cytological atypia and loose random arrangement is found. In the periphery more organized arrangement of mature fibroblast with transformation into mature osteoid is seen. This is in contrast to neoplastic lesion in which more mature cells are seen at the center.

Clinical features: Clinical features are divided into three phases:
1. *Acute phase*: After a few days to a few weeks of injury, patient develops pain swelling and stiffness of nearby joints.
2. *Pseudotumoral phase*: This comes after 2–3 weeks and characterized by painless hard mass.
3. *Resolving phase*: This comes after 3–6 months. Gradual resolution of the lesion may occur in this phase.

Radiology: Initial X-rays are normal. Calcification and mineralization are seen 2–3 weeks after the onset of symptoms and matures in next 3–6 months. Periosteal reaction is seen as laminations. There are three variants of the myositic mass. In stalked variant a peduncle is attached to the underlying bone. In sessile variant, the mass has a broad-based attachment to underlying periosteum. In a third variant bony mass is only attached to involved muscle.

Diagnosis: It can be made on clinical background in association with X-ray features. In doubtful cases diagnosis can be confirmed by biopsy. Biopsy also differentiates it from a bone-forming tumor like osteosarcoma due to the presence of zonal phenomena.

Treatment: In acute cases, treatment consists of nonsteroidal anti-inflammatory drugs (NSAIDs), ice, compression dressing, splintage for the involved limb and active range of motion physiotherapy. Passive stretching should be avoided, rather active exercises are to be encouraged. If required, excision of the ossified mass can be done after maturation which usually takes a year or so (indicated by decreased levels of alkaline phosphatase and mature bone deposition on X-ray).

Volkmann's Ischemic Contracture (Figs 4.37A and B)
It is a sequel of the missed compartment syndrome. There occurs ischemic necrosis of muscles and nerves of the forearm, which are

then replaced by fibrous tissue **(Flow chart 4.3)**. Any obstruction to brachial artery caused by tight plaster, improper use of a tourniquet can also lead to Volkmann's ischemic contracture (VIC). There are four compartments in the forearm: (1) dorsal, (2) superficial volar, (3) deep volar and (4) compartment containing the mobile wad of Henry (brachioradialis, extensor carpi radialis longus and brevis). Volar (flexor) compartment is most commonly involved compartment with flexor digitorum profundus (FDP) and median nerve being the most common involved muscles and nerve in VIC, respectively.

Clinical features: Picture varies with the severity of the injury:
- *Mild involvement*: Only the deep extrinsic finger flexors (FDPs) are involved and usually involve only two or three fingers. The middle and ring fingers are most frequently involved.
- *Moderate involvement*: After the FDP, flexor pollicis longus muscle is commonly involved. Other muscles, the flexor digitorum superficialis (FDS), flexor carpi radialis (FCR) and flexor carpi ulnaris (FCU) may also be involved later. Typical deformity is the intrinsic-minus hand deformity (claw hand) from extrinsic muscle contracture [hyperextension at MCP joint and flexion at interphalangeal (IP) joints]. Concomitant median and ulnar nerve neuropathy further contribute to claw hand deformity in addition to sensory changes.
- *Severe involvement*: Along with forearm flexor compartment extensors are also involved to varying extent. However, the clinical picture is still that of only flexor involvement because of strong and larger flexors. With severe cases there are elbow flexion, forearm pronation, wrist flexion, thumb flexion and adduction, digital MCP joint extension and IP joint flexion.

Treatment: Mild cases with intact sensation can be treated with range of motion and strengthening exercises and static and dynamic extension splinting. A turnbuckle splint **(Fig. 4.38)** is most commonly used for mild deformities. Turning the buckle distracts the contracted tissue gradually and corrects a mild deformity. In moderate cases the surgery of choice is the Maxpage's muscle sliding operation (excising the common flexor origin and translating it distally on to the interosseous membrane). Severe cases require neurolysis, excision of the infarcted muscle mass and bone shortening procedures.

HIGH-YIELD POINTS

- *Cubitus rectus:* This refers to a neutral alignment at the elbow (i.e. zero carrying angle). Best assessment of carrying angle is given by humeroulnar angle **(Fig. 4.30B)**.
- Supracondylar humerus fracture is the most common fracture associated with neurovascular injury (median nerve and brachial artery), compartment syndrome and VIC and myositis ossificans in a child.
- Ipsilateral radius fracture is most commonly-associated fracture with supracondylar humerus fracture.
- Posteromedial supracondylar humeral fractures are more common than posterolateral type. Radial nerve injury is more common in posteromedial type and median nerve injury is more common in posterolateral type, but posterolateral type is more commonly associated with nerve injury so median nerve is most commonly injured nerve in supracondylar fractures.

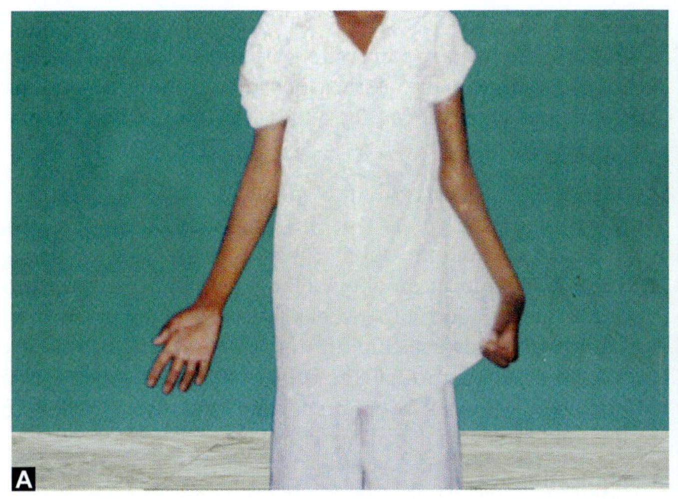
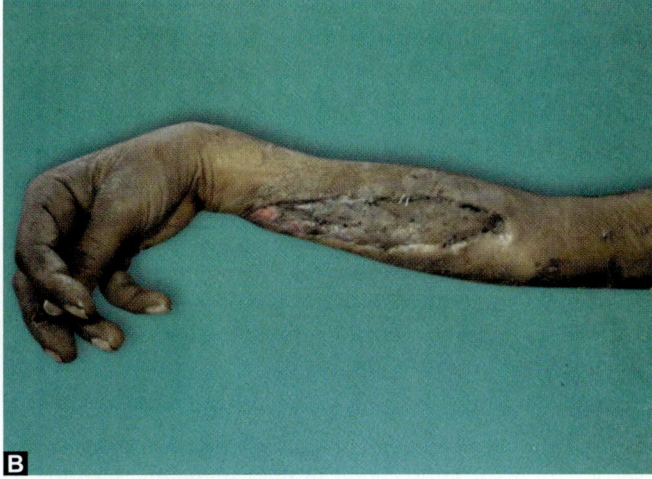

Figs 4.37A and B: Volkmann ischemic contracture of forearm muscles

Flow chart 4.3: Sequence of events in development of Volkmann's ischemic contracture

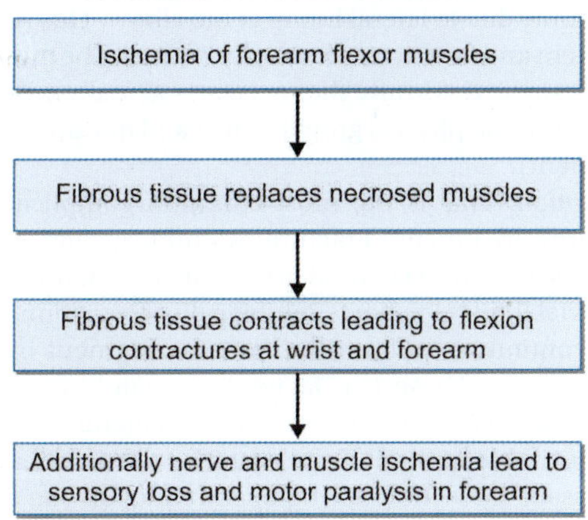

Ischemia of forearm flexor muscles

↓

Fibrous tissue replaces necrosed muscles

↓

Fibrous tissue contracts leading to flexion contractures at wrist and forearm

↓

Additionally nerve and muscle ischemia lead to sensory loss and motor paralysis in forearm

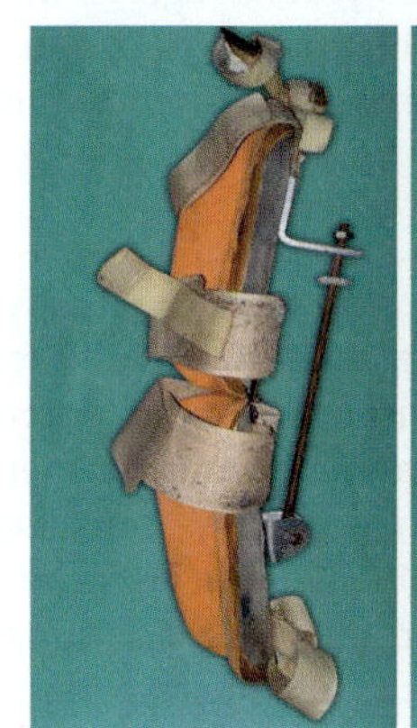
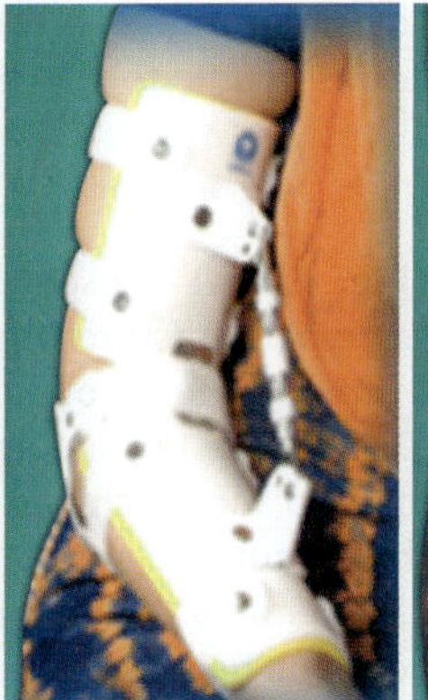
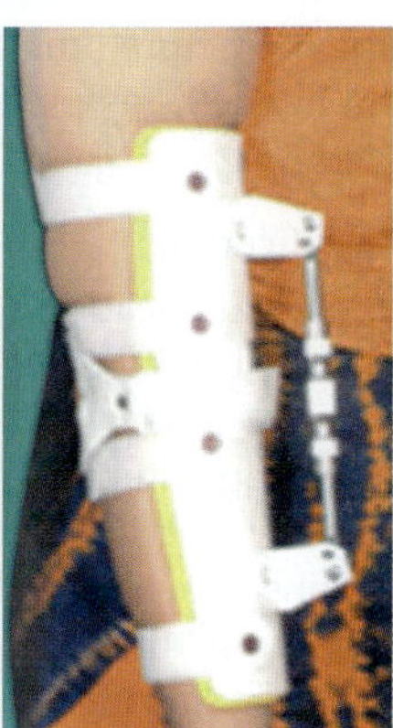

Fig. 4.38: Turnbuckle splint

- Although nerve injury is an early complication of supracondylar humerus fracture, a late presentation may also be possible. In such cases the median nerve gets entrapped in the fracture callus (Metev sign).
- Iatrogenic ulnar nerve injury is associated with medial pinning in supracondylar fracture. To prevent it, two lateral pins can be inserted to maintain reduction or medial pin should be inserted with the elbow in extension.
- Fish tail sign in supracondylar humerus predicts about the presence of abnormal horizontal rotation. However, fish tail deformity is seen in osteonecrosis of trochlea that may rarely be seen as complication of the fracture or may result from Hegemann's disease (osteochondritis of trochlea).
- Although a number of causes can lead to compartment syndrome like blunt injury, surgery, infection, snake bite, tight plaster/bandage, tourniquet and intravenous (IV) fluid administration, the most common cause is a fracture. In children, most common fracture that leads to compartment syndrome is supracondylar humerus fracture while in an adult it is a proximal tibia fracture. Overall, it is tibial fracture that is the most common cause and most often the compartment syndrome occurs in the leg.

- Although fasciotomy is a treatment option for compartment syndrome, it is also indicated in cases where there has been vascular disruption of a major vessel to a limb for more than 4 hours, as there are high chances of developing compartment syndrome after a vascular disruption.
- Elbow joint, followed by hip joint is most commonly involved joint by myositis ossificans.
- *Myositis ossificans progressiva*: It is a rare, autosomal dominant and fatal condition seen in children usually below 6 years. It is characterized by spontaneous or injury-induced progressive ossification of soft tissues including- muscle, tendon and ligaments at multiple sites, ultimately leading to death. Exact etiology is not known, but the presence of macrophages, lymphocytes and mast cells in early lesions with perivascular lymphocytic infiltration and response to corticosteroid may indicate towards involvement of the immune system. Microdactyly of the great toe is a characteristic association. Other common abnormalities include exostoses, dental and ear deformities, hypogonadism and short/broad neck. Sternocleidomastoid muscle is almost always involved to start with and torticollis is a common initial presenting complaint. Cardiac muscles, smooth muscles and many skeletal muscles like diaphragm, tongue and extraocular muscles are spared from heterotopic ossification. Initial

signs of disease are pain and swelling of involved muscle followed by ossification. Neck, spine and shoulder girdle are commonly involved. Death is usually due to respiratory failure and its complications.

LATERAL CONDYLE HUMERUS FRACTURE

After a supracondylar humerus fracture, this is the next most common fracture in children between 5 years and 10 years age. It is usually caused by a fall on an outstretched arm that causes impaction of the radial head into the lateral condyle (push off theory). It may also be caused by the pull of the common extensor origin (pull off theory). The fracture line runs between the attachment of ECRL and brachioradialis.

Pathoanatomy

Lateral condyle fracture fragment consists of lateral epicondyle and secondary ossification center of the capitellum. Secondary ossification center of the capitellum appears at around 2 years of age and that of lateral epicondyle at 12–13 years of age. At the time of fracture most of the structures involved are cartilaginous and hence X-ray picture is unable to give the exact extent of the fracture.

Classification

Milch classification **(Fig. 4.39A)** is used commonly to classify these injuries. A Milch type I fracture line extends laterally to trochlear groove and through the secondary ossification center of the capitellum. In Milch type II, fracture line extends farther medially (medial to or into the trochlear groove) and trochlea remains attached to the fracture fragment. Elbow joint becomes unstable in Milch type II fractures. X-ray interpretation concerning Milch classification is difficult because the fracture line extending through cartilaginous part is not seen in X-ray.

Milch type I fracture is considered as Salter-Harris type IV fracture as the fracture line extends through metaphysis, physis and epiphysis. Milch type II fracture is Salter-Harris type II fracture as the fracture line does not extend through the secondary ossification center of the capitellum (i.e. capitellar epiphysis).

Diagnosis

The child presents with pain and swelling of the elbow. Tenderness is present mainly on the lateral aspect of the elbow. Diagnosis can be confirmed with X-rays **(Fig. 4.39B)**.

Treatment

Treatment is based on the displacement of fracture. A nondisplaced fracture is one in which displacement is less than 2 mm on oblique views. These fractures can be managed by immobilization in an above elbow cast in 90° elbow flexion and internal rotation for 4 weeks followed by range of motion physiotherapy. However, majority of these fractures are displaced (also called as Fracture of Necessity, *see* Page 35) owing to pull off the common extensor origin and such fractures require open reduction and internal fixation with K-wires.

Complications

- *Lateral spur formation*: Lateral spur formation is the most common complication and usually results from ossification under the periosteum that gets raised due to displacement of fracture or during surgery, leading to cubitus pseudovarus deformity due to lateral bump at the elbow. This is a cosmetic problem and functions are usually normal. The most common problematic deformity that occurs is actually cubitus valgus (due to lateral physeal growth arrest and nonunion of fracture fragment).
- *Nonunion*: This is the most common complication which requires treatment. Fracture is intracapsular so there is continuous synovial fluid irrigation of fracture fragments. Synovial fluid is known to inhibit callus formation. Also, there is a continuous pull on the fracture fragment by extensors of the wrist. These two factors are mainly responsible for nonunion of lateral condylar fracture. Lateral condyle derives most of its blood supply from posterior soft tissues so extensive soft tissue dissection during open reduction can also lead to nonunion. A lateral condyle fracture which does not show signs of healing by 3 months is said to be in nonunion. Early nonunion fracture presents with pain and instability. These

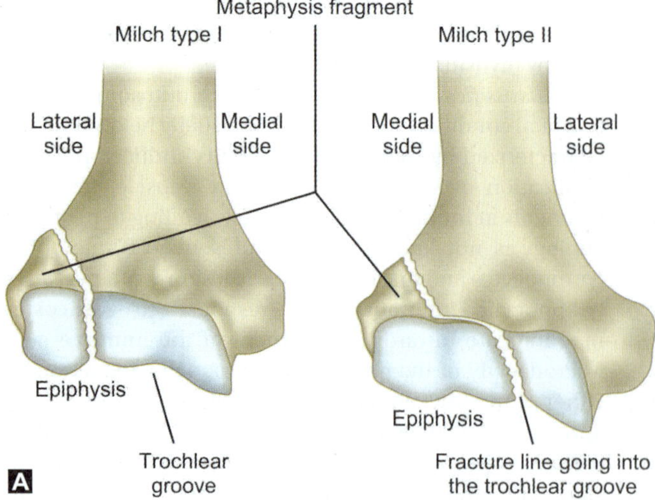

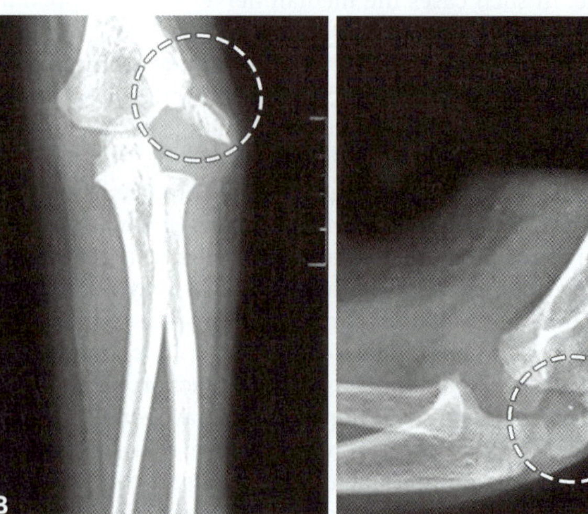

Figs 4.39A and B: (A) Milch classification of lateral condyle fracture; (B) X-ray of elbow anteroposterior and lateral views showing lateral condyle fracture (encircled)
Courtesy: Dr Sachin Ingole.

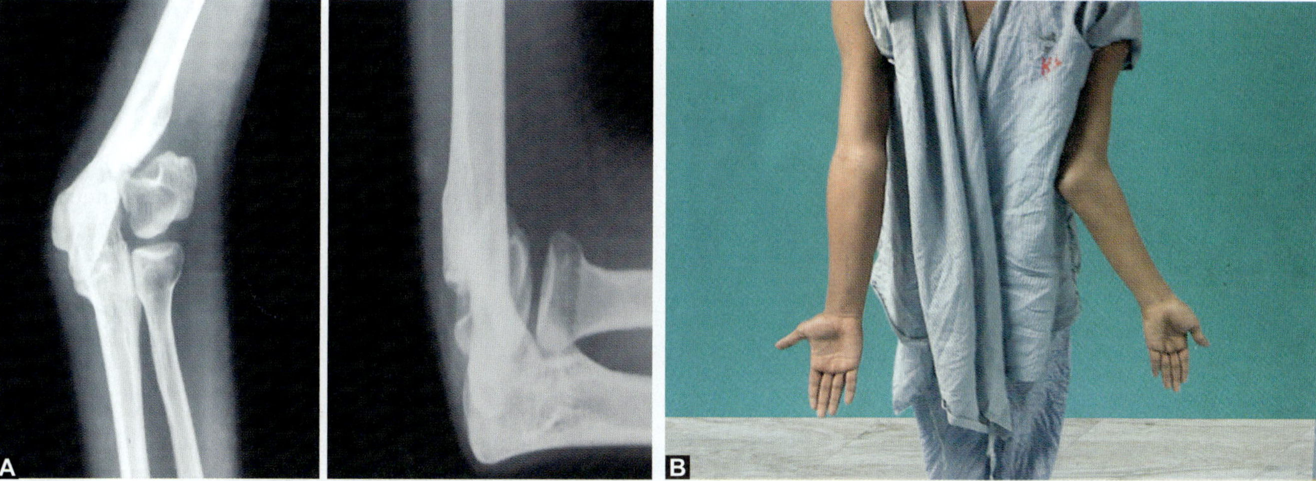

Figs 4.40A and B: (A) X-ray elbow anteroposterior and lateral views showing nonunion fracture lateral condyle; and (B) Cubitus valgus deformity following nonunion of lateral condyle fracture

patients are treated by open reduction and internal fixation with bone grafting. Late presentation of nonunion is either a painless mass or a cubitus valgus deformity **(Figs 4.40A and B)**. With increasing valgus, tardy ulnar nerve palsy may develop (due to stretching of ulnar nerve with increasing valgus). Severe cases are treated by corrective osteotomy (Milch osteotomy) with or without ulnar nerve transposition.

- *Angular deformities*: Cubitus valgus is more common than cubitus varus deformity due to lateral physeal arrest.
- Growth arrest and AVN are other rare complications.

MEDIAL EPICONDYLE FRACTURE

It is a common fracture in children between 5 years and 15 years of age. Ossification center of medial epicondyle appears about 5 years of age and unites with the humeral diaphysis between 16 years and 18 years. It is usually an avulsion injury and caused by falling on an outstretched hand when extended elbow is forced into valgus.

Diagnosis

The patient presents with pain, swelling and tenderness at the medial epicondyle. Diagnosis can be confirmed on X-ray **(Fig. 4.41)** but the findings may be difficult to interpret in young patients below 5 years of age as the ossification center is not yet ossified. Approximately 50% of medial epicondyle fractures are associated with elbow dislocation. X-rays may be compared with those of normal side to clinch the diagnosis.

Treatment

Undisplaced or minimally displaced (<5 mm) fractures are managed by immobilization in a sling for 2–3 weeks followed by range of motion physiotherapy. Intra-articular fragment should be removed urgently. Close extraction of entrapped fragment can be done by valgus stress on extended elbow and then supinating the forearm and extending the wrist. If close attempt fails open extraction should be done.

In displaced fractures good results have been obtained both by closed treatment and open reduction with internal fixation.

Complications

Joint stiffness is the most common complication and can be prevented by early range of motion physiotherapy. Ulnar nerve neuritis is also common, especially where the fracture fragment is entrapped in the joint. It is usually neurapraxia and improves with time. Nonunion may also occur and requires open reduction and fixation with K-wire with bone grafting.

DISTAL HUMERAL FRACTURE IN ADULTS

Distal humeral fractures account for 2% of all adult fractures. They are usually caused by direct fall on elbow. High-energy road traffic accidents are usually responsible for these fractures in young adults.

Classification

They are classified into three types [Arbeitsgemeinschaft Osteo-synthesefragen (AO)/Association for the Study of Internal Fixation (ASIF) classification, **Figs 4.42A to C**]:

1. *Type A*: Extra-articular supracondylar fracture
2. *Type B*: Partial articular (unicondylar) fracture
3. *Type C*: Complete articular (bicondylar) fracture.

Diagnosis

The patient presents with pain and swelling of the elbow. There is severe tenderness and crepitus of the distal humerus. A thorough neurovascular examination should be done. Diagnosis can be confirmed on X-ray **(Figs 4.43A and B)**.

Treatment

Undisplaced fractures are treated in an above elbow cast for 4 weeks, followed by range of motion exercises. Displaced supracondylar, unicondylar and bicondylar fractures in adults are treated with open reduction and internal fixation with plates **(Figs 4.43C and D)**. A severely comminuted distal humerus fracture in an elderly is best treated by elbow arthroplasty. An alternative in this situation is so called "bag of bones" treatment. The arm is held in a sling, till the pain diminishes. A hinged brace is applied and the patient is encouraged to move the joint. Fracture mostly

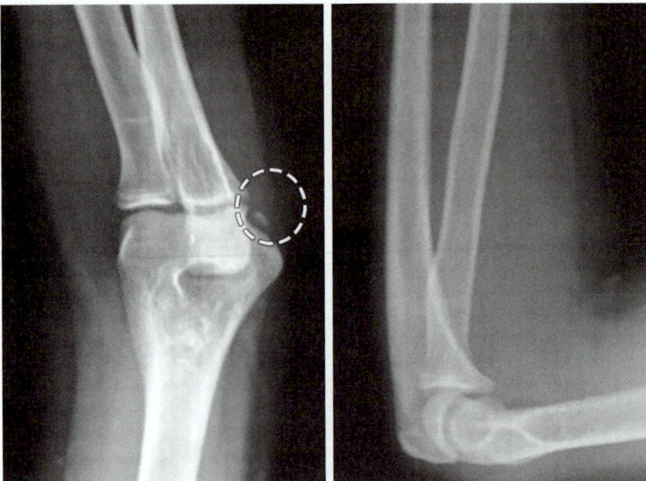

Fig. 4.41: X-ray elbow anteroposterior and lateral views showing medial epicondyle fracture (encircled)

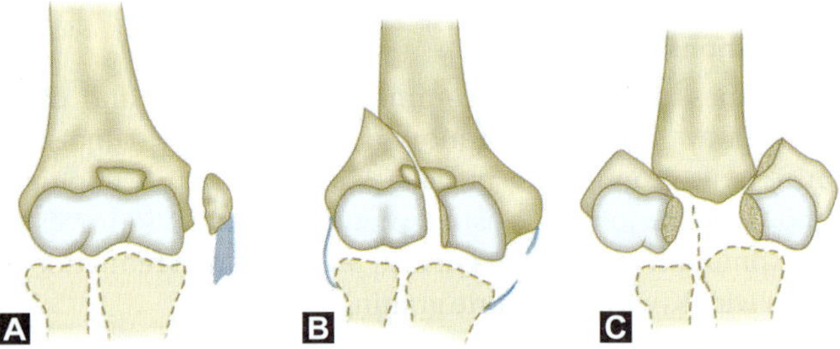

Figs 4.42A to C: Arbeitsgemeinschaft Osteosynthesefragen (AO)/Association for the Study of Internal Fixation (ASIF) classification of distal humeral fractures in adults

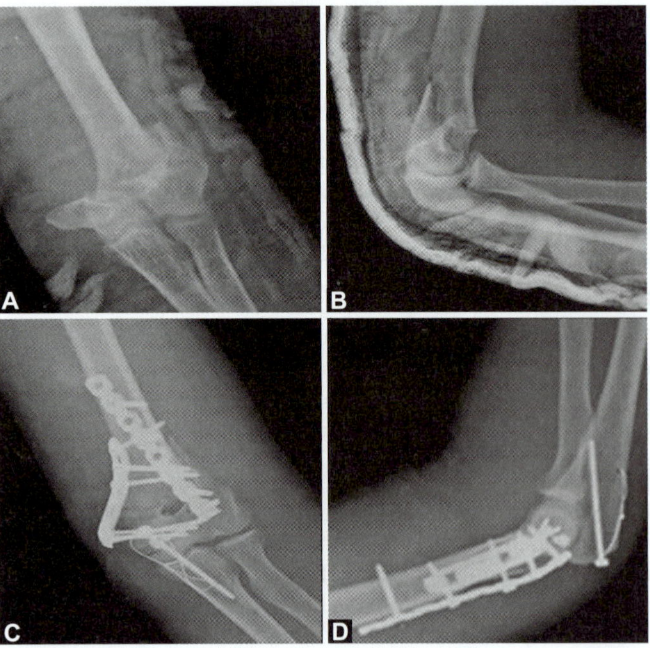

Figs 4.43A to D: (A and B) X-ray elbow anteroposterior (AP) and lateral views showing intercondylar fracture (type C) of humerus; and (C and D) AP and lateral views of the elbow after open reduction internal fixation (ORIF) with plates

unites in 6–8 weeks and a useful range of motion (45–90°) can often be attained.

Complications

Early

Neurovascular injury: Injury to the brachial artery, median and ulnar nerve may occur with fracture. A thorough neurovascular examination should always be done.

Late

Elbow stiffness: This is the most common complication of distal humerus fracture. Early range of motion should be encouraged to prevent it.

Myositis ossificans: This may occur following any fracture around the elbow and especially seen in fractures associated with severe soft tissue injury. Massage and aggressive movements should be avoided.

Malunion of fracture leading to cubitus valgus and cubitus varus may occur.

ELBOW DISLOCATION

Elbow dislocation is the second most common dislocation in orthopedic practice after shoulder dislocation. Although it is the most common dislocation in children, its incidence is particularly high in younger adults (10–20 years old). It is usually caused by a fall on the outstretched hand with the elbow in extension and forearm in supination. Posterior or posterolateral dislocation is more common (>90% cases) as the ulna is pulled back by the bulky triceps muscle inserted on the olecranon **(Fig. 4.28)**. It is associated with a tear of LCL and in more severe cases, both LCL and medial capsuloligamentous structures are torn. When associated with fractures of the radial head and coronoid process (Hotchkiss terrible triad of elbow), recurrent dislocation may result.

Classification

Elbow dislocation is classified as per the direction of displacement of ulna. Posterior or posterolateral dislocation is most common. Other types are posteromedial, lateral, medial, anterior and divergent type. Another way to classify is to divide into simple and complex types. A simple dislocation is one without a concomitant fracture while a complex dislocation is associated with a fracture around the elbow. Most commonly associated fracture is a fracture of the medial epicondyle of the humerus.

Diagnosis

The patient presents with swelling and obvious deformity of the elbow. Bony landmarks of the elbow (radial head, olecranon, etc.) are palpated at abnormal places. The ulna while translating posteriorly may button hole into the triceps causing bowstringing of the triceps. Diagnosis is confirmed with X-rays **(Figs 4.44A and B)**. A thorough neurovascular examination should be made.

Treatment

Dislocations without fracture are reduced by close maneuver. The patient is made in prone position with forearm hanging on the edge of the table. Traction is given on the forearm with the elbow in flexion. Forward pressure is applied on the olecranon

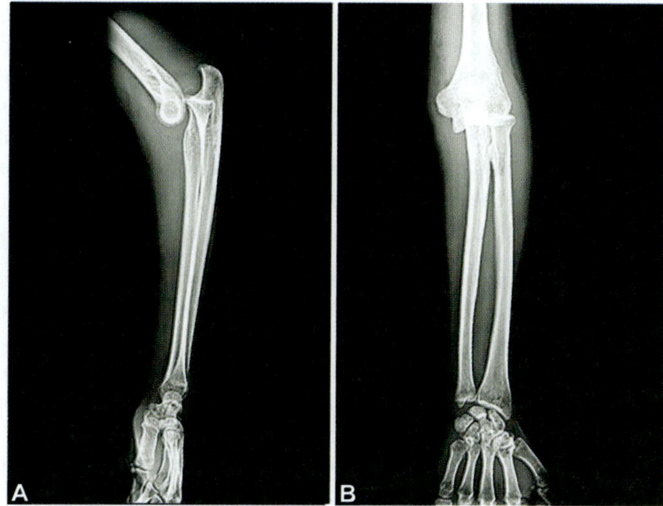

Figs 4.44A and B: (A) X-ray of elbow lateral; and
(B) Anteroposterior views showing posterior elbow dislocation

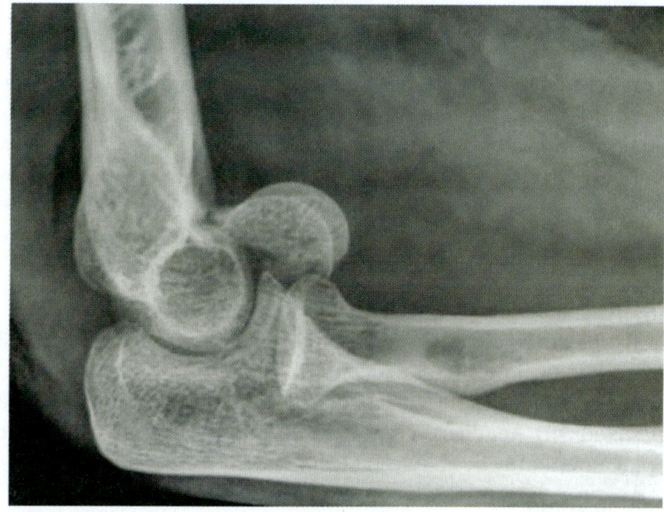

Fig. 4.45: X-ray lateral view of elbow showing capitellum fracture

and sideways deformity is corrected by direct pressure. After reduction, the elbow should be able to make full range of motion. It is put into cuff and collar sling for 3 weeks. For complex dislocations, ORIF of fracture and reconstruction of the torn capsuloligamentous structures are usually required.

Complications

Injury to the brachial artery, median and ulnar nerve should be looked for in all cases of elbow dislocations. The most common nerve injured in simple elbow dislocation is the median nerve while in complex elbow dislocations, it is the ulnar nerve that is generally injured.

Late complications are elbow stiffness, myositis ossificans and recurrent dislocations. Recurrent dislocations are often part of terrible triad and usually require ORIF with reconstruction of torn lateral capsuloligamentous structures. These surgeries usually involve reconstruction of the lateral ulnar collateral ligament.

HIGH-YIELD POINTS

- The elbow is the most common joint to dislocate in children (as shoulder dislocation is uncommon in children). Elbow dislocations are also very common in the second decade (13–15 years). However, in adults, it is the shoulder that is the most common dislocation while the elbow is the second most common major joint to dislocate.
- *Hotchkiss terrible triad of elbow injury*: Radial head fracture, fracture of coronoid process of ulna and a posterolateral dislocation of elbow.

PULLED ELBOW (NURSEMAID'S ELBOW)

Sudden subluxation of radial head out of the annular ligament occurs when traction is given on the hand of a child (aged 1–4 years) with extended elbow and pronated forearm. This commonly occurs when one tries to lift the child by holding his hand or distal forearm or when a child suddenly steps down while one of his parents holds him from the hand. Radial head comes out from the anterior portion of annular ligament upon pulling the pronated forearm. When traction is released annular ligament

gets interposed between the radial head and capitellum thus, prevents a spontaneous reduction. The injury is uncommon after 5 years of age as radial head by that age ossifies.

Diagnosis

A typical history and clinical examination clinch the diagnosis. The child starts crying immediately after having pulled or swung in the air by holding his hand. A click may be felt by the person while pulling the child. The child keeps his elbow flexed with forearm in pronation. He refuses to use his affected limb. If child allows examination, supination is found restricted. X-rays of the elbow are mostly normal.

Treatment

The radial head is reduced by flexing the elbow and rapidly supinating the pronated forearm. Again a click may be felt in the child's elbow while reducing it. The child stops crying and starts using his limb within minutes after reduction.

FRACTURE OF THE CAPITELLUM

This is a rare injury. The patient presents with swelling and tenderness in front of the elbow. Diagnosis is made on radiographs of the elbow **(Fig. 4.45)**. The fracture can present as either of two types. A Hahn-Steinthal type has a large osseous fragment of the capitellum while a Kocher-Lorenz type (aka uncapping of condyle) is predominantly a chunk of articular cartilage with minimal subchondral bone.

Undisplaced fractures are treated by immobilization in a sling for 2 weeks, followed by range of motion physiotherapy. Displaced fractures require open reduction and headless screw fixation. Joint stiffness is common, so early movement should be encouraged as soon as the pain subsides.

FRACTURE OF THE RADIAL HEAD

This is a common elbow injury in adults. A fall on the outstretched hand with the elbow in extension and valgus is the usual event which causes axial loading of radial head against capitellum leading to fracture of the radial head.

Diagnosis and Classification

The patient presents with swelling and ecchymosis of the elbow joint with painful elbow motion. Crepitation of the radial head may be felt with forearm supination and pronation movement. Diagnosis can be confirmed by anteroposterior and lateral views of the elbow joint **(Figs 4.46A to C)**. In case of doubt, a special view called as Greenspan view **(Fig. 4.46A)** can be taken to better visualize the radiocapitellar articulation. Based on the X-ray picture, the fracture can be classified by Mason's classification **(Table 4.3)**.

Treatment

Undisplaced fracture requires only sling immobilization for 3 weeks. Small nonarticular fragment (lateral one-third fragment) can be excised. The large articular fragment should be reduced and fixed with headless screw. In comminuted fracture prosthetic replacement may be required **(Table 4.3)**.

Complications

Joint stiffness is the most common complication and early motion should be encouraged to prevent it.

Osteoarthritis is a long-term sequel of intra-articular fractures of the elbow. It usually does not cause much disability.

Myositis ossificans is an uncommon complication.

FRACTURE OF THE RADIAL NECK

Fracture of the radial neck usually occurs in children. Falling on an outstretched hand with the elbow in extension and valgus is a common mechanism of injury. Diagnosis is made on X-ray.

Undisplaced or minimally displaced (<30° angulation) fracture is managed by rest in a sling or above elbow cast for 2 weeks. More displaced fractures require close reduction and cast immobilization. Percutaneous reduction using K-wire or open reduction with or without K-wire fixation may be required in severely displaced fracture where close reduction fails. Joint stiffness, shortening and cubitus valgus deformity due to physeal arrest or fracture malunion may complicate the fracture.

ESSEX-LOPRESTI FRACTURE

It is a fracture of the radial head with the splitting of interosseous membrane and distal radioulnar joint dislocation. This is also an unstable fracture and requires ORIF of the radial head with small headless Herbert screw or a radial head replacement to maintain the length of the radius. If in this fracture the radial head is excised, the radius will migrate proximally into the elbow restricting movements of the joint **(Fig. 4.47)**. If at all excision of the head is planned in such cases, it should always be delayed for 3 weeks to allow the interosseous membrane to heal up.

HIGH-YIELD POINTS

- For fixation of radial head fractures, screws are to be inserted in the nonarticulating zone (posterolateral part), called as a safe zone.
- In children, radial head excision should not be done as the radius may migrate proximally causing subluxation of inferior radioulnar joint and cubitus valgus deformity of the elbow.
- In Essex-Lopresti fracture and in terrible triad (fracture of the radial head and coronoid with elbow dislocation) radial head excision is contraindicated; rather it should be reconstructed.
- Metaizeau's technique is used for reduction of a displaced radial neck fracture. A wire is introduced through the medullary canal into the fracture fragment and rotated to reduce the fracture.
- Laugier's fracture refers to a fracture of the trochlea. It is an extremely rare injury often associated with elbow dislocation.

OLECRANON FRACTURE

This is a common fracture in adolescents and young adults. It is also called as Javelin throwers fracture as it is common in players involved in this sport. At other times it occurs due to direct fall on the tip of the elbow. Avulsion fracture of olecranon may occur in the fall on the hand with a partially flexed elbow with triceps muscle avulsing the fracture fragment.

Diagnosis

Pain, swelling and tenderness at the tip of the elbow are presenting features. Mostly it is a transverse displaced fracture as the proximal fragment is pulled away by triceps. In such cases often a gap can be felt at the fracture site. Active extension of the elbow joint may not be possible. Diagnosis can be confirmed on X-ray **(Figs 4.48A and B)**.

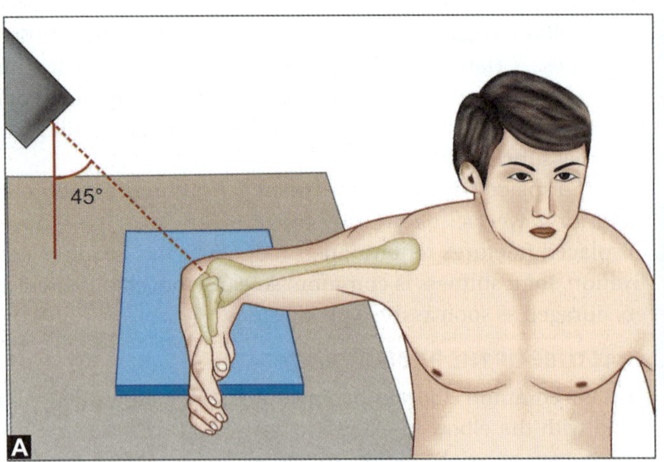

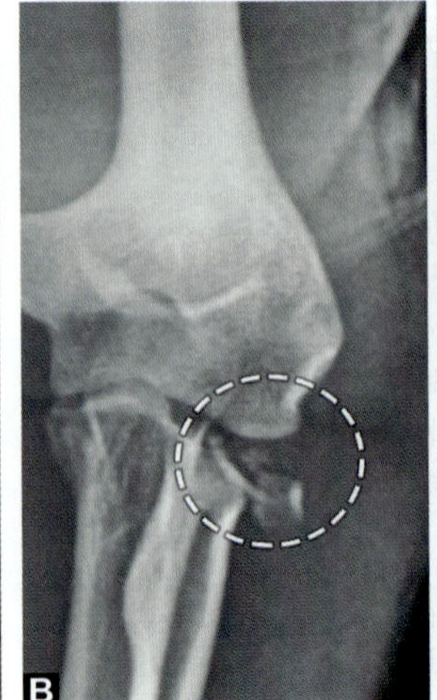
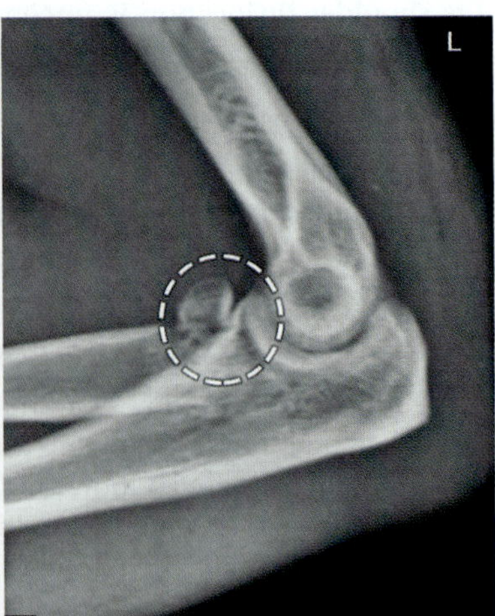

Figs 4.46A to C: (A) A patient being subjected to special Greenspan view for visualizing fractures of capitellum and radial head; (B and C) A fracture of the radial head (type III, circle) anteroposterior and lateral views

Table 4.3: Mason classification of radial head fracture and treatment

Type I	Undisplaced marginal fracture		Rest in a cuff and color sling for 3 weeks. Early active range of motion is allowed as soon as the pain subsides
Type II	Displaced fracture (fragment involving more than 30% of articular surface that is displaced more than 2 mm)		Open reduction and internal fixation with headless screws
Type III	Comminuted fracture		Radial head excision with or without prosthetic replacement
Type IV	Fracture associated with elbow dislocation		Repair of capsuloligamentous structure and ORIF of associated fractures

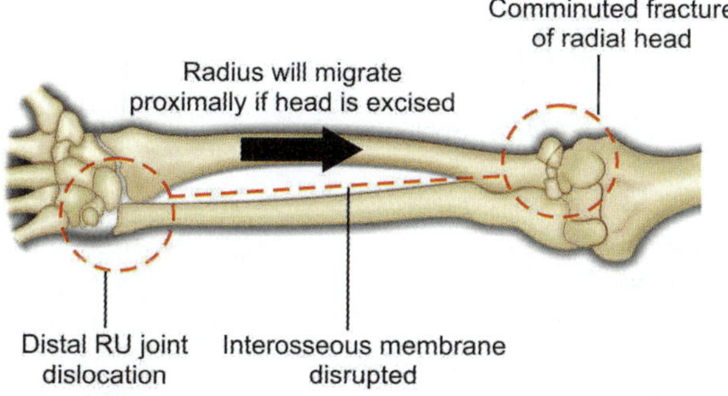

Fig. 4.47: Schematic depiction of Essex-Lopresti lesion

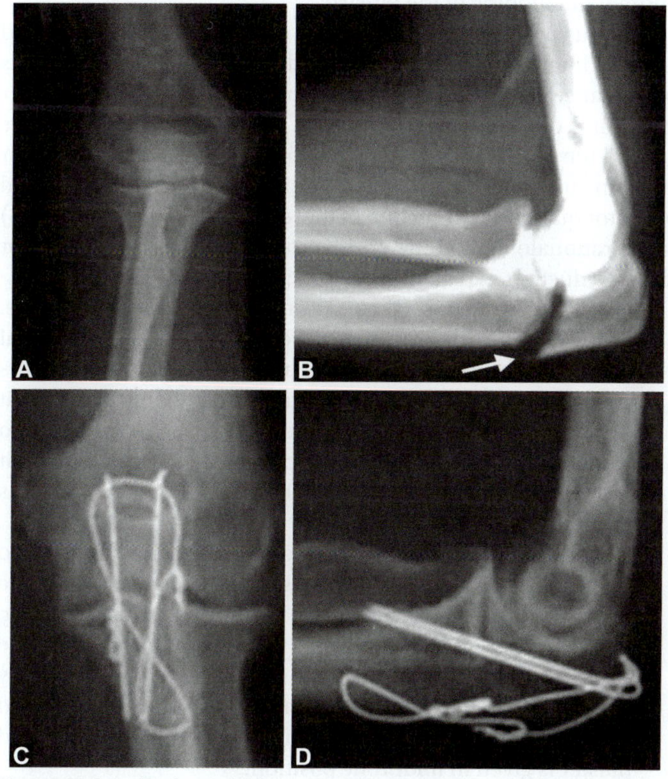

Figs 4.48A to D: (A and B) X-ray of elbow anteroposterior and lateral views showing fracture of the olecranon (arrow); (C and D) Open reduction and tension band wiring of olecranon fracture

Treatment

Olecranon fracture is classified into undisplaced, displaced and comminuted fractures. Undisplaced fractures require above elbow cast immobilization in 90° elbow flexion for 3–4 weeks, followed by a gentle elbow motion. Simple transverse displaced fractures require open reduction and internal fixation with tension band wiring (*see* Page 32) using screw and/or K-wires **(Figs 4.48C and D)**. Comminuted fractures require open reduction and plate fixation. An avulsion fracture of tip involving less than one-third of olecranon can also be excised in low-demand patients.

Complications

Elbow stiffness: As with other elbow fractures, it is common with prolonged immobilization. To prevent it, early elbow motion should be started after operative fixation. Treatment is range of motion physiotherapy.

Nonunion can result from inadequate reduction and fixation. Treatment is ORIF and cancellous bone grafting.

Osteoarthritis is a late sequel of imperfect reduction. Usually the patient can be managed symptomatically. In severe cases elbow replacement may be required.

HIGH-YIELD POINT

- The places where excision of bone is the treatment of choice—comminuted fracture of radial head, fracture tip of the olecranon, comminuted fracture of patella, etc.

INJURIES OF THE FOREARM, WRIST AND HAND

FRACTURE OF BOTH BONES OF FOREARM

Fracture of radius and ulna is a common diagnosis in orthopedic emergency. These are common in adults and are among the most common fractures found in children. The radius and ulna function as a unit and often fracture together. Most common mechanism of injury is falling on an outstretched hand. This usually causes a spiral fracture.

Relevant Anatomy

Radius and ulna are the two bones of the forearm. Radius has an apex lateral proximal curve and an apex medial distal curve. The ulna is relatively straight with apex posterior curve. In children deformity of these curves may occur without fracture (plastic deformity) and restoration of these curvatures is essential for optimal functioning of the forearm.

Radius and ulna are attached to each other at proximal and distal radioulnar joints and at the midportion by the interosseous membrane. Supination and pronation take place at the radioulnar joints and during these movements it is the radius that rotates around the ulna **(Fig. 4.49A)**. While biceps brachii and supinator assist in supination, pronation is achieved by pronator teres and pronator quadratus. Direction of these muscle forces **(Fig. 4.49B)** is the rationale behind the position of the forearm in a cast after closed reduction, explained as follows:

- In fractures, proximal to pronator teres insertion (i.e. fractures of the proximal third forearm), the proximal radius will be supinated by the attached supinators (biceps and supinator) while the distal radius will be pronated as it has only pronators (teres and quadratus) attached to it. So supinating the distal forearm in plaster is required to align it with a supinated proximal fragment and hence the plaster is given in supination.
- In fractures, distal to pronator teres insertion (but proximal to pronator quadratus), i.e. fractures of mid and distal shaft, the distal fragment is pronated by pronator quadratus. However, the proximal radius remains neutral (midprone) as the supinating forces of biceps and supinator get countered by attached pronator teres. Hence, the distal forearm is placed midprone in plaster, to align with the proximal fragment and plaster is given in midprone position.
- In fractures of the distal end (i.e. distal to pronator quadratus), the proximal radius fragment will be pronated by both the pronators attached to it. Hence, the distal fragment will have

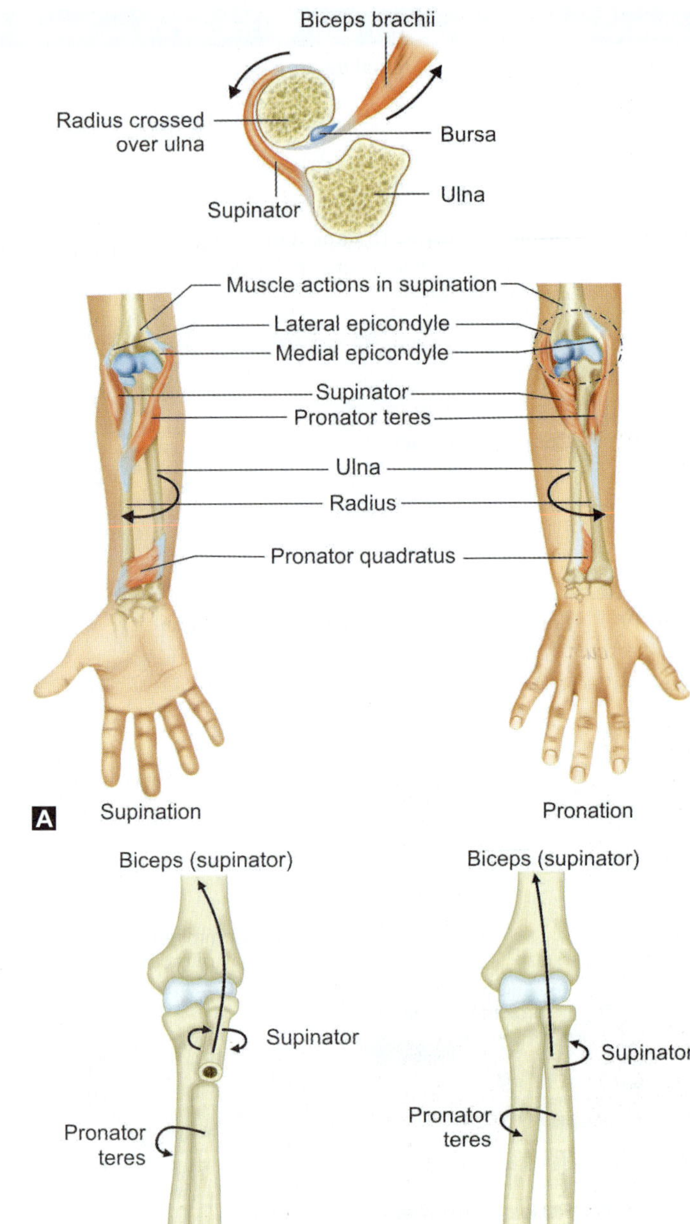

Figs 4.49A and B: (A) The anatomy of the forearm bones. See radius crossing over the ulna in pronation; (B) Muscle forces displacing forearm fractures. Only displacements of radius have been shown as it is radius that rotates around a stationed ulna

to be pronated as well, to align it with the proximal fragment. So, forearm in these cases is immobilized in pronation.

Clinical Features

Patients with both bones forearm fracture present with pain and swelling of the forearm. In displaced fractures, crepitus and obvious deformity may be present. In children, plastic deformation (bone bends without fracture) and green stick fractures are common and obvious signs of fractures may not be present. All patients with forearm fractures should be thoroughly assessed for neurovascular injuries. The diagnosis is easily confirmed on X-ray, AP and lateral views of the forearm **(Fig. 4.50A)**.

Treatment

In children, forearm fractures are mostly managed with close reduction and above elbow cast immobilization. Operative intervention (compression plating or flexible intramedullary nailing) is required only in irreducible fractures, open fractures or fractures with vascular injury and compartment syndrome.

In adults, an attempt may be given at closed reduction and plaster immobilization **(Flow chart 4.4),** but the same is difficult to achieve as reducing two bones simultaneously and maintaining reduction is very difficult. So mostly in adults, these factors need open reduction. Open reduction and internal fixation with compression plating **(Fig. 4.50B)** is the standard treatment of adult forearm fractures.

Complications

Early

Neurovascular injury: Nerve injury in forearm fractures is almost always iatrogenic (damaged during surgery by the surgeon). The posterior interosseous nerve is at risk in proximal radius fractures. Injury to radial artery may occur by displaced fracture fragment or during ORIF of radius fracture. However, due to presence of excellent collateral circulation, vascular injury to single forearm artery seldom causes any problem.

Compartment syndrome: Always keep an eye on the circulatory status of the forearm. The diagnosis should always be made on clinical ground of tense swelling and pain on passive stretching.

Late

Malunion: Inadequate reduction, loss of reduction or failure to maintain interosseous space in the cast may lead to angulation and rotational deformity. Rotational movements (supination and pronation) are worst affected in malunion. In severe functional deformity corrective osteotomy may be required.

Delayed and nonunion: Delayed union of one bone (usually ulna) is not uncommon. Immobilization may need to be extended in delayed union. Nonunion of one or both bone may occur. Inadequate reduction, insufficient immobilization and open fracture are more likely to end up with nonunion. Treatment of established nonunion is bone grafting and internal fixation.

Cross-union: A cross-union of the two bones may occur if fracture happens at the same level. An open fracture and a concomitant head injury to the patient further increase the risk of this complication (due to increased release of growth factors). It limits rotational movements and may require surgery to break the bony bridge between both bones.

MONTEGGIA FRACTURE DISLOCATION

It comprises of fracture of proximal third ulna with associated radial head dislocation (proximal radioulnar joint dislocation). This is more common in children and relatively rare in adults.

Mechanism of Injury and Classification

Based on the direction of the displacement of the radial head, Monteggia fractures are classified by Bado classification into four types **(Figs 4.51A and B)**. Type I is the most common (in children, young adults and overall). In adult, type II is the most common type. Although all these fractures are caused by a fall on an outstretched hand, the exact mechanism varies with the fracture type **(Table 4.4)**. Monteggia equivalents have also been described by Bado and some other authors for these fractures. Most common equivalents are fractures of the ulnar shaft with fracture of the radial proximal epiphysis or radial neck and anterior dislocation of the radial head.

Clinical Features

The patient presents with pain and swelling of the forearm. There is obvious deformity of the elbow. Radial head may be palpated at abnormal location. Elbow flexion, extension and rotational movements are painfully restricted. A thorough neurovascular examination should be done in all patients. The posterior interosseous nerve is the most commonly involved nerve by Monteggia fracture. Diagnosis is confirmed by X-rays. In X-ray, radial head should be carefully evaluated, if the fracture of ulnar shaft is seen. Normally in all degrees of flexion and extension a line passing through the longitudinal axis of radial head should pass through the center of the capitellum **(Fig. 4.52)**.

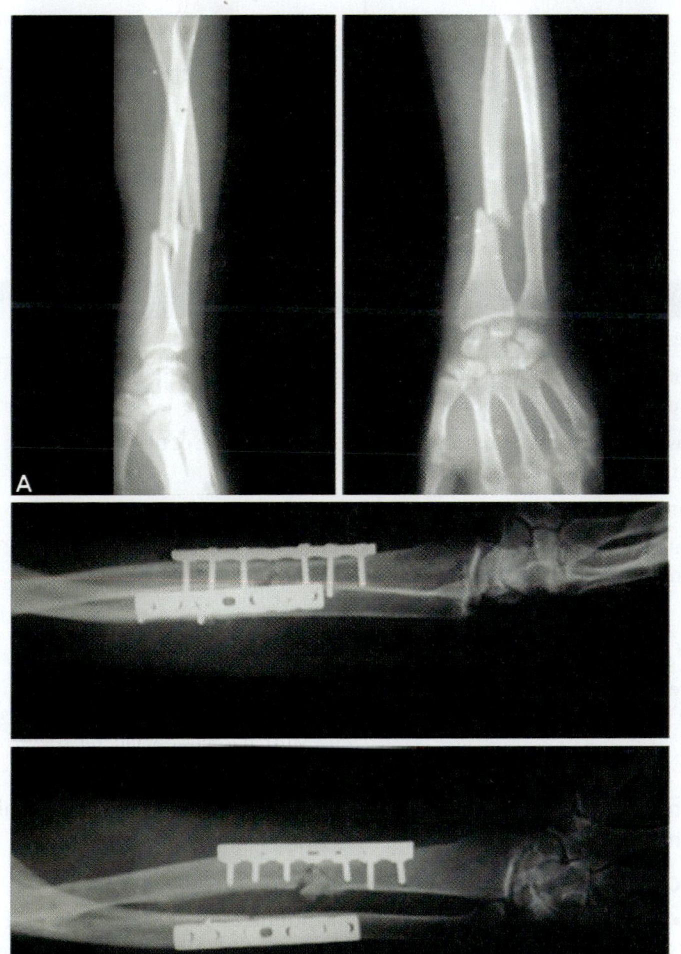

Figs 4.50A and B: (A) X-ray forearm anteroposterior and lateral views showing fracture in both bone forearm; and (B) Its fixation with compression plating

Flow chart 4.4: Closed reduction technique for both bone forearm fractures

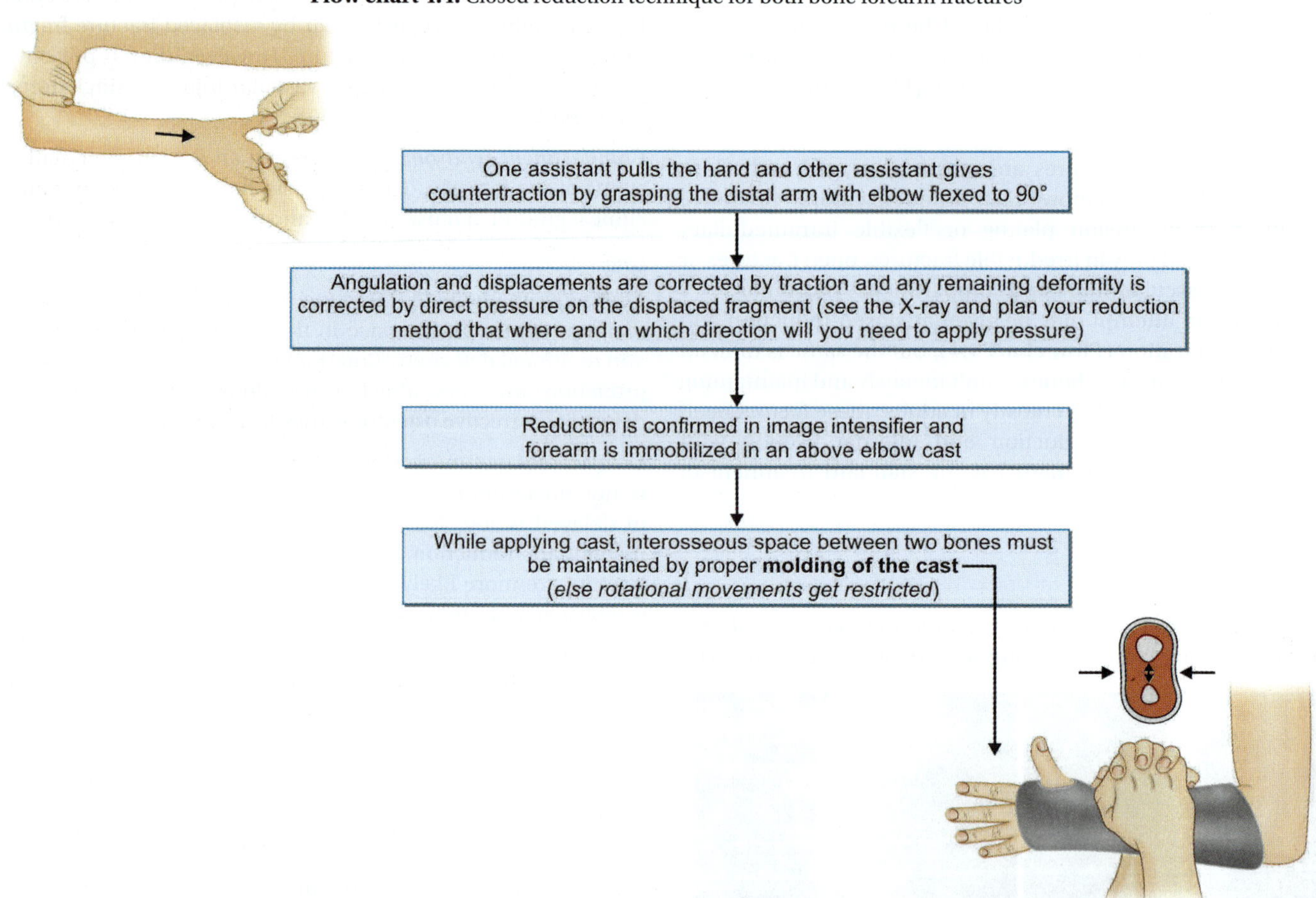

Table 4.4: Bado classification of Monteggia fracture

Bado type	Mechanism of injury	Description
Type I (most common in children and overall)	Forced pronation of the forearm	Anterior dislocation of the radial head with fracture of ulnar diaphysis at any level with anterior angulation
Type II (most common type in adults)	Axial loading of the forearm with a flexed elbow	Posterior dislocation of the radial head with fracture of ulnar diaphysis with posterior angulation
Type III	Forced abduction of the elbow	Lateral dislocation of the radial head with fracture of ulnar metaphysis
Type IV	Type I mechanism in which the radial shaft additionally fails	Anterior dislocation of the radial head with fractures of both radius and ulna within proximal third at the same level
Monteggia equivalents	(i) Isolated radial head dislocation	
	(ii) A proximal ulnar fracture with fracture of radial neck	
	(iii) Fracture of proximal third both bone forearm with radial fracture being more proximal	
	(iv) An ulnohumeral dislocation	

Treatment

Closed reduction and casting in Monteggia fractures is primarily reserved for pediatric population. The anatomical relationship of head of radius and capitellum should be achieved in all cases by concentric reduction of the radial head. Hence, in adults open reduction and internal fixation with plate and screws has become a standard practice (Fracture of Necessity, *see* Page 35). ORIF of ulna usually reduces radial head. If the radial head does not get reduced in place after ORIF of ulna then open reduction of radial head should also be done.

Complications

- Stiffness may result from immobilization or myositis ossificans. Early and active physiotherapy may restore range of motion after immobilization. Massage and aggressive, passive exercises should be discouraged as it may provoke the formation of myositis mass.

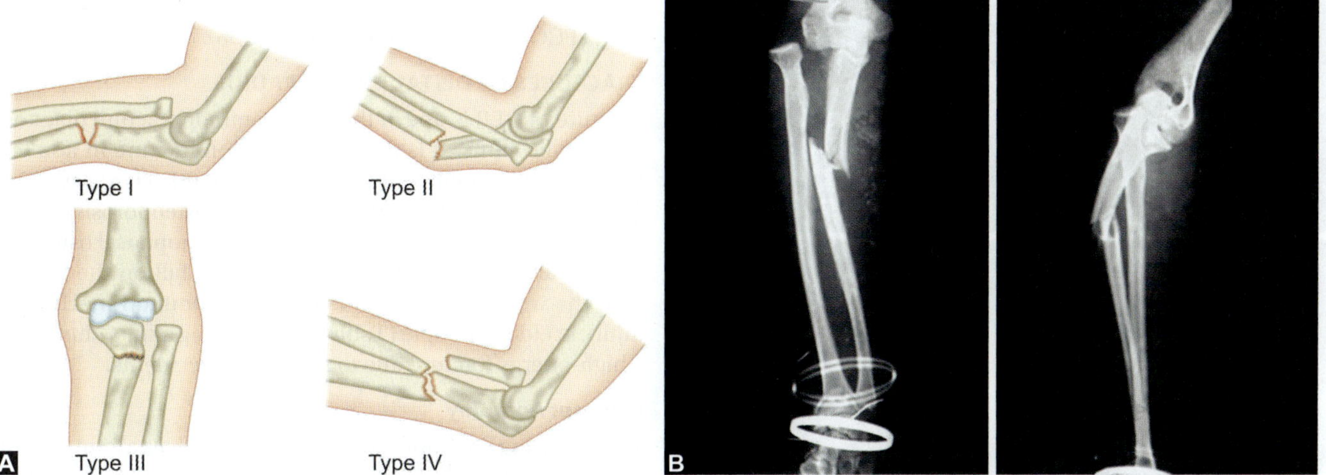

Figs 4.51A and B: (A) Bado classification of Monteggia fracture (types I to IV); and (B) X-ray forearm anteroposterior and lateral views showing Bado type I of Monteggia fracture

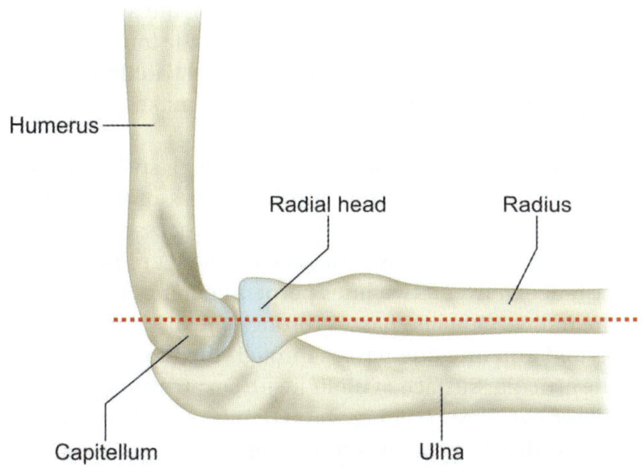

Fig. 4.52: Anatomical relationship of head of radius and capitellum (radiocapitellar line)

- Malunion is common in conservatively treated Monteggia fractures. Restoration of ulnar length and concentric reduction of radial head should be done in all cases. In malunited cases elbow flexion and rotational movements are restricted. Osteotomy of ulna with or without radial head excision may be required.
- Posterior interosseous nerve is the most commonly injured nerve, most commonly being involved in type II and III fractures. Fortunately, in most cases it is neurapraxia only and functions usually return within 3 weeks. If no recovery is seen by 3 months and electromyography and nerve conduction tests show no signs of innervation, the nerve should be explored.
- Compartment syndrome and Volkmann's ischemic contracture may occur following any forearm fracture. Diagnosis should be made on clinical ground. Urgent fasciotomy is the treatment of choice for established compartment syndrome.

GALEAZZI FRACTURE DISLOCATION (PIEDMONT'S FRACTURE)

A Galeazzi fracture refers to a fracture of the radial diaphysis at the junction of the middle and distal thirds with associated disruption of the distal radioulnar joint **(Fig. 4.53A)**. This is an unstable fracture and usually caused by a fall on an outstretched hand. It is almost three times more common than a Monteggia fracture dislocation.

Diagnosis

The patient presents with pain, tenderness, crepitus and deformity of the forearm. Instability of distal radioulnar junction (DRUJ) should be suspected in all patients with fracture of the distal one-third of radius. Fracture of the ulnar styloid process with large fracture fragment, difficulty in reduction and widening at the DRUJ in anteroposterior X-ray with or without balloting of distal ulnar end are indicative of unstable DRUJ that is a common association with this fracture. Diagnosis is confirmed on AP and lateral X-rays of the forearm.

Treatment

In children, these fractures can be treated by close reduction and above elbow cast application. Irreducible fractures in children and Galeazzi fracture in adults must be treated by open reduction and internal fixation with compression plating **(Fig. 4.53B)**. Since this fracture always requires open reduction and internal fixation, it is also called as Fracture of Necessity (*see* Page 35). During fixation it is imperative to ensure adequate reduction of DRUJ and restoration of radial length.

Complications

Malunion, nonunion and instability of the DRUJ are the usual complications.

HIGH-YIELD POINTS

- Monteggia first described the ulnar fracture in 1814 but the term was coined by Bado in 1967.
- Radial head dislocation in Monteggia fracture (or its equivalents) is traumatic. However, a congenital dislocation

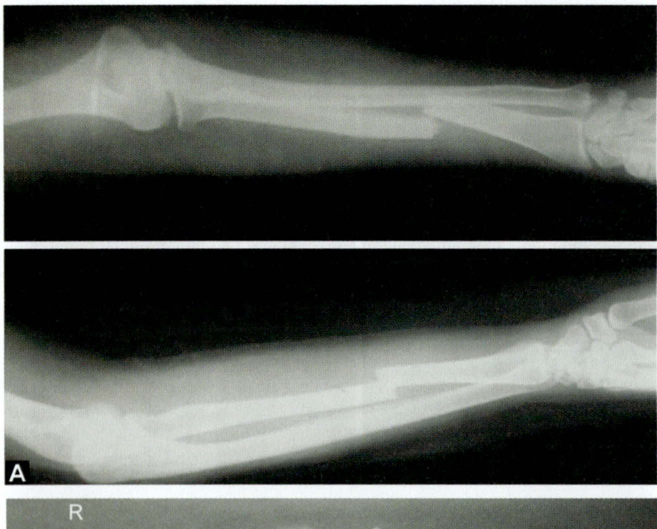

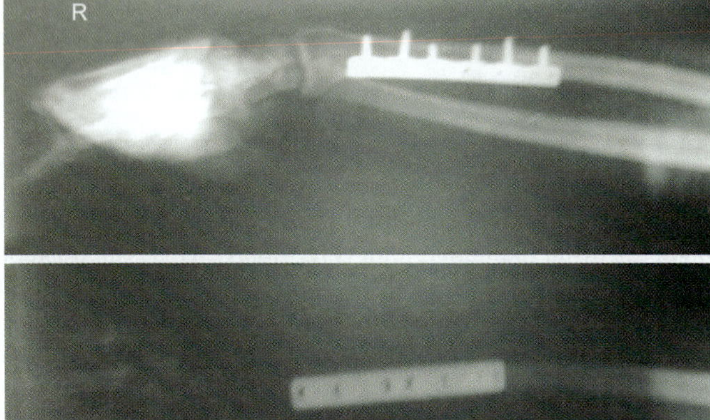

Figs 4.53A and B: (A) X-ray of forearm anteroposterior (AP) and lateral views showing Galeazzi fracture dislocation; (B) Open reduction internal fixation (ORIF) with compression plating of same fracture

of radial head is also known. While a traumatic dislocation of the radial head is mostly anterior, congenital dislocations of radial head are often bilateral and posterior. In X-ray radial head is seen enlarged and elliptical due to lack of modulation by capitellum. Capitellum may also be seen flattened in congenital cases.

- *Hume's fracture:* This is basically a Monteggia variant occurring in children where there is fracture of olecranon (i.e. proximal ulna) along with anterior dislocation of radial head.
- *Nightstick fracture*: It is isolated fracture of shaft of ulna that occurs in an attempt to resist a lathi blow to the forearm.
- *Reverse Galeazzi fracture*: This is a fracture of the distal ulna with associated disruption of the distal radioulnar joint.
- In irreducible Galeazzi fractures entrapment of the extensor carpi ulnaris tendon is a common cause and may require open reduction by a small separate incision at the wrist.
- *Piano key sign*: Ballotting (up and down movements as in pressing a piano key) of distal ulnar end can be demonstrated in instability of the DRUJ. It is seen in Galeazzi fracture dislocation, Madelung deformity (*see* Page 378) of distal end

radius (DER) and tear of triangular fibrocartilage complex (TFCC) injury (**Fig. 4.61** and Page 96).

FRACTURES OF DISTAL END OF RADIUS

Fracture of DER is one of the most common fracture diagnosis in orthopedic clinic. It is the most common fracture in adults who give a history of a fall on an outstretched hand. It is a very common fragility fracture (occurring secondary to osteoporosis) in elderly and its highest incidence is seen in postmenopausal osteoporotic women and it rises with age. Low-energy fall on the wrist joint with the wrist in extension is the most common mechanism of injury in elderly people (**Table 4.5**). In young adults, this is usually a high-energy fracture due to road traffic accidents.

Relevant Anatomy

The following are important anatomical indices around DER:
- *Volar (palmar) tilt:* Normally distal end of radius has a palmar or a volar, tilt i.e. in a lateral view of the wrist, the angle between the longitudinal axis of radius and a line tangential to the slope of the dorsal-to-volar surface of the radius makes an angle of 11° (**Fig. 4.54A**).
- *Radial inclination (RI)*: In PA view of the wrist, the angle between a line drawn perpendicular to the long-axis of radius and a line drawn from the tip of radial styloid process to the ulnar corner of distal end of the radius makes an angle of 22° (**Fig. 4.54B**).
- *Radial length (RL, Fig. 4.54C)*: Radial styloid process is about 1-cm distal to the styloid process of ulna (except in supination when the radial and ulnar processes come at same level). Radial length is measured on the PA radiograph as the distance between two lines perpendicular to the long-axis of the radius. One line passes through the distal tip of the radial styloid and one line passes through the most distal point on the articular surface of ulnar head. On an average it is 11 mm.
- *Ulnar variance (UV, Fig. 4.54D)*: It is the difference in levels of the distal articular surfaces of radius and ulna. Normal ulnar variance is negative, i.e. ulnar articular surface is slightly proximal to that of the articular surface of the radius. A positive ulnar variance means ulna projects more distally than radius.

Eponyms for Distal Radius Fractures

Many eponyms have been used to describe different types of distal end of radius fractures:
- *Colles' fracture*: This is the most common subtype. It is a fracture of the distal end of radius at the corticocancellous (metaphyseal-diaphyseal) junction with dorsolateral displacement of the distal fragment. It occurs due to a fall on an outstretched hand with a pronated forearm and dorsiflexed (extended) wrist.
  - *X-ray features*: AP and lateral views of wrist joint show transverse fracture of radius at corticocancellous junction. Typical displacements of distal fragment in Colles' fracture are supination, impaction into the proximal fragment, dorsal tilt and displacement and lateral tilt and displacement producing typical dinner fork deformity (**Figs 4.55A to C**).
- *Smith's fracture (reverse Colles' fracture, Figs 4.56A and B)*: It is caused by a fall on the dorsal aspect of the hand (flexed hand).

Table 4.5: Differences in distal end radius fracture in elderly and young adults

	Mechanism of injury	*Geometry of fracture*	*Sex distribution*
Elderly people	Simple fall on extended wrist	Usually extra-articular	Much more common in elderly females
Young adults	High-energy road traffic accident or sport	High incidence of intra-articular fracture	Equal sex distribution

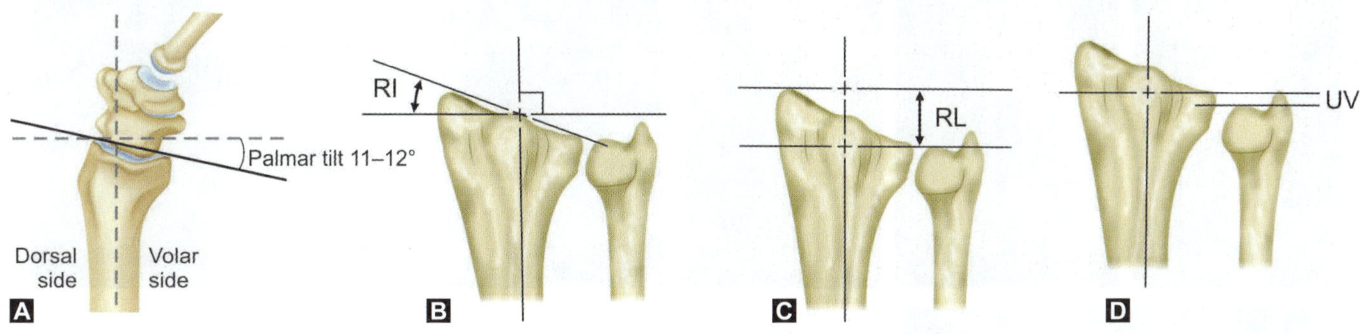

Figs 4.54A to D: Important indices around distal end radius

Abbreviations: RI, radial inclination; RL, radial length; UV, ulnar variance.

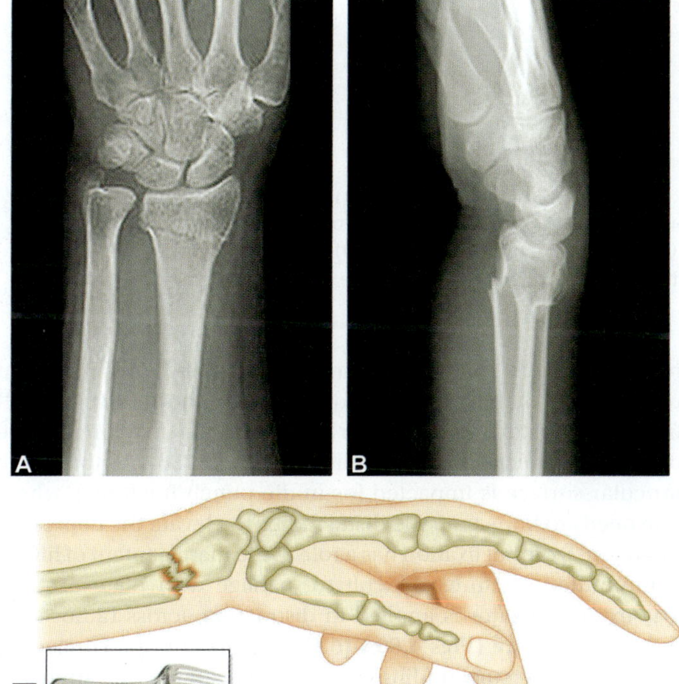

Figs 4.55A to C: (A and B) X-ray of wrist joint anteroposterior and lateral views showing—Colles' fracture; (C) Lateral view with resemblance to the dinner fork, hence the name "dinner fork deformity"

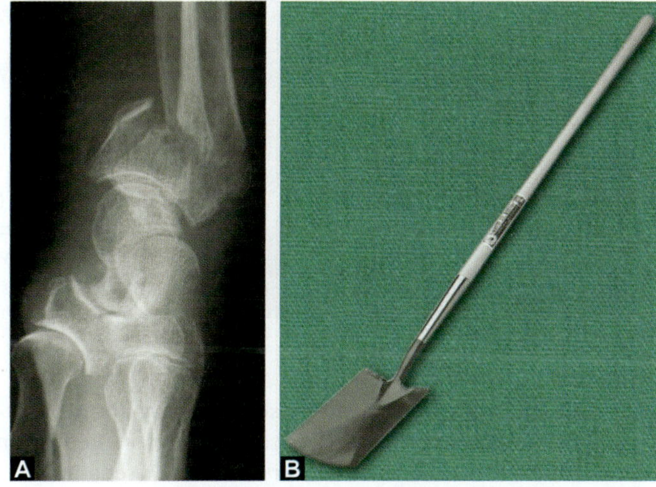

Figs 4.56A and B: (A) X-ray lateral views of wrist showing Smith fracture; and (B) Typical resemblance with a garden spade

It is similar to Colles' fracture except that the distal fragment is displaced anteriorly (volar/ventral displacement and tilt) producing garden spade deformity.

- *Barton's fracture (**Figs 4.57A and B**)*: Unlike the above two extra-articular subtypes, this is an intra-articular fracture through the distal articular surface of the radius, taking a margin of radius along with the attached carpals, either anteriorly (volar Barton) or posteriorly (dorsal Barton). Volar Barton is more common than Dorsal Barton fracture.
- *Chauffeur's fracture (**Fig. 4.57C**)*: Isolated fracture of the radial styloid process.
- *Di punch fracture (**Fig. 4.57D**)*: It is a comminuted impacted fracture of the distal end of radius resulting in a depressed fracture of only the lunate fossa of distal radius (lateral articular surface remains intact).

Diagnosis

Patients, usually osteoporotic postmenopausal females, present with pain, swelling and obvious deformity of the wrist joint. An AP and lateral X-ray views of the wrist confirm the diagnosis. The most common associated fracture visible in most X-rays is a fracture of the ulnar styloid process.

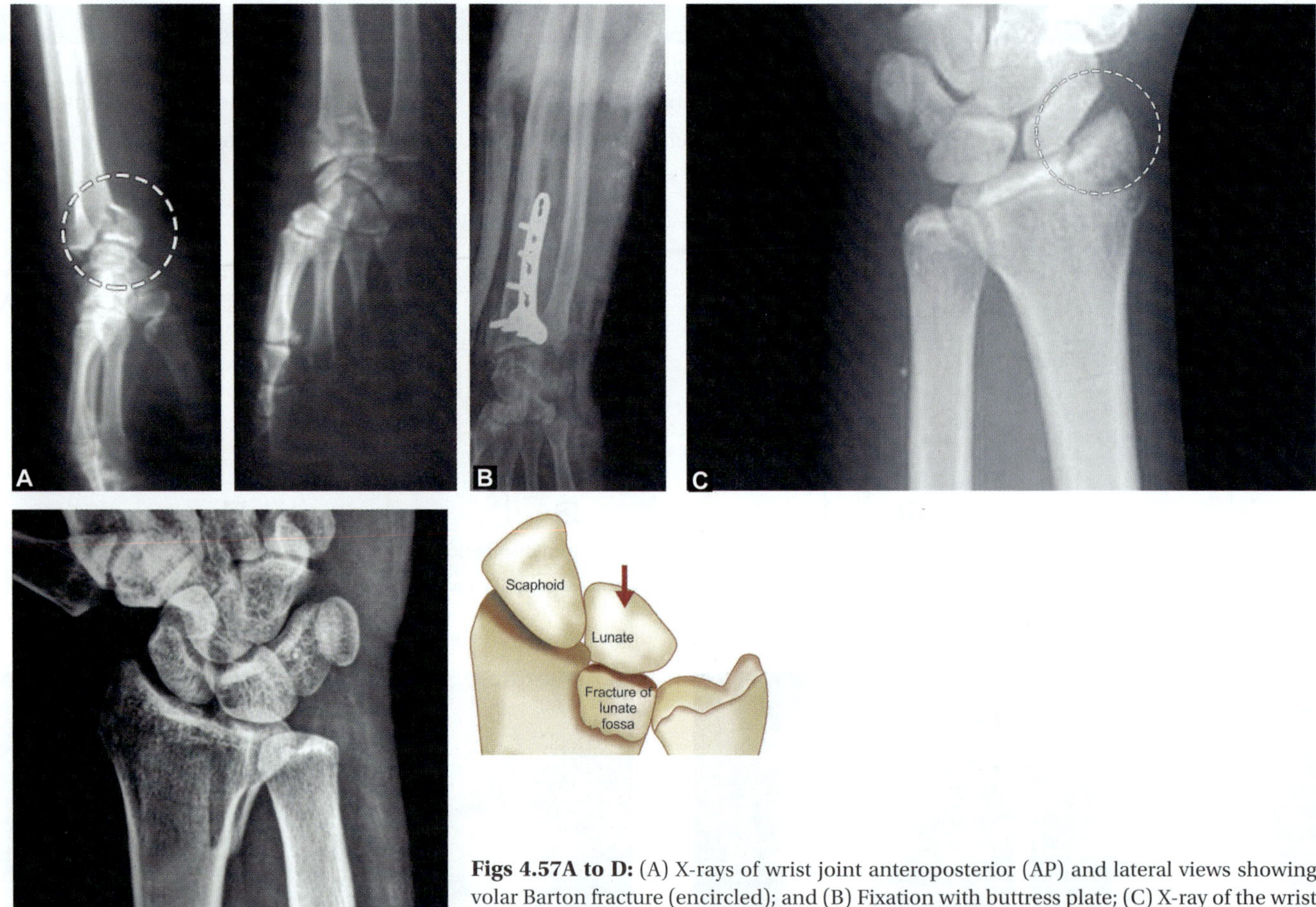

Figs 4.57A to D: (A) X-rays of wrist joint anteroposterior (AP) and lateral views showing volar Barton fracture (encircled); and (B) Fixation with buttress plate; (C) X-ray of the wrist joint AP view showing Chauffeur's fracture (encircled); (D) Schematic representation of a die punch fracture of the distal end of the radius (see the intact lateral part of the radial articular surface)

Treatment

Colles' fracture is mostly managed conservatively by closed reduction and below elbow plaster of Paris cast application. Reduction is done under hematoma block, axillary block or IV sedation.

One assistant holds the arm with elbow in 90° flexion and one assistant holds the fingers to give the longitudinal traction across the fracture (to disimpact the fracture). Reduction is achieved by direct pressure on the displaced fragment. The cast is traditionally applied in palmar flexion and ulnar deviation (handshaking pattern) and pronation to counteract the displacements **(Figs 4.58A to D)**. Excessive palmar flexion should be avoided. Many studies have shown no benefit of palmar flexion compared to neutral position. Recently there have been increasing trends towards immobilizing the Colles' fracture in neutral position. Conventionally cast is given for 6 weeks. The patient is encouraged to move his fingers, elbow and shoulder while in the cast to prevent stiffness, a very common problem with these fractures.

In Smith fracture, after disimpaction of distal fragment by longitudinal traction as in Colles' fracture, reduction is achieved by full supination and dorsiflexion of the wrist.

Operative Indications for Distal Radius Fracture

An unstable fracture where closed reduction is being difficult to maintain with cast can also be fixed percutaneously (closed reduction) with multiple K-wires **(Figs 4.59A and B)**. Open reduction is mainly required for displaced intra-articular DER fractures (Barton or Chauffeur) and internal fixation can be done with special buttress plates **(Fig. 4.57B)**. At times the articular surface is impacted (as in die punch fractures), where one needs to bone graft the distal radius to elevate the depressed fragment. External fixation has a role in the management of highly comminuted fractures difficult to manage with plate fixation. The external fixator is applied in distraction across radiocarpal joint and fracture **(Figs 4.60A to C)**. It works on the concept of ligamentotaxis (surrounding capsule and ligaments are stretched and indirectly reduce the fracture fragments).

Complications

Early Complications

- *Tear of triangular fibrocartilage complex (TFCC)*: TFCC is a group of ligamentous and cartilaginous structures that connect the ulnar styloid process to ulnar carpus and distal end of the radius **(Fig. 4.61)**. It acts as a cushion between the distal end of the ulna and the ulnar carpus. Components of TFCC complex are: volar and dorsal radioulnar ligaments, ulnotriquetral and ulnolunate ligaments, ulnar collateral ligament, articular disc and extensor carpi ulnaris tendon sheath. TFCC transmits 20% load across the wrist and serves as the main stabilizer of

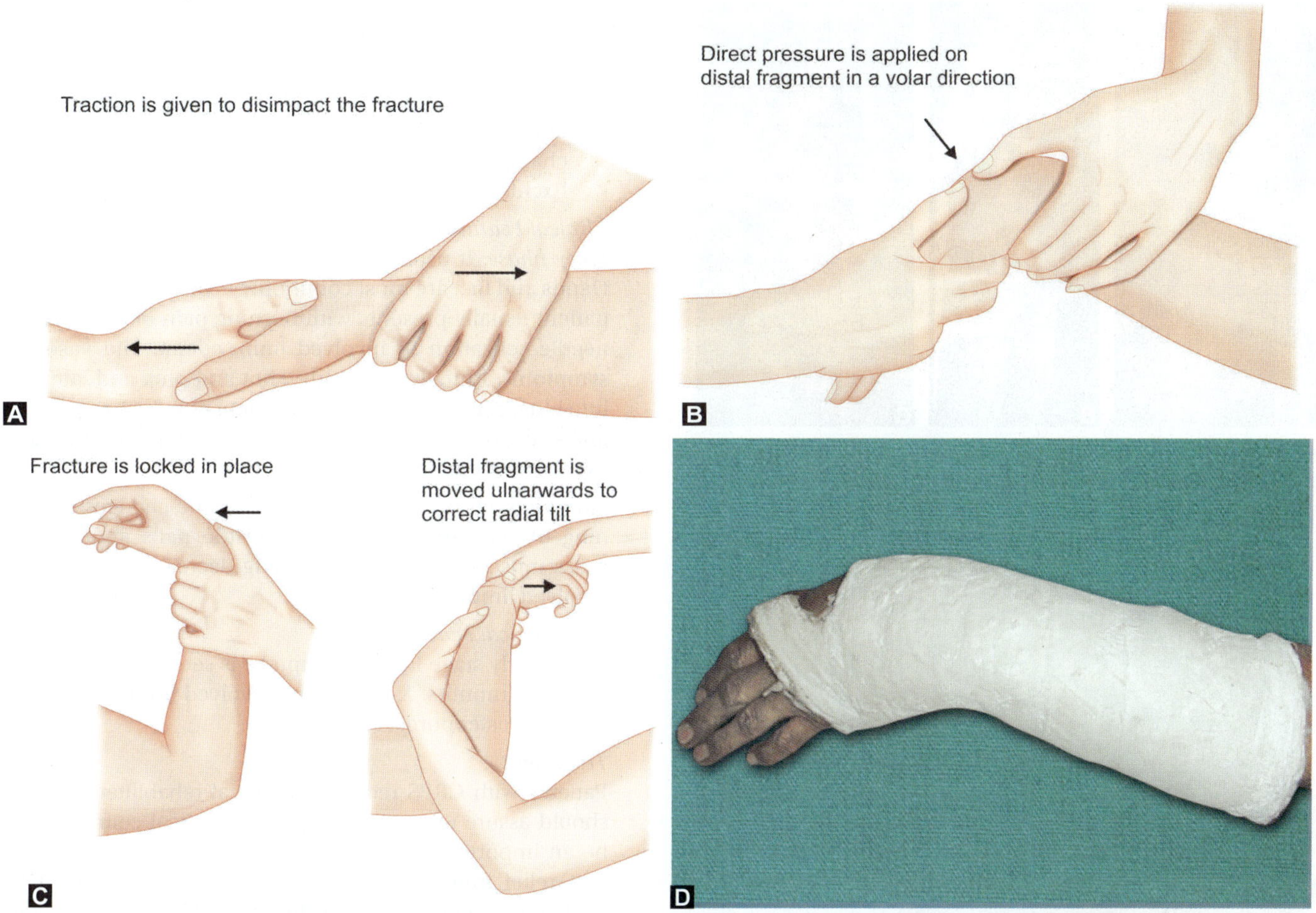

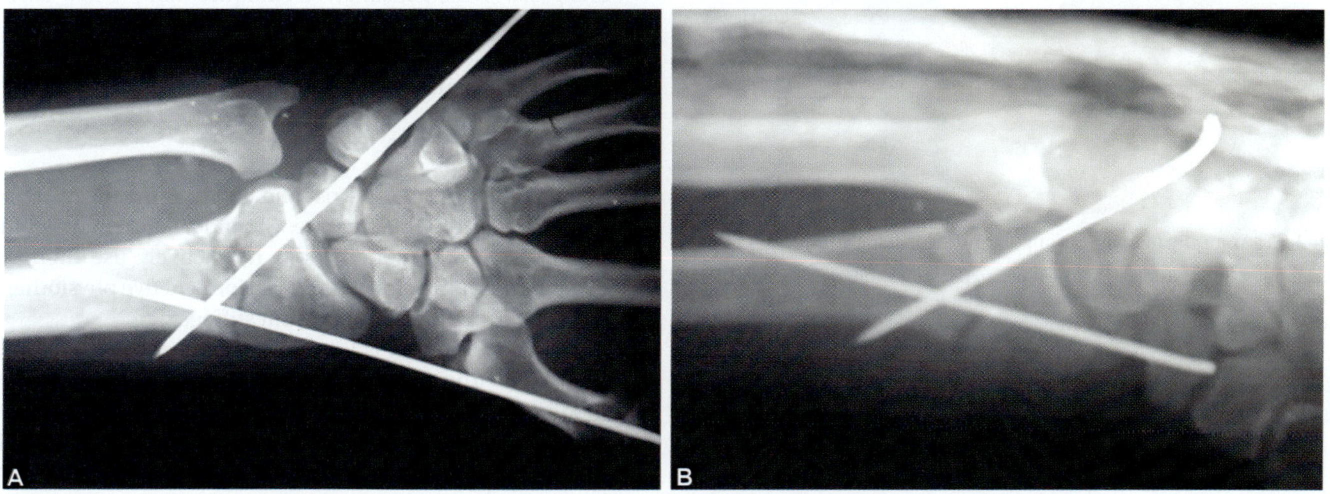

Figs 4.58A to D: Colles' fracture reduction. (A) Traction is given to disimpact the fracture; (B) Direct pressure on the distal fragment to reduce it; (C) Fracture is locked by palmar flexion and ulnar deviation; (D) Colles' cast in handshaking position

Figs 4.59A and B: X-ray wrist joint anteroposterior and lateral views showing percutaneous K-wire fixation of unstable distal end radius fracture

the DRUJ. Injuries to TFCC can lead to DRUJ instability and ulnolunate abutment causing wrist pain. Injuries to TFCC are seen in up to 40–70% intra-articular fractures of DER. In most cases there is an evident fracture of the ulnar styloid process.

Repair may be required when these injuries are associated with distal radioulnar joint instability.

- *Complex regional pain syndrome (CRPS):* Earlier this was known as reflex sympathetic dystrophy or Sudeck's dystrophy

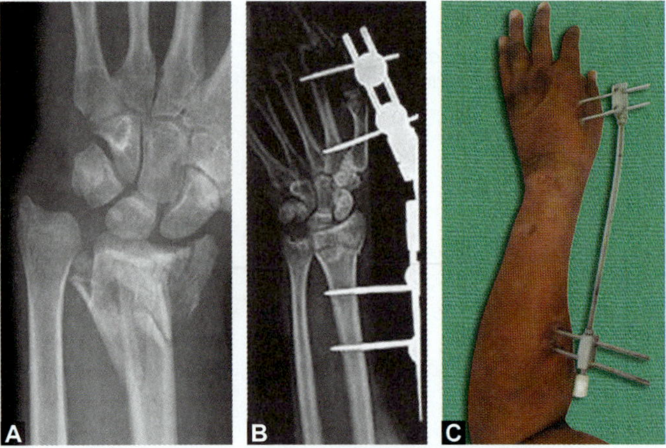

Figs 4.60A to C: (A) X-ray, anteroposterior view of the wrist joint showing comminuted fracture distal end of radius; (B) Fixation of same fracture by application of an external fixator in distraction mode (ligamentotaxis); and (C) Clinical picture of the use of external fixator for wrist fracture

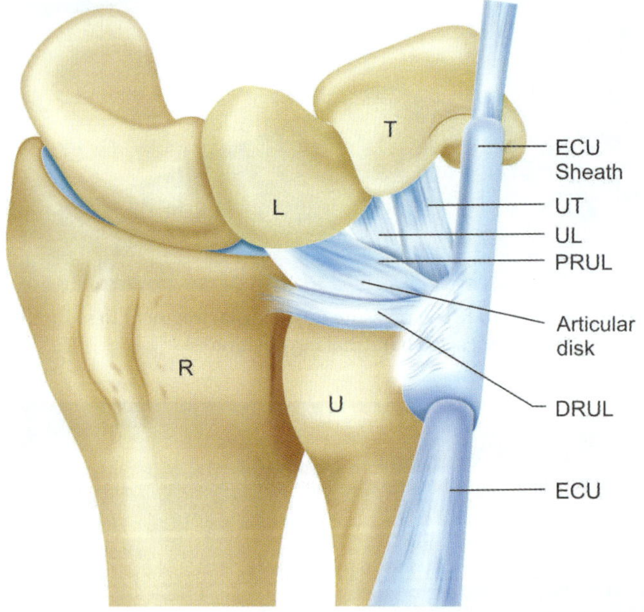

Fig. 4.61: Anatomy of tear of triangular fibrocartilage complex (TFCC)

Abbreviations: ECU, extensor carpi ulnaris; UT, ulnotriquetral ligament; UL, ulnolunate ligament; PRUL, proximal radioulnar ligament; DRUL, distal radioulnar ligament; L, lunate; T, triquetrum; R, radius; U, ulna.

or casualgia (meaning burning pain). It is a chronic pain syndrome usually involving one of the limbs that may follow a bony or soft tissue injury (CRPS type I) or a nerve injury (CRPS type II). The etiopathogenesis is not completely understood, but is thought to be an imbalance between the sympathetic and parasympathetic systems. Mild signs and symptoms of CRPS are seen in an approximate 40% of fractures and surgical trauma patients. However, the incidence of chronic and severe CRPS is less than 2%. Diagnosis is made primarily on clinical ground.

Diagnostic Criteria
- Presence of an inciting event
- Pain (burning in nature) disproportionate to this event
- Presence of signs and symptoms of autonomic imbalance like swelling, edema, vasomotor symptoms, trophic changes, etc.
- Exclusion of all other possible causes.

Clinical Features
Early phase: It usually begins weeks after an inciting event. Hands and feet are most commonly involved body parts. The patient usually presents with burning pain or with pins and needle sensation of involved limb, edema and vasomotor symptoms. Initially limb is dry, hot and pink and later turns into blue, cold and sweaty. The patient may have temperature and sweating abnormality (altered sensitivity to temperature, excessive sweating, etc.).

Late phase: It is characterized by trophic changes like thinning of skin, fragile hairs and brittle nails and in severe cases muscle contractures causing decreased movement of involved limbs.

Radiological Features
In the early stage increased uptake is seen in the bone scan. After 2–3 months, X-rays of the involved limb show marked localized osteoporosis.

Treatment
Patients with CRPS require functional rehabilitation. Doctor should assure the patient and psychological counseling may be an important part of treatment. The majority of patients gets relief from multidisciplinary approach treatment with analgesics, vitamin C, desensitization techniques and guided physiotherapy. A combination of NSAIDs and a centrally acting analgesic like amitriptyline may be given together for excellent analgesia. Desensitization techniques have been used to normalize sensation of the involved limb. Sympatholytic drugs, nerve blocks and surgical sympathectomy have also been used with variable success. Immobilization of the limb should be avoided.

Late Complications
- *Stiffness:* Stiffness of the wrist and fingers is the most common complication of DER fracture. Shoulder and elbow stiffness may follow if the patient does not actively use them after plaster immobilization of the wrist joint. Active physiotherapy should be encouraged to prevent stiffness.
- *Malunion:* Malunion is the second most common complication. It is particularly common following nonoperative treatment of distal radius fractures. Cosmetically Colles' fracture malunites to result in the classical Dinner fork deformity **(Fig. 4.55C)**. Loss of palmar tilt and radial inclination may cause loss of grip strength and pain in the DRUJ. Loss of rotational movement may occur with dorsal angulation. Corrective osteotomy may be required for symptomatic malunion with persistent DRUJ or midcarpal pain or weakness of grip.
- *Tendon injury:* Although rare, but extensor tendon injury, especially of extensor pollicis longus may occur at the time of Colles' fracture or later due to friction on callus or malunited

fracture. More often it is seen after 2–3 months of the fracture. Treatment is by tendon transfer.

HIGH-YIELD POINTS

- Most important deformity to be corrected while reducing Colles' fracture is radial length (impaction).
- Edema or swelling is most consistent sign of CRPS. Localized osteopenia (patchy osteoporosis) is characteristic X-ray finding.
- Although DER fracture is the most common cause of CRPS in upper limb the most common complication of DER fractures is stiffness followed by malunion.

FRACTURES AND DISLOCATIONS OF THE CARPAL BONES

RELEVANT ANATOMY

There are eight carpal bones in the hand arranged in two rows **(Fig. 4.62A)**. First row consists of scaphoid, lunate and triquetrum and pisiform. Pisiform is a sesamoid bone in the sheath of flexor carpi ulnaris tendon. Distal row is made up of trapezium, trapezoid, capitate and hamate. These carpal bones are kept in place by many intrinsic ligaments (interconnecting carpal bones) and extrinsic ligaments (connecting carpal bones to radius, ulna and metacarpals). Injury to these ligaments is also well known. A rupture of scapholunate ligament produces an abnormal gap (>3 m wide) between scaphoid and lunate. It appears on X-rays as the well-recognized Terry Thomas sign **(Fig. 4.62B)**, named after the famous British comic character who had a gap in between his central incisor teeth.

SCAPHOID FRACTURE

This is the most common carpal bone fracture. Scaphoid fracture is the most common fracture in young adults and adolescents with a history of falling on an outstretched hand and is rare in children.

Relevant Anatomy

Scaphoid bone consists of tubercle, waist and proximal and distal poles **(Fig. 4.63)**. In adults, fracture of waist followed by proximal pole is the most common while in children distal pole fracture is the most common. Scaphoid bone receives most of its blood supply from a single important blood vessel (branch of radial artery) that enters the scaphoid from distal pole and travels proximally across the waist to supply the proximal pole **(Fig. 4.63)**. Thus, vascularity of scaphoid bone reduces proximally

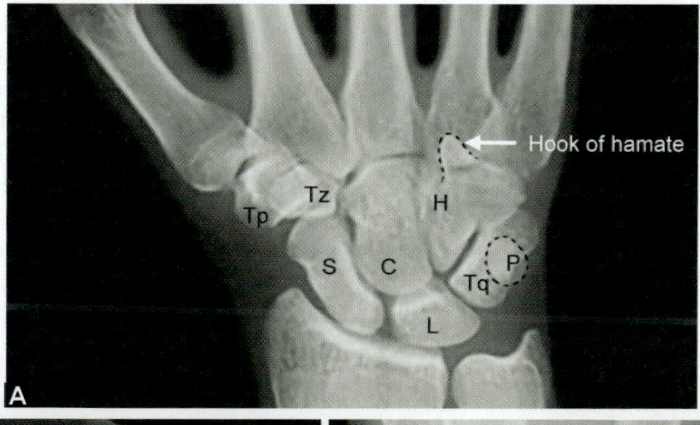

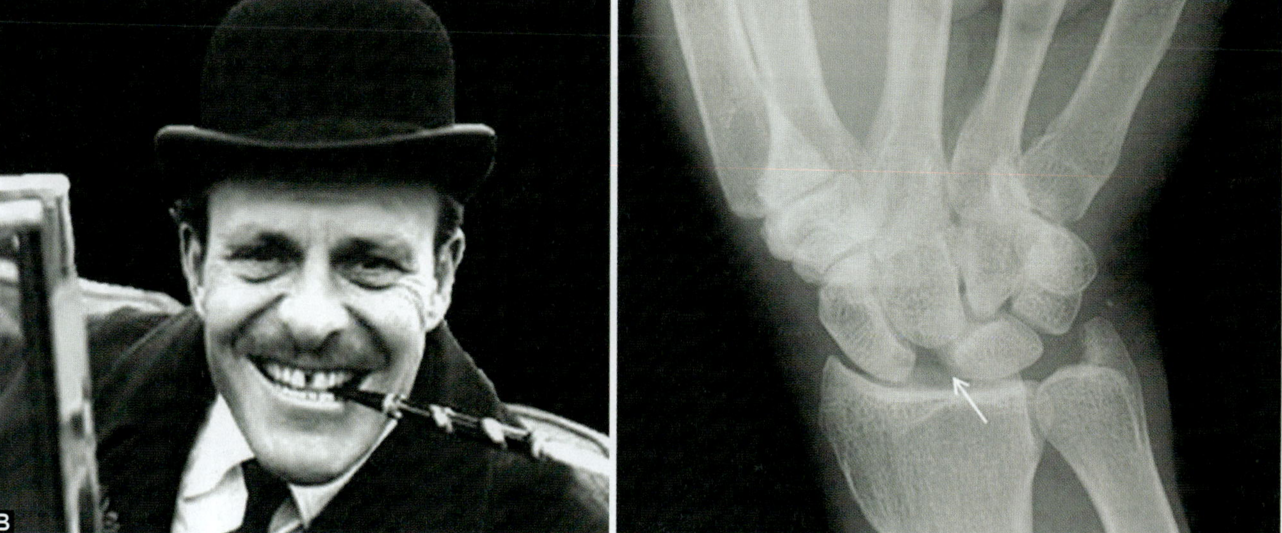

Figs 4.62A and B: (A) Carpal bones of hand; (B) Terry Thomas sign (arrow) as seen in rupture of the scapholunate ligament of wrist

Abbreviations: S, scaphoid; L, lunate; Tq, triquetrum; P, pisiform; Tp, trapezium; Tz, trapezoid; C, capitate; H, hamate.

Courtesy: Learningradiology.com.

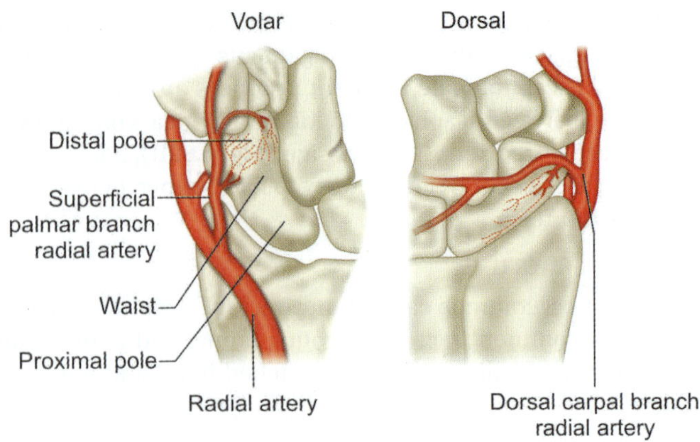

Fig. 4.63: Blood supply of scaphoid bone

(retrograde blood flow). Due to this precarious blood supply, fracture of waist of scaphoid can lead to AVN of the proximal pole of scaphoid.

Mechanism of Injury

It is usually a hyperextension injury caused by extreme dorsiflexion of the hand following a fall on an outstretched hand.

Clinical Features

The patient presents with wrist pain and swelling after acute fracture. Usually there is no obvious deformity. Tenderness in anatomical snuff box is a sensitive test for scaphoid fracture. Pain with axial compression of thumb, tenderness at scaphoid tubercle and painful thumb movements are other signs used for diagnosis of a scaphoid fracture.

Diagnosis

Diagnosis can be confirmed by AP, 45° oblique and ulnar-deviated AP X-rays of hand **(Fig. 4.64A)**. Undisplaced scaphoid fractures are often not visible on the initial X-rays. Therefore, X-rays should be repeated after 10–14 days if a fracture is suspected, by this time resorption occurs around the fracture ends and the fracture may become better defined. Magnetic resonance imaging (MRI) is the most sensitive and specific investigation to detect occult scaphoid fractures.

Treatment

Undisplaced scaphoid fractures are managed conservatively by cast immobilization. Scaphoid cast is given from below the elbow to just short of the MCP joints and also includes the proximal phalanx of thumb. The wrist is held in dorsiflexion and slight radial deviation and thumb forward in the glass holding position **(Fig. 4.64B)**. The cast should be given until a fracture unites which usually takes 6–12 weeks. In displaced scaphoid fractures (displacement with >1 mm step off or scapholunate angle >60°) percutaneous or open reduction and fixation with special headless screws (Herbert screw) is required. However, an important thing to remember is that since this fracture is often not visible in fresh X-rays, one has to apply the scaphoid cast if at all there is tenderness in the anatomical snuffbox.

Complications

Nonunion

It is seen in approximately 10% of cases and is more common in displaced and unstable fractures. A hump may form at the back of the wrist due to the angulation at the fracture site (hump back deformity). Factors associated with nonunion are fracture displacement greater than 1 mm, AVN and proximal pole fracture. If no radiological evidence of union is seen after 3 months of treatment, diagnosis of nonunion can be considered. X-ray features of nonunion of scaphoid fracture are subchondral sclerosis and resorption at the fracture site. Treatment of established nonunion is bone grafting (Matte Russe technique) and screw fixation. In unstable nonunion cystic changes, sclerosis and bony erosions lead to collapse of bone fragments and deformity. In Russe bone graft technique corticocancellous bone graft is wedged between fracture fragments and a compression screw is inserted.

Avascular Necrosis

It is a late and common complication of scaphoid fracture although slightly less common than nonunion. It is mostly seen

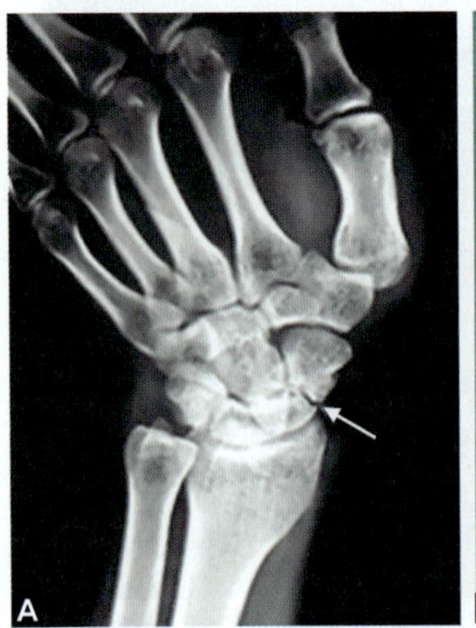

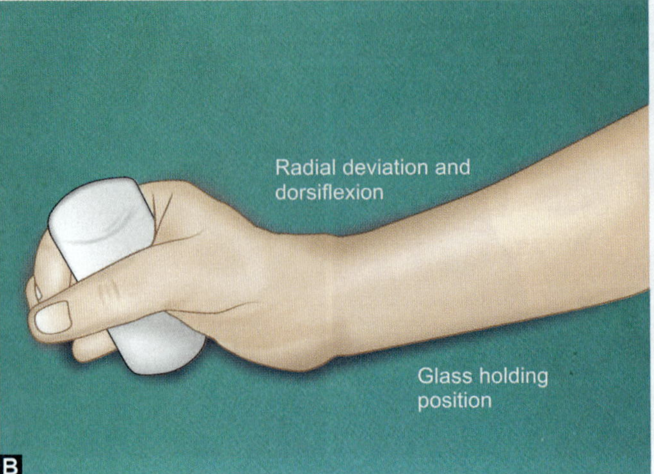

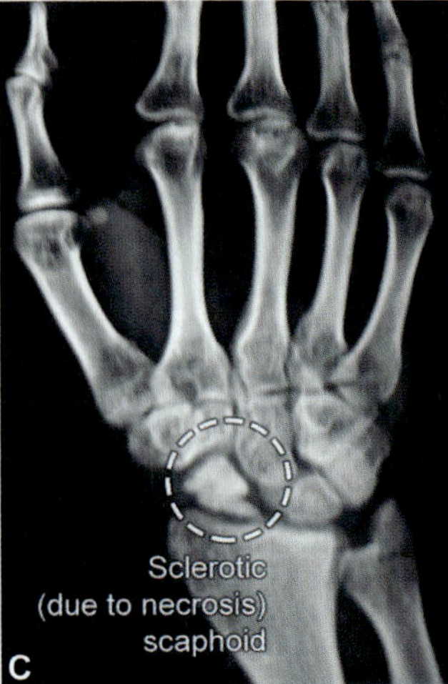

Figs 4.64A to C: (A) X-ray of hand (anteroposterior view) showing scaphoid fracture (arrow); (B) Position of scaphoid plaster, i.e. glass holding position (dorsiflexion and radial deviation); (C) Avascular necrosis of the scaphoid (in a different patient) following fracture (encircled)

in proximal pole fractures and least in tuberosity fractures due to its precarious and retrograde blood supply. Over 80% of the scaphoid surface is covered with articular cartilage and 70–80% of blood supply comes from the dorsal scaphoid branches entering along the dorsal ridge. This tenuous blood supply makes the scaphoid prone to AVN following fracture. Patient presents with increasing wrist pain and stiffness. X-ray shows sclerosis of fracture fragment, cystic changes, bone collapse and deformity **(Fig. 4.64C)**. MRI is the investigation of choice in a suspected case of AVN. This is a difficult condition to treat. Treatment options include vascularized bone grafting or excision of dead bone and carpal fusion.

Osteoarthritis

It is a late complication of a scaphoid fracture. Secondary osteoarthritis of wrist joint may occur following nonunion and AVN.

FRACTURES OF OTHER CARPAL BONES

Triquetrum followed by trapezium is most commonly fractured carpal bone after scaphoid (the order of carpal bone fracture in decreasing frequency is scaphoid, triquetrum, trapezium, lunate, capitate, hamate, pisiform and trapezoid). Fracture of other carpal bones like pisiform, trapezium, lunate, trapezoid, capitate and hamate is rare. Mostly these are avulsion injuries and treated with cast immobilization for 2–3 weeks. In displaced fractures ORIF or excision may be required.

LUNATE AND PERILUNATE DISLOCATIONS

Common dislocations at wrist joint are lunate and perilunate dislocation. In lunate dislocation the lunate dislocates out of the carpus while in perilunate dislocation, the lunate stays in its place while all other carpal bones dislocate out of the carpus. The more common of the two is the perilunate dislocation. Trans-scaphoid perilunate dislocation is the term used when there is a perilunate dislocation in association with a fracture of scaphoid.

Diagnosis

X-rays can reliably make the diagnosis. Normally in a lateral view of the wrist, radius, lunate, capitate and third metacarpal are in a straight line. In lunate dislocation long-axis of radius passes through the capitate and in perilunate dislocation long-axis of radius passes through the lunate **(Figs 4.65A and B)**. Some other important radiological signs that may guide the diagnosis include:

- Discontinuity of Gilula's arcs **(Fig. 4.66)**.
- *Spilled tea pot sign*: In cases with lunate dislocation, in a lateral view of the wrist, the lunate is seen primarily rotated and no longer articulates with the capitate **(Fig. 4.65C)**.
- *Piece of pie sign*: In cases with lunate dislocation, in AP view of the wrist, lunate appears triangular in shape, simulating a slice of a pie **(Fig. 4.65D)**.

Treatment

In reducible dislocations, close reduction and percutaneous K-wire fixation are recommended. Close reduction is achieved by Tavernier maneuver in Perilunate dislocation. For irreducible dislocations, open reduction, K-wire fixation and repair of torn ligaments is required.

HIGH-YIELD POINTS

- A 45° semisupinated oblique AP view is the best view for proximal pole fracture of scaphoid.
- Bones with retrograde blood flow (blood supply reduces from distal to proximal)—scaphoid, talus and head of femur. AVN is common in fractures of these bones.
- Avascular necrosis is a well-recognized complication of scaphoid fractures. Preiser's disease is the term used for an atraumatic AVN of the scaphoid, which is also a known clinical entity.
- Fractures of the hook of hamate can compress the median nerve in carpal tunnel and present as carpal tunnel syndrome. A special X-ray view called as the carpal tunnel view is used to make diagnosis in these fractures.
- The most common nerve injured in perilunate dislocation as well as in fracture of lunate is the median nerve.
- *Space of Poirier*: This is an area of the wrist capsule lying between the distal portion of radiocapitate and ulnocapitate ligaments. This is a weak spot in the floor of carpal tunnel and lunate displaces through this space into the carpal tunnel.
- Just like the shoulder and knee, instability can also occur at the wrist. Out of various types, rotatory subluxation of the scaphoid is the most common form of carpal instability.

METACARPAL FRACTURES

There are five metacarpals in the hand consisting of head, neck, shaft and base. Metacarpal bone fractures are common fractures and account for 40–50% of all hand injuries. The neck is the most common site of metacarpal fracture and fifth metacarpal is most commonly involved. Metacarpal fractures are usually caused by a direct blow to the hand, axial or torsional loading.

RELEVANT ANATOMY

Metacarpals are slender bones with slight dorsal convexity. The shaft of metacarpals gives origin to three palmar interosseous and four dorsal interosseous muscles. These muscle forces often pull the fracture fragment and cause apex dorsal deformity and shortening. The hand is immobilized in intrinsic plus position or functional or safe or James' position **(Figs 4.67A and B)** with MCP joint in 70–90° flexion, IP joint in full extension, thumb in abduction and wrist joint in slight extension. In this position IP joint volar plate and MCP joint collaterals are taut thus preventing shortening and flexion contracture.

CLINICAL FEATURES

Patients present with pain, swelling and usually apex dorsal angular deformity of the hand. Injury to the dorsal aspect of the hand is often associated with open wounds and damage to extensor tendons.

TREATMENT

Metacarpal head fractures are intra-articular fractures which often require ORIF with headless screws or K-wires. Metacarpal neck and shaft fractures are usually amenable to close reduction and cast immobilization for 3 weeks in functional position of the hand. Few degrees of angulation (up to 10° for second to third metacarpals and up to 40° for fourth to fifth metacarpals) is acceptable. Rotational malalignment is less tolerable and 10° is generally considered the upper limit. Unstable fractures

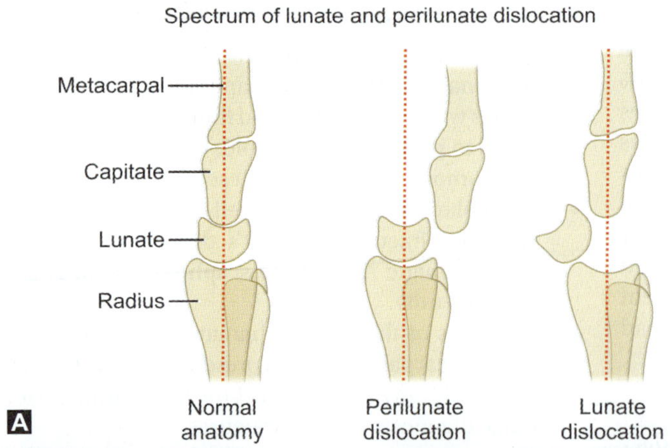

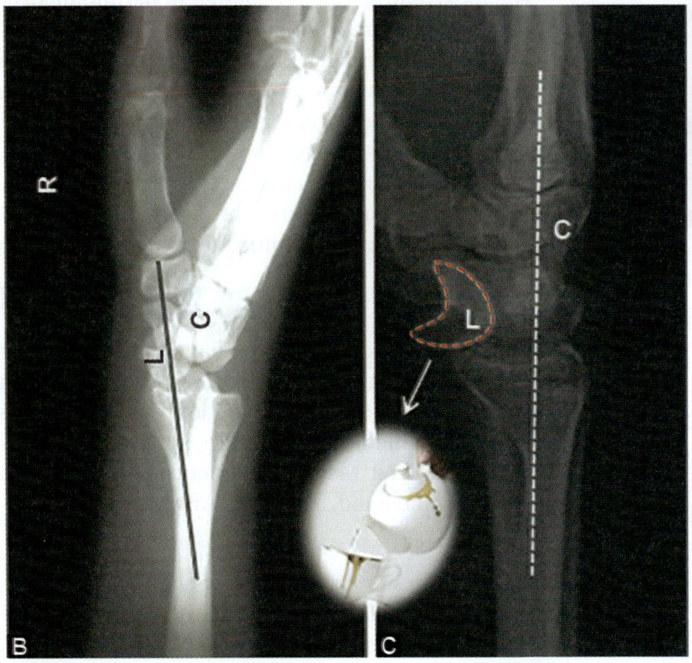

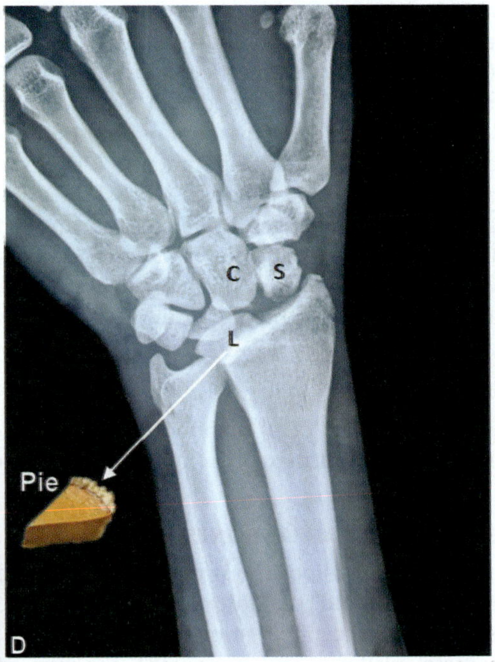

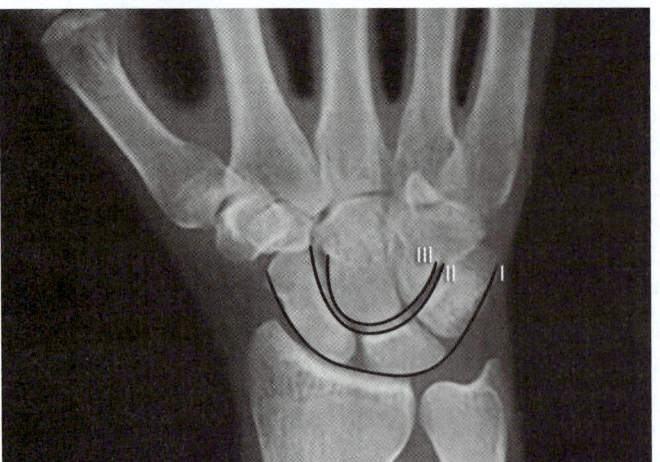

Spectrum of lunate and perilunate dislocation

Figs 4.65A to D: (A) Diagrammatical presentation of lunate and perilunate dislocation; (B) X-ray lateral view of wrist showing perilunate dislocation; (C) X-ray lateral view of wrist showing lunate dislocation and the spilled tea pot sign; (D) X-ray anteroposterior view of wrist showing a triangular-shaped lunate (simulating a piece of a pie) in a patient with lunate dislocation

Fig. 4.66: Gilula's arcs. These are three incomplete semicircles which outline the proximal and distal surfaces of proximal row carpal bones and proximal surface of distal row carpal bones. These semicircles are broken in carpal fracture dislocations and ligamentous instability

like spiral fractures require close reduction and K-wire fixation or open reduction and compression plating. Metacarpal base fractures are usually stable injuries (except for first metacarpal base fractures, discussed subsequently) and can be managed well with cast immobilization. A displaced intra-articular base fracture may require close reduction and percutaneous pinning.

COMPLICATIONS

Stiffness is most common complication of hand fractures. It is especially common after intra-articular fractures of head of the metacarpals. The hand should be splinted in the functional position as described earlier **(Figs 4.67A and B)** and early range of motion physiotherapy should be started to prevent it. Malunion of metacarpal fractures usually produce an apex dorsal deformity. Corrective osteotomy is required if it produces unacceptable cosmetic or functional deformity. Another common complication is hypersensitivity due to injury to small cutaneous nerves either due to injury or due to surgery. Post-traumatic arthritis is a delayed complication of intra-articular fractures of the head or base of the metacarpals.

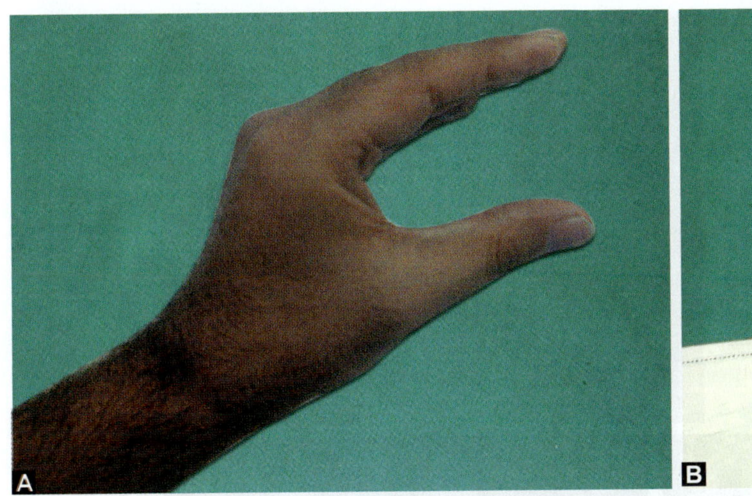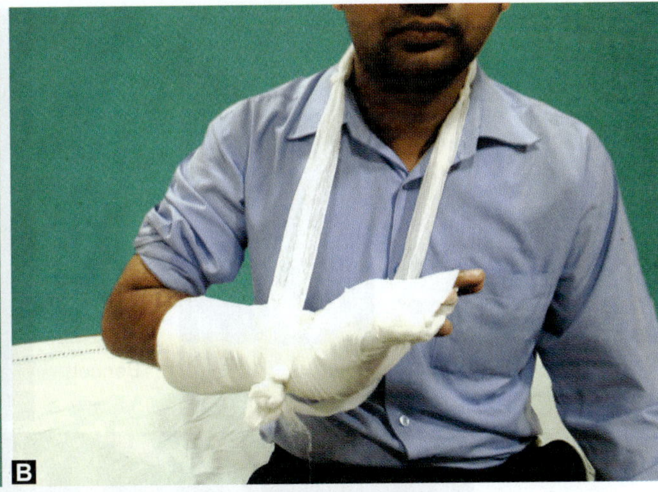

Figs 4.67A and B: Safe (intrinsic plus or functional) position of hand for immobilization

FRACTURES OF THE BASE OF FIRST METACARPAL

Fracture of base of first metacarpal may be extra-articular (transverse or oblique fracture) or intra-articular (Bennett's fracture—dislocation or Rolando's fracture dislocation).

Extra-articular Fractures

Extra-articular fractures **(Fig. 4.68A)** are usually caused by low-energy axial force or a bending or torsion of thumb. Patients present with pain and swelling at base of thumb and painful thumb movements. These are treated by close reduction and thumb spica immobilization for 3 weeks. Angulation up to 30° is acceptable. In unstable fractures, closed reduction and percutaneous K-wiring may be required.

Intra-articular Fractures

Two important intra-articular fractures that merit a mention are Bennett and Rolando.

Bennett's Fracture Dislocation

This is the most common fracture of base of thumb. It comprises of an oblique intra-articular fracture of base of first metacarpal, a kind of carpometacarpal fracture dislocation **(Fig. 4.68A)** in which distal diaphyseal fragment is displaced laterally, proximally and dorsally by a combined pull of abductor pollicis longus (primarily) and adductor pollicis **(Fig. 4.69)**.

Mechanism of injury: Carpometacarpal (CMC) fracture disloca-tions are usually high-energy injuries. These are caused by axial force to the partially flexed and adducted thumb as in while punching with a clenched fist.

Diagnosis: The patient presents with pain and swelling at base of thumb. Thumb movements are painful. Diagnosis is confirmed by anteroposterior and oblique X-rays (hyperpronated thumb view or Roberts' view best shows this fracture) of hand which show the oblique fracture line with a triangular fracture fragment.

Treatment: Small avulsion fractures can be managed by closing reduction and if a reduction is stable, thumb spica immobilization for 6 weeks. Most of these fractures are unstable injuries and

require close or open reduction, K-wire fixation and cast immobilization in a thumb spica for 4–6 weeks.

Complications: Post-traumatic osteoarthritis of the first CMC joint is a long-term complication due to the intra-articular nature of the fracture.

Rolando Fracture Dislocation

This is an intra-articular three-part fracture (V- or Y- or T-shaped fracture) of the base of the first metacarpal **(Figs 4.68A and B)** caused by axial loading of thumb which crushes the base of the first metacarpal. Base is split into triangular volar and dorsal fragments. Deforming forces are same as in Bennett's fracture dislocation **(Fig. 4.69)** but diaphyseal fragment is usually not displaced. Volar or palmar oblique ligament prevents displacement of volar fragment. Close or open reduction and K-wire or plate fixation is often required for these fractures.

BOXER'S FRACTURE

It is a transverse or short oblique fracture of neck of usually, the fifth **(Figs 4.70A and B)** or less commonly, the fourth metacarpal. It is the most common metacarpal fracture and commonly occurs in young people while punching with a clenched fist. AP and lateral X-rays of hand show apex dorsal angulation of fracture. It can mostly be treated by close reduction and cast immobilization or K-wire fixation.

FINGER CARPOMETACARPAL JOINT FRACTURE DISLOCATIONS

Although CMC joint of the thumb is the most common to be injured, among the fingers, it is the fifth metacarpal and the hamate CMC joint that is most commonly injured (as it is the most mobile of these joints). Treatment is usually close reduction and cast immobilization.

PHALANGEAL FRACTURES AND DISLOCATIONS

Phalangeal fractures and dislocations are the most common hand injuries. These are usually caused by a direct blow or axial loading, and often associated with open wounds. Distal phalanx is the

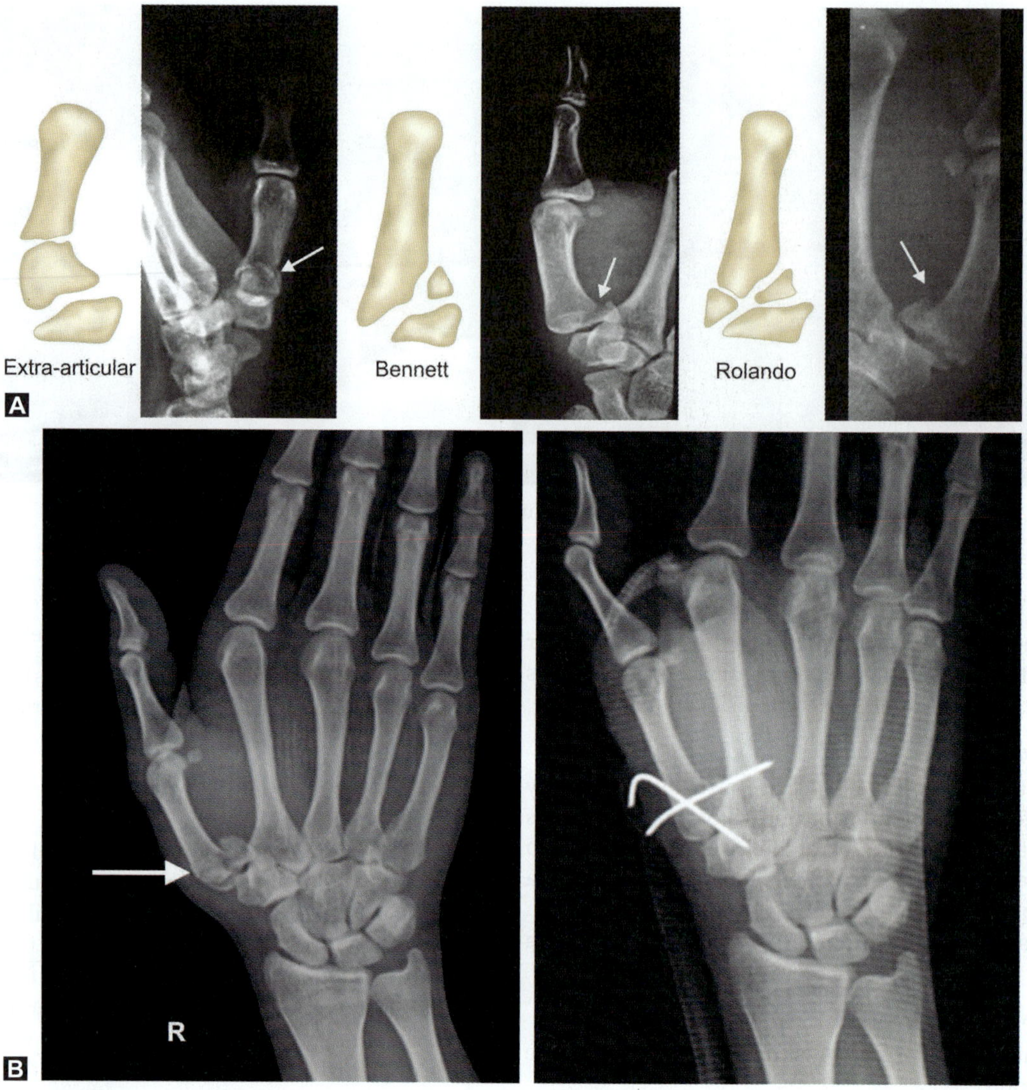

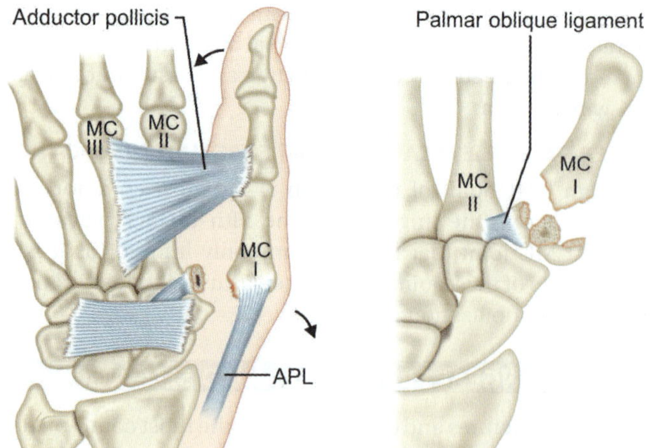

Figs 4.68A and B: (A) Bennett's fracture dislocation, Rolando fracture dislocation and extra-articular fracture of base of thumb; (B) X-ray hand oblique view showing Rolando fracture (arrow) and its closed reduction internal fixation with K-wires

Courtesy: Dr Rajat Kumar Garg.

Fig. 4.69: Deforming forces in Bennett and Rolando fractures are caused by the abductor pollicis longus and adductor pollicis

most commonly fractured bone in the hand. Thumb followed by fifth finger MCP joints are most commonly dislocated MCP joints. Proximal IP joint dislocations are more common than a distal IP joint dislocation.

Diagnosis

Phalangeal diaphyseal fractures can be transverse, oblique, spiral or multifragmentary. X-ray reliably provides the diagnosis in almost all cases.

Treatment

Most of the phalangeal fractures are stable undisplaced or minimally displaced fractures and can be managed by strapping to neighboring finger (buddy strapping, **Fig. 4.71**) for 2–3 weeks. Finger physiotherapy should be started after 2–3 weeks to prevent stiffness. Unstable fractures and intra-articular fractures of the base or head require close reduction and K-wire or small screw fixation. Close reduction and splinting is usually successful for most MCP joint and IP joint dislocations. After close reduction finger is buddy strapped and active range of motion physiotherapy is started soon.

KAPLAN INJURY

It is irreducible dorsal dislocation of fingers (most commonly index finger) at the MCP joint. The volar plate and joint capsule get interposed between the base of the proximal phalanx and the metacarpal head **(Fig. 4.72)**. It requires surgical reduction. Presence of sesamoid bone in MCP joint is pathognomonic of Kaplan injury.

TUFT FRACTURE

The ungual tuberosity of the distal phalanx is called tuft. Anatomy of the tuft is given in **Figures 4.73A and B**. Germinal matrix grows the nail while sterile matrix supports the nail. Tuft fracture is usually the crush injury of the tip of fingers (shattered by hammer or caught in the door). Fracture management is of secondary importance and soft tissues (pulp and matrix) should be taken care of first. Hematoma beneath the nail is drained and nail bed is repaired. The nail may be removed or reinserted depending on the amount of injury and finger is splinted.

HIGH-YIELD POINTS

- Brewerton view is used to see metacarpal head fractures and Roberts view is used for thumb CMC joint.

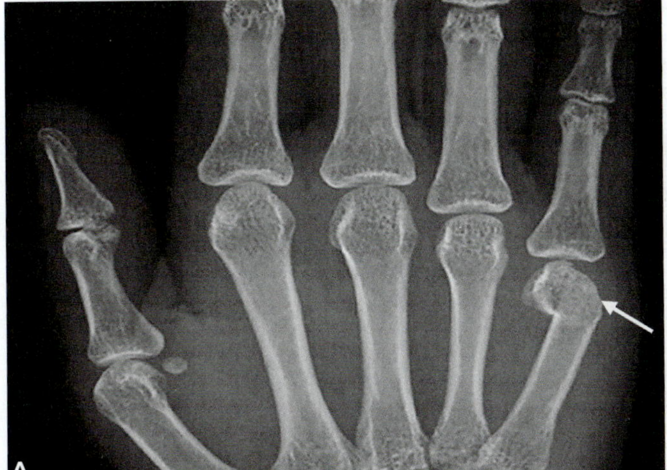

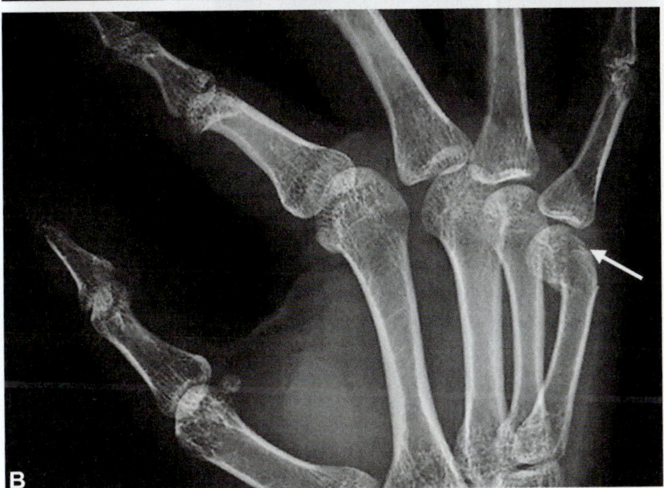

Figs 4.70A and B: X-ray hand. (A) Anteroposterior; and (B) Oblique view showing Boxer's fracture (arrow)

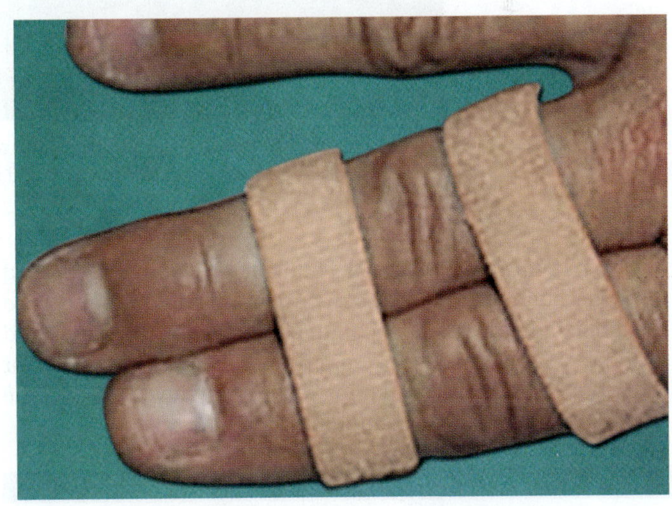

Fig. 4.71: Buddy strapping for phalangeal fracture

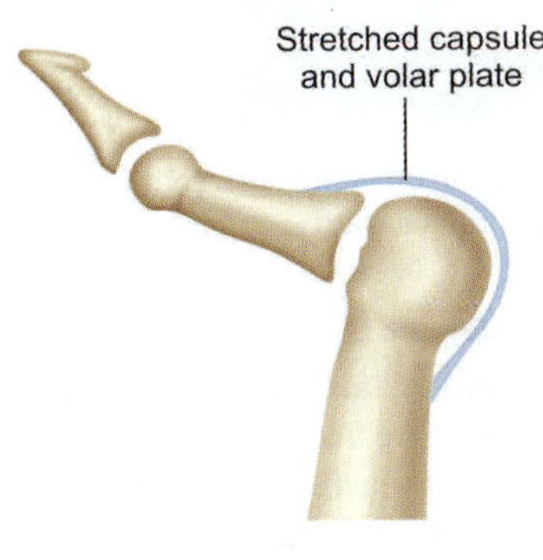

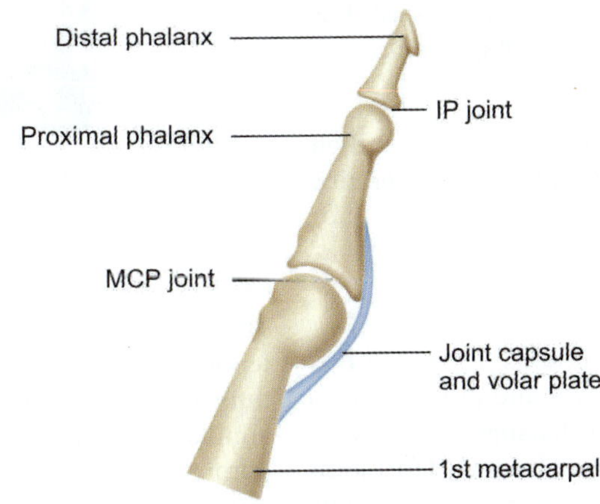

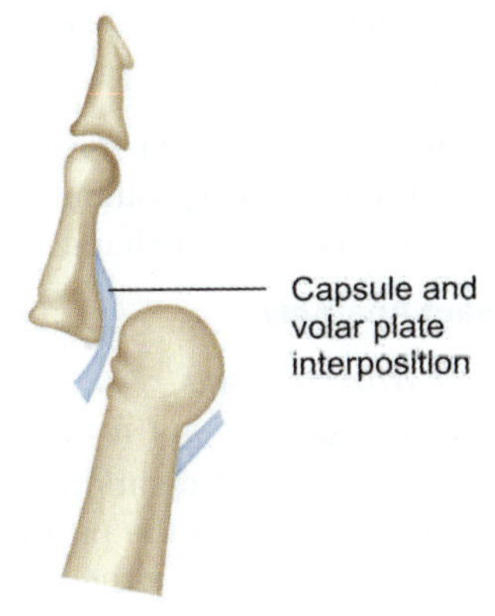

Fig. 4.72: Pathogenesis of a Kaplan dislocation
Abbreviations: IP, interphalangeal; MCP, metacarpophalangeal.

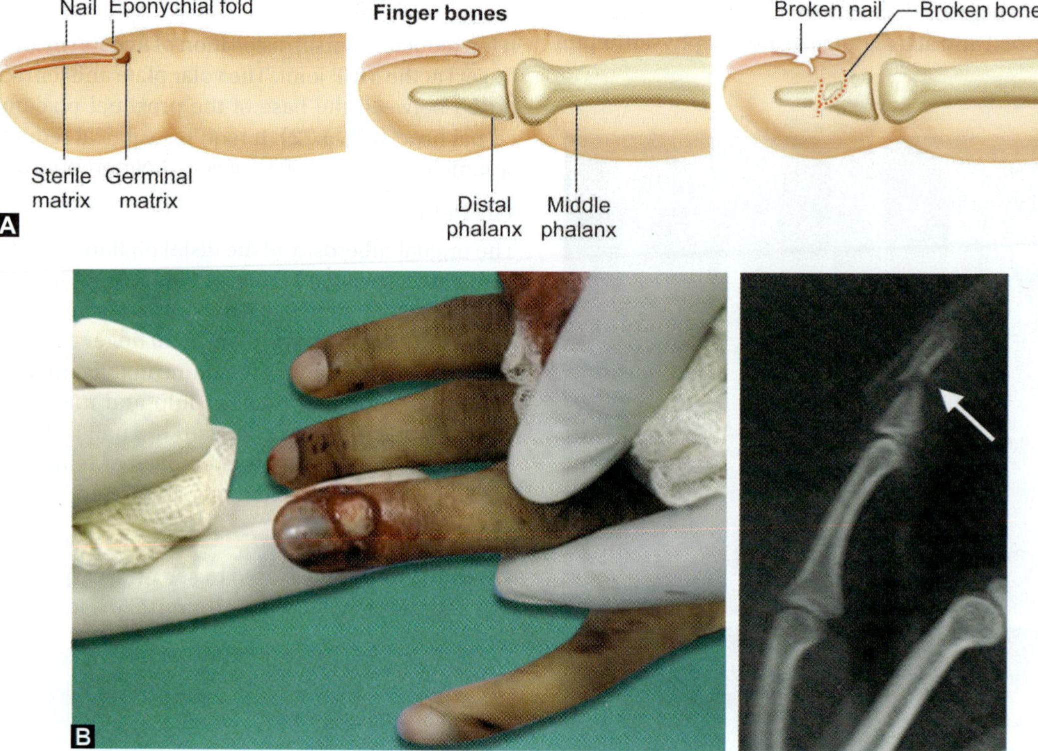

Figs 4.73A and B: (A) Anatomy of the tuft and pictorial description of tuft fracture; (B) Clinical picture of tuft fracture and underlying distal phalanx fracture in X-ray

- *Boxer's knuckle*: It is caused by injury to MCP joints (knuckles) of the hand. There occurs disruption of sagittal band (two stabilizing soft tissue slips attaching tendon to radial and ulnar sides of finger) leading to dislocation of the extensor tendon. Middle finger is most commonly involved and the radial sagittal band is commonly disrupted.

TENDON INJURIES OF THE HAND

Tendons attach the muscle to bone and serve to transmit the muscle force to bone thus helping joint movement. Tendon injuries of the hand are a very common occupational hazard **(Fig. 4.74)** and hence one needs to know the right management.

FLEXOR TENDON INJURIES

Flexor tendon injuries of the hand are common due to their vulnerable anatomical position. They are usually cut by lacerating injuries or crush injury of hand.

Relevant Anatomy

Flexors of Wrist and Hand

Flexor carpi radialis and FCU are wrist flexors. There are two flexor tendons (flexor digitorum superficialis and profundus) to each finger. FDS flexes the proximal interphalangeal (PIP) joint and FDP primarily flexes the distal interphalangeal (DIP) joint and assists FDS in flexing the PIP joint. Flexor pollicis longus flexes the IP joint of thumb and flexor pollicis brevis flexes the MCP joint of thumb.

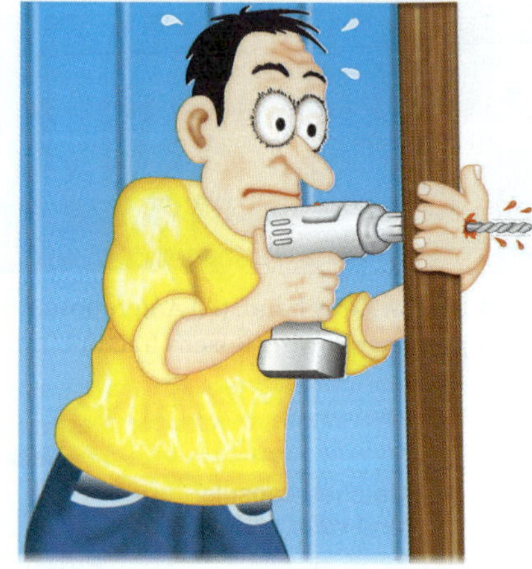

Fig. 4.74: Tendon injuries of the hand are a common occupational hazard

Flexor Zones and Pulleys (Figs 4.75A and B)

The hand is divided into five zones **(Table 4.6)** containing flexor tendons and several pulleys. There are five annular (A1 to A5) and three cruciate (C1 to C3) pulleys in each finger. Thumb has two annular (A1 and A2) and one oblique pulley. These are condensed fibrous tissues tunnels through which passes the flexor tendons, thus they help in proper tracking of tendons. A1 pulley is most commonly involved in trigger finger and A2 and A4 pulleys are biomechanically most important pulleys, the absence of which

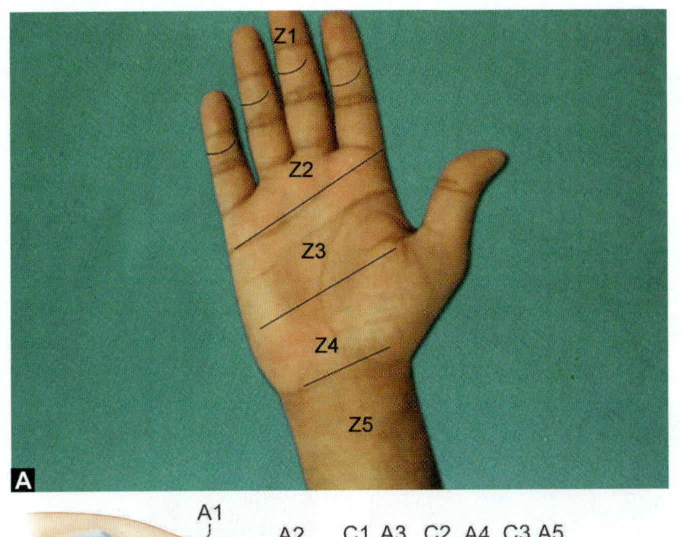

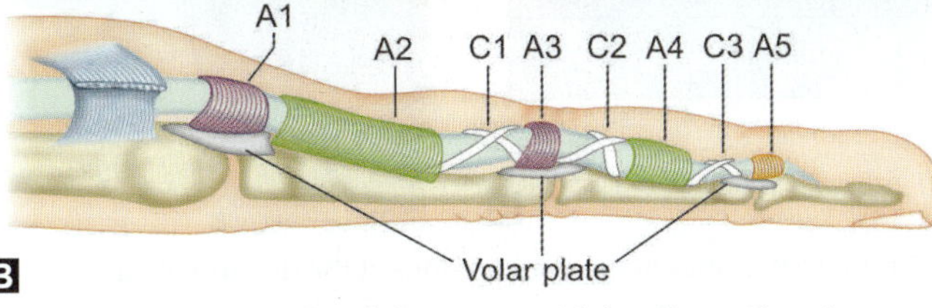

Figs 4.75A and B: (A) Zones; and (B) Pulleys of hand

Table 4.6: Zones of flexor tendon in hand	
Zone 1	Distal to the flexor digitorium superficialis (FDS) insertion at base of middle phalanx
Zone 2 (no man's land)	Between insertion of FDS and proximal margin of flexor tendon sheath
Zone 3	Between proximal margin of flexor tendon sheath and distal edge of carpal tunnel
Zone 4	Carpal tunnel
Zone 5	Forearm proximal to carpal tunnel

causes bowstringing of flexor tendons. A1, A3 and A5 pulleys are attached to palmar plate at MP, PIP and DIP joints, respectively.

Clinical Testing

If a patient presents with these injuries of the hand, a systemic examination of all flexor tendons should be done. To test the FDS patient is asked to actively flex the PIP joint, but FDP also causes the flexion of PIP joint so to remove the effect of FDP all adjacent fingers are held with all joints in extension **(Fig. 4.76)**. Since all FDPs are interlinked, blocking all fingers block all FDPs and the flexion of fingers at PIP joint is now by the action of FDS mainly. FDP is checked by stabilizing the PIP joint and asking the patient to actively flex the DIP joint of the finger to be tested. Flexor pollicis longus is checked by ability to actively flex the IP joint of thumb. FCR and FCU are wrist flexors. If FCR is cut, then wrist will deviate towards the ulna while active flexion is being performed and if FCU is cut, then wrist will deviate towards radius while active flexion of wrist is being done.

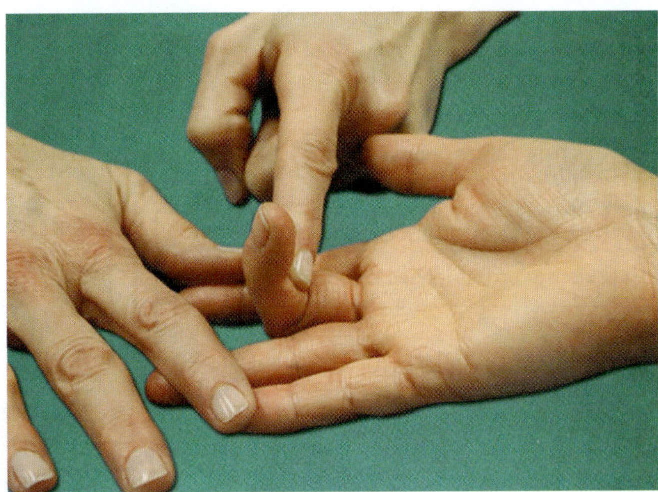

Fig. 4.76: Clinical examination for flexor digitorum superficialis

EXTENSOR TENDON INJURIES

Extensor tendon injuries are more common than flexor tendon injuries. Because of their location on back of hand, they are easily injured even by a minor cut. The extensor tendon of the middle finger is most commonly injured.

Relevant Anatomy

Extensor tendons are grouped in six compartments **(Fig. 4.77A)** at the wrist. The extensor digitorum communis, extensor indicis proprius and extensor digiti minimi insert at the base of the middle phalanges as central slips and to the base of the distal phalanges as lateral slips. Long extensors of the fingers are primarily responsible for MCP joint extension. Lumbricals and interossei are main extensors of IP joints.

Extensor Zones

Dorsum of hand is divided into eight zones **(Fig. 4.77B)** according to extensor tendon injuries. Zone IV (disruption over the metacarpals) is most commonly injured area.

TREATMENT OF TENDON INJURIES

Partially torn tendons can be treated by immobilization in extension splinting. Completely torn tendons require operative repair. In acute cases with clean wound primary (*primary repair* is within 24 hours) end-to-end repair can be done. In contaminated and dirty wound initial thorough debridement is done and a delayed primary tendon repair is done as soon as there is evidence of wound healing without infection (*delayed primary repair* is repair within 10–14 days). Some cases have gross contamination and need a secondary repair (*secondary repair* is between 2 weeks and 4 weeks). Infected cases will still have a longer rehabilitation and would require a *late secondary repair* (>4 weeks) and surgeon in such cases should be prepared to face consequences such as difficult delivery of the tendon through the digital sheath. CR and percutaneous pinning or extensor block pinning may be required for bony avulsions. In crush injury of hand, often primary repair is not possible and tendon graft from other tendons is used. Palmaris longus is commonly used graft in hand injuries. In chronic rupture

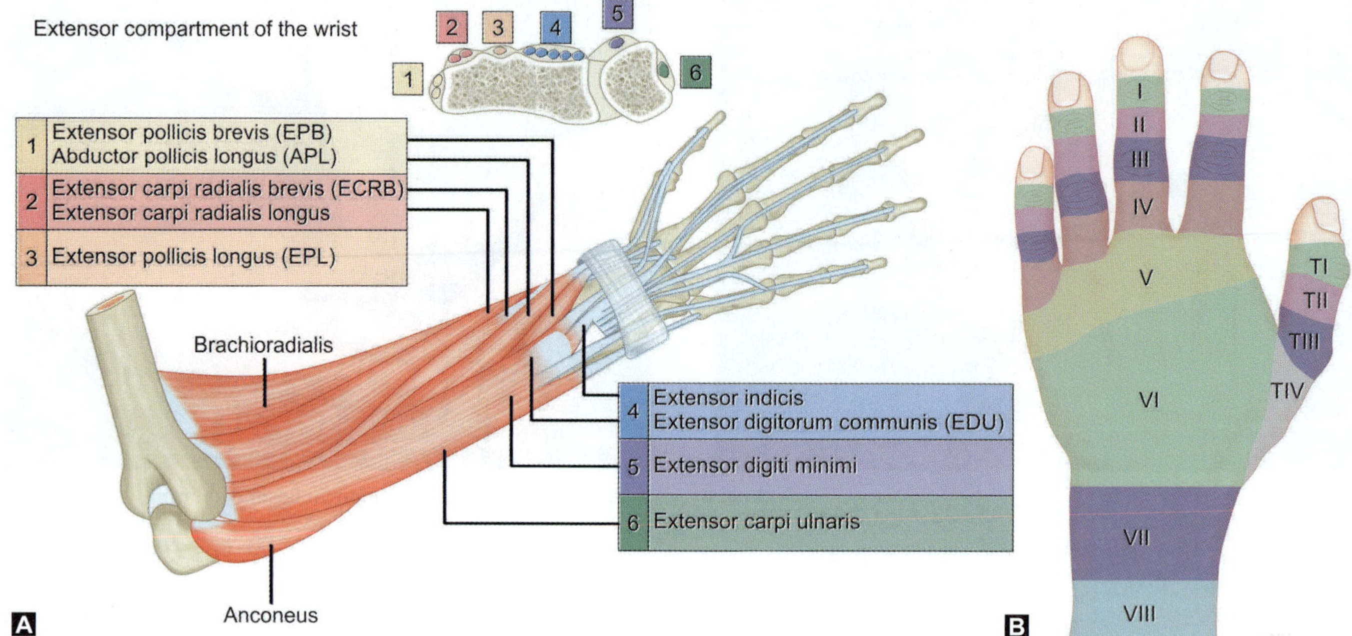

Figs 4.77A and B: (A) Extensor tendons at the wrist are divided into six groups; (B) Zones of extensor tendons at the dorsum of hand

cases, reconstruction is often not possible and then less needed tendon can be transferred to more useful positions. Postoperative adhesions and finger stiffness are common complications of tendon repair. In general worst outcome of flexor tendon repair is seen in zone II (dangerous area or no man's land) because both FDS and FDP run together in a common sheath.

CRUSH INJURY OF THE HAND

These are common patients in orthopedic emergency and are usually victims of occupational hazards like machines injury, road traffic accidents, animal bites or having the hand caught between two heavy objects. The optimal hand function is necessary for good quality of life, especially if dominant hand is affected.

Evaluation of Crush Injury of Hand in Emergency Department

Evaluation of the crushed hand should start from the vascular examination and proceed to assess soft tissue coverage, bone, nerves and tendons. Make sure that radial pulse is intact and check for capillary refill and active bleeding. Any catastrophic bleeding should be immediately stopped by a tight compression bandage. Absence of pulses, tense, swollen hand and severe pain on passive movement all indicate towards tense compartment and the need for an urgent fasciotomy.

Look at the soft tissue coverage of bone and tendons, skin condition and any foreign material and contamination. Hand fractures and dislocations may be quite obvious or may be masked in a swollen hand. Sensation (light touch, pinprick, etc.) and motor examination should be done. While doing radial nerve (wrist extension), ulnar nerve (finger IP joint extension, finger abduction/adduction, etc.) and median nerve (thumb opposition) examination lacerations of muscles and tendons should be kept in mind. The patient may not be able to move fingers with lacerated muscles and tendons. After splinting the injured limb patient should be sent for X-rays.

Management and Decision Making

Management of crushed limb, mostly requires a staged surgery. The first step is to perform a good debridement and reduce and stabilize the fractures. Tendons and nerves should be repaired primarily if conditions permit, for example, adequate soft tissue coverage is there and wound is not much contaminated, otherwise delayed repair can be done. Adequate soft tissue coverage, in fact, is the greatest priority and if required a skin graft or a flap should be done, else exposed tendons and tissues tend to dessicate. An intact vascularity should be the goal, but arterial injury is generally not a problem because single artery (radial or ulnar) is sufficient to provide adequate blood supply to hand in most cases (palmar arch receives contribution from both radial and ulnar arteries). In badly crushed hands repair or grafting may not be possible, then reconstruction using tendon transfers or arthrodesis may be required later.

REIMPLANTATION OF A TRANSECTED DIGIT (OR A LIMB)

A transacted limb means that the limb has separated completely from the rest of the body. With modern antisepsis methods and advanced technology, it is possible to replant some vital body parts provided some criteria are met. Because irreversible necrotic changes begin in muscles after 6 hours of ischemia (warm ischemia time), it is preferable to begin the replantation of parts with good muscular bulk (viz. parts proximal to palms and foot) within this time. With cooling (to 4°C), this time may be extended to 12 hours (cold ischemia time). For small parts with less muscle bulk (e.g. digits), warm ischemia time may be extended to 8 hours or more while the cold ischemia time may be as long as 30 hours. If the ischemia time is crossed, replantation is not advisable (especially of muscle rich parts) as there is a risk of revascularization injury that can end up with renal damage due to myoglobinuria, acidosis and hyperkalemia resulting

> **Box 4.1:** Some common fracture patterns in skull bones
>
> *Linear fracture*: Most common type of skull fracture. These fractures look like a thin line that involves either the inner or outer table or the full thickness of the skull. There is no displacement of bone
>
> *Depressed fractures or signature fractures*: In signature fractures the broken bones are displaced inward. They occur when a heavy object with small striking surface (e.g. hammer) hits the head. The outer table is driven inward while the inner table is fractured irregularly
>
> *Ring fracture*: These fractures, particularly occur following a fall from a height (with "feet first" impact) and involve the posterior fossa around the foramen magnum
>
> *Gutter fractures*: They are formed when part of the thickness of the bone is removed so as to form a gutter, e.g. oblique bullet wound
>
> *Spider web fractures or mosaic fractures*: These comprise of multiple comminuted fractures in the form of depressed fracture lines with radiating fissures
>
> *Hinge fracture or motorcyclist fracture*: This fracture is seen in patients with fall from height or seldom in motorcyclists who land up with high-velocity road traffic accidents that gives a blow to the side of the head. The force is transmitted via the helmet to the base of the skull, producing a transverse fracture of the floor. At autopsy the base of the skull is found to be divided into two halves, anterior and posterior, each moving independently of each other as if connected via a hinge, hence also called as "hinge fracture"
>
> *Pond or indentation fractures (ping pong skull)*: These are a type of shallow depressed fracture, which occur in infant skulls which are elastic and are able to be indented without a frank break in the bone. In a pond fracture, the inner table and the dura are intact. The fracture is usually caused by a fall when the skull hits the edge of a hard blunt object, such as a table. The skull appears deformed, with a shallow trench on the surface of the skull
>
> *Diastatic skull fractures*: Diastatic fractures occur when the fracture line traverses one or more sutures of the skull causing a widening across the sutures. These are also usually seen in infants and young children as the sutures are not yet fused

from metabolites released in significant amounts from necrotic muscles.

Transportation of the Amputated Part

The transacted part is first rinsed gently with sterile saline or ringer lactate to remove excess contamination. Then the part is wrapped with sterile gauze, then soaked in sterile ringer lactate or saline and placed in a plastic bag which is then sealed. The bag is placed on ice in an insulated container so that the part is not touching the ice to avoid freezing of the part. Cooling of the amputated part to about 4°C is imperative to prolong the viability of the transacted part.

Sequence of Repair in Reimplantation

Pneumonic "BE FAN of Virender Sehwag" is an easy way to remember the order of repair—bone, extensor tendons, flexor tendons, artery, nerve, vein and lastly skin closure. So, fractures and dislocations should be dealt with first, but the meticulous vascular repair is given the greatest priority to save the replanted digit or limb.

SKULL AND FACIAL FRACTURES

SKULL FRACTURES

Box 4.1 describes some common fracture patterns seen in the skull. The most common skull bone prone to fracture is the temporal bone. Fractures in the temporal bone can be longitudinal (more common) or horizontal. Longitudinal fractures can produce rupture of the tympanic membrane with bloody discharge from ear (hemotympanum). Transverse fractures on the other hand, are more known to produce a facial nerve paralysis as they extend into the petrous part of the temporal bone.

Apart from these, there can be fractures of the cranial fossa (anterior, middle and posterior). Anterior fossa fractures can lead to bilateral ecchymosis with swelling of the upper lids (Racoon's sign/Panda sign). Olfactory nerve is the commonly involved nerve

in these fractures. Middle fossa fractures can cause a cerebrospinal fluid (CSF) rhinorrhea apart from damaging the sixth, seventh and eighth cranial nerves. The posterior cranial fossa fractures on the other hand, tend to involve the 9th to 11th cranial nerves. Not uncommon in these fractures is to find the classical Battle's sign (delayed ecchymosis over the mastoid region).

MAXILLOFACIAL FRACTURES

The most common facial bone to fracture is the nasal bone followed by the zygomatic bone. Fractures that involve the middle third of the face (between supraorbital ridge and upper jaw) are classified by the Le Fort classification into three types. Type III fractures are the severe most causing complete disruption of the attachment of the facial skeleton to the cranium. Types II and III may also injure the cribriform plate causing CSF rhinorrhea. For details on the classification and these fractures kindly refer to ENT textbook.

MANDIBULAR FRACTURES

Mandibular fractures mostly result when there is a blow to the chin. The most common site is through the neck of the condyle. On clinical examination one may find Coleman's sign, i.e. hematoma on the floor of the mouth in fractures involving the body of the mandible. Most fractures are displaced because of the pull of masseter. Early reduction and fixation is the aim under a cover of broad spectrum antibiotics.

NASAL FRACTURES

A blow to the nose from front results in Jarjaway's fracture. The fracture line starts just above the anterior nasal spine and runs horizontally backward, ending near the junction of septal cartilage with vomer. A blow from below to the nose results in the Chevallet fracture. Here the fracture line runs vertically upward from the nasal spine to end at the junction of the bony and cartilaginous septum. For details on other fracture patterns and appropriate management of these areas, the reader is suggested to read ENT textbook.

Traumatology: Injuries of Pelvis, Hip and Lower Limb

FRACTURES OF PELVIS AND ACETABULUM

RELEVANT ANATOMY

Two innominate bones [each formed by the fusion of three ossification centers: (1) ilium, (2) ischium and (3) pubis] and sacrum constitute the pelvis. Both hip bones are attached anteriorly by pubic symphysis and posteriorly they articulate with sacrum at the sacroiliac joint (SI joint) to form the pelvic ring. Both hip bones and sacrum are stabilized by a number of ligaments. Posterior ligaments are stronger than anterior ligaments. These ligaments include sacroiliac ligaments (anterior, posterior and interosseous), sacrospinous ligaments, sacrotuberous ligaments and iliolumbar ligament. Anteriorly, pelvic ring is stabilized by relatively weak symphyseal ligaments.

Pelvic Inlet and Outlet

Pelvic inlet **(Figs 5.1A and B)** or brim is formed anteriorly by pubic crest and symphysis, posteriorly by sacral promontory and ala of sacrum, and on the sides by the iliopectineal lines. Below this is the true or lesser pelvis that contains the pelvic viscera and above this is the false or greater pelvis that represents the inferior aspect of the abdominal cavity. Pelvic outlet **(Figs 5.2A and B)** is formed anteriorly by pubic arch, laterally by ischial tuberosities, posterolaterally by sacrotuberous ligaments and posteriorly by coccyx.

Pelvis provides a room and protects pelvic viscera and traversing neurovascular structure. Bladder, urethra and vagina are important structure just behind the pubic symphysis whereas rectum is an important structure just anterior and in relation to the sacrum. Sciatic nerve, superior gluteal nerve and artery, inferior gluteal nerve and artery and internal pudendal nerve and artery pass through the greater sciatic foramen to exit pelvis. Obturator nerve and artery traverse through the obturator foramen to exit the pelvis.

PELVIC FRACTURES

These range from low-energy osteoporotic fractures in elderly to high-energy life-threatening pelvic ring injuries in young adults which occur usually in RTA. High-energy pelvic injuries are frequently associated with retroperitoneal and intraperitoneal visceral and vascular injuries. In most of the cases, pelvic hemorrhage pools into retroperitoneal space from venous damage (presacral and paravesical venous plexus) and bleeding from fractured bone. Damage to branches of internal iliac arteries may also occur and superior gluteal arteries and internal pudendal artery are most commonly damaged. Early death in pelvic injuries is due to heavy blood loss (1.5–2 liters or 4–8 units

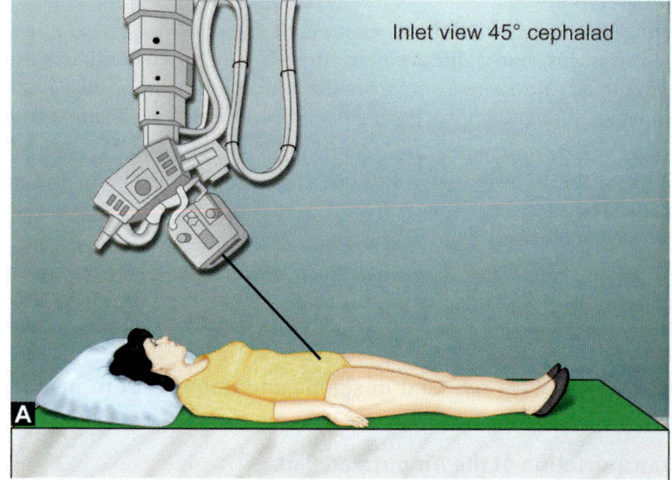

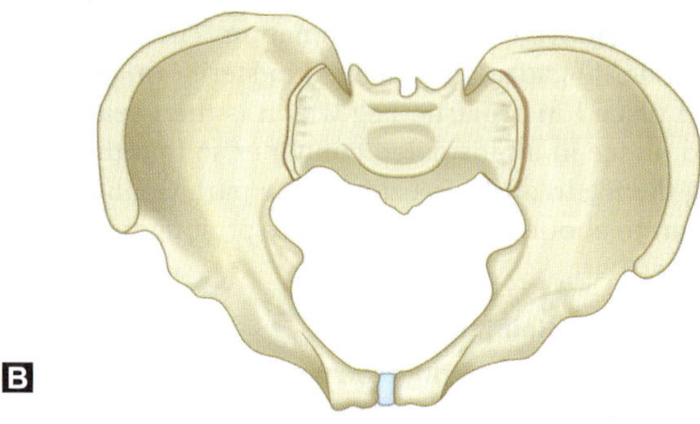

Figs 5.1A and B: Pelvic inlet view

on an average) and concomitant head injuries. Later sepsis and multiorgan failure are the main cause of patient loss.

Polytrauma patients who receive pelvic injuries are also likely to have other associated injuries. Chest injuries, fracture of long bones, head injuries and injury to the bladder and urethra are common in multiple injured patients who sustain pelvic trauma.

Classification

Pelvic injuries can be stable or unstable. A stable injury is one which can withstand normal physiological forces without any further deformation while an unstable injury would displace on a rotational or vertical force. Two classification systems are commonly used to classify these pelvic fractures. Young and Burgess classification is based on the mechanism of injury (direction of force) of pelvic fracture **(Table 5.1 and Fig. 5.3A)**.

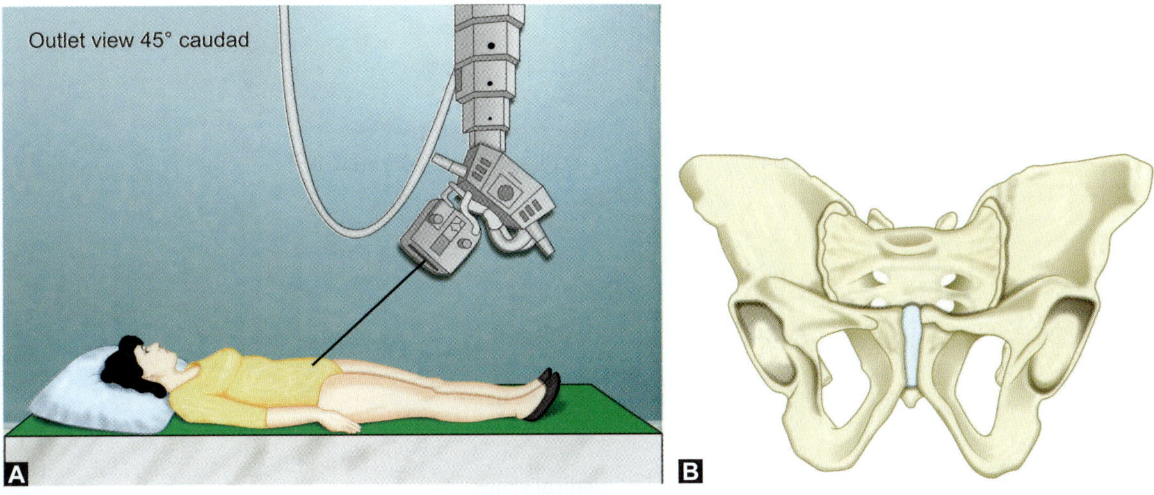

Figs 5.2A and B: Pelvic outlet view

Type I	Lateral compression (LC)	LC-I—Pubic rami fracture plus sacral ala fracture on side of impact LC-II—Crescent fracture on side of impact LC-III—LC-I or LC-II on side of impact with contralateral open book injury
Type II	Anteroposterior compression (APC)	APC-I—Slight opening of the pubic symphysis and SI joint anteriorly APC-II—Anterior opening of SI joint with intact posterior SI ligaments APC-III—Complete disruption of SI joint
Type III	Vertical shear (VS)	Symphyseal diastasis with vertical displacement of the hemipelvis
Type IV	Combined injury mechanism	A combination of two or more above-mentioned forces leading to complex fracture pattern

Tile's classification system **(Table 5.2 and Fig. 5.3B)** is based on rotational and vertical stability of the pelvis. Type A are mainly avulsion fractures where the pelvic ring disruption is not there (or if there, is minimal and stable). Type B and C are injuries that disrupt the pelvic ring. Type B fractures occur either in anteroposterior compression of the pelvis (open book injuries) or side to side compression of the pelvis (bucket handle fractures). Both are rotationally unstable injuries, but are vertically stable due to largely intact strong posterior ligamentous structures. Type C injuries involve massive displacements and disruption of all ligamentous restraints thereby displaying both rotational and vertical instability.

Initial Assessment and Management

Pelvic bone fracture is often a miniscule part of the major traumatic burden. Attending orthopedic surgeon should assess the pelvic trauma patient on the guidelines of ATLS (Advanced Trauma Life Support). Proper attention should be paid to ABCs of trauma assessment and rapid management of airway, breathing and unstable hemodynamic status and disability (neurological assessment) is lifesaving (*see* Chapter 3). A rapid assessment of the presence of an unstable pelvic fracture can clinically be made by compressing the pelvis from side to side (pelvic compression and distraction test). A crepitus or a springy feeling if elicited provides the clue to the presence of an underlying unstable pelvic injury. However, this test should not be done as it does not give reliable information; rather the maneuver may dislodge the clot and cause a retroperitoneal hemorrhage further worsening the shock. Not uncommon in vertical shear injuries is to find a limb length discrepancy.

In a hemodynamically unstable pelvic trauma patient with high-grade pelvic injury (LC-III, APC-III, VS or combined) shock is likely due to pelvic hemorrhage. In these patients pelvic hemorrhage should be controlled at earliest by use of noninvasive methods like pelvic binders/sheath wrapped tight around the pelvis **(Fig. 5.4A)** or military antishock trousers—MAST (inflatable trousers for exsanguinating pelvic blood) or invasive methods **(Fig. 5.4B)** like external fixators (anterior external fixator for anterior pelvic injury/open book fracture and pelvic C clamp for posterior pelvic ring injury, **Fig. 5.4C**), preperitoneal pelvic packing and angiographic embolization. Generally the first step in an emergency is to tie a pelvic binder, start I/V fluids (preferably Ringer lactate) and replace the binder at earliest with a more effective external fixator applied in compression mode (*see* **Flow chart 5.1** for sequence of steps).

Once the patient is hemodynamically stable, thorough physical and radiological examination should be done. Presence of blood at meatus or inability to void in a pelvic injury patient indicates urethral (10% incidence) or bladder injury (20% incidence). On suspicion these injuries should be dealt with in consultation with a urologist. Generally intraperitoneal ruptures of the bladder are repaired while the extra peritoneal ruptures can be observed. Urethral injuries can be attempted a delayed repair. In case there is blood at the meatus, a single gentle

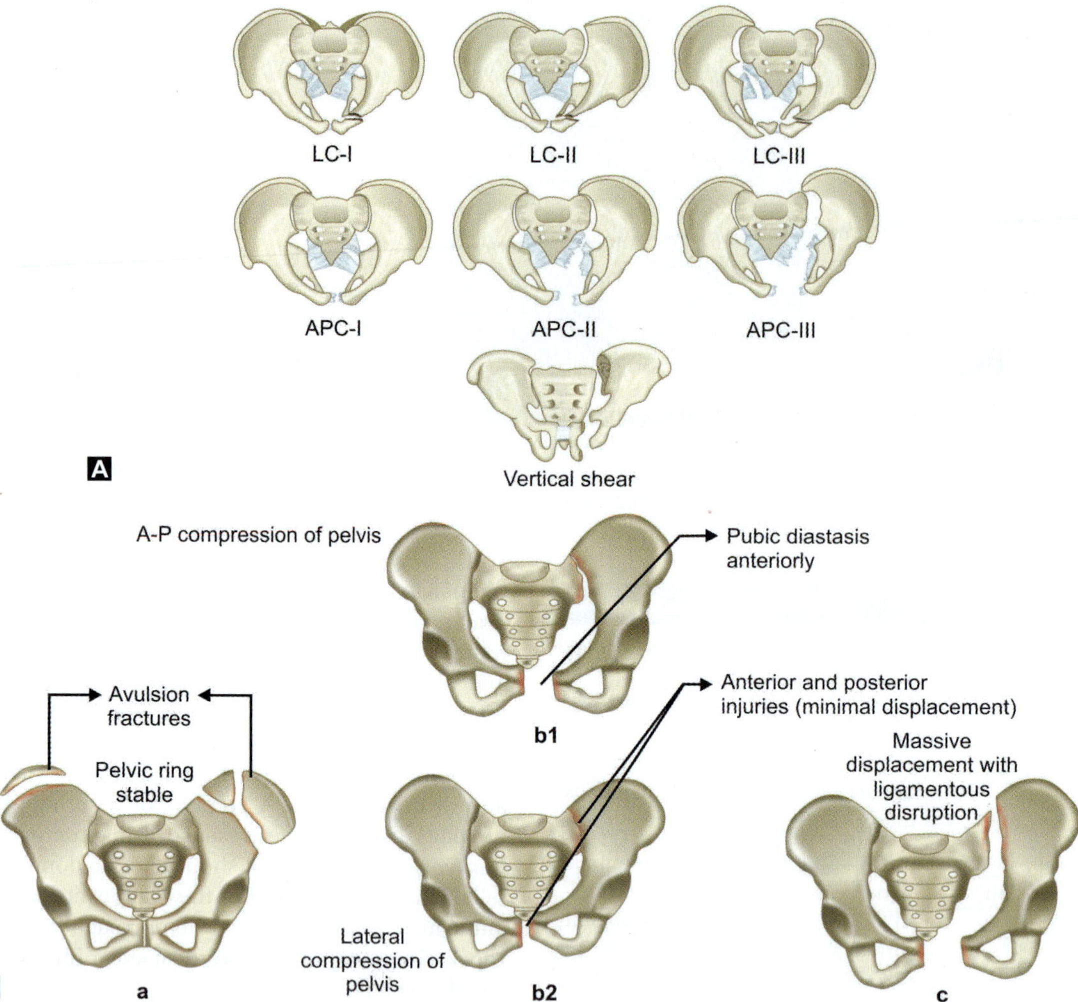

Figs 5.3A and B: (A) Young and Burgess classification and (B) Tile's classification of pelvic injuries

Table 5.2: Tile classification of pelvic fractures

Types	Subtypes
(A) Stable pelvic ring	A1—Fracture not involving the ring (avulsion fracture, crest fracture, etc.) A2—Stable fractures of pelvic ring
(B) Pelvic ring vertically stable, but rotationally unstable	B1—Open book type B2—Lateral compression, ipsilateral B3—Lateral compression, contralateral or bucket handle type injury
(C) Pelvic ring rotationally and vertically unstable	C1—Unilateral C2—Bilateral C3—Associated with acetabular fracture

catheterization attempt may be taken, but if difficult a suprapubic cystostomy should rather be opted. Abdominal palpation and rectal examination should be done. Rectal examination can identify high lying prostate suggesting urethral injury.

Definitive Treatment of Pelvic Fractures

Pelvic fracture is definitively dealt with after stabilization of the patient. Pelvic anteroposterior inlet and outlet views and computed tomography (CT) scan are helpful in better identification of pelvic fractures. Inlet view is better to demonstrate the anteroposterior

displacement, while an outlet view is better to demonstrate a vertical displacement. The goal of treatment should be the identification of instability and its management to prevent long-term functional impairment. Intraoperative stress radiographs and CT scan are useful in the assessment of instability.

Nonoperative Treatment

The most common type of pelvic fractures are rami fractures (due to lateral compression injuries) and are stable. These lateral impaction injuries with minimal displacement and pubic rami

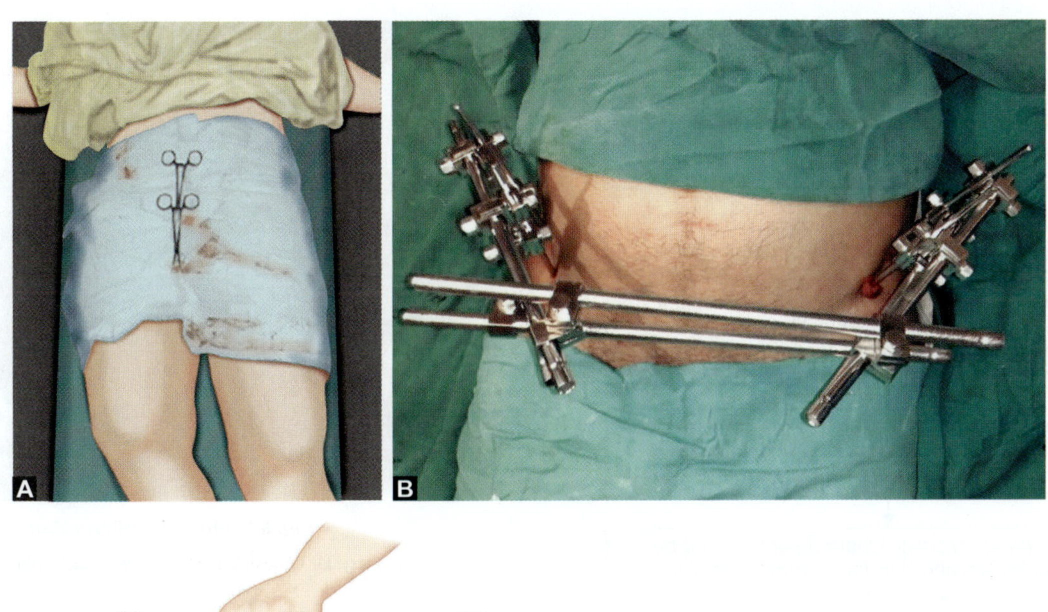

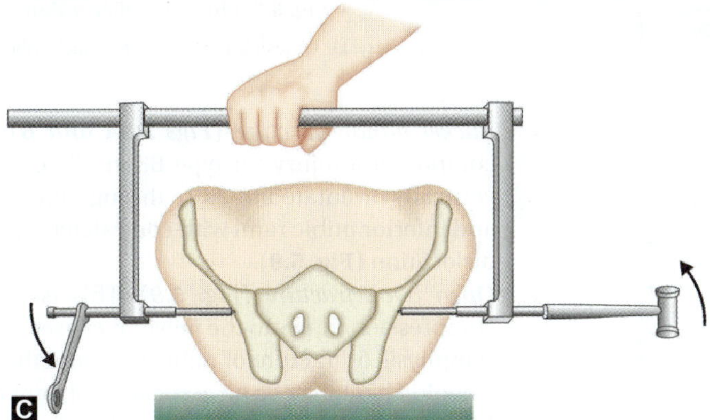

Figs 5.4A to C: (A) Pelvic sheath application for unstable pelvic fracture with suspected pelvic hemorrhage; (B) Anterior external fixator application for unstable pelvic fractures; and (C) Pelvic C-clamp for posterior stabilization of the pelvis

fractures with no posterior displacement (LC-I and APC-I) are treated conservatively with protected weight bearing. Walker or crutches are used for early mobilization. Open book fractures (Tile type B1) with pubic symphysis opening less than 2.5 cm also respond well to conservative treatment.

Operative Treatment

Unstable injuries, mostly need operative fixation. LC-II fractures require open reduction and internal fixation (ORIF) of ilium. APC-II or open book type fractures with opening more than 2.5 cm require open reduction and anterior symphyseal plate fixation or external fixator application. Both fixation methods give good results.

High-grade injuries LC-III and APC-III are difficult fractures to treat. Posterior ring integrity is important in transferring loads to lower limbs. APC-III fractures require anterior stabilization with a plate or external fixator and posterior stabilization with SI joint screw or plate. LC-III injuries are also unstable and require posterior stabilization with SI joint screw or plate.

Management of Open Pelvic Fractures

Open pelvic fractures are dangerous injuries that apart from routine management described above need special consideration in context of the genitourinary and fecal contamination risk. If there is a risk of fecal contamination of the wound, then colostomy is required. A thorough examination of pelvic organs and genitourinary system is mandatory in patients with open pelvic injuries.

Complications

Injury to the urethra and bladder, sexual dysfunction, thrombo-embolism (deep vein thrombosis and pulmonary embolism) and sciatic nerve injury are commonly encountered problems. Prophylactic anticoagulation may be warranted in high-risk trauma patients with unstable pelvic injury requiring surgical fixation. Sexual dysfunction is common in men after pelvic injury. Disruption of the pubic symphysis is frequently associated with temporary erectile dysfunction. Urethral injuries may lead to strictures, incontinence, and impotence. Urologist consultation is required for the management of these injuries. The sciatic nerve injury is usually neurapraxia and recovers within few weeks.

A notable complication that needs special mention is the Morel-Lavallée lesion **(Fig. 5.5)**. This is a post-traumatic closed degloving soft tissue injury in which the skin and subcutaneous tissue are torn away from the underlying fascia creating a potential space. This disruption may tear the perforating vessels and lymphatics and the potential space may be filled with blood, serosanguinous fluid, and necrotic fat. These lesions may complicate traumatic pelvic and acetabular injuries. Patients present with enlarging painful mass and anterolateral thigh (area around greater trochanter) is the most commonly involved area. Treatment options include aspiration, tube drainage, and the use

Flow chart 5.1: Management of the hemodynamically unstable patient with a pelvic fracture

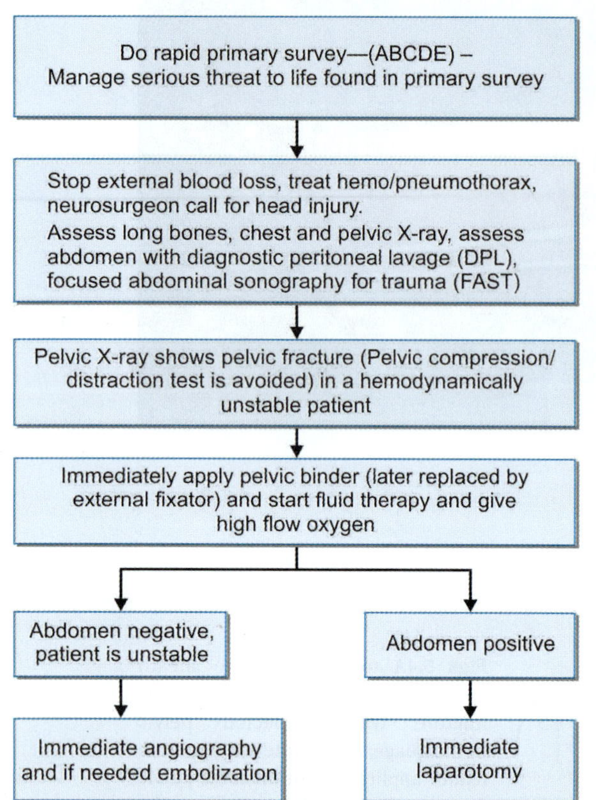

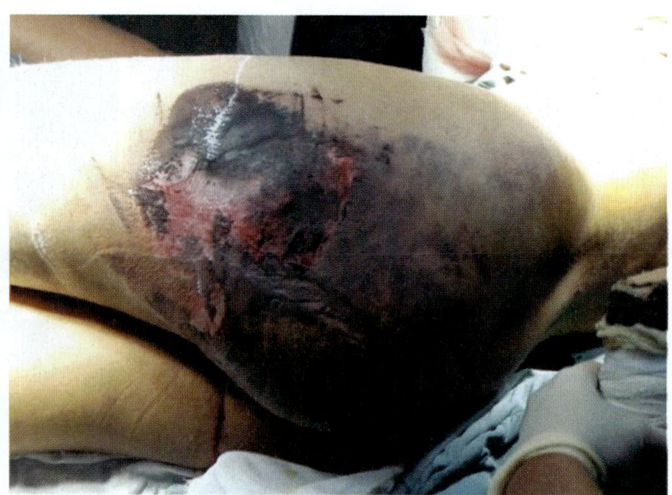

Fig. 5.5: Morel-Lavallée lesion

Courtesy: Dr Umesh Meena, SMS Medical College, Jaipur.

of sclerosing agent. In one-third cases the lesion may be infected in which case an incision and drainage may be required.

HIGH-YIELD POINTS

Learn the terminology of pelvic fractures

- *Straddle injury (Figs 5.6A and B):* Bilateral fracture of both superior and inferior pubic rami.
- *Duverney fracture*: Iliac wing fracture.
- *Malgaigne's fracture (Figs 5.7A and B)*: This is a lateral compression injury resulting in an unstable pelvic fracture which comprises two vertically oriented fractures in one hemipelvis.

- *Bucket handle fracture (Figs 5.8A and B):* This is a lateral compression injury (or type B3 in Tile classification). It is a vertically orientated fracture through the ipsilateral superior and inferior pubic rami with contralateral SI joint disruption/dislocation (**Fig. 5.9**).
- *Open book fracture (Fig. 5.9)*: This is an anteroposterior compression injury to the pelvis. It causes disruption of pubic symphysis or fracture of pubic rami and the pelvis opens like a book. There may be an associated SI joint disruption.
- *Windswept pelvis (Figs 5.10A and B)*: It is a lateral compression injury of ipsilateral hemipelvis and open book or external rotation type injury of contralateral hemipelvis.
- *Crescent fracture (Fig. 5.11A)*: This is an iliac wing fracture that enters into the SI joint, causing a SI joint fracture dislocation.
- *Suicidal Jumper's fracture*: This is a transverse fracture of sacrum seen in patients who have jumped from a height during a suicidal attempt. The fracture is characterized by an H- or U-shaped fracture line in the upper sacrum (**Fig. 5.11B**), usually involving the S1-S2 region. Typically, the anterior segment of the pelvic ring is not injured.

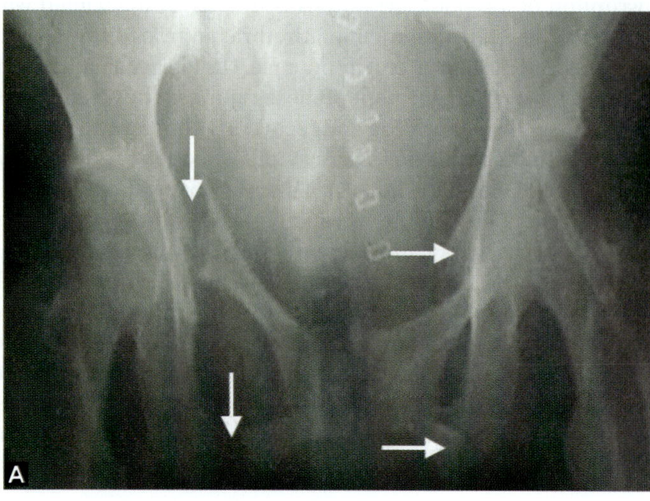

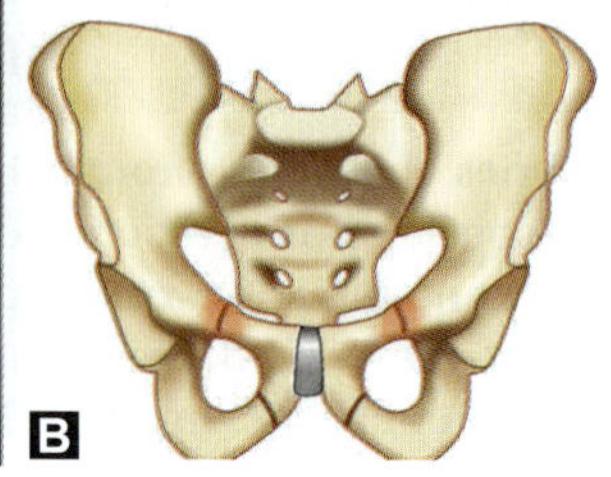

Figs 5.6A and B: X-ray of pelvis with both hips, anteroposterior view showing straddle injury

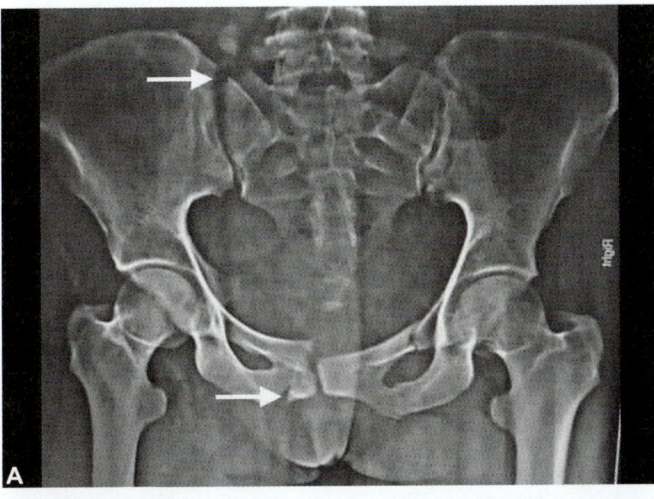

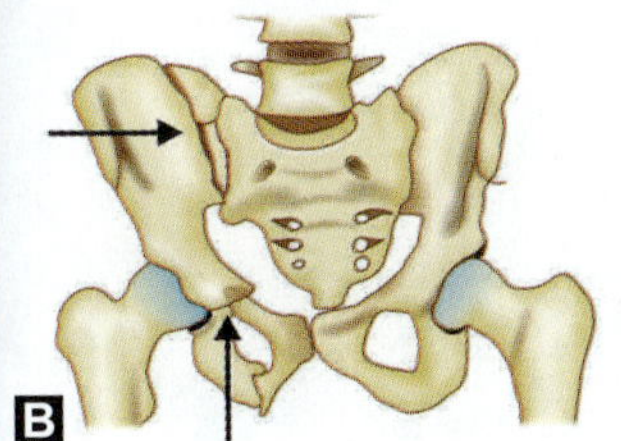

Figs 5.7A and B: Malgaigne's fracture

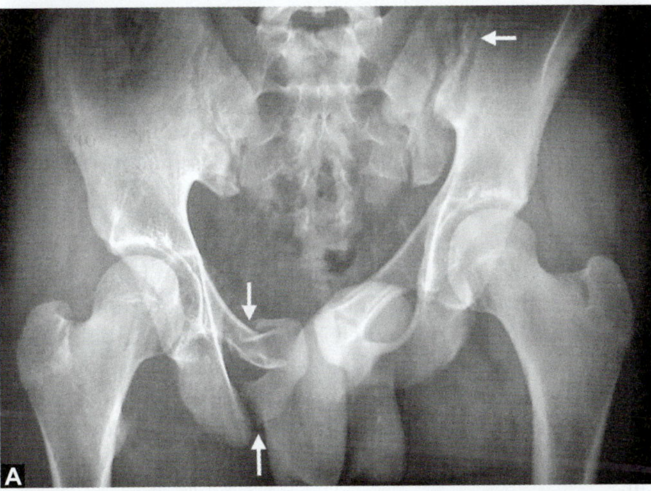

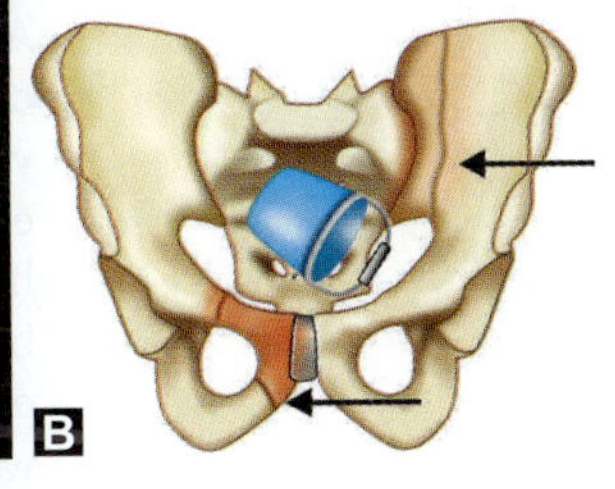

Figs 5.8A and B: X-ray of pelvis, anteroposterior view showing unstable bucket handle type pelvic fracture (right pubic rami fracture and left iliac wing fracture)

(lateral impact as in a fall from height) or in RTA when flexed knee (with flexed hip) strikes against a dashboard nipping off the posterior rim of the acetabulum.

Since, these patients are usually victim of high-energy injury a rapid primary survey should be done in all these patients to cinch any threat to life. If the patient is stable then detailed physical examination should include any associated soft tissue injury (Morel-Lavallée lesion), neurological examination (injury to the sciatic nerve is most common), limb deformity (concurrent posterior hip dislocation may be there), and other associated fractures.

Relevant Anatomy

Innominate bone is divided into two columns, anterior and posterior **(Figs 5.12A and B)**. Anterior column includes anterior half of the iliac wing, anterior half of the acetabular articular surface, and anterior pubis with symphysis. The posterior column begins at the superior aspect of greater sciatic notch and extends below to include the greater sciatic notch, posterior part of the articular surface of the acetabulum, lesser sciatic notch, and ischial tuberosity.

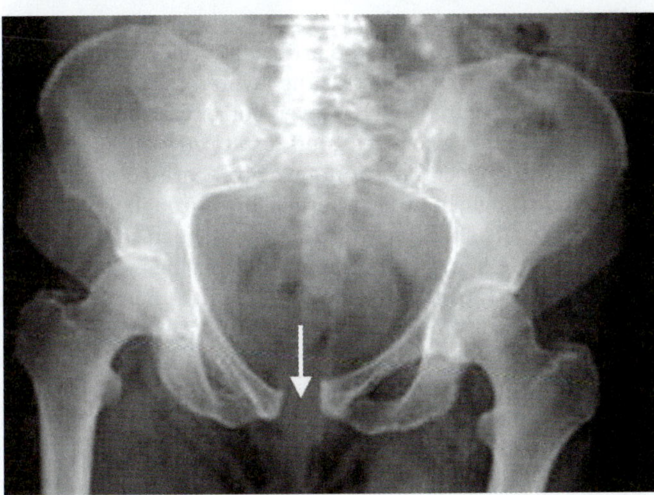

Fig. 5.9: X-ray of pelvis with both hips, anteroposterior view showing open book fracture

Classification

The traditional concept of a central fracture dislocation/traumatic protrusio acetabuli which occurs in a lateral blow to the trochanter

ACETABULAR FRACTURES

Acetabulum fractures are rare, but difficult to manage injuries. These are caused when the femoral head strikes the acetabulum. This may happen following a blow on the greater trochanter

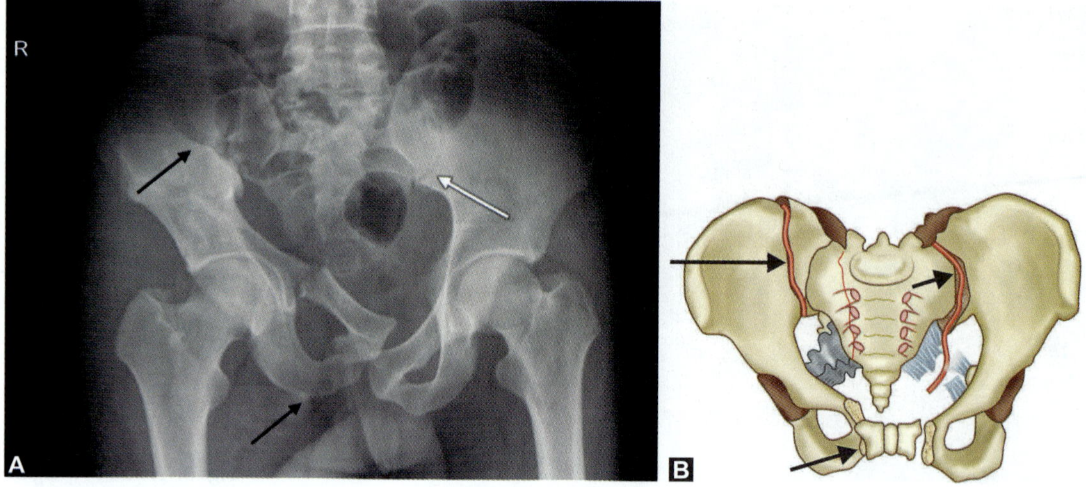

Figs 5.10A and B: X-ray, anteroposterior view showing a wind swept pelvis (fractures are indicated by arrows)
Courtesy: Dr Mike Cadogan.

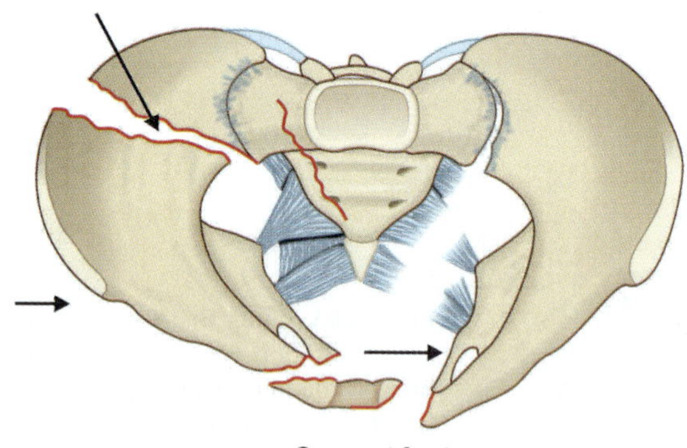

Fig. 5.11A: Schematic depiction of a crescent fracture of pelvis

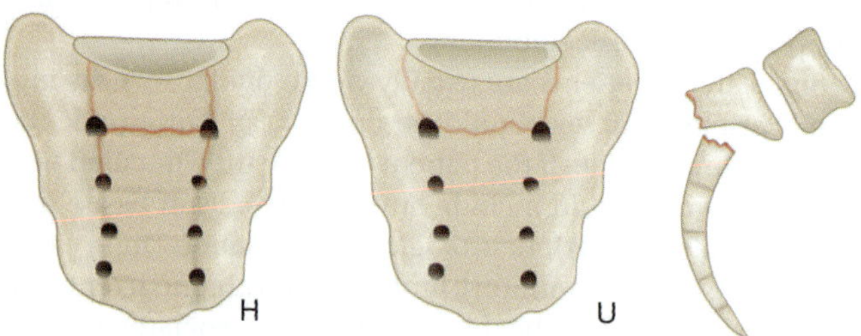

Fig. 5.11B: Suicidal Jumper's fracture
(sacrum fractures occur in H or U pattern)

(fall from a height with the lateral side of hip hitting the ground) that causes the acetabular floor to fracture and the head to migrate inside the pelvis is now a refuted concept. Based on two column principle Letournel and Judet have classified acetabular fractures into more descriptive patterns. These include five elementary and five associated fracture patterns **(Figs 5.13A to J)**. The position of the femoral head at the time of the injury, the magnitude of force, and the age of the patient determines the fracture pattern.

Posterior wall fractures are the most common type out of all. The central fracture dislocation as per this classification is a both column type of fracture.

Diagnosis

Anteroposterior view and special Judet views of the pelvis are conventionally prescribed to identify acetabular fractures. Judet views are oblique views of pelvis and include iliac oblique (45° external) and obturator oblique (45° internal) views and better help to delineate an acetabular fracture. While the obturator view better delineates the anterior column and posterior wall, the oblique iliac view better delineates posterior column and anterior wall.

Treatment

Acetabular fractures involve the articular surface so anatomical reduction and internal fixation is the favored treatment by most of the orthopedic surgeons. However, conservative treatment of acetabular fractures also gives good result provided the fracture is minimally displaced and of nonweight-bearing zone. Matta's roof arc angle (angle between a vertical line through the center of the femoral head and a line from the femoral head center passing through fracture site) is a special angle that helps in deciding between conservative and nonconservative management in acetabular fractures **(Fig. 5.14A)**. An angle >45° basically predicts the fracture is in the weight-bearing zone and needs operative fixation.

All the patients who are chosen for conservative treatment should be put on skeletal traction (above the knee, supracondylar skeletal traction) for 6–8 weeks. After that, patients are allowed to walk with crutches or a walker. Passive and active range of motion physiotherapy should be started early. Dislocation of the femoral head may be associated with acetabular fracture and requires urgent reduction to prevent avascular necrosis (AVN). Displaced fractures require congruent ORIF with plate and screws **(Figs 5.14B and C)**.

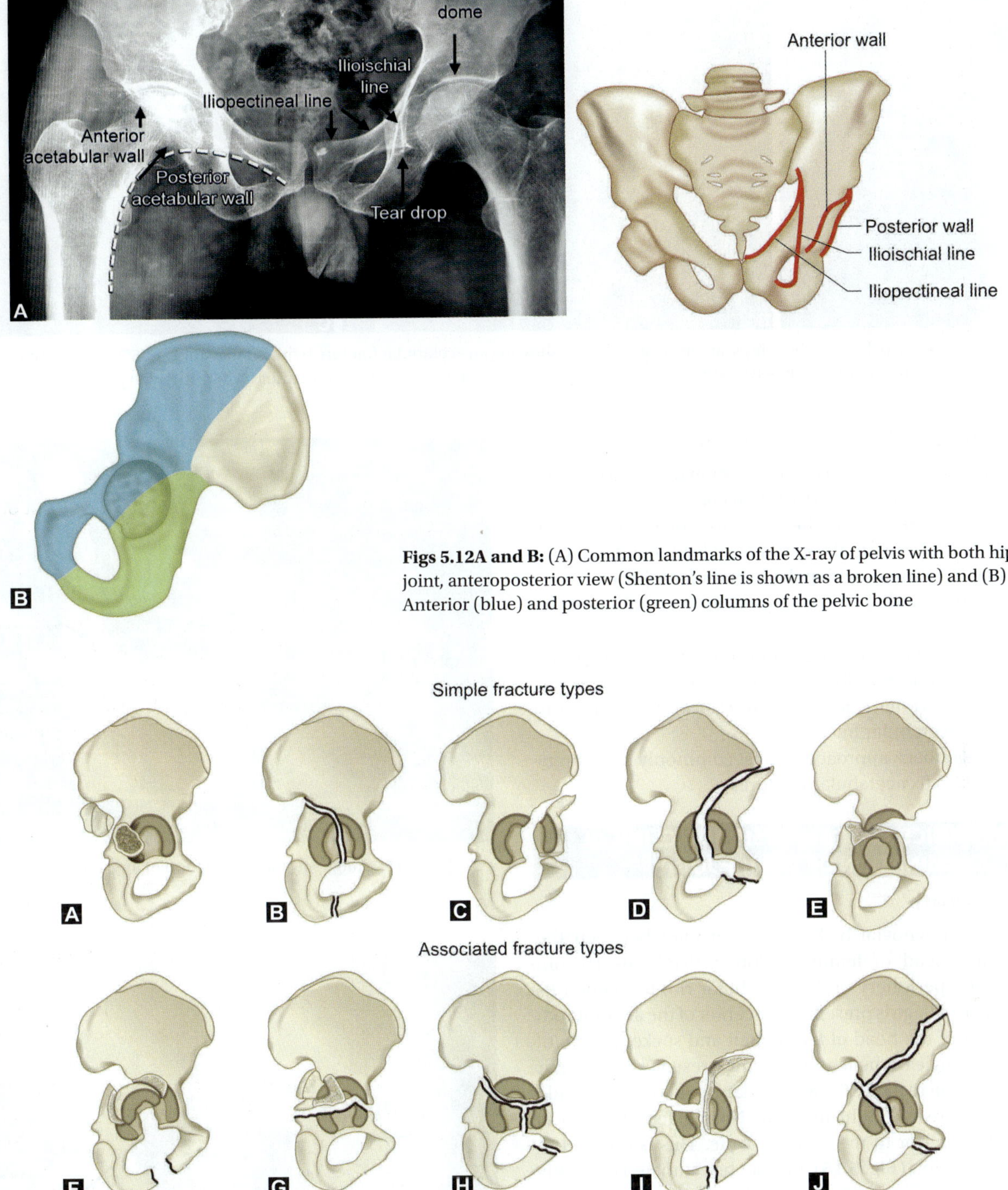

Figs 5.12A and B: (A) Common landmarks of the X-ray of pelvis with both hip joint, anteroposterior view (Shenton's line is shown as a broken line) and (B) Anterior (blue) and posterior (green) columns of the pelvic bone

Figs 5.13A to J: Judet and Letournel classification of acetabular fractures. (A) Posterior wall; (B) Posterior column; (C) Anterior wall; (D) Anterior column; (E) Transverse; (F) Posterior column + posterior wall; (G) Transverse + posterior wall; (H) T type; (I) Anterior column + posterior hemitransverse; (J) Both columns

Complications

The most common complication of acetabular fractures is secondary osteoarthritis of the hip joint. Heterotopic ossification, sciatic nerve injury (mostly iatrogenic), AVN of the femoral head, and venous thromboembolism are other notable complications of acetabular fractures.

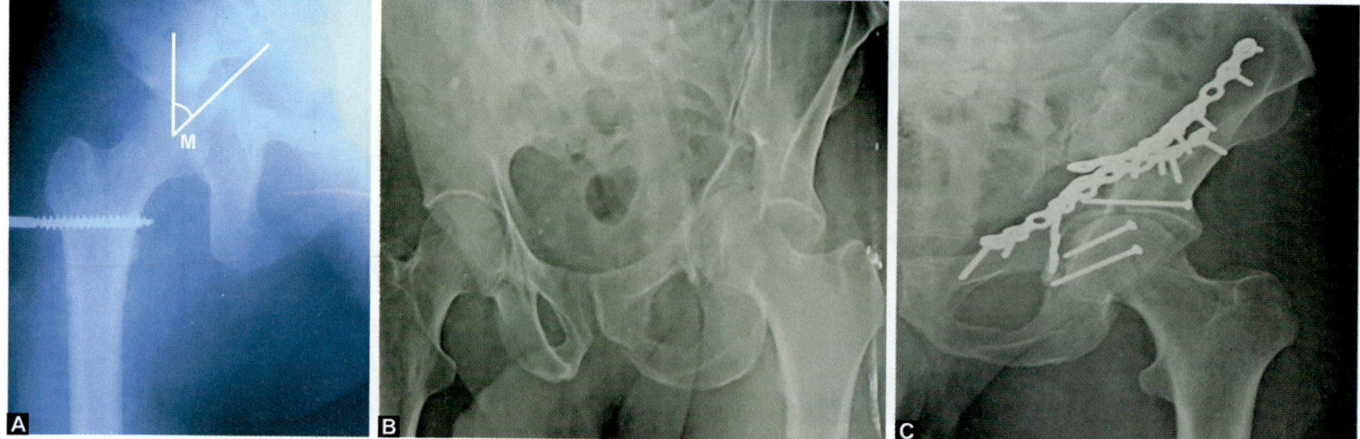

Figs 5.14A to C: (A) X-ray of pelvis with both hips, anteroposterior view showing an acetabular fracture (with Matta's angle > 45°) managed conservatively with lateral traction; (B) X-ray of pelvis with both hips showing T type fracture of acetabulum; and (C) its ORIF with plate and screws

HIGH-YIELD POINTS

- Corona Mortis is a vascular communication between external (inferior epigastric artery) and internal iliac (obturator artery) systems that is present just behind superior pubic rami in 85% of patients. Injury to the corona can lead to a dangerous hemorrhage in patients with pelvi-acetabular injuries.
- Some important radiographic signs seen in acetabular fractures are:
    - *Gull wing sign**: Seen in the anterior column plus posterior hemitransverse fracture of the acetabulum.
    - *Secondary congruence and Spur sign*: Seen in both column acetabular fractures.
- Kocher-Langenbeck approach is most commonly used surgical approach to fix acetabular fracture.

BIOMECHANICS, GAIT ANALYSIS AND CLINICAL EXAMINATION OF THE HIP JOINT

RELEVANT ANATOMY

The hip joint is a synovial ball and socket joint between the acetabulum and head of femur. A fibrocartilaginous labrum is attached to the periphery of the acetabular rim to deepen its cavity. Articular cartilage is present at the center of the acetabulum and covers most of the head of femur. Ball and socket nature of joint, neck-shaft angle of the femur, and the presence of articular cartilage beyond the reach of the acetabular rim allows for a wide range of motion possible at the hip joint. Normal femoral neck is rotated 15°–20° anterior to the coronal plane. This is referred to as femoral anteversion **(Fig. 5.15)** and can be estimated clinically by Craige's test (*see* **Fig. 5.15**). Femoral anteversion decreases from 40° at birth to 15°–20° in adults. Acetabulum also has 15°–20° anteversion and 45° inferior inclination. The neck shaft angle is deduced by measuring the angle between a line in the center of the femoral neck and a line in the center of femoral shaft **(Fig. 5.16)**. The normal neck shaft angle decreases from 140° at birth to 125° ± 5° in adult. Increase in neck-shaft angle greater than 130° is called coxa valga (as distal to the hip the limb moves

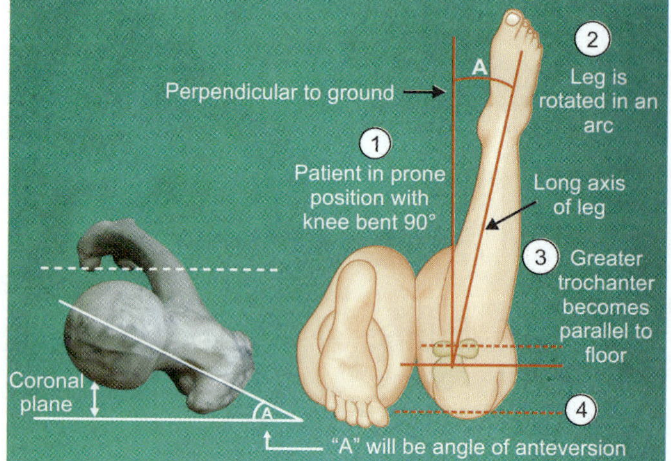

Fig. 5.15: Craige's test for estimation of angle of anteversion

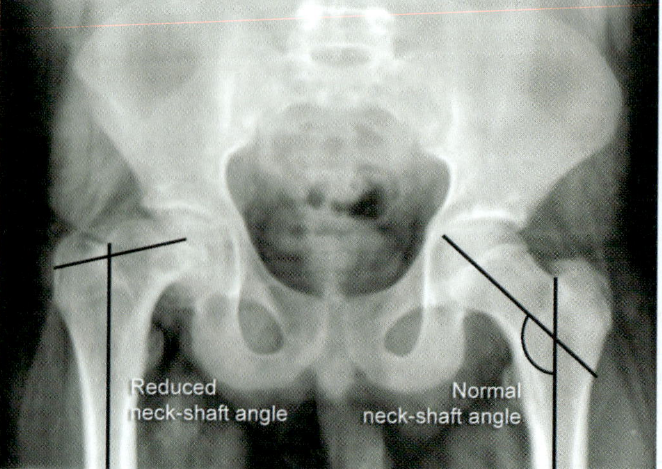

Fig. 5.16: Normal neck shaft angle and coxa vara

---

*Gull wing sign is also described for osteoarthritis changes in hand X-rays. See Chapter 16 for details.

laterally, *see* Page 6) and reduced neck-shaft angle less than 120° is known as coxa vara (as distal to the hip the limb moves medially, *see* Page 6).

Stability of hip joint depends upon the following factors:
- The depth of the acetabular cup and presence of labrum.
- Ligaments on both anterior (iliofemoral, pubofemoral) and posterior side (ischiofemoral). Iliofemoral ligament of Bigelow is the strongest ligament in the body. It prevents the pelvis from tilting posteriorly and limits adduction.
- The length and orientation of the neck of the femur.
- *Ligament of head of femur*: This band is called the ligamentum teres. It is implanted into the noncartilaginous area bearing fovea centralis on the head of the femur. A small artery runs along it to the head of the femur.
- Thick joint capsule and muscle cover.

Trabecular System of Femoral Neck (Fig. 5.17)

On radiographs, femoral neck can be observed to display two types of trabeculae. Horizontal set of tensile trabeculae is formed due to abductor muscle forces and vertical compressive trabeculae result of weight-bearing forces in the femoral head, both crossing each other at right angles. The knowledge of the trabecular anatomy is sometimes useful to decipher an impacted femoral neck fracture on a radiograph. Also, a special index (Singh's index) grades osteoporosis on the basis of this trabecular system.

Vascularity of Femoral Head and Neck (Fig. 5.18)

It can be divided into three main sources:
1. *Capsular vessels*: These arise from the medial circumflex femoral artery (MCFA) and lateral circumflex femoral artery (LCFA) which are in turn branches of profunda femoris artery. Branches from MCFA and LCFA form an extracapsular arterial ring at base of the femoral neck. Ascending cervical or retinacular vessels arise from extracapsular arterial ring and form a subsynovial intra-articular arterial ring at base of head. Epiphyseal arteries arise from the subsynovial arterial ring. Lateral epiphyseal vessels through lateral ascending cervical arteries (branches of MCFA) are the most important source of blood supply to the head and neck.
2. *Artery of ligamentum teres (medial epiphyseal artery)*: It is a branch of obturator artery. It makes a small contribution to the blood supply of the head.
3. *Intramedullary metaphyseal blood supply*: It makes least contribution to blood supply to the head.

HIP BIOMECHANICS AND ABNORMAL GAIT PATTERNS

When we stand on two legs the weight of the body is equally borne on both legs, the center of gravity (COG) is centered between the two hips (generally lying around 5 cm anterior to S2 vertebra) and the weight of the body (minus the weight of both legs) is equally distributed on the femoral heads. In single leg stance the COG is shifted distal and away from the supporting/loaded hip due to swing leg being considered as part of the body. As a result the supporting hip is subjected to the following three forces **(Fig. 5.19A):**
1. Body weight
2. Abductor muscle force
3. Joint reaction force.

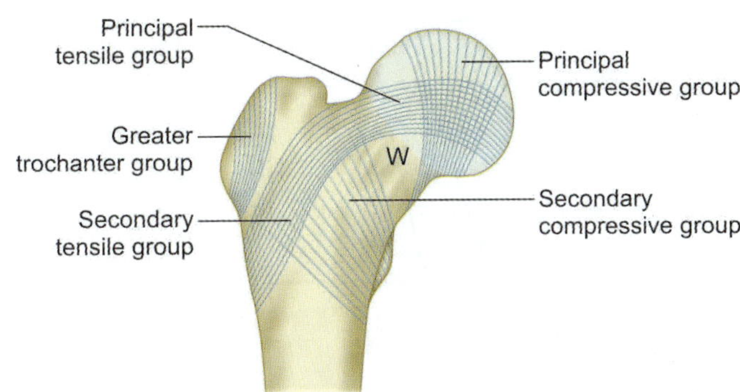

Fig. 5.17: Schematic representation of the trabecular system of femoral neck (W-Ward's triangle, a triangular shadow in trabecular system)

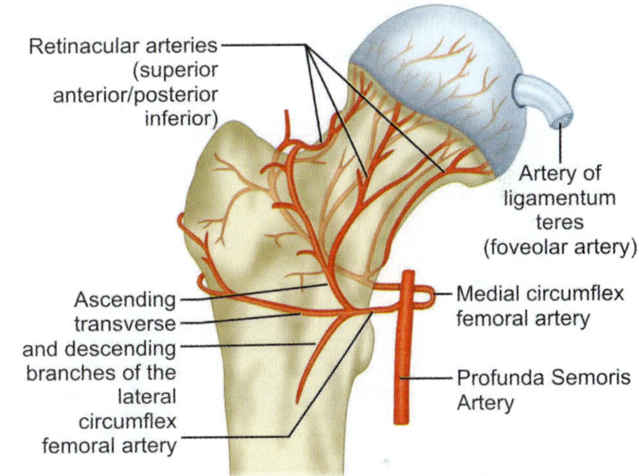

Fig. 5.18: Vascularity of femoral head

Joint reaction force is the force that generates within a joint in response to forces acting on the joint. In the hip joint these forces are body weight and abductor muscle force. To maintain a stable hip, torque produced by body weight should be countered by torque that abductor muscles can generate **(Fig. 5.19B)** with the femoral head acting as a fulcrum in this lever system.

How Does a Cane or Limp Help to Reduce the Hip Pain?

The joint reaction force across a painful hip can be reduced by either reducing the body weight (K) or its moment arm (A), or by increasing the abductor force (M) or its moment arm (B).

Cane in the opposite hand transmits part of body weight to ground and thus reducing the body weight (K) that needs to be countered by abductor muscle force (M). Hence, a cane is always prescribed in the opposite hand.

Limp toward the same side (of pathology) reduces the body lever arm (A) by shifting the COG toward loaded hip. Hence, when the abductors are paralyzed (from any cause) one bends toward the side of paralyzed abductors to shift the COG toward affected hip in an attempt to decrease joint reaction force in the hip.

Normal Gait Pattern

Normal gait comprises a series of rhythmical alternating movements of limb and trunk which result in forward progression of the COG of the body. Normal gait requires adequate muscle strength,

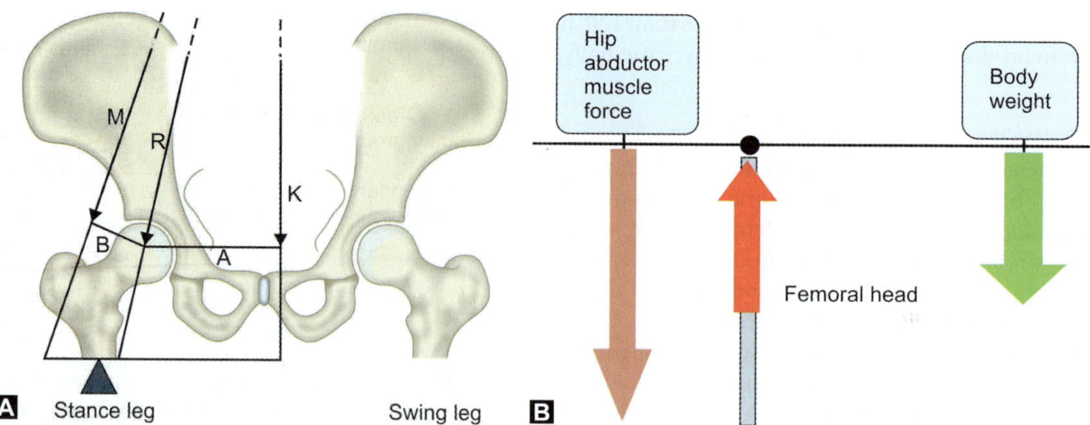

Figs 5.19A and B: (A) Free-body diagram for the calculation of the hip joint force while walking, where K is the body weight (minus the weight-bearing leg), M is the abductor muscle force, and R is the joint reaction force; (B) Hip joint is Class I lever with femoral head acting as a fulcrum in the center and forces (load or effort) distributed on either side. For a stable hip, load produced by body weight should be countered by abductor muscle effort

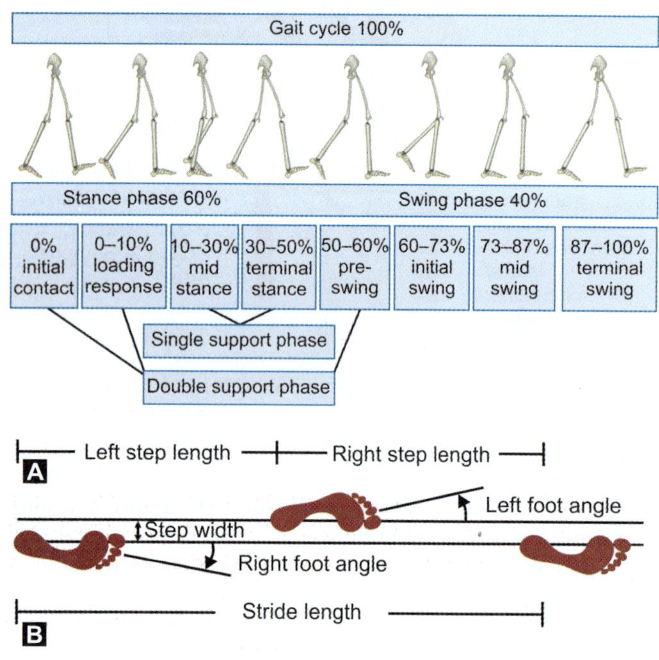

Figs 5.20A and B: (A) Normal gait cycle and (B) Various parameters of gait

full range of motion of all involved joints, good proprioception, and balance (alignment and length of the limbs). Identification of abnormal gait requires understanding of a normal gait cycle.

A "gait cycle" is defined as the time interval or a sequence of motions occurring between two consecutive initial contacts (heel strikes) of the same foot; each cycle lasting for 1–2 seconds. Gait cycle is divided into stance and swing phases **(Figs 5.20A and B)**. Stance phase is the period during which the foot is in contact with the ground while in the swing phase, the foot remains in the air. The stance phase usually accounts for 60% of the cycle and the swing phase accounts for 40% of the cycle.

The stance phase is subdivided into:
- Initial contact (heel strike)
- Loading response (flat foot)
- Mid stance (single leg support)
- Terminal stance (heel off), and
- Preswing (toe off).

The swing phase is subdivided into:
- Initial swing (acceleration)
- Mid-swing, and
- Terminal swing (deacceleration).

In a gait cycle there are two periods of single (60%) and two periods of double (40%) leg support. In single leg support phase only one foot is in contact with the ground. Double support is the period in normal gait cycle when both feet are in contact with the ground. With increasing speed the swing phase and single leg support becomes proportionately longer and the stance phase and double support phase becomes shorter. In running, the period of double support is absent (i.e. during no time are two feet simultaneously in contact with ground). Rather running is characterized by a phase called "double float", a period in which neither foot is in contact with the ground.

*Various Parameters of Gait (**Fig. 5.20B**)*
- Cadence is the number of steps taken per minute. Usually a person takes 90–120 steps/min that provides a comfortable walking speed of around 1.4 m/s or 5 km/h.
- The stride length is the linear distance between points of heel contact of the same foot. It is equal to sum of two step lengths, left and right. Its average value is about 150 cm.
- Step length is the linear distance between points of heel contact of the contralateral feet. Its average value is about 75 cm.
- Base of gait or step width is the distance between the medial aspect of the heels. Normally it is 6–8 cm.
- Angle of foot (syn. foot progression angle) is an angle between an imaginary line from heel to second toe and the line of progression. On an average it is 10°.

Abnormal Gait Patterns

Any deficiency or deviation from normal gait produces an abnormal gait pattern which is usually adapted to compensate for that deficiency.

Antalgic Gait

This is the most common pattern seen with painful hip (or presence of pain anywhere in the lower limb). It is characterized by slow walking speed, reduced stance phase on the painful limb, reduced joint excursion, and a limp toward the painful hip to reduce the moment arm of the body weight and thereby reduce the joint reaction force in the affected hip.

Trendelenburg Test and Gait (Duchenne de Boulogne)

Trendelenburg gait (syn. gluteus medius gait) is seen in weak abductor mechanism due to any cause. For an effective abductor mechanism one requires, an intact fulcrum (hip joint proper), lever arm (head and neck), and power (abductors). During one legged stance of the gait cycle, when one stands on a single leg (for instance left leg), the right side pelvis is lifted up to clear the ground. This is done by contraction of abductors on the left side (mainly gluteus medius that is running between ilium and the greater trochanter on the lateral aspect of the hip) acting via an intact lever arm and fulcrum. If the left side abductor mechanism is defective, the opposite side of the pelvis will dip down by virtue of gravity (positive Trendelenburg sign/test, **Fig. 5.21**). In this case, while walking, patient lurches to the same side, i.e. he shifts all his weight to the left side to prevent the right pelvis from dipping down and keep the pelvis leveled (Trendelenburg gait). When a patient lurches on both sides (positive Trendelenburg sign on both hips), it is known as "waddling gait".

Common causes of Trendelenburg gait are:
- *Defect in fulcrum:* Hip dislocation, advanced cases of TB hip and septic arthritis of hip joint, developmental dysplasia of the hip, Perthes disease, advanced cases of AVN hip.
- *Defect in lever arm:* Fracture head or neck of femur, coxa vara, and trochanteric fractures.
- *Defect in power:* Abductor paralysis due to poliomyelitis or superior gluteal nerve injury, tensor fascia lata and iliotibial tract palsy and L5 radiculopathy.

Short Limb Gait

The patient walks on toes of shortened limb by keeping a foot in equinus or may maintain flexion of the hip and knee of the lengthened limb to level the limbs. Often it is confused with Trendelenburg gait. The two can be differentiated by the fact that in short limb gait the "shoulders drop down" as patient walks, but the lurch (sway) toward the affected side is absent.

Foot Drop Gait (High-Stepping Gait)

It is seen in common peroneal palsy or sciatic nerve palsy where there is paralysis of the dorsiflexors. Patient lifts his leg more to clear the ground and he keeps his forefoot first than heel on the ground.

Stiff Knee Gait

It is characterized by decreased knee flexion (for instance, in tuberculosis of knee) in swing phase. Patient circumducts (excessively abducts) and brings the leg forwards to clear the ground.

Stiff Hip Gait

Here pelvis is lifted to bring the leg forward as in cases of tuberculosis of hip with ankylosed hip.

Crouch Gait

Patients walk with hip and knee flexion and ankle equinus. It is seen in cerebral palsy and polio.

Gluteus Maximus Lurch Gait

It is seen in polio, inferior gluteal nerve palsy, etc. Patients lurch backwards with every step to compensate for lack of hip extension.

Scissoring Gait

It is seen in cerebral palsy due to adductors spasm of both hip joints.

Hand-to-Knee Gait

It is seen in polio due to quadriceps weakness with inability to lock the knee while walking. The patient puts his hand on the knee to prevent it from buckling.

HIGH-YIELD POINTS

- Limp and Lurch are two interchangeably used terms. Ideally, "limp" is a symptom (usually pain) described by the patient that is causing change in his normal gait mechanics while "lurch" is an observation made by the clinician where he finds a sway of the patient's trunk or pelvis during the gait cycle.
- The head is never higher during normal gait than it is, when a person is standing.
- During normal gait body's COG describes vertical and horizontal displacements that simulate "figure of 8", confined within a square of 5 cm.
- Preswing is the only phase in the gait cycle where all muscle groups are silent.
- Phase with maximum kinetic energy is heel strike/loading response while the phase with maximum potential energy is mid stance.
- Cane in the opposite hand or limp toward the same side are an effective way to reduce the pain in ipsilateral hip or knee joint. So prescribe a cane always in the opposite hand, may the problem be in the hip or the leg.

EXAMINATION OF THE HIP JOINT

Hip examination starts from the point patient enters the clinician's room. Look at the gait pattern and attitude of patient

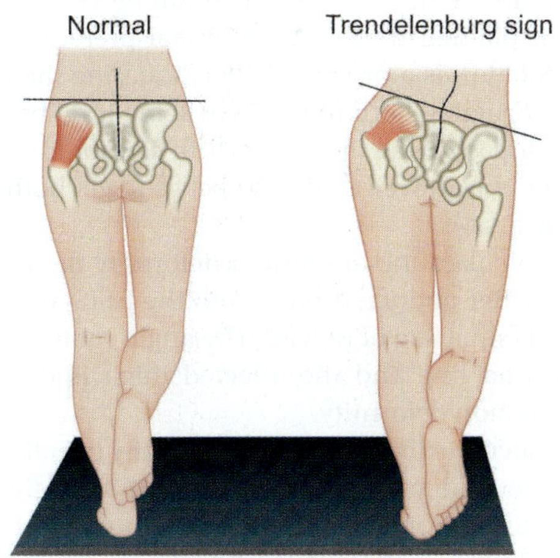

Fig. 5.21: Trendelenburg test

in standing and lying position. This gives an idea about the part of the lower limb which is diseased. Inspection should be done from the front, back, and side to see any wasting, swelling, deformity, and abnormal skin conditions. Palpate the all relevant bony points [GT, anterior superior iliac spine (ASIS)] and look for tenderness at base of Scarpa's triangle (syn. femoral triangle). Anteriorly femoral head can be located 1 cm below and out to the mid-inguinal point (located at the midpoint of a line between the ASIS and pubic symphysis). Palpate the inguinal group of lymph nodes and record range of motion at hip joint.

Understanding the fundamentals of hip examination require the reader to know two important concepts:
1. The concept of a fixed deformity
2. The concept behind true and apparent shortening.

Assessment of Fixed Deformity

Normally in the movements of the hip, the pelvis remains stable as movement occurs between femoral head and the acetabulum. A fixed deformity of the hip is one where the movement of the hip joint is lost in a particular direction either due to joint destruction or due to soft tissue contractures. Now on attempting that movement, the pelvis moves as a whole, rather than the movement occurring in the joint.

Pathological fixation of the hip joint in a fixed position of joint is one from where the limb can be moved further in the same plane but cannot be moved in the opposite direction as this moves the pelvis. So in a hip fixed in 15° adduction, abduction will not be possible as on abducting pelvis will tilt but further adduction may be possible.

Patients with fixed deformities of the hip joint, usually adopt compensatory postures to hide the deformity. The compensation depends on the type of fixed deformity as explained below.

- In fixed flexion deformity patient compensates for by excessive lumbar lordosis **(Fig. 5.22)**. Thomas test is used to assess this fixed flexion deformity of the hip joint.

  Thomas test (Fig. 5.23): Patient is positioned supine on a firm bed and then asked to flex the normal hip to bring the knee of normal side to his chest. Patients with fixed hip flexion deformity compensate by excessive lumbar lordosis (as explained in **Fig. 5.22**), so this is done to obliterate that compensatory lumbar lordosis so that the flexion deformity at affected hip can manifest. Hence, ensure that there is no space between the patient's back and the table before proceeding further. Now ask the patient to hold this normal limb in this position with his own hands. This automatically brings the diseased hip (with fixed flexion deformity) into some flexion (as obliteration of lumbar lordosis makes the masked deformity manifest). The examiner then passively lowers the affected limb to the bed. If the limb remains up off the table, a fixed flexion deformity of the hip is suspected. The angle subtended between the thigh and the bed is the angle of flexion deformity.

- In fixed adduction or abduction deformities, to ambulate normally, the body compensates by tilting the pelvis. In fixed abduction deformity ASIS is fixed at a lower level as compared to the other side (*see* **Fig. 5.24A** for an explanation) while in fixed adduction deformity ASIS will be at a higher level as

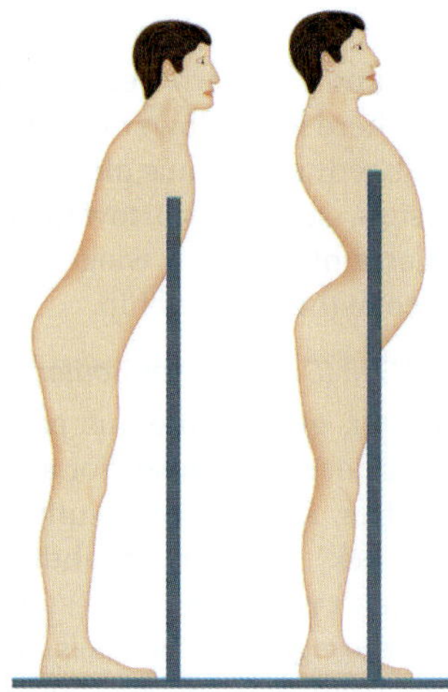

Fig. 5.22: Flexion at hip has been compensated by increasing lordosis at lumbar spine and the trunk has been leveled

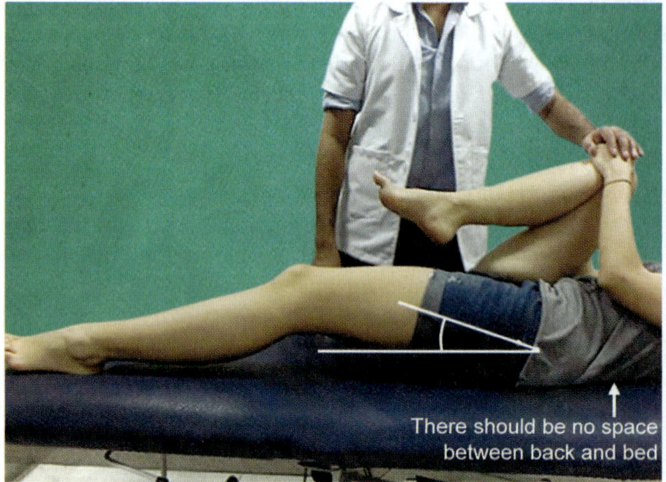

Fig. 5.23: Thomas test

compared to the other side (*see* **Fig. 5.24B** for explanation). The amount of either deformities can be very easily quantified as explained below. An essential prerequisite to make the calculation is a process called "squaring the pelvis". This involves bringing both the ASIS to same level by moving the affected hip (moving the normal hip cannot tilt the pelvis so affected hip is moved to tilt the pelvis to get both ASIS on to the same level).

- To calculate the amount of deformity the affected limb is further abducted until both the ASIS are at the same level (squaring of pelvis). The angle subtended between the mid line and the affected thigh is the amount of abduction deformity.

- To calculate the amount of deformity the affected limb is further adducted until both the ASIS are at the same level (squaring of pelvis). The angle subtended between the mid line and affected thigh is the amount of adduction deformity.

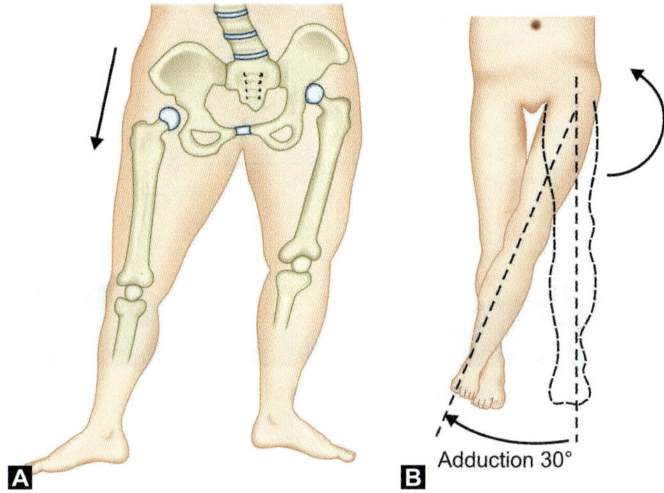

Figs 5.24A and B: (A) Right hip of this patient has fixed abduction. To place it flat on the ground, the ipsilateral ASIS has to be dropped down and thus over time it gets fixed at a lower level, and (B) Left hip of the patient has fixed adduction. To bring this leg into parallel alignment (dotted diagram), the ipsilateral ASIS has to be lifted up and thus it gets fixed at a higher level

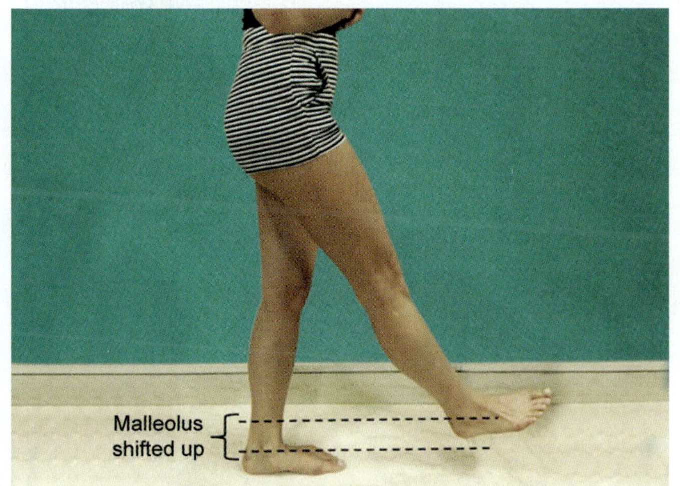

Fig. 5.25: Malleolus moves proximally when the hip is flexed apparently shortening the limb

Assessment of True and Apparent Length

Affections of the hip can lead to alterations in the limb length. The alteration can occur either due to real bone loss causing true change in length of limb or due to compensatory postures adopted by the patient causing apparent changes in length of limb. For example, if there is a fixed flexion deformity of the hip, the malleolus apparently moves proximally as shown in **Figure 5.25**, although the limbs are actually of the same length. Now the patient brings this hip to extension by developing compensatory lumbar lordosis but the malleolus stays proximally located giving a false impression of a short limb. Similarly, in fixed adduction, due to compensation the ASIS gets fixed proximally and the limb is apparently shortened while in fixed abduction, the ASIS goes lower and the limb is apparently lengthened (**Figs 5.24A and B**).

The true and apparent lengths can be measured as shown in **Table 5.3**. Remember that finally, true length = apparent length ± (compensation because of fixed deformity), where you add for flexion or adduction deformities that shorten limb while subtraction is done for abduction deformity that lengthens the limb.

Assessment of Supratrochanteric Shortening

Any pathology in the lower limb (hip, thigh, leg, etc.) can be a cause of limb length discrepancy. In case the clinical examination reveals true shortening (i.e. loss of bone length), the next step in such patients is to decipher the level of shortening. This can be deciphered by performing the Galeazzi's test.

*Galeazzi/Allis test (**Figs 5.26A and B**):* This test demonstrates whether the shortening is in the femur or tibia. The patient lies supine with the hips flexed to 45° and the knees flexed up to 90° and both the lower limbs placed side to side with malleoli touching together. The examiner assesses the position of both knees from the end of the bed and from the side. Normally both knees lie at the same level. When the normal knee projects farther forwards than the affected, the affected femur is shorter and when affected knee is lower than the other the tibia is shorter.

In patients with hip pathologies with Galeazzi's test the shortening can thus be localized to the femur. Next step is to localize whether the shortening is subtrochanteric (measure length from GT to lateral knee joint line and compares two sides) or is supratrochanteric (pathology located above the greater trochanter as in the destruction of the femoral head, neck, or a dislocation of the joint). From hip joint affection one would

Table 5.3: Measurements of true and apparent length				
True length	From ASIS* to medial malleolus	Limbs in identical position with respect to pelvis	Pelvis is squared	In fixed abduction deformity true shortening will be more than apparent shortening. In fixed adduction deformity true shortening will be less than apparent shortening
Apparent length (functional length)	From any central point on trunk (umbilicus or xiphisternum) to medial malleolus	Limbs parallel to each other	Pelvis is not squared	It is primarily a measurement of pelvic tilt

*ASIS (anterior superior iliac spine) is identified by first palpating the pubic tubercle and then following the inguinal ligament up and laterally. The first bony landmark encountered is the ASIS.

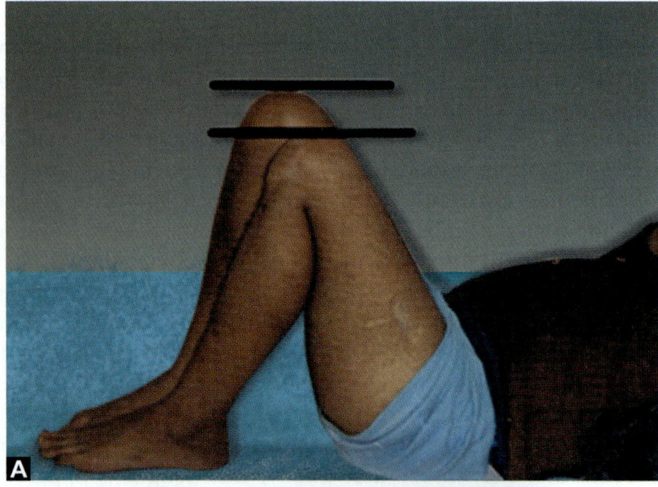

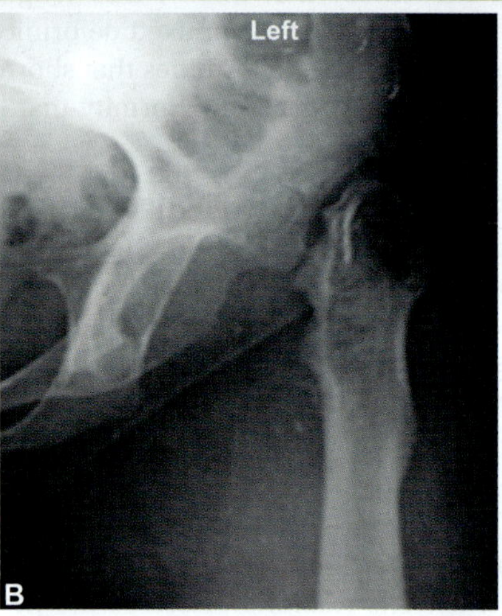

Figs 5.26A and B: Positive Allis/Galeazzi's test due to resorption of head and neck of femur, see X-ray (as a sequel of septic arthritis in this patient)

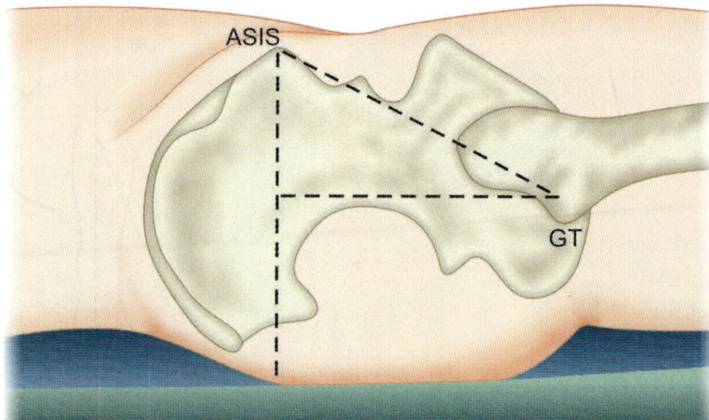

Fig. 5.27: Bryant's triangle

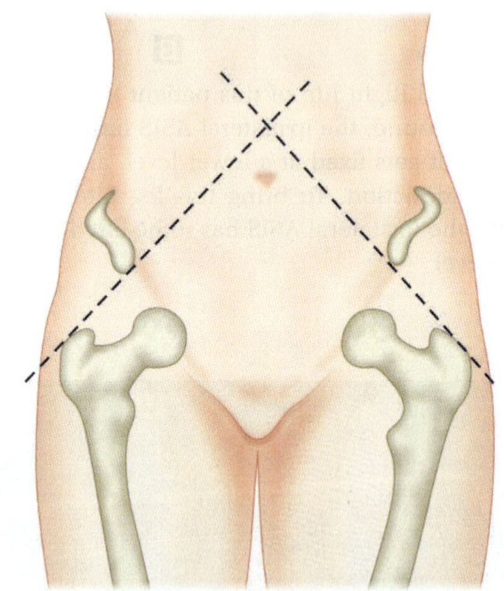

Fig. 5.28: Schoemaker's line

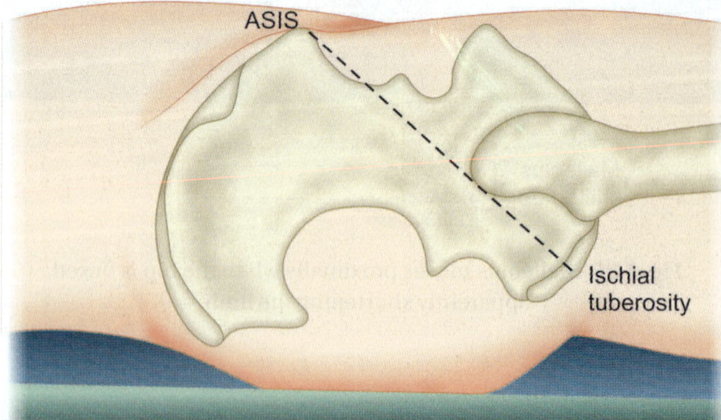

Fig. 5.29: Nelaton's line

expect to find supratrochanteric shortening. This can be deduced and measured in a number of ways as follows:

- *Bryant's triangle (**Fig. 5.27**)*: In a squared up pelvis in supine position a line is drawn from the ASIS perpendicular to the bed. Another line perpendicular to the first line is drawn from tip of GT. A third line from ASIS to tip of GT completes the triangle. This is compared to Bryant's triangle of normal side. Any shortening of the base indicates supratrochanteric shortening.
- *Schoemaker's line (**Fig. 5.28**)*: In supine position line joining the ASIS and tip of GT should meet the same line of opposite side at or above the umbilicus in the midline. In supratrochanteric shortening this line of affected side meets its counterpart below the umbilicus and the intersection is not centered at midline.
- *Chienes line*: With the patient lying supine, lines are drawn joining the two ASIS and the two greater trochanters. Normally, the two lines would stay parallel. In the case of one trochanter has migrated proximally, the lines will converge on that side.
- *Nelaton's line (**Fig. 5.29**)*: Patient is positioned in lateral position with the diseased side up. Flex the hip joint at 90°. Draw a line joining the ischial tuberosity to ASIS. In

supratrochanteric shortening the trochanter will be above this line. Normally, this line passes through the tip of GT. The advantage of Nelaton's line over the other methods is that it can measure supratrochanteric shortening in cases of bilateral hip pathologies as comparison with other side is not needed.

Special Tests around the Hip

*Telescopy (**Fig. 5.30**)*: With the patient in supine position, flex the hip and knee joint to 90° (or less if this much of flexion is not possible) and adduct the hip joint slightly (10°–15°). To test the right hip, stand on the right side of the patient, hold his flexed knee with right hand and put palm on the trochanter and extended fingers on the buttock. Now pull up and push down the knee. The push movement is more important to focus. An obvious excursion of the trochanter can be felt if telescopic test is positive.

This test indicates the instability of the hip joint and is positive in neglected posterior dislocation of hip joint, congenital dislocation of hip, paralytic hip, nonunion fracture neck of femur, advanced cases of AVN, and septic arthritis with resorption of head and neck.

Note: Stand on same side of affection. The clinician is standing on the opposite side to ensure good visibility to the reader.

HIGH-YIELD POINTS

- Lumbar lordosis can hide up to 30° of flexion deformity at the hip joint.
- Thomas test cannot detect bilateral hip flexion deformity. In such cases a prone test is used for detection.

INJURIES AROUND THE HIP JOINT AND FRACTURE SHAFT OF FEMUR

DISLOCATION OF THE HIP

Hip dislocations are orthopedic emergencies that require immediate diagnosis, evaluation, and treatment. The dislocation may be posterior, central, or anterior. 90% of hip dislocations are posterior type in both adults and in children owing to the classical mechanism of injury (*see* below). Anterior fracture dislocation is more common than central fracture dislocation which is rarely seen.

Mechanism of Injury

The hip is the most stable joint in the body with best articular configuration. The strongest ligament in the body (the Y-shaped iliofemoral ligament or the ligament of Bigelow) is also present around the hip. So in the majority of cases dislocation of the hip occurs due to a high-velocity motor vehicle injury. Posterior traumatic hip dislocations occur when axial force is applied to flexed, adducted, and internally rotated hip joint. Dashboard injuries in which person's flexed knee, with flexed hip strikes against the dashboard is a common mechanism of injury for posterior dislocation of hip. Thompson-Epstein classification is used to classify posterior hip dislocations **(Table 5.4)**. Anterior hip dislocation is classified by Epstein's classification into superior (pubic and subspinous) and inferior types (obturator and perineal).

Clinical Features

Patients present with a typical attitude of limb depending upon the type of dislocation **(Table 5.5)**, with inability to use the involved lower limb. Since the mechanism is mostly a dashboard injury, many a times these patients can have a concomitant fracture of posterior wall of the acetabulum, patellar fractures, and posterior cruciate ligament injury in the knee.

All hip movements are painful. Femoral head may be palpable at the ipsilateral gluteal region in posterior dislocation while it is palpable in groin in an anterior dislocation. In a central fracture

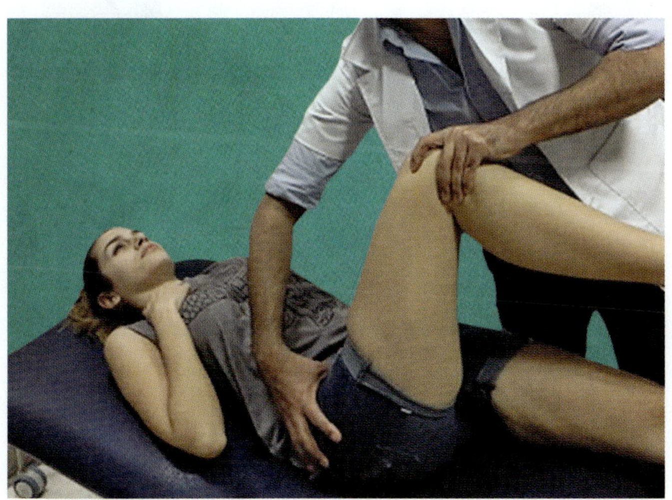

Fig. 5.30: Telescopy test of the hip joint

Table 5.4: Thompson-Epstein classification of posterior dislocation of the hip joint	
Type	*Description*
Type I	Posterior dislocation with no or minor fracture of posterior acetabular rim
Type II	Posterior dislocation with large single fracture of posterior acetabular rim
Type III	Posterior dislocation with comminution of acetabular rim, irrespective of the size of fragments
Type IV	Posterior dislocation with fracture of the acetabular floor
Type V	Posterior dislocation with fracture of the femoral head

Table 5.5: Mechanism of injury and limb attitude in hip dislocation		
Type of dislocation	*Mechanism of injury*	*Attitude of limb*
Posterior dislocation of hip	Axial force along the shaft of femur with hip flexed, adducted, and internally rotated	Flexion, adduction, and internal rotation, true shortening may be present **(Fig. 5.31)**
Anterior dislocation of hip	Hyperabduction and external rotation of flexed hip joint	Abduction and external rotation with flexion (with limb shortening, obturator type) or extension (with limb lengthening, pubic type) at hip joint
Central fracture-dislocation of hip joint.	Axial force on internally rotated and abducted hip, direct injury on the trochanter	Virtually any deformity possible. Mostly flexion, abduction and internal rotation or flexion, adduction and external rotation. True shortening may be present

dislocation (fracture of acetabular floor where head migrates into the pelvis), the head can often be palpated on a per rectal examination. Vascular sign of Narath (i.e. inability to feel femoral pulse against femoral head) is positive in posterior dislocations. However, in the anterior dislocation, head may be felt stays in the groin so despite a dislocation femoral pulsation may be palpable.

Immediate assessment of vitals, associated injuries, and distal neurovascular status is utmost important in patients with hip dislocation. Thorough neurological examination, especially of sciatic nerve must be done and recorded before reduction as sciatic nerve injury is the most common acute complication. Clinical examination may also reveal the classical deformity indicating the type of dislocation **(Fig. 5.31)**. Limb length discrepancy may be evident (shortening in posterior while lengthening in anterior dislocation). The diagnosis can be further strengthened on plain anteroposterior, iliac, and obturator views of the joint. X-ray **(Fig. 5.32)** shows the empty acetabulum proximally migrated femoral head due to pull by the gluteal muscles (in posterior

dislocation) and broken Shenton's line (normally a continuous line formed by the inferior margin of the superior pubic ramus and the medial margin of the neck, **Fig. 5.12A**). For visualization of the acetabular fracture and associated fracture head of femur, CT scan remains the modality of choice.

Management

Hip dislocation with or without acetabular or femoral head fracture is an emergency and must be reduced as early as possible else the head may undergo avascular necrosis (*see* below). Around 2–4% dislocations are irreducible, else most of the times closed reduction under general anesthesia is possible. Many methods of closed reduction of posterior hip dislocation have been described like Allis maneuver **(Figs 5.33A to D)**, Bigelow's maneuver (leverage method, can reduce both anterior and posterior dislocations, but not used due to high-risk of femoral neck fractures), Stimson's gravity method **(Fig. 5.34)** and modified east Baltimore lift **(Fig. 5.35)**. Allis maneuver is the most commonly used method for closed reduction of posterior hip dislocation. Anterior hip dislocations can be reduced with axial traction, direct lateral force on the proximal medial aspect of the thigh, and internal rotation of the hip.

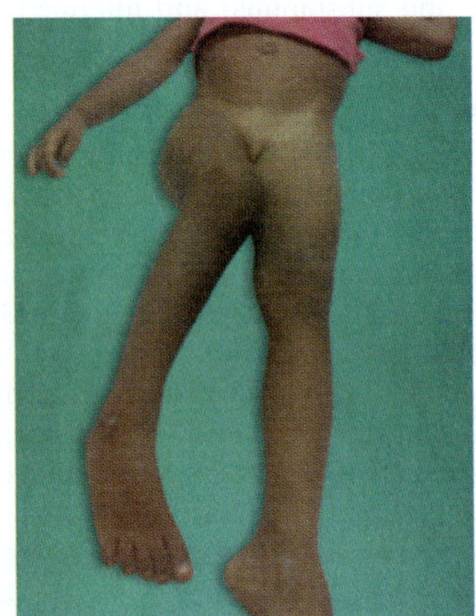

Fig. 5.31: Classical attitude of flexion, adduction, and internal rotation in a patient with posterior dislocation of right hip

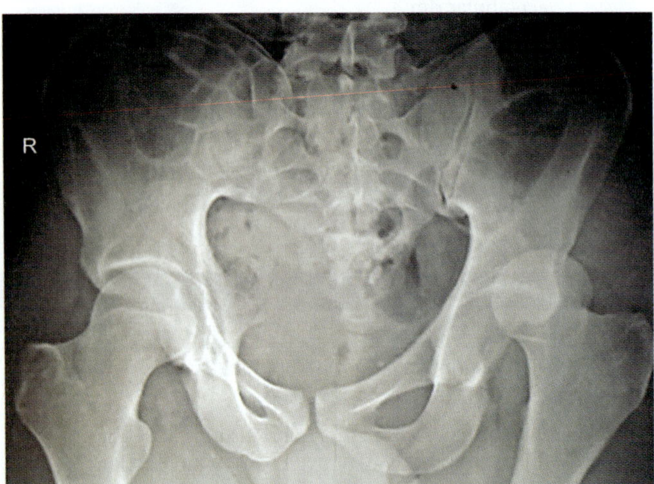

Fig. 5.32: X-ray of pelvis with both hips. Anteroposterior view showing posterior dislocation of hip joint—see adduction and internal rotation (lesser trochanter is not visible) of the femur also the Shenton's line is broken

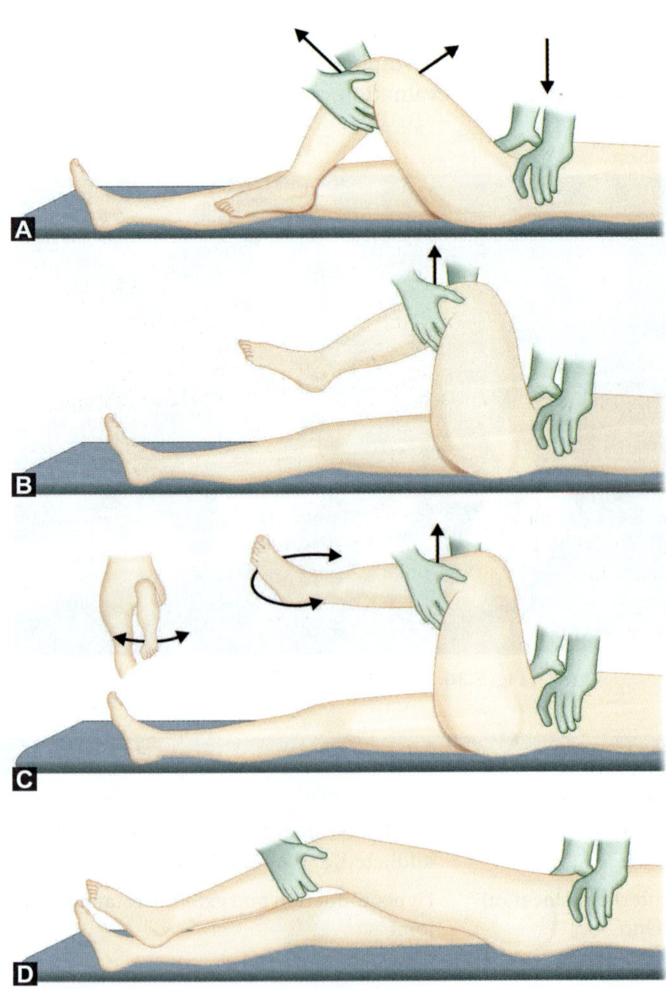

Figs 5.33A to D: (A) Affected hip is flexed and adducted; (B) Traction is given in line of femur; (C) Rotation movements are performed to achieve reduction; and (D) After reduction hip is abducted and extended

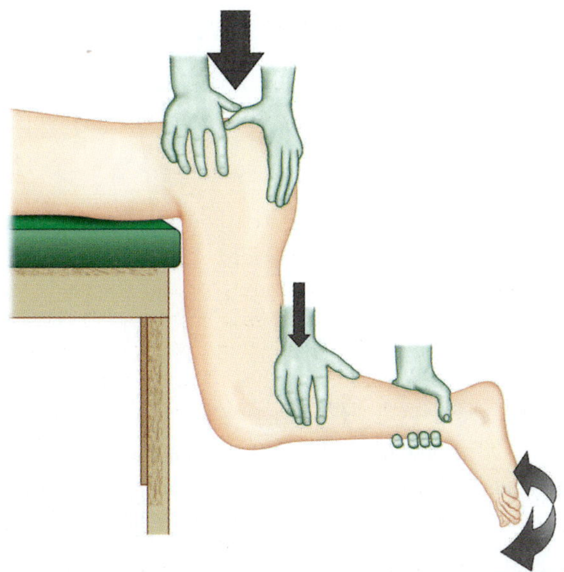

Fig. 5.34: Stimson's gravity method (gravity-assisted reduction by making anesthetized patient lie prone with hips left hanging at the edge of the table)

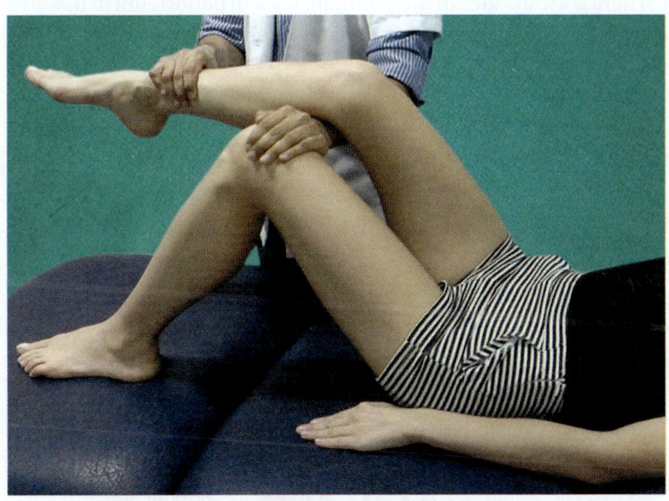

Fig. 5.35: Modified East Baltimore Lift (the examiner flexes the normal hip and passes his forearm under the flexed knee of the affected side to convert the system into pulley mechanism with his forearm acting as fulcrum. A downward force on affected leg will pull the dislocated hip anteriorly and reduce it)

Once a stable closed reduction is achieved, the patient can be mobilized with crutches. Weight bearing is allowed as tolerated and gradually progressed as pain allows. However, if a closed reduction fails (interposed labrum, osteocartilaginous loose body in the acetabulum or buttonholing of the head through the capsule and piriformis, etc.), patient should be urgently posted for an open reduction. Patients with concomitant femoral neck or head fractures also usually require primary open reduction.

Complications

Early Complications

Nerve injury: Sciatic nerve injury is the most common acute complication in posterior dislocation of the hip and chances is even more in fracture dislocation. Peroneal component affection is more common than complete loss as peroneal fibers are the outermost fibers in the nerve. Femoral nerve injury may occur in anterior dislocation. Mostly these cases are neurapraxia which spontaneously recover in 6–12 weeks. If a sciatic nerve injury appears after close reduction urgent exploration may be needed to rule out its entrapment by reduction maneuver.

Vascular injury: Superior gluteal artery may be injured. If suspected urgent exploration and vascular repair is required.

Associated fractures: Fractures of the femoral head and neck can be associated either due to injury or iatrogenic during reduction. The risk of avascular necrosis of the femoral head is greatly increased in such cases.

Delayed Complications

Avascular necrosis of the femoral head: Chances of AVN of hip increases with delay in reduction. If the hip is reduced within 6 hours of dislocation then AVN of the head occurs in up to 10% cases. The greater the duration of the delay in reduction, the greater is chances of development of AVN. Greatest chances of AVN postreduction are in type IV and III (up to 50% chance of AVN). Type I has the least complication rate postreduction. Changes of AVN first appear on MRI and it may take even 1–2 years to make a diagnosis on X-rays. The patient presents with pain in hip joint after a painless period postreduction. Ultimately the patient develops secondary osteoarthritis with the collapse of the head and may end up needing a total hip replacement.

Heterotopic ossification: This is a common complication of posterior fracture dislocation (maximum chances in type IV). It is particularly common after open reduction (more with anterior approach) of posterior dislocation and is associated with severity of trauma. Indomethacin and radiation therapy are used in the prophylaxis.

Osteoarthritis: Secondary osteoarthritis is the most common complication of hip dislocation (maximum chances in type IV). This happens due to articular cartilage damage at the time of dislocation or reduction, incongruent fracture reduction, or due to AVN of the head. Most suitable treatment of advanced cases is total hip replacement.

Recurrent dislocation: It is exceedingly rare, but known complication. Recurrent posterior dislocation is mostly seen in patients who have a decreased femoral anteversion while anterior one is common in patients with increased femoral anteversion.

Thromboembolism: Hip dislocation patients are high-risk patients and shoulder preferably be given DVT prophylaxis for at least 2 weeks.

HIGH-YIELD POINT

- Type V posterior hip dislocation (Thompson and Epstein), as mentioned above, is one where there is associated fracture of the femoral head. These femoral head fractures are further classified by Pipkin's classification.

PROXIMAL FEMORAL FRACTURES

Introduction

Proximal femoral fractures are broadly classified into two main categories: (1) the intracapsular and (2) the extracapsular fractures. Capsule in the neck of femur is attached anteriorly along the intertrochanteric line and posteriorly just a finger breadth proximal to the intertrochanteric ridge. So any fracture proximal to this attachment is classified as intracapsular while a fracture distal to the attachment of the capsule is classified as an extracapsular fracture **(Fig. 5.36)**. In other words, any fracture that would involve the two trochanters will be extracapsular, hence the other name of extracapsular fracture can be "intertrochanteric fracture". The term "fracture neck of femur", on the contrary is popular to indicate the intracapsular fracture.

This division of proximal femoral fractures is primarily based upon the varied behavior of the two fracture types. Both these fractures involve the cancellous metaphyseal bone with abundant blood supply, but behave in an entirely divergent manner. Extracapsular fracture displays a good union propensity and almost always unites, but at times if not appropriately treated, it malunites. The intracapsular fracture on the other hand is notorious to end up in nonunion, despite involving the cancellous part of the bone **(Table 5.6)**. The other important complication seen in the latter type is the AVN of the femoral head. This complication is limited to intracapsular variety, as the fracture line in intracapsular fracture cuts off the vascular supply from the extracapsular arterial ring formed at the base of the femoral neck by the circumflex femoral vessels **(Fig. 5.37)** while an extracapsular fracture does not. However, both fractures present in almost similar age group and with a similar deformity with only subtle differences **(Table 5.7)**.

FRACTURE OF NECK OF FEMUR

It is a common fracture in elderly (age group 40–60 years), particularly females. It is a significant burden on the health care system due to increasing elderly population. It usually results from a household fall and is uncommon in young people where generally this fracture results after the high-energy impact. These fractures are most common in white females of Europe and America and incidence increases with age.

Risk Factors

These are broadly divided into risk factors associated with decreased bone density and those risk factors which increase the risk of falls.

Risk of falling increases with advancing age due to multiple factors like weak eye sight, neurological diseases, weak muscle power, and gait abnormalities. Osteoporosis either due to advanced age or due to any disease (i.e. osteomalacia, drug induced, alcohol abuse, rheumatoid arthritis, etc.) increases risk of fracture of neck of femur.

Mechanism of Injury

In elderly people weak bone breaks with simple low-energy fall whereas high-energy trauma is more common mode of injury in young people. Rarely in runners and military recruits repetitive strain and cyclical loading may cause stress fractures of neck of femur.

Clinical Features

Patients present with moderate to severe pain in the hip joint with inability to use the involved lower limb. On examination limb is externally rotated and shortened (as neck fractures, the

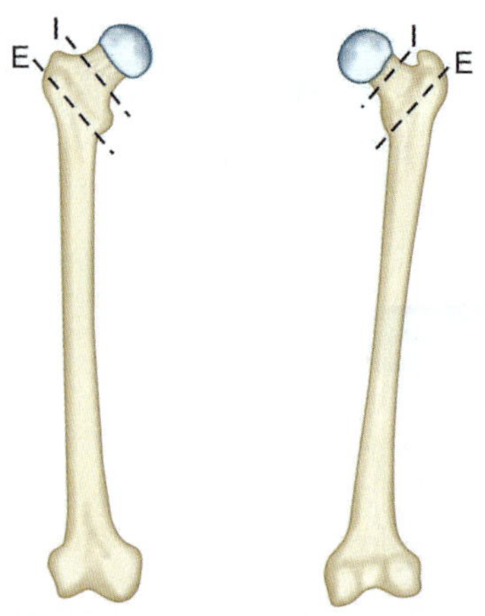

Fig. 5.36: Schematic depiction of intracapsular and extracapsular fracture (E, extracapsular, I, intracapsular)

Table 5.6: Reasons for nonunion in intracapsular neck femur fracture

- *Intracapsular nature:* Being intracapsular, the fracture is bathed in synovial fluid that has inhibiting factors to callus formation
- There is an absence of the cambium layer of periosteum in this area
- Blood supply to the area is precarious and often damaged during the injury
- Maintaining reduction is difficult as the head fragment is small and cancellous so it does not offer better purchase to the fixing implant
- Often there is posterior comminution that makes fracture highly unstable

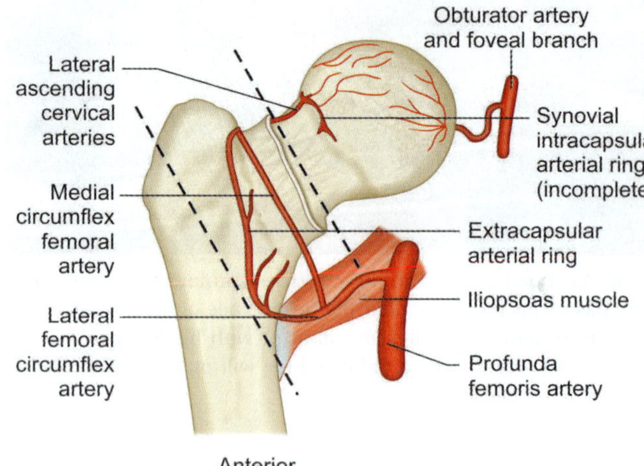

Fig. 5.37: Intracapsular fracture (I) is disrupting the supply from extracapsular ring to head while the extracapsular fracture (E) is not

femur falls into external rotation by virtue of gravity while the limb shortens due to trochanter being pulled proximally by the glutei). On palpation there is tenderness in Scarpa's triangle (femoral triangle) and the patient lacks an active straight leg raising (SLR). There may not be any obvious deformity in an undisplaced impacted fracture and patient might even be able to perform an active SLR. Such fractures can be traced on X-ray by a change in the trabecular pattern of the femoral neck or better by

Table 5.7: Comparison of extra- and intracapsular fractures of proximal femur*

	Fracture neck of femur (intracapsular)	*Intertrochanteric fracture (extracapsular)*
Definition	Intracapsular, fracture line is proximal to the insertion of capsule	Extracapsular, fracture line is distal to the insertion of capsule
Age profile	Common in elderly 40–60 years old	Seen in relatively older individuals (above 70–80 years)
Mechanism of injury	Low-energy fall, high-velocity trauma in young patients	Low-energy fall, high-velocity trauma in young patients
Clinical features	Moderate to severe pain in Scarpa's triangle, swelling, and ecchymosis are usually absent	Severe pain, swelling, and ecchymoses are usually present around greater trochanter
External rotation deformity**	Less	More, lateral border of foot almost touching the couch
Shortening**	Generally less than 2.5 cm	Generally more than 2.5 cm
Trochanteric palpation	Normal	Broadening and tenderness
Straight leg raising and walking	May be possible in impacted fracture	Not possible
Complications	AVN is the most common complication followed by nonunion	Malunion is the most common complication

*An easier way to remember the difference is that an extra capsular fracture has all extra: It is extra common, extra age (occurs in older people), extra deformity, and extra union chances (malunion).

**Although deformities are same, they are less exaggerated in intracapsular fracture as the capsule acts as a restraint to limit the displacements.

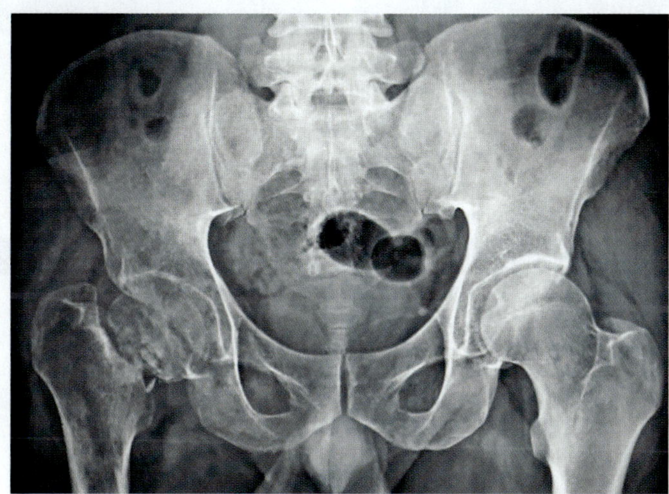

Fig. 5.38: X-ray of pelvis with both hips, anteroposterior view showing fracture neck of femur

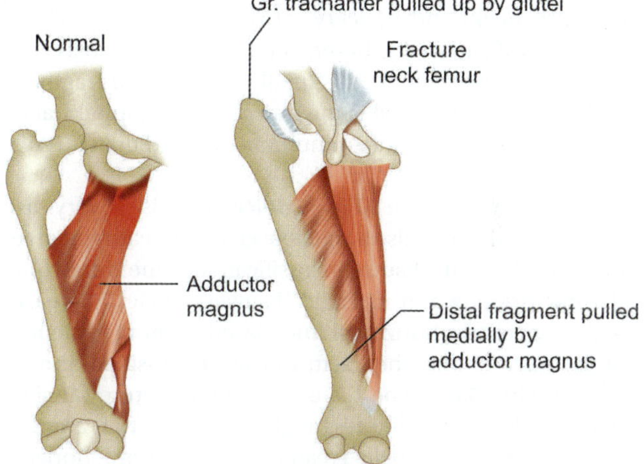

Fig. 5.39: Schematic representation of muscle forces producing the characteristic deformities after femoral neck fractures

an MRI (investigation of choice for occult fractures). Diagnosis in most cases however is confirmed on anteroposterior and lateral X-rays of the hip joint **(Fig. 5.38)**. X-ray shows the fracture line with a break in the trabeculae, broken Shenton's line, proximally migrated greater trochanter, and more prominent lesser trochanter due to external rotation of femur. The distal fragment is pulled medially by the adductor magnus **(Fig. 5.39)**, lessening the neck shaft angle (coxa vara), although the changes are subtle compared to an extracapsular fracture.

Classification

Three commonly used classification systems for neck femur fracture are as follows:

1. *Anatomical classification **(Fig. 5.40A)**:* As per the anatomical classification a fracture of neck femur can be subcapital

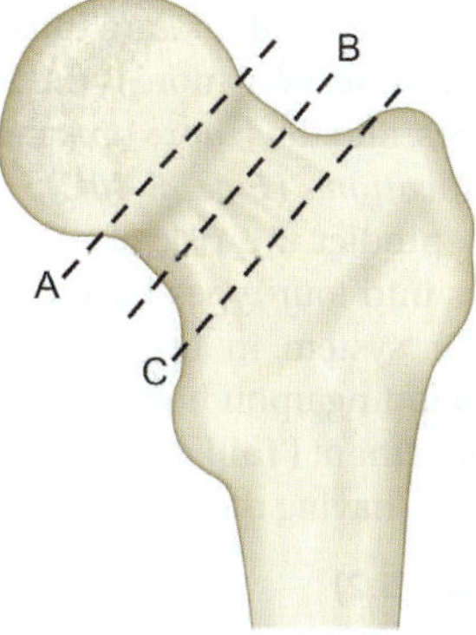

Fig. 5.40A: Anatomical classification (A–subcapital, B–transcervical, C–basicervical)

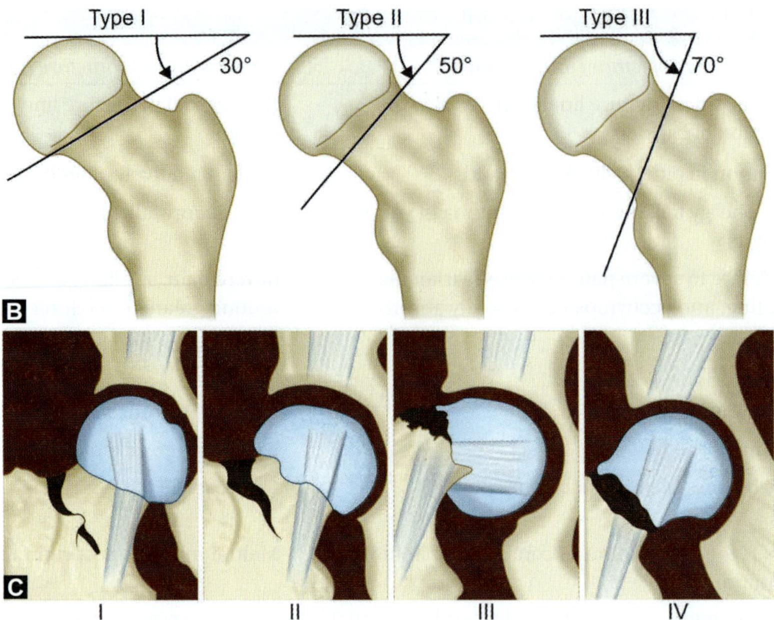

Figs 5.40B and C: (B) Pauwel's classification of fracture neck of femur and (C) Garden's classification

(fracture at femoral head and neck junction), transcervical (through neck) and basicervical (fracture at base of neck). This classification is based upon the prognosis. More proximal is the fracture, the smaller is the head fragment to be fixed and hence bad is the outcome. Subcapital fractures are most prone to go into nonunion and land up with AVN of the femoral head.

2. *Pauwel's classification* **(Fig. 5.40B)**: This is a very useful classification that is also a valuable guide to treatment of these fractures. As per the Pauwel's classification, a line is drawn along the fracture line and its angle (Pauwel's angle) is measured with respect to a horizontal line. Based upon the orientation of the fracture line, the fractures can be classified into three types **(Table 5.8)**. Type I is a horizontal fracture (angle less than 30° from horizontal, less angle) while type III is a vertically oriented fracture (angle greater than 50° from horizontal, greater angle). In type II fracture angle is between 30° and 50° from horizontal. The fundamental behind this classification is that vertical fractures will displace under load due to shear forces and hence be unstable while the horizontal fractures would compress under load and are thus stable fractures. So, as per Pauwel's classification, more is the Pauwel's angle, more are shearing forces, and thus more unstable is the fracture.

3. *Garden's classification* **(Fig. 5.40C)**: This is a useful classification to predict the risk of AVN. This classification divides fractures into four types based upon the orientation of the trabecular system in the femoral head, neck, and acetabulum depending upon how it changes with increasing degrees of displacement **(Table 5.9)**. Type IV is most severely displaced fractures having the maximum risk of AVN.

Treatment (Flow Chart 5.2)

The treatment varies with the age of the patient, the level of the fracture and displacement of fragments. It also depends upon the

Table 5.8: Pauwel's classification of fracture neck of femur

Pauwel's classification—based on the orientation of the fracture line

Type I	<30° from horizontal
Type II	30°–50° from horizontal
Type III	>50° from horizontal

Table 5.9: Garden's classification of fracture neck of femur

Garden classification—based on fracture displacement on anteroposterior radiograph		*Description*
Type I	Incomplete fracture, valgus impacted	This is a valgus impacted incomplete, subcapital fracture. Fracture line does not break the medial cortex. Trabecular line in head forms an angle with those of the acetabulum
Type II	Complete fracture, undisplaced	This is a complete but an undisplaced fracture so trabecular lines of head, neck, and the acetabulum are collinear
Type III	Complete fracture, partially displaced	This fracture is complete so all set of trabeculae is out of line with each other
Type IV	Complete fracture, completely displaced	This is completely displaced fractures so there is no contact between head and neck. Head returns to its normal position in the acetabulum and trabeculae of the head and the acetabulum are collinear, but head and neck trabeculae are not aligned

Flow chart 5.2: Treatment algorithm for fracture neck of femur

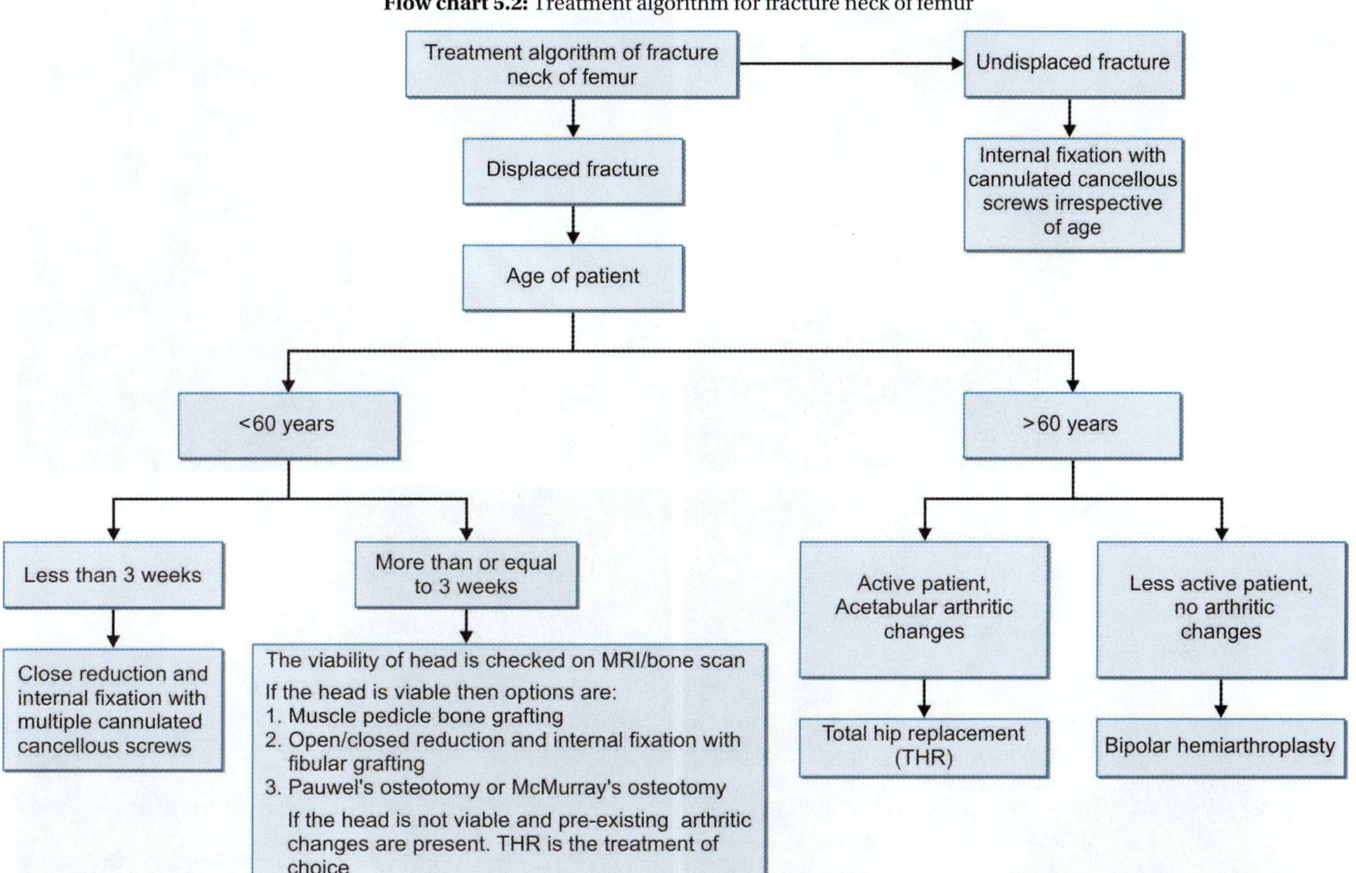

duration of the fracture and level of activity. Biological rather than chronological age should be taken into consideration.

Nonoperative treatment may be an option in undisplaced fractures with medical contraindications to surgery or in elderly patients with advanced cognitive impairment and psychiatric problems. These patients are kept immobilized usually in a Thomas splint for 6–8 weeks until the fracture heals. In all other patients with undisplaced fracture neck of femur closed reduction and internal fixation with cannulated cancellous screw is advocated.

In displaced fractures in patients with less than 60 years closed reduction and internal fixation with cannulated cancellous screws is recommended **(Figs 5.41A and B)**. If close reduction fails, then ORIF with cannulated cancellous screws is done. In the basicervical type of fracture, dynamic hip screw **(Fig. 5.54)** can also be used for fracture fixation.

Replacement arthroplasty is the treatment of choice in fracture neck of femur in patients older than 60 years. In less active older patients with no arthritic changes in the acetabulum, bipolar hemiarthroplasty is a rational option **(Fig. 5.41C)**. Total hip replacement **(Fig. 5.41D)** is recommended in active, ambulatory patients with fracture neck femur with concomitant degenerative changes in the acetabulum.

Management of Late Presentation of Fracture Neck of Femur

There is a lack of consensus on the best option for treatment of these cases. Definition of late presentation arbitrarily includes patients presenting 3 weeks or more after fracture neck of femur. A closed reduction is generally not possible in these patients and open reduction involves tissue dissection and is associated with high rates of complications like AVN. In tertiary centers the surgeons mostly prescribe an MRI to see the status of the femoral head. If the head is vascular, an attempt is made by the methods mentioned below to salvage it. If the head is avascular a replacement arthroplasty is done. In other centers where MRI is difficult to get treatment is dictated by age. In patients above 60 years a replacement arthroplasty (bipolar or THR) is the preferred choice. However, in young patients a salvage attempt is made by opting for one of the following methods that can hasten union:

- Muscle pedicle bone grafting (Meyer's procedure)
- Open reduction and internal fixation with fibular grafting (free or vascularized)
- Valgus intertrochanteric osteotomy/Pauwel's osteotomy
- McMurray's osteotomy.

Meyer's Procedure

In neglected fracture neck of femur blood supply of the femoral head may have been compromised. In Meyer's procedure the fracture is opened from behind and is fixed with cancellous screws. A vascularized (artery intact) quadratus femoris-based muscle pedicle bone graft is rerouted to be attached at the fracture site **(Fig. 5.42)**. These osteomuscular grafts provide an additional source of blood supply and promote healing.

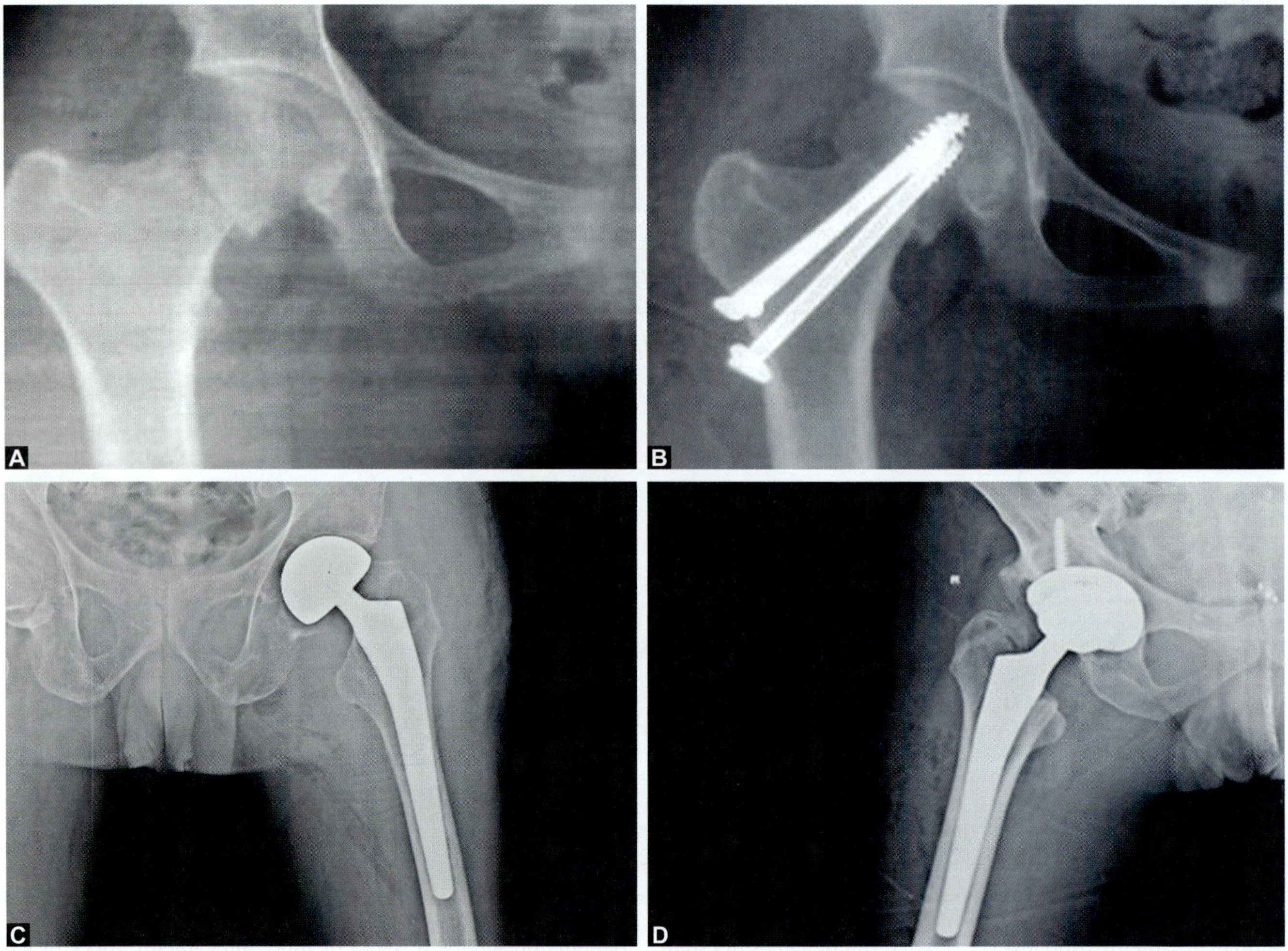

Figs 5.41A to D: (A and B) X-ray showing fracture neck of femur in 40-year-old male fixed with multiple cannulated screws; (C) X-ray of pelvis with hip joint showing bipolar hemiarthroplasty (see acetabulam is not replaced); and (D) X-ray of pelvis with hip joint showing total hip replacement (see both head and acetabulam are replaced)

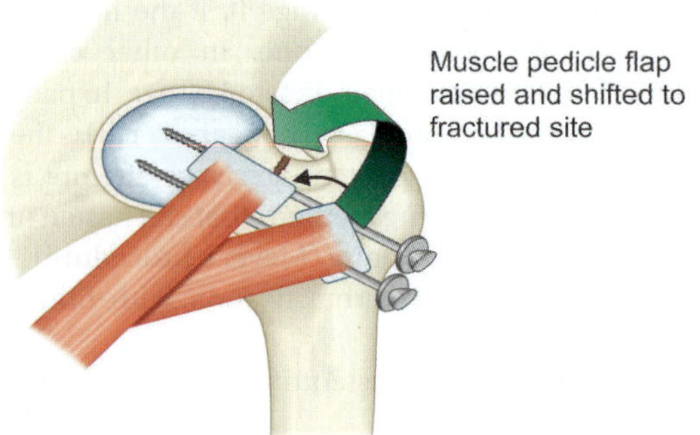

Fig. 5.42: Meyer's procedure

Bone Grafting with Free or Vascularized Fibular Graft

Open reduction and internal fixation with added fibular bone grafting **(Figs 5.43A to C)** is done to hasten union. Cortical fibular bone grafts provide mechanical strength to the weak osteoporotic bone in elderly in addition to stimulating the fracture union. Vascularized fibular grafting (with intact blood supply, **Fig. 5.44**)

is a technically demanding procedure as it requires microvascular anastomosis but is biologically superior and speeds up union even better.

Pauwel's Osteotomy

Pauwel's osteotomy works on converting a vertical unstable fracture into a horizontal stable fracture so that shear stress turns into impaction force on weight bearing **(Figs 5.45A and B)**. In this procedure a laterally based wedge of bone is removed from the area of lesser trochanter and the proximal fragment is rotated down to close the wedge-shaped gap and fixed with an implant, such that after fixation, a vertically oriented fracture eventually assumes horizontal orientation. Although a bit demanding procedure, it is one of the favored treatment options today.

McMurray's Osteotomy (Displacement Osteotomy or a Pelvic Support Osteotomy)

This was once a popular procedure in the past, but is not favored nowadays because of difficulty in future hip replacement and some unavoidable complications like shortened limb and limp. The osteotomy works on a "biomechanical" principle called as "arm chair effect" that basically describes the fact that the osteotomy

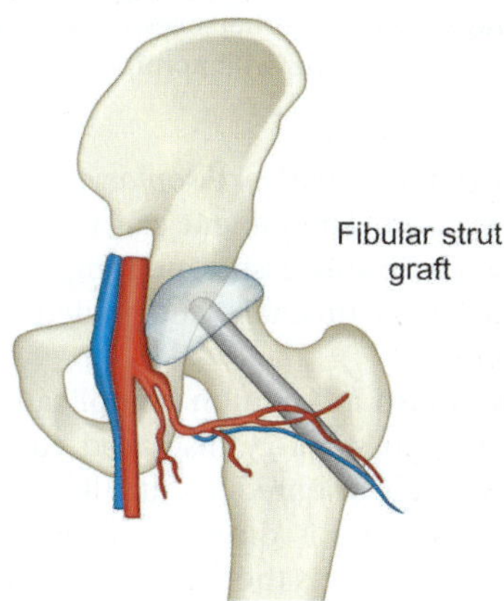

Figs 5.43A to C: (A) Neck femur fracture (arrows) reconstructed with (B, C) fibular grafts (vascularized fibular grafts, arrows)

Fig. 5.44: Diagrammatic depiction of vascularized fibular graft

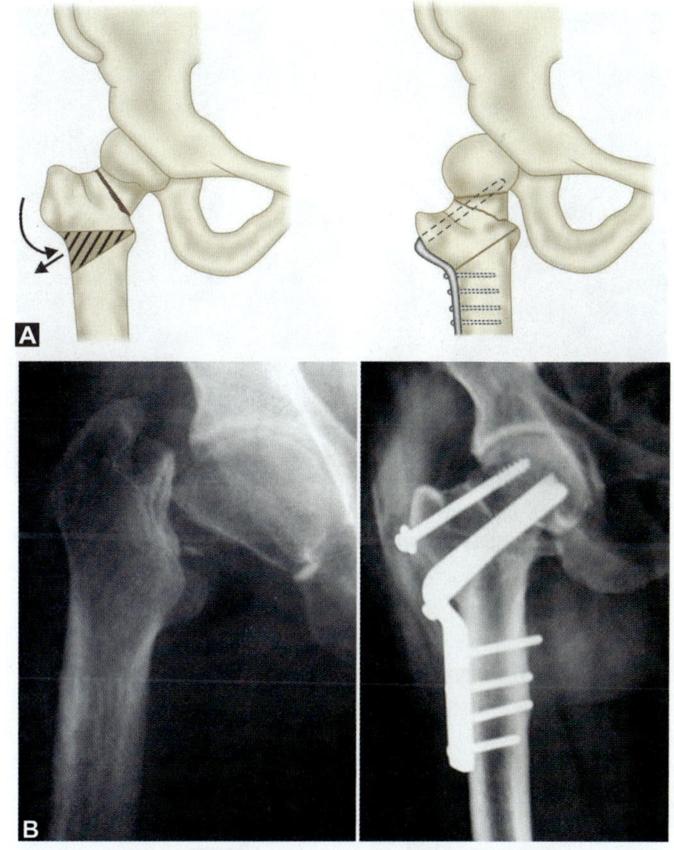

Figs 5.45A and B: (A) Concept of valgus intertrochanteric (Pauwel's) osteotomy; and (B) Pauwel's osteotomy for a vertical fracture to convert it into a horizontal pattern

bypasses the fracture site and redistributes the forces around it (like putting weight on arms while getting up from a chair bypasses legs and redistributes the forces from knee to elbows).

The osteotomy is done from the base of the greater trochanter to the top of lesser trochanter and the distal fragment is abducted and displaced medially **(Fig. 5.46)**. The new line of weight bearing now passes from the acetabulum to the head, directly to distal fragment, bypassing the fracture site. Thus, the mechanics are altered as a line of weight bearing has been mobilized. Also, abducting the distal fragment causes the fracture line to become more horizontal which redistributes the forces making tensile forces become impaction forces under the stress of weight bearing. This creates a biological environment that hastens union, and hence describes the biomechanical effect of the osteotomy.

Complications

- Avascular necrosis of the femoral head **(Fig. 5.47)** is the most common complication of fracture neck of femur followed by nonunion [incidence AVN (25%) and nonunion (20%) in displaced fractures]. It may take a long time (1–2 years) for the signs of AVN (increased density of the head, segmental collapse) to appear on plain X-rays. MRI can detect the problem well before the X-rays. In the early stage (before the

collapse of the head) it can be prevented by performing a muscle pedicle grafting (Meyer's procedure) to increase the vascularity. However, once collapse sets in, lost head cannot be recovered. In this stage patient is offered three options:

1. *Arthrodesis/fusion of joint* **(Fig. 5.48)**: Relieves pain, provides a stable construct, but movement at the joint is lost.
2. *Replacement arthroplasty*: Movement good, but in young chances of loosening of prosthesis.

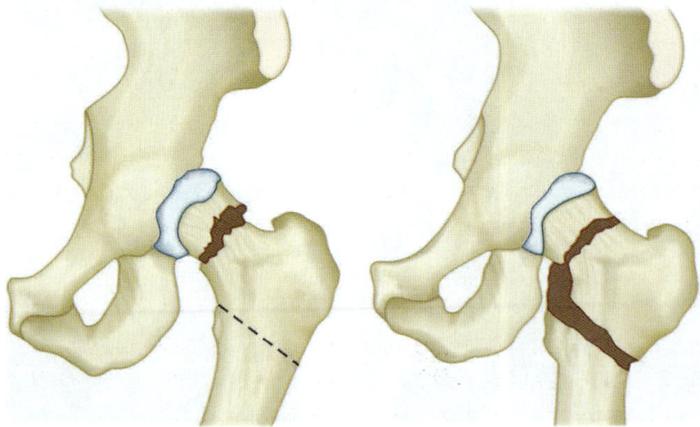

Fig. 5.46: McMurray's osteotomy

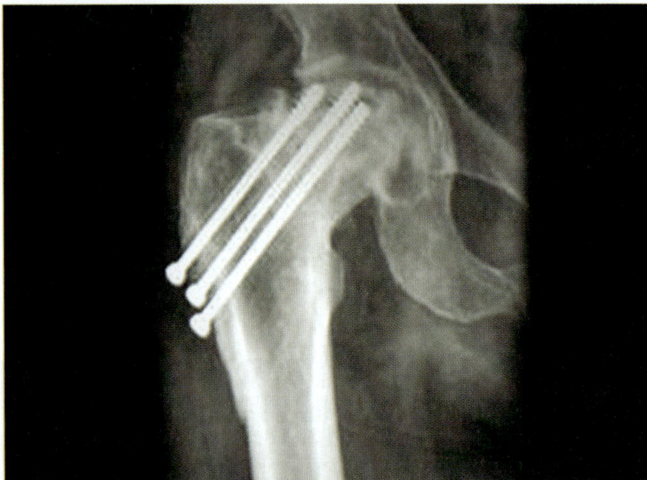

Fig. 5.47: X-ray showing sclerosed and collapsed femoral head (postsurgery) having undergone avascular necrosis

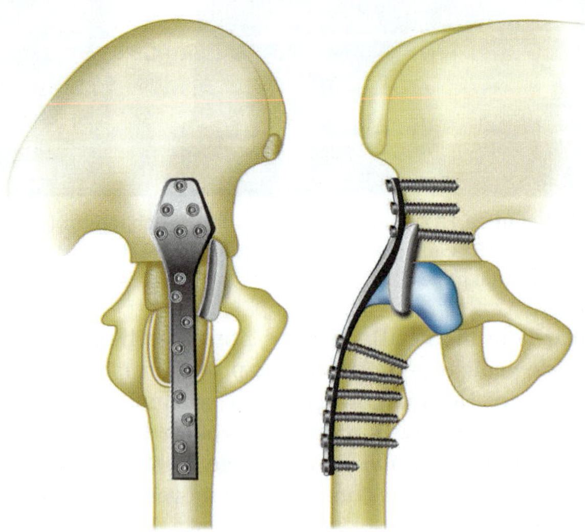

Fig. 5.48: Diagrammatic depiction of fusion (arthrodesis) of the hip performed using a special "Cobra plate"

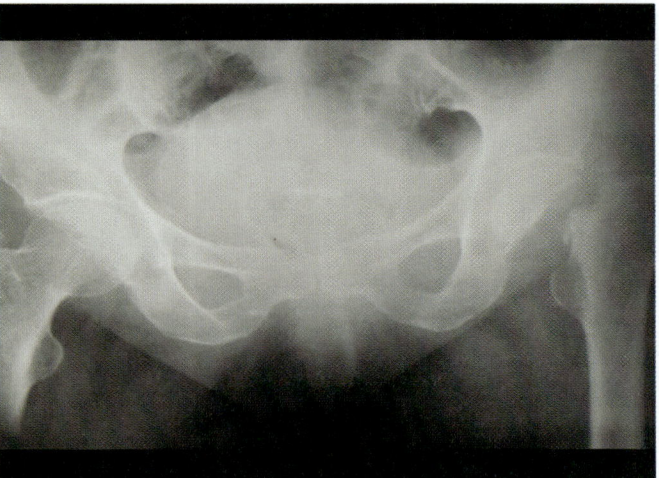

Fig. 5.49: X-ray showing resorbed neck in a case of neglected neck femur with nonunion

3. *Excision (Girdelstone) arthroplasy*: Head and proximal neck is excised. The patient can walk as the space fills with a tough fibrous tissue and range of motion is excellent, but hip is unstable and patient cannot perform heavy work.

- *Nonunion*: It is also a common complication. Chances are particularly high in severely displaced subcapital fractures that have a vertically oriented fracture line. Delay in reducing and fixing the fracture is directly related to nonunion and hence urgent treatment is the key in prevention.

  Management in a patient greater than 60 years old remains hemiarthroplasty or THR. In a young patient union can be hastened and head can be salvaged by those same procedures discussed above:
  - *Meyer's procedure (vascularized muscle pedicle bone grafting)*: Increases blood supply to hasten union
  - *Neck reconstruction (bone grafting with fibula)*: Neck in prolonged cases is mostly resorbed **(Fig. 5.49)** and fibular grafts can be effectively used for reconstruction.
  - Pauwel's osteotomy
  - McMurray's osteotomy (can be used, but is not a preferred option nowadays)

- Osteoarthritis of the hip joint is a late sequel of fracture neck of femur. It is usually secondary to AVN and collapse of the head. In advanced stages total hip replacement may be needed.

HIGH-YIELD POINTS

- Chances of AVN of head and nonunion of fracture neck of femur are maximum for subcapital fracture (subcapital → transcervica → basal → intertrochanteric).
- Risk of AVN is directly related to delay in fixation, so urgent treatment is the utmost priority.
- Screw fixation in neck femur generally involves putting at least three cancellous screws in an inverted triangle pattern.
- Bakshi's procedure also involves vascularized muscle pedicle bone grafting, but the muscle used is tensor fascia lata (unlike Meyer where quadratus femoris is used).

FRACTURE NECK FEMUR IN CHILDREN

Fractures of proximal end of the femur in children **(Fig. 5.50)** are rare and usually result from high-velocity trauma (fall from height, RTA, etc.). Delbet classification **(Table 5.10)** is the commonly used classification to classify these injuries.

Treatment

Conservative treatment (immobilization in hip spica/Thomas splint) is associated with a high rate of complications and often result in failure of reduction so internal fixation should be done whenever feasible. Undisplaced fracture in children below 3 years can be managed with hip spica in abduction.

Closed reduction internal fixation (CRIF) with percutaneous pinning using smooth Moore's pins or Knowles pins **(Fig. 5.51)** and postoperative spica application in abduction and internal rotation is done in displaced fractures. Pediatric

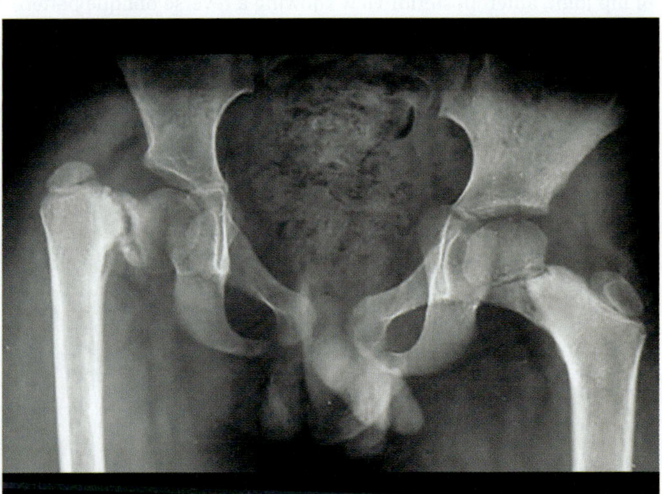

Fig. 5.50: X-ray of pelvis with both hips, anteroposterior view showing fracture neck of femur in a 8-year-old child

Table 5.10: Delbet classification of pediatric hip fractures	
Types	
I. Transepiphyseal	Least common
II. Transcervical	This is most common
III. Cervicotrochanteric	Second most common
IV. Intertrochanteric	

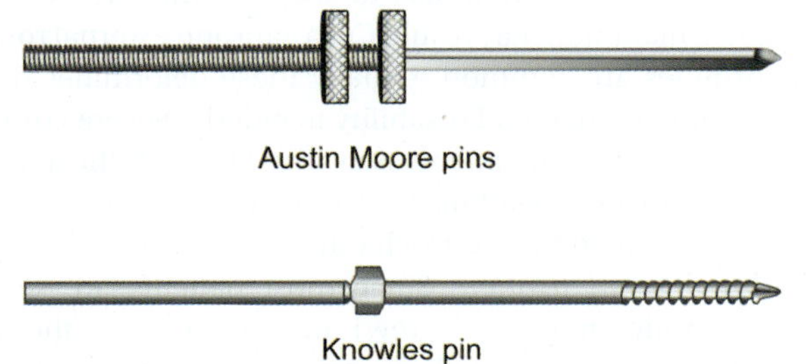

Fig. 5.51: Moore's pins and Knowles pins: fixation devices used for pediatric neck femur fractures

hip screw/[dynamic hip screw (DHS)] can be used in type IV cervicotrochanteric fractures.

Complications

Avascular necrosis of the hip is the most common complication. Coxa vara is the next most common complication. Other complications include chondrolysis, premature physeal closure, and limb length discrepancy.

INTERTROCHANTERIC FRACTURE OF FEMUR

This is an extracapsular fracture of proximal femur seen mostly in people above 70 years of age. Like fracture neck of femur these also usually result from a low-energy simple fall. Young people usually sustain these injuries in a road traffic accident.

Classification

Based on the fracture pattern the fracture can be classified as stable and unstable (Evans classification). Unstable fracture patterns involve the comminution in the posteromedial part of the proximal femur **(Fig. 5.52A)**, subtrochanteric extension of fracture line or a special pattern called reverse oblique pattern (a fracture line extending downwards from medial to lateral cortex, **Fig. 5.52B**).

Clinical Features

Patients present with severe pain in the hip joint with inability to bear weight on the involved hip. Swelling and ecchymoses around trochanter are common findings. All hip movements are painful and tenderness can be localized over the greater trochanter. Deformity is same as in the intracapsular fracture (shortening and external rotation) but it is far more apparent due to the absence of a restraining capsule. In fact, the leg is often so much externally rotated that the lateral border of the foot touches the couch.

Diagnosis is confirmed by anteroposterior X-ray of involved hip. X-ray **(Figs 5.52A and B)** shows the fracture line in the trochanteric region, which may involve greater or lesser trochanter or both.

Treatment

Treatment of intertrochanteric fracture is essential surgery in all patients except those with untreatable medical conditions who are too ill to tolerate surgery and in patients with advanced dementia and psychiatric illness. Conservative treatment of intertrochanteric fracture requires limb to be stabilized by below the knee skeleton traction in bed until fracture unite and pain subsides (usually 6–8 weeks). Hamilton-Russell traction **(Fig. 5.53)** is most commonly used for conservative treatment of intertrochanteric fractures.

Operative treatment of intertrochanteric fracture is anatomical reduction of fracture and internal fixation. Fracture is reduced closed under the guidance of X-ray image intensifier and fixed with internal fixation implant. DHS is most commonly used internal fixation device for intertrochanteric fracture **(Fig. 5.54)**. It consists of a screw that can slide inside a barrel plate. As the patient bears weight, the screw slides inside the barrel and it produces compression at fracture site that encourages the union (sliding compression/controlled cancellous collapse). An intramedullary fixation device like a proximal femoral nail (PFN), Gamma nail, or Recon nail is recommended in unstable fracture pattern **(Figs 5.55A and B)**.

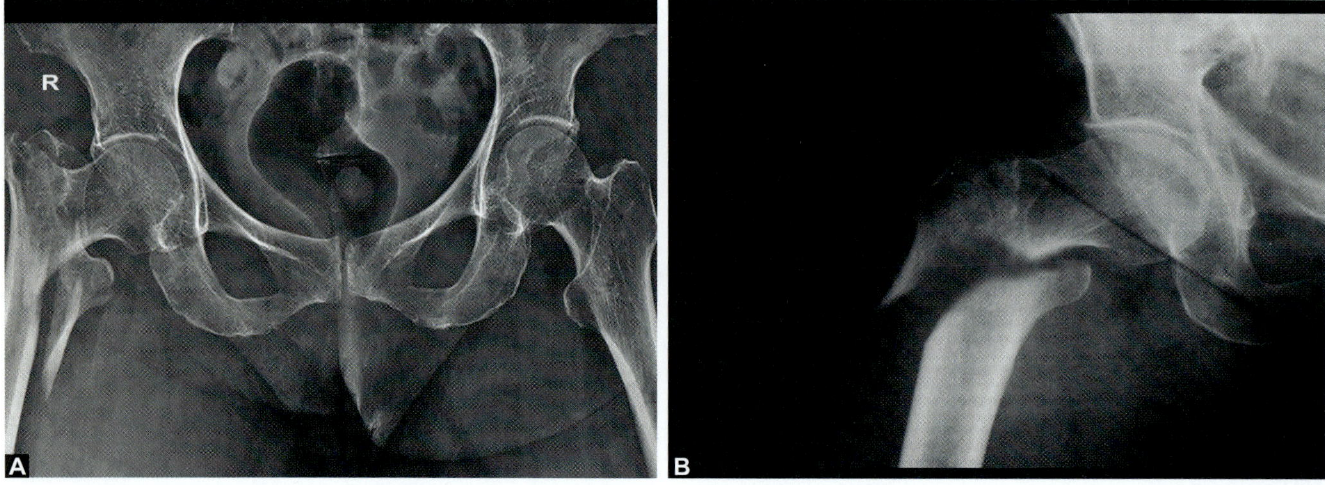

Figs 5.52A and B: (A) X-ray of pelvis with both hips, anteroposterior view showing intertrochanteric fracture of right femur. Note comminution in region of lesser trochanter (posteromedial part of proximal femur); (B) X-ray of hip joint, anteroposterior view showing a reverse oblique pattern of intertrochanteric fracture

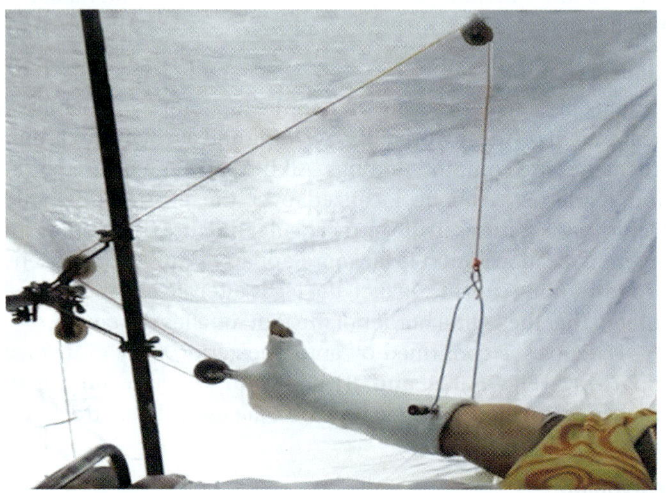

Fig. 5.53: Hamilton-Russell traction for intertrochanteric fracture femur

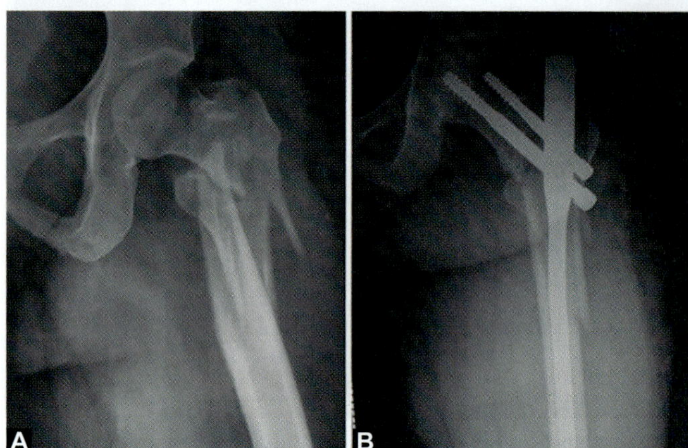

Figs 5.55A and B: Unstable intertrochanteric fracture with posteromedial comminution fixed with a proximal femoral nail

Surgery should be done as soon as possible as prolonged recumbency in the elderly may cause decubitus ulcers (bed sores) and chest problems like pneumonia and thromboembolic complications.

Complications

- *Malunion*: Since these fractures involve cancellous metaphyseal bone, they rarely fail to unite, but if not properly reduced or if reduction fails to keep the fracture fragments aligned, malunion may result. Coxa vara and external rotation deformities are common. Usually these deformities do not cause much functional disability in elderly. Severe coxa vara deformity in young patients may interfere with the abductor muscle function, leading to Trendelenburg gait (*see* Page 121). It is treated by intertrochanteric osteotomy.
- *Failed internal fixation*: Since most patients are severely osteoporotic, implant (screw) may cut-out of the bone superiorly leading to failure. An eccentric placement also

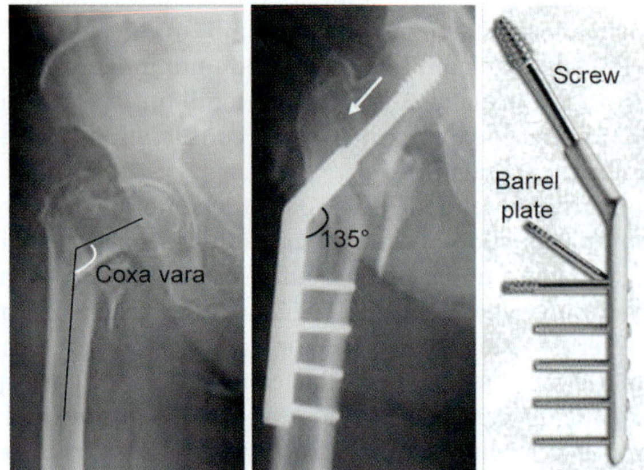

Fig. 5.54: X-ray, anteroposterior view of hip joint showing intertrochanteric fracture and its fixation with DHS. Note the neck shaft angle is restored

leads to this end result (ideally screw should be either in the center or in the posteroinferior aspect of the head). This usually occurs before union (3–4 months) and may necessitate a revision surgery. Some surgeons prefer using a special DHS with a helical screw **(Fig. 5.56)** to lessen the risk of screw cut-out in severely osteoporotic patients.

- Osteoarthritis rarely may be a late complication of malunited trochanteric fractures due to change in hip biomechanics.

SUBTROCHANTERIC FRACTURE

These fractures occur below the lesser trochanter and up to 5 cm distal to it **(Fig. 5.57A)**. In the elderly, these fractures usually result from a low-energy fall whereas a young person sustains these injuries in high-velocity injuries. These are less common than fracture neck femur and intertrochanteric fractures. Patients present with severe pain in hip and inability to use involved limb. The limb is externally rotated and shortened. Diagnosis is confirmed by X-rays. The treatment is essentially surgical. CRIF/

ORIF with intramedullary nail (i.e. PFN, recon nail, Enders nail or Gamma nail) or plate (dynamic condylar screw, condylar blade plate or DHS) is required **(Figs 5.57B and C)**. The failure rate is high owing to high stresses in the subtrochanteric area.

FRACTURE SHAFT OF FEMUR

The shaft is the area between 5 cm distal to the lesser trochanter and 5 cm proximal to the adductor tubercle. Although femur is the longest and strongest bone of the body which is surrounded by a thick muscle mass all around, its fractures span all age groups. In children below walking age femur fracture usually results from child abuse. In older children high-velocity road traffic accidents accounts for majority of fractures. In young adults femoral shaft fractures are usually the result of high-velocity road traffic accidents. And in elderly with severely osteoporotic bones, low-energy fall may be sufficient to cause femoral shaft fracture.

Displacements

Muscle forces causing fracture displacement in femoral shaft fracture are depicted in **Figure 5.58** and **Table 5.11**.

Classification

Fractures can be classified based on the geometry. Fracture geometry largely depends upon the type of applied force. Geometry of fracture, according to type of force is tabulated in **Table 5.12** (common to fractures of all long bones). The more useful in management and decision making is the Winquist and Hansen classification **(Table 5.13, Fig. 5.59)** which is based on the amount of comminution at the fracture site.

Clinical Features

All patients with femoral shaft fractures should be assessed on the basis of ATLS guidelines as most of them are high-velocity road traffic accidents victims so have multiple injuries. Diagnosis of femoral shaft fracture is usually straightforward. Patients present with pain, swelling, deformity and shortening of the thigh. A careful examination of the involved limb should be done as concomitant ipsilateral hip dislocation, knee injuries and tibia

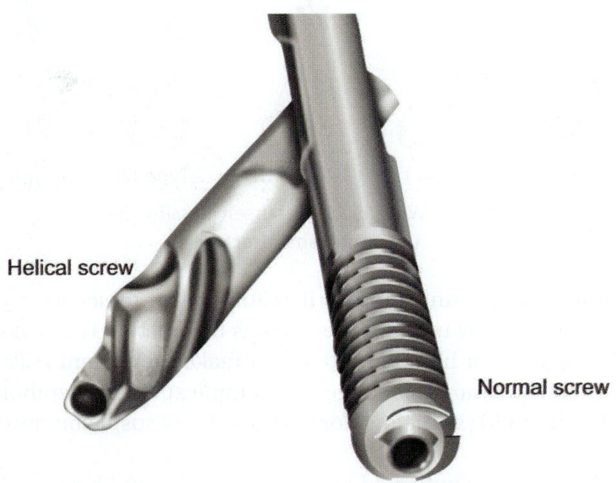

Fig. 5.56: Helical screw versus a normal screw of a dynamic hip screw

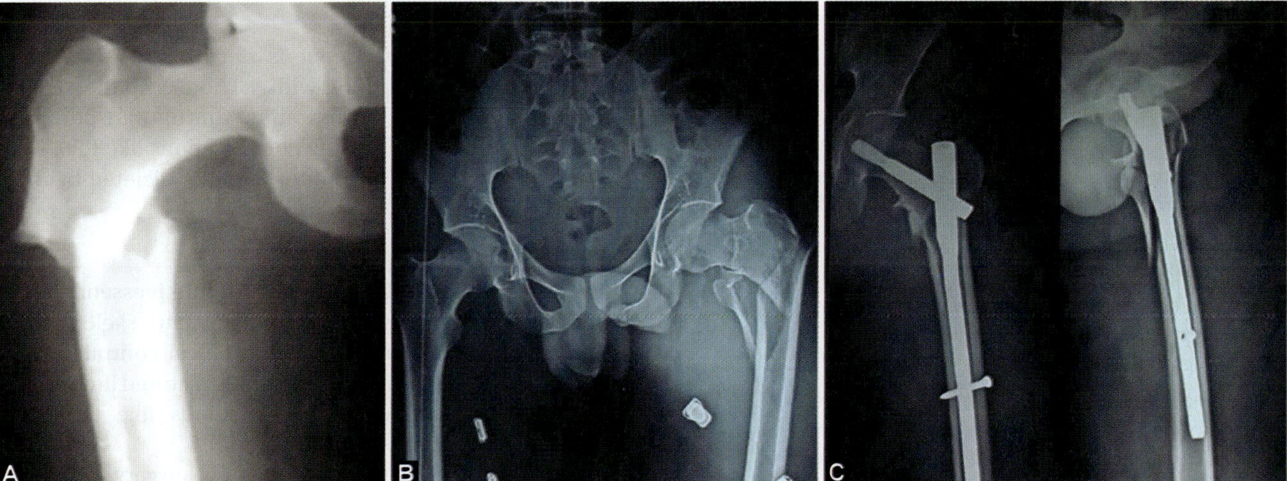

Figs 5.57A to C: (A) X-ray of hip, AP view shows subtrochanteric fracture; (B) X-ray, pelvis with both hips AP view showing trochanteric fracture with subtrochanteric extension and (C) CRIF with PFN
Abbreviations: AP, anteroposterior; CRIF, closed reduction internal fixation; PFN, proximal femoral nail.

Table 5.11: Deforming forces in the fracture shaft femur

Fracture site	Proximal fragment	Distal fragment
Proximal third	Abducted and flexed by the abductors and flexors of the hip joint (iliopsoas)	Displaced upward and medially by the adductor and hamstring group of muscles
Middle third	Abducted but less as compared to proximal third fractures and flexed due to the iliopsoas muscle	Externally rotated by the weight of the foot and displaced upward and posteromedially due to the adductors and hamstring muscles
Distal third or supracondylar	Pulled in flexion and adduction by the iliopsoas and adductor muscles	Flexed posteriorly by the pull of the gastrocnemius muscle

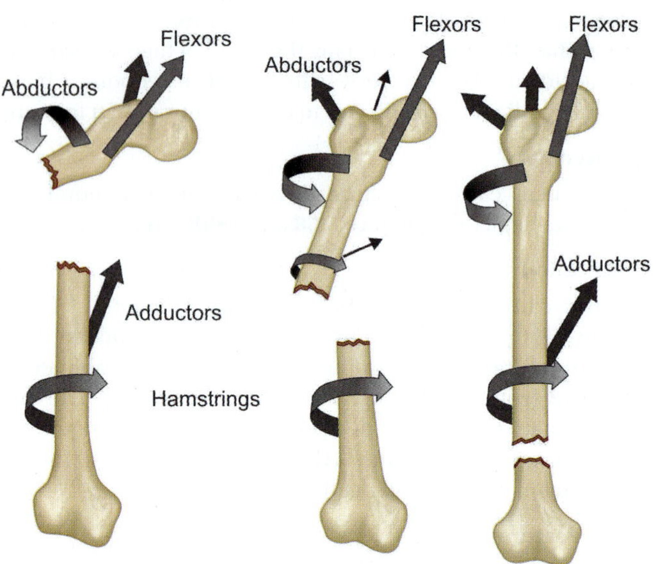

Fig. 5.58: Deforming forces in a fracture shaft of femur

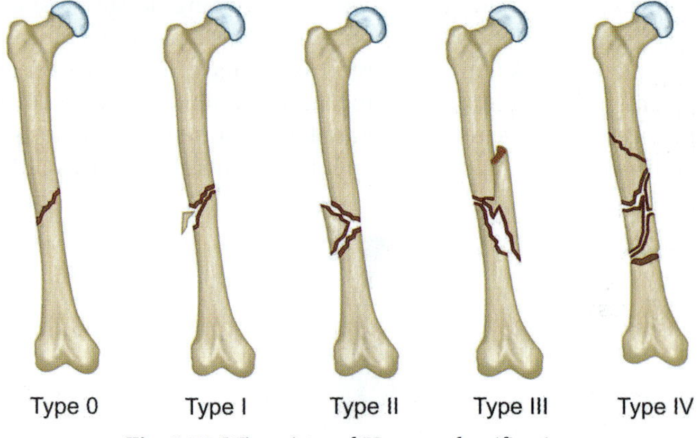

Fig. 5.59: Winquist and Hansen classification of femoral shaft fracture

Table 5.12: Common mechanisms of fractures

Type of force	Geometry of fracture
Bending	Transverse/oblique
Twisting/torque	Spiral
Moderate axial compression combined with bending and torsion	Oblique
High-energy force and direct impact	Comminuted

Table 5.13: Winquist classification of femoral shaft fracture

Type 0	No comminution
Type I	Minimal comminution at fracture site
Type II	More comminution than that in type I but more than 50% of the circumference of the cortices of two major fracture fragments remains intact
Type III	Comminution involves more than 50% of the circumference of the cortices of fracture fragments. Only a small area of contact is left between fracture fragments
Type IV	Comminution of entire bony circumference over a segment of bone, no contact between cortices

fractures are not uncommon. It is imperative to secure an i/v access and closely monitor the vitals as the fracture is associated with a significant blood loss that can make the patient collapse due to shock. A rare but dangerous complication is fat embolism syndrome (FES) (*see* below) for which index of suspicion must be high.

Diagnosis is confirmed by anteroposterior and lateral X-rays of the injured thigh. Anteroposterior view of the pelvis and anteroposterior and lateral views of the ipsilateral knee should also be done.

Treatment

Before a definitive treatment is decided, it is imperative to splint the fracture. Splinting with a Thomas splint (*see* Page 20) avoids additional soft tissue trauma during transportation, and lessens risk of life-threatening complications like FES. Definitive treatment of fractures of shaft of femur is dictated by the age of the patient.

Age Greater than 10 Years

Treatment of fracture shaft of femur in adults is essentially surgical. Nonoperative treatment (cast bracing and skeleton traction) is indicated only in patients with medical contraindications to anesthesia or surgery. In these patients fractured limb is stabilized with different skeletal traction methods like the Hamilton-Russell's traction (*see* **Fig. 5.53**).

In patients who are candidates for surgery, fractured limb is stabilized on the Thomas splint until the patient is shifted to operation theater for surgery. Operative treatment of choice for femoral diaphyseal shaft fracture in this age group is closed intramedullary interlocking nailing. Kuntscher revolutionized the management of diaphyseal fracture of shaft of femur by developing V-shaped intramedullary nail in early 40s and later cloverleaf model (*see* Page 469) of intramedullary nail in the late 40s **(Fig. 5.60)**. The present form of modern interlocking intramedullary nail has passed through several stages. In the 1950–60 surgeons used to do open nailing of femoral shaft fractures. In 1960 development of image intensifier allowed surgeons for close intramedullary nailing.

Close intramedullary interlocking nailing **(Fig. 5.61)** is minimally invasive technique in which close reduction of fracture is done under guidance of an image intensifier. Medullary cavity is reamed with reamers and the nail is placed into the medullary cavity. Modern interlocking nails have holes for proximal and distal interlocking screws which provide rotational stability of the fracture.

The external fixator is indicated in open femoral shaft fractures and as temporary stabilization in severely injured patients who cannot tolerate intramedullary nailing (Damage Control Orthopedics, *see* Page 58). ORIF with plate is indicated in fractures extending into metaphyseal region.

Age 5–10 Years

In children below 10 years of age interlocking nails cannot be used for fixation. These nails use greater trochanter as the entry portal and in children this may damage the growth plate in the region that is open till 10–12 years of age. Shaft fractures in these patients are preferably fixed by smooth nails (Rush nails) or elastic nails [Ender's nail and TENS (titanium elastic nailing system)] **(Fig. 5.62)**. The elastic nails are bendable nails and need not be inserted via the trochanteric portal. They are inserted from the sides of metaphysis above the growth plate and two or three nails can be stacked inside the medullary cavity to provide stability. Those who are unfit to undergo the surgical procedure are managed with different forms of traction like the 90–90 traction **(Fig. 5.63)**, particularly employed in proximal femoral shaft fractures in children 2–10 years of age.

Age 6 Months to 5 Years

In stable fractures, after acceptable closed reduction a hip spica, the cast is applied to the hip in flexion (60°–90°) and abduction (30°–45°) and knees in 90° flexion **(Fig. 5.64)** after well padding of the child. In case shortening is more than 3 cm skeletal traction may be given for a short period to distract and align and then a spica is applied. Acceptability criteria for fracture shaft femur below 5 years are no more than 2 cm of shortening, less than 10° of coronal plane and less than 20° of sagittal plane deformity and less than 10° of rotational malalignment.

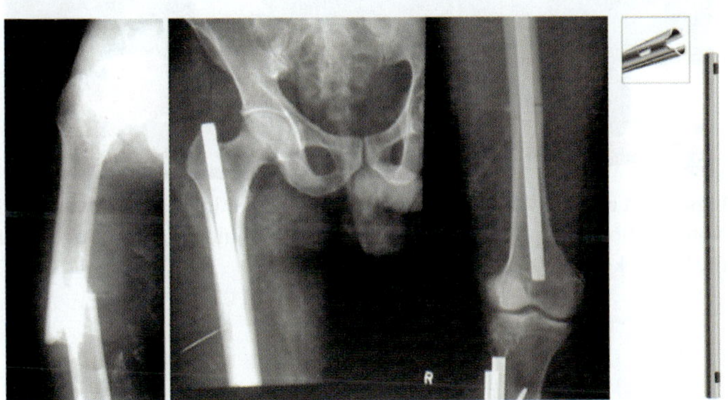
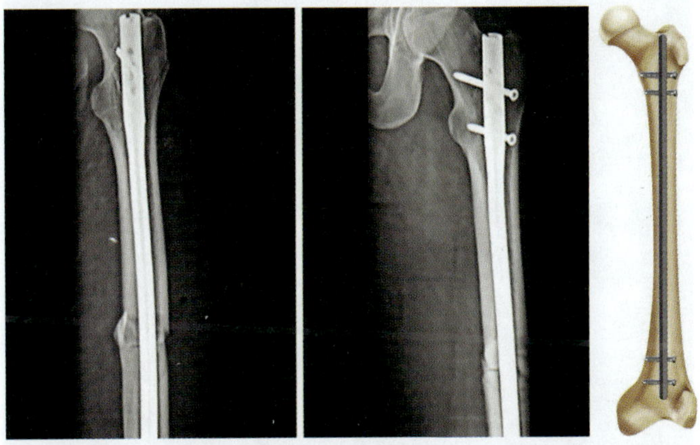

Fig. 5.60: Fracture shaft femur fixed with a K nail (rarely used nowadays)

Fig. 5.61: X-ray of hip with thigh AP and lateral views showing CRIF of femoral shaft fracture with a femoral interlocking nail
Abbreviations: AP, anteroposterior; CRIF, closed reduction internal fixation

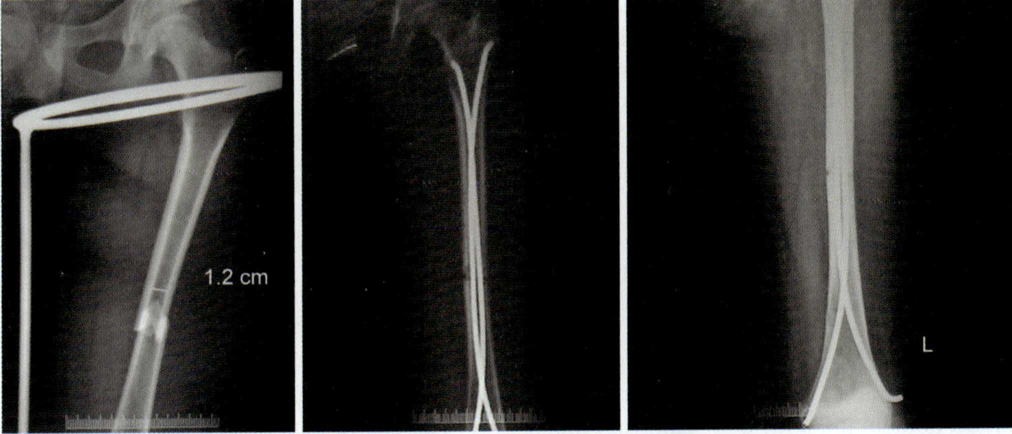

Fig. 5.62: Fracture shaft of femur in 9-year-old girl and its fixation with elastic nails

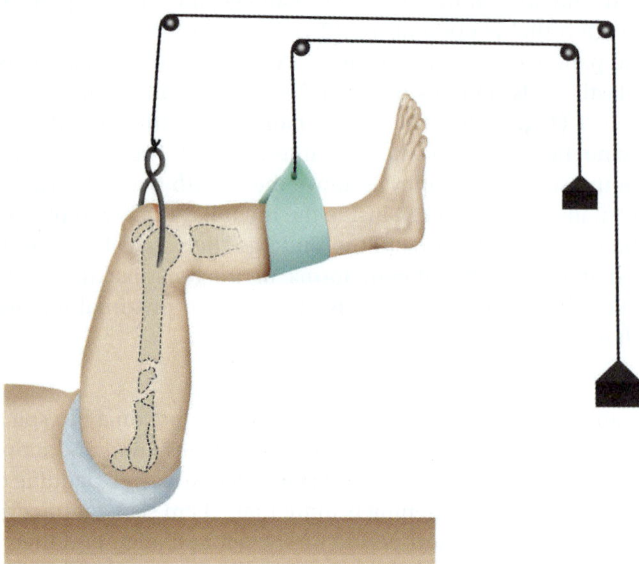

Fig. 5.63: Schematic depiction of 90–90 traction used in managing proximal femoral fractures in children (2–10 years of age). In adults flexion contracture of the knee can result so not preferred

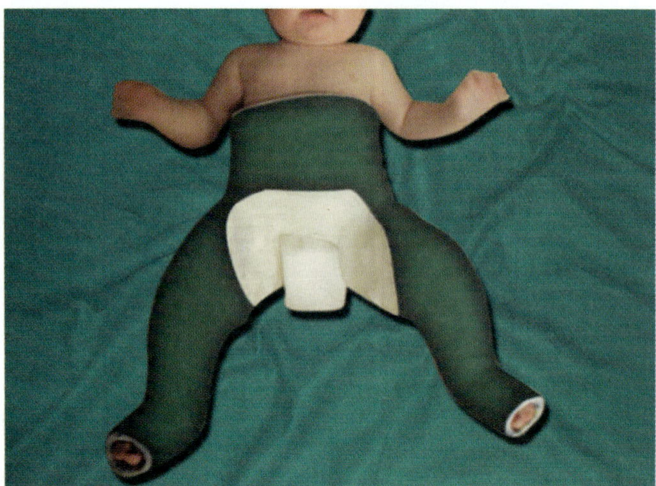

Fig. 5.64: Hip spica for fracture shaft of femur in children less than 5 years

In children under the age of 2 years applying a spica directly is often difficult as the child is not cooperative. These children are initially managed with Gallow's **(Figs 5.65A and B)** or Bryant's traction **(Fig. 5.66)** for 2–3 weeks till fracture becomes sticky or some callus is seen on X-rays and then a hip spica can be safely applied.

Age up to 6 Months

Pavlik harness (*see* Page 366) is applied in 80°–90° hip flexion and around 45° hip abduction. It does not require any anesthesia and allows for easy nursing and toilet care.

Complications

Blood Loss

The femur is the largest bone in the body and significant blood loss (1–1.5 liter or 2–4 units) may occur even in a close fracture

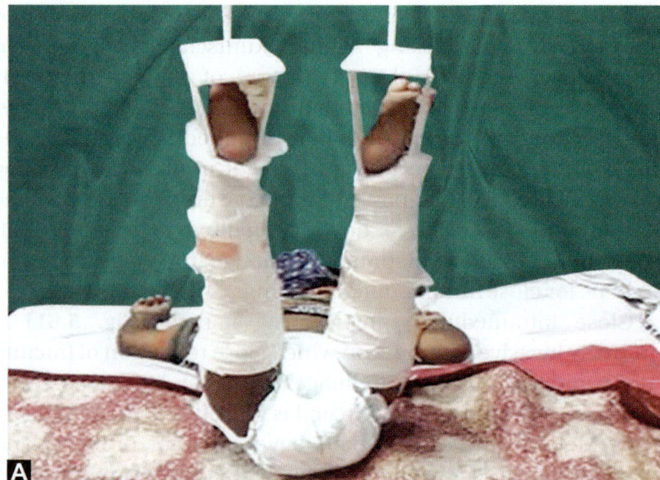

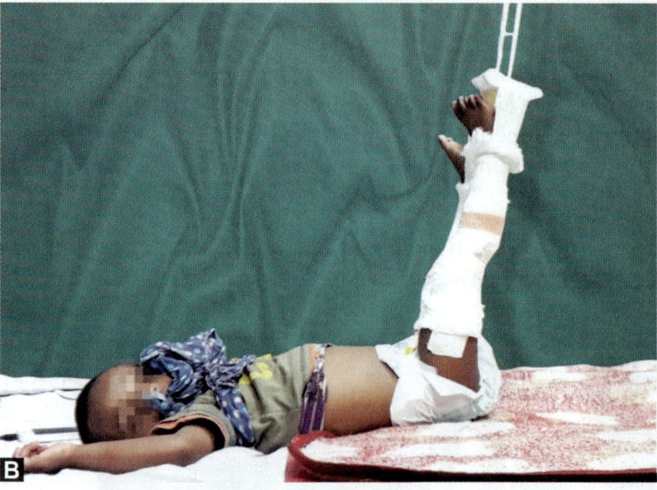

Figs 5.65A and B: Gallow's traction for shaft femur in less than 2 years old. Note traction is applied on both legs. Weight should be just enough to lift the buttock off the bed

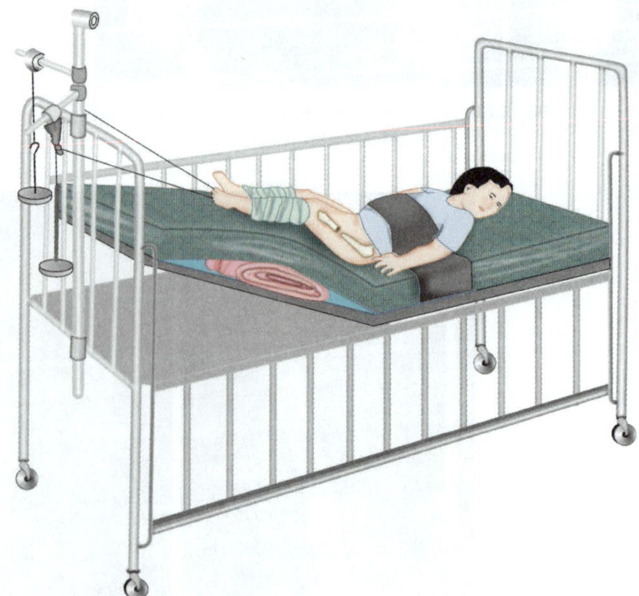

Fig. 5.66: Bryant's traction (a modified form of Gallows traction where the mattress is raised for counter traction)

shaft of femur. Almost 40% of these patients eventually require preoperative blood transfusion. However, in patients of fracture shaft femur with hypotensive shock other causes of blood loss (intra-abdomen hemorrhage, intrathoracic hemorrhage, head injury, etc.) should also be ruled out as very often these patients have multiple injuries.

Fat Embolism Syndrome

First described by Von Bergman in 1873, FES is a rare (less than 4% incidence) but a dangerous complication (mortality 7–15%). Fat emboli occurs in all patients with long bone fractures, but only small numbers of patients (1–2%) develop the FES (i.e. symptomatic fat emboli). Minimum amount of fat needed to cause FES should be around 100 mL and bones like the femur and tibia have 70–130 mL fat. Hence, FES can be seen after fractures of femur, pelvis and tibia and postoperatively, after hip and knee arthroplasty. This is more common in closed fractures (can occur in open fractures with severe soft tissue damage) and in patients with multiple fractures.

Pathophysiology: It is not clear, but two main theories have been put forward. According to the "mechanical theory", fat emboli are released from the injured site into the blood. These emboli (20–40 μm) get lodged into the pulmonary vasculature and from there they travel to the brain or cutaneous sites. Their lodging into microvessels causes ischemia and inflammation. According to the "biochemical theory", hydrolysis of embolized fat by pneumocytes into free fatty acids causes toxic injury and inflammation in the lungs, leading to acute lung injury and acute respiratory distress syndrome (ARDS). Trauma-induced hormonal changes may cause systemic release of chylomicrons into the circulation, which coalesce and get deposited into blood vessels.

Clinical features: Symptoms of FES usually develop by 24–72 hours of injury and the risky period spans for over a week. The syndrome characterized by the triad of pulmonary dysfunction, cerebral dysfunction and axillary and sub- conjuctival petechiae. The latter is nonthrombocytopenic and result from occlusion of dermal capillaries by fat globules and subsequent extravasation of RBCs. Respiratory signs and symptoms appear earliest and include dyspnea, tachypnea, cyanosis and hypoxemia. Cerebral dysfunction manifests as confusion, drowsiness and may progress to convulsions or coma. Nonpalpable petechial rashes may appear in the chest, axilla and conjunctiva.

Investigations: Blood gas analysis (most important investigation) shows features of hypoxia and hypocapnia. Serial chest X-ray may show diffuse bilateral pulmonary infiltrates (Snow storm appearance). Fat globules may be detected in urine, blood and sputum on cytological examination. A formal way of establishing the diagnosis is by applying the Gurd's criteria **(Table 5.14)**.

Treatment: The first step in treatment is prevention. Early splinting of fracture (by Thomas splint or external fixator) reduces the chances. In case the syndrome is established, then treatment of FES is only supportive. Treatment aims at maintaining adequate oxygenation, ventilation and normal hemodynamics. I/V alcohol to dissolve fat, heparin (activates lipase and block thromboxane), aspirin and corticosteroids all have been tried with doubtful success but are best avoided as of today. Mechanical ventilation to maintain oxygenation is the best form of therapy today. With time, the fat dissolves and the emboli are washed off. Corticosteroids may be useful in the setting of ARDS but most studies do not support much role. The early fracture fixation should be considered to prevent further embolism. Caution is to be exercised in nailing these patients. Unreamed nailing is preferred to prevent the fat emboli from dislodging from bone marrow.

Table 5.14: Gurd's criteria* for diagnosis of fat embolism syndrome	
Major criteria	Signs of CNS depression
	$PaO_2 < 60$ mm Hg
	Axillary and subconjunctival petechiae
Minor criteria	Pyrexia > 38.5
	Pulse > 110/min
	Retinal embolism
	Reduced platelet count
	Fat globules in urine
	Fat globules in sputum
	Increased ESR

*Fat embolism syndrome is diagnosed when at least one major plus four minor criteria are present.

Neurovascular Injury

Excessive traction during nailing may cause pudendal nerve palsy and presents with numbness of the penis, scrotum or labia. Mostly it is neurapraxia only and recovery occurs within 3 months. Sciatic and peroneal injuries may also occur. Usually these are traction injuries (excessive stretching) and recover fully. Vascular injury is rare, but femoral artery may be damaged by fracture fragment particularly at the junction of the middle and distal third of femur.

Infection

Infection may occur following surgery of the close fracture shaft of femur. The incidence is low as intramedullary nailing is a minimally invasive surgery. Open contaminated fractures are at increased risk of infection and risk increases with increase in Gustilo grading of open fractures.

Knee Stiffness

Some degree of loss of flexion and extension lag is common after nailing fracture shaft of femur. Scarring of quadriceps due to injury by fractured fragment or missed knee ligament injury is the most common cause. Treatment is dedicated postoperative physiotherapy. If knee stiffness persists even after 6 months of treatment, knee manipulation under anesthesia or arthroscopic arthrolysis of intra-articular adhesions of the knee joint or quadricepsplasty may be required.

Malunion

Angular deformities are more common in fractures of proximal third of femur. Valgus or varus angulation less than 10° are usually clinically insignificant. Arthritis can rarely develop in a malunited weight-bearing long bone due to the change of the anatomical axis of the limb and unequal load distribution of the joint. Rotational malunion may also occur following intramedullary nailing. External rotation deformity is more common, although internal rotation deformity is more problematic. Significant malunion (greater than 15° of rotational deformity and greater than 10° of angular deformity) may require osteotomy. In adults after femoral shaft fracture reduction, angulation and rotation should be less than 10°. In children below 12 years up to 25° of angulation and rotation are acceptable.

Delayed and Nonunion

With appropriate treatment a shaft femur fracture generally unites in about 100 days (3–4 months); however, there is no uniformly accepted definition of delayed and nonunion in a fracture shaft of femur. Most surgeons agree for 6 months, beyond which a fracture shaft femur can be labeled as having gone into nonunion. Incidence of delayed and nonunion is low with modern interlocking intramedullary nailing. Treatment of delayed union is bone grafting. Nonunion after intramedullary nailing requires removal of the nail and overreaming of the medullary canal and placement of the larger nail (exchange nailing) with bone grafting.

Heterotopic Ossification

Heterotopic bone formation is not uncommon after intramedullary nailing and most common sites are at the entry point of the nail and around GT. Head injury is the most common associated risk factor. Surgical excision is rarely required.

HIGH-YIELD POINTS

- Fracture of middle third and transverse fracture (caused by bending load) is the most common location and type of femoral shaft fracture, respectively.
  However, in children the fractures most commonly involve the upper third, while pathological fractures, especially in the elderly involve the relatively weak metaphysiodiaphyseal junction.
- Nails used for femur can be inserted antegrade (from greater trochanter or pyriform fossa) or retrograde (from the intercondylar area of distal femur). Mostly antegrade nailing technique is used to avoid opening the knee joint. However, retrograde nails are easier to insert owing to easy identification of entry point and are used in obese patients, floating knees (simultaneous lower femur and upper tibia fractures as both bones can be nailed from one incision) and periprosthetic fractures in a TKR patient.
- The diameter of the nail that can be inserted in the femur is decided by measuring the diameter of the isthmus, the narrowest part of the medullary cavity of femur. The length of the femoral nail to be inserted correlates well with the length from olecranon to tip of little finger.
- Knee ligament injuries are most common associated injury and fracture neck femur is the most commonly missed concomitant fracture with fracture shaft of femur.
- *Waddell's triad*: Femoral fracture plus head injury plus intrathoracic/intra-abdomen injury. It is seen in pediatric pedestrian in road traffic accidents.
- The most common fracture associated with FES is femur fracture. Bilateral fractures and multiple fractures are associated with greater incidence.
- Lower limb fractures are almost inevitably associated with shortening. Sequence of decreasing amount of shortening is: posterior dislocation of hip → femoral shaft fracture → subtrochanteric femur fracture → intertrochanteric fracture → intracapsular neck femur fracture.

DISTAL FEMUR FRACTURES

Distal femur fractures, accounting for about 6% of all femur fractures, include the supracondylar and intercondylar fractures and involve the femur extending distally from the diaphyseal-metaphyseal junction (around 10–15 cm of length). These have a bimodal age distribution with fractures commonly occurring in young males (below 40 years) with good quality bone after high-velocity trauma and in elderly females (above 50 years) with osteoporotic bone with minor falls.

Mechanism of Injury

In both age groups axial force is the most common mechanism of injury. Young people sustain these injuries in high-energy trauma, such as road traffic accidents and fall from height, whereas in elderly females a simple fall is responsible for the majority of these fractures.

Types (Fig. 5.67A)

- *Supracondylar*: Extra-articular fracture involving distal femoral metaphysis.
- *Unicondylar*: Fracture involving either the medial or lateral femoral condyle. Commonly unicondylar distal femoral fractures occur in the sagittal plane. Fracture of any femoral condyle in coronal plane is called Hoffa's fracture **(Fig. 5.67B)**.
- *Intercondylar*: Intra-articular fracture, it can be simple (T or Y type) or complex (comminuted intra-articular fractures).
- The combination of all/any of these.

Clinical Features

Patients present with severe pain and swelling around the knee. Weight-bearing is not possible on the injured limb. In displaced fractures obvious deformity may be present. Abnormal mobility and crepitus can be elicited at the site of fracture. Always assess vascular status, because of the proximity of the fracture to the popliteal artery, which may get damaged during the injury. In high-energy injuries significant soft tissue damage may occur and open injuries are common in intra-articular fractures. Diagnosis is confirmed on anteroposterior and lateral X-rays of knee **(Figs 5.68A to D)**.

Management

Undisplaced fractures can be treated in a long leg nonweight-bearing cast for 6 weeks, but, it leads to recumbency-related complications and secondary joint stiffness and risks secondary displacement. ORIF are required for all displaced distal femoral intra-articular fractures. Unicondylar fractures can be fixed with multiple cancellous screws (lag screw) or a buttress or a locked compression plate (LCP) can be used. Intercondylar fractures require ORIF with LCP (locking compression plate, **Figs 5.68E and F**), dynamic condylar screw (DCS) or condylar blade plate. Supracondylar fractures can be fixed with ORIF with LCP or retrograde intramedullary nailing (distal femoral nail, **Figs 5.68G and H**). LCPs (*see* Page 471) are especially advantageous in osteoporotic bone in elderly. Open fractures may require temporary fixation with external fixator till soft tissue injury heals (damage control surgery).

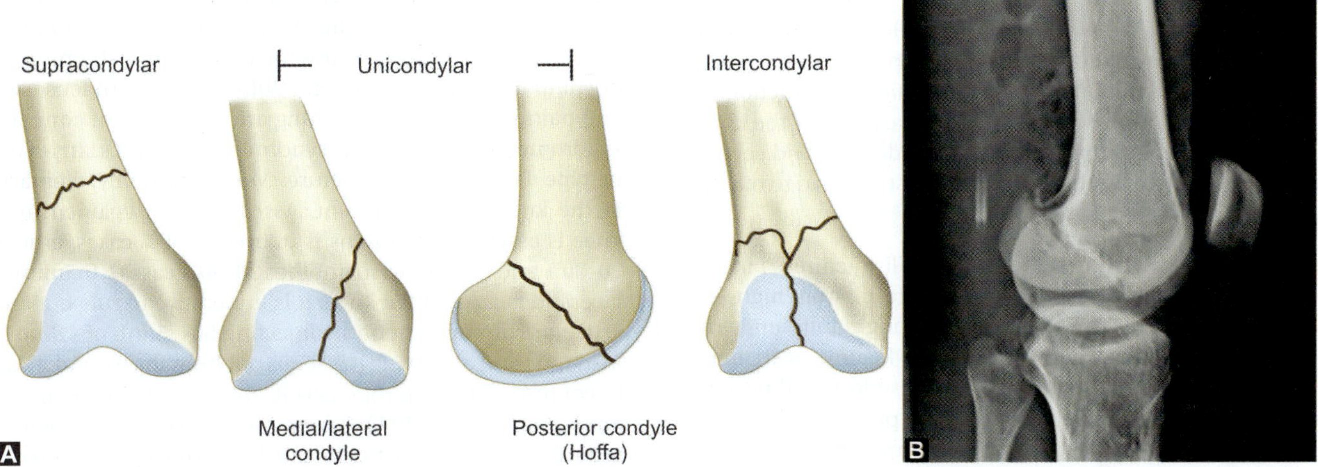

Figs 5.67A and B: (A) Types of distal femoral fractures; and (B) X-ray of lateral view of knee showing a Hoffa fracture

Courtesy: Dr Rajat Kumar Garg.

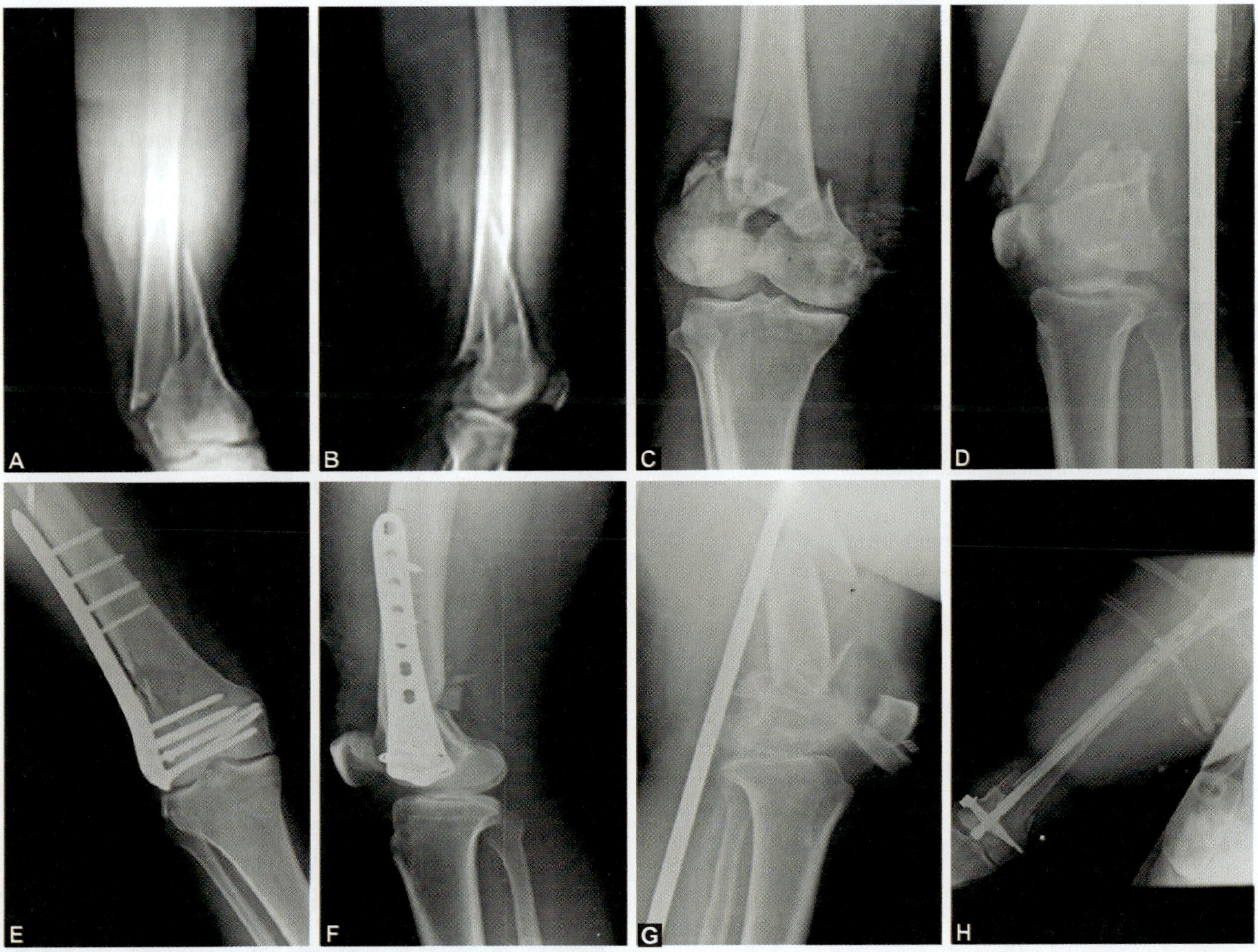

Figs 5.68A to H: (A and B) X-ray, knee AP and lateral views showing supracondylar fracture femur and (C and D) X-ray, AP and lateral views showing intercondylar fracture and (E and F) its fixation with LCP; (G and H) X-ray of knee with proximal thigh and leg lateral view showing comminuted supracondylar femur fracture with fracture shaft of femur and its CRIF with retrograde (distal femur nail) nail

Abbreviations: AP, anteroposterior; LCP, locked compression plate; CRIF, closed reduction internal fixation.

Complications

- *Knee stiffness*: It may arise due to prolonged immobilization and lack of postoperative physiotherapy.
- *Osteoarthritis*: Inappropriate intra-articular reduction of the fracture can result in secondary osteoarthritis of the knee.
- *Malunion*: Inappropriate operative reduction and secondary displacement of the fracture as in a cast can lead to malunion.

TIBIAL PLATEAU FRACTURES

These fractures constitute about 1% of all fractures. Like distal femoral fractures, tibial plateau fractures result from high-energy injuries (RTA or fall from height) in young adults and from a low-energy simple fall in elderly. Axial loading with bending forces (varus/valgus) are usually responsible for tibial plateau fractures. Less commonly direct hit to the proximal tibia (by a car bumper) may lead to these fractures (bumper fractures).

Classification

Schatzker's classification **(Table 5.15 and Fig. 5.69)** is the most commonly used system to classify these fractures. Isolated fractures of lateral condyle comprise one-third of these fractures (medial condyle being stronger, fractures less commonly).

Clinical Features

Patients present with severe pain and swelling around the knee with inability to bear weight on the injured limb. Crepitus, abnormal mobility at fracture site is usually present. In displaced fractures obvious deformity is present. Neurovascular assessment of the involved limb should always be done as there is a high incidence of injuries to the popliteal neurovascular

bundle. Peroneal nerve may also be injured, but it is mostly the stretching of the nerve leading to neuropraxia. Always look for the compartment syndrome as this fracture is the most common cause of compartment syndrome in adults. Presence of tense swelling and pain with passive stretching are suggestive of compartment syndrome. Compartment syndrome is particularly common in type IV Schatzker fracture. Very commonly, hemarthrosis in the knee may be present. Assessment of ligament injury to knee is essential (meniscus is injured in 50% cases, cruciates in 20–30% and collaterals in another 20–30% cases). In injuries with lacerations around the knee, it is imperative to rule out an intra-articular communication by injecting 50–75 mL of saline (saline load test) and observing if it seeps out from the wound. Diagnosis is confirmed by anteroposterior and lateral X-rays of involved knee joint **(Fig. 5.70A)**. Stress views (with the patient under sedation) can be done to assess injury to the ligaments (collateral ligament injury).

Management

As usual, undisplaced fractures can be managed in a long leg, nonweight-bearing cast for 6 weeks, but it risks joint stiffness and secondary displacement. So many surgeons prefer to go with percutaneous screw fixation to achieve early mobilization. There is a general consensus for ORIF (with buttress or LCP) of all displaced intra-articular fractures of the tibial plateau **(Fig. 5.70B)**. The depressed fragment is elevated with instruments and metaphyseal defect is filled with bone grafts before fixation. Bicondylar (type V) and type VI fractures are best fixed with a LCP. Sometimes dual plating (both medial and lateral side) is required for these. In open injuries and where there is massive soft tissue damage posing a risk for compartment syndrome, a knee spanning external fixator is applied for temporary stabilization. Once the soft tissue condition allows definitive fixation can be pursued.

Complications

Knee stiffness, malunion and osteoarthritis are a common complication like distal femoral fractures. Neurovasular injuries

Table 5.15: Schatzker's classification for tibial plateau fracture	
Type I	Split in lateral plateau
Type II	Split and depression of lateral plateau
Type III	Only depression fracture of lateral plateau
Type IV	Fracture of the medial plateau
Type V	Bicondylar fracture
Type VI	Intra-articular fracture with metaphysiodiaphyseal dissociation

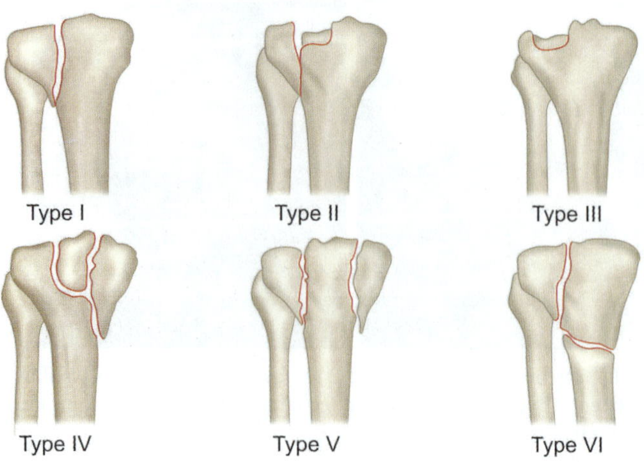

Fig. 5.69: Schatzker's classification of tibial plateau fracture

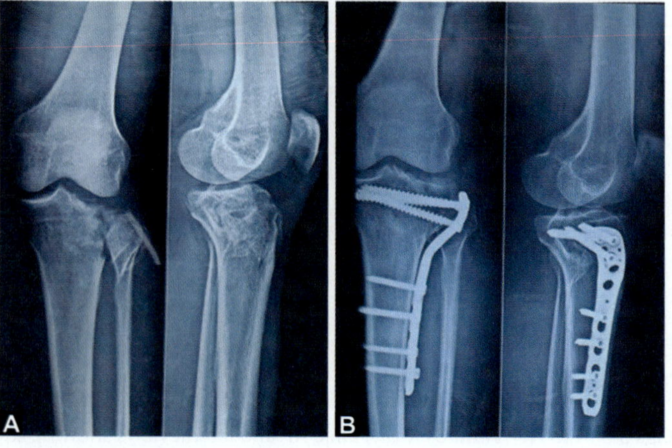

Figs 5.70A and B: (A) X-ray of knee, AP and lateral views showing tibial plateau fracture (Schatzker's type II) and (B) ORIF with LCP

Abbreviations: AP, anteroposterior; ORIF, open reduction and internal fixation; LCP, locked compression plate.

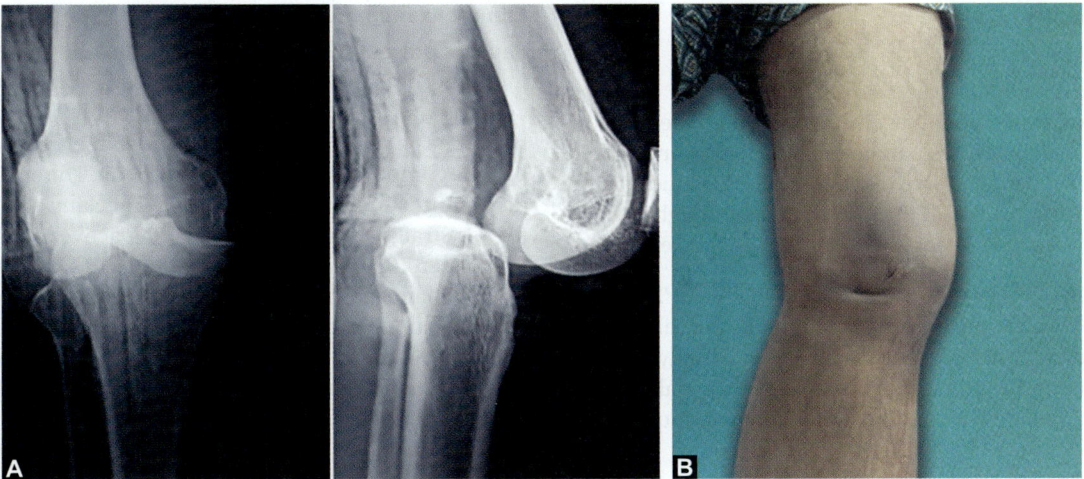

Figs 5.71A and B: (A) X-ray of knee, anteroposterior and lateral views showing posterior knee dislocation. Note tibia displacing posteriorly; (B) Dimple (syn. Pucker) sign of posterolateral knee dislocation. Note puckering of the skin over the medial femoral condyle

can involve the popliteal neurovascular bundle and the peroneal nerve. The latter is usually a neuropraxia. Compartment syndrome is always to be ruled out in fractures of the tibial plateau.

Compartment Syndrome

Forewarned is forearmed, patients with proximal tibial fractures should be kept on strict limb elevation and ice packs to reduce the swelling. Extravasation of blood, soft tissue swelling and fracture itself increase the pressure in the tight ungiving fascial compartments of the leg leading to compartment syndrome. Treatment is emergency fasciotomy of all compartments of the leg.

DISLOCATION OF THE KNEE

These are one of the rare, but one of the most dangerous dislocations that result from dashboard injuries and high-energy motor vehicle accidents. The true incidence is unknown, as almost 50% of these spontaneously reduce. Hyperextension injuries of the knee joint are the most common mechanism of injury. Anterior knee dislocation (tibia displacing anteriorly) is the most common type followed by posterior type **(Fig. 5.71A)**. A posterolateral dislocation often presents with the characteristic Dimple or Pucker sign **(Fig. 5.71B)** where the medial femoral condyle button holes through the medial capsule-ligamentous structures and becomes irreducible.

Popliteal artery and peroneal nerve are at particular risk in knee dislocation and neurovascular examination is vital in all cases as the reported incidence is although variable but high (20–60%). Posterior knee dislocation is most commonly associated with popliteal artery injury. If vascular injury is suspected (diminished pulses or ankle-brachial index < 0.9) urgent CT angiogram or duplex ultrasound is warranted. Vascular injury should be repaired before 6–8 hours of injury.

A knee dislocation without fracture or vascular injury should be reduced closed immediately and supported by a hinged knee brace in 20–30° of knee flexion (do not immobilize in extension as it may inadvertently tighten the posterior capsule). An irreducible dislocation often manifests with Dimple/Pucker sign and requires urgent open reduction. Multiligamentous knee injury is the sequel of knee dislocation and three or more major ligaments (ACL,

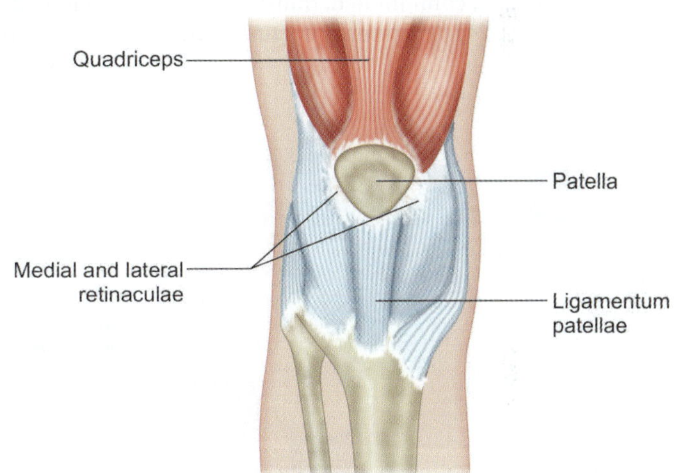

Fig. 5.72: Anatomy of the extensor apparatus of the knee

PCL, MCL and LCL) are usually torn. MRI is the investigation of choice to detect ligament injury to the knee. Definitive treatment involves reconstruction of torn ligaments (*see* Chapter 6).

FRACTURE OF PATELLA

Although a sesamoid bone, patella is an important part of the extensor apparatus of the knee joint. Quadriceps tendon inserts on the superior pole of patella and ligamentum patellae extends from the lower pole of the patella to the tibial tuberosity. Thus, patella transmits the tensile force of quadriceps contraction to the patellar tendon enabling the patient to extend the knee and perform a straight leg raise. Patella increases the moment arm of the quadriceps extensor mechanism and allows knee extension with a lesser quadriceps force. Medial and lateral retinaculae are condensations of fascia and are attached to the medial and lateral margins of patella **(Fig. 5.72)**.

Patellar fractures account for 1% of all skeletal injuries. They are more common in males between 20 years and 50 years of age. In high-energy injuries, distal femoral and proximal tibial fractures are commonly accompanying fractures with fracture of patella.

Mechanism of Injury

Indirect Mechanism

This is the most common mechanism. This occurs following sudden and strong knee flexion against a fully contracted quadriceps muscle. It usually causes a transverse fracture or avulsion of the inferior pole of patella. Force often continues beyond fracture and also tears the retinaculae **(Fig. 5.73)** so active "straight leg raising (SLR) test" is usually not possible as knee cannot be extended.

Direct Blow to Anterior Knee (Fall on Knee or Dashboard Injury)

Its subcutaneous position makes it vulnerable for direct blow injury. After direct blow injury, displacement is usually minimal due to preservation of retinacular expansions. It usually causes comminuted or stellate type fracture. The patient can usually do active SLR.

Classification

Patella fracture may be classified on basis of displacement, viz. undisplaced or displaced; or depending upon the fracture pattern, viz. stellate, comminuted, transverse, vertical (marginal) and polar **(Fig. 5.74)**. Transverse fracture is the most common fracture pattern.

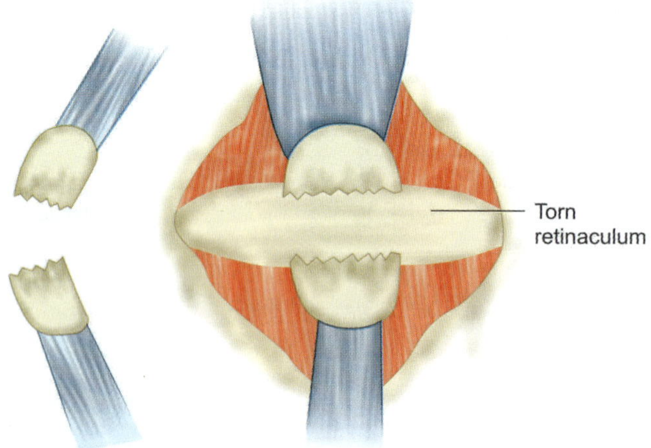

Fig. 5.73: Diagram showing torn retinacular extensions in a transverse fracture of patella

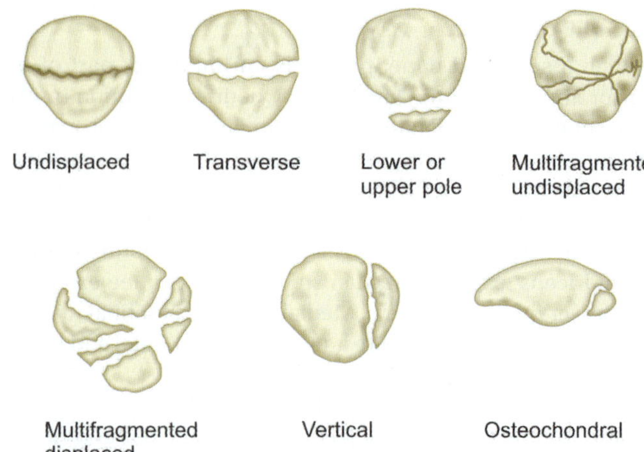

Fig. 5.74: Types of patellar fracture

Clinical Examination

Patients present with anterior knee pain and swelling of the knee joint and difficulty in walking. On examination tenderness and crepitus are present. In two part fracture, the gap may be felt between the patellar fragments. Due to the subcutaneous nature of bone compound fractures are common. The extensor apparatus disruption should be evaluated by checking the ability to raise the leg straight. If the patient is doing active SLR, despite patella fracture, retinacular expansions are likely intact, and fracture can be managed conservatively provided no significant step on articular surface. A patellar fracture patient may not be compliant with examination if a tender and large hemarthrosis (blood in the joint) is present. In this situation aspiration of hemarthrosis, and injection of local anesthetic into the knee joint may be helpful. Diagnosis is confirmed with anteroposterior and lateral **(Fig. 5.75A)** radiographs of the involved knee. Occasionally, a patella skyline view **(Figs 5.76A and B)** may be required in undisplaced fractures.

Management

Conservative

Nonsurgical management is usually successful in fractures with minimal displacement and no articular step-off with an intact extensor mechanism (patient doing active SLR). These patients can be managed with extensor splinting/bracing or with a cylindrical cast **(Fig. 5.77)** for 4–6 weeks. Straight leg raises and quadriceps physiotherapy is encouraged early in the cast. Early partial weight-bearing is encouraged with help of crutches.

Operative

Displaced fractures and disruption of the extensor mechanism requires surgical repair. The options of surgery depend upon the fracture configuration and salvage potential of the patella. Whatever surgery is performed, retinacular disruption, if found, should always be repaired at the time of surgery. Various surgical options are as follows:

- *ORIF with tension band wiring [(TBW)*, **Fig. 5.75B**]: Two part fracture of the patella is fixed with TBW. It allows early knee bending. TBW converts the tensile forces at the anterior

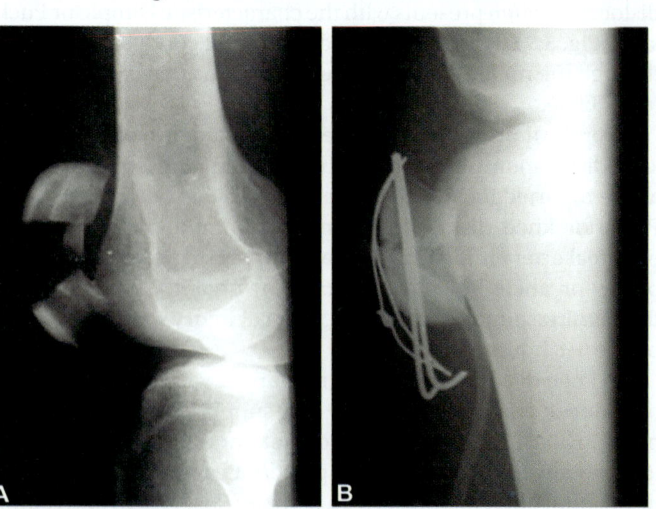

Figs 5.75A and B: (A) X-ray of knee, lateral view showing patellar fracture and (B) Tension band wiring of patella

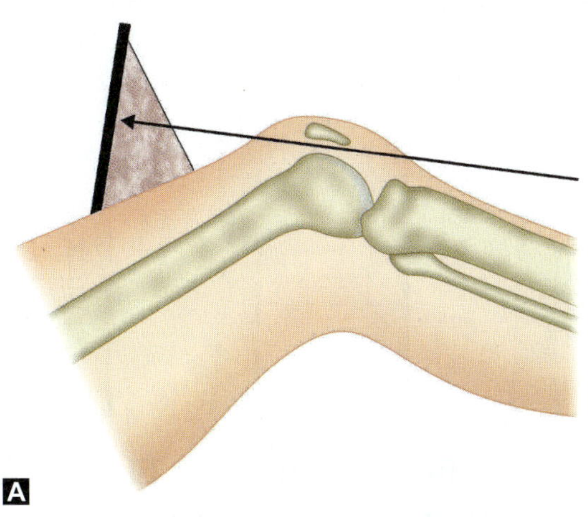

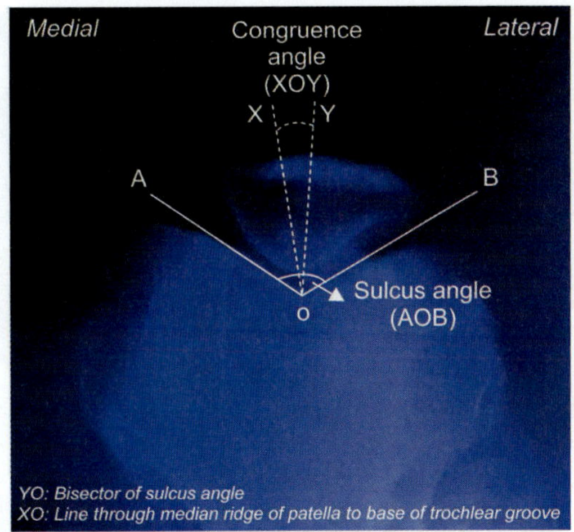

Skyline view-positioning

Skyline view of normal patella

Figs 5.76A and B: (A) Diagram showing how a skyline view of the patella is taken and (B) Skyline view showing a normal patella centered well in the trochlear sulcus (On an average, Sulcus angle is normally 138° while Congruence angle is 6°)

cortical surface of the patella into compressive forces at the articular surface (*see* Chapter 2 for details).

- *Cerclage wiring*: If the fracture is comminuted/stellate fracture, cerclage wiring of the patella may be performed to hold the fracture fragments in place.
- *Partial patellectomy*: It is indicated in comminuted fractures of the inferior pole of patella. In patellar tendon avulsion, the inferior pole fragment is excised and patellar tendon is reattached.
- *Complete patellectomy*: Every attempt should be made to preserve the patella. Total patellectomy may be indicated in severely comminuted fracture where internal fixation is not possible. The patella is excised and the extensor mechanism is repaired end-to-end. In patients with complete patellectomy, there remains an extensor lag (inability to fully extend the knee).

Complications

- *Knee stiffness and quadriceps atrophy*: This is a common complication. To prevent it early range of motion physiotherapy and strengthening exercises should be started.
- *Painful retained hardware*: This is common due to the subcutaneous location of the patella. It may necessitate removal of implant for adequate pain relief.
- *Extensor lag*: It is mostly seen after complete patellectomy. It may also be due to quadriceps atrophy or due to inadequate extensor mechanism repair.
- *Post-traumatic patellofemoral arthritis:* This is a late complication of patellar fracture.

HIGH-YIELD POINTS

- The patella is the largest sesamoid bone in the body and has thickest articular cartilage in the body which covers proximal three-fourths of the patella. The distal pole is entirely devoid of articular cartilage and distal pole fractures are extra-articular.
- *Bipartite patella*: Patella ossifies from a single ossific nucleus. In a bipartite patella a secondary ossific nucleus (mostly

on the superolateral aspect) fails to unite with the primary nucleus **(Fig. 5.78)**. It should not be confused with a fracture.

- Partial rupture/avulsion of patellar tendon from the lower pole of patella leads to a traction tendonitis and calcification in the patellar ligament—the Sinding-Larsen-Johansson syndrome (classified under osteochondritis).
- Tendinitis of the patellar ligament is referred to as Jumper's knee.
- The most common joint to sustain open injuries is the knee joint.

EXTENSOR MECHANISM DISRUPTIONS

These injuries include tear of patellar or quadriceps tendon ruptures and patellar dislocations. Details have been discussed in Chapter 6.

FRACTURES OF THE SHAFT OF TIBIA AND FIBULA

Tibial fractures are very common long bone fractures. Tibial shaft fractures are commonly associated with fracture of shaft of fibula as the energy of trauma is transmitted along the interosseous membrane to fibula also. Like distal femoral and tibial plateau fractures these fractures also have a bimodal age distribution. The first age group is young adults with age less than 40 years who sustain these fractures in high velocity road traffic accidents or fall from height. The second age group consists of elderly women over 70–80 years of age with osteoporotic bones who sustain these fractures due to a simple fall mostly at home.

Anterior and medial aspect of the tibia is covered by a thin, soft tissue cover of skin and subcutaneous tissues. Therefore, open fractures are extremely common.

Classification

Fractures can be classified based on the fracture geometry. Like any long bone fracture, tibial shaft fracture may be spiral, oblique, transverse, comminuted and segmental fracture **(Figs 5.79A to E)**.

Toddler's fracture **(Fig. 5.80)** is a special variant seen in children below 3 years. It is a nondisplaced/minimally displaced

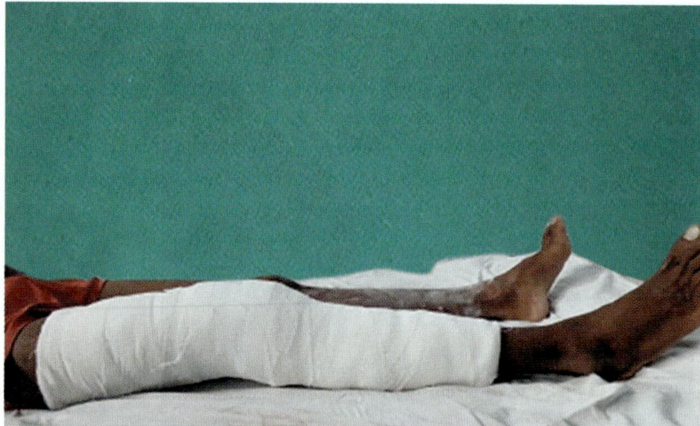

Fig. 5.77: Cylindrical plaster for managing an undisplaced fracture of patella

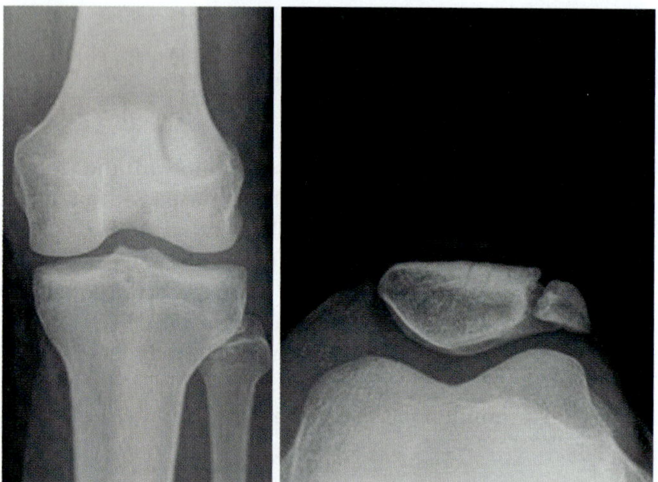

Fig. 5.78: Anteroposterior and skyline views showing a separate ossicle present on the superolateral aspect of the patella (bipartite patella). Note the rounded edges, unlike a fracture

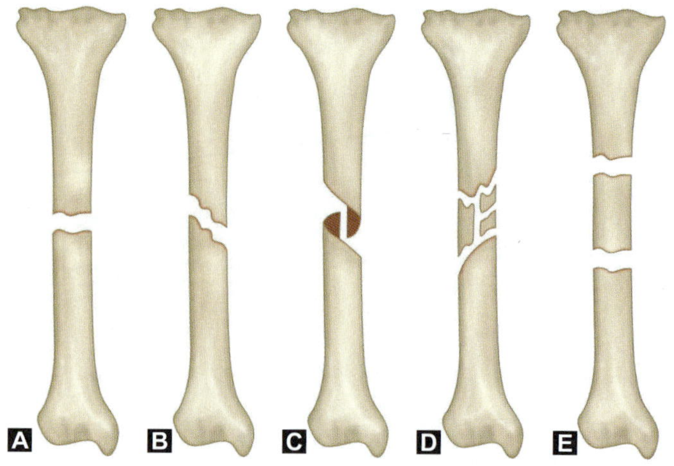

Figs 5.79A to E: Fracture geometry. (A) Transverse; (B) Oblique; (C) Spiral; (D) Comminuted; (E) Segmental

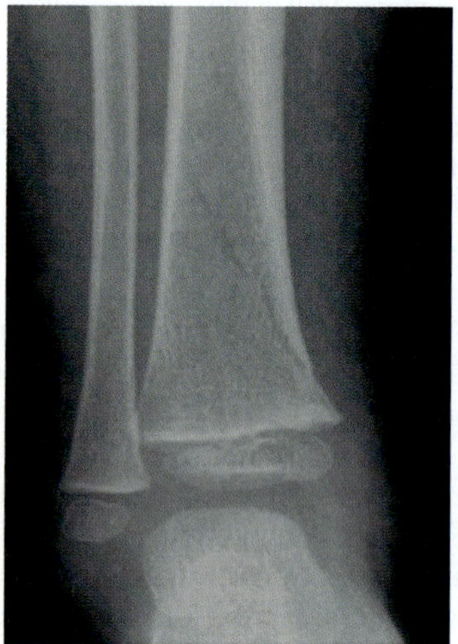

Fig. 5.80: Toddler's fracture

spiral or oblique fracture of tibial shaft only and fibula remains intact. It is also known as childhood accidental spiral tibial (CAST) fracture.

Clinical Features

Patients present with pain and swelling of leg and inability to bear weight on the injured limb. Crepitus, abnormal mobility and deformity are present on site of fracture. High-energy injuries are often associated with open fractures and compartment syndrome. Diagnosis of compartment syndrome should be made on clinical grounds of tense compartment and pain on passive stretching of muscles. Neurovascular examination should be done and recorded in all patients of fracture of shaft of tibia and fibula who are victim of high-energy injuries. Peroneal nerve is particularly at risk in fibular neck fracture.

Diagnosis is confirmed by anteroposterior and lateral X-rays of the involved leg **(Fig. 5.81A)**. All patients of the suspected fracture of tibia should be splinted before transporting the patient for radiological examination. This avoids additional trauma to the soft tissues. Ankle and knee joints of the involved leg should also be X-rayed, as there may be intra-articular extensions and associated dislocation of proximal or distal tibiofibular articulation.

Management

High-energy tibial shaft fractures should be assessed on the basis of ATLS guidelines. If the patient does not have any life-threatening injury fractured limb should be splinted and patient can be planned up for definitive management. All open fractures with bone ends protruding outside the skin should be reduced to avoid desiccation of bone. If reduction is not possible in the emergency room, then protruded bone ends should be covered with saline gauze pieces.

Conservative

A low-energy undisplaced/minimally displaced fracture can be treated in a nonweight-bearing long leg cast in 10° knee flexion for 4 weeks, followed by a patellar tendon bearing cast **(Figs 5.82A and B)** or functional brace for another 4–6 weeks.

Acceptability criteria for reduction of tibial shaft fracture are:
- Varus/valgus angulation < 5°
- Anterior/posterior angulation <10°
- Rotation <10°
- Shortening <1.5 cm.

Weight-bearing and range of motion exercises are started at 4 weeks. In children the majority of fractures of shaft of tibia and fibula is treated with close reduction and long leg cast application. Functional bracing is relatively contraindicated in tibial shaft fractures with intact fibula, due to higher chances of varus deformity.

Operative

For closed diaphyseal tibial fractures close reduction and intramedullary nailing **(Fig. 5.81B)** is the gold standard treatment. Reduction is achieved under the guidance of an image intensifier and fixed with intramedullary nail. Fibula is nonweight-bearing bone (transmits just 10–15% of load) and no internal fixation is usually required for fibular fracture. In children, unstable tibial shaft fractures may require close reduction and percutaneous pinning or flexible intramedullary nailing (elastic nails like Enders nail or TENS).

Metaphyseal tibial fractures are best treated with ORIF with plating. Minimally invasive plate osteosynthesis (MIPO, *see* Chapter 19) is a relatively new technique of plating of metaphyseal fractures of long bones in which fracture site is not opened and reduction is achieved by indirect technique and confirmed under C-arm. Small incisions are given just on the screw insertion sites and at the site of insertion of a plate.

Open tibial shaft fractures are most common open fractures. In low-grade open injury (all Gustilo type I and some most type II) thorough surgical wound debridement and primary closure of wound can be done simultaneously with definitive fixation of fracture with intramedullary nail or plate.

High-grade open injuries (all Gustilo type III and some type II) require thorough surgical wound debridement and temporary fixation of fracture with an external fixator. Serial debridement is required until the wound becomes healthy. The external fixator is converted to definitive fixation (intramedullary nail or plate) after optimization of patient health and when the wound becomes healthy for closure (delayed primary closure or skin graft or flap). In rare situations even an external fixator can be continued till bone union.

Complications

- *Delayed union/nonunion **(Figs 5.83A and B)**:* There is no consensus on the definition of delayed union, which differentiates it from nonunion. Factors which favor nonunion include open fractures, infection, high-energy trauma, comminuted and segmental fractures, bone loss, conservative treatment of displaced and unstable fractures, inadequate reduction and postoperative fracture gap, delayed surgery, smoking, diabetes and alcohol consumption. Fractures of the distal third of the tibia are more prone to undergo nonunion than proximal fractures due to precarious blood supply and constitute the most common site where nonunion is seen in clinical practice.

Intramedullary nailing with bone grafting is done for nonunion of diaphyseal tibial shaft fractures. If a nonunion occurs with previous intramedullary nailing then removal of the nail, overreaming of the canal and insertion of a larger diameter nail is required (exchange nailing).

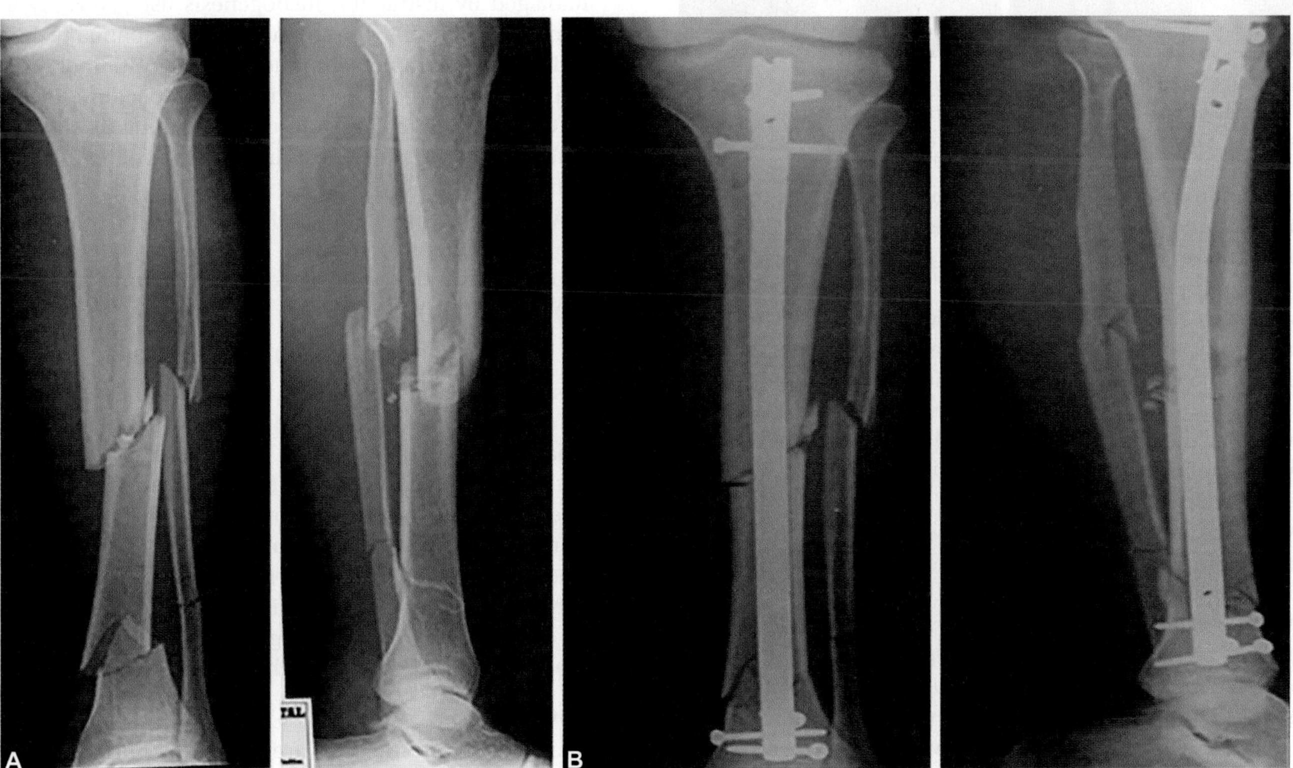

Figs 5.81A and B: (A) X-ray of knee with leg, AP and lateral views showing segmental fracture of the tibia and fibula; (B) CRIF with tibia interlocking nail
Abbreviations: AP, anteroposterior; CRIF, closed reduction internal fixation.

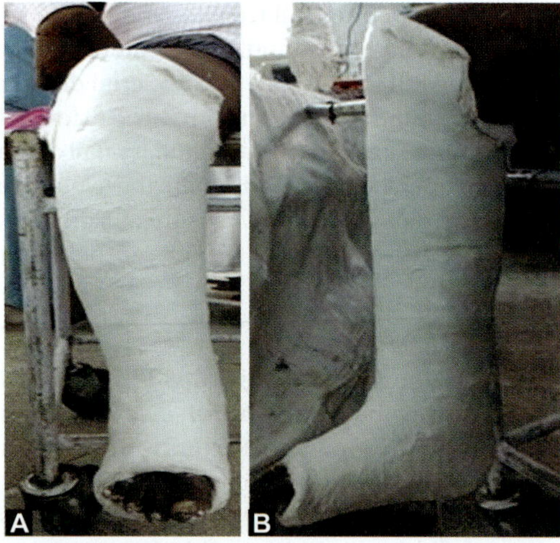

Figs 5.82A and B: PTB cast applied in case of a tibia fracture

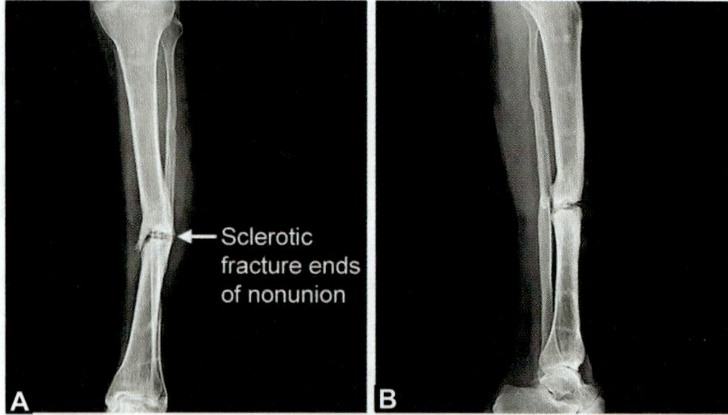

Figs 5.83A and B: X-ray of leg anteroposterior and lateral views showing nonunion of midshaft fracture of the tibia

Nonunion due to small segmental bone loss can be treated by fibular bone grafting. Larger segmental bone defect requires either bone lengthening by Ilizarov technique or vascularized bone graft.

- *Malunion*: Angular and rotational deformities and shortening may occur following inadequate reduction or loss of reduction in the cast. In general varus deformity is more troublesome than valgus deformity. Malunion most commonly occur in the distal third of tibial shaft fractures. Patients with significant deformity causing functional disability may require correction by osteotomy.
- Anterior knee pain is a common complication of intramedullary nailing. With time pain decreases, but in few patients it may be persistent and problematic.
- *Neurovascular injury and compartment syndrome*: Victims of high-velocity road traffic accidents should be thoroughly assessed for associated neurovascular injury. Peroneal nerve is most commonly injured nerve by intramedullary nailing. Usually it is transient and recovers with time. A compartment syndrome may occur following both close and open tibial shaft fractures. Diagnosis should be made on high index of suspicion. Pain out of proportion and pain on passive stretch are the earliest symptoms of compartment syndrome. Anterior compartment is most commonly involved compartment. Treatment is urgent fasciotomy of the involved compartment.
- *Infection*: Superficial and deep infections may complicate the surgical treatment of tibial shaft fracture. Increased risk is seen in open fractures and risk increases with increase in Gustilo grading of open fractures. Superficial infection often responds to IV antibiotics. Deep infection presents with increasing pain and wound drainage. Treatment of deep infection is serial debridement and irrigation of the wound and IV antibiotics. Removal of intramedullary nail and placement of antibiotic impregnated cement nail may be needed in recalcitrant cases.

HIGH-YIELD POINTS

- Open tibial fractures do not preclude the possibility of the development of a compartment syndrome. Compartment syndrome should be suspected in all tibial shaft fractures. (Open fracture does not mean decompressed compartment).
- *Dynamization*: It is a method of accelerating bone union in cases of delayed union. The interlocking nails have two types of holes—static (circular) and dynamic (oval). In dynamization statically locked screw (placed in circular holes) is removed, leaving only dynamic screw in the nail (*see* Page 470 for details). This increases compression at the fracture site on weight-bearing as bone can now translate by a few millimeters on the nail and promotes healing.
- Not uncommon is to find gap non-union in tibia where a large segment of bone is missing. Such cases can be managed by distraction histiogenesis using Ilizarov fixator, bone grafting using massive allografts (Capanna technique), Induced membrane technique or transposition of ipsilateral fibula (if intact) to tibia (Huntington procedure, **Figs 5.84A to C**). In the latter procedure, as the fibula is subjected to loads, it hypertrophies over time to replace the lost segment of tibia.
- Newer nonsurgical methods of treating delayed and nonunion are low intensity pulsed ultrasound, electromagnetic stimulation and use of osteoinductive bone morphogenic proteins (BMPs).

TIBIAL PLAFOND FRACTURES (PILON FRACTURE)

The distal tibial articular surface is referred to as tibial plafond. Pilon fracture of the tibia is a fracture of tibial plafond with proximal extension **(Figs 5.85A and B)**. These fractures are usually caused by high-energy axial force such as fall from height. High-velocity pilon fractures are often associated with severe soft tissue injury **(Fig. 5.86)** and fracture comminution.

Patients present with pain, swelling, ankle deformity and inability to bear weight. Diagnosis is confirmed by anteroposterior, lateral and mortise view (*see* **Figs 5.92A and B**) of the ankle. Involved leg and foot should also be X-rayed.

Management

Minimally displaced fractures are treated by nonweight-bearing short leg cast for 6 weeks. Time of surgical intervention is largely guided by the condition of the soft tissues. Edema, bruises, blisters, etc. indicate significant soft tissue injury, and surgical intervention

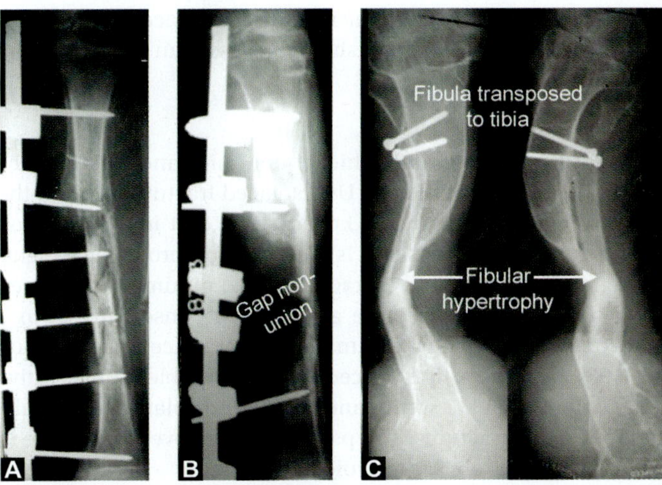

Figs 5.84A to C: Huntington procedure. X-rays showing fibula undergoing hypertrophy after tibialization under weight-bearing loads in a patient who had gap non-union in tibia secondary to bone loss after an open fracture

Courtesy: Dr.Zile Singh Kundu, Professor, Orthopedics, PGIMS Rohtak.

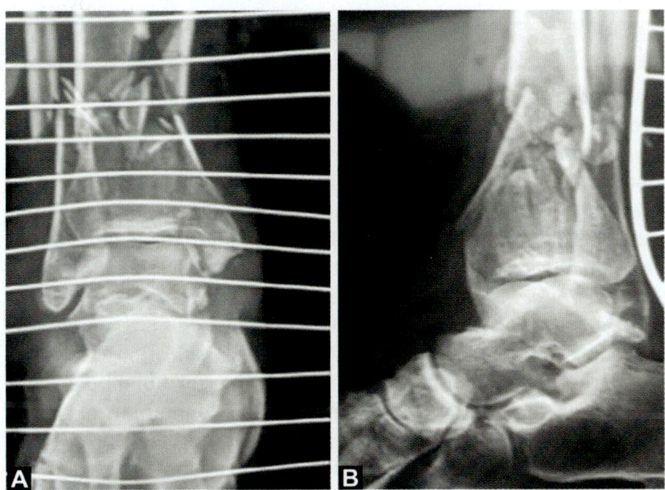

Figs 5.85A and B: X-ray of ankle, anteroposterior and lateral views showing pilon fracture

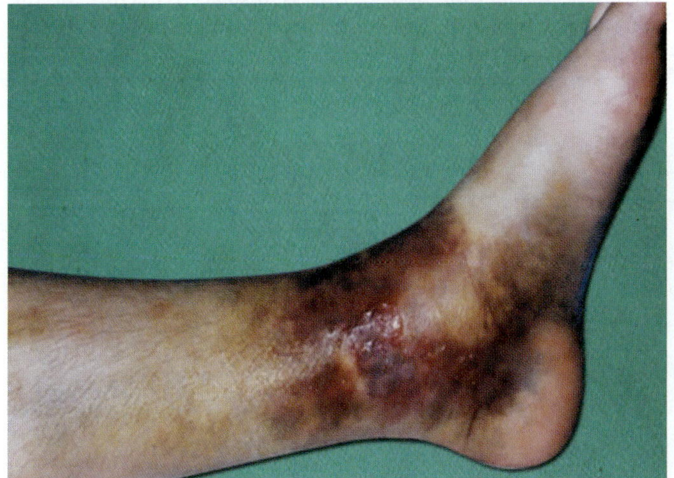

Fig. 5.86: Severe soft tissue injury is usually seen with pilon fracture

in these cases is associated with a high rate of complications like wound breakdown and infection. Temporary fixation of fracture by an external fixator in distraction mode (ligamentotaxis, *see* Page 34) is done in this situation and definitive surgery should be delayed until the wrinkles appear around the ankle (wrinkle sign) which indicates subsidence of edema. Once soft tissue injuries recover definitive internal fixation is done using locked compression periarticular distal tibial plates.

Complications

Superficial skin necrosis and sloughing are the most common complications of pilon fracture. Sloughing of full thickness skin and wound dehiscence is also not uncommon in high-energy injuries. It requires wound debridement, irrigation and IV antibiotics. Post-traumatic arthritis is also common due to the intra-articular nature of the fracture. One should also look for signs and symptoms of increased compartment pressure by serial evaluation and maintain a high index of suspicion for development of compartment syndrome in these high-velocity ankle injuries.

INJURIES AROUND THE ANKLE AND FOOT

RELEVANT ANATOMY

Normal ankle joint is required for rhythmic effortless gait and to withstand up to 1.5 times body weight while walking and more than it during running. Three bones [(1) tibia, (2) fibula above and (3) talus below] together constitute the ankle joint which is a modified hinge joint. The distal articular surface of the tibia along with the medial and lateral malleoli forms a convex surface proximally referred to as ankle mortise. The dome of the talus (convex) fits into the mortise (concave) formed by the tibia and fibula to make a hinge **(Fig. 5.87)** and form the ankle joint. The subtalar (talocalcaneal) joint lies distal to the ankle joint and is formed by the talus above articulating with the calcaneum below. While ankle joint is primarily responsible for the dorsiflexion and planter flexion movements **(Fig. 5.88A)**, prime movements at the subtalar joint, **(Fig. 5.88B)** include inversion (inward twisting of the foot, i.e. varus) and eversion (outward twisting of the foot, i.e. valgus). Supination refers to the combination of inversion plus plantar flexion and adduction at foot while pronation refers to the combination of eversion plus dorsiflexion and abduction at foot.

FRACTURES AROUND THE ANKLE

These are common fractures, especially in young, active persons involved in sports and in elderly females. These fractures can be unimalleolar, bimalleolar or trimalleolar. Various eponyms are used to describe some common fractures in this area as given in **Box 5.1**. These fractures are usually caused by low-energy twisting injury (mechanism of injury is same to that of ankle sprain). Direction of force and position of foot at the time of injury determines the fracture pattern as described by Lauge and Hansen.

Classification

Lauge-Hansen classification, based on the mechanism of injury, is the most popular way to classify these injuries. Four main types are described. The first word in each type describes the position of the foot at the time of injury and the second word in each type describes the direction of the deforming force. Different combinations can lead to a different sequential injury pattern, the final injury depending upon the magnitude of deforming force. The classification has been summarized in **Table 5.16**. The most common type out of all is the supination-external rotation injury (foot is supinated at time of injury and deforming force pushes it into external rotation), comprising 40–75% of all malleolar fractures.

Clinical Features

The patient usually gives a history of a twisting injury followed by severe pain, swelling and inability to bear weight. On examination the ankle will be swollen and tender with crepitus. Condition of skin and neurological status should be assessed. Open fractures and dislocations require urgent intervention.

Anteroposterior and lateral view of the ankle are mostly sufficient to make the diagnosis. Fracture pattern, the amount of displacement, comminution, articular congruity, and disruption of syndesmosis (normally there is a small overlap between distal tibia and fibula; in syndesmotic injury the overlap is decreased) are the things which should be noted in the radiograph. Mortise view or anteroposterior view of ankle in 15° internal rotation of the ankle (to offset the posterior shadow of the fibula) is the best view to see the ankle articular surfaces. Normally, in mortise view medial clear space should be equal to superior clear space

and equal to or less than 4 mm. Lateral clear space changes with rotation and in mortise view it should be less than 6 mm (*see* **Fig. 5.92A**).

Management

The aim of the treatment is to achieve bone union and maintenance of tibiotalar joint congruency. Undisplaced fractures around the ankle are managed by below knee plaster cast immobilization for 6 weeks. After 6 weeks cast is removed and protected weight-bearing can be allowed in a brace. Isolated minimally displaced lateral malleolus fractures are also treated conservatively in a below knee cast. Recently pneumatic walking braces (Aircast boot, **Fig. 5.93**) have been introduced for comfortable, conservative management of ankle sprain and stable undisplaced/minimally displaced ankle fractures. The patient can remove them while in bed for periodic exercises to avoid joint stiffness.

Operative Treatment

Displaced fractures that disrupt the articular part of mortise, fractures with syndesmotic widening (decreased tibiofibular overlap to less than 6 mm on the AP views and less than 1 mm

---

Box 5.1: Some common fracture eponyms around ankle

Pott's fracture: A bimalleolar (medial and lateral malleolus) fracture around ankle

Cotton's fracture (**Fig. 5.89A**): A trimalleolar fracture (in addition to both malleoli the posterior malleolus of the tibia is also fractured)

Maisonneuve fracture: A fracture of medial malleolus in association with a fracture of the proximal third of fibula. This is an external rotation type of ankle injury (see Lauge-Hansen classification)

Le Fort Wagstaffe fracture: Avulsion fracture of the anterior tibiofibular ligament from the anterior surface of fibula. This is a supination-external rotation injury (*see* Lauge-Hansen classification)

Tillaux-Chaput fracture: Avulsion of the anterior tibiofibular ligament from the anterior tibial margin (tibial counterpart of the Le Fort fracture). This is a Salter-Harris type III injury (**Fig. 5.89B**). This is generally seen in adolescents and rarely in adults

Bosworth fracture dislocation: It is a fracture of distal fibula with entrapment of proximal fibular fracture fragment behind the tibia. It is difficult to reduce and ORIF is often required to treat this injury

Pronation-dorsiflexion injury: This is displaced fracture of the anterior articular surface of the tibia. It is thought to be a variant of pilon fracture

---

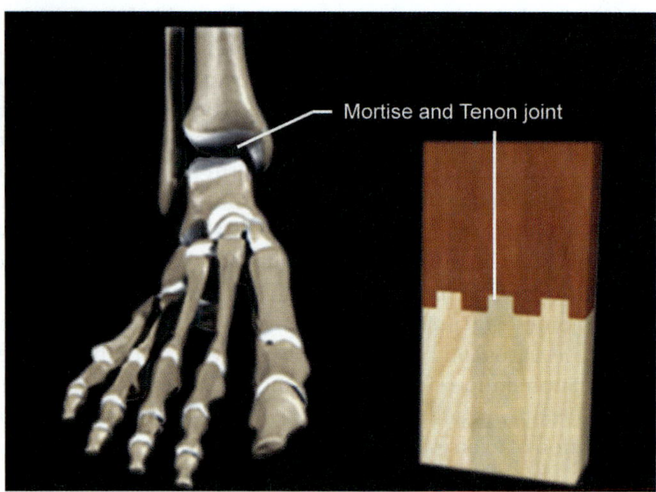

Fig. 5.87: Ankle mortise

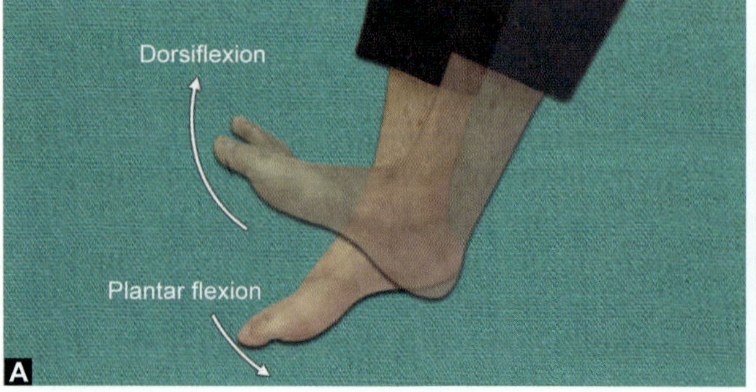

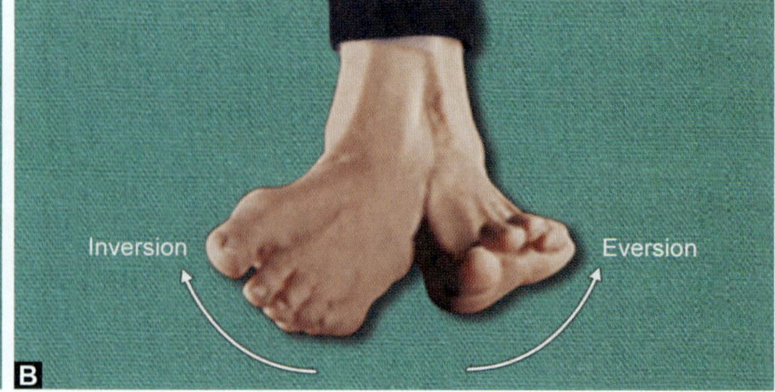

Figs 5.88A and B: (A) Dorsiflexion and plantar flexion and (B) Inversion and eversion

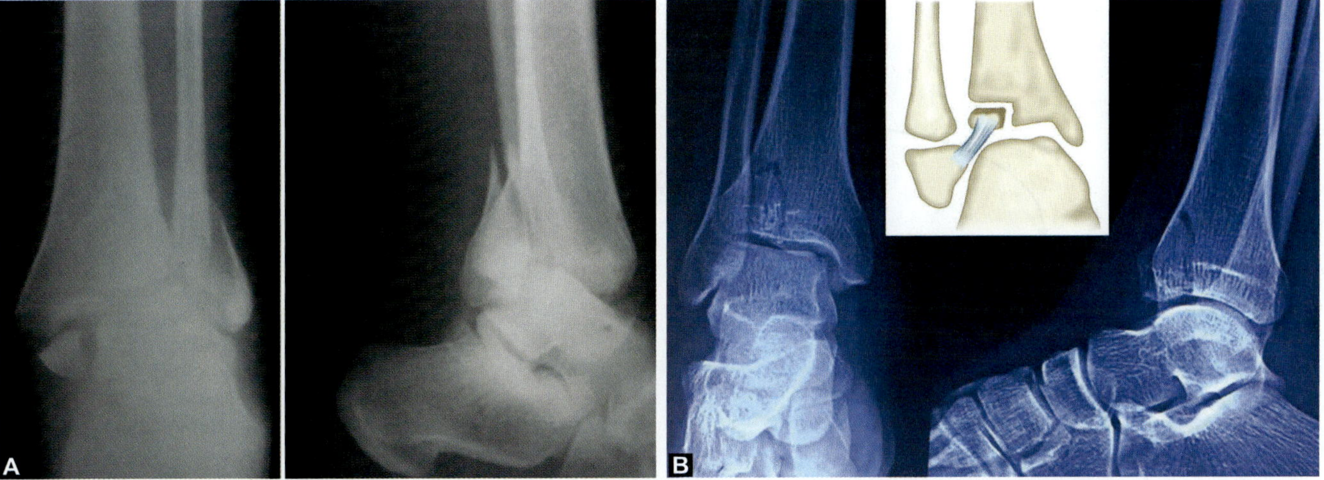

Figs 5.89A and B: (A) X-ray of ankle, anteroposterior view showing both malleoli fractured and lateral view showing the posterior malleolus of tibia fractured additionally (Cotton's fracture); (B) X-ray of ankle anteroposterior and lateral views showing Tillaux-Chaput fracture

Table 5.16: Lauge-Hansen classification **(Figs 5.90 and 5.91)**

I. Supination-adduction (SA)
- *Stage I:* Avulsion fracture of fibular tip
- *Stage II:* Vertical fracture of medial malleolus

II. Supination-external rotation (SER) (most common type)
- *Stage I:* Sprain of anterior tibiofibular ligament
- *Stage II:* Spiral fracture of distal fibula (fracture line runs from anteroinferior to posterosuperior)
- *Stage III:* Tear of posterior tibiofibular ligament ± fracture of posterior malleolus
- *Stage IV:* Transverse fracture of medial malleolus or tear of deltoid ligament

III. Pronation-abduction (PA)
- *Stage I:* Tear of deltoid ligament or transverse fracture of medial malleolus
- *Stage II:* Rupture of syndesmotic ligaments
- *Stage III:* Transverse fracture of the fibula above the level of the syndesmosis

IV. Pronation-external rotation (PER)
- *Stage I:* Tear of deltoid ligament or transverse fracture of medial malleolus
- *Stage II:* Tear of anterior tibiofibular ligament
- *Stage III:* Spiral fracture of fibula above the level of the syndesmosis (fracture line runs from anterosuperior to posteroinferior)
- *Stage IV:* Tear of posterior tibiofibular ligament or avulsion fracture of posterior malleolus

on the mortise view and increased clear space more than 5 mm on both the AP and mortise views measured 1 cm above the plafond between the medial border of the fibula and the lateral border of the posterior tibia, **Fig 5.92B)** or obvious subluxation or dislocation are candidates for surgical fixation. In displaced fractures open reduction of the fracture is done and fracture is fixed internally using plates and screws. Anatomical reduction of the fracture is must to maintain the congruity of the ankle mortise. Any subluxation of the joint should be accurately reduced. Intraoperatively reduction is assessed under image intensifier. Medial malleolus fractures are fixed with compression screw (malleolar screws) or tension band wiring **(Figs 5.94A and B)**. Displaced lateral malleolus fractures are managed with buttress plating (for spiral or oblique or comminuted fractures) and compression screws or tension band wiring (for transverse fracture).

It is imperative to look for syndesmotic injury in all cases after fixing the fracture. The fibula is pulled laterally using a hook, the joint will open up in case of syndesmotic disruption (known as Cotton's test). A syndesmotic injury should be fixed with a syndesmotic screw (a transverse screw from the fibula to the tibia). Posterior malleolus (fracture of the posterior lip of tibial plafond) fracture is usually a part of trimalleolar fracture (Cotton's fracture). If posterior fracture fragment involves more than 25–30% of articular surface operative fixation with compression screw is required.

Caution is to be exercised in the presence of marked edema or blisters. In such cases, operative fixation should be delayed. The leg is splinted and elevated until the skin condition improves.

Complications

- Wound breakdown and infection is particularly common in diabetics. Superficial wound breakdown (stitch line necrosis) may be treated with wound cleaning (removal of devitalized tissue and dry crust) and moist dressing. Deep tissue infection requires serial irrigation and debridement.
- Nonunion is less common with operative intervention. Inadequate reduction, loss of reduction or soft tissue or periosteum interposition (most common cause) between fracture fragments during reduction may lead to nonunion. Asymptomatic nonunion does not need treatment. Painful nonunion requires ORIF with compression screw with bone grafting. Fibular nonunion is rare.
- Joint stiffness may occur following prolonged immobilization in plaster. The plaster should be applied in correct (neutral) position and physiotherapy should be started after removal of plaster.

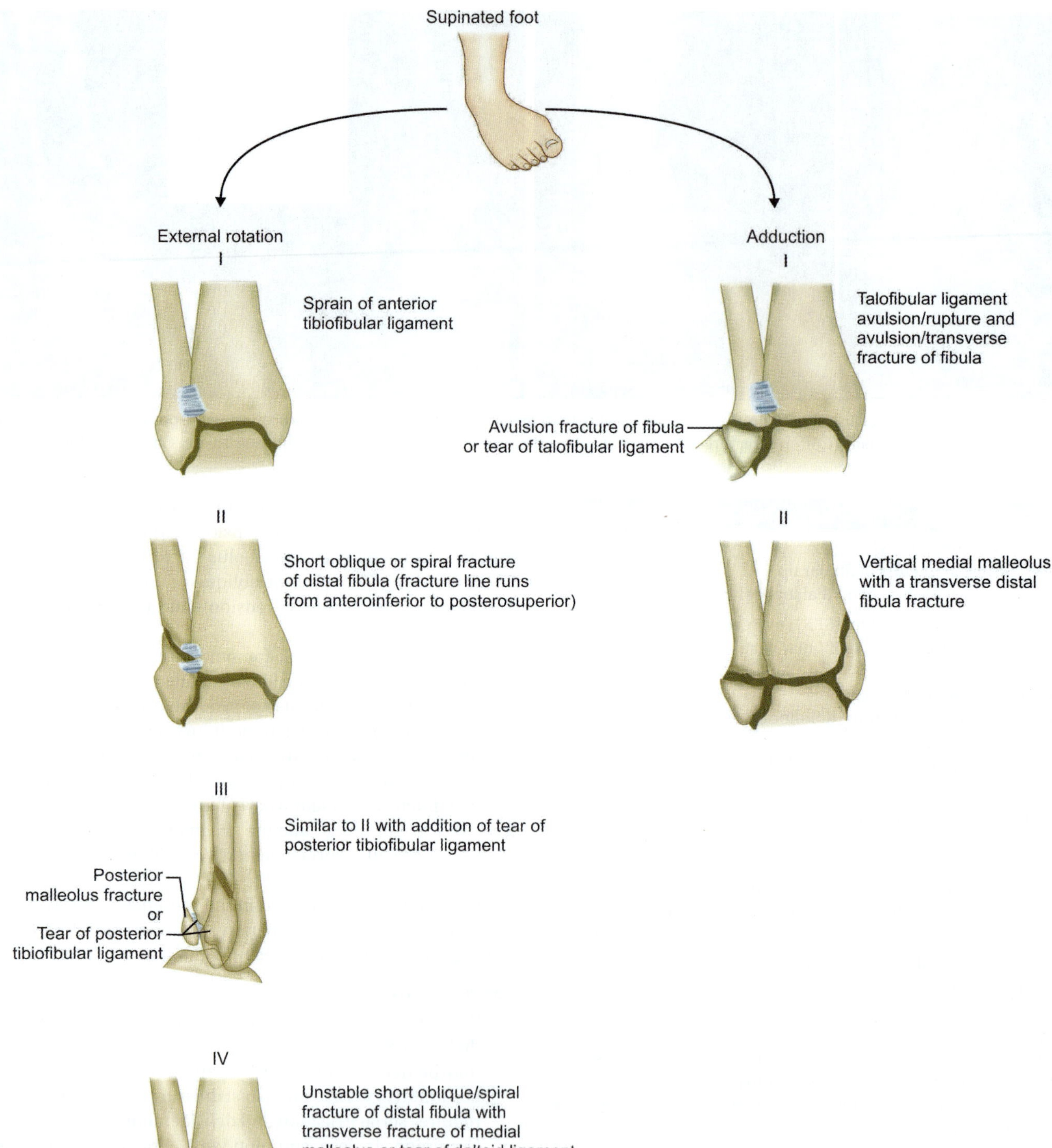

Fig. 5.90: Schematic depiction of stages of supination injuries around ankle

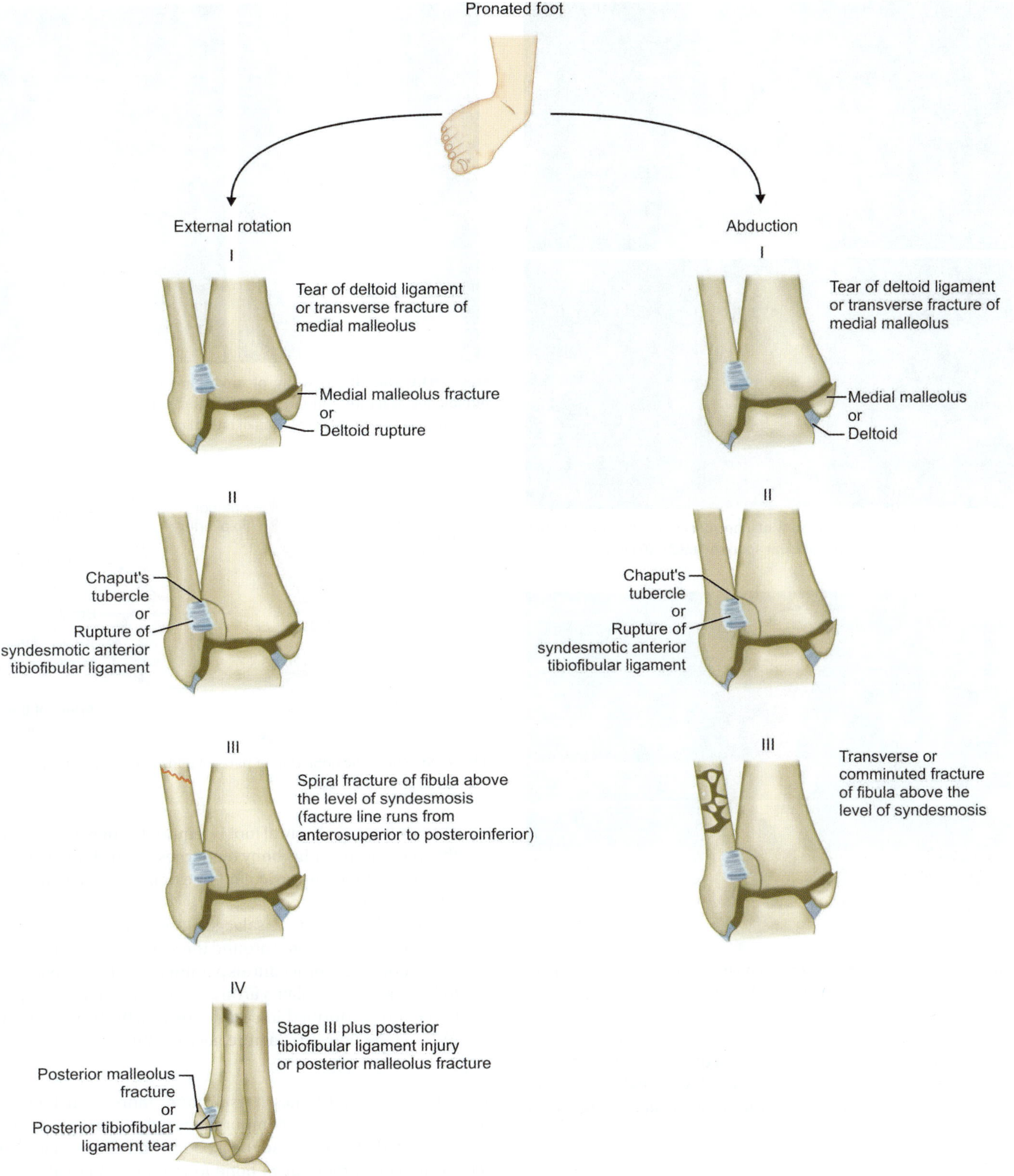

Fig. 5.91: Schematic depiction of pronation injuries around ankle

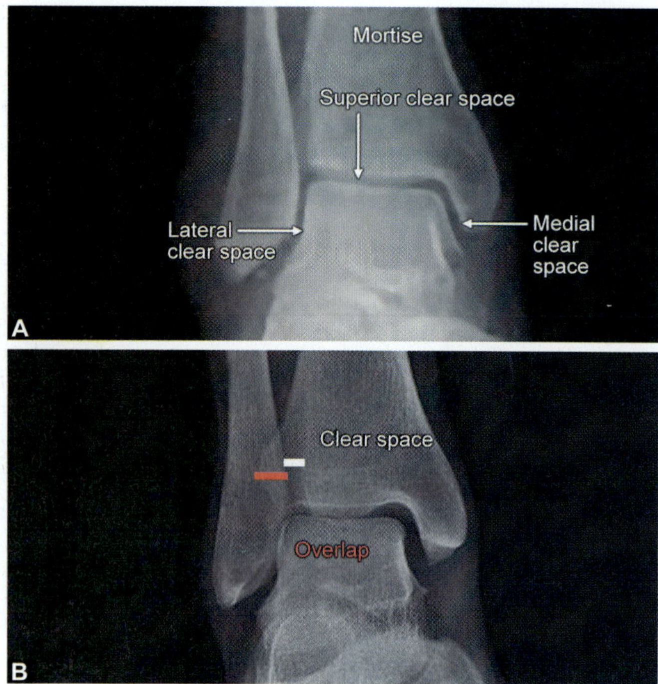

Figs 5.92A and B: (A) Mortise view of a normal ankle; (B) Normal tibio-fibular overlap and clear space in ankle AP view

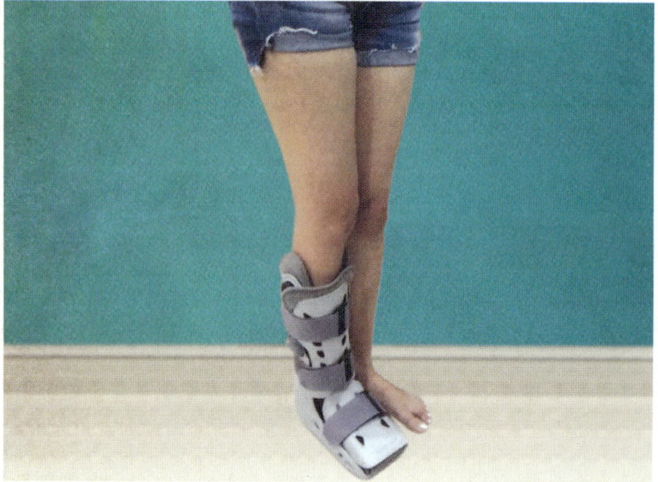

Fig. 5.93: Modern Aircast boot (pneumatic walking brace) used in the management of ankle sprains and undisplaced ankle fractures

- Osteoarthritis is a late complication of malunion/inadequate reduction. Usually it can be managed with analgesics, severe cases may require ankle arthrodesis (fusion of talus and tibia).

- *Ottawa ankle rule*: It is used to avoid unneeded radiographs after ankle injury (i.e. which patient needs X-ray after ankle injury?). An ankle X-ray is required if there is pain in malleolar region, plus bony tenderness along the distal posterior edge (or tip) of medial or lateral malleolus or inability to bear weight for four steps.

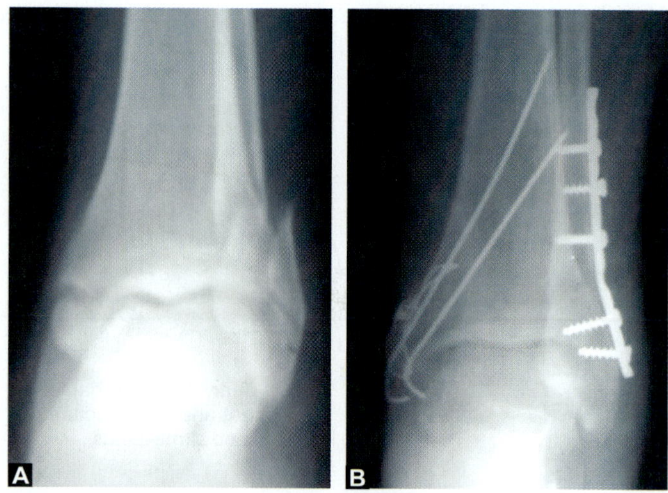

Figs 5.94A and B: (A) X-ray of ankle, anteroposterior view showing bimalleolar fracture and (B) Tension band wiring of medial malleolus fracture and compression plating of lateral malleolus fracture

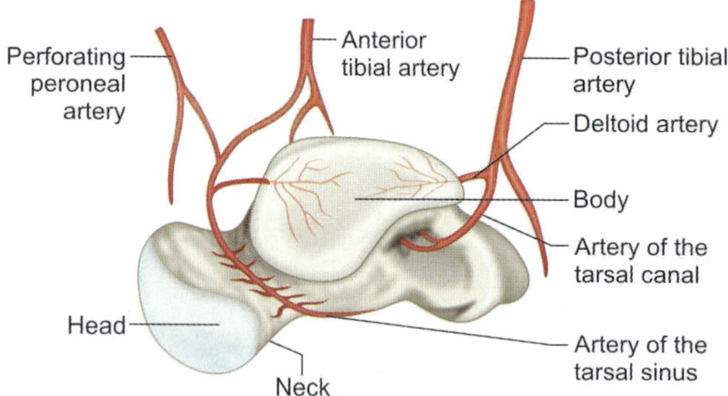

Fig. 5.95: Schematic depiction of parts of talus and blood supply of talus

- *Ottawa foot rule*: X-ray of foot is required if there is any pain in the midfoot zone plus bony tenderness at the base of the fifth metatarsal or at the navicular bone or inability to bear weight for four steps.
- Ankle arthrodesis is a salvage option in cases of painful arthrosis (syn. arthritis) around the ankle. The most common indication for the procedure is painful secondary osteoarthritis following trauma. Blair's arthrodesis of the ankle is a special procedure performed in cases of osteoarthritis secondary to AVN of talar body (in fracture neck of talus).

FRACTURE OF TALUS

Talus is the second largest tarsal bone. More than half of its surface is articular as it is an important weight-bearing bone in the foot. It is divided into a head, neck, body and dome. Talus is the second most common tarsal bone to fracture (after calcaneum) and fractures mostly involve its neck (*see* below). A major blood supply to the body of the talus is contributed by artery of tarsal sinus, the branches of which enter via the neck **(Fig. 5.95)** and travel proximally to supply the body. Thus, talus has a precarious retrograde blood supply and a fracture of the talar neck can cause a break in the blood supply resulting in AVN of the body.

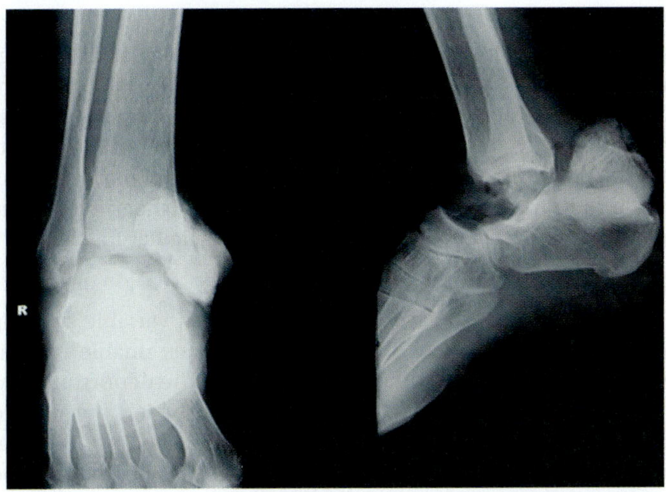

Fig. 5.96: X-ray of ankle, anteroposterior and lateral view showing talus fracture with ankle dislocation

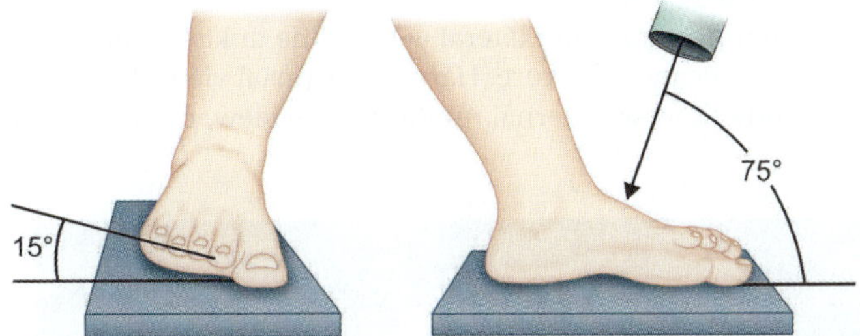

Fig. 5.97: Positioning for Canale view, specialized view for talar neck

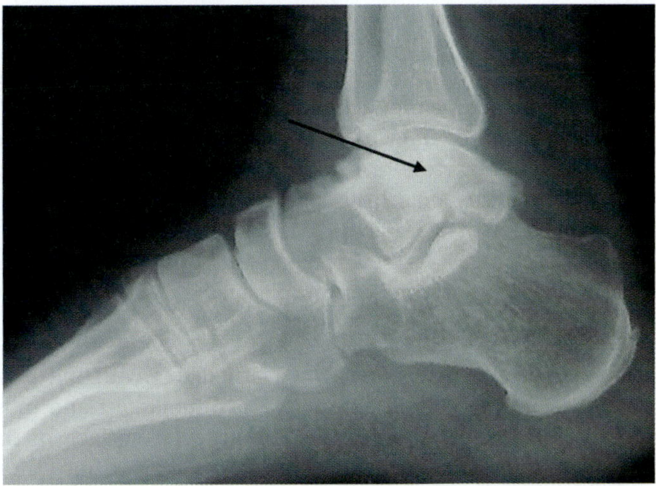

Fig. 5.98: Avascular necrosis of the body of talus [note dense sclerosis (arrow) in the body of talus]

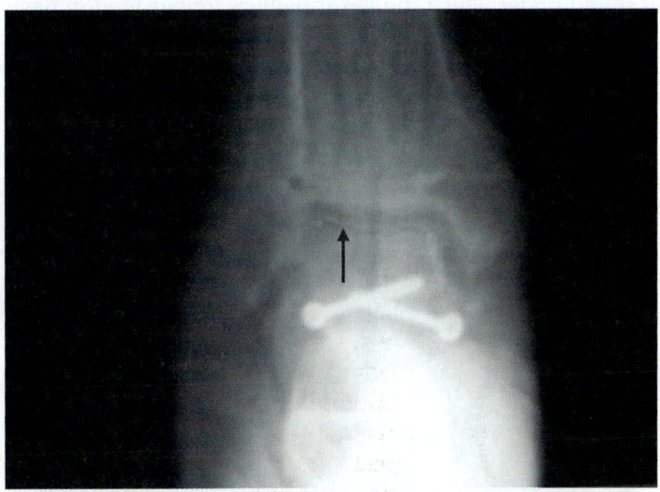

Fig. 5.99: Anteroposterior view of talar fracture after ORIF with screws. Note the zone of lucency in the subchondral area beneath the dome of talus. It indicates viability and goes against the development of AVN (Hawkin's sign)

Mechanism of Injury

Talus is fractured by forced dorsiflexion (in hyperdorsiflexion talar neck abuts against the anterior tibia) of the foot when the weak talar neck gives way. High-energy motor vehicle injuries and fall from height are common mechanisms of injury. Talus fractures are most commonly seen in young adults. This fracture has been described as Aviator's fracture because in pilots who rest their feet at the rudder bar, forced dorsiflexion may cause talus fracture on impact.

Clinical Features

Talar fractures usually present with swelling and pain in the hind and midfoot. In displaced fractures gross deformity may be present. Ankle movements are painful and weight-bearing is not possible. Diagnosis is confirmed by anteroposterior, lateral and oblique X-rays of foot and ankle **(Fig. 5.96)**. Canale view **(Fig. 5.97)** is the specialized X-ray view that provides the most optimum view of the talar neck.

Management

Undisplaced fractures can be managed with a plaster cast (applied in equinus) for 8–10 weeks. After 4 weeks X-ray is repeated to see the reduction and fracture position. If fracture displaces in cast in follow-up X-rays, ORIF should be considered. Displaced fractures are primarily managed by ORIF with screws. Treatment should be urgent to minimize the chances of development of AVN.

Complications

- *Avascular necrosis of the body of Talus* **(Fig. 5.98)**: This is a common and dangerous complication of talar neck fracture. Talar neck fractures are classified into four types by Hawkin's classification based on displacement. Chances of AVN increase with severity of displacement of fracture. On X-ray between 6 weeks and 8 weeks necrosed bone shows increased density (the earliest sign on X-ray) compared to the surrounding bone. Actually, this is due to viable surrounding bone, which becomes porotic (due to loss of calcium) with disuse. By this time if a subchondral lucency is seen in the talar dome instead of increased density it indicates viability of bone and excludes AVN (Hawkins sign, **Fig. 5.99**).
- *Malunion*: Displaced fracture if not adequately reduced and fixed may lead to malunion commonly in the varus position. This leads to excessive weight-bearing on the lateral side of

the foot, making condition often painful and ending up at times in osteoarthritis of the subtalar and ankle joint.

- *Nonunion*: This may complicate 15% of cases and may necessitate an open reduction and bone grafting.
- *Osteoarthritis of the ankle*: Damage to articular cartilage, malunion of fracture or osteonecrosis of the talus can lead to secondary osteoarthritis of the subtalar (most common complication of talar fractures) and the ankle joint. Advanced arthritic changes with severe pain may require ankle/subtalar arthrodesis or total ankle arthroplasty.

CALCANEUM FRACTURE

Calcaneum is the heel bone which articulates with the talus superiorly and the cuboid anteriorly. It is the largest and most commonly fractured tarsal bone. The articular surface of the calcaneum that articulates with the talus is divided into three facets: (1) anterior, (2) middle (formed over the sustentaculum tali) and (3) the posterior. Sustentaculum tali is an eminence on the medial side of calcaneum that supports the middle articular facet and under which the flexor hallucis longus tendon passes **(Figs 5.100A and B)**. The extra-articular posterior part of the calcaneum forms the tuberosity where the tendo-Achilles inserts.

Mechanism of Injury

It is usually a fall from a height with landing on heel (axial loading) and hence also called as Lover's fracture or Don Juan fracture (named after persons who jumped from balcony after being caught in a love affair). Less commonly motor vehicle accidents may be the cause when the brake pedal impacts the plantar aspect of the foot. Axial loading causes crushing and shearing of bone and up to 75% calcaneal fractures are intra-articular fractures.

Clinical Features

Patients present with severe pain in heel with variable swelling and broadening of heel. The patient becomes unable to bear weight. Always look for other associated fracture of dorsolumbar spine, pubic rami and atlantoaxial injuries which are caused by the same mechanism of injury, i.e. axial loading. Bilateral fractures are present in 5–10% cases so the other side must also be examined. Prior to surgery look for skin wrinkles on dorsiflexion and eversion of the ankle. It is a rough guide to indicate that swelling has reduced to an acceptable level and surgery can be done (Wrinkle test).

Anteroposterior and lateral view of the ankle is sufficient to diagnose calcaneal fracture. Harris view (axial view of hind foot) and Broden's view (internal rotation of leg view, used mostly for

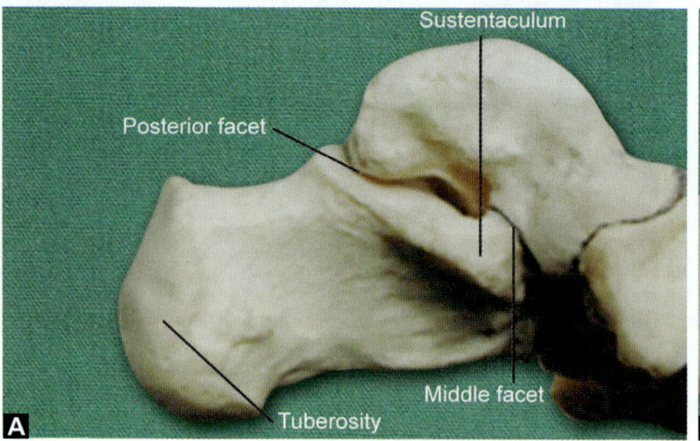

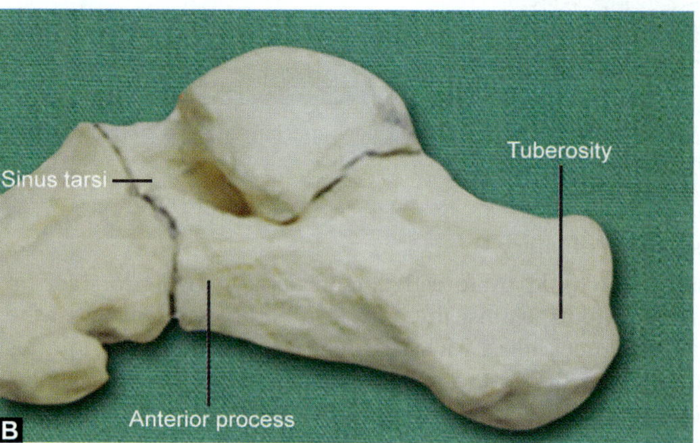

Figs 5.100A and B: Calcaneal anatomy. (A) Medial view; (B) Lateral view

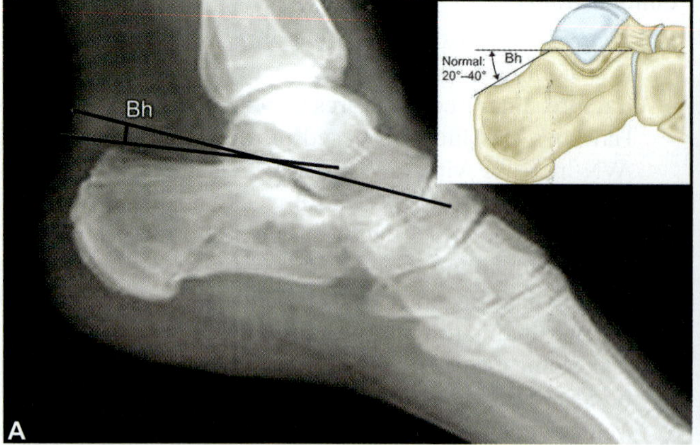

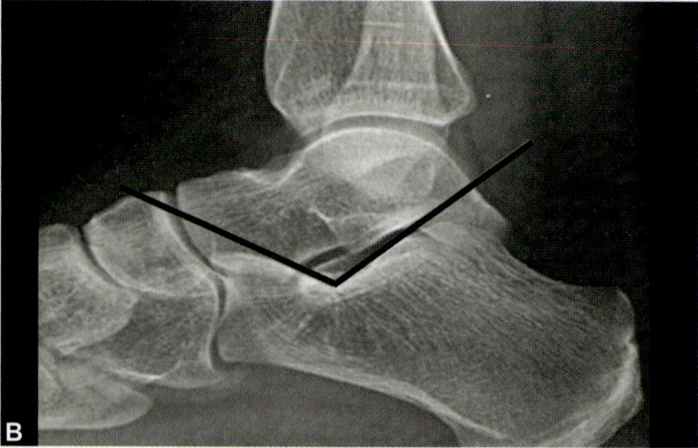

Figs 5.101A and B: (A) Bohler's angle (Bh) decreased in a patient with fracture of the calcaneum (see inset image for normal angle) and the collapse of posterior facet; (B) X-ray showing a depiction of angle of Gissane

intraoperative assessment) are special views to look into finer details of the tuberosity and articular surface, respectively.

The lateral view demonstrates two important angles and a triangle:

- *Bohler's angle (normal is 20°–40°)*: It is formed between two lines, one line joins the highest point of the anterior process to the highest point of the posterior facet and another line is drawn tangent to the superior edge of the tuberosity. A decrease in Bohler's angle indicates the collapse of the posterior facet **(Fig. 5.101A)**.
- *Angle of Gissane (normal is 100°–145°)*: It is formed by a line along the lateral margin of the posterior facet and another line extending anterior to the beak of the calcaneus **(Fig. 5.101B)**. An increase in this angle represents the collapse of posterior facet.
- *Neutral triangle of calcaneum **(Fig. 5.102)***: It is an area of sparse trabeculations within the calcaneum trabeculae. This is the weakest area of the calcaneum and fractures usually occur through this area. The triangle is distorted in calcaneal fractures.

CT scan is the investigation of choice for calcaneal fractures. Saunders classification is used to classify these fractures and is based on the number and location of articular fragments on a coronal CT image.

Management

Undisplaced/minimally displaced extra-articular fractures and undisplaced intra-articular fractures can be managed with nonweight-bearing in a cast for 6–8 weeks. Range of motion exercises should be started as soon as the pain subsides. Conservative treatment is also indicated in calcaneal fracture in insulin-dependent diabetics and severe peripheral vascular disease due to risk of wound-related complications. Displaced extra-articular and collapsed/displaced intra-articular fractures need ORIF with plate **(Figs 5.103A and B)**. The aim of the treatment is to maintain anatomy of the articular facets. If the facet is collapsed, it should be lifted and should be supported with bone grafts and fixed with plate.

Complications

- Widening of heel and some degree of heel pad pain are almost always present after calcaneal fracture. It may occur following both operative and conservative treatment of calcaneal fractures.
- *Stiffness of the ankle and subtalar joint*: This is common after plaster immobilization. Early range of motion exercises should be started to prevent it.
- Calcaneal malunion is common following conservative treatment of displaced intraarticular fractures and may end up in subtalar and/or calcaneocuboid arthritis.
- *Wound dehiscence*: This is the most common complication following operative management of calcaneal fractures. Diabetics, smokers and patients with severe peripheral vascular diseases are particularly at risk of wound-related complications.
- Malunited calcaneal fracture with lateral protuberance may cause peroneal tendinitis. It is more commonly seen following nonoperative treatment. Bony spurs after malunion may also compress the posterior tibial nerve in the tarsal tunnel causing tarsal tunnel syndrome. Operative reduction of mass may be required if pain persists and conservative treatment fails. A displaced fracture of calcaneal tuberosity that malunites may lead to tendoachilles slackening.

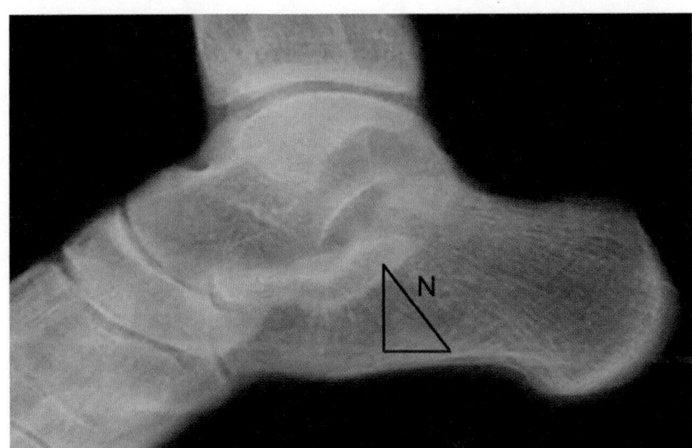

Fig. 5.102: X-ray depicting the neutral triangle in calcaneum

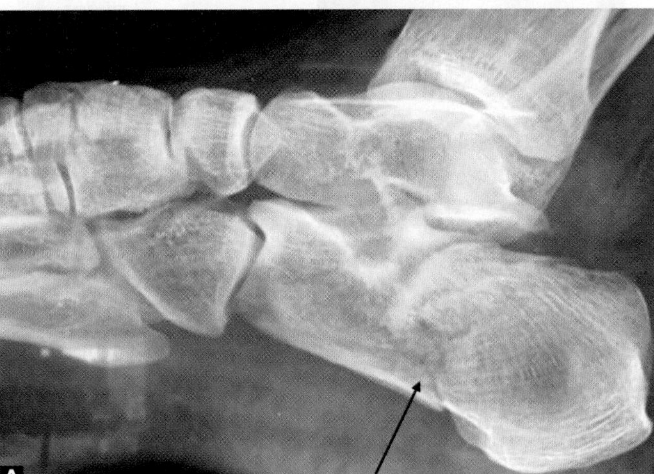

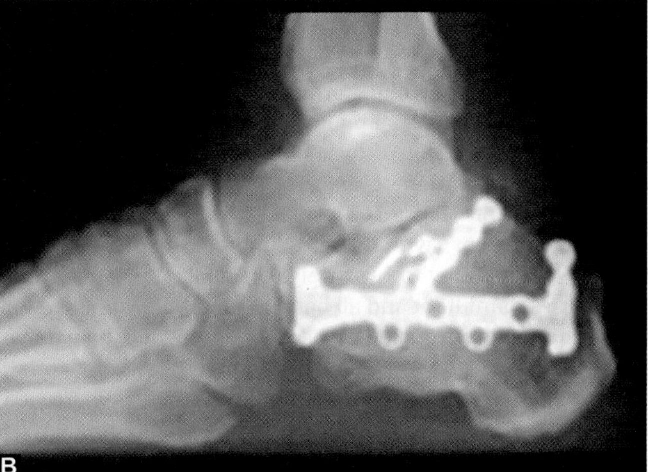

Figs 5.103A and B: (A) X-ray of ankle lateral view showing calcaneal fracture (arrow) and (B) Its fixation with calcaneal plate

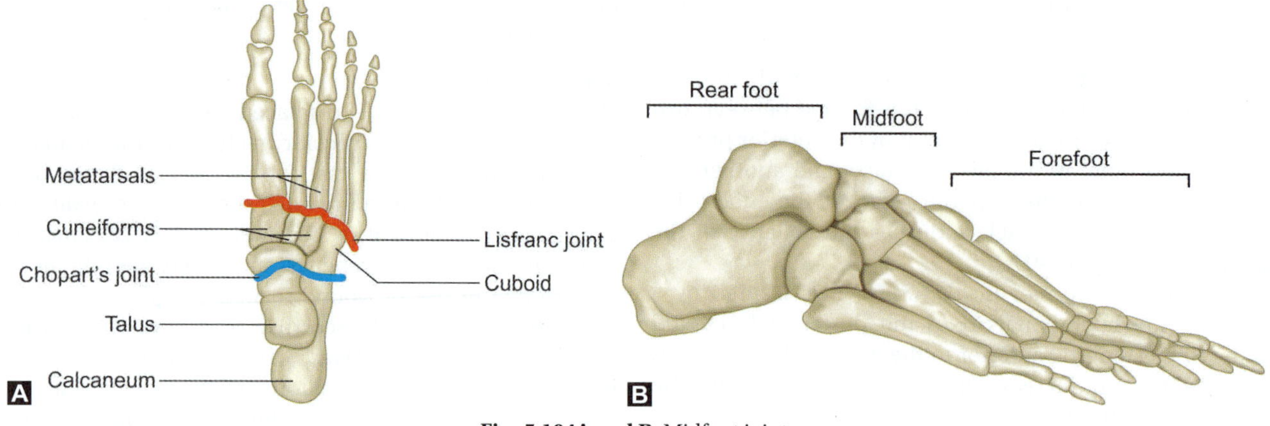

Figs 5.104A and B: Midfoot joints

MIDTARSAL INJURIES

The midfoot **(Figs 5.104A and B)** consists of the calcaneocuboid joint, talonavicular joint and the lesser tarsal bones, i.e. navicular, cuboid, and medial, middle and lateral cuneiform bones. Injuries to midfoot are uncommon and range from a simple sprain to displaced fractures and frank dislocation. Midtarsal (or transverse tarsal) joints, i.e. calcaneocuboid and talonavicular are also called Chopart's joint and Chopart's dislocation is plantar dislocation of calcaneocuboid and talonavicular joints. Isolated fractures of navicular are rare injuries but more common than those of cuboid and cuneiforms.

Clinical Features

Patients present with swollen and tender midfoot. Foot movements and weight-bearing are painful. Fracture and dislocations may produce obvious deformity. Diagnosis is confirmed by anteroposterior, oblique and lateral X-rays of the foot.

Management

Undisplaced fractures and fracture sprain (avulsion fractures of tarsal bones) are treated by below knee walking cast for 4–6 weeks. Displaced fractures and fracture dislocations require close reduction (open reduction if close attempt fails) and internal fixation with K wires or screws.

LISFRANC DISLOCATION (TARSOMETATARSAL DISLOCATION)

The Lisfranc joint consists of the tarsometatarsal joint complex, which includes the three cuneiforms, cuboid and their articulations with the five metatarsal bones. Dislocations of the Lisfranc joint are the most common dislocations of the foot. These injuries usually result from high-energy injuries like forced hyperflexion in road traffic accidents **(Fig. 5.105)** and fall from height.

Patients present with severe midfoot pain, swelling, deformity, and inability to bear weight. This is one of the most severe injuries of midfoot and all patients should be assessed for compartment syndrome of foot (tense foot, severe pain on passive toe movement). Diagnosis is made with anteroposterior, lateral, and oblique radiographs of the foot. On X-ray, there is increased space between the medial cuneiform and the second metatarsal (due to rupture of Lisfranc ligament that runs between these points) called as Fleck sign **(Figs 5.106A and B)**. This dislocation

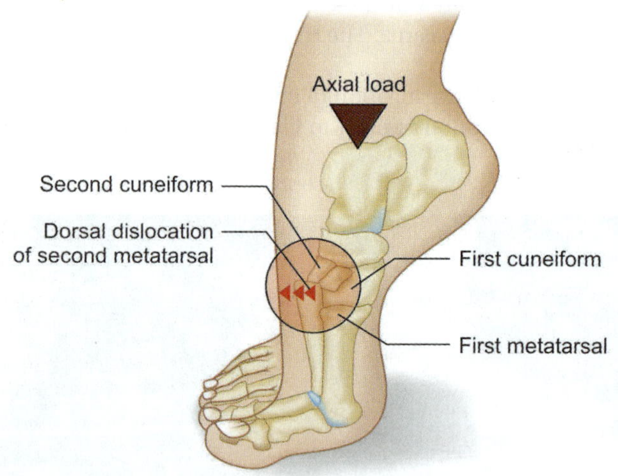

Fig. 5.105: Forced hyperflexion causing Lisfranc injury in the foot

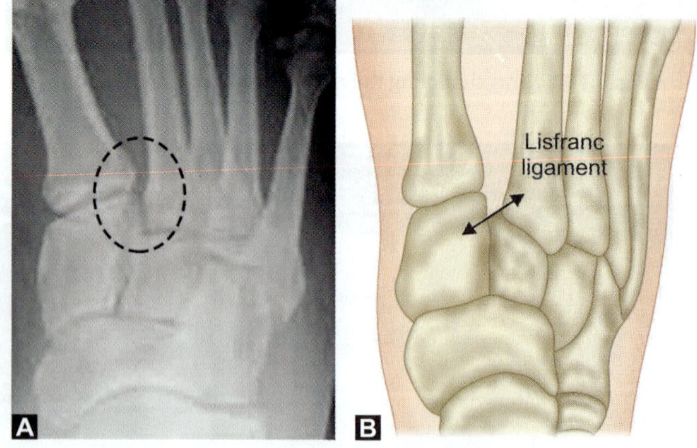

Figs 5.106A and B: X-ray of Lisfranc dislocation showing Fleck sign (encircled) due to rupture of Lisfranc ligament

has to be reduced accurately either by closed or open means and has to be fixed with K wires or screws. Secondary midfoot arthritis (due to articular damage) is a common complication.

METATARSAL FRACTURES

These are common fractures of the foot. These are usually caused by a direct blow (fall of heavy object) and twisting of the foot. Patients usually present with pain and swelling of foot and painful weight-bearing. Diagnosis is made on anteroposterior, lateral and oblique X-rays of the foot.

The foot becomes swollen and tender. Anteroposterior and oblique X-ray views of the foot is sufficient for the diagnosis. Most single metatarsal fractures are usually minimally displaced. Undisplaced and minimally displaced metatarsal fractures are managed with splint/below knee cast for 3–4 weeks with progressive weight-bearing as tolerated. Open fractures, multiple metatarsal fractures, and displaced fractures are treated with CRIF/ORIF with K wires.

Fractures of Base of Fifth Metatarsal

These are common injuries. Peroneus brevis tendon and lateral band of plantar fascia insert onto the base of the fifth metatarsal. Sudden inversion of the foot may cause traction at the base of fifth metatarsal due to pull by peroneus brevis tendon or the band of plantar fascia resulting in fractures involving three different zones **(Fig. 5.107)**. Jones fracture is a fracture of the base of fifth metatarsal at junction of the metaphysis and diaphysis **(Fig. 5.108)**. It is caused by a direct blow on base of fifth metatarsal of a plantar flexed foot. Pseudo-Jones or Dancer's fracture is an avulsion fracture of the tip of the fifth metatarsal (Tuberosity avulsion fracture, **Fig. 5.109**).

Patients present with pain and tenderness at base of fifth metatarsal at the lateral border of foot with painful weight bearing. Diagnosis is confirmed on X-rays. Nondisplaced avulsion fractures are treated by walking cast for 3–4 weeks with weight-bearing as tolerated. Acute undisplaced Jones fractures may be managed with nonweight-bearing cast for 6–8 weeks. Since the rate of nonunion is high, many surgeons prefer to treat these injuries with close/open reduction and internal fixation with compression screw.

March Fracture

It is a stress fracture of the distal part of the shaft of the metatarsals. The second followed by third metatarsals are most commonly involved. It is common in military recruits, dancers, etc. due to repetitive stress of the foot striking on the ground. The patient presents with pain which is activity related and often point tenderness at the site of stress fracture can be elicited. Initially X-rays rarely show any sign, but over the time incomplete subperiosteal fracture or a slight area of periosteal reaction is seen **(Fig. 5.110)**. MRI (investigation of choice) and bone scan are modalities to show the stress fracture when they are negative on X-rays. Treatment is the cessation of the offending activity. A nonweight-bearing short leg cast is given for 3–4 weeks.

FRACTURES OF PHALANGES

These are usually caused by fall of heavy objects on the foot. No immobilization is required. The injured toe is usually strapped (buddy strapping) with the adjacent toes and the patient is encouraged to walk.

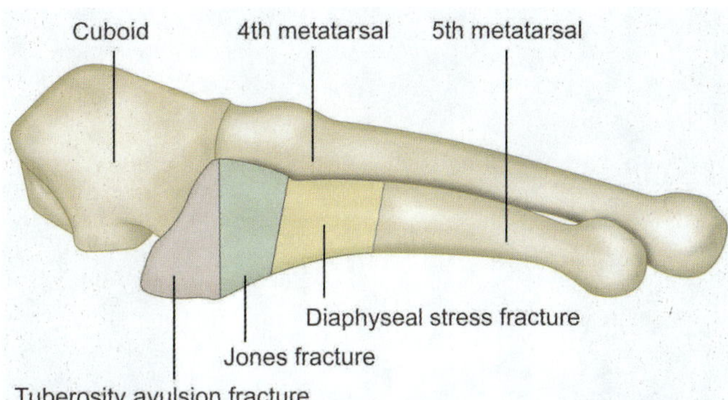

Fig. 5.107: Fractures of base of fifth metatarsal

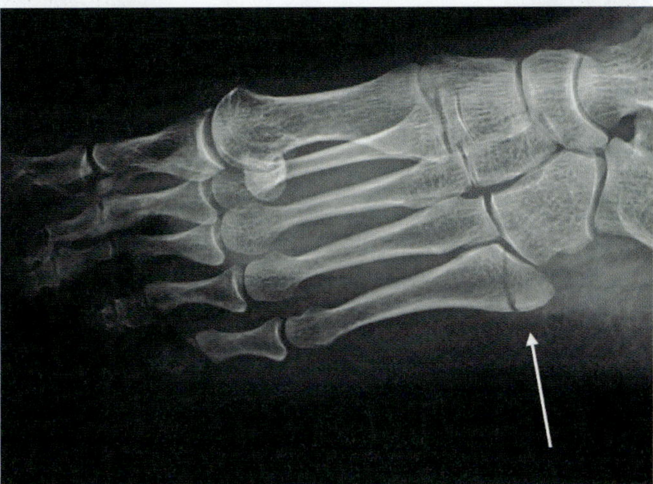

Fig. 5.108: X-ray of foot showing Jones fracture involving metadiaphyseal junction of the base of the fifth metatarsal

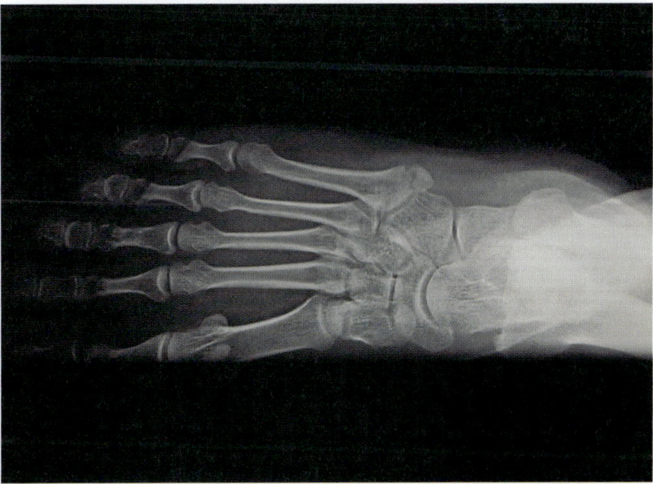

Fig. 5.109: X-ray of foot showing avulsion of the fifth metatarsal base (pseudo-Jones or Dancer's fracture)

HIGH-YIELD POINTS

- Talus is the only bone which does not have any muscular attachment.

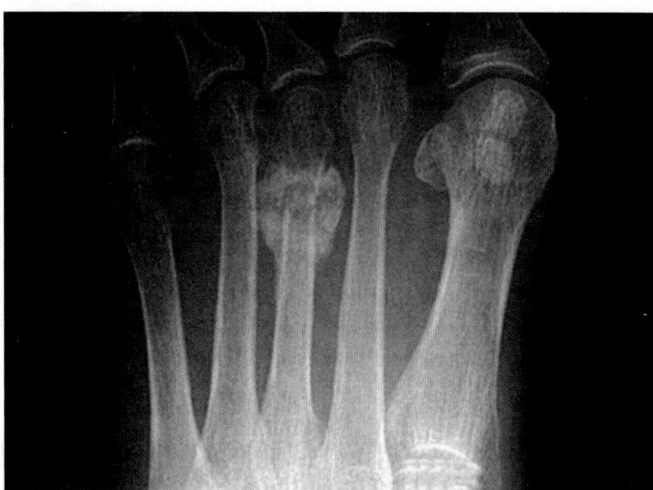

Fig. 5.110: X-ray of foot, anteroposterior view showing stress fracture of the third metatarsal (see callus formation due to the healing of the fracture)

Source: Courtesy by Learning Radiology.com.

- Second metatarsal is the longest of all metatarsals and most common site for a stress fracture in the foot. Traumatic fractures most commonly involve the fifth metatarsal, which is the most common metatarsal to fracture.
- Peri-talar dislocation/subtalar dislocation refers to the dislocation of talus from its distal articulations, viz. subtalar joint and talonavicular joint. In total talus dislocation the talus is dislocated from all articulations including the ankle joint.
- *Nutcracker injury:* Forceful abduction of the foot may lead to fracture-dislocation of the second metatarsal base with an associated cuboid crush fracture known as "nutcracker" injury.
- Navicular stress fractures are common in runners. Patients present with mid-dorsal pain. Treatment is nonweight-bearing cast immobilization for 6 weeks.
- Calcaneum is the second most common site for stress fractures in the foot after metatarsals.
- Although calcaneal fractures are common in fall from height, but the most common fractures in fall from height are D12 > L1 vertebra.

6

CHAPTER

Sports Injuries and their Rehabilitation

Sports medicine is an upcoming orthopedic superspeciality that encompasses the following elements: physical fitness and training of a sports person, sports injury prevention and treatment, rehabilitation, exercise for health, nutrition and drug recommendations for sports persons. This chapter mainly deals with sports injuries and their treatment.

Sports injuries are injuries that occur while playing or exercising resulting in inability to practice or compete normally. Many sports injuries, if not effectively treated, can end a professional career of an athlete.

CLASSIFICATION OF SPORTS INJURIES

Sports may be contact, noncontact, collision or combat. In non-contact sports, players are not expected to come in direct contact against other players, e.g. tennis, cricket, swimming, etc. In contact sports, players come in direct contact with each other, but intentional blow is not a part of the game, e.g. soccer, basketball, etc. The injury rate is higher in contact sports compared to noncontact sports. In some sports like rugby and *kabaddi*, intentional blow to the body is an expected part of the game. These are called collision sports. In combat sports, like wrestling and boxing, players are directly involved in fight with each other, although with rules and regulations. Hand and face injuries are particularly common in combat sports.

Depending upon the type of sport one is involved in, different athletes are at risk of different injuries.

1. *Acute sports injuries:* Since the collisions involved in sports are generally low to medium velocity trauma, soft tissue damage (muscles and ligaments) is generally the cornerstone. Acute sports injuries are hence mostly musculoskeletal injuries caused by low velocity forces which are not usually enough to fracture a bone. As a result the soft tissue envelope surrounding a bone or a joint gets injured. Examples are hamstring strain, ankle sprain or an anterior cruciate ligament (ACL) tear in the knee.
2. *Overuse injuries:* Around 45–60% of all injuries treated in a sports medicine clinic are sufferers of overuse injuries. These are "cumulative trauma injuries" caused by repetitive stress to bone, muscle, ligament or tendon without allowing time to heal. Typical examples are medial tibial stress syndrome, tennis elbow or a stress fracture. Overuse injuries are common in noncontact sports due to repetitive action while playing such as running, throwing/bowling in cricket or serving a ball in tennis. In some sports like gymnastics, overuse injuries are particularly common due to high demand of the game for unusual positions and repetitive strain on muscles, tendons and joints. Since repetitive movements are not limited to sports, overuse injuries can also be related to occupation or work. This is why tennis elbow is also commonly seen in washer women, drivers and housewives. Some risk factors that increase the chances of getting overuse injuries include anatomical malalignment, muscle weakness or imbalance.
3. *Heat and cold illnesses:* Not all sports conditions are injuries per se. Sporting activities in hot weather predispose the athlete for dehydration, heat stroke, cramps, exercise associated collapse and exercise associated hyponatremia while exercises at the extremes of cold and altitude may cause hypothermia and frostbite. A sports physician is expected to deal even with these conditions effectively.

PREVENTION OF SPORTS INJURIES

"Do not merely play a sport to get in shape; get in shape to play a sport." One of the most effective ways to avoid sports injuries is to stay fit. Health promotion by proper training methodology among sports people who have never had a sports injury is primary prevention. Early diagnosis and treatment of sports injuries also limits the disability due to injury and fastens the recovery. This is called secondary prevention.

Core principles of primary prevention of sports injuries are as follows:

1. *Identification of risk factors and their management:* Many injuries have specific risk factors that may be modifiable (body weight, body mass index, level of fitness, etc.) or nonmodifiable (age, sex, anthropometric or anatomical abnormalities). Recognizing them and designing programs to neutralize them may lower the injury rate amongst playing sportsmen. For example, a sex-related risk factor is high rate of ACL tear in female athletes due to their small intercondylar notch, wider pelvis and greater Q angle. Hence, many targeted programs have been instituted towards ACL injury prevention in female athletes.
2. *Appropriate training:* Instructions should be provided for a proper warm up, stretching, an appropriate sports technique and a cool down.
   Warm-up: Warm-up within half an hour before the event or exercise, prepares the body for the training. Warm-up can consist of general exercises like stretching of trunk and limbs, aerobics like jogging and sports specific exercises, intense enough to result in just initiation of sweating but not result in fatigue. During the warm-up, blood flow to the muscles increases, which enhances body temperature, oxygen delivery to muscles, cellular metabolism and sensitivity

of nerve receptors. Increased range of motion (ROM) and decreased stiffness also reduces the chances of ligament sprains and tendon and muscle strains.

Stretching: Pre-exercise stretching of muscles in isolation does not reduce the injury rate but regular stretching of muscles, reduces the chances of muscle, ligament and tendon injury. Gentle stretching exercises reduce muscle soreness, increases ROM and decreases the likelihood of sports injury. Stretching should be to the point of tension but never pain.

Good sports technique: Good sports technique is a key to prevent overuse injuries in sports. For example, in racquet sports, major factor producing elbow pain is an incorrect stroking technique especially the backhand drive. If the ball is not hit from the center (eccentric hit), it transfers greater shock to elbow and shoulder compared to hit from the central portion. Grip size (neither too large nor too short) and string tension (the stiffer the racquet the larger the force transmitted to arm) should also be appropriate.

Cool down: After exercises high amounts of lactic acid accumulates in the body and the muscles are exhausted, and stiff. Cool down exercises are light exercises which are done after an intense activity (such as a training session) to allow the body to remove lactic acid and get back to resting state. This overcomes the fatigue and speed up the recovery process. Cooling down usually consists of stretching exercises which slows down heart rate and improve flexibility.

3. *Use of Protective Equipment, Taping and Bracing and Suitable Playing Surfaces*

   Protective equipment: Protective equipment are used by players to protect various body parts against injury like a helmet in cricket, groin protector in ice hockey and shin pad in field sports like cricket, soccer and hockey. They are designed in such a way that they do not interfere with sports activity. In certain sports they are mandatory like a helmet in cycling.

   Taping and bracing (Figs 6.1A and B): Taping (a type of strapping) and bracing are used to restrict harmful joint motions (excessive motion or motion in unwanted directions). They are also thought to increase the proprioceptive feedback from joints reducing injury chances. They are mainly used during rehabilitation phase following injury but can also be used as a primary prevention in high risk sports.

4. *Maintenance of appropriate fitness:* A fittest athlete is less likely to get injured. Optimal physical fitness relies on adequate muscular strength and balance, power, endurance, neuromuscular control, joint flexibility, cardiovascular endurance and good body composition.

SPORTS INJURIES AROUND THE SHOULDER

RECURRENT DISLOCATION OF SHOULDER

First episode of dislocation of the shoulder is mostly traumatic in nature, the mechanisms, clinical presentation and management of which have already been discussed in chapter 4. Thereafter, in most of these patients (90% of patients under the age of 25 years) the joint dislocates recurrently even with minimal trauma due to failure of important stabilizing restraints to heal up. The younger the age at first dislocation, the higher the chances the patient

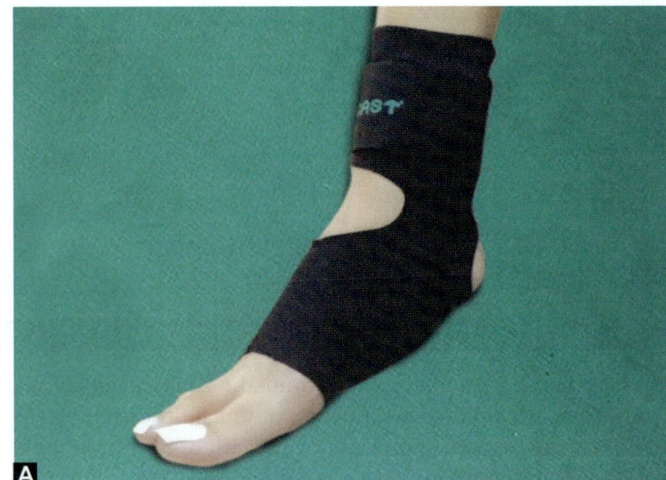

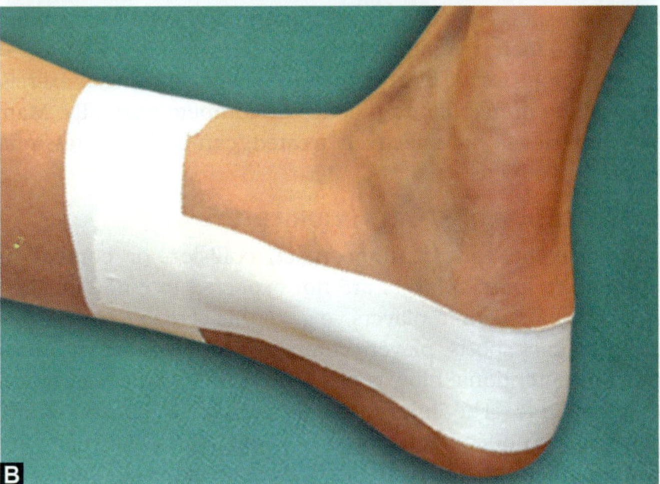

Figs 6.1A and B: (A) Ankle brace; (B) Ankle taping

may come back with recurrence. Hyperlaxity of shoulder capsule, usually associated with hyperlaxity of other joints (as may occur in conditions like Marfan syndrome, Ehler-Danlos syndrome, etc.) may additionally contribute to recurrent dislocations (read shoulder instability here).

Pathological Changes in Recurrent Dislocation of Shoulder

Recurrent dislocations are mostly the anterior and rarely posterior, and associated with following pathological changes in the glenohumeral joint.

(A) Pathological lesions associated with recurrent anterior dislocation:

- *Bankart's lesion:* This is the most common lesion being present in almost 90–98% cases. Glenoid cavity is deepened by the presence of a fibrocartilagenous rim called labrum **(Fig. 6.2A)** which is attached at its circumference all around. Bankart's lesion **(Fig. 6.2B)** is a detachment of the anteroinferior labrum from the margin of glenoid that produces recurrent anterior dislocations.
- *Humeral Avulsion of Glenohumeral Ligaments (HAGL) lesion:* Here the glenohumeral ligament (a static restraint) is avulsed from the humeral neck **(Fig. 6.2C)** with the failure of the ligaments to heal up.

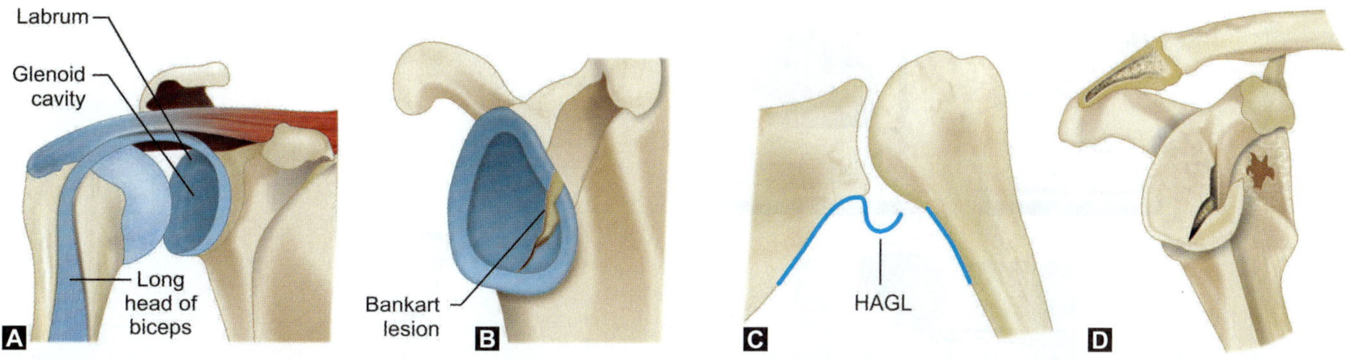

Figs 6.2A to D: (A) Shoulder joint with intact labrum; (B) Bankart's tear of the labrum; (C) HAGL lesion; (D) 3D CT showing Bony Bankart's lesion

- *Bony Bankart's lesion*: This refers to avulsion fracture of the anteroinferior glenoid rim **(Fig. 6.2D)**.
- *Hill-Sachs lesion*: A defect is excavated on the posterolateral aspect of humeral head **(Fig. 6.3)** due to repeated impact against the anterior glenoid rim in patients who have had several episodes of dislocations. In throwing positions (90° abduction and external rotation) this defect engages (confronts) the glenoid rim and instability may result.
- *Glenoid bone defects*: These may also result following dislocation and if the loss is more than 20% of the glenoid, it may give rise to recurrent dislocation.

(B) Pathological lesions associated with recurrent posterior dislocation:

- *Reverse Bankart's lesion*: It refers to detachment of the posteroinferior labrum from the glenoid margin.
- *Reverse Bony Bankart's lesion*: In this there is an avulsion fracture of the posteroinferior glenoid rim.
- *Reverse Hill Sachs lesion*: This comprises a defect in the anteromedial aspect of the humeral head (Trough sign).

Management of Recurrent Dislocation of Shoulder

Management of recurrent dislocation involves first and foremost identifying the lesions with suitable investigations. Special X-ray views of the shoulder like can demonstrate the bone defect in the head of the humerus or glenoid. While the West point axillary view **(Fig. 6.4A)** is the popular view for spotting a glenoid bone defect, Hill-Sachs lesion is better delineated in Internal rotation view of shoulder or the Stryker notch view **(Fig. 6.4B)**. The investigation of choice for Bankart's lesion is magnetic resonance imaging (MRI) **(Fig. 6.5A)** but to visualize bone loss in either humerus (Hill-Sachs lesion) or glenoid, a computed tomography (CT) scan of the affected shoulder **(Fig. 6.5B)** is the preferred method.

Once the diagnosis has been made appropriate surgical procedures are to be offered to the patients as per the pathological lesions causing the recurrence. Following are the surgical procedures commonly employed:

For Bankart's Lesion

Bankart's repair **(Fig. 6.6)** is currently the mainstay of treatment. Here the torn labrum and the detached capsule are reattached back to the anteroinferior glenoid rim with suture anchors (anchors are special fixation devices capable of fixing soft tissue

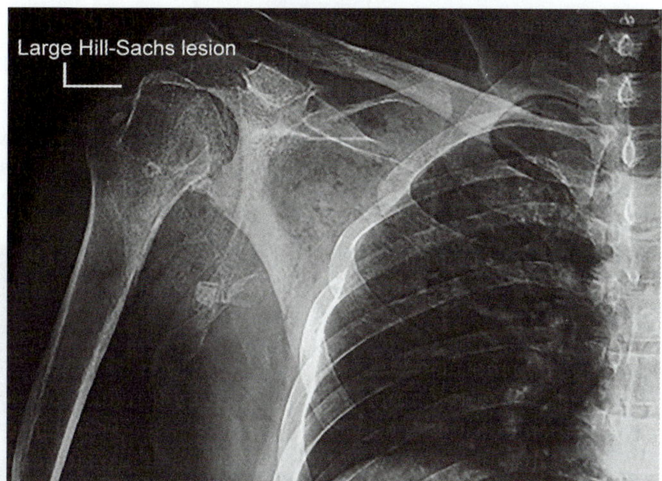

Fig. 6.3: X-ray, AP view of shoulder joint showing large Hill-Sachs lesion

to bone). The procedure nowadays is done arthroscopically and arthroscopic Bankart's repair is the treatment of choice.

For Humeral (Hill-Sachs Lesion) or Glenoid Bone Defects

Although small bone defects (humeral head defect < 10% or glenoid defect < 25%) may be neglected, larger ones may require intervention.

Putti-Platt operation (double breasting of subscapularis tendon, **Fig. 6.7A**) is one of the methods in managing a Hill-Sachs lesion. Double breasting of this tendon shortens it and limits external rotation of humerus thereby preventing the humeral bone defect to engage the glenoid. However, this procedure is only of historical importance and is no longer preferred as it limits significant movement.

The preferred surgery in patients with small Hill-Sachs lesion (10–30% of bone loss) is Remplissage **(Fig. 6.7B)** where infraspinatous tendon is tacked into the humeral head defect to prevent it from engaging the glenoid. In a large Hill-Sachs lesion (more than 30% bone loss from head) or where glenoid bone loss is more than 25% or when there are bipolar lesions (both humeral head and glenoid bone defects), the Bristow-Latarjet operation **(Fig. 6.7C)** is the preferred method. During this surgery the coracoid process along with the attached muscles (conjoint

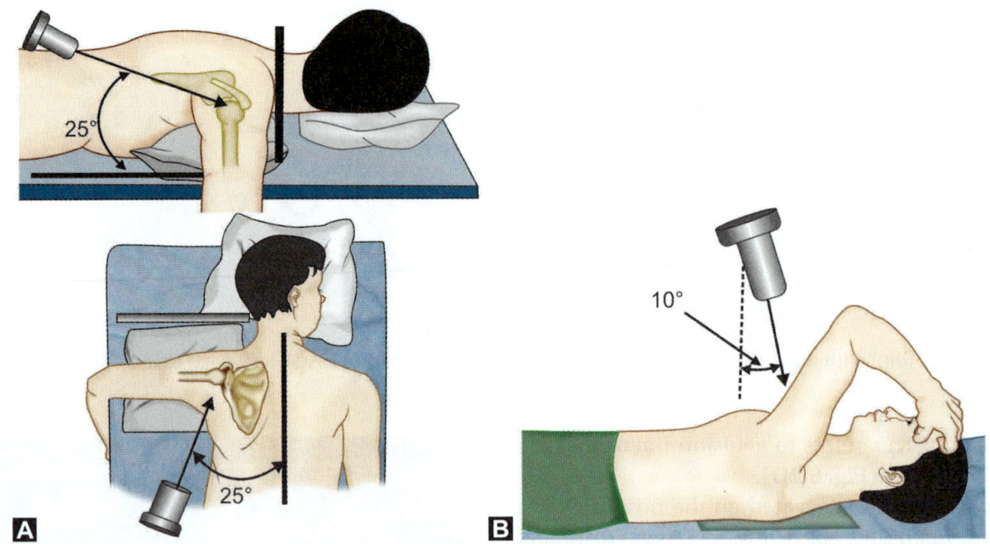

Figs 6.4A and B: (A) Position for the west point prone axillary view to see glenoid bone loss or bony Bankart's lesion; (B) Position for the Stryker notch view to see bone loss from the head of humerus (Hill-Sachs lesion)

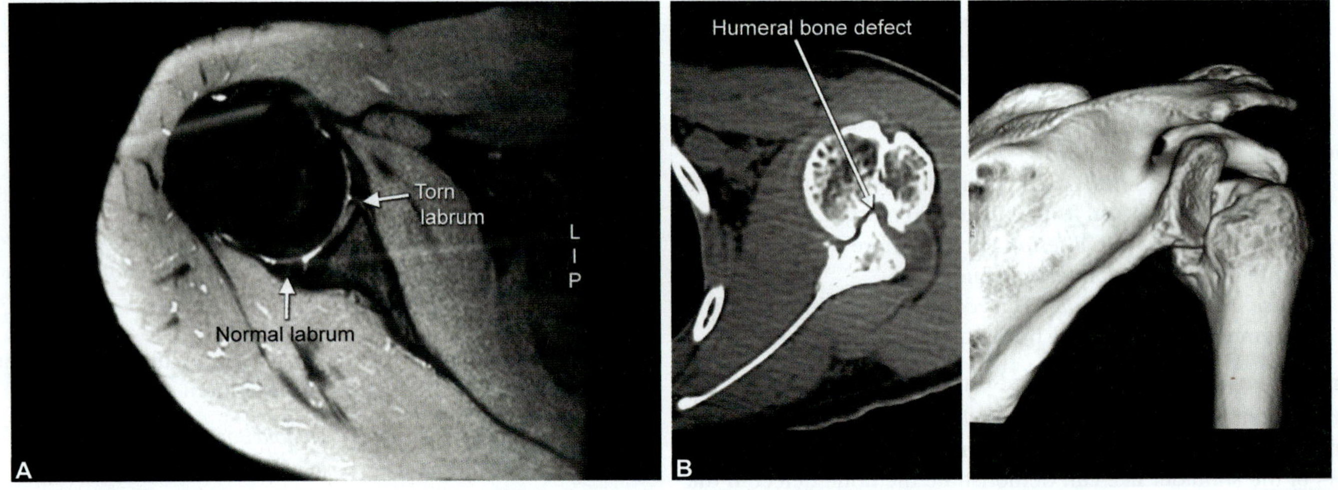

Figs 6.5A and B: (A) MRI axial section showing Bankart's lesion (Note the torn labrum); (B) CT axial cut and 3D CT reconstruction demonstrating Hill-Sachs lesion (defect in humeral head) that is engaging against the glenoid rim as the shoulder dislocates anteriorly

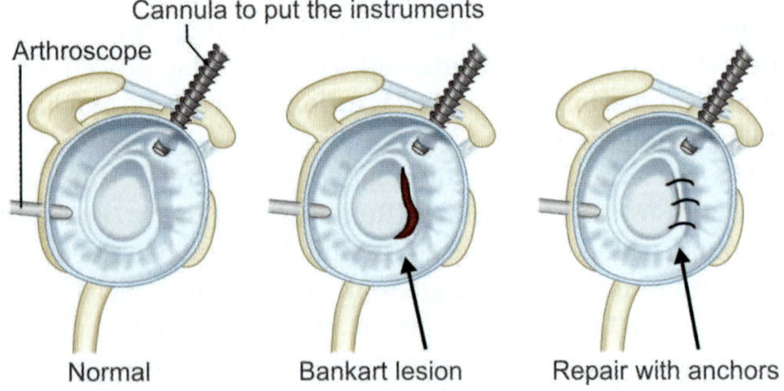

Fig. 6.6: Arthroscopic Bankart's repair is now standard treatment for anterior shoulder instability

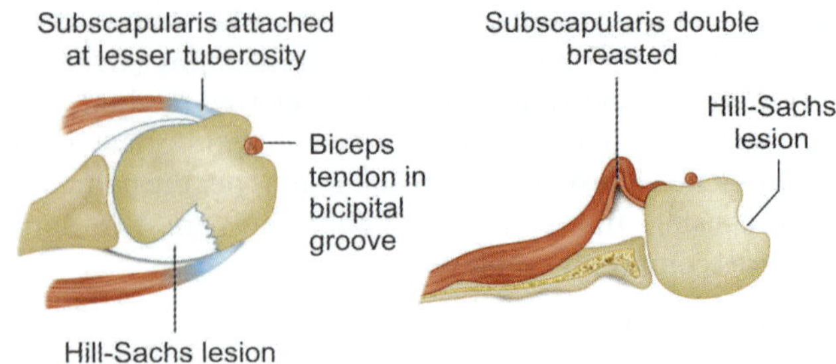

Fig. 6.7A: Putti-Platt operation. Subscapularis has been double breasted (overlapped) in front to make Hill-Sachs move more laterally preventing it from engaging the glenoid

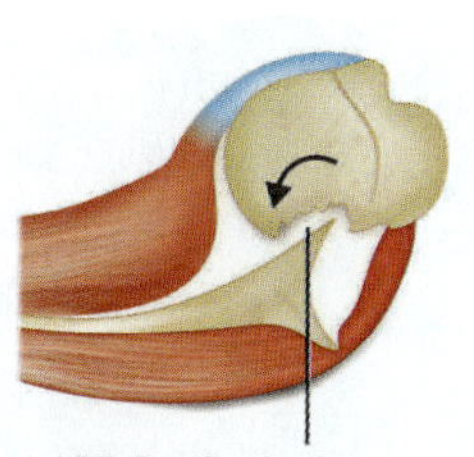
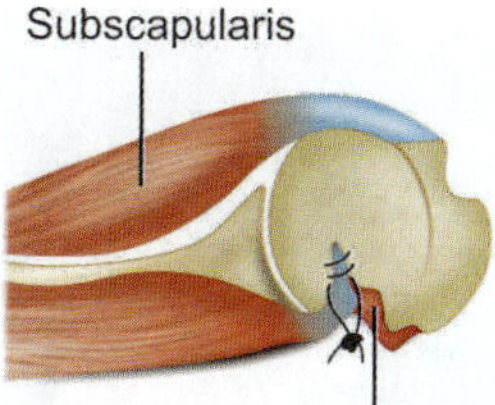

Fig. 6.7B: Remplissage procedure. Infraspinatous has been tacked into the Hill-Sachs defect to prevent it from engaging

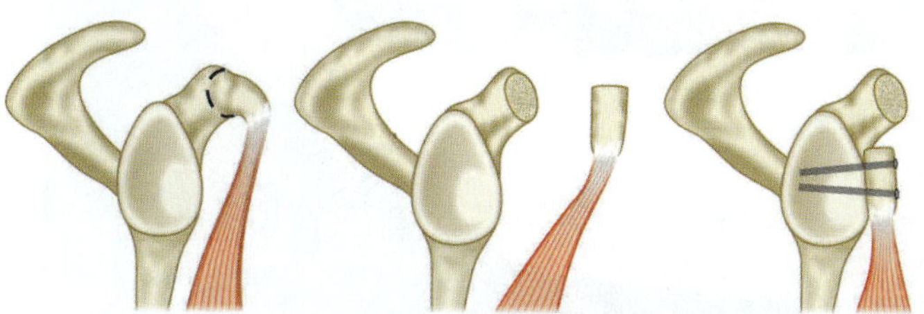

Fig. 6.7C: Bristow-Latarjet operation

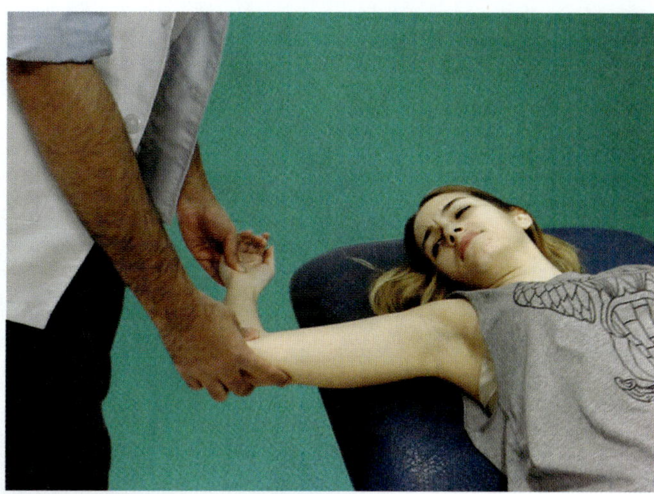

Fig. 6.8: Apprehension test in anterior glenohumeral instability

tendon) is osteotomized at its base and transferred down to be fixed to the anteroinferior margin of the glenoid to prevent the head from subluxating anteriorly as the conjoint tendon forms a muscular sling in front. The procedure also lengthens the articular arc (by adding bone to glenoid) and prevents a Hill-Sachs lesion from engaging.

SHOULDER INSTABILITY

It is essential to understand that since the shoulder is a joint entirely stabilized by soft tissue, the patients who tend to have lax ligaments from any cause can exhibit abnormal pathological motion in the joint. The reason for the ligament laxity can be multifold appropriately coated as torn loose (ligament laxity after trauma when the native ligaments fail to heal up), born loose (ligament laxity secondary to genetic defects) or microtrauma (players involved in throwing sports who gradually stress their shoulder stabilizers due to repetitive external rotation and abduction). Lax ligaments or capsule from any cause makes these patients more prone to dislocation with minimal trauma and also predisposes them to more chances of recurrent dislocations. However, at times they may not experience a frank dislocation, rather have a minimal extra motion that manifests as a subluxation. Such subluxations withhold them from participating in sporting activities or at times may even interfere with their daily routine.

Tests for Glenohumeral Instability

Patients with shoulder instability can be tested for the instability concerned, by following clinical tests.

For Anterior Instability

Jobe's Apprehension test (Fig. 6.8): In supine position patient's arm is abducted to 90 degrees and externally rotated to behind the coronal plane (elbow flexed to 90 degrees). The patient becomes apprehensive and resists the examiner.

Jobe's relocation test: In apprehension test when the patient feels apprehension the examiner applies a posterior force against the proximal arm. This relieves the patient's apprehension as the humeral head moves from an anteriorly subluxed position to a centered position in the glenoid.

Anterior drawer test (Fig. 6.9A): The patient is placed supine and the arm is abducted 60°. Axial force is applied to the humerus with the arm in neutral rotation. Now examiner translates the humeral head anteriorly. Translation of the head to the glenoid rim is grade I, translation over the rim that spontaneously reduces is grade II, and dislocation without spontaneous reduction is grade III.

For Posterior Instability

Jerk test/Jahnke test (Fig. 6.9B): This can be performed with the patient standing or sitting. The examiner holds patient's elbow with one hand and stabilizes the scapula with the other hand. The shoulder is flexed to 90°, internally rotated and adducted, and an axial load is applied to the elbow. The shoulder may subluxate or dislocate posteriorly with a sudden jerk. Now the arm is gradually abducted, the humeral head may reduce back onto the glenoid.

Gerber-Ganz posterior drawer test: Same as anterior drawer except with posterior force.

Posterior apprehension test: Examiner pushes the adducted, flexed and internally rotated arm (elbow 90 degrees flexed) posteriorly—apprehension positive.

For Inferior Instability

Sulcus sign (Fig. 6.10): The arm is pulled distally in 0 degree and 45 degrees of abduction. The shoulder is observed for a sulcus or dimple between the acromion and the humeral head.

Management of Recurrent Shoulder Instability

The patients who tend to have recurrent instability secondary to generalized ligamentous laxity, i.e. born loose patients (as those with Marfan or Ehler-Danlos syndrome, etc.) mostly present with multidirectional instability (inferior instability plus either anterior or posterior instability or both) while the patients who tend to be in the other two categories (torn loose or microtrauma) tend to present with unidirectional instability. The

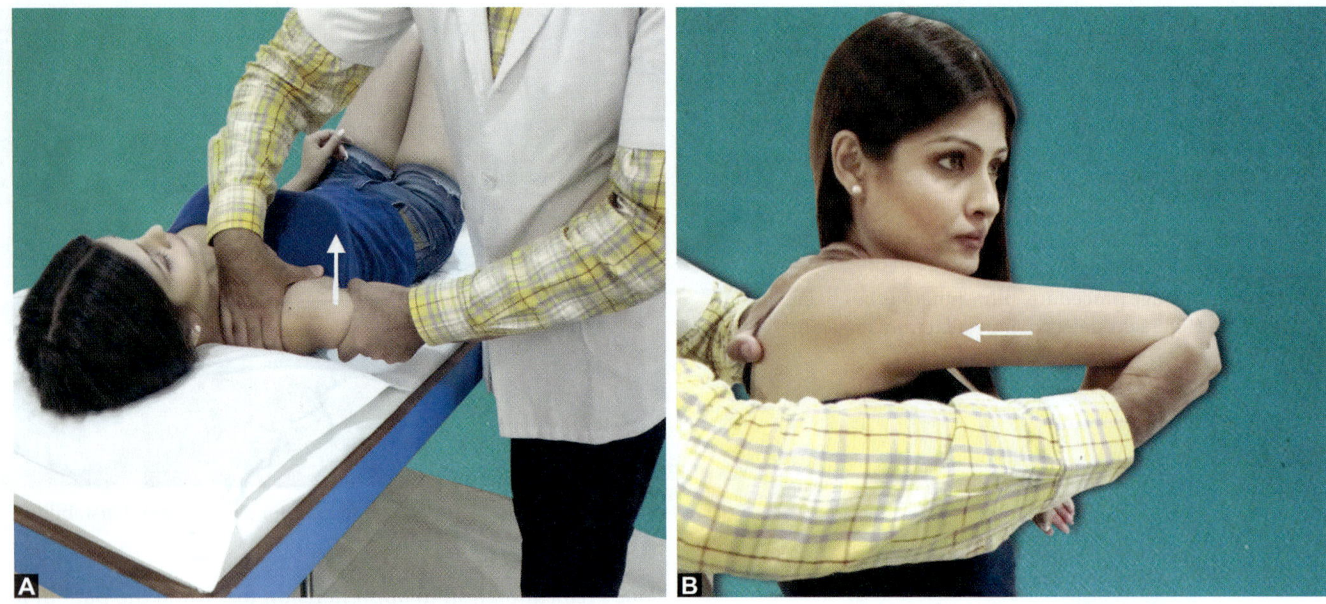

Figs 6.9A and B: (A) Schematic representation of anterior drawer test at shoulder; (B) Schematic representation
of the Jerk test/posterior drawer test at shoulder

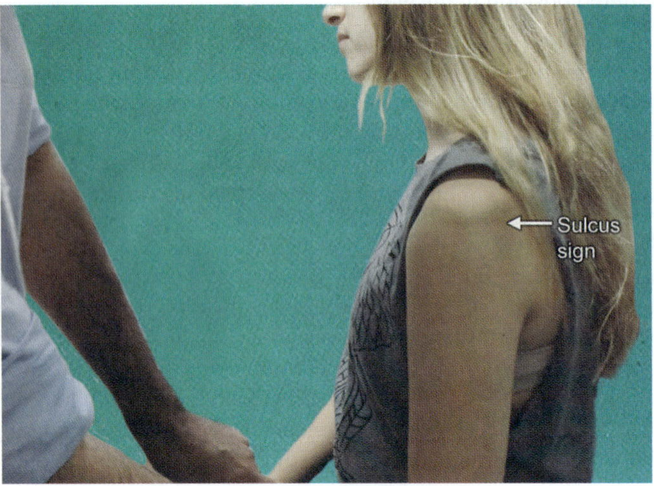

Fig. 6.10: Sulcus sign

- Shoulder is also the most common site for recurrent dislocation followed next in frequency by the patella.
- *Voluntary dislocater*: A small proportion of patients are able to dislocate and relocate their shoulders in one or more directions at will. This condition is very difficult to treat as a majority of these patients have underlying psychiatric illness. Surgery is preferably avoided in these patients and treatment usually consists of skillful neglect or strengthening the rotators and deltoid.
- The most common joint to show voluntary dislocation is also the shoulder, followed next in frequency by the patella.
- Although the weakest part of the shoulder joint capsule is the inferior part, the most common dislocation type in shoulder is anterior (subcoracoid subtype), as the injurying mechanism is mostly abduction and external rotation (as in a throwing motion).

ROTATOR CUFF TEARS AND ARTHROPATHY

Relevant Anatomy

Rotator cuff comprises of four tendons that surround and stabilize the shoulder joint **(Fig. 6.11A)**. These include: subscapularis, supraspinatus, infraspinatus and teres minor.

Subscapularis: It originates from the costal surface of scapula and goes laterally crossing the humeral head anteriorly to insert on the lesser tuberosity of humerus. It is mainly an internal rotator of the shoulder and assists in actions performed with hand behind the back (since these actions are not used in routine, it is also sometimes called "forgotten muscle" of cuff).

Supraspinatus: Originates from supraspinous fossa, travels under the acromion and attaches to greater tuberosity. It is involved in the first 15° of shoulder abduction (15–90° of shoulder abduction is carried out by deltoid and overhead abduction occurs by action of the trapezius and serratus anterior). Another major role of supraspinatous is to compress the humeral head into the glenoid

management in the latter group is similar to lines of managing a recurrent dislocation. Same surgical procedures are offered after identifying the direction of instability and the cause. The former ones, however, seldom benefit from surgery and are better managed with stringent physiotherapy to strengthen the shoulder stabilizers. Surgery (inferior capsular shift, a capsular tightening procedure to reduce capsular volume) in such patients is offered only in nonresponding cases.

Mathysen gave a useful physiological classification of recurrent instability that guides the treatment. He advocated the use of mnemonics *TUBS* and *AMBRI* to guide treatment in cases of recurrent instability of the shoulder as explained in **Table 6.1**.

HIGH-YIELD POINTS

- Shoulder is the most mobile joint in the body, but also the most common joint to dislocate in the body (followed next in frequency by the elbow).

Table 6.1: Mathysen classification of recurrent shoulder instability

TUBS	*AMBRI*
T—Traumatic dislocation leading to recurrent instability	**A**—Atraumatic dislocation (minimal trauma)
U—Unidirectional instability is usually present	**M**—Multidirectional instability would be there
B—Bankart's lesion is the most common lesion in such patients	**B**—Most patients will have bilateral problem
S—Surgery is the mainstay of treatment in such cases	**R**—Rehabilitation (physiotherapy) is to be tried initially
	I—In nonresponders inferior capsular shift procedure is to be done

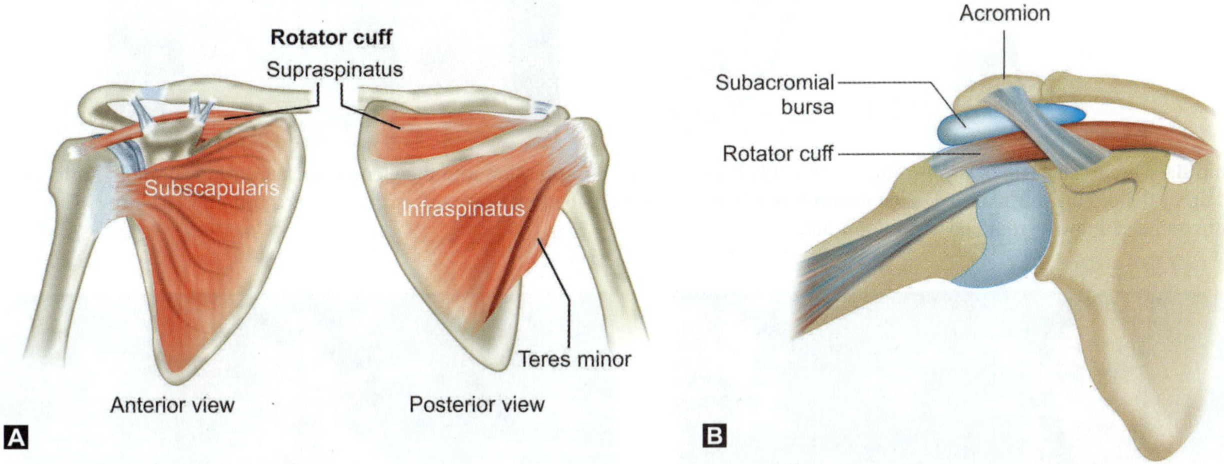

Figs 6.11A and B: (A) Rotator cuff; (B) Subacromial bursa and rotator cuff below it

socket (owing to direction of its pull) as the deltoid elevates the shoulder into abduction.

Infraspinatus and teres minor: Both these muscles come from the lower part of the dorsal surface of scapula and go laterally on the posterior aspect of shoulder to insert on the greater tuberosity. Both are primarily involved in external rotation.

Rotator cuff passes through the subacromial space beneath the subacromial bursa and above the glenohumeral articular surface **(Fig. 6.11B)**. Bursa provides for smooth gliding of rotator cuff tendons during shoulder movement.

Pathomechanics of Rotator Cuff Deficient Shoulder

Trauma to shoulder during unaccustomed athletic activity at times may lead to tears in these muscles. More commonly, in older individuals age-related fatty degeneration may result in spontaneous ruptures in these tendons, with supraspinatous being involved in majority of cases.

Long standing cuff tears, result in loss of subacromial space. Since an important function of supraspinatous is to compress the humeral head into the glenoid as the deltoid abducts the shoulder, absence of this compression effect causes upward migration of humeral head with deltoid contractions, making it abut against the undersurface of the acromion **(Fig. 6.12A)**. With time this superior migration leads to damage in articular cartilage of head giving rise to degeneration of the shoulder joint, referred to as cuff tear arthropathy **(Fig. 6.12B)**.

Classification

Rotator cuff tear can be partial or full thickness tear.

Full thickness tears are further classified based on the length of the greatest diameter of the tear into:
- Small (less than 1 cm)
- Medium (1–3 cm)
- Large (3–5 cm)
- Massive (greater than 5 cm)

Partial thickness tears are classified by
- *Location*: (A) articular surface (tear is on articular side), (B) bursal surface (tear is on subacromial bursa side), or (C) interstitial (a mid-substance tear).
- *Depth*: (I) <3 mm, (II) 3–6 mm, or (III) >6 mm. Cuff is almost 12 mm thick, so a grade III tear is supposedly involving more than 50% of the cuff thickness.

Clinical Testing

For Subscapularis

Belly-press test (Gerber)/Napoleon sign: Patient is asked to place the hand on the belly (with elbow in front of the trunk) and press the abdomen or apply pressure against the examiner's hand **(Fig. 6.13A)**. If subscapularis is normal, the patient presses the abdomen by hand by internal rotation of the shoulder and elbow remains in front of the trunk. If the subscapularis is weak, then internal rotation cannot be maintained and the patient

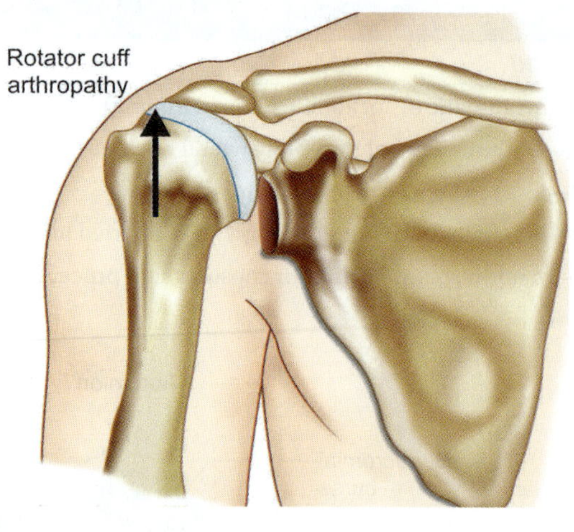

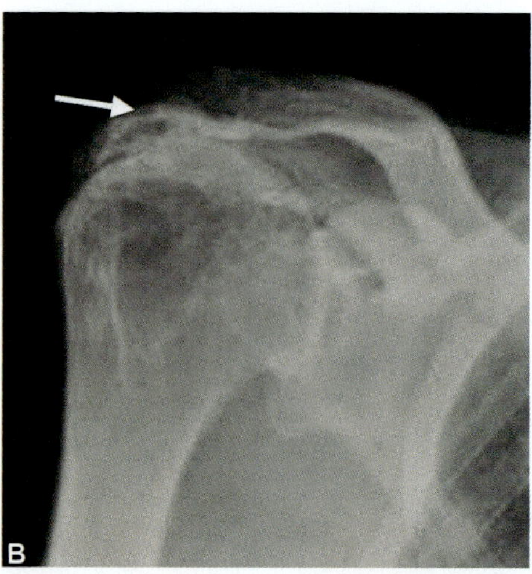

Figs 6.12A and B: (A) With absence of supraspinatous, head fails to maintain compression into the glenoid socket during shoulder abduction and is rather pulled up by deltoid making it abut against the undersurface of acromion, leading to genesis of cuff tear arthropathy; (B) X-ray of a patient with massive rotator cuff tear showing reduced acromiohumeral space

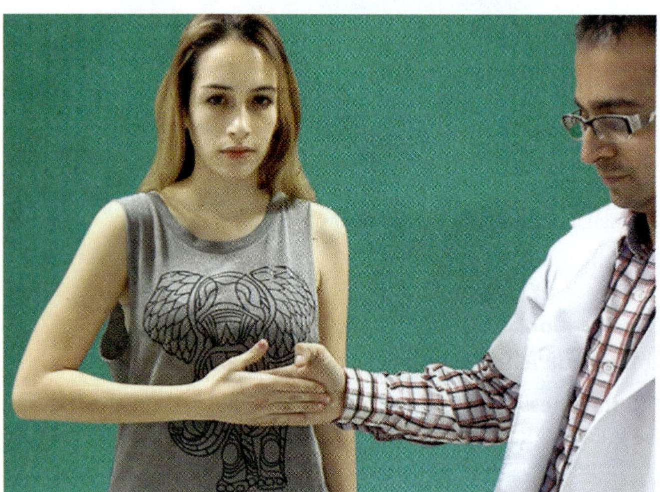

Fig. 6.13A: Belly-press test

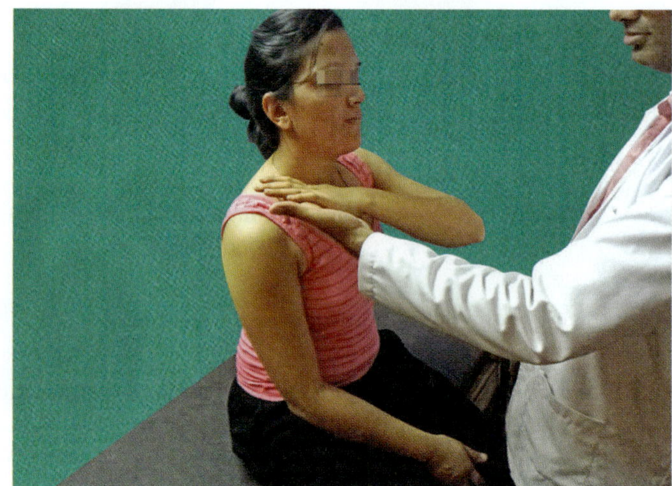

Fig. 6.13C: Bear Hug test

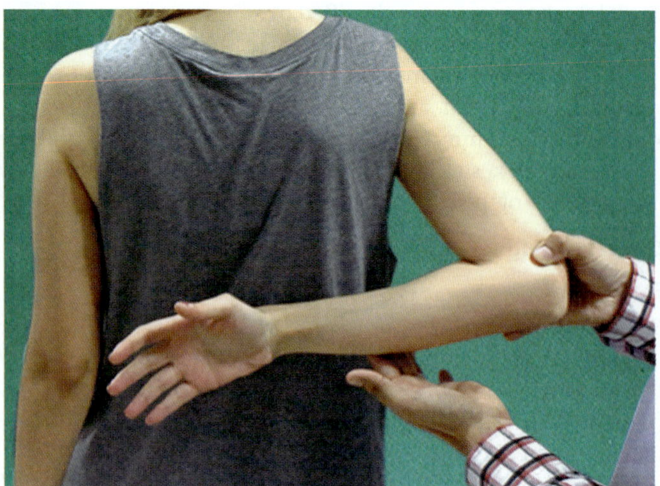

Fig. 6.13B: Lift-off test

presses the abdomen by extending the shoulder and dropping the elbow behind the trunk (Belly press test) or by flexing the wrist (Napoleon sign, named after the peculiar posture in which Napoleon is depicted in many photographs).

Lift-off test (Gerber): Patient's arm is internally rotated with dorsum of the hand touching the back. If the patient is able to lift his hand off the back, subscapularis function can be presumed to be normal **(Fig. 6.13B)**.

Bear hug test (Burkhart and De Beer): Both the earlier tests fail to recognize subscapularis tears when less than 50% of the muscle may be torn (especially when only the upper third fibers are torn). In such situations more sensitive is the Bear Hug test. Patient places the hand on the contralateral shoulder. Examiner supports the elbow in front of the body. Now examiner tries to raise the hand off the shoulder and patient resists it **(Fig. 6.13C)**. A positive test is indicated by failure of the patient to resist the examiner.

For Supraspinatous

Jobe's empty can sign: Elevate the shoulder to 90° abduction in scapular plane (30° forward flexion from coronal plane of body) and internally rotate so that the thumb points toward the floor (as if emptying a can). Now ask the patient to elevate his arm against a resistance. Weakness suggests a tear of supraspinatus **(Fig. 6.14A)**.

Drop arm test (Codman): Patient's arm is elevated overhead and then he is asked to move it down slowly in reverse motion. Test is considered positive if there is sudden onset acute pain or if the patient is unable to smoothly control the lowering motion **(Fig. 6.14B)**.

For Infraspinatus and Teres Minor

External rotation resistance stress test: The test is performed to check the integrity of external rotators (infraspinatous and teres minor). Patient keeps his arms by his side in 0° abduction-flexion with elbows bent to 90°. Now the shoulders are externally rotated to 60°. Next, the examiner tries to internal rotate the shoulders by applying pressure on dorsum of patient's hands which the patient is asked to resist **(Fig. 6.15A)**. Pain or weakness suggests insufficiency of external rotators.

*External rotation lag sign (ERLS, **Fig. 6.15B**)*: This tests the integrity of infraspinatous mainly. To elicit the ERLS, patient is seated on a chair with elbows bent to 90°. The examiner elevates the patient's shoulder by 20° in scapular plane and rotates them externally to full extent. The patient is asked to maintain this position. The test is positive when angular drop occurs.

Drop sign: This sign also tests the integrity of infraspinatous. The procedure is absolutely similar as in ERLS, however, in this test the shoulders are elevated to 90° in scapular plane. Sensitivity as well as specificity has been reported to be slightly more with the ERLS.

*Hornblower sign (Patte, **Fig. 6.15C**)*: This sign predicts more accurately the integrity of teres minor. With elbows bent to 90°, patient's arm is elevated to 90° in scapular plane. The patient is then asked to laterally rotate the shoulder. Weakness or pain on trying to do so suggests insufficiency of teres minor.

Diagnosis

X-rays are usually normal but in massive cuff tears they may show reduction of acromiohumeral distance to less than 6 mm (due to superior migration of humeral head, **Fig. 6.12B**). Ultrasound is a highly sensitive and specific modality for full thickness rotator cuff tears. However, it is operator dependent and less accurate for detecting partial thickness tears and tear size itself compared to MRI. MRI is the investigation of choice for rotator cuff tears as it is comparable to ultrasonography (USG) for full thickness rotator cuff tears and superior than USG in detecting partial thickness rotator cuff tears. Another advantage offered by MRI is that it can quantify the amount of fatty degeneration (replacement of muscle with fat) that may occur in a torn cuff it is neglected for a long time. Arthroscopy remains the gold standard for all cases and is a diagnostic tool as well as a treatment modality.

Management

Treatment is mainly conservative in old people and in those with low demand. NSAIDs for pain relief along with stretching and cuff strengthening exercises are instituted. If strength improvements

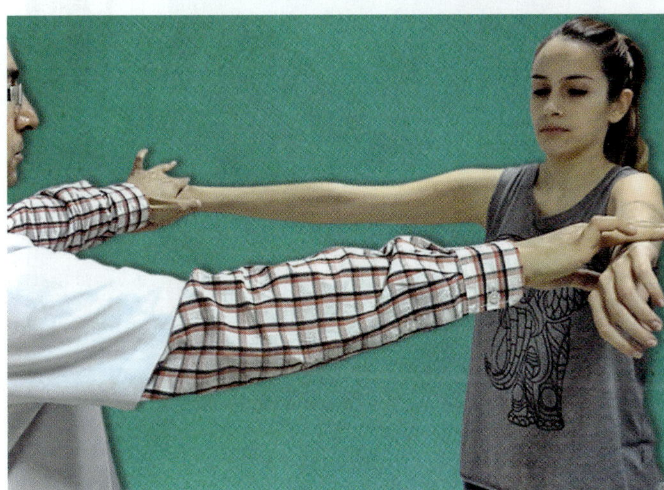

Fig. 6.14A: Empty can sign

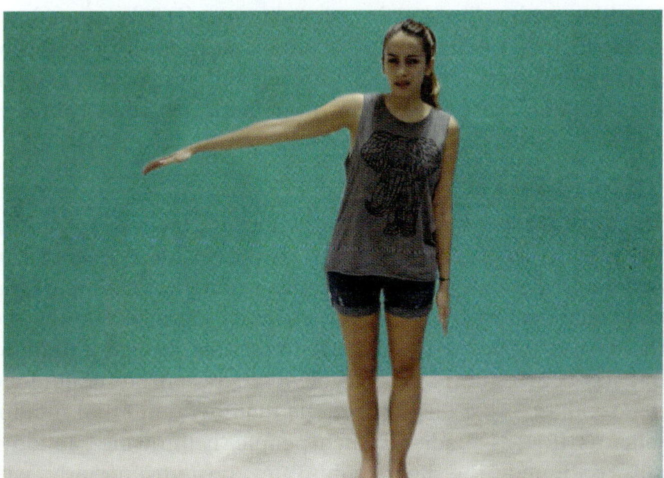

Fig. 6.14B: Drop arm test

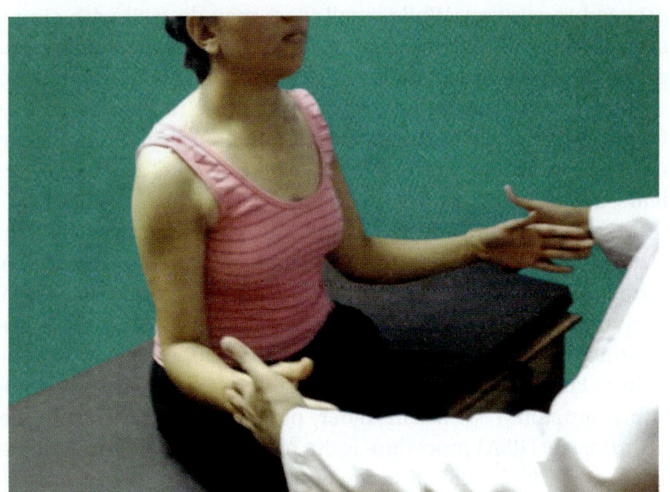

Fig. 6.15A: External rotation resistance stress test

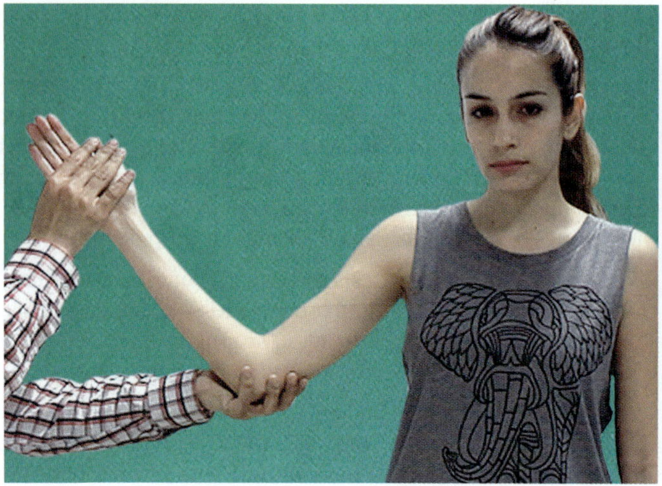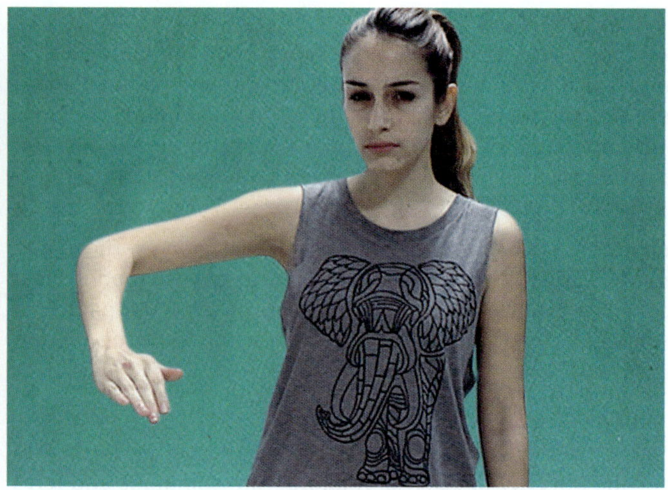

Fig. 6.15B: External rotation lag sign

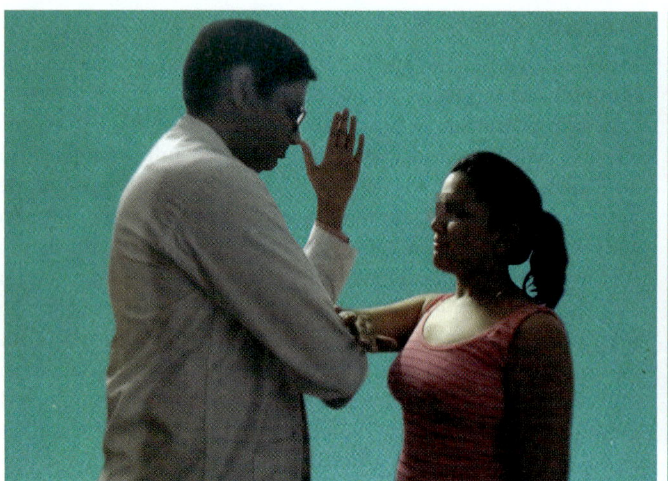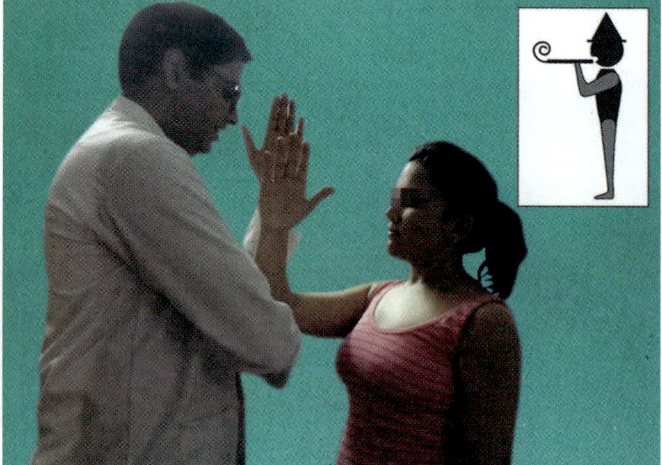

Fig. 6.15C: Hornblower sign

are minimal or a pain relief is not noticed by 6 weeks, one may proceed to surgery. While small tears may do well with simple arthroscopic debridement procedure, full thickness tears and grade III partial thickness tears (i.e. involving more than 50% of cuff thickness), mostly need an arthroscopic repair. There is an increasing trend toward early arthroscopic surgical repair of tears in young high demand patients, especially the articular sided tears, as vascularity of cuff on articular side is relatively poor.

However, there may be some late presentations in all age groups where the patient comes late and the torn cuff has retracted, has fatty degeneration (muscle replaced by fat) and is irreparable. In such cases, in patients less than 70 years of age, treatment is appropriate tendon transfers (donors like pectoralis major, latissimus dorsi, trapezius, etc. are used to substitute supraspinatous) while in older patients, a reverse shoulder arthroplasty (RSA) procedure is the recommended treatment (*see* Page 481). The latter is also the option to opt in cases of patients who land up with cuff tear arthropathy.

DISABLED THROWING SHOULDER AND SLAP LESIONS

An athlete with a disabled throwing shoulder (DTS) cannot throw overhead or hit a ball without discomfort and pain. This condition is commonly encountered in throwing athletes such as bowlers in cricket and those who are involved in hitting a ball as in lawn tennis, etc.

Pathomechanics of DTS

Repetitive throwing action involves forceful internal rotation at the shoulder as the ball is released. This stretches the capsule on posterior side of shoulder repeatedly leading to micro tears that eventually heal with fibrosis and posterior capsular contracture. This results in loss of internal rotation at the throwing shoulder and when the side to side difference between both shoulders is more than 25°, a diagnosis of glenohumeral internal rotation deficit (GIRD) is made. In such people, if throwing motion is still continued, the head subluxates posterosuperiorly with every throw, contacting the posterosuperior cuff (*see* internal

> **Box 6.1:** Common pathological lesions seen in patients with disabled throwing shoulder (DTS)
>
> 1. SLAP tears
> 2. Rotator cuff injuries and biceps tendon injuries
> 3. Shoulder instability
> 4. Range of motion deficits (GIRD)
> 5. Muscle strength imbalance
> 6. Scapular dyskinesia

Abbreviations: SLAP, superior labral tear anterior to posterior; GIRD, glenohumeral internal rotation deficit.

impingement, *see* Page 457) and taking down the posterosuperior labrum. The resultant pathological lesions, i.e. an articular sided cuff tear and a SLAP tear (read later) finally lead to loss of speed and control while throwing, causing DTS. With further progression and damage to shoulder stabilizers, instability at shoulder may develop. Common pathological lesions that are seen in people who have DTS have been listed in **Box 6.1**.

SLAP Tears

SLAP (superior labral tear anterior to posterior) tear is a tear of superior labrum that occurs at the attachment of the long head of biceps to the labrum **(Fig. 6.16)**. These labral tears are a common cause of DTS in throwing athletes. Patients with a SLAP tear are usually below 40 years age and present with pain and often a popping and clicking sound while throwing that result in loss of throwing speed and control.

Clinical examination in these cases may reveal increased external rotation and decreases internal rotation (GIRD). A number of clinical tests **(Table 6.2, Figs 6.17A to E)** have been devised for diagnosis of SLAP tear as none is highly specific and sensitive, so diagnosis should likely be considered if a battery of tests is positive rather than a single test. MRI may aid in diagnosis as well **(Figs 6.18A and B)**, however, MR arthrography (MRI after injection of contrast material in joint) is considered the investigation of choice.

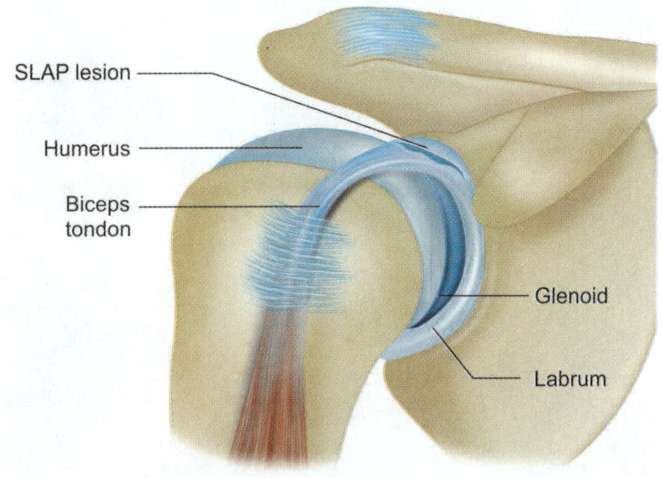

Fig. 6.16: Schematic representation of a SLAP tear

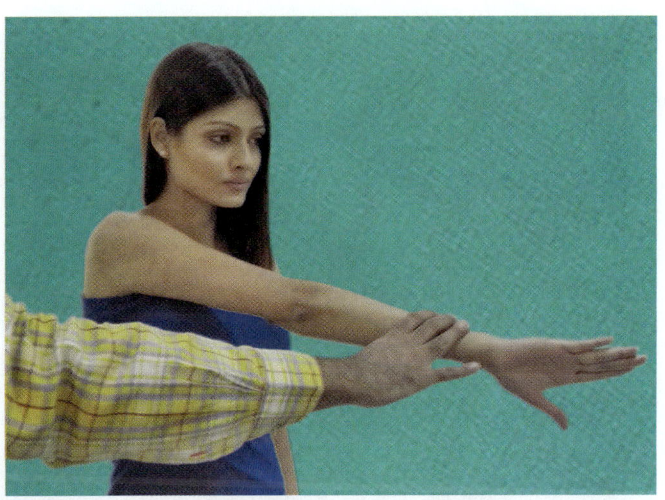

Fig. 6.17A: O Brien's test

Table 6.2: Common clinical tests for SLAP tear	
1. O Brien's test **(Fig. 6.17A)**	The arm to be tested at 90° of flexion and about 10° of adduction and in full internal rotation, pointing the thumb to the ground. The patient is now asked to resist downward force by examining at distal forearm. The test is then repeated but with the arm in external rotation. Pain in the shoulder in internal rotation, but no pain in external rotation indicates a SLAP tear
2. Biceps load test I **(Fig. 6.17B)**	The patient's arm is abducted to 90°, externally rotated and the forearm is supinated. This produces pain in case of a SLAP tear. Now active elbow flexion against resistance should decrease the patient's discomfort
3. Biceps load test II **(Fig. 6.17C)**	In the supine position, the arm is elevated to 120° and externally rotated to its maximal point, with the elbow in the 90° flexion and the forearm in the supinated position. The patient is asked to flex the elbow against resistance. The test is considered positive if the patient complains of pain during the resisted elbow flexion
4. Modified dynamic labral shear test (MDLS) **(Fig. 6.17D)**	In a standing patient the shoulder is abducted to 120°, arm kept in the scapular plane, elbow flexed to 90°, and their shoulder externally rotated. The examiner then lowers the arm while maintaining the external rotation. A positive test is indicated by a painful clicking at the posterior joint line when the arm is lowered between 120° and 90°
5. Uppercut test **(Fig. 6.17E)**	With the shoulder in neutral rotation, elbow flexed to 90° and the forearm supinated and hand in a fist, the patient rapidly brings the fist toward the chin (as in a upper cut punch) against examiner's resistance. Pain in the shoulder indicates a SLAP tear

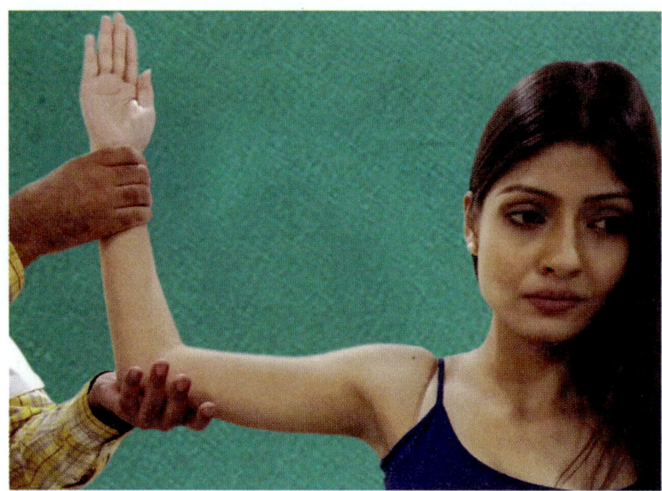

Fig. 6.17B: Biceps load test I

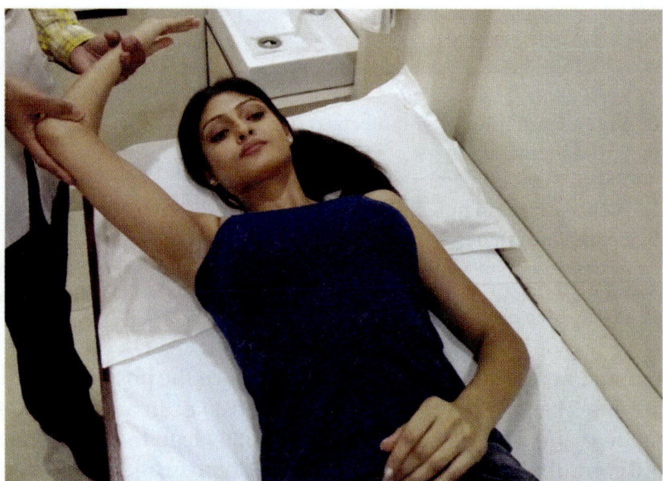

Fig. 6.17C: Biceps load test II

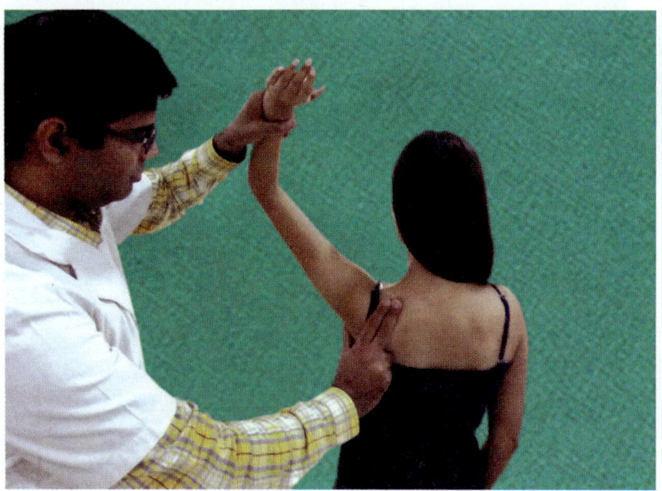

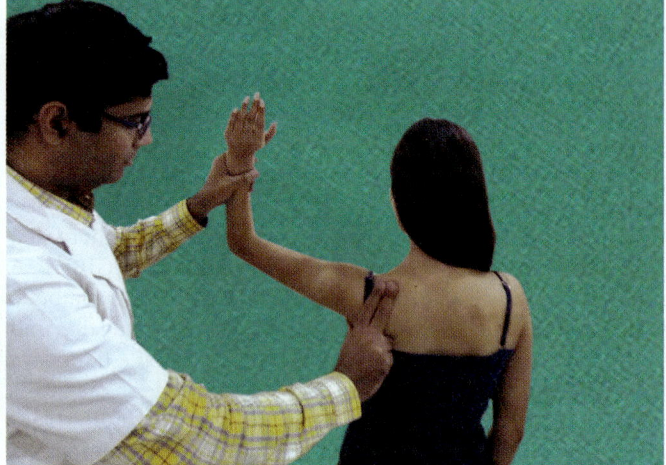

Fig. 6.17D: Modified dynamic labral shear test

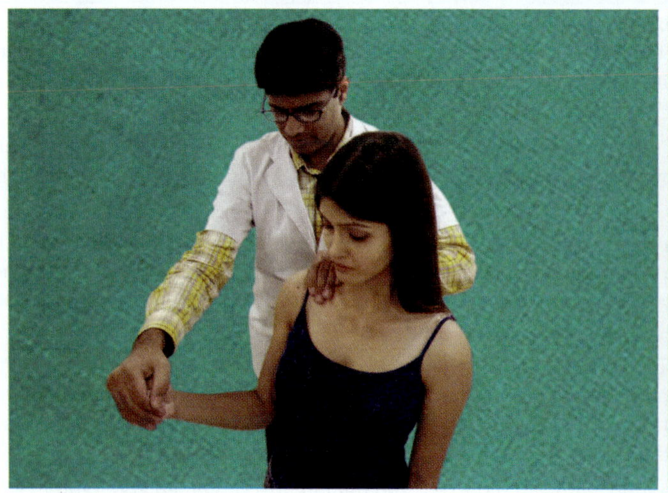

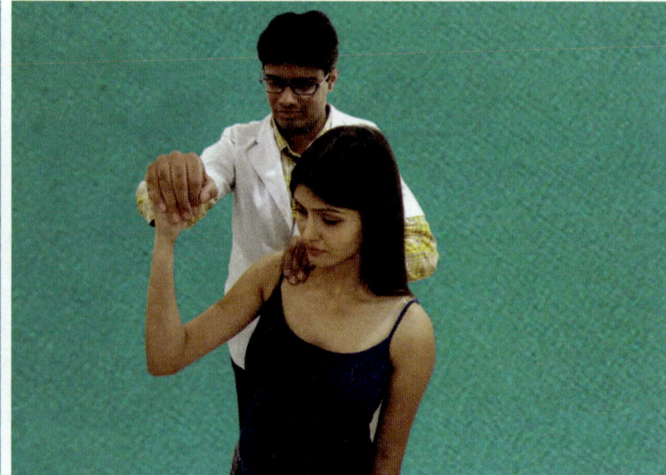

Fig. 6.17E: Uppercut test

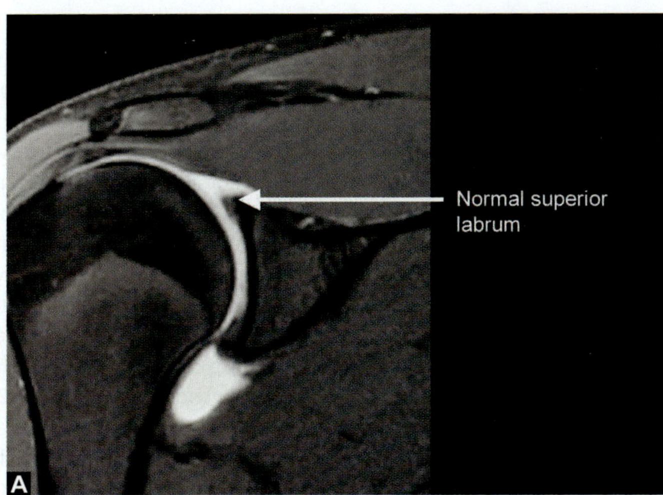

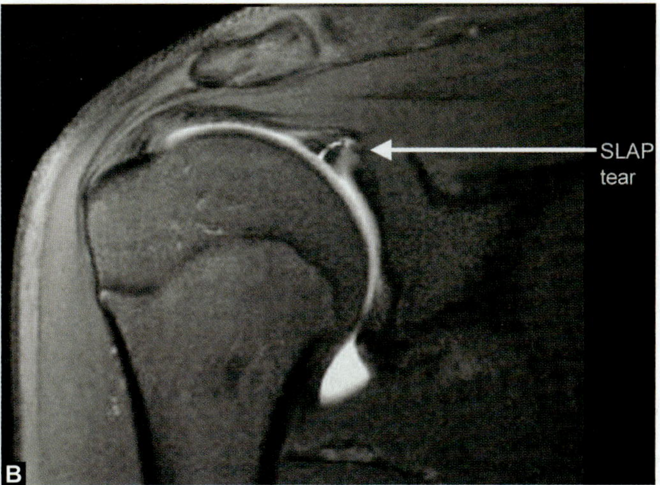

Figs 6.18A and B: (A) MRI shoulder showing normal superior labrum (arrow); (B) MRI shoulder depicting torn superior labrum (arrow)

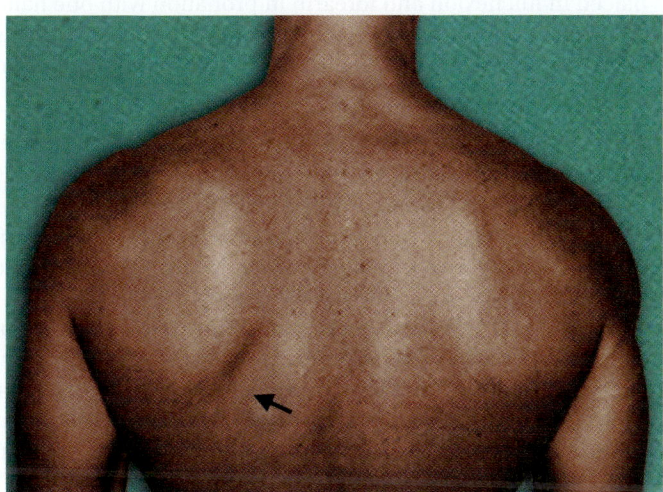

Fig. 6.19: Prominent medial border of left scapula indicating scapular dyskinesia

Treatment of a symptomatic SLAP tear generally requires an arthroscopic labral repair with suture anchors. However, isolated SLAP tears are uncommon and usually associated with other shoulder pathologies. Chances of coexistent pathology increase with age of presentation and must be taken care of simultaneously.

Scapular Dyskinesia

Scapular dyskinesia in this acronym refers to an altered static position as well as dynamic motion of the scapula that alters the efficiency of throwing motion. Alterations in muscle activity secondary to overuse and fatigue or balance issues concerning flexibility result in scapular dyskinesia. Patients may present with winging of medial and inferior scapular borders, medial border prominence **(Fig. 6.19)** and lack a smooth, coordinated movement (normally with every 90° of shoulder abduction there is 30° upward tilt of scapula). An acronym SICK scapula (Scapular malposition, Infero-medial scapular border prominence, Coracoid region pain and dysKinesis of scapular movement) is often used to refer to this clinical scenario.

Scapular dyskinesia can be diagnosed by checking the normal and symmetrical scapular movement (scapulo-humeral rhythm) during shoulder elevation and by scapular assistance test (*see* Page 455). Most patients with scapular dyskinesia can be treated conservatively with exercise programs designed to strengthen the scapular muscles.

SPORTS INJURIES AROUND THE ELBOW

LATERAL EPICONDYLITIS (TENNIS ELBOW)

Tennis elbow, also called lateral epicondylitis, is chronic tendinitis of the common extensor origin [more specifically extensor carpi radialis brevis (ECRB)], seen mostly in patients between 30 years and 50 years of age. It is hypothesized that chronic stress (overuse) causes small tears (micro-tears) that lead to fibrocartilaginous metaplasia, calcification and painful vascular reaction in the tendon fibers close to the site of origin on the lateral epicondyle. Most commonly it affects individuals (male and female ratio almost equal) whose work profile involves repetitive wrist extension against resistance and twisting activities. It may be seen in tennis players (those using the back hand stroke) or at times even in nonplayers as those involved in activities like hammering, squeezing clothes, carrying loads like a bucket or suitcase in hand, etc.

Clinical Testing

One may classically find tenderness localized to the lateral epicondyle of the humerus or just distal to it. The important diagnostic tests are:

- *Cozen's test*: Pain in the region of the lateral epicondyle during resisted extension of the wrist **(Fig. 6.20A)**.
- *Maudsley's test*: Pain in the region of the lateral epicondyle during resisted extension of the middle finger **(Fig. 6.20B)**.
- *Mill's test:* In a sitting posture with the shoulder slightly abducted, elbow flexed to 90°, the forearm pronated and wrist flexed, examiner supports the arm of the patient with one hand and maintain the flexed position of the wrist and pronation of the forearm with the other hand **(Fig. 6.20C)**. Now the elbow is extended slowly. Pain over the lateral aspect of the elbow joint indicated a positive test.

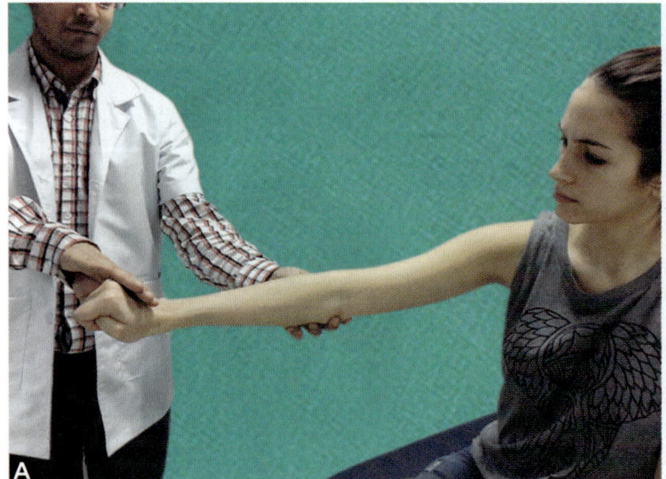

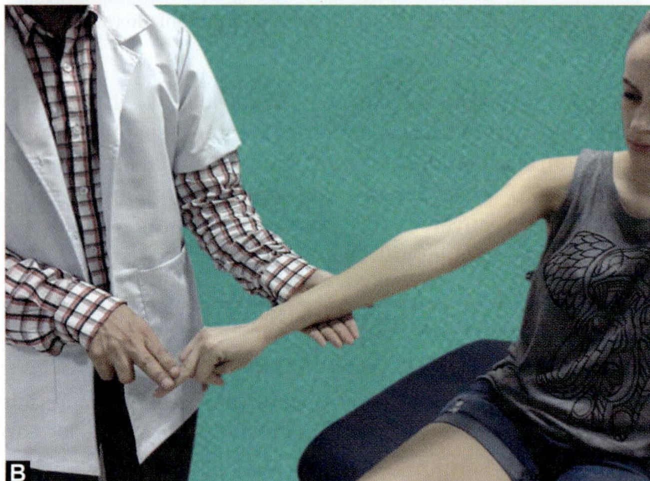

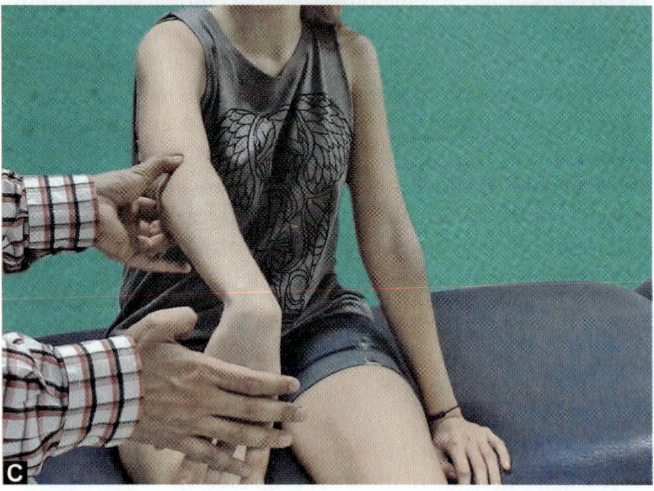

Figs 6.20A to C: (A) Cozen's test; (B) Maudsley's test; (C) Mill's test

X-ray

X-ray is usually normal. Rarely one may find calcification adjacent to the lateral epicondyle.

Differential Diagnosis

Radial tunnel syndrome (*see* Page 274).

Management

Initially management is conservative (NSAIDs and activity modification). Forearm eccentric extensor strengthening exercises (read later) are very effective and should be advised early in the treatment. A wrist strap may be given to provide local support and restrict activities. Local heat therapies and intralesional steroid injections are useful in resistant cases. Some other treatment options involve injecting blood at the site to cause fibrosis or injecting platelet rich plasma (PRP) to provide growth factors and promote healing of the lesion. Only in recalcitrant cases is surgery needed where the origin of ECRB is debrided and if needed released. In still non-resolving cases of epicondylitis, the end resort remains epicondylectomy (but no more than 25% of the epicondyle should be removed).

Several manipulation techniques have also been described for the treatment of lateral epicondylitis. Mill's manipulation is most commonly used. The affected extremity is kept at 90° of abduction and internal rotation of the shoulder. Patient's wrist is placed in full flexion and forearm in pronation with one hand, and clinician applies high velocity, low amplitude varus thrust at the elbow with the other hand. One or two manipulations are given per week for total of 6 weeks.

MEDIAL EPICONDYLITIS (GOLFER'S ELBOW)

This condition, much less common than tennis elbow, is just its medial counterpart, where chronic overuse tendinitis involves the common flexor pronator origin (especially flexor carpi radialis). The tenderness in these cases is localized to the medial epicondyle of humerus. The affected people generally have a work profile that involves squeezing actions or swinging action of the forearm (such as golfers, cricketers, baseball players, etc.) or frequently have to perform overhead motions (e.g. persons involved in racquet sports). The diagnostic and management aspects are basically the same as in the above condition except that here eccentric strengthening of forearm flexors is helpful.

HIGH-YIELD POINTS

- Even in Golfer's, the more common epicondylitis is lateral (Tennis elbow).
- *Baseball pitcher's elbow/Little leaguer's elbow*: This is basically medial epicondylar apophysitis, counterpart of the Golfer's elbow seen in young players before or around the age of puberty.
- *Little Leaguer's shoulder*: This is a Salter-Harris Type I injury of the proximal humerus in children.
- *Javelin throwers' elbow*: The term refers to painful elbow in a javelin thrower. Two etiologies are described—a sprain of ulnar collateral ligament of the elbow or a tendinitis of triceps insertion at olecranon **(Fig. 6.21)**.

COMMON SPORTS INJURIES OF THE HAND

BOWLER'S THUMB

It is digital nerve neuroma (strictly speaking, it is perineural fibrosis and not a true neuroma) of thumb seen in those involved in spin bowling. Thickening of the nerve occurs due to constant friction as the ball rubs against the lateral thumb surface during bowling. The ulnar digital nerve of thumb is involved.

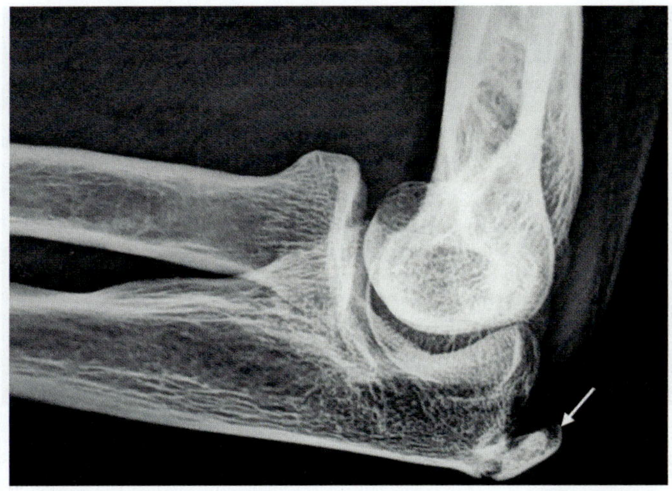

Fig. 6.21: Triceps tendinitis with calcification at triceps insertion

SKIER'S/GAMEKEEPER'S THUMB

This is the most common injury pattern at the first metacarpo-phalangeal (MCP) joint and refers to rupture of ulnar collateral ligament (UCL) of the MCP joint of thumb. On most occasions, UCL is avulsed from the base of proximal phalanx **(Figs 6.22A and B)**. It is named so because it was a common injury observed in Scottish gamekeepers (gamekeeper here refers to Scottish fowl hunters and game word refers to their prey which were rabbits) who used to kill small rabbits (game) by breaking the animal's necks between their thumb and index finger. Hyperabduction or extension of thumb is the usual event causing injury. The most common cause nowadays is a skier's hand landing on a ski pole **(Fig. 6.23)**, causing a valgus force on the thumb and injury to UCL. However, while skier's thumb is an acute injury, gamekeeper's thumb is more of chronic nature (occurs with repetitive trauma).

Diagnosis: Patients present with valgus instability at thumb and with pain and swelling of the MCP joint. Tenderness can be localized to the medial aspect of the MCP joint of thumb. X-ray may **(Fig. 6.22B)** show avulsion fracture at the ulnar corner of the base of the proximal phalanx and widening of MCP joint on stress views. MRI guides the diagnosis in doubtful cases.

Treatment: In partial ruptures thumb is unstable in flexion only and these injuries are treated with immobilization in a thumb spica plaster for 4 weeks. For complete tears (thumb is unstable in both extension and flexion) operative repair is required.

MALLET/BASEBALL FINGER

Mallet finger injury is the disruption of the extensor tendon (Extensor digitorum communis) insertion at the base of the distal phalanx and consequent inability of active extension of the distal phalanx. It is the most common closed tendon injury in athletes.

Classification: Terminal extensor tendon inserts at the base of distal phalanx so three types of mallet finger injuries are possible.
1. The rupture of the extensor tendon
2. Avulsion of the extensor tendon from its insertion into distal phalanx
3. Avulsion of the tendon from distal phalanx with a chip of bone **(Fig. 6.24A)**.

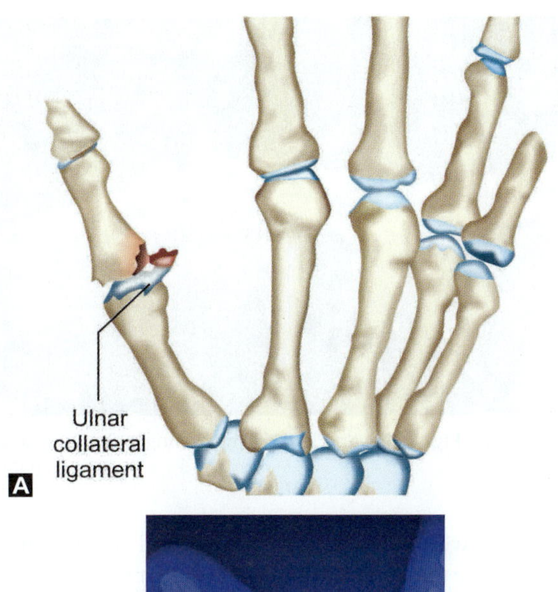

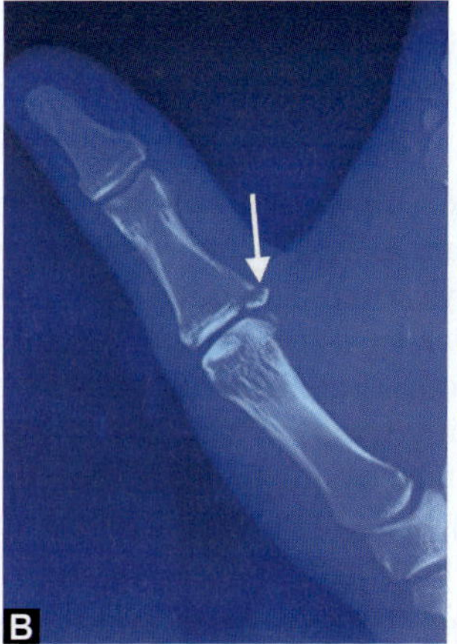

Figs 6.22A and B: (A) Diagram showing ulnar collateral ligament (UCL) avulsed from base of proximal phalanx in Gamekeeper's thumb/skier's thumb; (B) X-ray of hand oblique view showing avulsion of UCL (arrow) from base of proximal phalanx of thumb

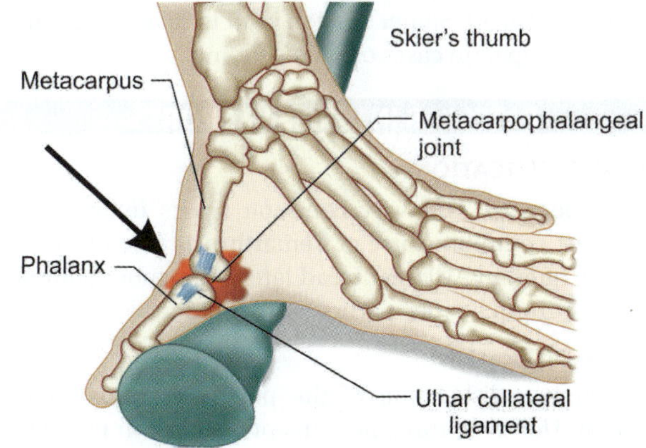

Fig. 6.23: Schematic depiction of mechanism of injury in Skier's thumb

Mechanism of injury: Axial loading and sudden, violent flexion of the distal phalanx is the usual cause of injury. This occurs when fingertip violently strikes to a hard object.

Treatment: Simple avulsion with or without a small bony piece is treated by extension splinting **(Fig. 6.24B)** for 8 weeks. Extension

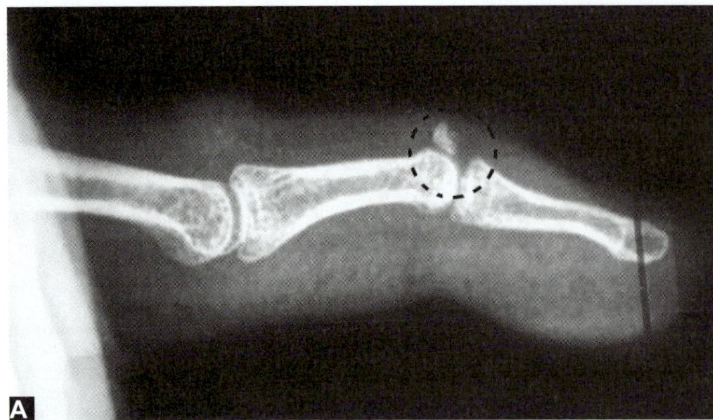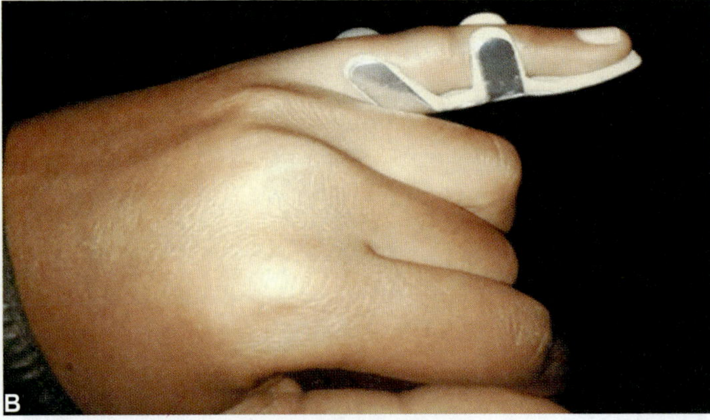

Figs 6.24A and B: (A) X-ray of finger showing avulsion fracture of the dorsal base of the distal phalanx (encircled); (B) Extension splitting for mallet finger

block pinning with K wires may be required if bony avulsion constitutes more than one-third of the articular surface.

JERSEY FINGER

Disruption of flexor digitorum profundus (FDP) tendon from its insertion at the palmar aspect of the distal phalanx is called jersey finger. It is usually caused by sudden and violent hyperextension of a forcefully flexing finger. This mechanism is common in contact sports and ring finger is most commonly involved finger. The patient presents with pain and swelling of the palmar aspect of distal finger with inability to actively flex the distal interphalangeal joints (DIP) joint. The treatment is essentially surgical repair of flexor tendon in all cases.

HIGH-YIELD POINT

- Stener's lesion is the avulsion of UCL from the base of proximal phalanx of thumb and its displacement above the adductor pollicis aponeurosis. Adductor aponeurosis gets interposed between retracted ligament and proximal phalanx of the thumb **(Fig. 6.25)**, thus prevents its healing with closed treatment. Stener's lesion is an indication for an open operative repair in cases of Skier's thumb.

PATELLAR INJURIES IN SPORTS

PATELLAR DISLOCATION

Patellar dislocation is a very common sports injury. It is the second most common cause of hemarthrosis (blood in a joint) in the knee after an ACL tear (read later). It is more common in younger age group people, particularly women.

Patterns of Dislocation

By and large a dislocation of the patella is always a lateral dislocation. However, three patterns of dislocation may be seen at this joint:

- *Acute traumatic dislocation*: Single episode after a significant trauma
- *Recurrent dislocation (most common)*: Multiple episodes of subluxation/dislocation of patella from the trochlear groove of femur after minor magnitude of trauma (usually a forceful flexion of the knee)
- *Habitual dislocation*: Patella subluxates laterally with every flexion and extension of the knee.

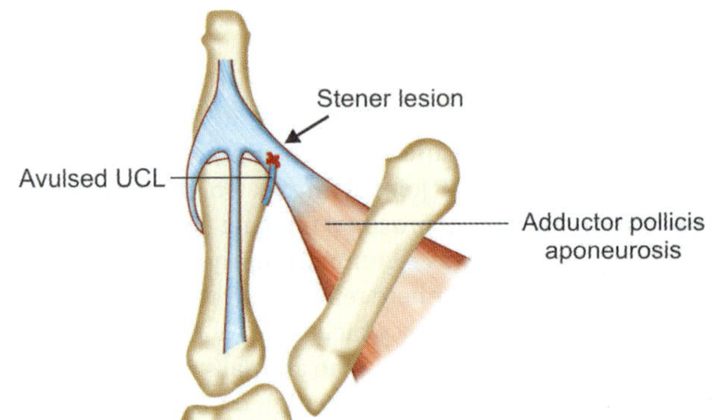

Fig. 6.25: Diagrammatic depiction of Stener's lesion. Note adductor aponeurosis interposing between torn and retracted ulnar collateral ligament (UCL) and proximal phalanx thumb

Surgical Anatomy

Patellofemoral joint is a synovial joint in which patella glides over femoral trochlea with knee movements. Patella has the least contact with the femur in extension where only lowest patellar facet contacts with femur. With increasing flexion this contact area increases (maximum contact is at 90° of flexion). Patella moves upwards on extension of the knee and rides down within the trochlear groove in knee flexion. It is best centered in the trochlear groove at about 30° of knee flexion.

The superior pole gives attachment to the tendon of the quadriceps femoris (the three vasti and the rectus femoris) while from the lower pole, arises the ligamentum patellae to attach on to the tibial tuberosity. Considering a normal valgus of 6–7° at the knee joint one can well imagine that the origin of the quadriceps (rectus femoris arises from the anterior inferior iliac spine) and its insertion (on the patella) lie in a line placed laterally with respect to the center of the patella **(Fig. 6.26)**. Hence, the resultant vector of pull with quadriceps contraction is directed laterally, making patellofemoral joint an intrinsically unstable joint.

There are two mathematical ways of measuring the lateral pull of the quadriceps on the patella:

1. *Quadriceps angle (Q-angle):* It may be defined as the angle subtended between a line drawn from the anterior superior iliac spine to the center of the patella, and a line from the center

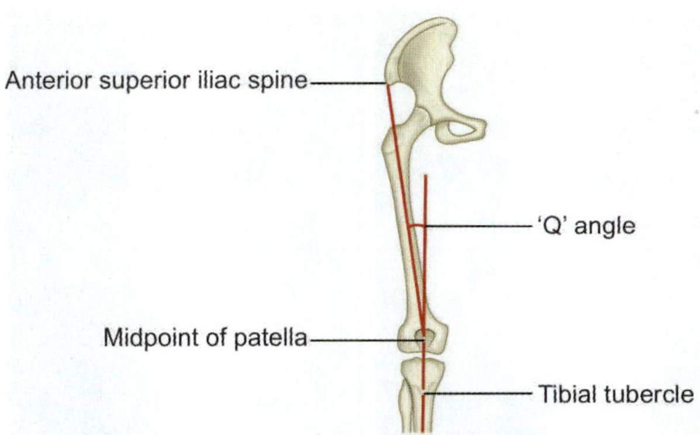

Fig. 6.26: Measurements of Q-angle

Pathophysiology of Patellar Dislocation

In acute dislocation a traumatic injury (usually a sudden, violent contraction of the quadriceps in a flexed knee with externally rotated tibia) ruptures one of the restraint (a soft tissue restraint is usually torn, most commonly being the MPFL) so that the patella subluxates laterally.

A recurrent or habitual dislocation occurs in those in whom a pathological factor exists such that one or more of the restraints are compromised. This may occur either due to nonhealing of a restraint torn during acute injury or due to a genetic or developmental factor like ligament laxity, trochlear dysplasia, patella alta **(Figs 6.27A and B),** etc. The list of factors that predispose to recurrent dislocations are given in **Table 6.3**; the most common of these is patella alta.

of the patella to the tibial tubercle **(Fig. 6.26)**. Normally the angle is 14° in males and 17° in females (on a standing radiograph). More is the Q angle (as when the tibial tuberosity is laterally shifted), more would be the lateral pull of the quadriceps and more unstable would be the patellofemoral joint.

2. *TT-TG distance (Tibial tuberosity to trochlear groove distance):* This is measured on CT scan/MRI and expresses lateral deviation of tibial tuberosity with respect to trochlear groove. Normally, it is less than 20 mm. A higher value predisposes the patient to lateral patellar instability and recurrent dislocation of patella.

Now, to stabilize this unstable joint and counter balance the lateral pull of the quadriceps, following static and dynamic stabilizers are there:

Static stabilizers: The shape of the trochlea (it is groove shaped with lateral edge elevated to contain the patella once it is fully seated, i.e. after 30° knee flexion), shape and position of the patella, the medial retinaculae and the presence of a medial patellofemoral ligament (MPFL) that binds medial side of the patella to the medial epicondyle of femur (and stabilizes in the first 30° knee flexion when patella is not fully engaged in the trochlear groove).

Dynamic stabilizer: Vastus medialis [its oblique fibers called vastus medialis obliquus (VMO)] stabilizes patella during initial phases of knee flexion in conjunction with static stabilizers.

Table 6.3: Predisposing factors for recurrent dislocation of patella
I. Problems in soft tissue restraints
a. Deficient medial restraints
i. MPFL insufficiency (not healed after previous trauma), generalized ligament laxity
ii. VMO insufficiency (wasting due to any pathology around knee)
b. Tight lateral restraints (e.g. Tight lateral retinaculum or iliotibial band)
II. Problems in bony restraints
a. Trochlear dysplasia (produces a shallow trochlear groove identified by some special X-ray signs, **(Figs 6.27A to C)**
b. Patella alta (high riding patella not well seated in trochlea) **(Fig. 6.28B)**
III. Increased lateral force vector of the quadriceps (increased Q angle)
a. External tibial torsion (inborn external twist in the tibia that shifts tibial tuberosity outwards, increasing Q angle)
b. Genu valgum (tibial tuberosity shifts outwards in a valgus leg and Q angle increases)
c. Increased femoral anteversion (such people have a femur that is more in internal rotation that increases the Q angle)

Abbreviations: MPFL, medial patellofemoral ligament; VMO, vastus medialis obliquus.

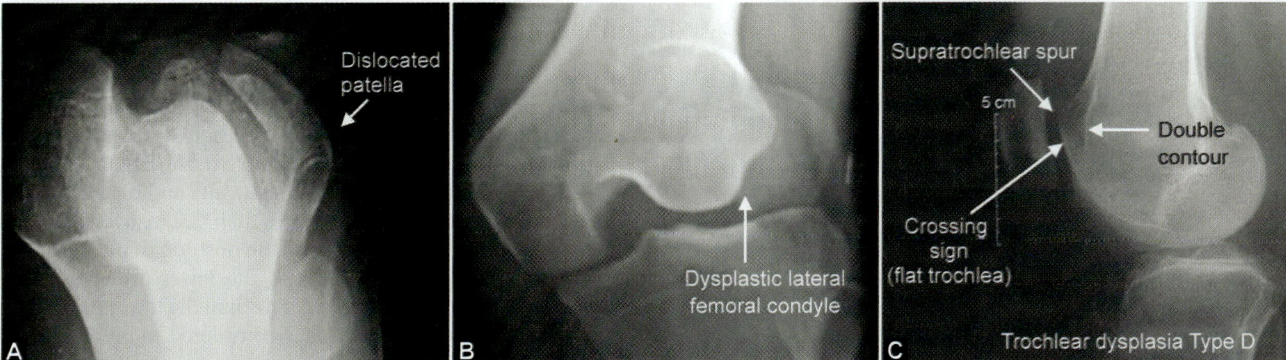

Figs 6.27A to C: (A and B) X-ray knee skyline and AP views showing dislocated patella due to trochlear dysplasia (dysplastic lateral femoral condyle); (C) X-ray knee signs seen in recurrent patellar dislocation. Crossing sign represents an abnormally elevated trochlear floor (i.e. flat trochlea) projecting anterior to femoral condyles and double contour is a double line seen in the anterior aspect of femoral condyles due to presence of a hypoplastic medial femoral condyle in patients with RDP
Source: Dr Ravish Chabra (JN Medical College, AMU).

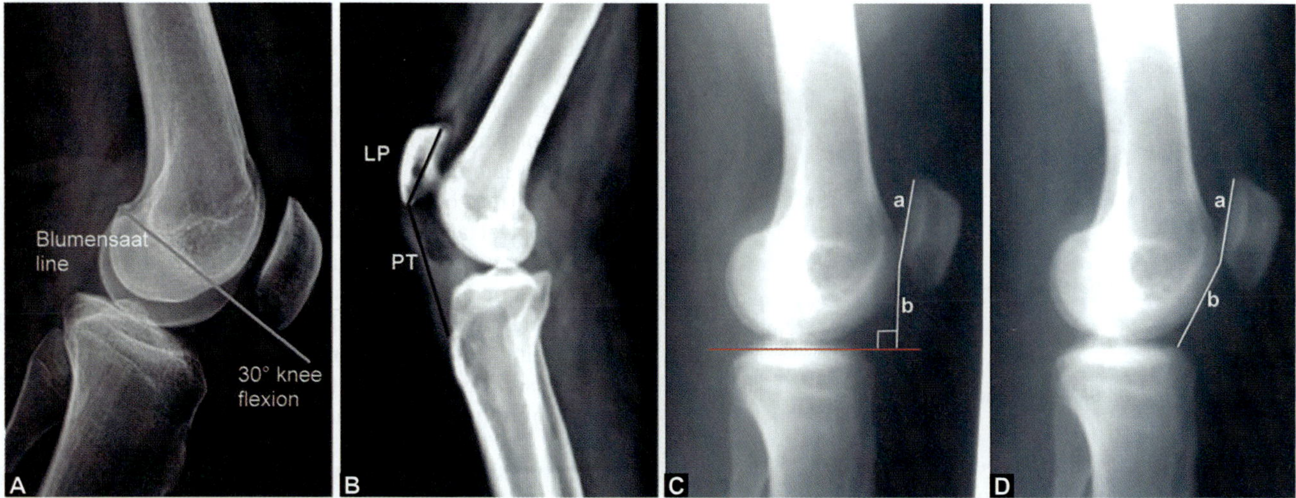

Figs 6.28A to D: (A) X-ray lateral view of knee showing the normal position of the patella in relation to Blumensaat line; (B) Insall-Salvati ratio (PT/LP) showing patella alta; (C) Blackburne-Peel ratio; (D) Caton-Deschamps ratio (*see* **Box 6.2**)
Abbreviations: LP, length of patella; PT, patellar tendon.

Clinical Presentation and Diagnosis

After the acute dislocation, patient presents with painful and swollen knee due to hemarthrosis. Tenderness can usually be elicited on medial aspect of the knee (due to torn MPFL). By the time a patient comes to the hospital patella has usually been spontaneously reduced. Skyline view (*see* Page 147, **Figs 5.76A**) may be ordered in doubtful cases (and sulcus and congruence angles can be calculated, *see* Page 147, **Fig 5.76B**) where dislocation still seems to be persisting. Merchant's view (a variant of skyline view taken in 45° knee flexion weight bearing position) may show an osteochondral fracture of the medial facet of patella.

In case this patient gives a history of previous dislocation, he must be assessed for hyperlaxity of joints. Patellar apprehension test **(Fig. 6.29)** is done to assess patellar stability. With knee in 30° flexion a lateral force is applied to the patella. Apprehension is noticed in patients with recurrent dislocation. There is increased passive lateral translation of the patella compared with the normal side in both 0° and 20° knee flexion (Patellar glide test). Tightness of the lateral retinaculum can be assessed by patellar

tilt test performed at 20° knee flexion. Lateral structure tightness should be considered when lateral patellar margin cannot be lifted up to atleast horizontal position. "J-sign" may be positive. It refers to the lateral patellar deviation during terminal knee extension.

MRI is the investigation of choice in cases with recurrent dislocations. It can not only assess the integrity of medial patellar stabilizers (MPFL, medial retinaculum and VMO), but also reveal trochlear dysplasia and calculate the lateral pull of quadriceps by estimating the TT-TG ratio.

> **Box 6.2:** Procedure to check for high (patella alta) or low (patella baja) situated patella
>
> 1. *Blumensaat line*: Blumensaat line is a line drawn on lateral X-ray of knee along the roof of intercondylar notch. Normally, in lateral X ray at 30° knee flexion, the lower pole of the patella is at the level of blumensaat line **(Fig 6.28A)**, if it is above this line it is patella alta, or if it is below the line, it is patella baja
> 2. *Insall-Salvati ratio*: This is the ratio of the patellar tendon length (PT) to the length of the patella (LP) in 30° flexion lateral X ray of the knee **(Fig. 6.28B)**. Normal ratio is between 0.8 and 1.2. Ratio more than 1.2 is suggestive of high riding patella (patella alta). Ratio less than 0.8 is suggestive of low lying patella (patella baja)
> 3. *Blackburne-Peel ratio*: It is the ratio of b/a in a 30° flexion lateral X-ray of the knee, where "b" is the shortest distance between distal most point of patellar articular surface and a line perpendicular to proximal tibial articular surface and "a" is the length of the patellar articular surface **(Fig. 6.28C)**. Patella alta and baja are diagnosed when b/a is more than 1 and less than 0.5, respectively. This is a more accurate method to know the position of patella compared to Insall-Salvati ratio, as it uses the lower articular margin of patella that is more easier to define than the lower pole
> 4. *Caton-Deschamps ratio*: This is considered to be the best index. It is defined as **(Fig. 6.28D)** the ratio between the distance from lower articular margin of patella to anterior articular margin of tibia (b) and the length of articular surface of patella (a). Normally this ratio (b/a) is 1. In patella alta > 1.3 while in patella baja it is < 0.6

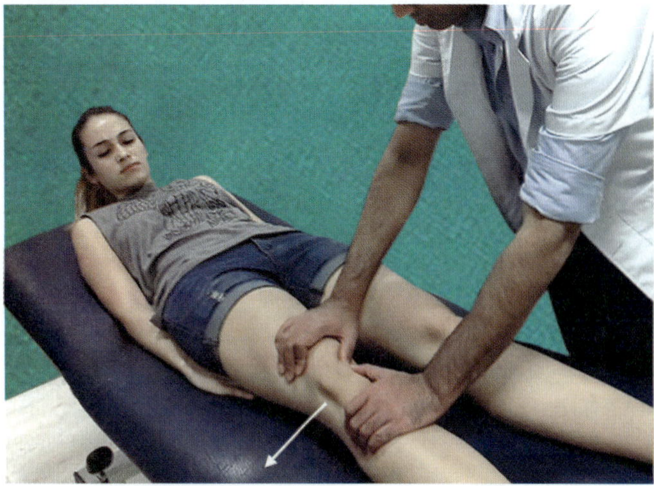

Fig. 6.29: Patellar apprehension test

Flow chart 6.1: Management algorithm for patellar dislocation

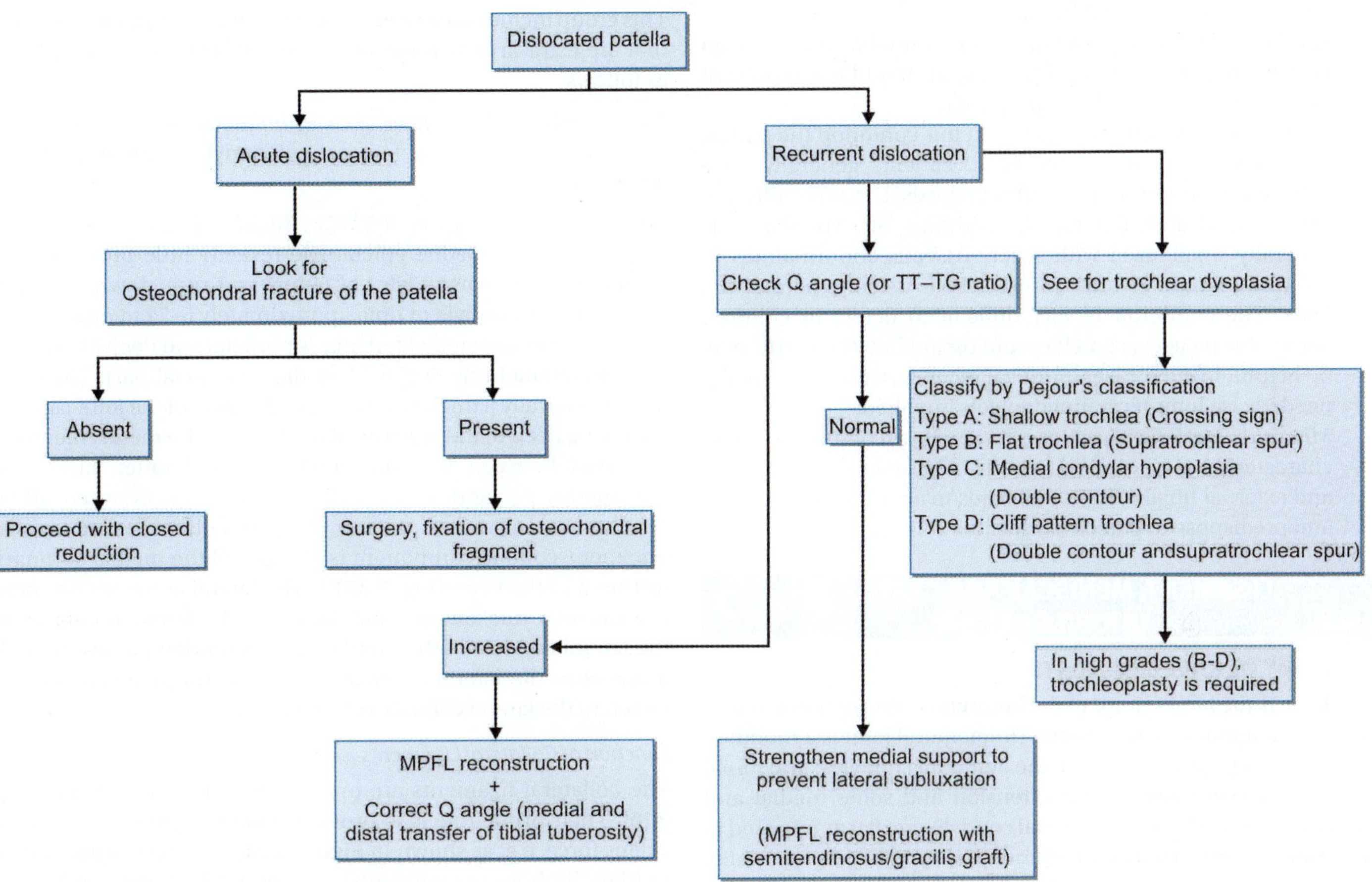

Management (Flow Chart 6.1)

Acute Dislocation Episode

If the patella is still dislocated at presentation, closed reduction should be done by simply pushing it medially. Patients after an acute episode of first patellar dislocation should be immobilized initially in knee extension brace for 3–4 weeks and ice should be applied to the knee for 10–15 minutes every 2 hours to allow soft tissue structures to heal. Weight bearing as tolerated with the help of crutches should be started. With the subsidence of pain, VMO strengthening exercises should be started.

Surgery for first time patellar dislocation is indicated in following cases:

- If there is a concomitant osteochondral fracture seen on Merchant's view.
- If merchant view shows still subluxated patella even after a closed reduction attempt.

Recurrent Dislocation Patient

Management of recurrent/habitual dislocation of the patella is essentially surgical **(Flow chart 6.1)**. The procedures that are employed are broadly categorized into three categories:

I. *Proximal realignment procedures (procedures performed proximal to lower pole of patella)*: These procedures aim at reconstruction of soft tissues restraints (e.g. MPFL reconstruction with a semitendinosus or gracilis tendon graft) and are indicated in all patients to strengthen the medial supports and prevent a lateral dislocation.

II. *Distal realignment procedures (procedures performed distal to the lower pole of patella)*: These procedures are added in patients with increased Q angle acting as a predisposing factor. They aim at realigning the extensor mechanism so as to produce a mechanically more favorable angle of pull of Quadriceps (i.e. they aim at decreasing the Q angle). This is done by transferring the tibial tuberosity to a distal and medial location (modified Elmslie-Trillat procedure).

III. *Trochleoplasty*: Patients in whom severe trochlear dysplasia is acting as a predisposing factor (Type B, C and D dysplasia as per Dejour's classification) require additionally reconstruction of the trochlea, a procedure called trochleoplasty.

HIGH-YIELD POINTS

- Patella is the largest sesamoid bone in the body within the quadriceps tendon. It has the thickest articular cartilage (8 mm thick) and still is the most frequent site of articular cartilage degeneration.
- In the initial knee flexion (<30°) soft tissue structures, mainly the MPFL and VMO play crucial role in stabilizing the patella but after 30°, patellar stability depends mainly on the shape of the trochlea.

- First time dislocation also predisposes to recurrent dislocation due to disruption of MPFL.
- Supratrochlear spur, crossing sign and double contour sign **(Fig. 6.27C)** are the X-ray signs (lateral view of knee) present in patients having trochlear dysplasia.
- *Congenital dislocation of patella:* In this condition the patella is laterally dislocated since birth. Patients generally have associated syndromes like Arthrogryposis, Larson syndrome, Down's syndrome, nail patella syndrome, etc. The patella is generally small sized with severe osseous abnormalities in the distal femur. Flexion contracture is usually there at the knee. The condition is very difficult to detect in children below 3 years age as patella is not ossified till then. MRI may be helpful in such cases. Surgical reconstruction is generally needed else long-term function gets impaired.
- *Miserable malalignment syndrome:* It encompasses three characteristics—increased femoral anteversion, genu valgum and external tibial torsion that leads to an increased Q-angle and predispose to patellar dislocation.

LIGAMENT, MENISCAL AND CARTILAGE INJURIES OF KNEE

ANATOMY OF KNEE LIGAMENTS

The knee is the largest joint of the body consisting of tibiofemoral and patellofemoral articulations. Tibiofemoral joint is a modified synovial hinge joint between the femoral condyles and tibial plateau, allowing flexion and extension and some medial and lateral rotation in flexion. The tibial condyles are flat as opposed to the femoral condyles that are rounded. Hence, like the shoulder, knee joint is inherently unstable and stability is largely dependent on surrounding capsule-ligamentous complex.

Ligaments and menisci primarily stabilizing the knee joint **(Fig. 6.30A)** are:
- Collateral ligaments (medial and lateral)
- Cruciate ligaments (anterior and posterior)
- Menisci (medial and lateral).

Collateral Ligaments

This group includes the medial and the lateral collateral ligaments that are extra-articular and extrasynovial. Their attachments are as follows:

Lateral collateral ligament (LCL)/fibular collateral ligament: It extends from the lateral femoral epicondyle to the apex of the head of the fibula.

Medial collateral ligament (MCL)/tibial collateral ligament: It begins from the medial epicondyle (exactly little proximal and posterior to the epicondyle) of femur and runs down to attach on the medial condyle of tibia approximately 6–7 cm distal to the joint line. It is further divided into superficial and deep fibers. The main functional role is played by the superficial part. The deep MCL is basically a thickening of medial aspect of the joint capsule only lying deep to the superficial MCL. It has the meniscofemoral (the part between femoral attachment and outer surface of the meniscus) and meniscotibial (the part between tibial attachment and outer surface of the meniscus) components. The meniscotibial component is also called the medial coronary ligament of the knee **(Fig. 6.30B)**. The lateral coronary ligament is a capsular thickening which connects the lateral meniscus to the lateral condyle of the tibia. Popliteus tendon passes through a hiatus in the lateral coronary ligaments (popliteus hiatus) to attach to the lateral condyle of femur.

Function of Collateral Ligaments

The collateral ligaments are present on either side of the knee joint. Their prime role is to provide stability against a varus or a valgus force, e.g. as shown in **Figure 6.31**, if a valgus stress (distal to joint, limb moves outwards) is given to the knee, the MCL is stretched and torn and vice versa. So, collateral ligaments basically stabilize the knee joint in the coronal plane (varus stability—LCL and valgus stability—MCL).

Cruciate Ligaments

These include the anterior and the posterior cruciate ligaments (PCLs) that classically cross centrally in the joint in the shape of

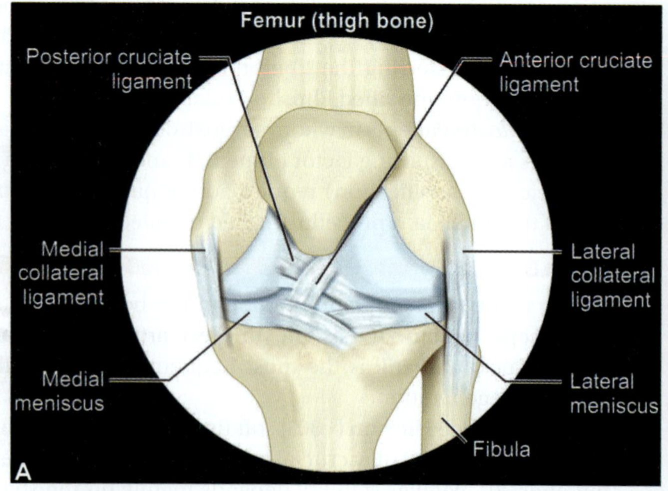

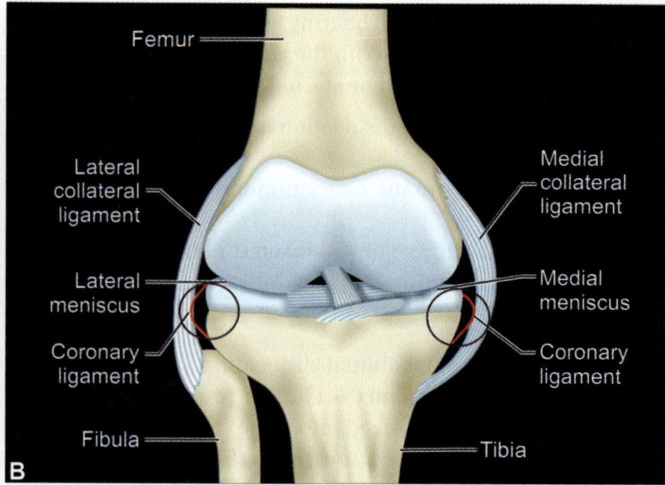

Figs 6.30A and B: (A) Ligaments stabilizing the knee joint; (B) Coronary ligaments in the knee

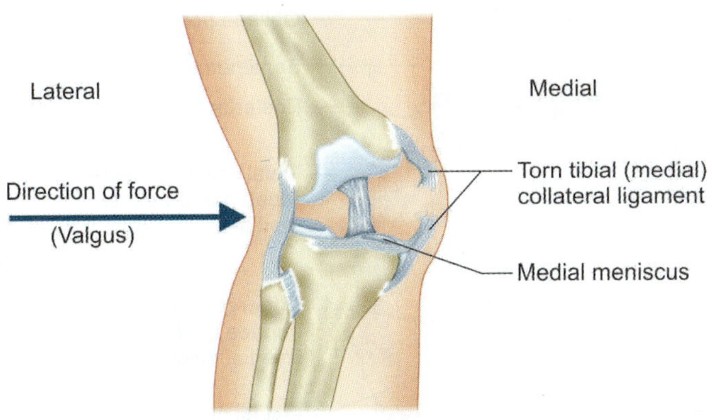

Fig. 6.31: Medial collateral ligament (MCL) getting stretched and torn in valgus stress to the knee

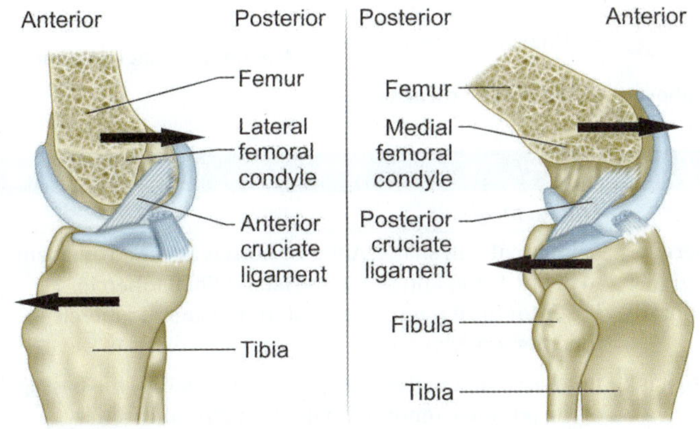

Fig. 6.32: Schematic representation of anterior cruciate ligament (ACL) and posterior cruciate ligament (PCL) on a sagittal section of knee

an "X" when viewed from the front. Both these are intra-articular ligaments but are considered to be extrasynovial in nature (as they have their own synovial sheath that contains their neurovascular supply and hence do not derive their nutrition from synovial fluid). Their anatomy and course is as follows:

Anterior cruciate ligament: It takes origin from the medial wall of lateral femoral condyle (posteriorly in the area of the intercondylar notch) and courses anteriorly and medially to insert on the intercondylar area of the tibia. In other words, it starts anteriorly from the intercondylar area of tibia and goes back to insert on the lateral condyle of femur **(Fig. 6.32)**. In a more detailed description, ACL is portrayed to consist of two bundles anteromedial bundle (bulkier), which is tight in flexion, and a posterolateral bundle, which is tight in extension.

Posterior cruciate ligament: This ligament (1.5 times thicker than ACL) has a course entirely opposite to that of ACL. It takes origin from the lateral wall of medial femoral condyle (anteriorly in intercondylar notch) and courses posteriorly and laterally to insert on an area that is around 1.5 cm posterior and inferior to the posterior articular margin of the tibia. In other words, it starts posteriorly on the tibia and courses in front to attach on the medial condyle of femur, running exactly opposite to the course of ACL **(Fig. 6.32)**. It also consists of two bundles anterolateral,

which is tight in flexion and a posteromedial bundle (bulkier) which is tight in extension.

Function of Cruciate Ligaments

Since the ACL runs from front on tibia coursing back to attach on femur, it will be stretched when the tibia moves forwards on femur while the PCL would stretch when the tibia is forced back on the femur. Hence, these ligaments function to provide the knee stability in the anteroposterior direction. ACL prevents the tibia from displacing forwards on femur while the PCL prevents the tibia from displacing backwards on the femur **(Fig. 6.32)**. Thus, their prime role is to stabilize the knee in the sagittal plane of the body. However, these ligaments also have a minor accessory function. The ACL is a secondary restraint to internal rotation of the tibia and resist varus displacement at full extension while the PCL is a secondary restraint to external rotation of the tibia and resists valgus displacement at full extension.

Menisci

The menisci are the wedge shaped semilunar fibrocartilaginous disks (made primarily of type I collagen) that are sandwiched between the opposing femoral and tibial condyles. These are intra-articular and intrasynovial structures that derive their nutrition primarily from synovial fluid. Each meniscus has a posterior horn, a body and an anterior horn. Anterior horn is attached anteriorly to the intercondylar tibia and the body courses back along the outer margins of the tibial condyles to insert as the posterior horn on the back of the intercondylar tibia **(Fig. 6.33)**. Also, they attach to the tibia via the coronary ligaments. The medial meniscus is elliptical and larger in size than the lateral, but lateral meniscus being more circular in shape has the greater surface area. Detailed comparison of medial and lateral meniscus has been given in **Table 6.4**.

Functions of the Menisci

Their prime role is to convert the flat tibial condyles into sockets so that the femoral condyles fit nicely into them. They also have a few accessory functions. They are elastic structures and hence act as the shock absorbers in the knee on axial loading and protect the articular cartilage by dissipating the forces (hence the absence of menisci leads to arthritis). They also play some role in the nutrition in the joint as they are involved in the distribution of the synovial fluid.

Miscellaneous Knee Ligaments

Meniscofemoral ligaments **(Fig. 6.34)**: Two meniscofemoral ligaments attach the posterior horn of the lateral meniscus to the intercondylar wall of medial femoral condyle. The ligament of Humphrey passes anterior to the PCL, whereas the ligament of Wrisberg passes posterior to the PCL.

Posterior oblique ligament (POL) and oblique popliteal ligament (OPL): POL is a condensation of the posteromedial capsule that strengthens the knee on the posteromedial aspect. The knee is also strengthened on the medial side by a slip from the semimembranosus as it inserts on the posteromedial tibia. This is called the oblique popliteal ligament.

Posterolateral corner ligaments (PLC): Posterolateral corner of knee **(Figs 6.35A and B)**, refers to structures that stabilize the

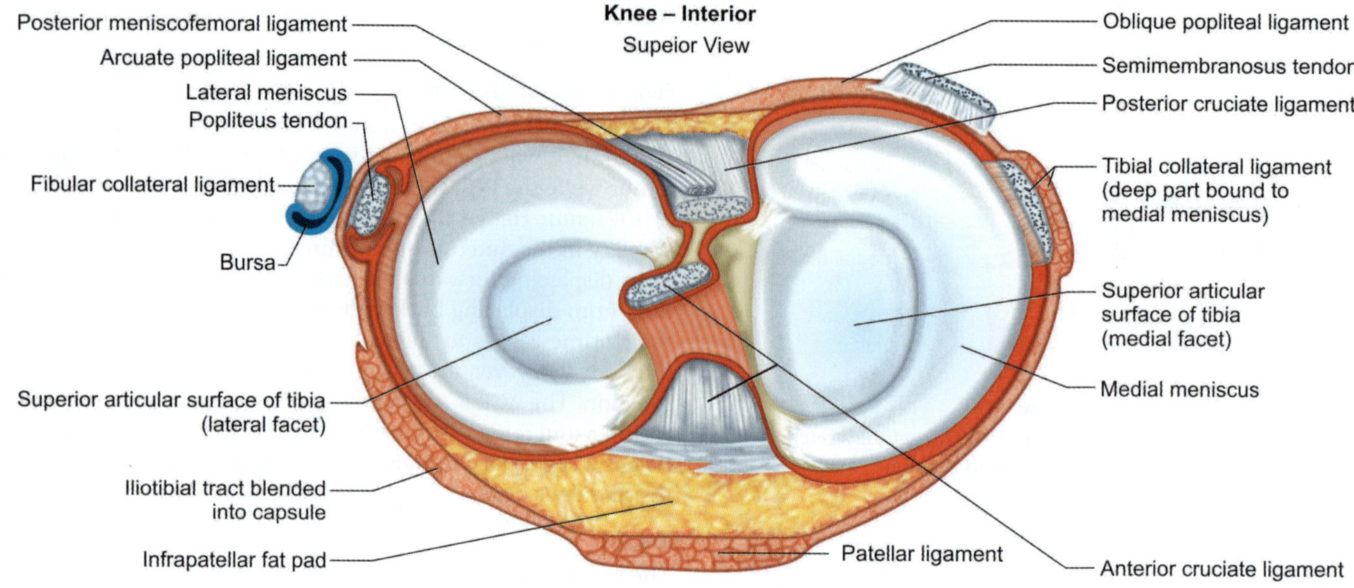

Fig. 6.33: View of the tibial plateau from above showing the two menisci

Table 6.4: Comparison of medial and lateral menisci

Features	Medial meniscus	Lateral meniscus
1. Shape and attachment	C-shaped, but more elliptical. Wider of the two. Anterior horn is attached anterior to the ACL insertion in intercondylar fossa. Posterior horn is attached anterior to the PCL in the posterior part of intercondylar fossa	Semicircular in shape. Anterior horn is attached adjacent to the ACL and anterior to the lateral tibial tubercle. Posterior horn is attached posterior to lateral tubercle in the intercondylar fossa
2. Fixity	Peripherally attached to medial capsule and MCL, so it is less mobile	Its attachment to the capsule is interrupted by the passage of the popliteal tendon (popliteus hiatus in coronary ligament), hence it is more mobile

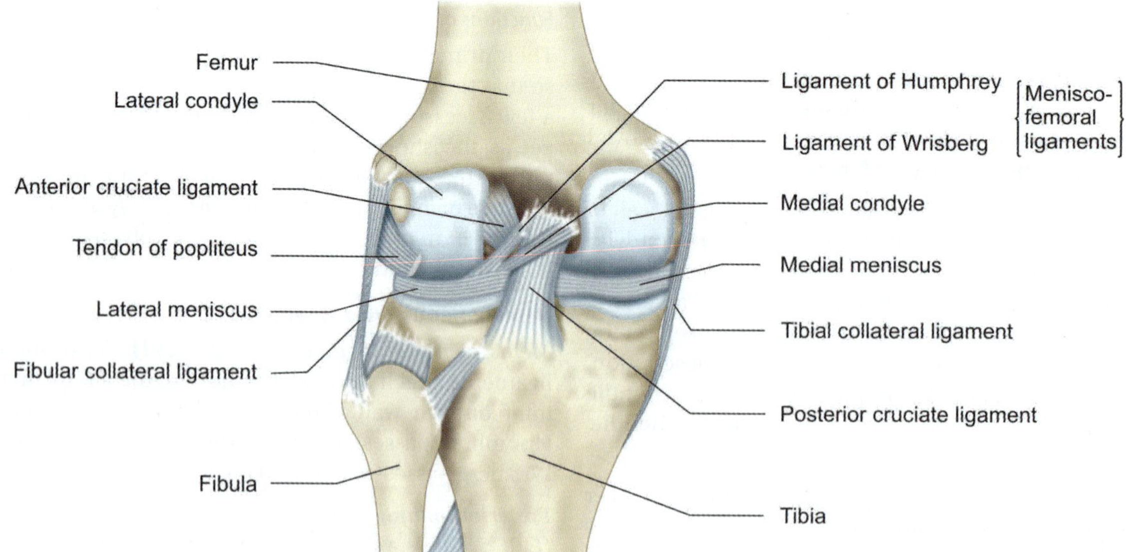

Fig. 6.34: Posterior view of knee joint showing meniscofemoral ligaments

posterolateral aspect of the knee. The main components are the LCL, popliteus tendon and popliteal fibular ligament. Some stability is also added by arcuate ligament (Y-shaped thickening of the capsule on the posterolateral side between popliteus muscle and lateral gastrocnemius muscle) and the fabellofibular ligament. The PLC works in coordination with PCL to strengthen

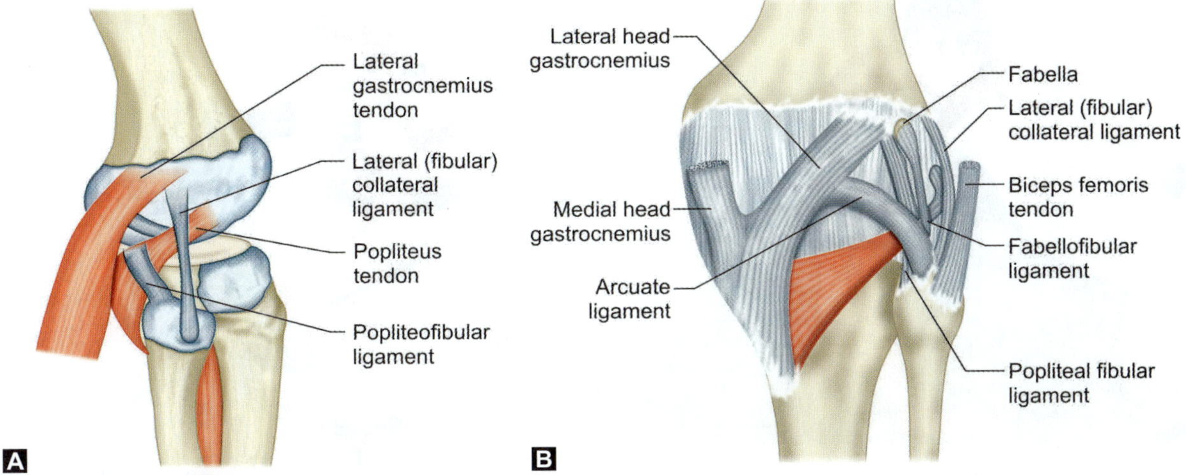

Figs 6.35A and B: Structures making up the posterolateral corner of the knee as viewed from the (A) lateral, and (B) posterior aspect

the knee from the posterolateral aspect and prevents excessive hyperextension of the knee, varus angulation and tibial external rotation.

HIGH-YIELD POINTS

- ACL and PCL are supplied by the middle geniculate artery (branch of popliteal artery) and posterior articular nerve (branch of tibial nerve).
- Menisci move with knee movements. They move forward in extension of the knee and move backward during flexion of the knee.
- Fabella is a sesamoid bone present in the tendon of the lateral head of the gastrocnemius muscle. The ligament that extends from the fabella to the fibular head (fabellofibular ligament) is called the ligament of Valloise.
- Posterolateral corner of the knee is also sometimes referred to as the "dark corner" of the knee, as missing these ligament injuries is often the foremost cause of failure in treatment of other major ligament injuries.
- *Screw home mechanism*: Tibia externally rotates in extension while in flexed knee it internally rotates such that the tibial tuberosity comes to lie in line with the patella. This is called screw home mechanism. It is due to the specific bony anatomy of the knee (condyles are unequal) and relative differences in lengths of the two cruciate ligaments.

MECHANISMS OF INJURY

Knee ligament tears are very common injuries amongst sports persons. The following forces can act to disrupt these ligaments during sports injuries:

- Valgus or varus force
- Hyperextension or hyperflexion force
- Rotational force
- Combined forces.

Valgus or Varus Injury to the Knee

Valgus injury to the knee occurs when there is a blow to the outside of the knee **(Fig. 6.36A)**. The tibia is forced outwards with respect to the femur stretching and tearing the MCL, mostly from

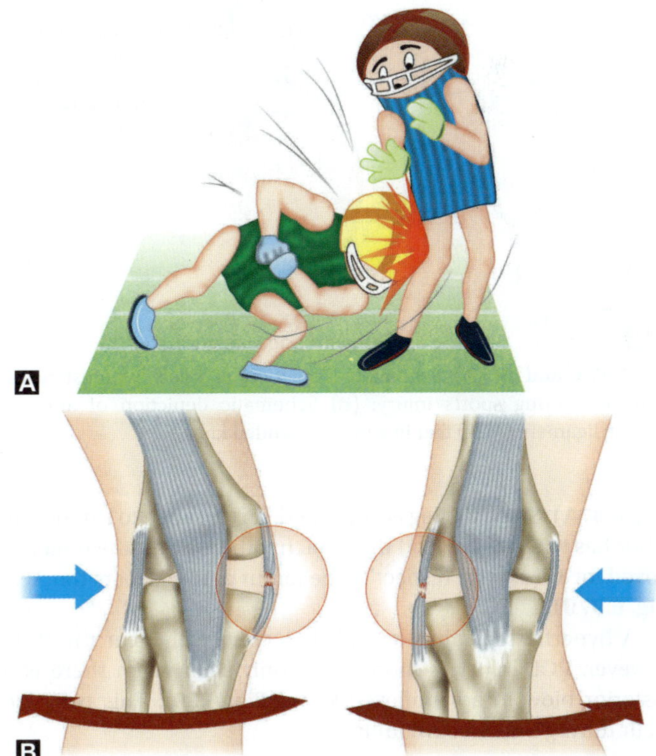

Figs 6.36A and B: (A) Schematic depicting of valgus injury to the right knee (note distal to knee leg going laterally); (B) Diagram depicting torn medial collateral ligament (MCL) in valgus injury and torn lateral collateral ligament (LCL) in varus injury

its femoral attachment **(Fig. 6.36B)**. An exact opposite situation can be expected in a varus injury that would injure the LCL. As the likelihood of varus force is less, LCL is torn less often, especially in isolation.

Hyperextension and Hyperflexion Injury

A hyperextension injury is a very common injury that occurs when a grounded leg gets stuck and knee hyperextends

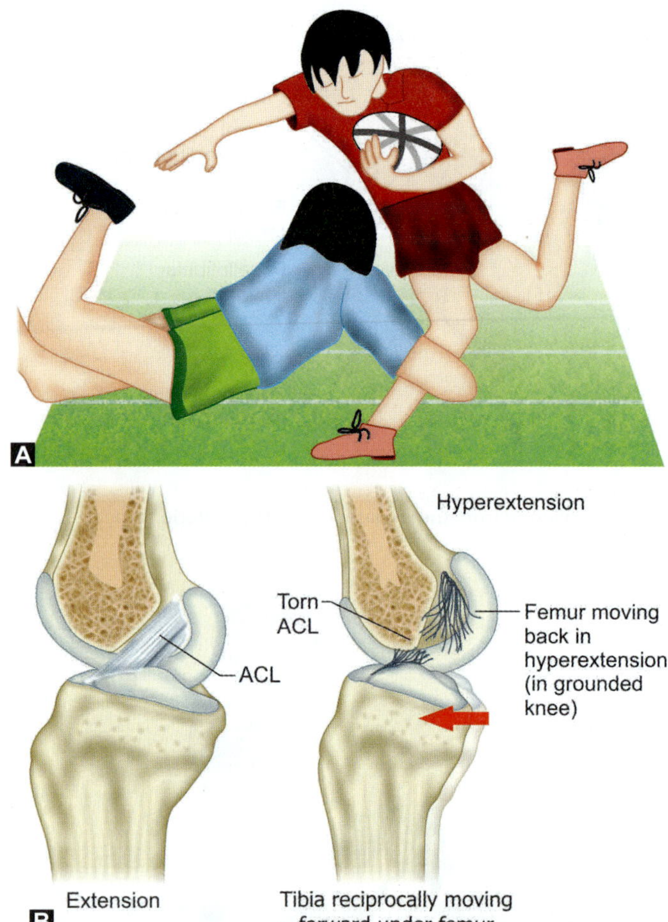

Figs 6.37A and B: (A) Schematic depiction of knee hyperextension occurring during sports injury; (B) Schematic depiction of anterior cruciate ligament (ACL) tear in a hyperextended knee

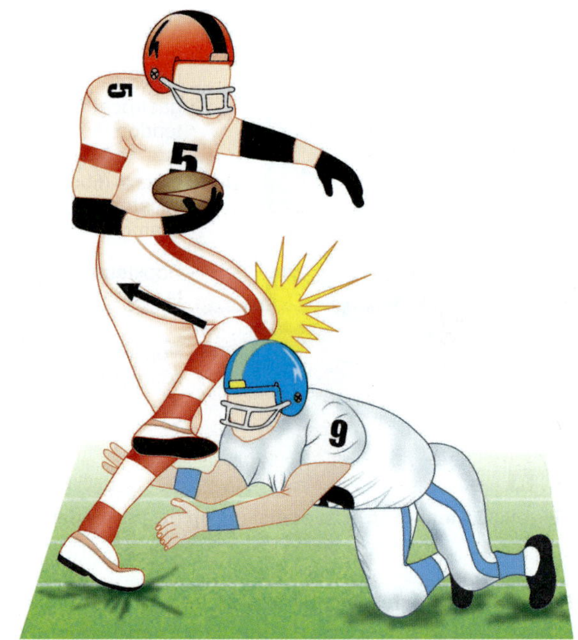

Fig. 6.38: Schematic depiction of posterior cruciate ligament (PCL) injury mechanism

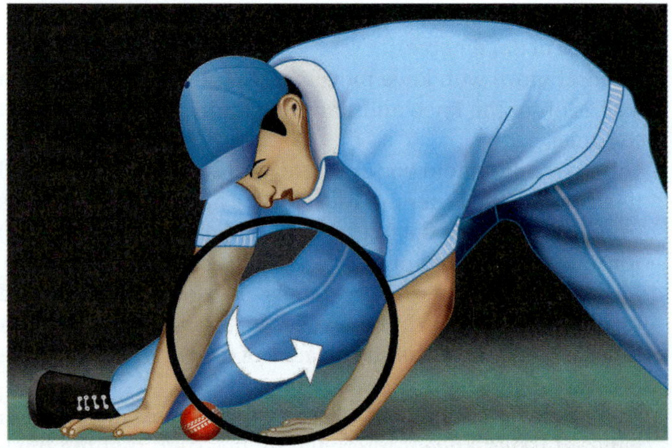

Fig. 6.39: Mechanism involved in producing the unhappy O'Donoghue's triad at the knee. Note as the player loses balance, the femur goes into valgus, flexion and internal rotation (with respect to tibia) to produce a pivoting at knee that ruptures the anterior cruciate ligament (ACL), medial collateral ligament (MCL) and medial meniscus

(Fig. 6.37A). Since the leg is grounded, for the knee to extend the femur has to move back on the tibia. In other words, the tibia has moved forwards with respect to the femur and this tears the ACL **(Fig. 6.37B)**.

A hyperflexion injury would thus conversely, tear the PCL. However, PCL injury is more commonly seen when there is a posterior blow to a semiflexed knee **(Fig. 6.38)**. This can also occur during a dashboard injury.

Rotational Injury to the Knee

When a rotation force is applied to the knee, the menisci are churned in between the rotating condyles tearing them. Hence, in a twisting injury to a semiflexed (rotation is not possible in an extended knee as it is physiologically locked) weight-bearing knee, the meniscus is sucked in and nipped off between femur and tibial condylar surfaces, the medial meniscus tearing much more often than the lateral.

Combined Forces

More commonly in practice the forces that disrupt the knee ligaments tend to act in combination and thus isolated ligament tears are rarely seen. In fact, it is argued that isolated tears reported are cases where the other ligaments have healed up.

Thus, on most occasions the orthopedic surgeon is confronted with different patterns of knee injuries where different forces tend to tear a different set of ligaments. The most common pattern that presents to the orthopedic clinic is the well-known, "O'Donoghue's unhappy triad of knee injury" where the ACL, MCL and the medial meniscus all three are torn simultaneously. It usually occurs when a combination of forces result in valgus, flexion and internal rotation of 'femur on tibia', as when a running athlete abruptly changes his direction **(Fig. 6.39)** leading to a non-contact pivoting (rotation) of the knee. Both MCL and medial meniscus are adherent structures and hence tear out very easily forming a part of this complex.

CLINICAL PRESENTATION

Most patients present with complaints of knee pain and swelling following a knee injury. Swelling is abrupt in case of cruciate ligament tears as there is hemarthrosis from tearing of vessels that stretches the capsule, the most pain sensitive structure in the joint. However, in meniscal tears the swelling appears after a night as it is mainly a synovial reaction to the injury, the menisci primarily being avascular.

When these patients present a few days after the injury, one can inquire about a history of a pop or a click. Often a torn piece of meniscus entrapped in the joint gives a clicking sound on flexion, extension of knee as would occur in climbing up or down the stairs. At times, the torn part is large. It can get trapped in between the condyles restricting the knee from full extension, a condition called locking of the knee. The locking usually gets resolved with subsidence of swelling, but it may occur from time to time, either resolving itself or requiring manipulation by the patient or the doctor.

The patients with cruciate ligament tears tend to have an extra sagittal motion in their knee that can present with a sensation of giving way of the knee. They express a feeling of buckling or instability in the knee (as the knee would dislocate) if they try to run or stress their knees. An indirect way is to inquire the comfort while climbing uphill or downhill. In going downhill one has to put a hyperextended knee on the ground and hence patients with ACL injury are troubled while the reverse occurs in patients with PCL injury.

In patients with any clinical signs suggestive of ligament disruption, a good clinical examination is mandatory.

CLINICAL EXAMINATION

Following clinical tests are done to test the integrity of the knee ligaments.

Testing for Collateral Ligaments

Collateral ligaments are best tested by the stress tests. Examiner keeps one hand on the knee of the patient and with other hand holds the leg to give a varus or valgus stress to the knee. Varus and valgus tests are shown in **Figures 6.40A and B** and the interpretation of these tests is given in **Table 6.5**. Performing the tests at 30° knee flexion relaxes other structures in the knee and one can specifically isolate the testing to the collateral ligaments.

Testing for Cruciate Ligaments

The conventional test for anterior cruciate ligament injury is the anterior drawer test **(Fig. 6.41)** while a more sensitive and a better test is the Lachman test **(Fig. 6.42)**. PCL on the other hand can be tested by the posterior drawer test, by Godfrey's posterior sag or by the Quadriceps active test. A complete description of all the tests is given in **Table 6.6**.

Testing for the Menisci

Although a number of tests are described for meniscal injuries as shown in **Table 6.7** here, the best test for meniscal injury today is considered to be the Joint line tenderness.

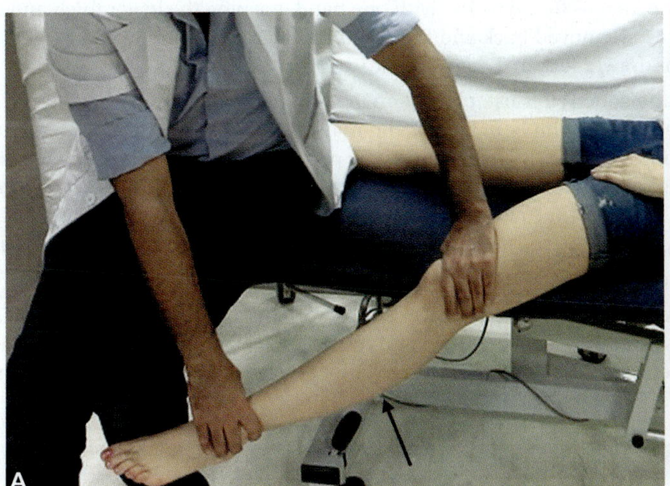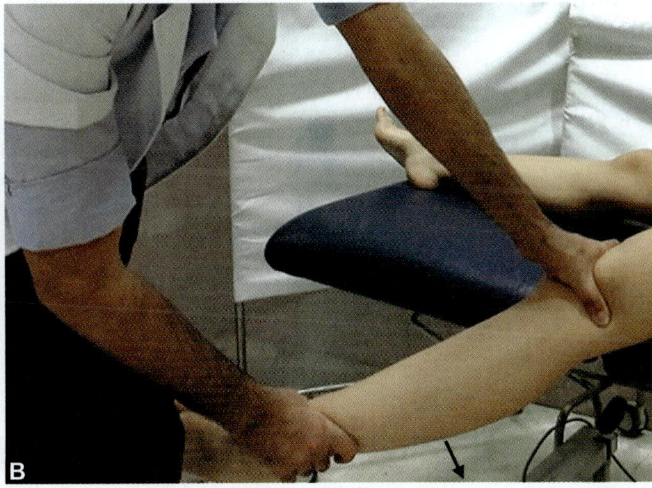

Figs 6.40A and B: (A) Varus stress test; (B) Valgus stress test

Table 6.5: Varus and Valgus stress tests for collateral ligament injury*		
	In 30 degree knee flexion	*In full knee extension*
Varus stress test **(Fig. 6.40A)**	If lateral joint opening occurs, it indicates LCL injury	If lateral joint opening occurs, it indicates PLC and PCL injury in addition to LCL injury
Valgus stress test **(Fig. 6.40B)**	If medial joint opening occurs, it indicates MCL injury	If medial joint opening occurs, it indicates concomitant posteromedial capsule, posterior oblique ligament (POL) and PCL injury in addition to MCL injury

More than 10 mm opening, indicates a complete tear of a ligament.

Abbreviations: LCL, lateral collateral ligament; PCL, posterolateral corner ligaments; MCL, medial collateral ligament.

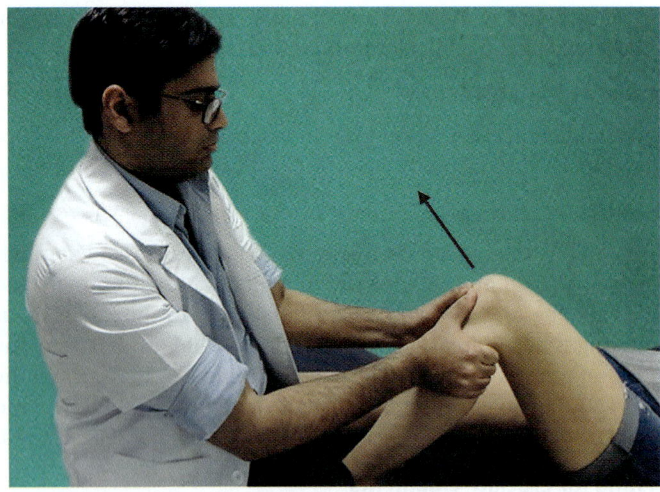

Fig. 6.41: Anterior drawer test for anterior cruciate ligament (ACL) injury

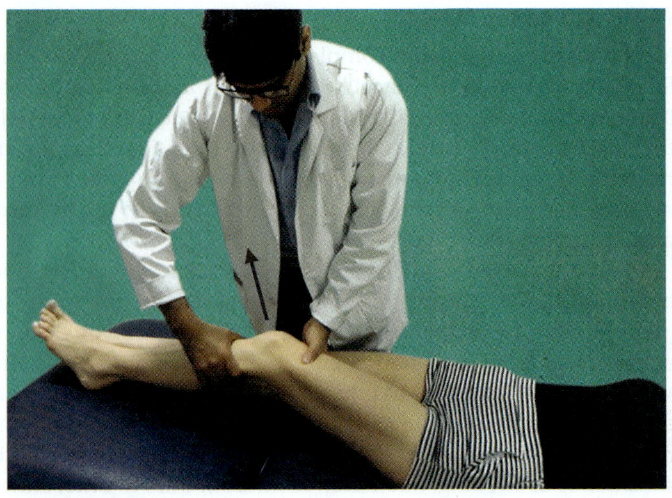

Fig. 6.42: Lachman's test for anterior cruciate ligament (ACL) injury

Table 6.6: Testing for the cruciate ligaments

Test for ligament injury

Anterior drawer test **(Fig. 6.41)**	With the knee flexed to 90° and feet resting on the couch (it is useful to sit on the foot of the patient to prevent the feet sliding forward), the examiner grasps the upper tibia with both hands, and making sure the hamstrings are relaxed, pushes the upper tibia anteriorly. Up to 3 mm of forward movement of the tibia is considered normal. The Grading for the test is: Grade 1 = 5 mm, Grade 2 = 5 to 10 mm, Grade 3 > 10 mm The anterior drawer test has low sensitivity, especially after an acute injury (with large swelling in the knee) as flexion of knee to 90° results in protective spasm of the hamstring muscles that alter the results. Also, the posterior horns of the menisci block the anterior translation (acting as "door stoppers") when knee is in 90° flexion. Hence, more sensitive way of testing for ACL is at 20° knee flexion, i.e. Lachman's test
Lachman test **(Fig. 6.42)**	This test was originally described by JS Torg. The knee is flexed to 20°, with one hand grasping the lower thigh and the other the upper part of the leg; the joint surfaces are moved back and forth. If the ACL is torn there would be gliding. Lachman test is more sensitive than the anterior drawer test, in diagnosing ACL tears
Posterior drawer test **(Fig. 6.43)**	With the knee flexed to 90° and feet resting on the couch (it is useful to sit on the foot of the patient to prevent the feet sliding backwards), the examiner grasps the upper tibia with both hands, and making sure the hamstrings are relaxed, pushes the upper tibia posteriorly. If the tibia glides posteriorly against the femur posterior drawer test is positive. Grade I is when the tibia slides posteriorly but still anterior to femur, in grade II anteromedial tibial plateau flushes with femoral condyle and grade III is when tibial plateau goes posteriorly to femoral condyle
Godfrey's posterior sag **(Fig. 6.44)**	The hips and knees of both limbs are flexed to 90° and both the limbs are suspended by holding them by the toes. If PCL of any side is torn, the leg on that side sags posteriorly
Quadriceps active test	In PCL tears, at 90° of knee flexion, when viewed from the side, backwards displacement of the upper tibia is visible (Posterior Sag). In this position, the examiner's hand supports the thigh and resists knee extension by keeping a hand at the ankle. The patient is then told to actively contract the quadriceps. A posterior sag caused by torn PCL is corrected when the quadriceps contracts

Table 6.7: Tests for meniscal injuries

McMurray's test **(Figs 6.45A and B)**	With the patient supine, and the knee is acutely flexed, grasp the heel in one hand. Place the other hand, over the knee, with the thumb and fingers on the joint line. Gently externally rotate the tibia **(Figs 6.45A and B)** and passively extend the leg from flexion. A palpable painful clicking at the medial joint line is considered a positive test for medial meniscus tear. For lateral meniscus tear internally rotate the leg while extending the knee. Painful clicking along the lateral joint line is considered to be a positive test
Apley's test **(Fig. 6.46A)**	With the patient prone the knee is flexed to 90° and rotated while applying a compression force, if symptoms are reproduced meniscal tear is present. (Apley's grinding test) The same maneuver is now repeated, but with leg pulled up (thigh pressed down with other hand), if symptoms are reproduced ligament tear is present (Apley's distraction test)
Thessaly test **(Fig. 6.46B)**	In this test patient is asked to stand on test leg with knee 5° flexion (other leg is in the air with flexed knee). The patient may hold the hands of the examiner for balance during the test. Now patient rotates the knee and the body medially and laterally three times. The same test is now repeated in 20° knee flexion. A positive test is indicated by joint line discomfort or locking/catching sensation. This test is claimed to have a high diagnostic accuracy (in 20° flexion) and is being used as a first-line screening test. This test reproduces the active dynamic loading of the knee joint

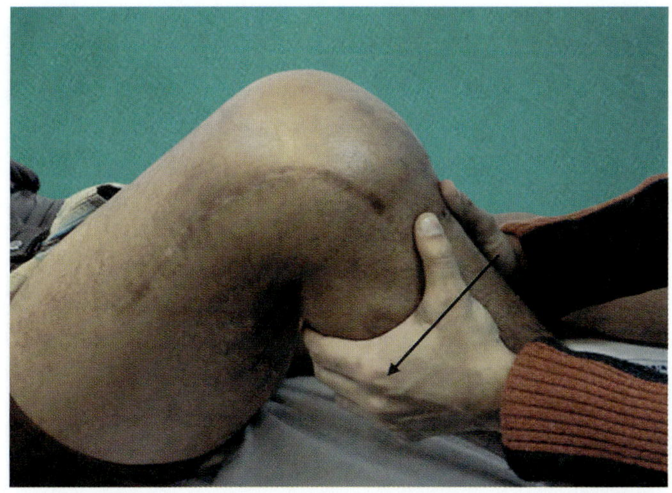

Fig. 6.43: Posterior drawer test for posterior cruciate ligament (PCL) tear

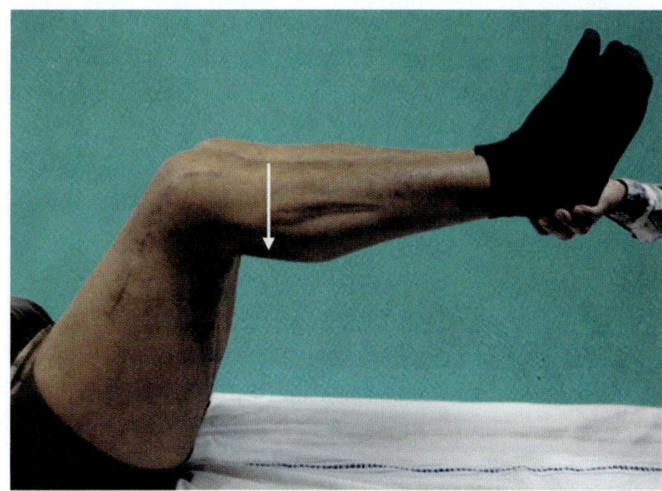

Fig. 6.44: Godfrey's posterior sag

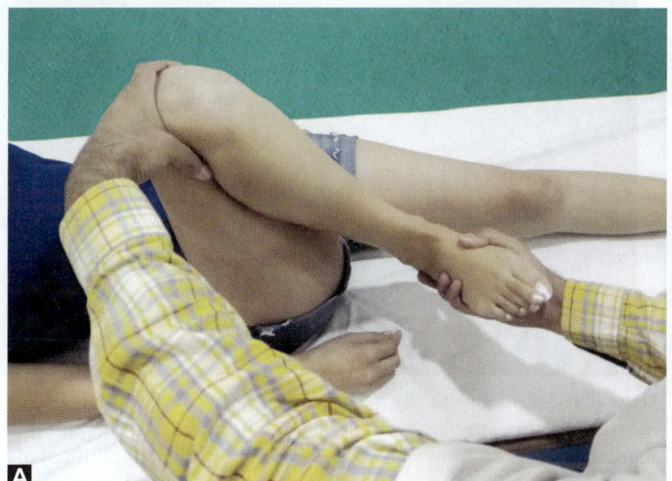

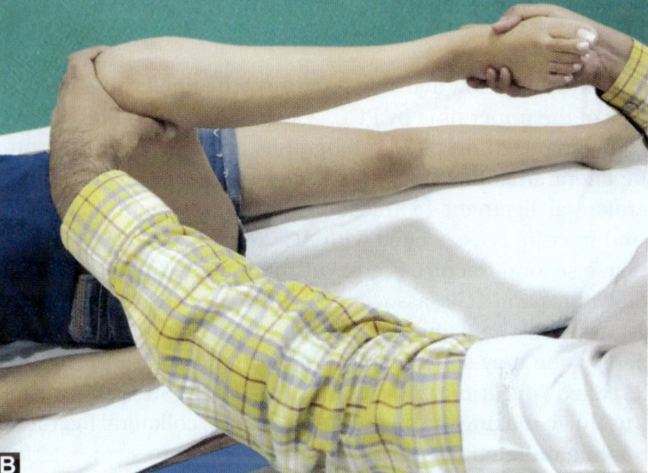

Figs 6.45A and B: Mcmurray's test for medial meniscus. For lateral meniscus tear internally rotate the leg

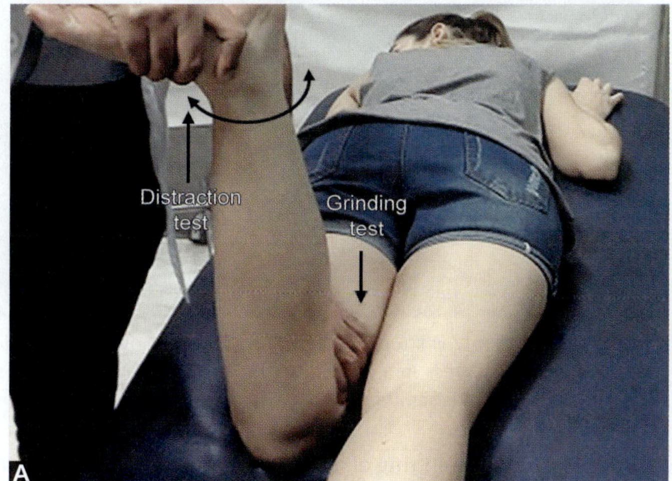

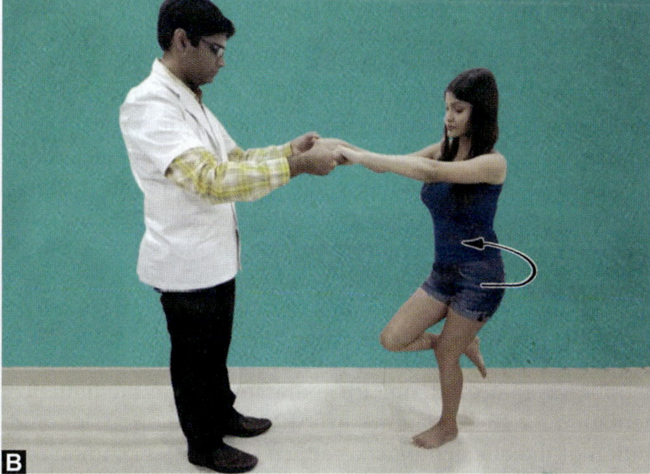

Figs 6.46A and B: (A) Apley's test; (B) Thessaly's test

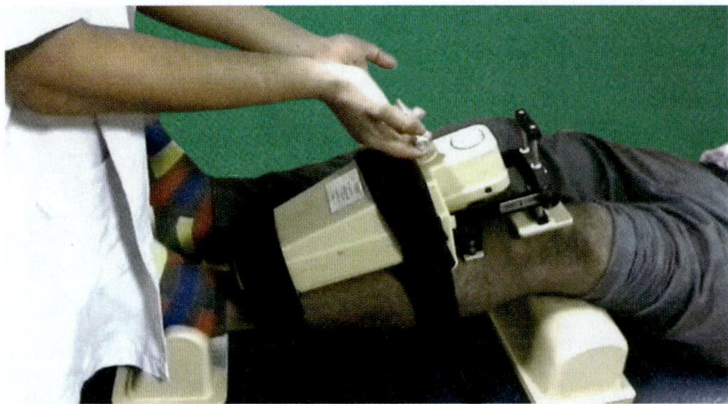

Fig. 6.47: KT-1000 arthrometer being used to quantify anterior translation in a patient with ACL tear

Knee Ligament Arthrometry

Arthrometers are special equipment that are capable of quantifying the amount of laxity. KT-1000 **(Fig. 6.47)** and KT-2000 are commonly used to measure anterior tibial translation in millimeters in cases of suspected ACL tear to support clinical diagnosis.

IMAGING

Plain X-rays may show avulsion fracture of the tibial spine by ACL or back of the upper tibia by PCL. A segond fracture **(Fig. 6.48A)** can be recognized on plain radiographs as an avulsion fracture of the lateral proximal tibia. It is actually a bony avulsion of the anterolateral ligament (a thickening in anterolateral capsule). Segond fracture is associated with ACL tear in 75–100% of cases. A reverse segond fracture is an avulsion fracture of the proximal medial tibia, and it is associated with PCL tear. It is actually avulsion of tibial attachment of deep MCL. In chronic cases of MCL tear one may spot calcification at the femoral insertion of MCL, called Pellegrini Stieda lesion **(Fig. 6.48B)**. Stress X-rays are very useful in making the diagnosis of PCL and collateral ligament tear. While radiography posterior stress is given to see posterior displacement of the tibia and valgus/varus stress is given to see medial and lateral opening of the knee joint on X-ray **(Fig. 6.49)**.

The imaging modality of choice (IOC) is the MRI **(Figs 6.50A and B)**. However, arthroscopic evaluation of the knee is considered the gold standard for diagnosing intra-articular, knee ligament tears (but it is not IOC as it is invasive) and the final treatment decision is based on that. However, the diagnosis of PCL tear is mainly based on the clinical examination (positive posterior drawer test). Best time to prescribe an MRI for suspected ligament and cartilage injury of the knee is in the acute setting, because blood in the joint provides a good contrast making identification easier, however, with progression of healing and resolution of edema injuries become less conspicuous.

MANAGEMENT

The patients who present with acute knee injuries tend to be in pain and an examination is often difficult. In such a situation a wise option is to institute the RICE therapy (rest to the limb, ice fomentation for 15–20 minutes every 2 hours, compression and elevation of the affected part to reduce swelling). Lachman test is particularly useful to reach a diagnosis in the acute setting, as it requires only 20° of knee flexion which is attainable in acutely

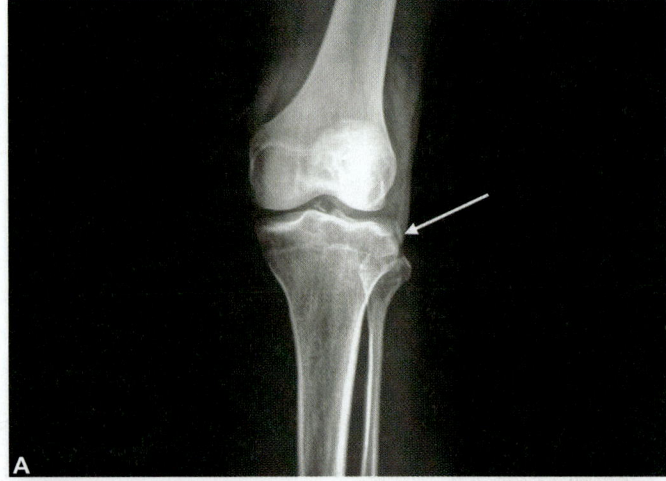

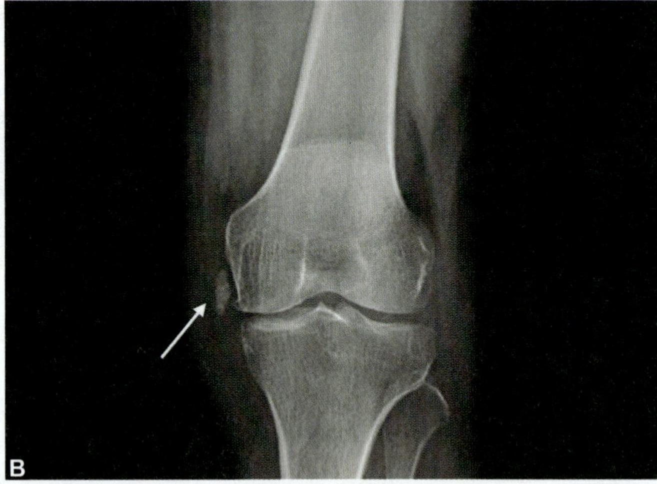

Figs 6.48A and B: (A) X-ray showing Segond fracture where the ACL is torn in the intercondylar area and a chip of bone (anterolateral ligament avulsion from tibia) has avulsed from the lateral tibial plateau (arrow); (B) X-ray knee showing calcification at the femoral attachment of medial collateral ligament (MCL) (Pellegrini Stieda lesion) (arrow)

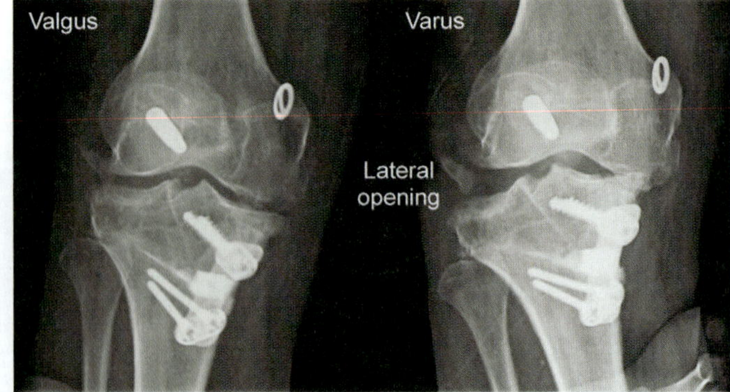

Fig. 6.49: Varus-valgus stress radiographs of knee showing lateral joint opening on varus stress in a patient with tear of LCL (*Note:* Side to side difference of >3 mm is significant)

injured knee in the setting of a knee hemarthrosis. Once pain and swelling subside, the patient can be re-examined. Once clinico-radiological diagnosis is made further management is based on it.

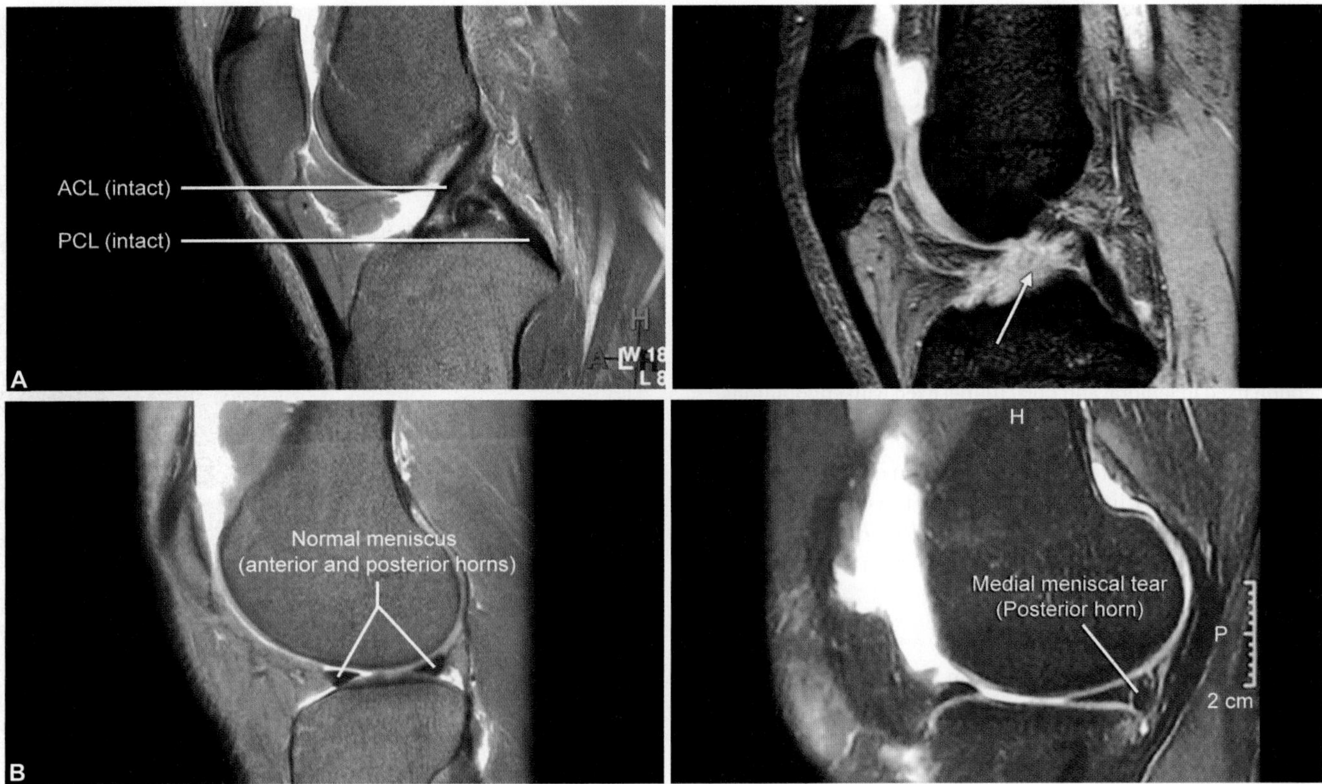

Figs 6.50A and B: (A) MRI showing intact (A1) and torn (A2) ACL; (B) MRI showing normal (B1) and torn (B2) meniscus

Collateral Ligament Tears

Most isolated collateral ligament injuries, particularly the MCL injury heal excellently with conservative treatment only. Knee is braced and the patient is instructed for protected weight bearing with crutches. Once the pain improves, ROM exercises are started. When patient gains full ROM crutches are discarded (usually in 4–6 weeks). A surgical repair (end to end suture) or reconstruction (avulsion fixation using suture anchors or reconstruction using an autogenous graft) is indicated in nonhealing complete tears of MCL or when the ligament is avulsed with a bony chip from femur or when there is a 'stener type' lesion (*see* Page 178) of MCL (tear of MCL from tibia with interposition of pes anserinus tendons). Lateral collateral ligament tears occurring in association with ACL or PCL tears are also mostly managed operatively.

Cruciate Ligament Tears

Partial ACL tears are managed conservatively. The knee is kept in a long brace and partial weight bearing is allowed with an ambulatory aid gradually progressing to full weight bearing. With dedicated physiotherapy the patient usually returns to sports by 6–8 weeks. Both hamstring and quadriceps exercises are advised in the rehabilitation of a torn ACL. Although quadriceps is an antagonist to ACL (as it pulls tibia anteriorly on contraction), but its atrophy sets in very rapidly after ACL tear so its strengthening exercises are also important. Isolated complete tears of the ACL in athletes should be managed by early (once knee is clinically silent and ROM > 0–90°) arthroscopic reconstruction (reconstruction refers to replacement of the torn ligament with a tendon graft), however, in old aged population and non-sports persons a trial

of neuromuscular rehabilitation (knee brace, quadriceps and hamstring exercises) may be given. Those who complain of residual instability after conservative management are then managed by arthroscopic ACL reconstruction.

Isolated partial PCL tears (grade I/II posterior drawer) are given a conservative trial. Patients with a complete PCL tear (grade III posterior drawer), patients complaining of instability after conservative management and patients having PCL tear in association with another ligament tear (e.g. PCL tear with postero-lateral corner injury) need arthroscopic PCL reconstruction.

Arthroscopic cruciate ligament reconstruction: In arthroscopic cruciate ligament reconstruction tendon grafts are harvested from the patient (most commonly hamstrings, i.e. semitendinosus and gracilis, less commonly part of quadriceps or patellar tendons) and fixed in tibial and femoral tunnels with screws (interference screws, *see* Page 493) and buttons (endobuttons) to replace the native ligament **(Fig. 6.51)**.

Meniscal Tears

Although meniscal tears are mostly seen in young patients who sustain a twisting injury to the knee, meniscal tears become more prevalent with age due to degenerative changes in the ageing meniscus. Underlying pathology in a meniscus, such as a discoid meniscus (more common on lateral side, read later) or a meniscal cyst (most commonly seen in posterior horn of lateral meniscus) also makes it more prone to injury.

Medial meniscus is less mobile due to its peripheral capsular attachment and attachment to MCL. Also popliteus sends few fibers into the posterior margin of the lateral meniscus, thus

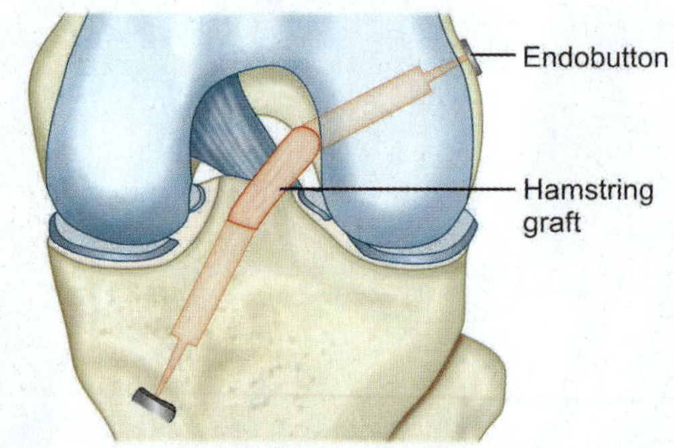

Fig. 6.51: Anterior cruciate ligament (ACL) reconstruction—hamstring tendon fixed in femoral and tibial tunnel fixed with endobuttons

withdrawing it posterolaterally during flexion of the knee, thereby preventing it from getting caught between the condyles of femur and tibia. Hence, overall medial meniscal tears (particularly of posterior horn) are much more common than lateral meniscal tears.

Classification of Meniscal Tears

Meniscal tears are classified based on tear pattern or by their proximity to the blood supply.

1. *Based on tear pattern:* Various tear patterns have been described in **Table 6.8**. Longitudinal tears are the most common variety and are mostly seen in posterior horn of medial meniscus. Lateral meniscus more commonly sustains radial tears.

2. *Based on blood supply pattern:* Only the peripheral 10–30% of the meniscus is vascularized (red-red zone) and has pain fibers. Meniscal tears can also be classified by their proximity to the meniscal blood supply, namely, whether they are located in the "red-red," "red-white," or "white-white" zones **(Fig. 6.52)**. A peripheral meniscal tear in the red-red zone has the maximum healing chances whereas central meniscal tear in the white-white zone almost never heals.

Treatment

Peripheral tears in a red-red zone may heal by conservative therapy. Other tears rarely heal due to poor vascularity and need to be treated surgically.

Following surgical options are available:

a. *Meniscus repair:* Acute (< 6 weeks old) and simple meniscal tears, in the peripheral zone (red-red and red-white) can be repaired by suturing (stitching) the torn pieces together.

b. *Arthroscopic meniscectomy:* A degenerative tear, complex tear or a tear in the inner margin of the meniscus (white-white zone) is not amenable to repair and is trimmed away. Depending on the size of tear meniscectomy may be partial or subtotal.

ROTATORY INSTABILITIES OF KNEE

Just as in the shoulder, instability can also exist at the knee. In patients with chronic ligament tears, over time the capsule and the surrounding ligaments get stretched and knee develops abnormal motion in various planes which, if untreated leads to abrasion of cartilage and the development of early arthritis.

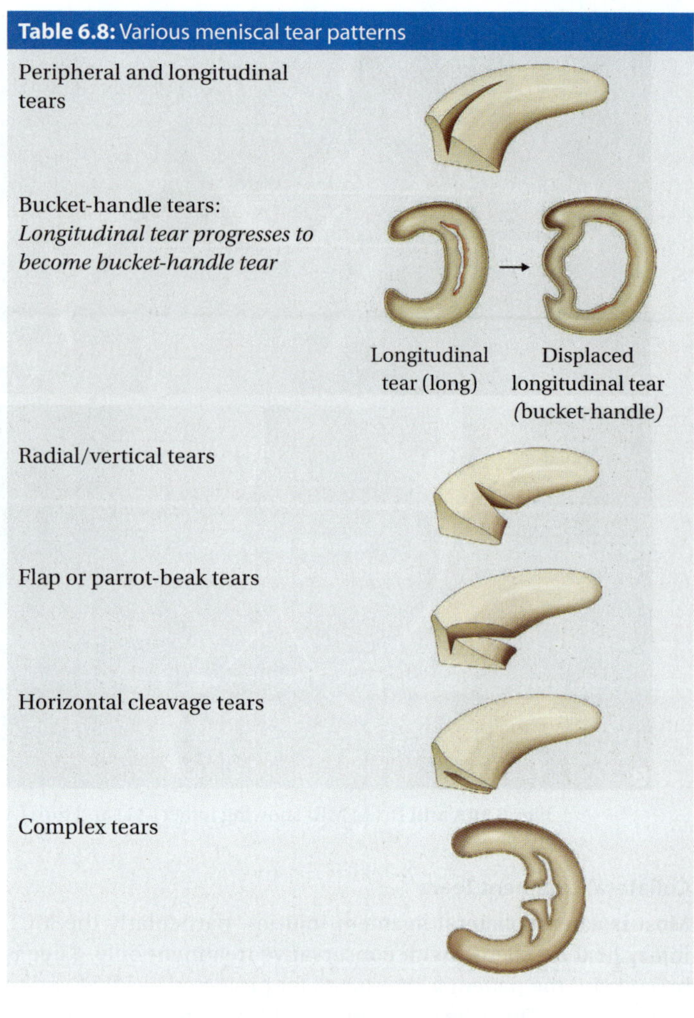

Table 6.8: Various meniscal tear patterns	
Peripheral and longitudinal tears	
Bucket-handle tears: *Longitudinal tear progresses to become bucket-handle tear*	Longitudinal tear (long) Displaced longitudinal tear (bucket-handle)
Radial/vertical tears	
Flap or parrot-beak tears	
Horizontal cleavage tears	
Complex tears	

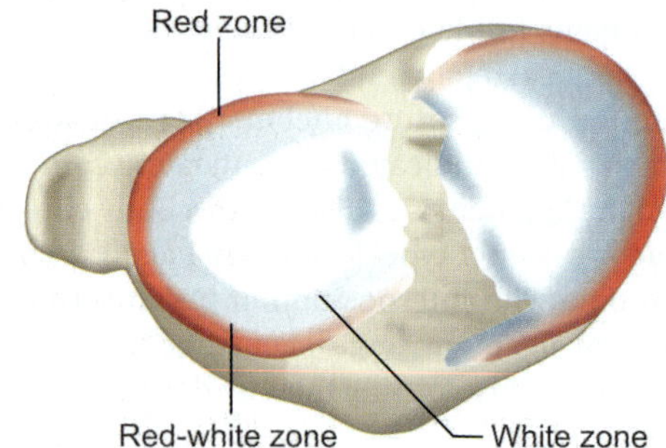

Fig. 6.52: Zones of meniscus according to blood supply

Important rotatory instabilities that can exist at the knee are the anterolateral (most common) and the posterolateral instability. The former is tested by the Pivot shift test while the latter can be detected by the Dial test or a reverse Pivot shift test (*see* **Table 6.9** for details of the test).

DISCOID MENISCUS

Discoid meniscus, i.e. disk shaped meniscus is the most common meniscal variant **(Fig. 6.54)**. It is almost exclusively seen on the lateral side. In this condition the meniscus is disk-like (rather than being wedge shaped). Due to its abnormal shape discoid meniscus is more prone to tearing. Discoid lateral menisci are classified into three types—Type I or complete is stable as it has normal tibial attachments, and spans the entire lateral tibial plateau; Type II or incomplete type also has normal tibial attachments, but covers less than 80% of the lateral tibial plateau; Type III (or Wrisberg variant) is rare. It is a most unstable type because it lacks a posterior meniscotibial (coronary) ligament and has only one posterior attachment, the posterior meniscofemoral ligament, or Wrisberg's ligament. Wrisberg variant meniscus is hyper mobile, tears often and can cause the snapping knee syndrome due to its hypermobility.

ARTICULAR CARTILAGE INJURIES

Articular cartilage (a hyaline cartilage) is smooth and glistening tissue that covers the articulating ends of bones and allows them

to glide over each other with very little friction. It can be damaged by injury or normal wear and tear. While the latter is mostly an irreparable diffuse damage, the former is generally a focal lesion and often reparable. Patients with traumatic cartilage injuries present with pain in knee and tenderness can often be localized to the site. Point of tenderness shifts with the condylar movement as opposed to meniscal injuries where tenderness remains

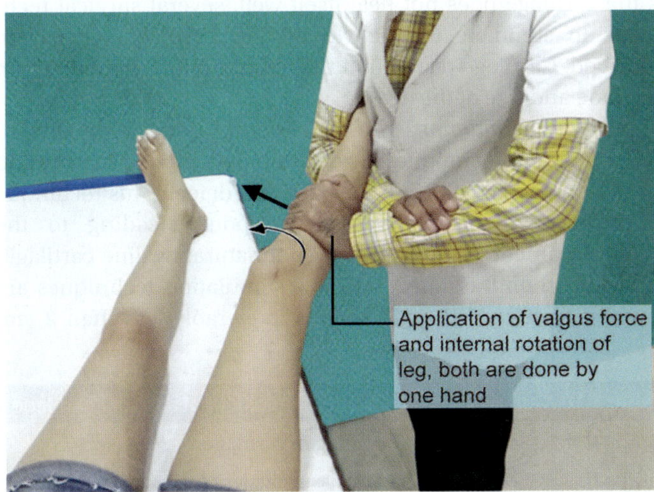

Fig. 6.53A: Easy method of doing Pivot shift test

Table 6.9: Tests for rotatory instabilities of knee	
Pivot shift test **(Fig. 6.53A)**	With the patient supine, and knee fully extended the examiner lifts the leg and internally rotates the tibia. The knee is gradually flexed along with application of valgus force. A sudden posterior movement of the tibia is seen and felt as the joint is fully relocated. The test is quite painful and is therefore performed under anesthesia. A positive test is suggestive of anterolateral instability (signifies torn ACL, LCL and lateral capsular laxity/tear)
Reverse Pivot shift test	The same as a pivot shift test, but the tibia is externally rotated. A positive test is suggestive of posterolateral instability (signifies torn PCL and the PLC structures of the knee)
Dial test **(Fig. 6.53B)**	With the leg dangling over the edge of the couch, one hand of the examiner stabilizes the distal femur and the other hand holds the heels. The examiner flexes the knee to 30°, and externally rotates the leg maximally, holding it through the heel, and notes the position of the tibial tuberosity. Same maneuver is repeated on the other side. If external rotation is more by 15° as compared to the other side, a posterolateral corner injury (PLC) is suspected The test is repeated with the knee flexed further to 90°. Increased external rotation indicates (as compared to 30°) concomitant PLC with PCL injury

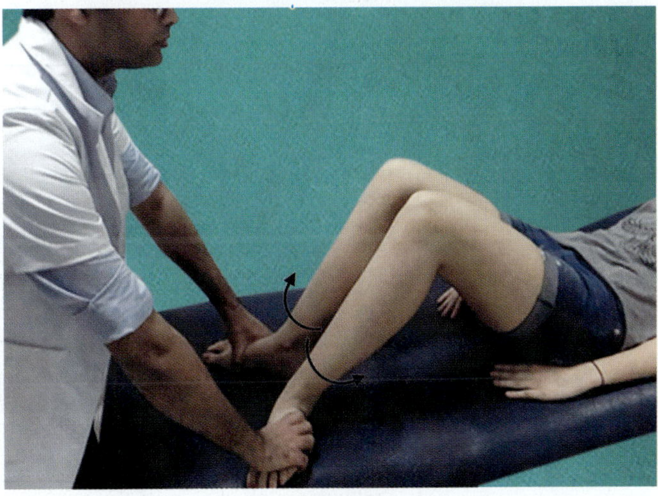

Fig. 6.53B: Dial test

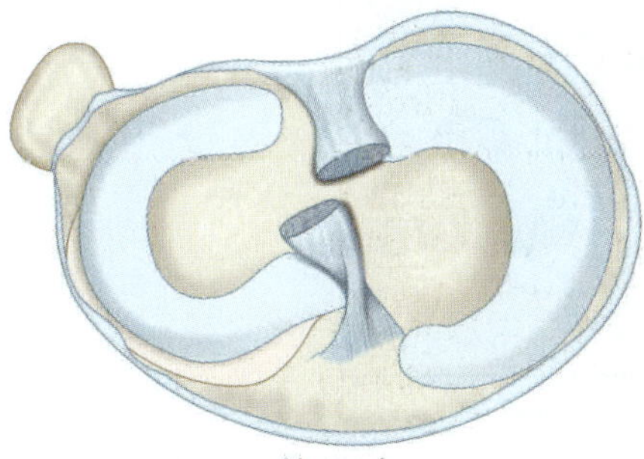

Normal

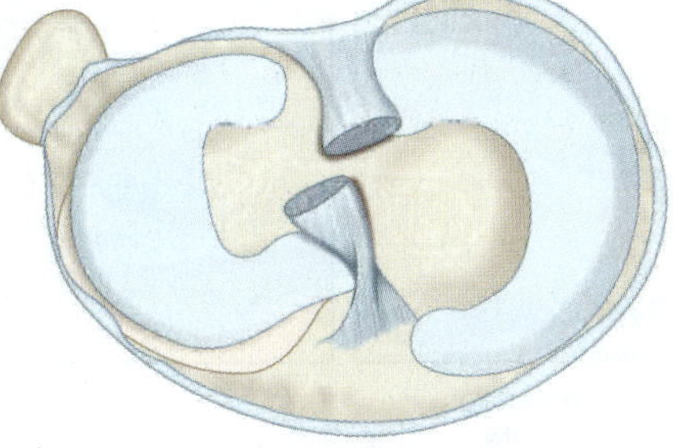

Incomplete

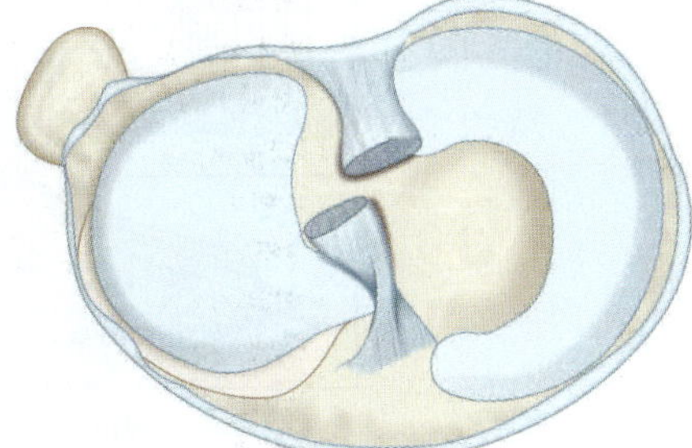

Complete

Fig. 6.54: Discoid meniscus

localized to posterior joint line. Rarely these patients may have symptoms of locking when the cartilage fragment lies as a loose body in the joint. MRI (specifically with gadolinium enhanced cartilage mapping) may pick up some lesions but arthroscopy is the investigation of choice and the gold standard for classification **(Table 6.10)**, diagnosis as well as treatment of chondral lesions.

Management

As the cartilage does not heal itself well, several surgical techniques to stimulate the growth of new cartilage have been described. Cartilage restoration treatment options depend upon the grade and size of the defect.

- *Marrow stimulation*: The subchondral bone is penetrated by different techniques to release blood, growth factors and mesenchymal cells into the chondral defect. This technique produces a healing vascular response leading to the development of fibrocartilage (not natural hyaline cartilage) in the chondral defect. Marrow stimulation techniques are used for Grade II or III lesions, preferably less than 2 cm² in size. They are used in larger lesions only in low demand population. Following techniques are in practice:
  - *Abrasion chondroplasty*: Motorized burr is used to remove 1–3 mm of subchondral bone.
  - *Subchondral drilling*: Motorized smooth wire is used to perform subchondral drilling.
  - *Microfracture technique (current preferred method)*: In this method an arthroscopic tapered awl perforates the subchondral bone at sites least 2–3 mm apart.
- *Osteochondral grafting*: Cartilage transfer procedure that involves moving healthy cartilage from an area of the knee that is nonweight bearing to a damaged weight-bearing cartilage area of the knee **(Fig. 6.55)**. The two procedures for this are—mosaicplasty and osteochondral autograft transfer system (OATS®). In mosaicplasty, multiple tiny dowel shaped plugs of healthy cartilage and bone are taken from a healthy cartilage area and moved to replace the damaged cartilage area of the knee. Since multiple tiny plugs used, once embedded, give a mosaic pattern, hence the name.

Table 6.10: Outerbridge classification (modified) of articular cartilage injury

Grade I	Softening and swelling of cartilage
Grade II	Fragmentation and fissuring, less than 50% of cartilage thickness
Grade III	Fragmentation and fissuring, greater than 50% of cartilage thickness
Grade IV	Full thickness cartilage loss with exposed subchondral bone

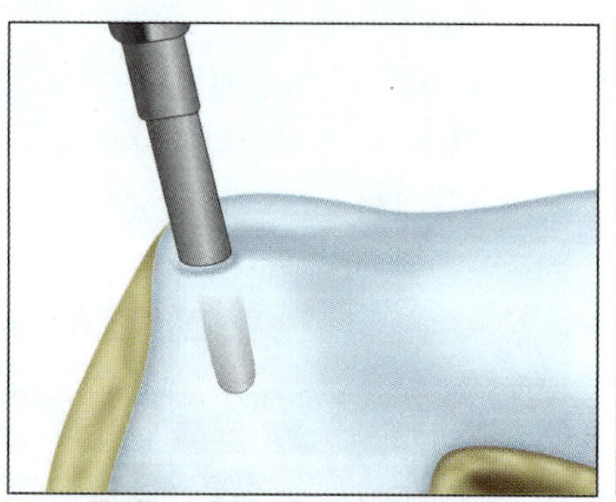
Graft are taken from a nonweight bearing part of the cartilage

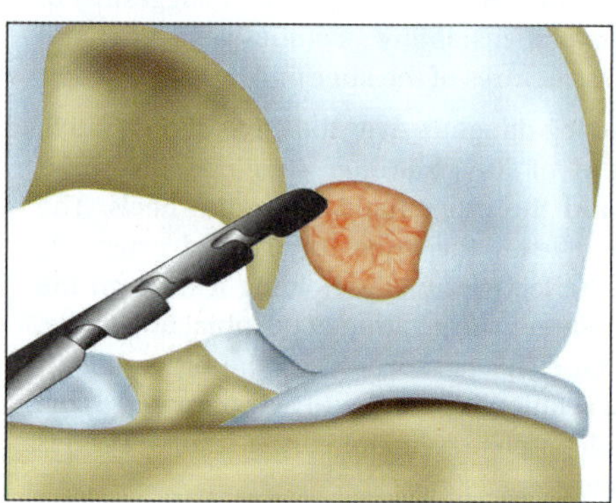
Holes drilled at defect site

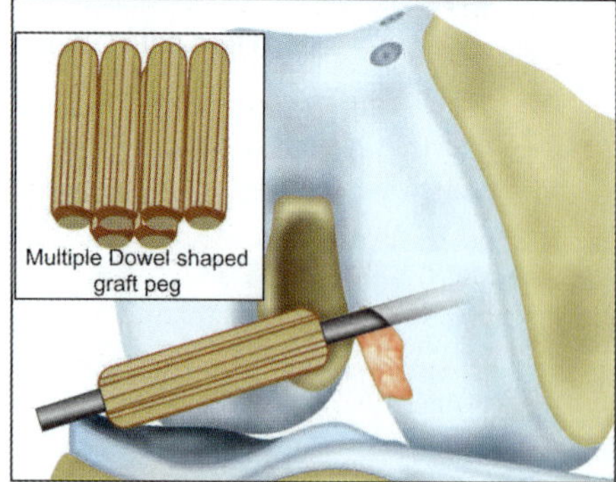

Dowel-shaped graft peg inserted at hole at chondral lesion site

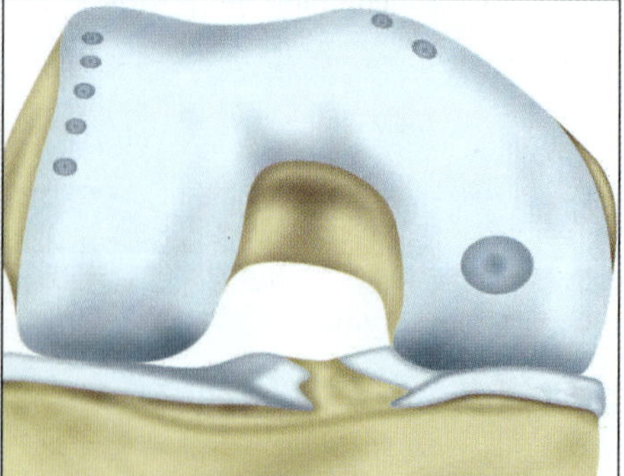
Lesion and donor sites

Fig. 6.55: Osteochondral autograft transplantation surgery (OATS®)

With OATS® procedure, the plugs are larger. Therefore, the surgeon only needs to move one or two plugs of healthy cartilage and bone to the damaged area of the knee. Full thickness defects (grade IV) of 1–2.5 cm² are ideal for osteochondral grafting when autograft is to be used while with availability of allografts, grade IV defects of up to 5 cm² can be grafted.

- *Autologous chondrocyte implantation (ACI)*: This articular resurfacing method is the first and only technique that uses true tissue engineering. The procedure requires two surgeries. During the first, the articular lesion is evaluated and normal host articular cartilage is harvested and cultured. The second procedure involves implanting the cultured cells into the chondral defect. Large grade IV osteochondral defects (2–10 cm²) can be treated by ACI.

LOOSE BODIES IN THE KNEE JOINT

A loose body is a free floating piece made of bone or cartilage or it can be a foreign object in a joint. The knee is the most common site for loose bodies. They can cause catching and locking (pseudo locking) sensation in the joint. Causes of loose bodies are as follows:

- *Osteoarthritis*: Most common cause of loose body in the knee joint.
- *Osteochondritis dissecans*: Most common cause of loose body in the knee joint in adolescents and young population.
- *Synovial chondromatosis*: Most common cause of multiple cartilaginous loose bodies.
- Charcot's joint.
- Trauma or iatrogenic injury leading to an osteochondral fracture.

Treatment, of symptomatic loose body, is arthroscopic removal.

HIGH-YIELD POINTS

- The most pain sensitive structure in the joint is the capsule and least pain sensitive structure in the joint is the articular cartilage.
- Internal derangement of knee is a vague term that is used sometimes by the clinicians to refer to ligament injuries of the knee.
- The most common meniscus tear associated with ACL tear at the time of initial injury is lateral meniscus, though in the chronic cases medial meniscus is torn more often than the lateral meniscus due to abnormal loading on medial side in the ACL deficient knee.
- Although medial meniscus tears are more common, a meniscal cyst and a discoid meniscus (that increase chance of meniscal tear) are much more commonly seen in lateral meniscus.
- Meniscal cysts clinically appear as swellings along the posterior joint line which disappear within the joint on knee flexion (Pisani sign).
- The best clinical test for meniscal injury is considered to be joint line tenderness, but recently Thessaly test has been shown to have high sensitivity and specificity in diagnosing meniscal tear. Other less commonly used tests for meniscal injuries are duck walk test, Payr's test and Helfet test.

- Bounce home test of the knee was earlier used to look for meniscal tear. The knee is flexed and allowed to fall and the endpoint is noted. The endpoint is firm (tear) or soft (intact) but never empty.
- Physiological locking refers to internal rotation of femur over a fixed/grounded tibia in extended knee. Unlocking occurs when popliteus externally rotates the femur and knee can then flex. However, in orthopedics, locking (pathological) refers to the restriction of terminal few degrees of extension of the knee. It can occur due to a torn meniscus (most common), loose bodies in the knee, osteochondral fractures and from fractured osteophytes lying in the joint.
- MCL followed by ACL is the most commonly injured knee ligament but most commonly operated knee ligament is the ACL (as most MCL injuries heal conservatively).
- ACL tears most commonly in the mid-substance while PCL tears more commonly from its femoral attachment.
- ACL injuries are more common in female athletes than male athletes due to smaller size of intercondylar notch, hormonal influences and increased ligamentous laxity.
- The most sensitive clinical test for an ACL injury is the Lachman test while the most specific test is the Pivot shift test (when the Pivot shift test is positive, ACL injury is must exist).
- PCL injury is often associated with injury of posterolateral corner ligaments of the knee. The clinical test to detect both these injuries is the Dial test.
- Investigation of choice for knee ligament injury is MRI (gold standard is arthroscopy) but for cartilage injury is arthroscopy.
- The ligament best seen on MRI is the PCL.
- Double PCL sign on MRI is seen in the presence of a bucket handle tear of the meniscus and not PCL tear.
- The grafts usually harvested for cruciate ligament reconstruction are the hamstring tendons (gracilis and semitendinosus) or part of the patellar tendon. The latter is harvested along with small chip of bone from the attachment site to enhance fixation and hence called bone-patellar tendon-bone graft.
- The most common tendon graft used in orthopedics is semitendinosus.
- The femoral attachments of cruciate ligaments are rich in mechanoreceptors involved in joint proprioception; hence in reconstruction of these ligaments the native ligament stump should preferably be preserved.
- Celery stalk appearance is seen on MRI in cases of chronic ACL tears (due to mucoid degeneration) while a celery stalk metaphysis is seen on X-ray in cases of congenital rubella.
- Multiligament knee injuries are defined as a disruption of at least 2 of the 4 (ACL, PCL, MCL, LCL) major knee ligaments as a result of trauma.
- ACL tear followed by dislocated patella are the most common causes of hemarthrosis in the knee joint.
- Fluid (effusion) in the knee joint can be tested by following tests:
  - Bulge sign (positive with even 4–8 mL of fluid)
  - Patellar tap
  - Ballottement of patella.

ANKLE INJURIES IN SPORTS

RELEVANT ANATOMY

Three groups of ligaments (medial, lateral and syndesmosis) play a fundamental role in providing stability to the ankle (tibiotalar) and subtalar (talo-calcaneal) joint. Lateral ligament complex **(Fig. 6.56A)** consists of the anterior talofibular ligament (ATFL), posterior talofibular ligament (PTFL), and calcaneofibular ligament (CFL). The medial ankle joint is stabilized by deltoid ligament complex (medial ligament complex). Deltoid ligament is the strongest ankle ligament and consists of two parts, superficial (crosses both ankle and subtalar joint) and deep (crosses only ankle joint). The superficial part consists of tibiocalcaneal, tibionavicular, posterior superficial tibiotalar and tibiospring ligaments. The deep part consists of anterior tibiotalar and posterior deep tibiotalar ligaments **(Fig. 6.56B)**. Syndesmosis between distal tibiofibular joint consists of anteroinferior tibiofibular ligament (AITFL), posteroinferior tibiofibular ligament (PITFL), transverse tibiofibular ligaments (TTFL), the interosseous ligament and the interosseous membrane. Anatomy is not consistent and all structures are not always present.

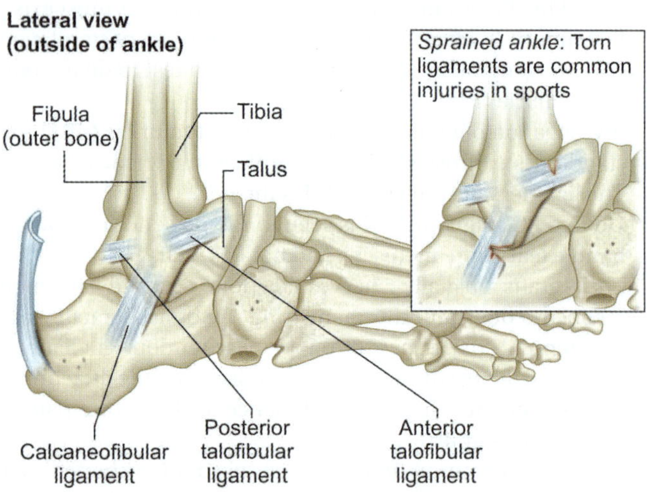

Fig. 6.56A: Lateral ligament complex of ankle joint

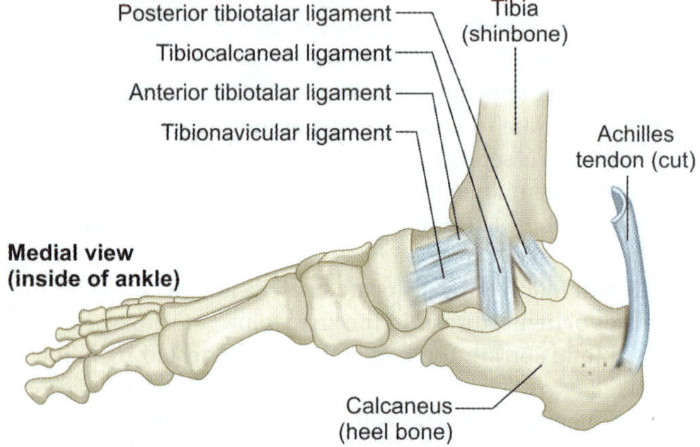

Fig. 6.56B: Diagrammatic representation of the deltoid ligament (medial ligament) of ankle joint

ANKLE SPRAIN

The ankle joint is the most common site for a ligament injury (sports injury) in the body and ligament injury at the ankle is called ankle sprain. More than three-fourths cases of ankle sprain involve lateral ligament complex (inversion ankle sprain) and it is ATFL (being the weakest of lateral ligament complex) that is most often torn. CFL is the second most commonly injured ligament in ankle sprains. Medial ankle sprains (eversion sprain) and syndesmotic sprains (high ankle sprain) are much less common.

Mechanism of Injury

The ATFL is the primary restraint against plantar flexion and internal rotation (inversion) of the foot. So the most common mechanism of injury in lateral ankle sprains occurs with forced plantar flexion and inversion of the ankle joint (inversion ankle sprain) as in stepping in a hole or jumping on uneven surface. Medial ankle sprains are less common and occur when the foot is turned outwards (eversion ankle sprain, i.e. deltoid ligament injury). Syndesmotic sprain is caused by excessive external rotation and dorsiflexion of the foot.

Clinical Presentation and Examination

Patients with ankle sprain present with pain and swelling around the ankle joint following a twisting injury of the foot. In lateral ankle sprain swelling, bruises and tenderness are present on the lateral aspect and front of the ankle. Medial ankle sprain presents with pain around the deltoid ligament and swelling and tenderness around the medial joint capsule. Patients with high ankle sprains present with tenderness over the anterior aspect of the ankle joint over the anterior or PITFL. The deltoid ligament serves as a secondary stabilizer to the distal ankle syndesmosis and may therefore be injured along with the syndesmotic ligaments in high ankle sprain injuries resulting in tenderness over the medial ankle as well. Walking is mostly difficult for these patients.

Lauge-Hansen grading method is commonly used to grade these injuries and abnormal motion and instability may be elicited in completely torn ligament injury **(Table 6.11)**. Clinical tests specific for ankle ligaments are given in **Table 6.12**.

Management

Diagnosis is made on clinical grounds. X-rays may be required if bony tenderness is present. High ankle sprains often pose a diagnostic difficulty and need identification of abnormal tibiofibular relationship on ankle X-rays **(Box 6.3)**. MRI is the best diagnostic modality to confirm any of these ligament injuries.

Treatment of an acute ligament sprain is RICE therapy (rest, ice, compression and elevation). Ice should be applied for 15–20 minutes every 2 hours for first 48 hours after an ankle sprain. This helps in reducing swelling and pain and fastens the healing of ligaments. Weight-bearing may be allowed as tolerated. Braces which limit inversion/eversion may be helpful in early course.

Table 6.11: Lauge-Hansen grading of ligament injury

Grade I injury	Grade II injury	Grade III injury
Ligaments are stretched only	Partial tear of ligaments	Ligaments are completely torn

Table 6.12: Clinical tests for ankle sprain **(Figs 6.57A to C)**

S.No.	Name of test	Method	Comments
1.	Anterior drawer test of the ankle joint	The examiner stabilizes the anterior distal leg with one hand and grasps the patient's calcaneus and rear foot with the other hand. Then the examiner pushes the rear foot anteriorly with a foot in slight plantar flexion. A positive test is indicated by the forward talus translation	A positive test indicates ATFL tear
2.	Inversion stress test (Talar tilt test)	Keep the ankle in 10° of dorsiflexion. Grasp the calcaneum (heel) with one hand and stabilize the leg with the other hand. Now invert the heel, if talus tilts* or gaps more compared to uninjured side or pain is produced, the test is considered positive	A positive test is highly sensitive for CFL injury or tear
3.	Eversion stress test	Keep the ankle in neutral position and grasp the heel and stabilize the distal leg with the other hand. Now evert the calcaneum. If the talus tilts* or gaps more compared to uninjured side or pain is produced, the test is considered positive	A positive test indicates deltoid ligament sprain
4.	External rotation stress test	Stabilize the distal leg with one hand and other hand grasp the medial aspect of the foot while supporting the ankle in neutral position. Now foot and talus are externally rotated	Medial joint pain indicates deltoid ligament injury while pain at the anterolateral ankle indicates injury to distal tibiofibular syndesmosis

*Talar tilt is noted on X-rays during these tests and is measured as angle between the dome of talus and the tibial plafond **(Fig. 6.57B)**. Difference of more than 10° between two sides is considered significant.

Box 6.3: X-ray criteria for "normal" tibiofibular relationship

1. Clear space between tibia and fibula (tibiofibular clear space) of ≤ 6 mm on anteroposterior and mortise views of ankle
2. Tibiofibular overlap of at least 6 mm on the anteroposterior view and 1 mm on the mortise view

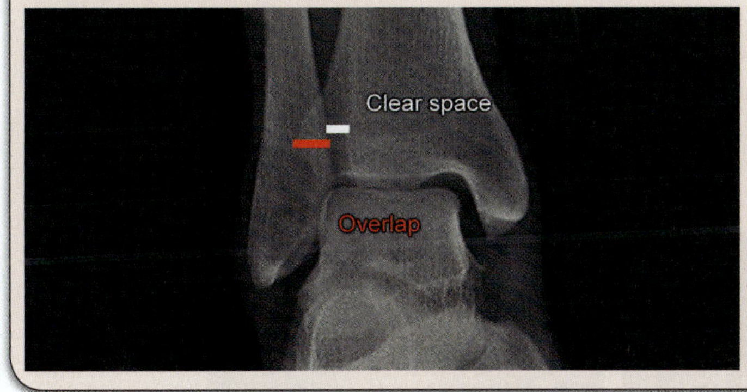

More severe injuries are best benefitted by immobilization in a below knee cast for 3–4 weeks.

Although majority of the patients can be managed conservatively, surgery (reconstruction of the torn ligament with tendon graft) may be needed in patients:

- Who do not respond to a fair trial of conservative treatment
- In whom persistent instability remains after conservative treatment trial
- In whom disruption of normal tibiofibular relationships is seen on radiographs.

IMPORTANT TENDON AFFECTIONS

INTRODUCTION

Rupture of a tendon is not an uncommon injury, especially in elite sportsmen. The most common site for a tendon rupture in the body is the supraspinatus (part of rotator cuff) followed by the tendo-Achilles (TA), while the rupture of the biceps, quadriceps/patellar tendon (knee extensor mechanism), pectoralis major have also been reported.

Most commonly these ruptures are secondary to an overuse injury, although purely traumatic ruptures can also occur. Some general risk factors for all tendon ruptures include an increasing age, history of smoking, comorbidities like diabetes, SLE, gout, uremia due to any cause and drugs (steroids, fluoroquinolones, etc.). Few important tendon ruptures are discussed here.

TENDO-ACHILLES RUPTURE

Although TA is the longest and strongest tendon in the body, it is also a very frequently ruptured tendon. The classical site of rupture is generally 3 cm proximal to its insertion into the calcaneal tuberosity, as there is a hypovascular zone present in this area of the tendon. The rupture is mostly seen in 30–40 years aged athletes who have excessive hind foot valgus/varus, excessive pronation (subtalar hyperpronation), increased femoral anteversion, a limb length discrepancy, high body mass index or have a stretched running schedule or when they are training on the unfamiliar running surface. If one TA ruptures, the chances of contralateral TA rupture also increase.

Clinically, these patients present with a weak plantar flexion causing difficulty in the push off phase of the gait cycle. Clinical tests for TA rupture are given in **Table 6.13**.

Important radiological signs include—decrease in size and obliteration of Kager's triangle (a space filled with fatty tissue, bordered by the margins of the anterior surface of the Achilles tendon, the upper part of the calcaneus, and the posterior surface of the deep flexor tendons), decreased Toygar angle (angle of the posterior skin surface adjacent to the TA; less than 150° is indicative of TA rupture) and thickened TA. X-ray may also show an avulsion fracture from the calcaneum **(Fig. 6.59)**. USG is another useful investigation to make the diagnosis in doubtful cases but MRI is the investigation of choice.

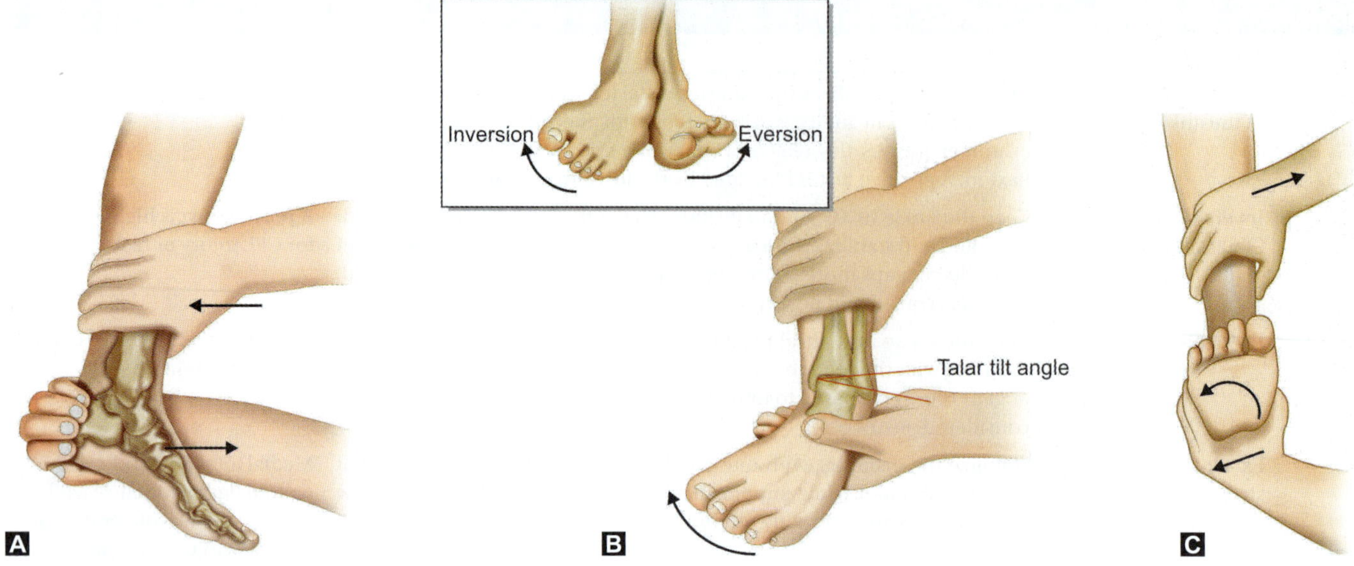

Figs 6.57A to C: (A) Anterior drawer test; (B) Talar tilt test; (C) External rotation stress test

Table 6.13: Clinical tests for tendo-Achilles (TA) rupture	
Name of the test	*Procedure*
Simmonds- Thompson test **(Fig. 6.58A)**	Normally, squeezing the calf irritates the gastrocnemius-soleus and the muscle contracts causing visible plantar flexion of the foot; however, when TA is torn, this maneuver is not followed by any noticeable plantar flexion of the foot
O Brien's needle test	With the patient prone, a small gauge needles is inserted (tip is just within the tendon) at a right angle through the skin of the calf, just medial to the midline, 10 cm proximal to the superior border of the calcaneum (i.e. proximal to common site of rupture). If the tendon is intact needle will move proximally on passive plantar flexion and distally on passive dorsiflexion of the ankle
Matles knee flexion test **(Fig. 6.58B)**	The patient is made in the prone position and asked to actively flex the both knees to 90°. Normally with knee flexion foot goes into plantar flexion but if TA is torn foot will remain in slight dorsiflexion compared to the normal side

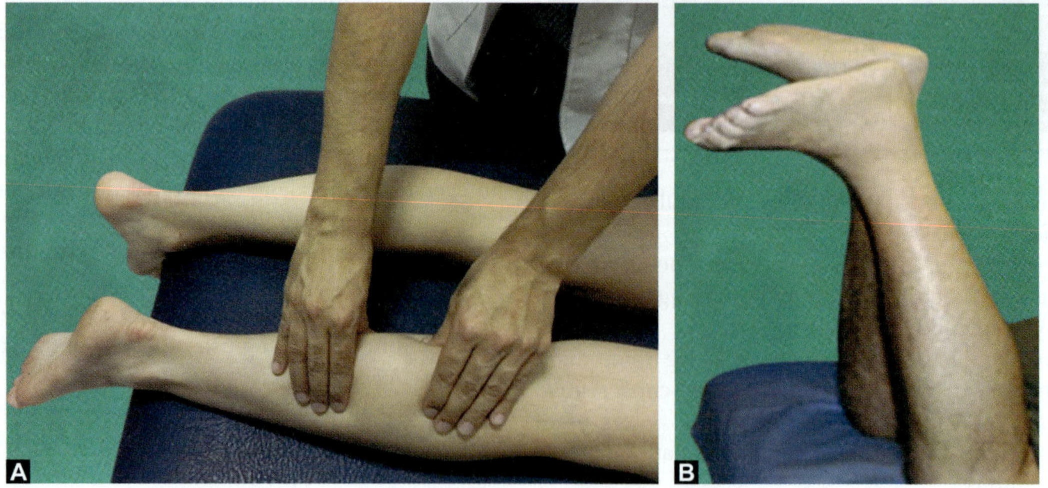

Figs 6.58A and B: (A) Simmonds-Thompson test; (B) Matles knee flexion test

Treatment of fresh ruptures (< 4–6 weeks old) is a primary repair, however, in neglected cases, one needs to go for augmentation by using a free fascia tendon graft (fascia lata or hamstring graft), local tendon transfer (peroneus brevis, flexor hallucis longus) fascial advancement (gastrocnemius soleus fascia turn down graft) or by V-Y plasty through gastrocnemius aponeurosis.

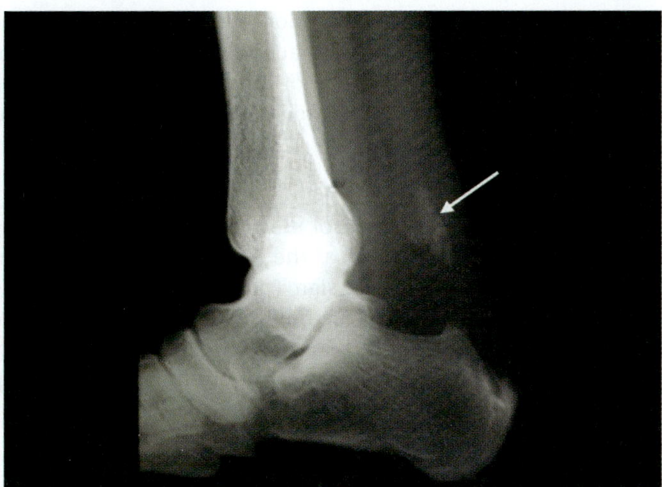

Fig. 6.59: X-ray ankle lateral view showing avulsion fracture of calcaneum at the insertion of TA. TA has retracted and calcified (arrow).

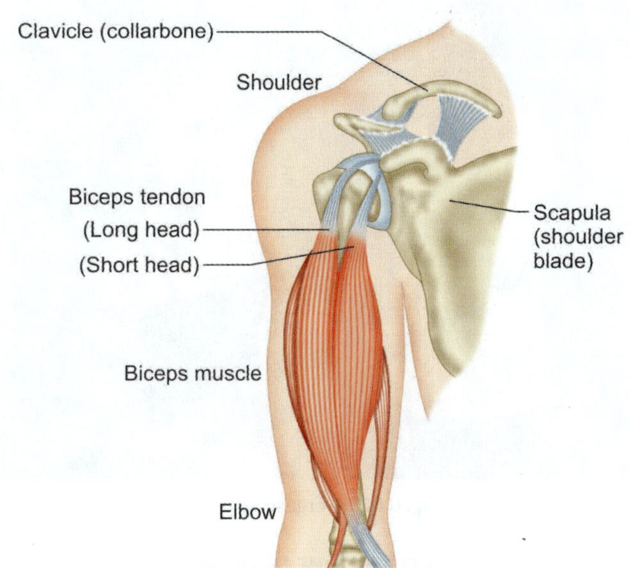

Fig. 6.60: Diagrammatic depiction of the biceps anatomy

BICEPS TENDON RUPTURE

The ruptures of the biceps tendon (**Fig. 6.60** for biceps anatomy) most commonly involve the long head of biceps with most common site of rupture being inter tubercular sulcus followed by myotendinous junction and glenoid attachment site. Hence, proximal tendon ruptures are far more common than distal tendon ruptures. Most of the tears are either traumatic injuries or overuse injuries in people who are in professions involving heavy overhead work or an overuse of the shoulder.

The proximal tendon ruptures are more common in fourth to sixth decade of life and are clinically almost indistinguishable from rotator cuff tears presenting with pain around the shoulder. The distal tendon ruptures are particularly common in young weight lifters and may present with the classical Popeye sign (**Fig. 6.61**). The tendon ruptures near the distal attachment and retracts and bunches up in the arm. This is most visible on contraction of the muscle (as on elbow flexion against resistance). Distal tendon ruptures may present with significant loss of supination strength (40–50% loss).

Treatment in cosmetically conscious or high demand sports persons involves surgical tenodesis of tendon (fixation of avulsed tendon back to bone) but low demand/aged patients generally have minimal functional loss and they can be willfully neglected.

Bicipital Tendinitis

This refers to inflammation of the long head of biceps tendon seen mostly in patients involved in overhead activities. Most of these patients present with pain anteriorly in the shoulder and tend to have concomitant rotator cuff disease or labral tears in the shoulder. Two important clinical tests that are used in identifying this pathology are the Speed's and the Yergason's test. Speed's test (**Fig. 6.62A**) is performed by asking the patient to resist the downward pressure at the wrist while the arm is in 60–90° forward elevation, elbow extended and forearm supinated. The maneuver produces pain in shoulder in cases with the biceps pathology. In Yergason's test (**Fig. 6.62B**) patient's elbow is flexed to 90° and the patient is asked to supinate the forearm against resistance while examiner looks for pain along the proximal biceps.

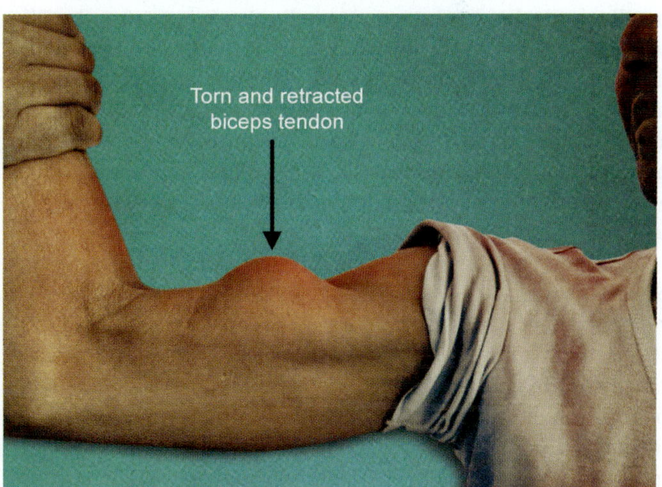

Fig. 6.61: Left biceps of the patient is torn at distal attachment and has retracted and bunched up in the arm (Popeye sign) (arrow)

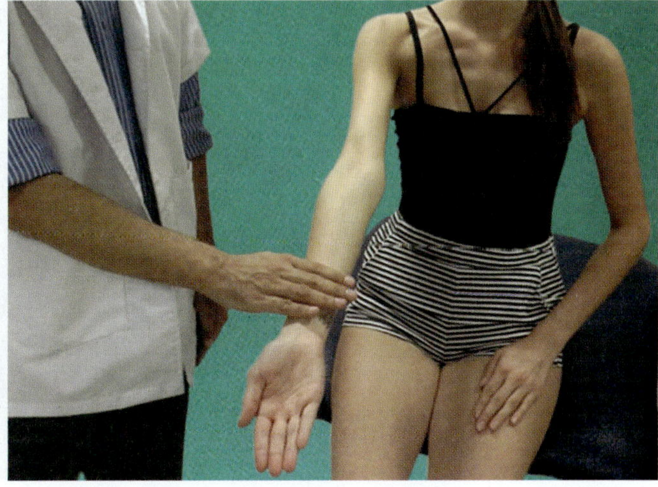

Fig. 6.62A: Speed's test

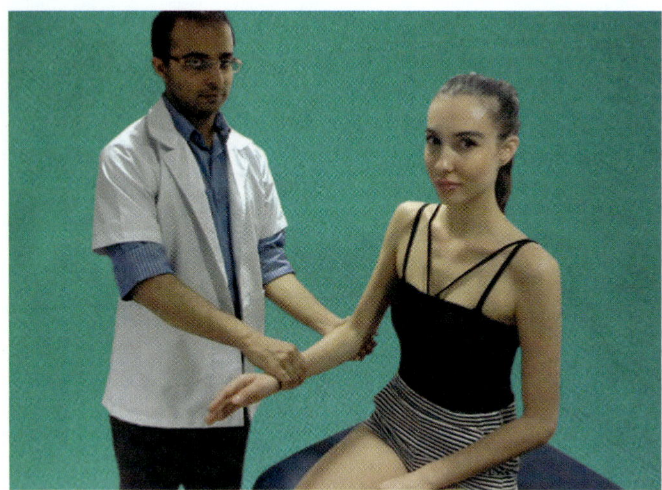

Fig. 6.62B: Yergason's test

RUPTURE OF KNEE EXTENSOR MECHANISM

Knee extensor mechanism includes the quadriceps femoris (the rectus femoris and the three vasti) inserting on the patella, the patella and the ligamentum patella inserting into the tibial tuberosity. The most common cause of disruption is actually a fracture of patella followed by the quadriceps tendon (ruptures mostly at the myotendinous junction, especially in older people) and then by the patellar tendon (ruptures mostly in young people). Quadriceps and patellar tendon may rupture following a violent and forceful contraction of the quadriceps in flexed knees in a jump or fall from a height.

Patients present with pain and tenderness around distal or the proximal pole of patella. On examination, there is an extension lag. A hemarthrosis may be present and if painful it should be aspirated. Plain X-ray may show avulsion fracture of patella or tibial tuberosity. In patellar tendon rupture patella may be abnormally high (patella alta) due to the unopposed pull of the quadriceps. Similarly, it may be low lying (patella baja) in quadriceps rupture. Diagnosis is confirmed on USG or MRI.

Treatment depends on whether tear is partial or complete. Partial tear with full active knee extension can be effectively managed conservatively with extension bracing/cast. The limb is immobilized in cylindrical cast/brace with full knee extension for 4–6 weeks, followed by range of motion and strengthening exercises. Operative repair is required in all cases of complete tear with extension lag.

Jumper's Knee (Patellar Tendinitis)

It is tendinitis of the knee extensor mechanism usually occurring at the tendo-osseous junction of the lower pole of patella. On X-rays one may find a tooth sign (periosteal reaction of the anterior patellar surface). Treatment is mostly conservative and involves refraining from jumping, relative rest (activity modification), stretching of lower extremity musculature, deep transverse friction massage of the patellar tendon, cryotherapy and eccentric quadriceps exercises.

ILIOTIBIAL BAND FRICTION SYNDROME

The iliotibial band (also known as Maissiat's band or iliotibial tract) is a longitudinal fibrous reinforcement of the fascia lata present on lateral side of the thigh. It inserts at the lateral condyle of the tibia at Gerdy's tubercle.

Iliotibial band friction syndrome (ITBFS) is one of the most common causes of lateral knee pain in sports people. Sports persons who are involved with sports which require a greater amount of flexion and extension activities, such as runners and cyclist are at a higher risk for iliotibial band syndrome. The exact pathogenesis is not known but it is believed that repetitive cycles of tightening of the lateral fascia exert a compression effect on connective tissues lying deep to the ITB and this compression generates the pain syndrome. Tight iliotibial band and weak hip abductors may predispose to ITBFS.

Clinical presentation is characteristic. A patient who is mostly a runner complains of a sharp pain, slight proximal the lateral joint line during running. Pain subsides with the cessation of activity. Noble compression test **(Figs 6.63A and B)** typically produces pain in ITBFS. In this test affected knee and hip are flexed to 90° in a supine patient. Now examiner compresses the ITB 2 cm proximal to the lateral femoral condyle and asks the patient to extend the knee and hip slowly. In ITBFS, this will typically produce pain.

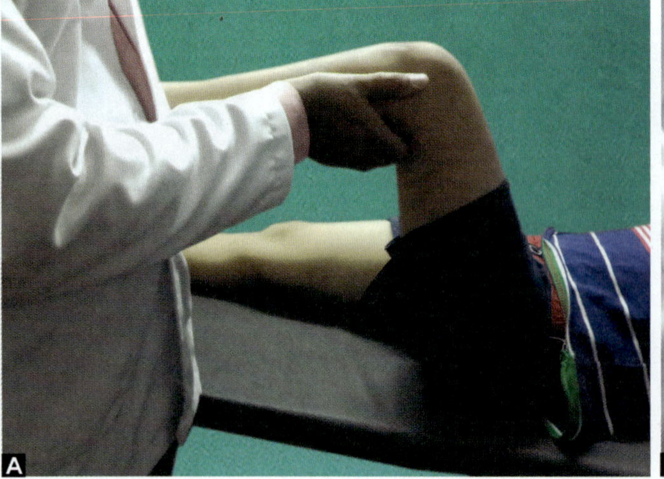
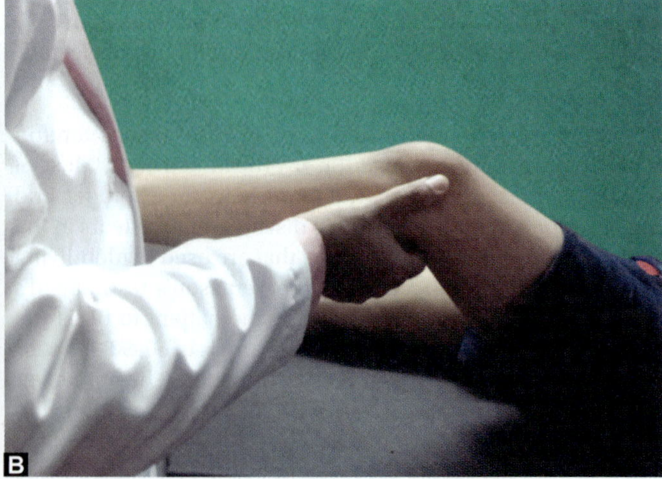

Figs 6.63A and B: Noble's compression test

Treatment involves rest and abstinence from the offending activity. Ice, NSAIDs and ITB stretching exercises help. Local corticosteroid injection may also help in acute cases. Many surgical options have been tried in nonresponders and surgery involves resection of the posterior half of band along with arthroscopic resection of the lateral synovial recess.

ILIOPSOAS TENDINITIS

Iliopsoas tendinitis is inflammation of the iliopsoas tendon resulting from acute trauma or more commonly from overuse injury (sports which requires repetitive hip flexion). Iliopsoas tendinitis is usually seen in ballet dancers, runners, jumpers and other athletes. Patients present with activity related groin pain following running, walking, etc. There may be complaint of snapping about the hip joint. On examination passive hip extension and active hip flexion (supine patient raises the heel 15° off the bed) are painful. Ludloff test (In sitting position on the chair, patient raises his thigh against resistance) often exacerbates pain. Treatment is almost always conservative with rest, ice and NSAIDs. Recalcitrant cases may require a corticosteroid injection in bursa or tendon sheath or rarely tendon release.

HAMSTRING STRAIN

The three muscles at the back of the thigh—semitendinosus and gracilis medially and biceps femoris laterally, are called the hamstrings **(Fig. 6.64A)**. They originate at ischial tuberosity and insert on upper leg such that they cross two joints (hip and knee), which makes them prone to injury.

Hamstring muscle strain is a very common sports injury in field and track games like running, jumping, etc. and infact it is the single most common injury in professional football. Two common mechanisms implicated are a high speed running and overstretching of the muscle. Running related hamstring strains (type I strains) generally occur during terminal swing phase of the gait cycle and typically involve the long head of biceps femoris near its muscle-tendon junction in lower thigh. Overstretching of the muscle (type II strains) may occur in movements that simultaneously involve hip flexion and knee extension (thus placing the muscle in a position of extreme stretch) such as kicking **(Fig. 6.64B)** or dancing. The stretching-type hamstring injury typically involves the semimembranosus (proximal free tendon) close to the ischial tuberosity.

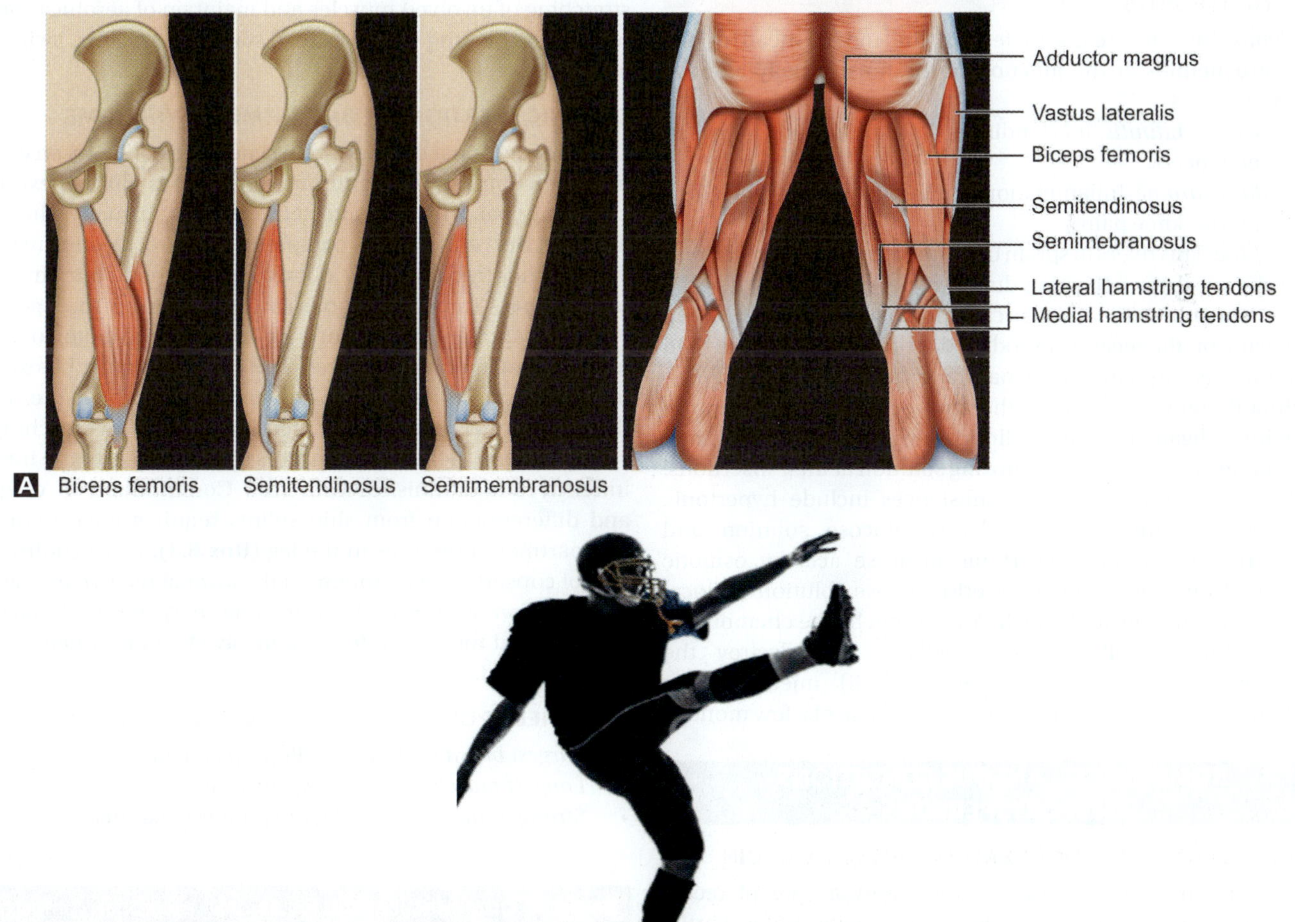

Figs 6.64A and B: (A) Anatomy of the hamstring muscles; (B) A common mechanism behind hamstring strain

Clinically, majority of these patients present with a sudden onset of posterior thigh pain after high speed running or other sport activity. Active knee flexion against resistance in the prone position is painful. USG and MRI (better in detecting muscle edema hemorrhage and tear) are commonly used to support the diagnosis.

Treatment immediately after a muscle strain consists of RICE therapy. Once the patient becomes pain free, rehabilitation program is started to include stretching, strengthening and functional exercises. Stretching and strengthening (concentric and eccentric exercises, read later) of the hamstring muscles should be followed by neuromuscular control exercises of the lumbopelvic region (core muscles) for optimal function of the hamstrings. Full recovery is very important before getting back to sports as the hamstring strains have the highest recurrence rate (residual scar tissue reduces extensibility of the musculotendon unit) among all sports injuries. Injuries involving biceps femoris that occur during high-speed running take less time to recover compared to those involving proximal semimembranosus, during dance and kicking. Thus, the proximal the site of injury (maximum pain), the greater the time patients mostly take to return to sports.

HIGH-YIELD POINTS

- *Tennis leg*: This refers to tear of the medial head of the gastrocnemius at the junction of the muscle belly and the aponeurosis.
- *Dancer's tendinitis*: It is tendinitis of flexor hallucis longus in ballet dancers.
- *Hoffa syndrome*: Inflammation in infrapateller fat pad leading to anterior knee pain.
- *Turf Toe*: This refers to sprain of the metatarsophalangeal joint of the great toe occurring due to hyperextension classically seen in professional American footballers who have been playing on the recently introduced artificial turf (a more rigid surface as compared to the natural grass).
- Prolotherapy (proliferant therapy) refers to treatment of painful, ligament and tendinopathies by injecting a small volume of an irritant or sclerosing solution at their insertions. The most commonly used substances include hypertonic dextrose solution, phenol-glycerin-glucose solution and morrhuate sodium. Hypertonic dextrose acts by osmotic lysis of the cells, phenol-glycerin-glucose solution by local cellular irritation, and morrhuate sodium by the chemotactic attraction of inflammatory mediators that destroy the pathologic neovascularity. Several (3–6) injections are delivered in 2–6 weeks interval over a course of a few months.

SOME MISCELLANEOUS CONDITIONS IN SPORTSPERSONS

SPORTS HERNIA/ATHLETIC PUBALGIA/GILMORE'S GROIN

This condition refers to strain at the insertion site of rectus abdominis (an abdominal muscle) on the pubic bone. Partial tear occurs in the muscle and when the abdominal organs, press against this muscle, it causes pain. The conjoint tendon insertion and the adductor longus insertions on the pubis may also be involved.

The patient is usually an athlete who presents with pain in the groin region noted mostly on exertion. There is no visible swelling, compared to the more common inguinal hernia, although uncommon in late cases a true herniation might occur. Hip movements mostly are unaffected, but one may find tenderness localized to the pubic tubercle.

Management is usually conservative with strengthening exercises and rest. Resistant cases may need inguinal myorrhaphy (Nesovic's operation).

MEDIAL TIBIAL STRESS SYNDROME (SHIN SPLINTS)

This is a condition where the patients complain of exertion related pain in the shins, mostly bilateral. It is believed to be a repetitive stress injury of tibialis posterior or soleus muscle, seen mostly in runners and athletes in response to repetitive muscle contractions causing a tibial strain. Patients present with exertional pain located at the posteromedial aspect of the leg (mostly distal one-third of leg). As the condition progresses, a frank stress fractures may become evident in the posteromedial cortex of the tibia. However, X-rays initially are usually negative. Technetium pyrophosphate bone scan and MRI help to differentiate periostitis (seen in medial tibial stress syndrome) from a frank stress fracture. Treatment is mainly conservative and involves a strict activity modification, stretching of involved muscles and maintain of aerobic fitness by nonweight-bearing exercises (e.g. stationary cycling, swimming, etc.).

CHRONIC EXERTIONAL COMPARTMENT SYNDROME

Chronic exertional compartment syndrome (CECS) is an exercise induced compartment syndrome that causes chronic exertional cramping pain in the affected extremity usually the lower leg (anterior and lateral compartments are mostly involved). The pathophysiology is poorly understood but increased muscle mass (muscle volume can increases up to 20% during exercise) and noncompliant soft tissues contribute to elevate intracompartmental pressures. The condition must be excluded in any young athlete (especially endurance athlete, i.e. a long distance runner) or a military recruit who comes with aching and cramping pain in the leg that occurs after a fixed exercise interval/ intensity but diminishes with rest. Confirmation of diagnosis and differentiation from shin splints requires measurement of compartment pressures in the leg **(Box 6.4)**. Once confirmed, a trial of conservative treatment in the form of relative rest, activity modification and muscle stretching may be undertaken; if unsuccessful then fasciotomy of involved compartments should be considered.

HIGH-YIELD POINTS

- *Largest bursa in the body:* Iliopsoas bursa.
- *Longest muscle in the body:* Sartorius.
- *Strongest muscle in the body:* Gluteus maximus.

Box 6.4: Diagnostic criteria for chronic exertional compartment syndrome (CECS)

- Pre-existing resting compartment pressure > 15 mm Hg
- Compartment pressure > 30 mm Hg × 1 minute after exercise
- Compartment pressure > 20 mm Hg × 5 minutes after exercise

- *Strongest ligament in the body:* Iliofemoral ligament (ligament of Bigelow).
- *Weakest ligament in the body:* ATFL.
- *Most common ligament to rupture in the body:* ATFL.
- *Strongest tendon in the body:* Tendo-Achilles.
- Most common tendon to rupture is supraspinatous followed by tendo-Achilles.
- Most common cause of tendon ruptures is overuse.
- The most common congenitally absent muscle is the pectoralis major.

REHABILITATION OF AN INJURED SPORTS PERSON

INTRODUCTION

Not only correct diagnosis and prompt treatment, but comprehensive rehabilitation also plays a key role for an injured athlete to get back to the field again. The goal of rehabilitation is to achieve the same or higher level of performance in competition. Lack of proper rehabilitation, not only results in functional deficit but also poses risk of reinjury.

PHASES OF REHABILITATION

Rehabilitation can be divided into four phases:
- *Phase I*: Targets control of pain and swelling.
- *Phase II*: Target is to achieve back joint ROM.
- *Phase III*: Focus is on building muscle strength and power, patient's endurance (stamina), bring back muscle flexibility and joint proprioception sense.
- *Phase IV*: Functional exercises and sports specific skills are introduced to prepare patient for return to sport.

Phase I (First Week)

This is phase of inflammation and goals here are to achieve control of pain and swelling by RICE principle (rest, ice, compression, elevation). Ice application (cryotherapy) reduces hematoma, tissue inflammation and necrosis and promotes faster healing. It can be applied as continuous (20 minutes continuous application every 2 hours) or intermittent (10 minutes ice, then 10 minutes rest and again 10 minutes ice every 2 hours) therapy for first 48–72 hours. Heat (hot bath) and massage should be avoided for 3–4 days after injury (as it may exacerbate swelling by vasodilatation). Analgesics (NSAIDs) can be given for short-term (<5 days) but prolonged treatment with NSAIDs should be discouraged. A joint injury or a surgery is always accompanied by some degree of reflex inhibition of joint muscles (e.g. quadriceps inhibition occurs after ACL reconstruction), so muscle conditioning (i.e. activation of muscle contraction) is started immediately by introducing at this stage isometric exercises (read here). These exercises do not need joint movement so are appropriate for this stage.

Phase II (1–8 Weeks)

Target in this early phase of rehabilitation is to restore full ROM of the joint so that strengthening exercises can be instituted. ROM exercises can initially be passive (where a therapist moves the joint through ROM) but later can be active assisted (patient self assists in joint movement by using normal limb) or fully active (patient moves the joint actively through full ROM). With return of ROM, target shifts to building muscle strength and power **(Figs 6.65A and B)**.

Phase III (8–16 Weeks)

This is the mid-phase where re building back the muscle strength and power are the key focus. While strength is returning, patient's cardiovascular fitness (endurance/stamina) is maintained by aerobic exercises (such as stationary cycling), joint flexibility by periodic stretching and joint position sense by special proprioceptive exercises.

Restoring Muscle Strength

Strength is the amount of force a muscle can exert against an external load. Three types of exercises are used to restore muscle strength: isometric, isotonic and isokinetic **(Table 6.14)**.

Isometric exercises: These are best exercises to introduce in the beginning phase as they do not require joint movement **(Fig. 6.66)**. However, they cannot build a muscle mass; they can only maintain it. Also they are relatively contraindicated in hypertensives.

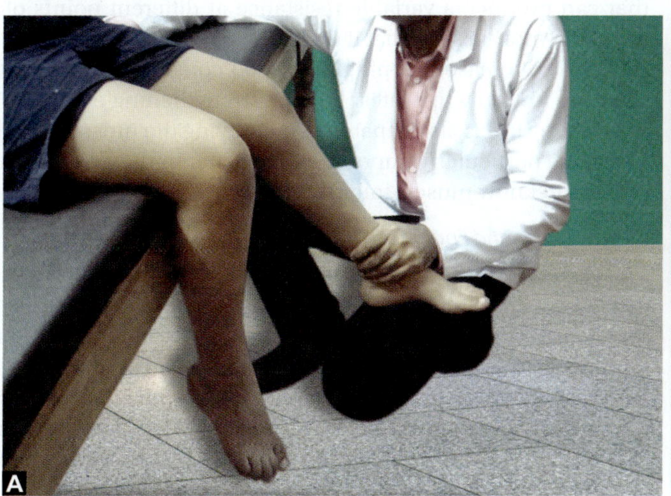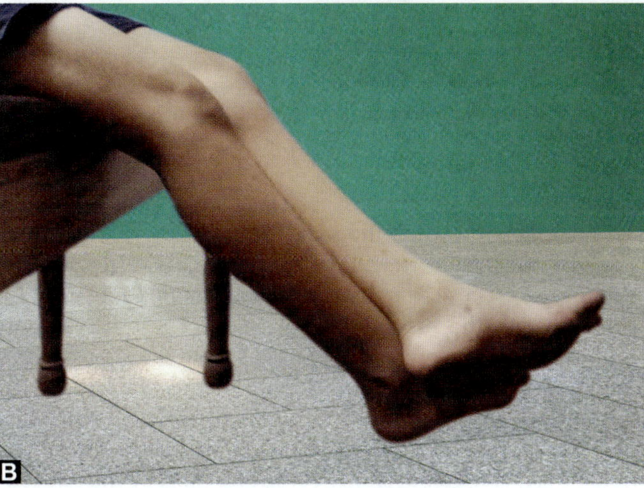

Figs 6.65A and B: Range of motion (ROM) exercises—(A) Passive exercises; (B) Active assisted exercises

Table 6.14: Types of strengthening exercises

Types of exercises	Results
Isometric exercises	Here muscle length remains constant during exercise, i.e. muscle contracts, but no joint movement occur
Isotonic exercises	Here muscle contracts against a "constant resistance" and joint moves through range of motion
Isokinetic exercises	These exercises are performed on a device at a fixed speed, but with "variable resistance", i.e. resistance varies throughout the range of motion to maintain a "constant speed"

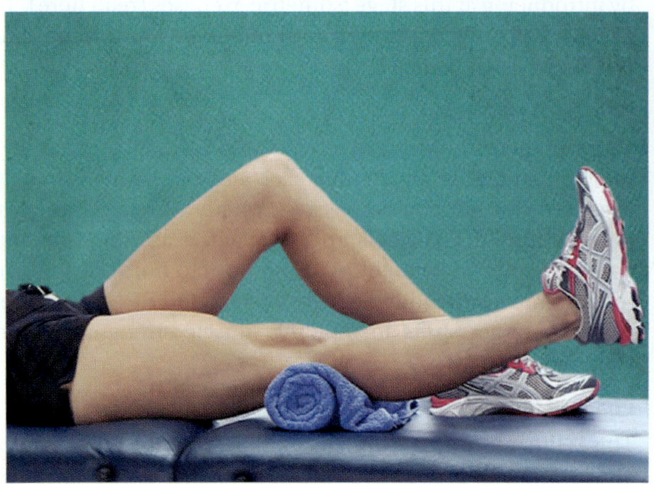
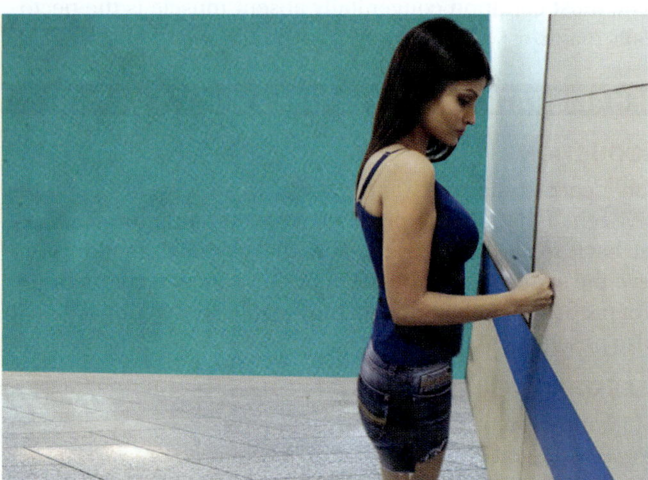

Fig. 6.66: Isometric quadriceps and deltoid contraction

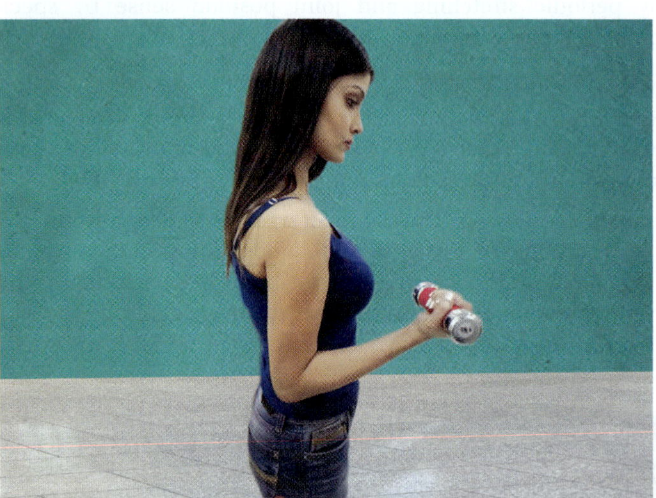

Fig. 6.67: Isotonic biceps contraction

Isotonic exercises: Isotonic exercises **(Fig. 6.67)** are performed later in rehabilitation when the joint is able to move through a ROM against a constant weight or resistance (e.g. a free weight like a dumbbell). These exercises are capable of building muscle mass and restore the preoperative strength. These can either by closed chain or open chain exercises **(Table 6.15)** or can be grouped into concentric or eccentric contractions **(Table 6.16)**.

Isotonic exercises can also be grouped into concentric or eccentric (details in **Table 6.15**) exercises. Initially concentric strengthening is started but slowly eccentrics must be introduced because eccentric exercises are pivotal to promote tendon remodeling and reduce the chances of recurrence of injury (as eccentric contractions are produced by the body to make muscles act as splint around the joint when movements occur during sporting activities). The demerits of isotonic exercises are a difficulty in quantifying the muscle strength gains achieved and slight risk of injury associated (since for resistance a weight is used against which speed cannot be controlled). These demerits are better tackled by isokinetic exercises.

Isokinetic exercises: Isokinetic exercises are done on a device **(Fig. 6.68)**, which works at a constant velocity throughout the ROM. To ensure constant speed, the device has an electric motor that can produce a variable resistance at different points of the arc of the motion such that if the patient applies greater force, the resistance increases keeping the speed constant and vice versa. They are not only the safest form of strengthening exercises, the device they use is also capable of quanifying the muscle strength. These are particularly important in the later part of rehabilitation process to know muscle imbalance.

Muscle Power and Endurance Training

Muscle power is the ability of muscle to generate as much force as fast as possible while muscle endurance (stamina) is the muscle's ability to perform repeated contractions. Once adequate strength has been gained, power can simply be upgraded by increasing the intensity of contractions (e.g. incrementing from 5 biceps curls in one set to 10 curls in same set timing) while endurance can be maintained by starting patient on aerobic exercises (stationary cycling, fast walking on treadmill, etc.).

Table 6.15: Concentric and eccentric exercises explained with example of biceps curl with a dumbbell

Concentric exercises	Eccentric exercises
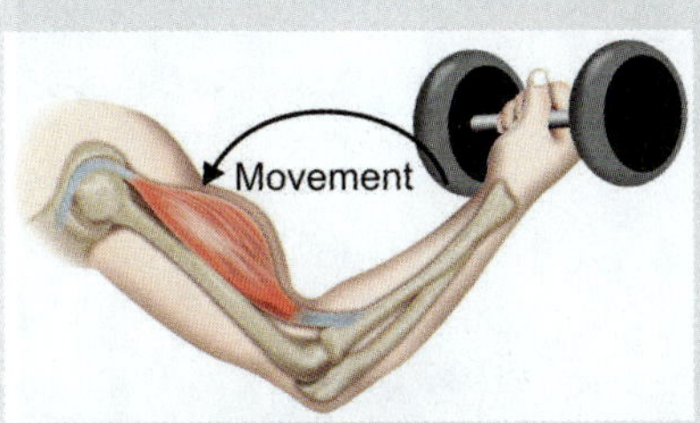 *Muscle fibers shorten during contraction*	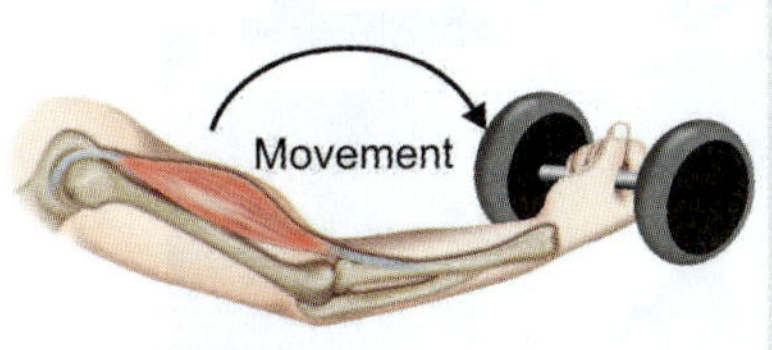 *Muscle fibers lengthen during contraction*
When one lifts the dumbbell during biceps curls it causes concentric contraction of the biceps (biceps contracts and shortens) as the origin and insertion of the biceps come closer to each other	During biceps curls at the end of the concentric movement *the weight is brought down to its initial position.* The biceps remains contracted to maintain control as forearm drops. This causes eccentric contraction of the biceps (biceps contracts yet lengthens) as the origin and insertion of the biceps separates
Tension in muscle fibers is lower as intramuscular force produced per motor unit is lower than eccentric contraction. So these are relatively safe	Tension in muscle fibers is high as intramuscular force produced per motor unit is higher than concentric contraction. Can be at times damaging to muscle and are particularly responsible for causing delayed onset muscle soreness (diffuse muscle aches that develop a day or two after exercise)

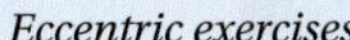

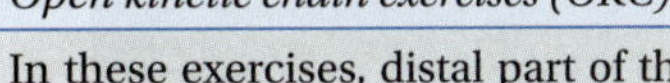

Table 6.16: Open and close kinetic chain exercises

Close kinetic chain exercises (CKC)	Open kinetic chain exercises (OKC)
In these exercises, foot (for lower limb exercises) and hand (for upper limb exercises) remains in contact with the surface (ground, wall or machine) and cannot move	In these exercises, distal part of the limb (foot or hand) freely moves in the space
Examples are leg press, squatting or pushup exercises	Examples are leg extension and flexion or straight leg raising
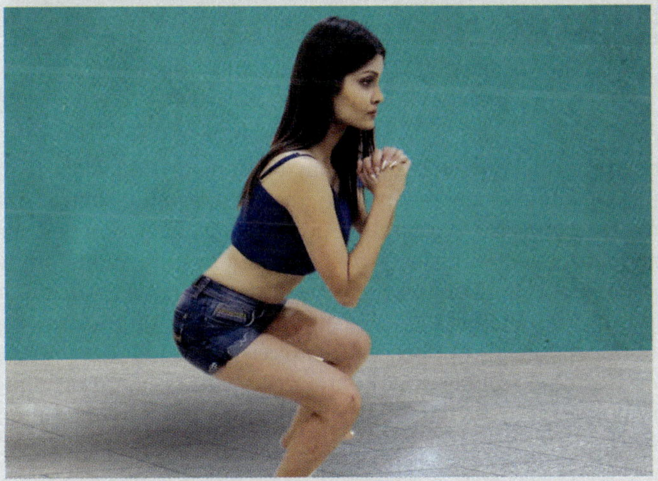	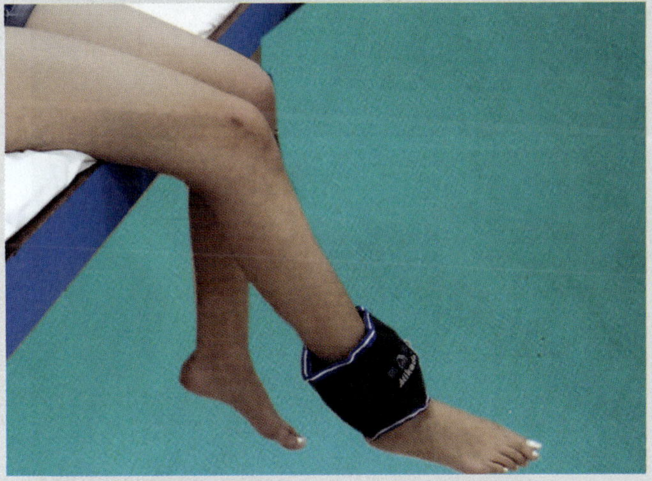
These exercises are weight-bearing exercises. These are more functional and involve multiple joints. These are considered safe for early rehabilitation. Their main drawback is that they cannot be centered to single joint of interest	These are nonweight-bearing exercises. These are less functional and often involve single joint. OKC exercises generate more shear joint forces and should be avoided in early rehabilitation. Their main advantage is that they can be centered to the single joint of interest that needs to be exercised

Flexibility

After injury, muscle flexibility (limits of ROM) often decreases due to inflammation and spasm of muscles. This often limits range of motion. Muscle flexibility and thus the range of motion can be maximized by a regular stretching program (**Figs 6.69A and B**) before every exercise session. Stretching decreases chances of getting muscle soreness after exercise and promotes muscle relaxation and joint flexibility.

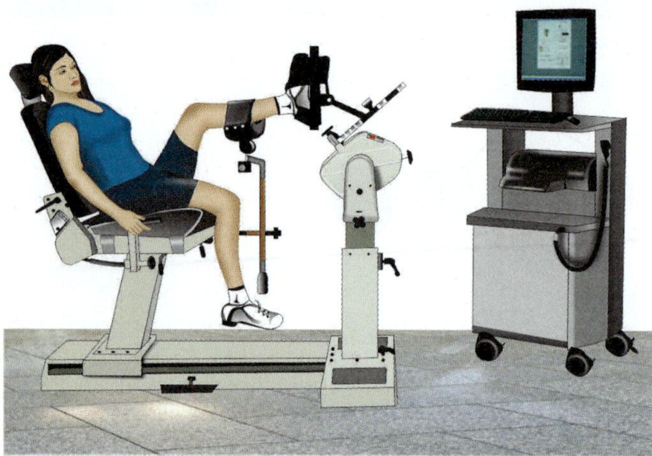

Fig. 6.68: Isokinetic strengthening being performed on isokinetic machine

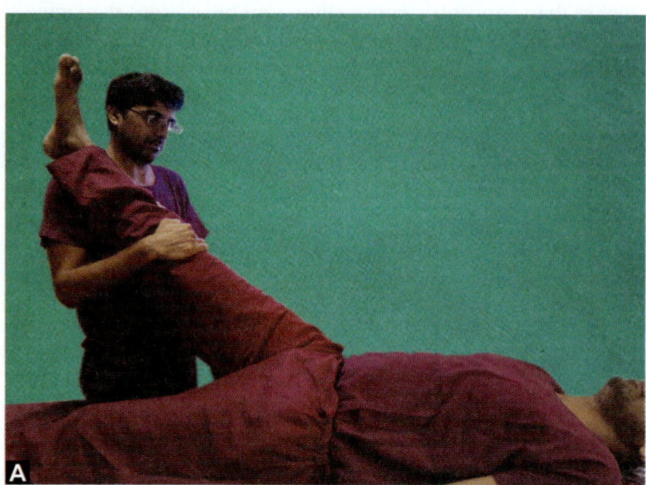

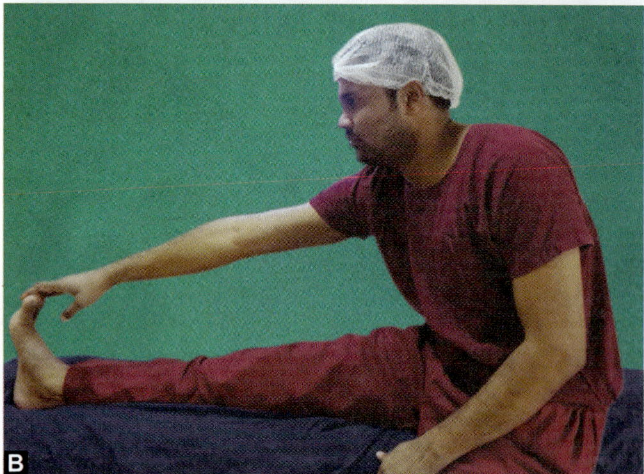

Figs 6.69A and B: Muscle stretches being performed

Proprioception, Balance and Neuromuscular Coordination

Proprioception is the ability of a joint to sense the position of the limb and hence maintain balance during a sporting activity.

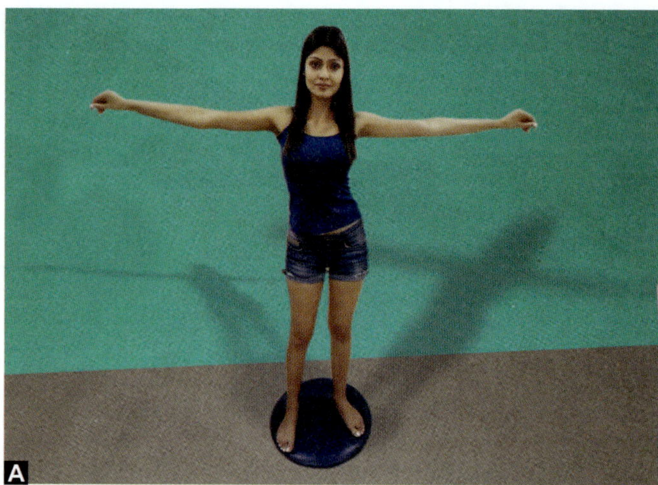

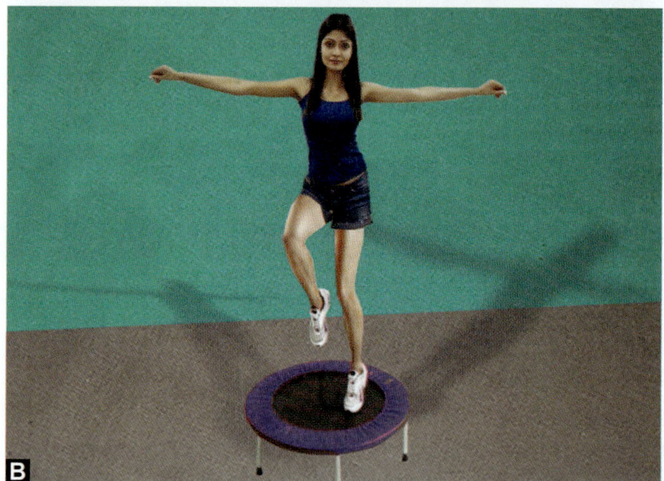

Figs 6.70A and B: (A) Dura disk; and (B) Mini trampoline exercises to increase proprioception

Since proprioceptive receptors may be damaged during a joint injury or surgery, patients have an impaired postural control and decreased muscle reaction time postoperatively. Sports persons with dampened proprioception are significantly more prone to reinjury. Proprioception exercises should be started rather early during rehabilitation as it may take long time to restore proprioception. Proprioception exercises include balancing exercises on a wobble board, dura disks, rocker board or mini-trampolines **(Figs 6.70A and B)** that aim to improve joint position sense and neuromuscular coordination.

Phase IV (16 Weeks Onwards)

Once the player has gained adequate muscle power, strength, flexibility, endurance, motor control and proprioception, advanced phase of rehabilitation begins that includes functional exercises and sport specific skills. The proper sporting technique can reduce the risk of reinjury significantly. Examples of sport specific exercises include kicking in football and bawling in cricket. Gradually a sports person progresses from simple to more complex sports activities such as from simple kicking to kicking for a goal and thereafter a return to sport can be planned usually by 6–9 months.

HIGH-YIELD POINTS

- *Plyometric exercises*: These exercises are used in all types of sports training and during advance rehabilitation to increase power (i.e. explosiveness). Plyometric exercises are a combination of eccentric action (rapid muscle stretching) followed by a concentric action (isotonic muscle shortening) of the same muscle, as occurs in activities like jumping, hoping, etc. This produces more force than produced by concentric muscle contraction alone. Plyometric exercises increase agility, speed, power and strength and are incorporated in later stages of rehabilitation.

- *Exercise-associated muscle cramps (EAMC):* These are painful, spasmodic involuntary skeletal muscle contractions that occur during or immediately after an exercise bout, mostly commonly in the calf. The etiology is unclear but an imbalance in neuromuscular control due to alterations in muscle spindle and motor neuron activity is thought to be responsible. Immediate treatment involves NSAIDs and passive stretching of involved muscle. There are no proven strategies for prevention but regular passive stretching works by altering spinal reflex activity. Correction of posture, proper muscle conditioning by exercising especially eccentric exercises, maintaining carbohydrate and electrolyte reserves, all may be beneficial.

- *Pedobarography:* This is the science of sports medicine that studies the pressure changes taking place between the plantar surface of foot and the supporting surface during exercise or sport. A special equipment called as 'Force Platform' is used to record these changes and perform an assessment of sport biomechanics and gait biometrics.

7

CHAPTER

Spine

RELEVANT ANATOMY (FIGS 7.1A AND B)

Spinal cord is approximately 45 cm long neural structure extends from the foramen magnum, where it is continuous with medulla oblongata and terminates mostly at the lower border of L1 as "Conus Medullaris", which technically refers to the sacral segments of the cord. Cauda equina (or Horse's tail) refers to the hanging nerve roots in the canal that are arising from respective spinal cord segments. Filum terminale is the fibrous septum that extends from the distal end of conus and then closely adhering to the dura mater it inserts into the first coccygeal segment.

Now, in an adult the spinal cord generally ends at the lower border of L1. However, in the fetus, the situation is quite different **(Fig. 7.2)**. Here, the cord is as long as the vertebral column. But due to differential growth between the vertebral column and the spinal cord, in an adult the cord ends earlier as the vertebral column grows more.

Each segment of spinal cord gives rise to a nerve, called a spinal nerve. Each nerve would leave the vertebral column through the intervertebral foramen beneath the corresponding vertebrae (e.g. L1 nerve root leaves beneath L1 vertebrae). Now, since the cord is ending at the lower border of L1, the nerve roots generally have to descend a bit of distance in the canal before they can exit; and this gives rise to the hanging nerve roots lying in the canal below L1 which arose from corresponding spinal segments but had to descend down their corresponding vertebral levels to exit the column and hence the "Cauda equina" formation.

Cross-sectional Anatomy of Spinal Cord (Fig. 7.3)

On cross-section, the core of the spinal cord has a butterfly like pattern that comprises the gray matter that is surrounded by the white matter. The gray matter comprises cell bodies of the neurons and hence is unmyelinated while the white matter comprises axons and is the myelinated component. In other words, gray matter is the thinking part of the cord while white matter has the connecting ascending and descending tracts that relay the information between higher centers and the end organs.

LOCALIZING A SPINAL LESION

Three concepts are pivotal to localization of any injury in the spinal cord:

1. The concept of upper and lower motor neuron (LMN) lesion
2. The understanding of a reflex
3. The knowledge of dermatomes and myotomes.

Upper and Lower Motor Neuron Lesions

Upper motor neurons (UMNs) refer to the nerve cells that extend from brain cortex to the anterior horn cells of the spinal cord

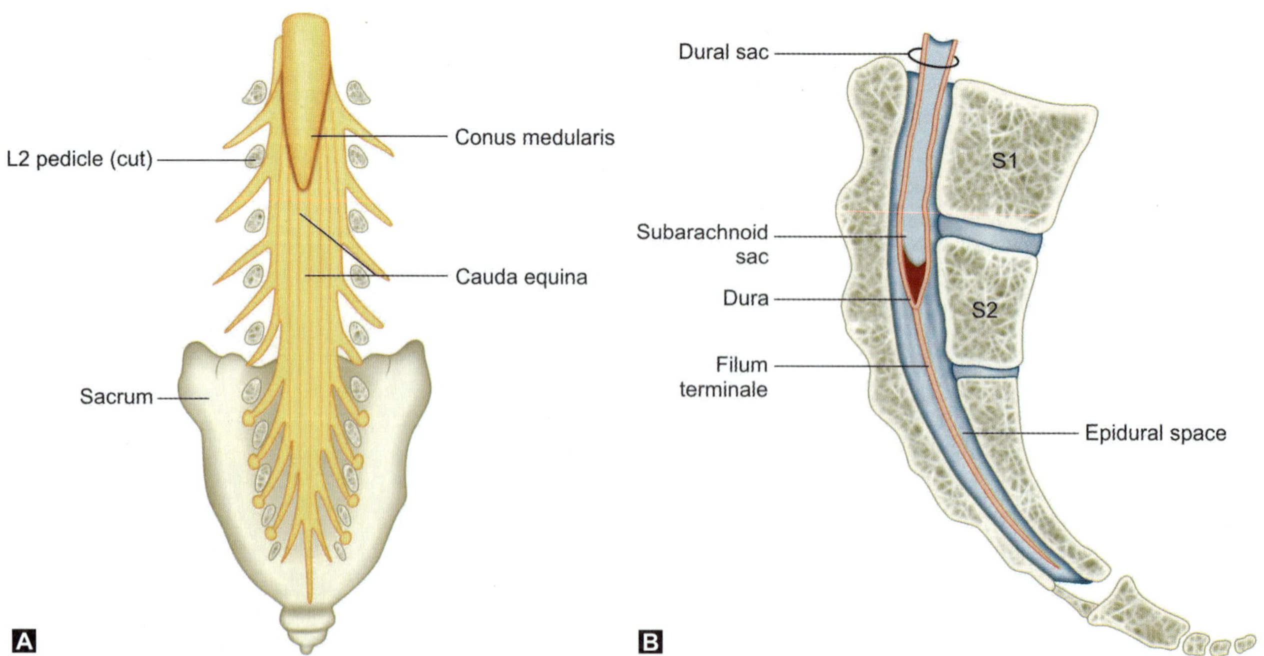

Figs 7.1A and B: Diagram depicting the terminal anatomy of spinal cord. (A) Coronal view; (B) Sagittal view

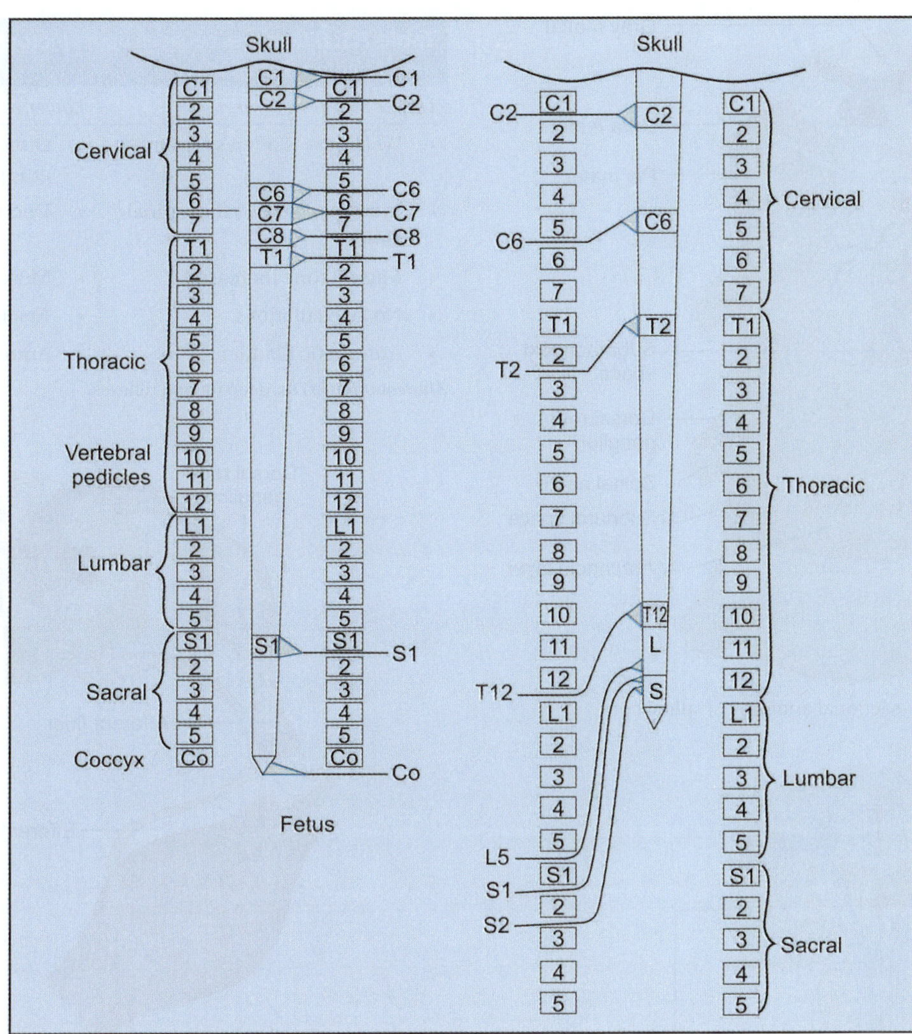

Fig. 7.2: Variable lengths of vertebral column and spinal cord

while the LMNs refer to the cells extending from the anterior horn of cord to the neuromuscular junctions. To simplify one may say that UMNs are basically the brain and spinal cord while the LMNs are the nerves **(Fig. 7.4)**. The features of both types of lesions are depicted in **Table 7.1**. Thus, one would find exaggerated reflexes and hypertonia when the injury involves the central nervous system while areflexia and flaccidity is a prime feature of peripheral nervous system lesions.

The concept behind such a presentation is very simple. Let us assume that the spinal cord is transected at C6 level, then the inhibitory impulses generated by the higher centers are unable to reach the lower cord and the neurons distal to the injury level start firing (owing to their innate excitatory tone). As a result, below the level of injury the muscles get hypertonic and reflexes become exaggerated. However, one must note that even in UMN lesion, at the level of the cord lesion, the reflexes are absent and the muscles are atonic. This is the complete presentation of UMN lesion. LMN lesion is absolutely different. In this, there is an injury to a nerve **(Fig. 7.4)** and the reflex contributed by the injured nerve or the muscle supplied by that nerve undergoes flaccid paralysis. However, in LMN lesion, the spinal levels below

the level of nerve injury are going to remain unaffected unlike UMN lesions, where the lower levels get hypertonic.

Reflexes

Most people would think of a reflex as an involuntary muscular contraction to a stimulus. Technically, a reflex is a simple sensory-motor pathway that involves a single spinal segment, which means in a reflex the stimulus is carried to the spinal cord via the dorsal root and the action returns to the contracting muscle by only involving the single spinal segment **(Fig. 7.5)**. A reflex does not need relaying with the higher centers and can function on its own. As opposed to this, the pathway for voluntary motion is absolutely different. The stimulus is carried from cord to brain via the white matter ascending tracts, processed in the brain and then relayed down to the appropriate muscles via the descending corticospinal tracts. Hence, the crux difference between a reflex and voluntary motion is that reflex does not need the ascending or descending tracts of the white matter of cord to function, unlike voluntary actions which rely on these connecting tracts. Imagine a patient with cord injury at D12 level. The cord below D12 will demonstrate UMN lesion and hence the knee reflex that arises

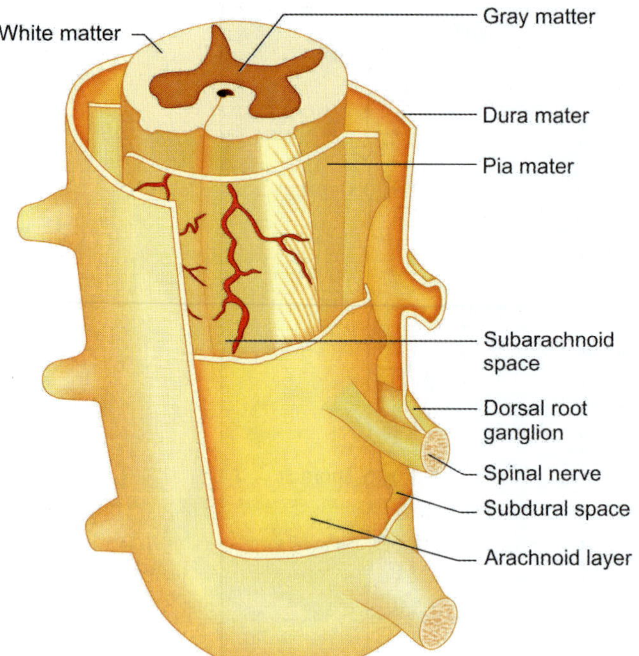

Fig. 7.3: Cross-sectional anatomy of spinal cord

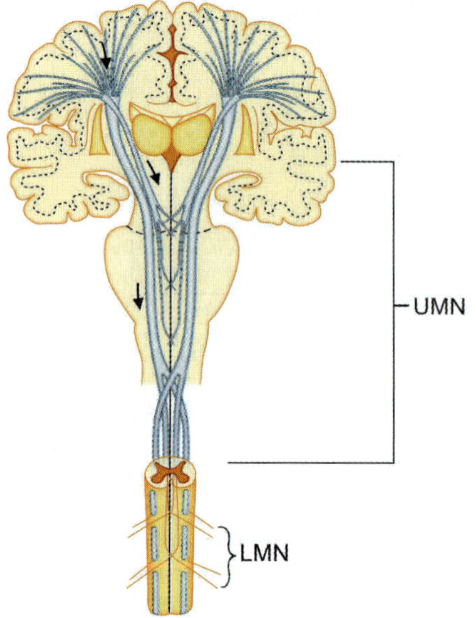

Fig. 7.4: The upper motor neurons (UMN) and
lower motor neurons (LMN)

Table 7.1: Differences between upper motor neuron (UMN) and lower motor neuron (LMN) lesion

Upper motor neuron	Lower motor neuron
• Weakness is often symmetric	• Often a single muscle group (with atrophy)
• Increased DTRs (after spinal shock)	• Decreased DTRs
• Muscle tone increased	• Muscle tone decreased
• No fasciculations	• Fasciculations
• Automatic bladder	• Autonomous bladder

Abbreviation: DTRs, deep tendon reflexes.

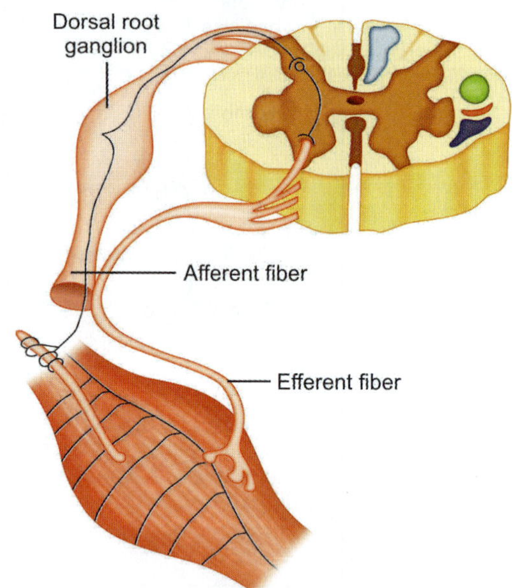

Fig. 7.5: Reflex arc

Hence, the moral is that if we know the level of various reflexes, and their behavior in response to injury, we can locate any spinal lesion. At the level of cord transection (UMN lesion), the reflexes are absent, but below that level the reflexes are present (because they traverse single spinal segment) and in fact, exaggerated. However, when a nerve is transected (LMN lesion), the reflex innervated by that particular nerve is absent, while the distal reflexes remain elicitable and are normal. Levels of some important reflexes are given in **Table 7.2**.

Note: The concept of a reflex discussed earlier holds true for deep tendon reflexes (DTRs) only as these are monosynaptic. The superficial reflexes are polysynaptic having multiple interconnections in the cord itself and they do not behave in the same manner. Superficial reflexes above the level of injury are spared while those at and below the level of injury are absent.

Dermatomes/Myotomes

A myelomere is a segment of the spinal cord that gives rise to a pair of dorsal and ventral roots that join to form a spinal nerve, total being 31 pairs. Let us understand how this spinal nerve is different from a peripheral nerve (e.g. median nerve, radial nerve,

from L2 to L3 will be exaggerated, which means if one strikes the ligamentum patellae with a knee hammer, the quadriceps contracts or more appropriately hypercontracts (exaggerated reflex). However, if you ask this person to voluntarily contract his quadriceps he cannot, because in this situation the impulse goes to the brain and is sent down by the connecting white matter tracts. But since the cord is transacted at D12 level, no information can go down that level, which means the patient voluntarily cannot contract quadriceps. This is what paraplegia is, i.e. when voluntary motion is not possible below the level of the lesion but reflexes will be intact because they involve a single spinal level.

etc.). Consider the T4 spinal nerve. The nerve arises from the spine and divides into ventral and dorsal rami and then the rami divide into motor and sensory branches. The sensory branches would supply the skin over the nipples and the motor branches would supply the intercostal muscles. However, the situation is very different for the spinal nerves that have to supply the limbs. The spinal nerves C5–C8, T1 leave the cord and then join in front of the scapula to form the brachial plexus for the upper limb while it is the lumbosacral plexus formation that takes place for the lower limbs. The nerves that leave the plexus are the peripheral nerves, although these peripheral nerves actually are carrying the fibers of spinal nerves only. So technically the plexuses mix up the spinal nerve fibers and redistribute them into peripheral nerves. For example, "Deltoid" is supplied by C5 spinal nerve, but the fibers reach the muscle via the axillary nerve which is a peripheral nerve. Similarly, although the sensation over little finger is supplied by C8 spinal nerve, the fibers actually are traveling via the ulnar nerve.

A dermatome refers to that area of skin which is supplied by a single spinal nerve, may the fibers travel via any number of peripheral nerves, and a myotome refers to that muscle which is supplied by a single spinal nerve. If we know the level of various dermatomes and myotomes and their behavior to injury, we can localize any spinal lesion. Understanding their behavior is very simple. Since sensory information is detected by peripheral receptors and then ascends across cord to be deciphered at appropriate centers in brain, in case of cord injury (UMN lesion), all dermatomes, may it be one at the level of injury or all below the level of injury demonstrate sensory loss, as no information can cross and ascend above the level of transection. However, in case of injury to a nerve (LMN lesion), the sensory loss is restricted only to the dermatome of the affected nerve, as cord is intact to relay information from other nerve roots.

Behavior of myotomes is different from dermatomes. In case of cord lesion (UMN), the myotomes at the level of cord injury end up in flaccid paralysis while those below the level of the injury show spastic paralysis due to cessation of inhibitory impulses from higher centers. But in nerve lesions (LMN), the myotomes supplied by the nerve only are paralyzed and demonstrate flaccid paralysis. The distal muscles remain normal.

Caution: Remember, paralysis refers to loss of voluntary control. Hence, spasticity and flaccidity, both are paralysis. Although a spastic muscle has good tone, can contract, it is considered paralyzed as it is out of voluntary control.

The levels of some important dermatomes **(Fig. 7.6)** and myotomes **(Table 7.3)** are shown later.

Deciding the Level of Spinal and Vertebral Lesion

After knowledge of the earlier discussed concepts, localization of spinal cord lesion becomes very simple. If a patient has exaggerated reflexes and hypertonia, there is an injury to the spinal cord. One should look for the absent reflex to locate the uppermost level of injury to the cord and would find all reflexes distal to that level to be exaggerated as would be the tone. An injury to a nerve root should be suspected when there is an isolated absent reflex or flaccid paralysis of a single level myotome with distal functions preserved.

Caution: Remember spinal cord ends at the lower border of L1, so there is no cord below that level and hence, if there is a lesion in the vertebral column below that level (for example, disk prolapse L4–L5), one can never have exaggerated reflexes or UMN lesion. It would present as a LMN lesion, which means that the involved reflex will be absent, muscle flaccidly paralyzed and sensation in the affected dermatome absent. However, everything below that level would be unaffected. The UMN lesion is generally common with vertebral injuries above L1, because most of the canal in this region is occupied by the spinal cord.

Identifying the Affected Vertebra

Once the level of cord lesion is elucidated, one can make out the likely vertebra that is involved as well, by a simple formula mentioned in **Table 7.4**. The level can further be confirmed by identifying **(Table 7.5)** and palpating the vertebra.

NEUROLOGICAL DEFICITS AT VARIOUS SPINAL LEVELS

Cervical Spine

Here injury to vertebral column generally causes injury to the spinal cord that occupies the greater part of the canal, thereby

Table 7.2: Levels of some important reflexes
1. C5: Biceps
2. C6: Supinator (Brachioradialis)*
3. C7: Triceps
4. L3, L4: Knee reflex (Quadriceps)
5. L5, S1: Plantar reflex**
6. S1, S2: Ankle reflex (Gastrosoleus)

*The term "supinator reflex" is a misnomer. It is actually brachioradialis reflex as we strike the tendon of brachioradialis muscle at the radial styloid process. The older name for brachioradialis was supinator longus and hence the term.

**Plantar reflex is elicited by striking the lateral border of the sole of the foot. In normal reflex there is plantar flexion of the great toe and all toes come together. When the reflex is exaggerated, there is great toe dorsiflexion and fanning of all toes. This is called as Babinski sign. When the reflex is absent, there is no toe movement and the reflex is said to be mute.

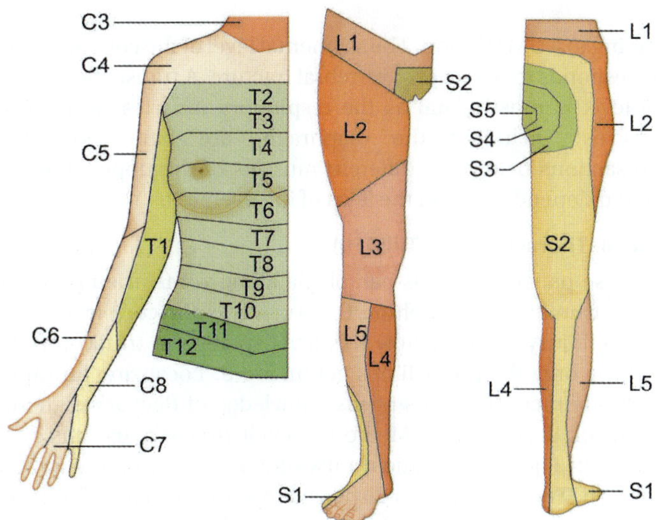

Fig. 7.6: Dermatomes of upper and lower limbs

Table 7.3: Important myotomes of upper and lower limbs

1. C5: Deltoid
2. C6: Wrist extensors
3. C7: Wrist flexors/elbow extensors
4. C8: Finger flexors
5. T1: Finger abductors
6. L1, L2: Hip flexor (Iliopsoas)
7. L3: Knee extensor (Quadriceps)
8. L4: Ankle dorsiflexor (Tibialis anterior)
9. L5: Long toe extensor (Extensor hallucis longus)
10. S1: Ankle plantar flexor (Gastrosoleus)

Table 7.4: Relationship between vertebral level and cord level

Spinal level	Cord level
Cervical vertebrae	Add 1 to vertebral level
Upper dorsal (D1 to D6)	Add 2 to vertebral level
Lower dorsal (D7 to D9)	Add 3 to vertebral level
D10	All dorsal segments over
D12	All lumbar segments over
L1	All sacral segments over
Below L1	Cauda equina

Table 7.5: Landmarks for identifying important vertebral levels

1. C2: First palpable spinous process C3: Hyoid bone
2. C4, 5: Thyroid cartilage C6: Cricoid
3. C7: Vertebra prominens (Longest cervical spinous process) T3, 4: Sternal notch
4. L3, 4: Umbilicus
5. L4, 5 disks: Highest point of iliac crest
6. S2: Posterior superior iliac spine

leading to a UMN lesion. The segmental level of the cord generally corresponds to the level of vertebral fracture. A transection above C5 level is mostly fatal as the respiratory muscles (intercostal muscles) including the diaphragm are paralyzed while transactions below C5, different muscles of the upper limb get spared depending upon the level of involvement.

Dorsal/Thoracic Spine (Till D10)

In these patients there is paraplegia along with varied paralysis of the trunk muscles. Behind D10 vertebrae the cord level is L1, so any injury at and below this level spares the trunk muscles and the only the lower limbs get involved. Localizing an injury in the thoracic segments needs knowledge of Beevor's sign and the trunk dermatomes. Method to elicit *Beevor's sign* has been shown in **Figure 7.7**. Patient raises the head from a recumbent position. The umbilicus is displaced toward the head. This is the result of paralysis of the inferior portion of the rectus abdominal muscle, so that the upper fibers predominate pulling upwards the

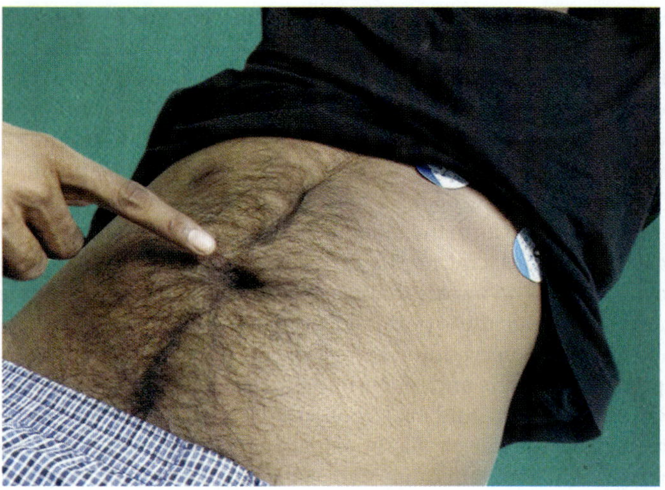

Fig. 7.7: Eliciting Beevor's sign

umbilicus, signifying injury distal to D10 cord level (remember, umbilicus lies at D10 spinal level).

D11–L1 Lesions

Behind these vertebral segments lie the lumbar and sacral cord segments. Injuries at these levels can involve both the cord as well as the nerve roots, and mixed pictures often result.

Lesions below L1 Vertebrae

Below L1, there is no spinal cord and the canal is occupied only by nerve roots the so called "cauda equina". Thus, injury in this area can only damage nerve roots and hence an upper motor picture is never possible. There is a lower motor lesion as per the number of nerve roots involved.

Nerve Root involved in a Prolapsing Disk

While a vertebral lesion (e.g. fracture, tumor, tuberculosis) by convention, involves the corresponding nerve root (for instance, L4 root in L4 fracture), the case is not same in disk prolapse. Disk prolapse is generally seen in lower lumbar spine with most common site being L4–L5 followed by L5–S1. We already know that every spinal nerve exits the canal by passing through the intervertebral foramen present on the sides of the corresponding vertebrae, e.g. L4 nerve root will pass out of the canal by exiting through the intervertebral foramen on the side of the L4 vertebrae. Now, consider the situation when there is a disk prolapse L4–L5. The disk is present below the L4 vertebrae and if this disk goes back, it cannot compress the L4 nerve root as the same has already exited **(Fig. 7.8)** from the foramen present on the sides of the vertebrae. However, the L5 nerve root is coming from the L1 level, where the cord has already ended and thus L5 is the traversing nerve root in the canal which is traveling down to exit on the side of the L5 vertebrae. Henceforth, if the disk between L4 and L5 prolapses, it would be the L5 nerve root that would be affected **(Fig. 7.8)**. The same applies to all lumbar nerve roots and it is always the lower level nerve root that is involved by a prolapsing disk.

Caution: Even in cervical disk prolapse where the nerves actually exit from the top of the corresponding vertebrae rather than below it, the lower nerve root is involved. This is because while in lumbar spine the disk involves traversing nerve root, in cervical spine the disk involves exiting nerve root due to a varied anatomy (*see* Page 240).

However, in cervical disk prolapse isolated nerve involvement occurs only if the disk prolapse is far lateral, as most other disks tend to indent cord present in the cervical area.

Cauda Equina and Conus Medullaris

We already know that if L4–L5 disk will prolapse, it will compress the L5 nerve root as the latter is the traversing nerve root in the canal. But one can well imagine that all distal nerve roots, viz. S1–S5 will also be the traversing roots at this level **(Fig. 7.8)**, although more central in location. When a single nerve root is compressed by any lesion (most often a disk), the condition is called as "radiculopathy". But many a times a compressing lesion (like a large sized disk) involves compression of multiple nerve roots that are hanging in the canal. This condition is referred to as "cauda equina syndrome" (c.f. Cauda equina—Hanging nerve

roots). This multilevel radiculopathy is manifested clinically as a LMN lesion as it is a nerve root compression and presents as a triad that includes asymmetric (since disks generally herniate posterolaterally to one side), areflexic (lower motor lesion) motor paralysis, bladder bowel involvement (S2–S4 involvement) and saddle anesthesia (anesthesia in distribution of S3 and S4 roots that involves the periphery of buttocks but initially spares the perianal area as perianal dermatome S5 is involved the last). One must remember that "cauda equina" is an orthopedic emergency and must be treated urgently.

An important differential of Cauda Equina syndrome is the Conus Medullaris syndrome. The latter results due to compression of the conus (sacral part of spinal cord). When the sacral part would be compressed, at the level of the lesion, there would be lower motor picture and below exaggerated picture. But this is an exception, because there is nothing below sacral level for exaggeration, the lesion turns out to be LMN type, thereby closely resembling Cauda Equina syndrome. However, the two can be differentiated on the following basis **(Table 7.6)**.

Grading of motor weakness is done according to standardized motor examination rating scale **(Table 7.7)**. Sensory examination should include pin prick, light touch and compared with other side.

ACUTE SPINAL CORD INJURY

The behavior discussed earlier is the behavior shown by the spinal cord in chronic long-term cases. In case there is an acute

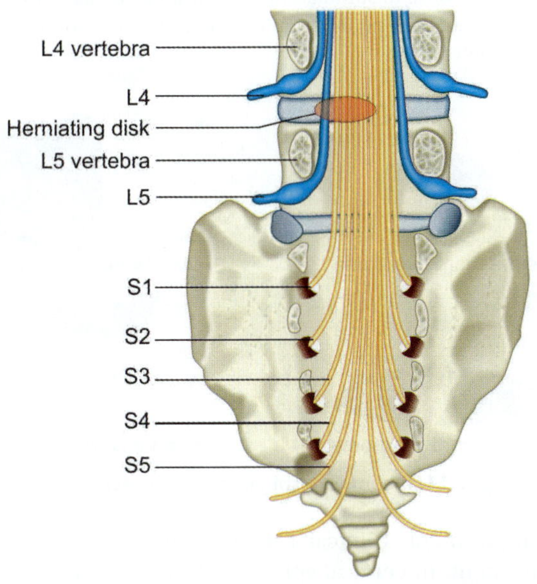

Fig. 7.8: Relation of nerve root and corresponding disk

Table 7.7: Grading of motor weakness, according to standardized motor examination rating scale

1.	Grade 0: Total paralysis
2.	Grade 1: Palpable or visible contraction
3.	Grade 2: Active movement through a full range of motion, gravity eliminated
4.	Grade 3: Active movement through full range of motion, against gravity
5.	Grade 4: Active movement through a full range of motion, against gravity and provides some resistance
6.	Grade 5: Active movement through a full range of motion, against gravity and provides normal resistance

Table 7.6: Differentiating features of cauda equina and conus medullaris syndrome

Features	Cauda equina syndrome	Conus medullaris syndrome
Presentation	Asymmetric	Symmetric
Radicular pain	Severe	Usually not present
Sensory involvement **(Fig. 7.9)**	Saddle anesthesia (S2–S4) with perianal sparing initially (S5 sparing)	Perianal anesthesia (S5) as sacral cord compression involves loss of S5 cord segment
Motor involvement	Asymmetrical flaccid paralysis	Symmetric usually flaccid sometimes hyper-reflexive paralysis
Reflexes	Areflexia is classical knee reflex is lost if L3 and L4 roots involved	Knee reflex is always preserved
Bladder bowel involvement	Late feature	Early feature
Level of causative lesion	Compression of nerve roots usually by vertebral lesion L1 vertebra	Compression of conus (sacral part) by D12–L1 vertebral lesions
Sensory dissociation	Not found	Sensory dissociation can occur

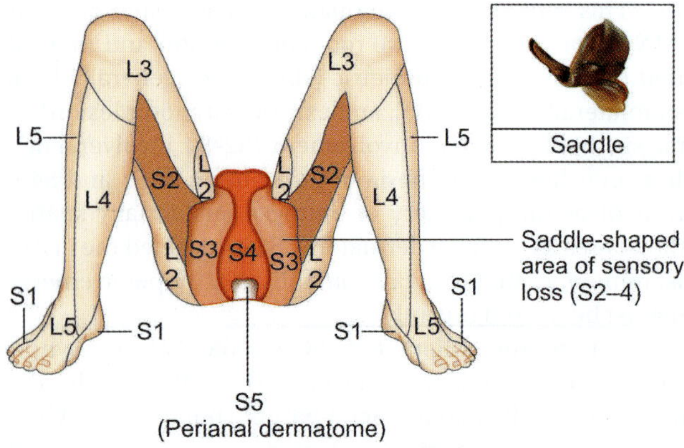

Fig. 7.9: Diagrammatic depiction of saddle and perianal anesthesia

traumatic injury to the cord, the initial behavior is slightly different till the classic patterns discussed above become evident.

Just after an acute cord injury there is cessation of all activity at and below the level of lesion. This stage of physiological disruption is referred to as "spinal shock". The stage persists for 24–48 hours after which recovery starts and the classical UMN pattern starts evolving. The first reflex to return once the spinal shock is over is the Bulbocavernosus reflex **(Fig. 7.10)**, hence the presence of this reflex heralds the end of the stage of spinal shock and onset of recovery.

COMPLETE VERSUS INCOMPLETE SPINAL CORD INJURY

Once the bulbocavernosus reflex returns, it signifies that spinal shock is over and recovery has started. Complete spinal cord transaction is characterized by complete absence of sensations as well as voluntary motor activity caudal to the level of spinal injury after the spinal shock is over, i.e. an elicitable bulbocavernosus reflex.

If any evidence of neurological function (motor or sensory) can be demonstrated distal to the level of lesion, the injury is termed incomplete. Incomplete injury means that at least sacral nerve root function is preserved since it is the central most part of the spine. This "sacral sparing" is represented by intact perianal sensations, voluntary rectal motor function and great toe flexor activity. It indicates at least partial continuity of white matter long tracts thereby signifying incomplete injury and potential for a greater return of cord function.

Incomplete Spinal Cord Injury Syndromes (Fig. 7.11)

Incomplete injury to the spinal cord may present in either of the following commonly encountered patterns:

Central Cord Syndrome

This is the most common incomplete spinal cord injury (SCI) syndrome. It results from hyperextension injury in older person with pre-existing osteoarthritis of spine. The spinal cord is pinched between the vertebral body anteriorly and the buckled ligamentum flavum posteriorly with pressure getting concentrated around the cord area lying in the vicinity of the central canal. Due to typical arrangement of spinal tracts (the arm fibers medially, and the leg fibers laterally, **Figs 7.12A and B)**, the arms are more severely affected than the legs, resulting in a disproportionate

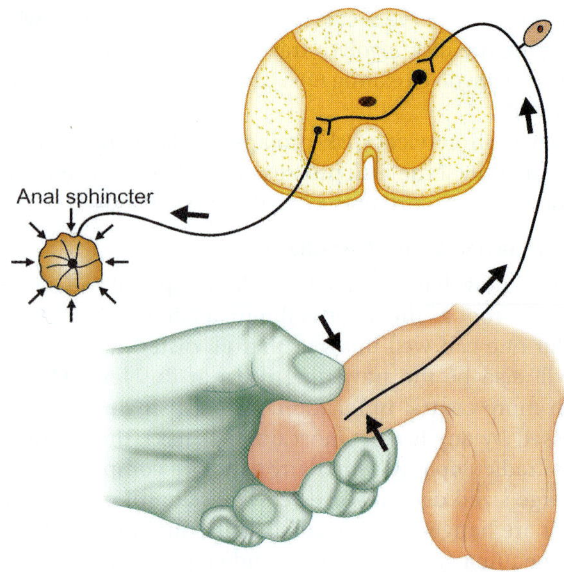

Fig. 7.10: Bulbocavernosus reflex refers to contraction of the anal sphincter in response to stimulation of the trigone of bladder with either a squeeze on the glans penis, a tap on the mons pubis or a pull on the uretheral catheter

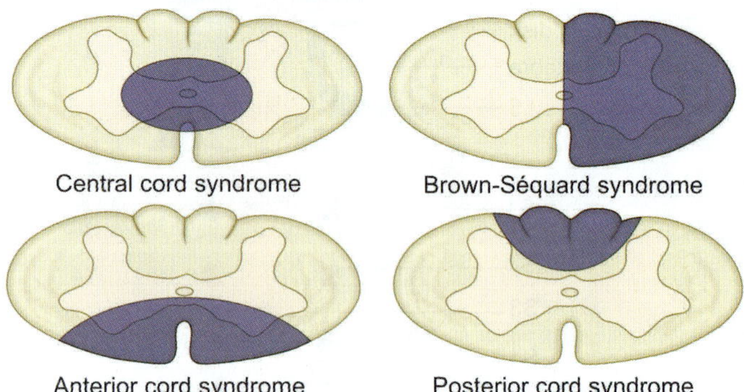

Fig. 7.11: Incomplete spinal cord injury syndromes

motor impairment. Clinical presentation depends on the site of involvement. In cervical spine involvement (most commonly affected area) patients present with quadriparesis with weakness involving the upper limbs (flaccid paralysis, due to a LMN type lesion at the level of spinal injury) more than lower limbs (spastic paralysis due to a UMN type lesion below the level of injury), varying degree of sensory loss below the level of spinal injury with or without bladder involvement. Prognosis is good with more than 50% patients recovering bladder, bowel function and ambulation.

Brown-Séquard Syndrome

It refers to hemitransaction of spinal cord characterized by ipsilateral loss of muscle power, proprioception and sense of vibration and contralateral loss of pain and temperature sensation. Prognosis for recovery is very good.

Anterior Cord Syndrome

Anterior cord syndrome typically results after hyperflexion injuries to the cord. It is characterized by predominantly motor loss, loss of pain and temperature. Dorsal column (sensations) function is preserved. The recovery rate is the poorest.

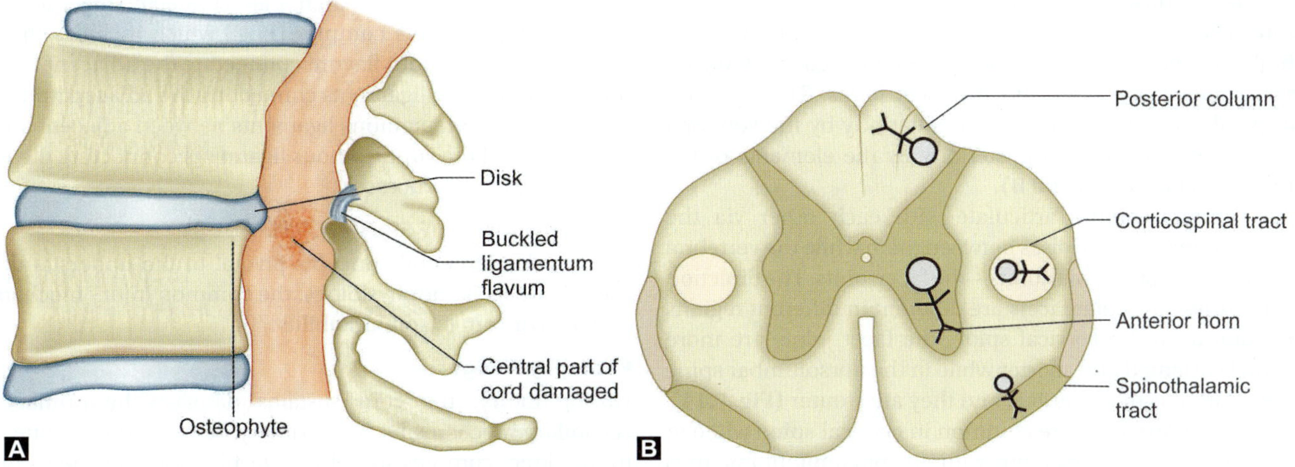

Figs 7.12A and B: Mechanism of central cord syndrome

Posterior Cord Syndrome

It is caused by extension injury and involves the dorsal column. There is loss of dorsal column function (proprioception and vibration). Motor and other sensory functions (pain and temperature) are generally spared. Recovery rate is poor.

COMPLICATIONS OF ACUTE SPINAL CORD INJURY

Two notable complications that may arise when the patient is in the stage of spinal shock are: (1) neurogenic shock, and (2) autonomic dysreflexia.

Neurogenic Shock

Neurogenic shock is seen in cases with SCI above T6 level. It results from impairment of the descending sympathetic pathways in the spinal cord resulting in loss of vasomotor tone and loss of sympathetic innervations to the heart.

The result is the classic hemodynamic triad consisting of hypotension (due to loss of vasopressor tone causing peripheral vasodilatation), bradycardia and hypothermia. An important differential is hypovolemic shock, but the latter is characterized by hypotension with tachycardia.

Management: Unlike hypovolemic shock where the prime treatment is fluid replacement, in neurogenic shock vasopressors have to be given to counteract hypotension and atropine to counteract bradycardia. The condition almost always resolves within 24–48 hours.

Autonomic Dysreflexia

Autonomic dysreflexia also occurs in people with a SCI at or above T6 level, but results in severe hypertension, bradycardia and symptoms such as profuse sweating and headache. The exact mechanism is unclear, but seems to be related to a large sympathetic outflow from the injured cord or increased responsiveness of organs to catecholamines after SCI.

Management

Management involves removing a potential trigger like a blocked catheter or administering drugs like antihypertensives (nitroglycerin), lidocaine to block afferent signal or spinal anesthetics.

HIGH-YIELD POINTS

- *Inverted reflex:* Here contraction of opposite muscle occurs than expected on performing the reflex. This is usually seen when there is radiculomyelopathy as when a degenerative disk presses both nerve root and cord. Nerve root compression leads to absent segmental reflex while cord compression leads to hyper-reflexia that causes antagonist muscle contraction. For example, in inverted radial reflex (C5 > C6) tapping the distal brachioradialis tendon produces diminished brachioradialis contraction but hyperactive finger flexion.
- *Hoffman reflex:* It is upper extremity variant of Babinski reflex. Flickering of terminal phalanx of 3rd–4th finger produces flexion of terminal phalanx of thumb.

SPINAL INJURIES

INTRODUCTION

Spinal cord injury remains the most devastating injury for patients and spine surgeons alike. Despite several basic science and clinical advances in the study of cord injury, there is still no effective cure. Hence, research continues and treatment principles continue to evolve as our understanding of the biomechanics is increasing.

Vertebral fractures span through all age groups and affect four times more commonly the males than the females. Almost one out of every five patients lands up with a neurological deficit, in the form of either paraparesis or quadriparesis. The most common mode of injury leading to spine fractures in the developing world remains fall from height while in the developed world the road traffic accidents have taken the precedence. Cases are also being increasingly reported in athletes and sportsmen (15%). The overall mortality from spinal fractures has been reported to be as high as 20% at initial hospitalization which signifies the catastrophic potential of SCI.

RELEVANT ANATOMY

The vertebral column is composed of 33 vertebrae (7 cervical, 12 dorsal, 5 lumbar, 5 sacral and 4 coccygeal; the last five segments being generally fused together). Each vertebra has a similar structure being composed of a vertebral body anteriorly and a vertebral arch posteriorly. The arch is composed of pedicles, laminae, spinous processes and the facet joints. The cord lies in the spinal canal being surrounded anteriorly by the vertebral body's posterior margin and posteriorly by the elements of the vertebral arch **(Figs 7.13A and B)**.

The vertebral bodies articulate with each other via the intervening intervertebral disks between them while the vertebral arches articulate via synovial joints—the facet joints. The direction and size of these articular facets are different in different regions of the column. In the cervical spine, the facet joints are more horizontally oriented and shorter while in the dorsolumbar spine their orientation is more vertical and they are stouter **(Fig. 7.14)**. Hence, dislocations are more common in cervical spine while in the lower spine, pure dislocations without concomitant fractures are rare.

Apart from these bony articulations, a number of ligaments play vital role in providing stability to the spine **(Fig. 7.15)**. The anterior and posterior longitudinal ligaments run longitudinally along the anterior and posterior margins of the vertebral body respectively. The vertebral arches are connected together via the posterior ligamentous complex (PLC) which includes the thick but elastic ligamentum flavum connecting the adjacent laminae, the intertransverse ligaments connecting the adjacent transverse processes, the interspinous ligaments between adjacent spinous processes and the supraspinous ligaments connecting the tips of adjacent spinous processes.

BIOMECHANICS OF SPINAL CORD INJURY

The key fundamental concepts pivotal to the understanding of the SCI are its pathophysiology, the common injury mechanisms and the concept of spinal stability.

Pathophysiology

During injury, the cord sustains damages by primary and secondary mechanisms. The primary damage to the spine refers to the direct compression of the cord by bony fragments or disk material leading to hypoxia of both white and gray matter. This acute primary damage initiates a cascade of vascular and metabolic events consisting of oxidative free radical damage and reperfusion injury to the cord. This post-traumatic cord ischemia (secondary damage) is directly proportional to the severity of injury.

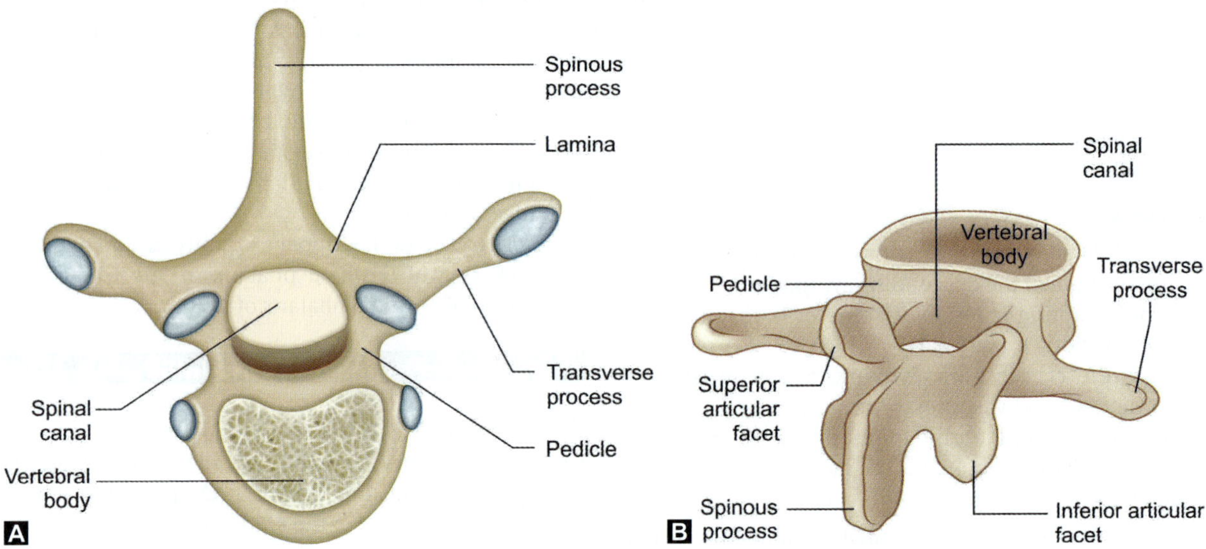

Figs 7.13A and B: Parts of a vertebral body

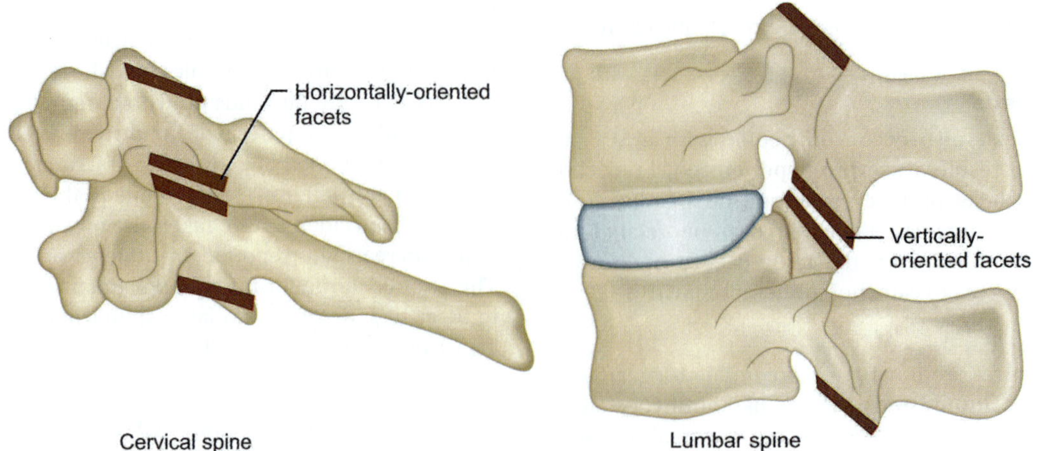

Fig. 7.14: Orientation of the facet joints

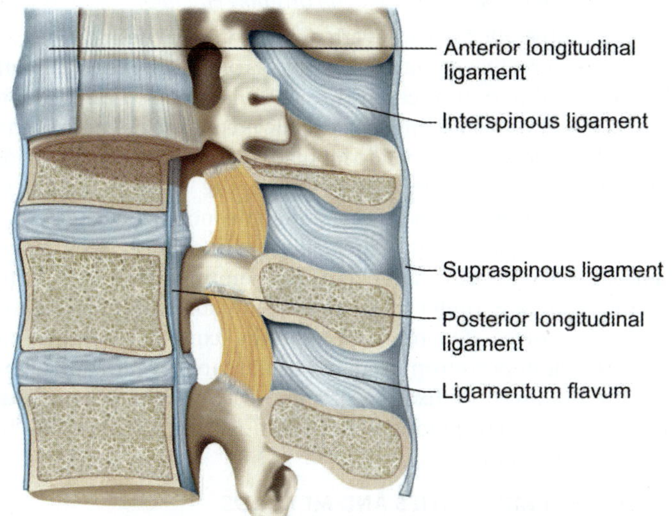

Fig. 7.15: Diagrammatic depiction of the spinal ligaments

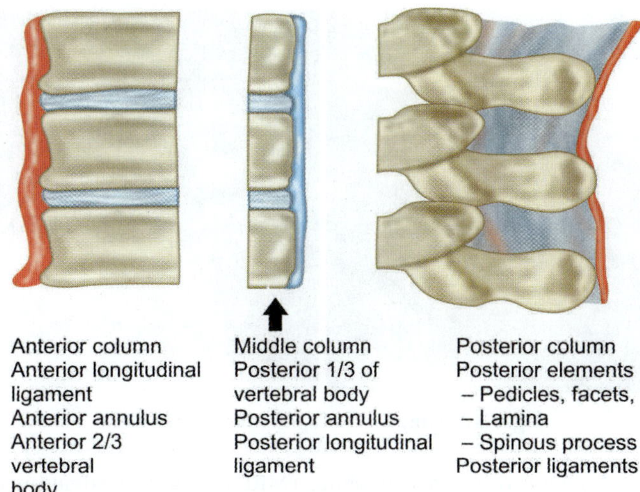

Fig. 7.16: Denis three column concept of spinal stability

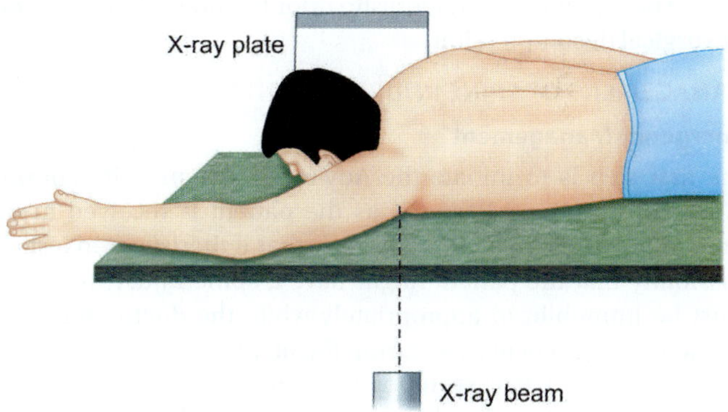

Fig. 7.17: Patient positioning in swimmer's view

Mechanisms of Spinal Cord Injury

Many types of forces act either in isolation or more commonly in combination to cause spinal injury. Basically there are four categories of forces relevant to spinal injuries:
1. Axial compression or distraction
2. Hyperflexion (most common) or hyperextension
3. Rotation
4. Shear/translation.

These forces mostly act in varied combinations to produce bony and ligamentous injury of spine. Due to the different shape and orientation of vertebrae in different parts of spine same forces may produce different patterns of injury in different parts of the spine (*see* later).

CONCEPT OF SPINAL STABILITY

A stable injury is one where the vertebral fracture would not displace further by normal movements of the spinal column. So if the neurological structures are not damaged, there is little risk of any damage occurring further. An unstable injury is one where there is a risk of further displacement of the fracture during the normal spine movements, thereby posing significant risk of further neurological deterioration.

To define spinal instability, Denis gave the three column concept of spinal stability **(Fig. 7.16)**. He divided spine into three columns—(1) anterior, (2) middle, and (3) posterior.

Injuries that involve two or more than two columns are considered unstable. Also injuries that do not involve the middle column are termed "minor injuries" and are considered stable.

A recently proposed concept is by Punjabi and White for quantifying the spinal stability for cervical as well as thoracolumbar region. It is a complex scoring based on the amount of displacement in spinal fracture, presence of neurological damage and the response of the spine on physiological loading.

DIAGNOSTIC ASPECTS

Clinical Assessment

A meticulous clinical examination is must for ruling out the presence of a neurological involvement. A thorough neurological assessment (as described earlier in behavior of the spine) should answer the three important questions:
1. What is the level of vertebral and cord involvement?
2. Whether the spinal cord injury is complete or incomplete?
3. If there is any associated injury (e.g. head injury).

The examination is particularly difficult in an unconscious patient in whom a spinal injury must be assumed unless proven otherwise. Alarming signs include absence of a painful stimulus, a flaccid anal sphincter, diaphragmatic breathing, concomitant head injury and hypotension with bradycardia (neurogenic shock).

Imaging

It is mandatory to get both AP and lateral radiographs of spine in every polytrauma patient who complains of pain or stiffness around neck or back. A lateral X-ray can identify lesion in 85% cases of cervical spine fractures. Open mouthed views may be required for visualizing the upper two cervical vertebrae. Swimmer's view **(Figs 7.17 and 7.18)** is useful to obtain visualization of all cervical vertebrae and sometimes it may also show the upper half of T1 vertebrae.

For imaging difficult areas like the upper cervical spine or the cervicothoracic junction, CT scan is the preferred modality. CT is ideal for identifying any structural damage to the vertebra or displaced vertebral fragments into the spinal canal.

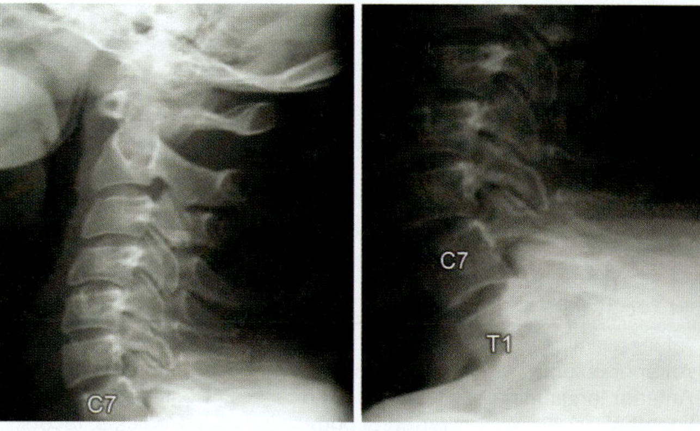

Fig. 7.18: X-ray cervical spine: Swimmer's view

Magnetic resonance imaging (MRI) is the investigation of choice for displaying the intervertebral disks, ligamentum flavum and the neural structures. It can best identify compression of the cord or nerves and is a prerequisite prior to undertaking a patient for surgical decompression.

MANAGEMENT OF SPINE INJURY PATIENTS

Emergency Management

The first step is to initiate the Advanced Trauma Life Support (ATLS) protocol (*see* Page 52) as the patient is received in the emergency. The essential principle is that if there is even a slight possibility that the patient might have a spine injury, the spine must be immobilized appropriately while the doctor starts the resuscitation protocol by securing the airway (airway with cervical spine control). In case intubation or an airway patency procedure is required to be performed, manual in line stabilization (*see* **Fig. 3.8**, Page 54) of the cervical spine must be maintained. In case one needs to examine the back, the log rolling technique (*see* **Fig. 3.11**, Page 55) should be used to turn the patient. Thereafter, other serious injuries should be identified and appropriately treated. Details regarding emergency management have already been discussed in Chapter 3. Immobilization of the spine should be discontinued only after the spine has been cleared after thorough clinical and radiological assessment.

The most commonly used treatment strategy during emergency management to prevent the secondary injury to the spinal cord is "methylprednisolone". Although as per current literature the benefit is dubious, some surgeons prefer to give this steroid in a dose of 30 mg/kg IV bolus followed by a maintenance infusion of 5.4 mg/kg/hour over the next 23 hours, preferably in patients who present within 8 hours of injury.

Definite Management

Definitive management of these lesions is guided by two important factors—(1) the stability of the spine, and (2) the presence of a neurological deficit.

No Neurological Deficit and Stable Fractures

The management in such cases largely is conservative. A period of spinal immobilization (with collars, halo or braces) is all that is needed to give rest to the healing tissues and ligaments. Neurological deficit in stable fractures develops only occasionally, which could be an indication for decompression of the cord and fusion of the unstable spine.

Presence of Neurological Deficit or an Unstable Fracture

In case of unstable fractures with no neurological deficit, one can opt for conservative management but it is practically very difficult. A substantial period of cervical traction is required for patients with cervical spine fractures. A specialized team is needed to turn the patient every 2 hourly, care for bladder and bowel and provide appropriate physiotherapy. Over time the fracture stabilizes spontaneously and the patient can then be mobilized.

In most other cases, especially the ones with progressive neurological deficit (or significant cord compression on MRI), the doctors generally prefer to go ahead with surgical intervention. Surgery involves decompression of the cord (by removal of fracture fragments retropulsed into spinal canal), reduction of the fracture, followed by fixation of spine with special instruments (e.g. pedicle screws) along with fusion of the unstable spine by inserting bone grafts.

TREATMENT MODALITIES AND METHODS

For Cervical Spine

Cervical Collars (Figs 7.19A to D)

A wide variety of cervical collars are available for providing immediate spinal support in patients suspected of having a cervical spine injury. Soft collars provide only minimal support and hard/rigid collars are thus preferred. A still better option is the Philadelphia collar.

Crutchfield Tongs and Cervical Traction

Cervical traction is a conservative method of achieving reduction and maintaining it in unstable cervical spine fractures. Crutchfield tongs **(Fig. 7.20)** are fixed to the skull and a weight of minimum 10 kg is applied. Check X-rays are performed every 12 hours and weight adjusted as per needed. Once acceptable reduction is achieved, light traction is continued for 6 weeks and then a halo vest (*see* later) or a four postcollar is applied for another 6 weeks. A close watch must be kept on the neurological status during traction as, at times, it may even be deteriorating, in that case a surgical intervention is generally warranted.

Halo Vest (Figs 7.21A and B)

The halo ring is fixed to the forehead and connected to a vest applied to the chest to achieve immobilization of the neck. The stability of the system is very good. Proper positioning and checking torque pressure on the pins used for fixation of the halo ring regularly is essential.

Decompression and Fixation

Unstable fractures with neurological deficit need decompression in the form of removal of the fractured vertebral body (corpectomy) followed by spinal fusion with bone grafting and instrumentation. Surgical fusion of the unstable fractures allows early mobilization and is widely gaining popularity. The cervical spine is generally approached via the anterior approach (anterior cervical corpectomy).

For Thoracolumbar Spine

Spine Board

Spine board (*see* **Fig. 3.12**, Page 56) is used for transporting patients suspected of having fractures in thoracolumbar spine. It must be available in all emergency departments.

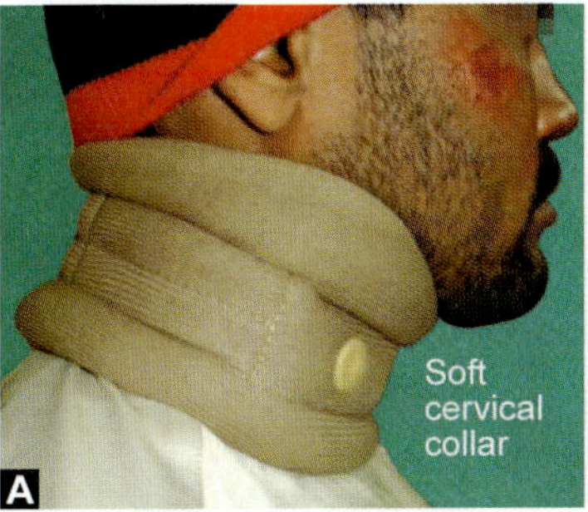

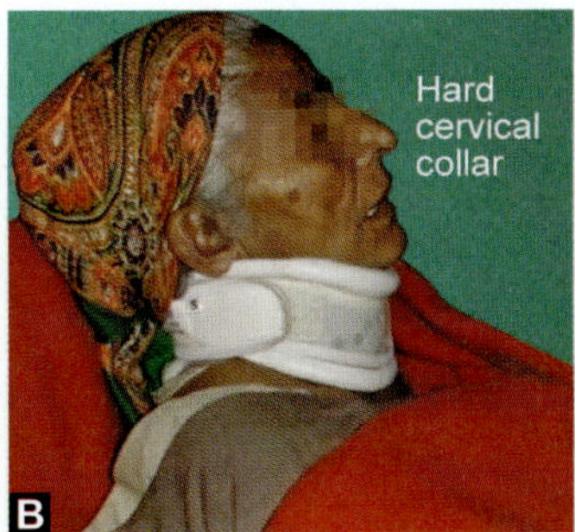

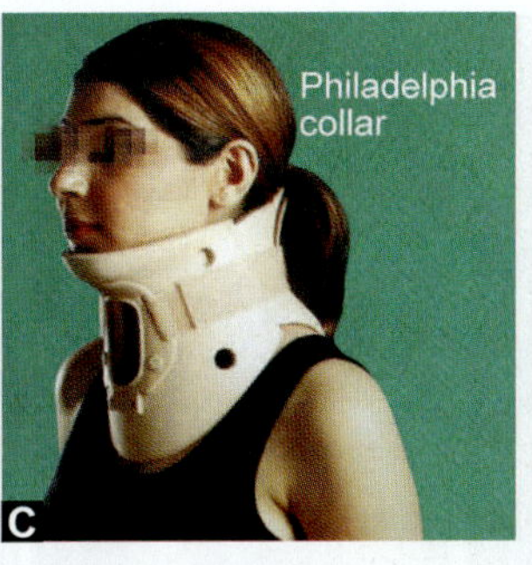

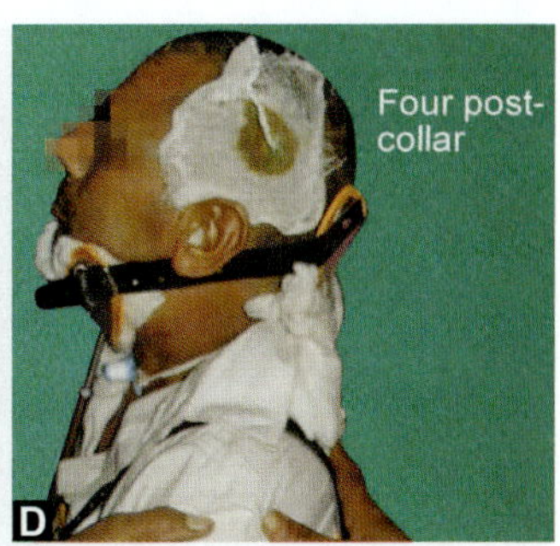

Figs 7.19A to D: Cervical spine immobilization with cervical collars

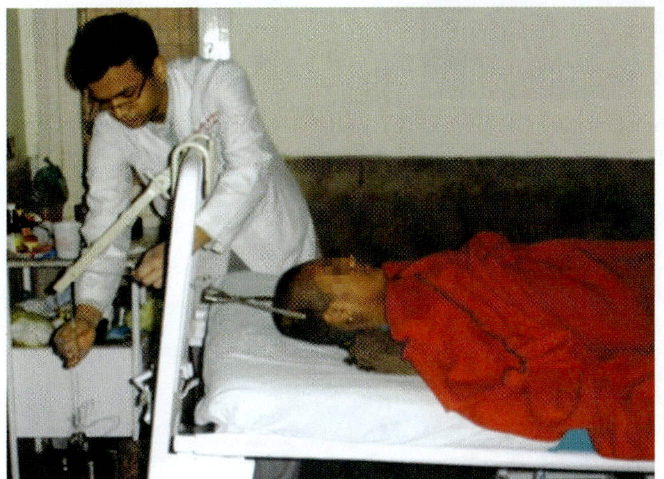

Fig. 7.20: Cervical traction via the crutchfield tongs

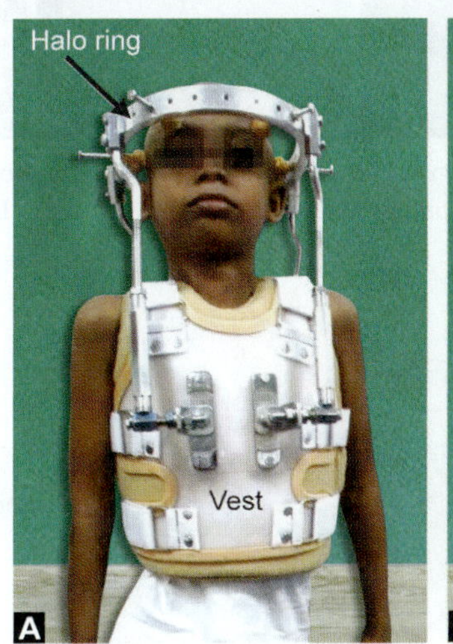

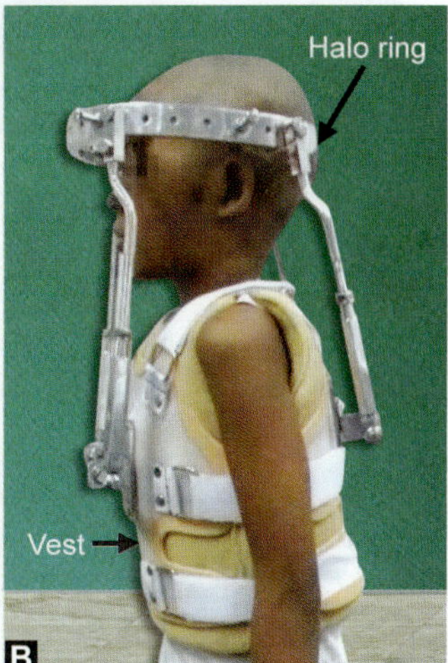

Figs 7.21A and B: (A) Halo vest—front view; (B) Halo vest—side view

Braces

Many types of thoracolumbar braces are available. Anterior spinal hyperextension (ASHE) brace **(Fig. 7.22)** provides three-point fixation and avoids inadvertent flexion that can be damaging. It is particularly used in some burst fracture and compression fracture cases where the patterns are stable and the patient has no neurological deficit.

Decompression and Fixation

For patients presenting with neurological deficit and unstable fracture, surgery in the form of decompression of cord (i.e. removal of retropulsed fracture fragments), instrumented fixation and spinal fusion (with bone grafts) is the preferred treatment.

For fusion, the graft is placed enclosed in a metal or plastic cage kept in place of intervertebral disk (called interbody fusion) followed by fixation performed mostly by the use of the special pedicle screw system **(Figs 7.23A to D)**. For surgery, the spine can be approached both by anterior and posterior approaches. The anterior approach is preferred for burst fractures where body fragments have retropulsed into the canal while the posterior approach being more surgeon-friendly is preferred in most other situations.

CERVICAL SPINE INJURIES

Distribution

The prevalence of injuries to the cervical spine has a bimodal distribution; they are most often encountered in adolescents

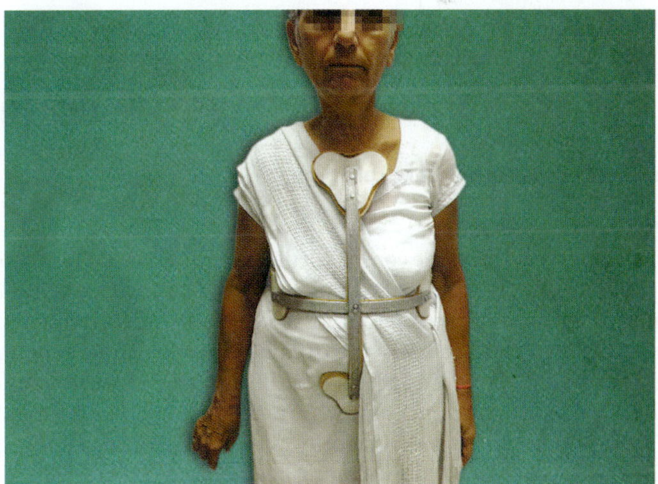

Fig. 7.22: Anterior spinal hyperextension (ASHE) brace

and young adults (15–25 years) and in those older than 60 years of age. Upper cervical spine injuries (C1 and C2) are responsible for the majority of these, with C2 being the most common site of injury. Head injury is the most common associated injury which occurs in conjunction with cervical spine injuries in up to 53% of these cases.

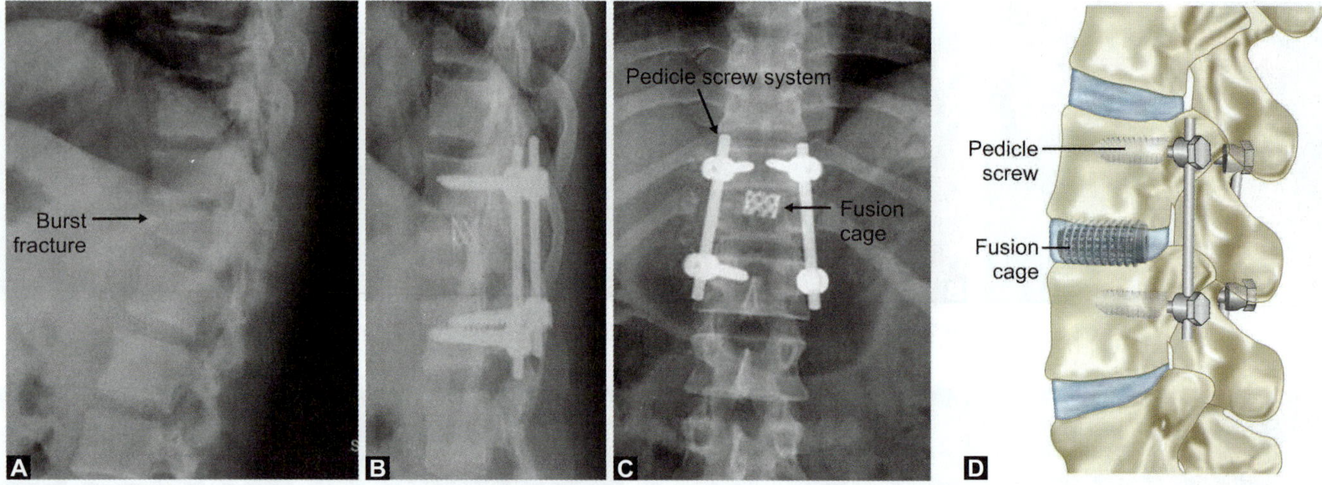

Figs 7.23A to D: (A) X-ray of thoracic spine lateral view showing burst fracture; (B) AP view; (C) Lateral views of thoracic spine of the same patient after pedicle screw fixation; (D) Diagrammatic representation of pedicle screw fixation

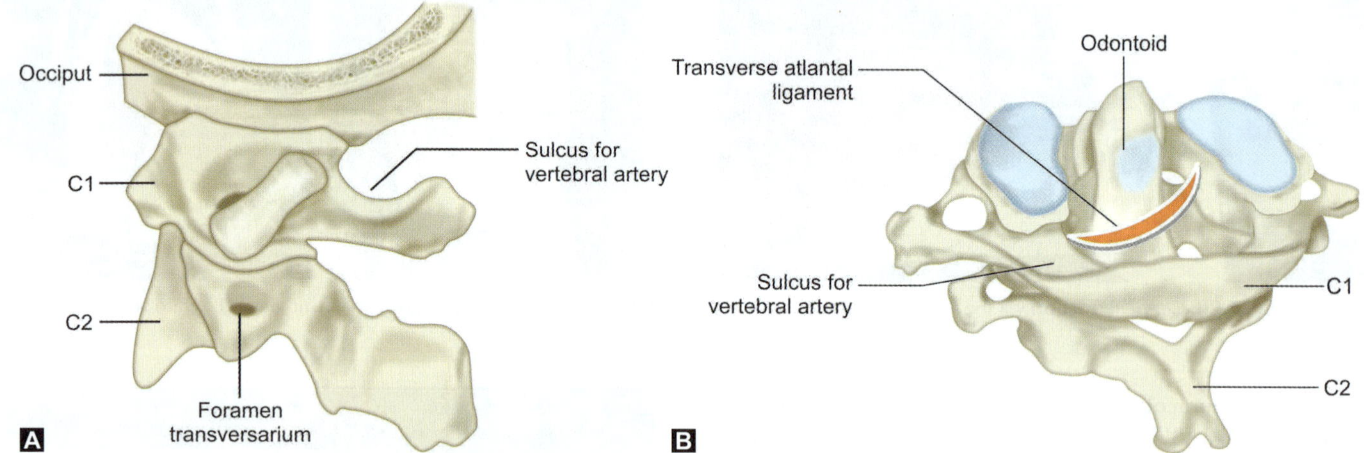

Figs 7.24A and B: Craniocervical junction. (A) Lateral view; (B) Posterior view

Injuries of the Upper Cervical Spine

Relevant Anatomy

The upper cervical spine consists of the occiput, atlas (C1) and axis (C2). These three structures along with their strong ligamentous attachments are often referred to as the craniocervical junction (CCJ) **(Figs 7.24A and B)**. The occiput-C1 articulation supplies approximately 50% of total cervical flexion and extension, and the C1–C2 articulations supply 50% of total cervical rotation. Corresponding to this, the majority of the mechanical stability at the CCJ is provided by the investing ligamentous structures.

Clinical Presentation

Patients with upper cervical spine injuries can present with complete ventilator dependent quadriplegia to incomplete lesions including central cord syndrome (*see* Page 214) or as Bell's cruciate paralysis (due to compression of crossed upper limb and uncrossed lower limb tracts). In these injuries, there is a high chance of a vertebral artery rupture, which can cause fatal ischemic damage to the brainstem. So, patients with upper cervical injury can also present with features of cranial nerve injury (CN VI, VII, IX, X, XI and XII). A classic example is Wallenberg's syndrome, which is a lateral medullary infraction resulting from occlusion of the vertebral artery (more common) or posterior inferior cerebellar artery. Delayed cortical blindness and recurrent quadriparesis can also occur from occult vertebral artery injury after cervical trauma.

Imaging

Plain radiographs are the first modality with anteroposterior (AP), lateral and the open mouth view as the standard series of X-rays. The sagittal alignment of the spine should be evaluated by four imaginary lines: (1) anterior vertebral line, (2) posterior vertebral line, (3) spinolaminar line, and (4) the spinous process line and the atlantodens interval (ADI) and posterior atlantodens interval (PADI) **(Figs 7.25A and B)**. In a perfect lateral view these lines should be unbroken. The ADI is the distance between the posterior surface of the anterior C1 ring and anterior surface of the odontoid. The PADI is the distance between the posterior surface of odontoid surface and anterior surface of the posterior C1 ring. ADI should be less than 3 mm in adults. PADI less than 13 mm indicates critical canal compromise. Computed tomography (CT)

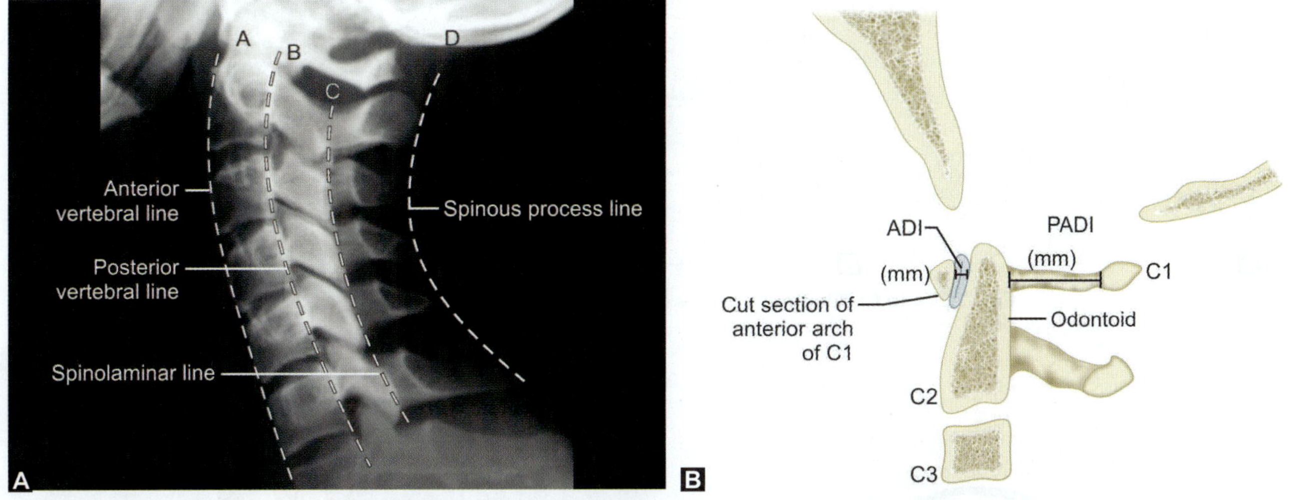

Figs 7.25A and B: (A) Cervical spine lateral X-ray showing important radiological indices;
(B) Atlantodens interval (ADI) and posterior atlantodens interval (PADI)

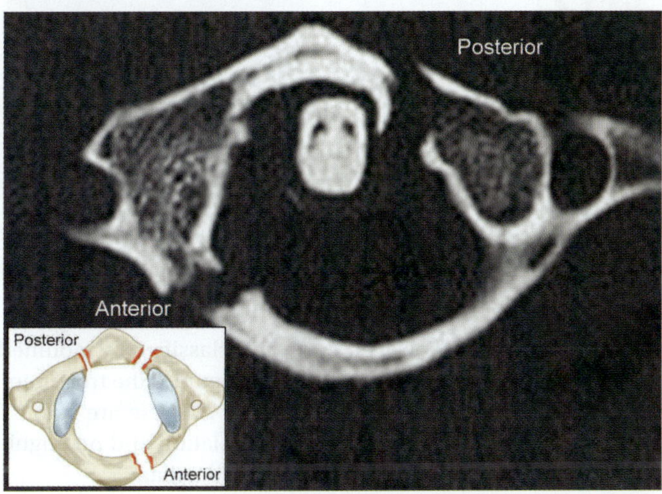

Fig. 7.26: Jefferson fracture

remains the most sensitive imaging modality to evaluate fractures of the upper cervical spine, subaxial spine and cervicothoracic junction. A clue to the presence of a cervical spine injury is given by the detection of abnormal thickness of prevertebral space. If it is more than 7 mm at the C2–C3 level and 21 mm at the C6–C7 level, it is indicative of cervical spine injury.

HIGH-YIELD POINTS

- Spinal canal is widest at C2 level.
- Vertebrae that are always constant in number are the cervical while most variable in number are coccygeal.
- Nontraumatic conditions associated with increase in atlantodens interval are—Down's syndrome, rheumatoid arthritis, osteogenesis imperfecta, Morquio syndrome, Grisel syndrome, neurofibromatosis, etc.

Some Specific Fractures of C1 and C2

Jefferson Fracture

This is a burst fracture of C1 vertebra (Atlas) caused by an axial loading force. There is fracture involving both anterior and posterior ring of the atlas **(Fig. 7.26)**. It has an extremely high association (up to 50%) with other cervical spine fractures. Patients will often complain of severe suboccipital discomfort and a sense of instability. At C1 level only 35% of the canal is occupied by the cord with plenty of space as opposed to 50% occupancy in the lower spine, hence, neurologic injury is uncommon.

However, when it occurs, the greater occipital nerve is most frequently injured, followed by the lower cranial nerves. Undisplaced fractures can be managed on collar while displaced ones are managed by the application of halo vest.

Odontoid/Dens Fractures

Fractures of the dens constitute approximately 10% of all cervical spine injuries. However, these are the most common types of Axis (C2) fractures (more common than Hangman's fracture). Hyperflexion results in anterior displacement of the dens fracture and hyperextension results in posterior displacement of the dens fracture. A displaced fracture is actually a fracture dislocation of the atlantoaxial joint.

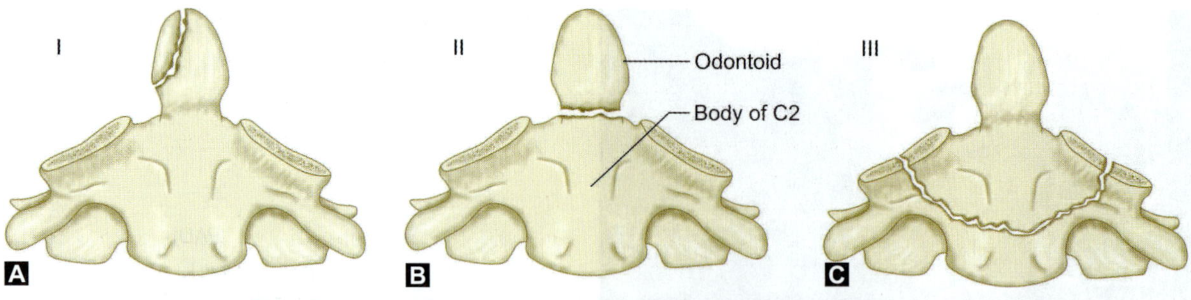

Figs 7.27A to C: Odontoid fractures classified by Anderson and D'Alonzo

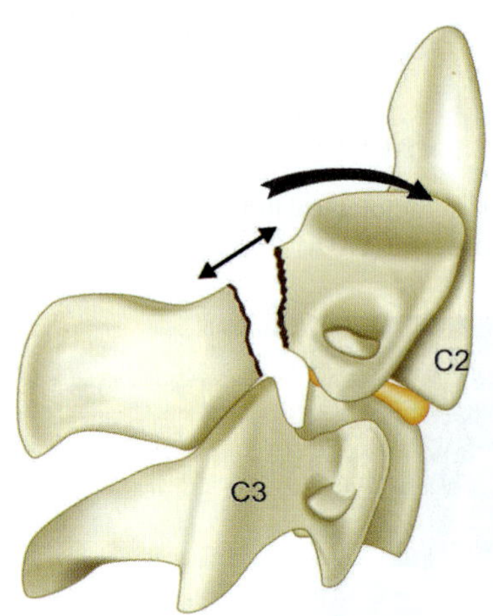

Fig. 7.28: Diagrammatic representation of Hangman's fracture

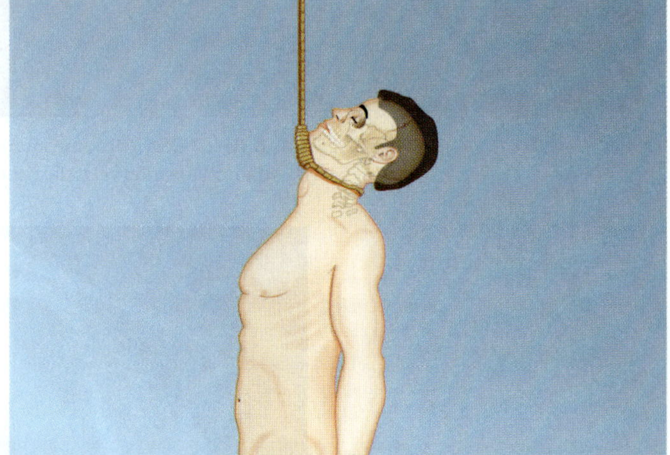

Fig. 7.29: Schematic depiction of injury mechanism in judicial hanging

An open mouth odontoid view aids in diagnosis. However, MRI is the preferred modality as it can also identify tear of the transverse atlantal ligament (*see* **Fig. 7.24B**) that can contribute to instability.

These fractures are classified by Anderson and D'Alonzo classification **(Figs 7.27A to C)** into three types:
1. Avulsion of apex of odontoid
2. Fracture at junction of body and neck (high nonunion rate)
3. Fracture extends into the vertebral body of C2.

Treatment: Type 1, type 3 and minimally displaced type 2 fractures are treated by halo vest immobilization. Displaced type 2 fractures which are not adequately reduced by traction or not maintained in immobilization require surgery (screw fixation and/or fusion).

Hangman's Fracture (Traumatic Spondylolisthesis of Axis)

Hangman's fracture **(Figs 7.28 and 7.29)** is a fracture of the isthmus part of the axis (pars interarticularis) characterized by forward slipping of C2 over C3 (spondylolisthesis), originally described in patients subjected to judicial hanging. The mechanism in judicial hanging is an extension of the spine with distraction.

Hangman's fracture is more commonly seen in road traffic accidents where it is caused by extension, of the spine with axial loading (when the head strikes to dashboard). Mostly there is no neurological deficit as the fracture of the posterior arch tends to decompress the spinal cord and acute postadmission mortality is low (2–3%).

It is classified by modified Levine and Edward's classification that also guides the treatment:
- *Type I*: These are stable fractures that have less than 3 mm translation and no angulation. These fractures are treated in a rigid collar.
- *Type II (most common subtype)*: These fractures have greater than 3 mm of displacement and angulation of C2 on C3. A variant of type II fractures has been described. This type IIA fracture shows significant angulation, but has minimal translation. It results from a flexion-distraction injury. Traction is contraindicated in such fractures as the mechanism is distraction. Type II fractures are reduced by traction and immobilized in a halo vest for 3 months. Type IIA fractures are reduced manually by extension and slight compression and immobilized in halo vest.
- *Type III*: These are unstable injuries associated with unilateral or bilateral facet dislocations of C2 on C3 and are usually the result of flexion-distraction followed by hyperextension. All type III fractures should be treated with surgical reduction and posterior C2–C3 fusion. Most of these fractures heal rapidly and union is almost never a problem.

Injuries of Lower/Subaxial (C3–C7) Cervical Spine

The osseous-ligamentous complex that surrounds and protects the upper cervical spinal cord, the brainstem, and lower cranial nerves is anatomically and functionally distinct from the motion segments in the subaxial cervical spine (C3–C7).

*Relevant Anatomy (**Fig. 7.30**)*

The spinous processes project posteriorly, angling downward, and are progressively larger from cranial to caudal direction. The spinous process of C3–C5 is always bifid, whereas C6 may be and C7 is never bifid. The vertebral body is short and connects to the next vertebra by a disk, uncovertebral and facet joints. The facets are oriented horizontally and hence the chances of pure dislocations in the subaxial cervical spine are more (*see* **Fig. 7.14**).

The vertebral artery ascends from the subclavian artery to pass within the foramen transversarium at C6. It exits the foramen transversarium of C2 turning anteriorly and medially in C2 and then again laterally into C1.

Classification of Subaxial Cervical Spine Injuries

These injuries are classified by Allen and Ferguson classification (**Table 7.8**). This is based on the mechanism of injury. Each of these has a subclassification of injury types based upon their characteristic patterns. The important fractures caused by these mechanisms in isolation or in combination have been discussed here.

Specific Fractures of Subaxial Spine

Wedge Compression and Tear Drop Fractures (Flexion-compression Injuries)

Flexion-compression injuries are common cervical spine injuries which range from mild wedge compression fracture to severe tear drop fractures. The most severe pattern results in posterior subluxation of the posterior vertebral body into the canal and disruption of posterior ligaments.

Wedge compression fractures (**Fig. 7.31A**) involve the anterior column and usually are stable injuries with no neurological involvement. Teardrop fractures are hyperflexion compression injuries, involving middle and anterior column. Teardrop fracture dislocation (**Fig. 7.31B**) is characterized by shearing of a tear drop bone fragment from the anteroinferior edge of the vertebral body and the protrusion of the posteroinferior edge into the spinal canal.

Treatment: Mild wedge compression injury without neurological involvement requires nothing more than collar immobilization. Severe injuries require corpectomy (removal of the vertebral body) and anterior column reconstruction using bone graft (in a metal cage) and fixation (with plating).

Facet Dislocations (Flexion-distraction Injuries)

Flexion-distraction injuries (in cervical spine, flexion-rotation is a part of this mechanism only) are the most common pattern of subaxial cervical spine injury. C5–C6 is the most common site.

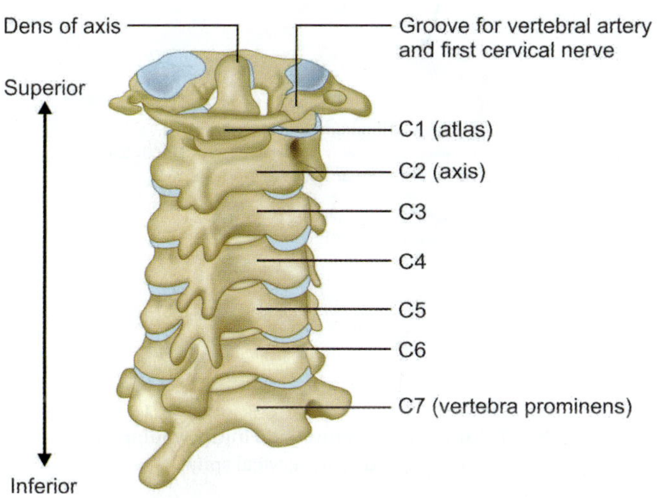

Fig. 7.30: Cervical spine anatomy

Table 7.8: Allen and Ferguson classification
1. Compressive flexion
2. Vertical compression
3. Distractive flexion
4. Compressive extension
5. Distractive extension
6. Lateral flexion

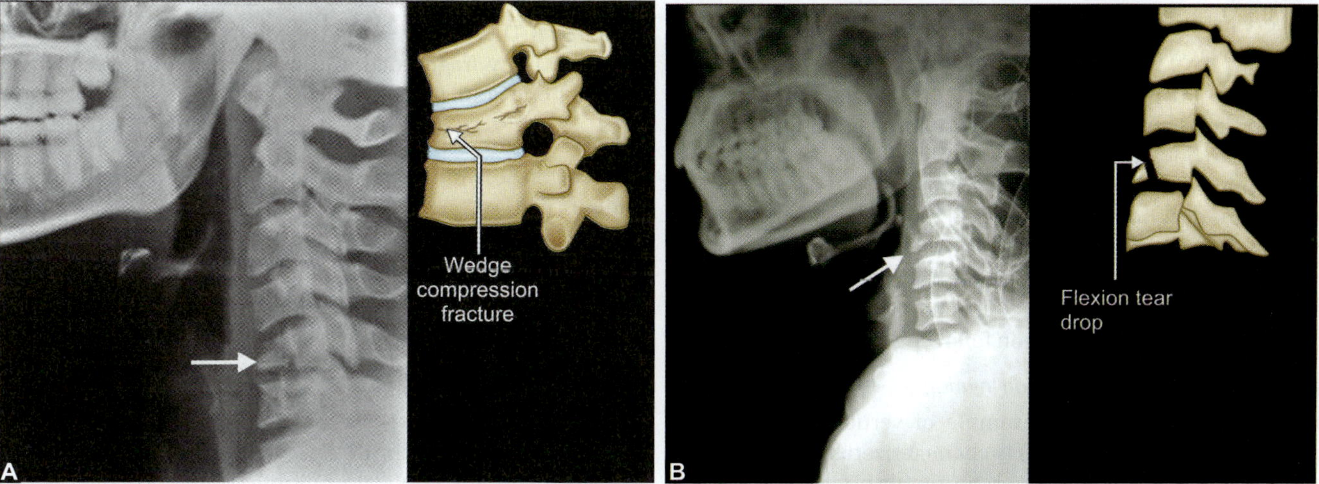

Figs 7.31A and B: Common fracture patterns following flexion compression injuries of lower cervical spine injury.
(A) X-ray showing wedge compression fracture (arrow); (B) X-ray showing teardrop fracture (arrow)

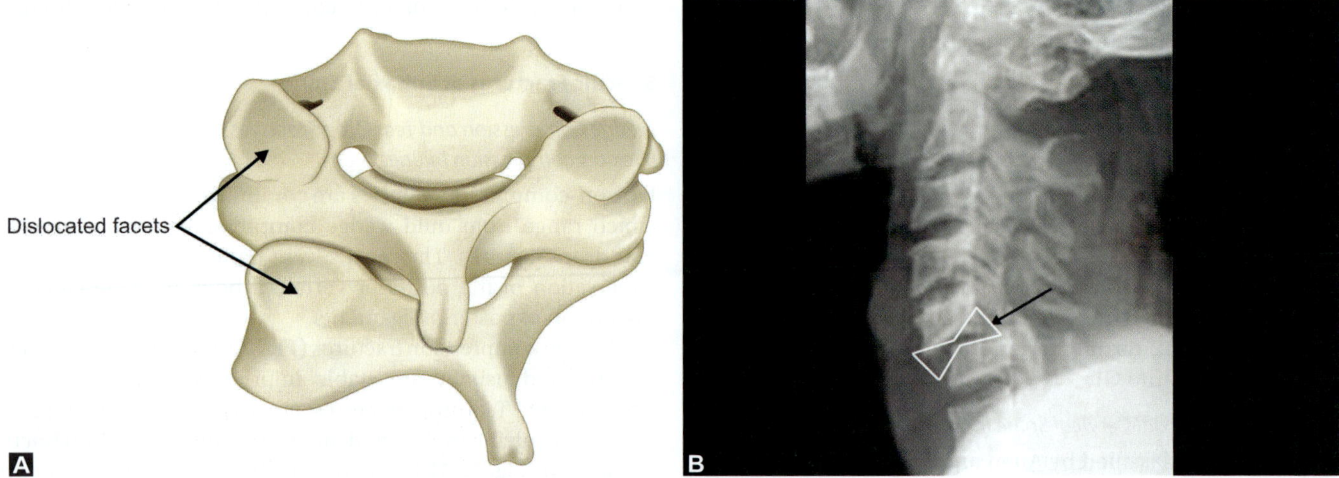

Figs 7.32A and B: Flexion distraction injury. (A) Facet dislocation; (B) X-ray cervical spine lateral view showing bow tie sign of facet dislocation (arrow)

Spectrum of flexion distraction injuries ranges from a posterior ligamentous sprain to unilateral or a bilateral facet dislocation.

In unilateral facet dislocations **(Fig. 7.32A)**, flexion and simultaneous rotation of vertebra around a facet joint causes the superior facet on the contralateral side to slip forwards over the tip of an inferior facet of the joint leading to dislocation of a single facet joint (called as locked facet). A fracture of the facet joint may be associated. Only the posterior ligaments are disrupted while the anterior ones remain intact. There can be up to 25% anterior subluxation at the involved level. In bilateral facet dislocations, there is flexion injury anteriorly and severe distraction posteriorly causing bilaterally locked facets. There is tear of all spinal ligamentous structures. Typically, there are no associated facet fractures as the posterior column is distracted. The anterior subluxation at the involved level can be up to 50%.

The diagnosis in unilateral facet dislocations can be difficult and caution should be high. In fact, a unilateral facet subluxation is one of the most frequently missed injury after an initial evaluation. Unilateral facet dislocations and facet fracture dislocations present typically with a bow tie or sail sign **(Fig. 7.32B)** in a lateral view of the cervical spine. Disk herniation can occur in up to 10% of patients with facet dislocations and should be evaluated by MRI.

Treatment: If MRI shows significant disk herniation anterior cervical diskectomy with fusion with bone grafting is done. Reduction can be achieved preoperatively (with skeletal traction) or at the time of anterior cervical diskectomy. If MRI demonstrates no significant disk herniation, a closed reduction via crutchfield traction may be achieved. In case closed reduction fails, then open posterior reduction with stabilization (fixation with instruments) is the treatment of choice. A bilateral facet dislocation has increased chances of redislocation following reduction.

Burst Fractures (Vertical Compression Injuries)

A burst fracture is a typical example of vertical compression injury. Burst fracture **(Fig. 7.33)** is characterized by involvement of anterior and middle column and shortening of vertebral height. Status of posterior column decides the stability of burst fracture. In unstable burst fracture vertical compression or axial loading

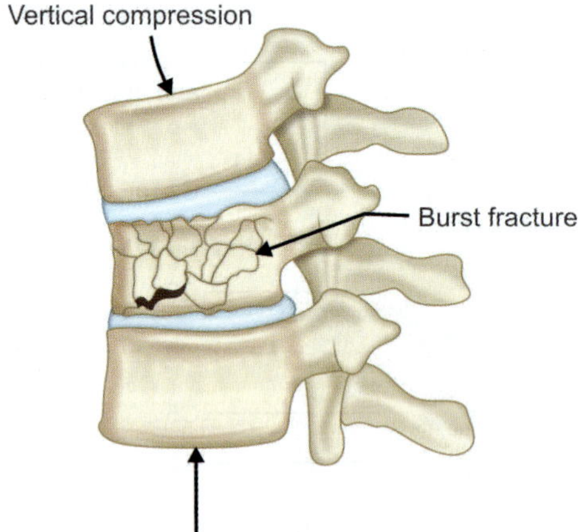

Fig. 7.33: Vertical compression injury leading to Burst fracture in cervical spine

of cervical spine causes comminution of the vertebral body and retropulsion of the vertebral body fragments into the spinal canal.

Treatment: These injuries are treated by corpectomy (removal of vertebral body fragments) and anterior column reconstruction using a bone graft/metal cage with plating.

Extension Injuries

Hyperextension injuries of the cervical spine are common in older patients with stiff neck. Loss of neck movement causes failure of dissipation of energy of trauma, thus patients with ankylosing spondylitis and disseminated idiopathic skeletal hyperostosis (*see* Page 416) are at particular risk of hyperextension injury. These injuries are characterized by anterior widening of disk space and/or disruption of posterior ligaments and posterior displacement of the vertebra. Central cord syndrome (*see* Page 214) is also an example of extension type cervical spine injury which is common in elderly with osteoarthritic changes in the cervical spine.

For treatment, cervical immobilization in a collar is usually all that is required. If MRI shows significant disk disruption, then anterior diskectomy, fusion with bone graft and plating is done.

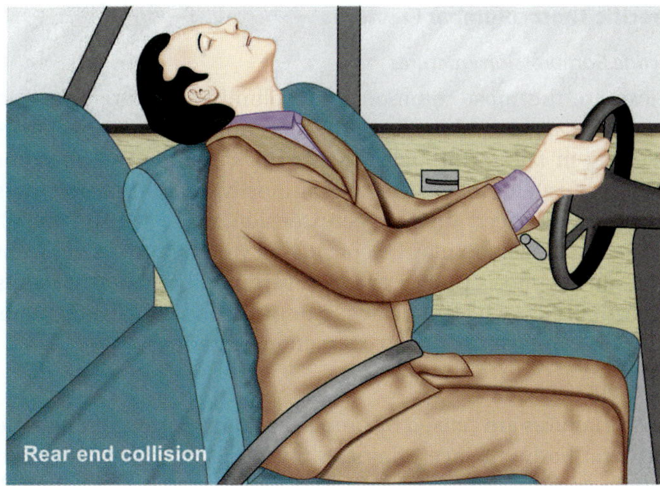

Fig. 7.34: Diagrammatic depiction of mechanism of whiplash injury after rear end collision of a vehicle

Whiplash Injury (Sprained Neck)

Whiplash describes a range of injuries in the neck seen after rear end collision of vehicles. Before the invention of the car, whiplash injuries were called "railroad spine/Erichsen's disease" as they were noted mostly in connection with train collisions and had been described by John Erichsen.

Although the exact mechanism in these injuries is debatable, the accepted theory is that the patient's body is thrown forwards from the car seat while his head flips back wards and then recoils in flexion (hyperextension followed by flexion) **(Fig. 7.34)**. Nevertheless the hyperextension force causes the prime damage. Mostly there is a sprain of the capsular ligaments of the facet joints and the neck muscles, in rare instances there could be an unstable fracture.

Women more commonly, land up with whiplash owing to their weaker muscles. Patients mostly present with pain and stiffness in the neck. There could be paresthesias in the ulnar nerve distribution due to nerve root compression by a spasmodic scalenus muscle. On examination, neck muscles are usually tender and movements often restricted. Neurological deficit is uncommon. The Quebec Task Force grading of the severity of whiplash injury lesion has been depicted in **Table 7.9**.

X-rays may be normal or show straightening of the normal cervical curvature, a sign of muscle spasm.

Treatment is largely symptomatic. Collars are avoided as they hinder recovery more than helping. Isometric exercises are encouraged and most of the patients fair well.

Clay-shoveler's Fracture

Clay-shoveler's fracture usually occurs in laborers who perform activities involving lifting weights rapidly with the arms extended **(Fig. 7.35)**. Violent muscle forces in these persons often lead to avulsion fractures of the spinous process of vertebra (C7 >D1). The fracture is absolutely stable and treatment is mainly symptomatic; neck exercises are encouraged as symptoms permit.

HIGH-YIELD POINTS

- The most common mode of cervical spine injury is fall from height.

Table 7.9: Quebec task force grading of whiplash injury
1. Grade 1: No neck symptoms or signs
2. Grade 2: Neck pains and stiffness, but no physical signs
3. Grade 3: Musculoskeletal signs
4. Grade 4: Neurological signs
5. Grade 5: Fracture dislocation present

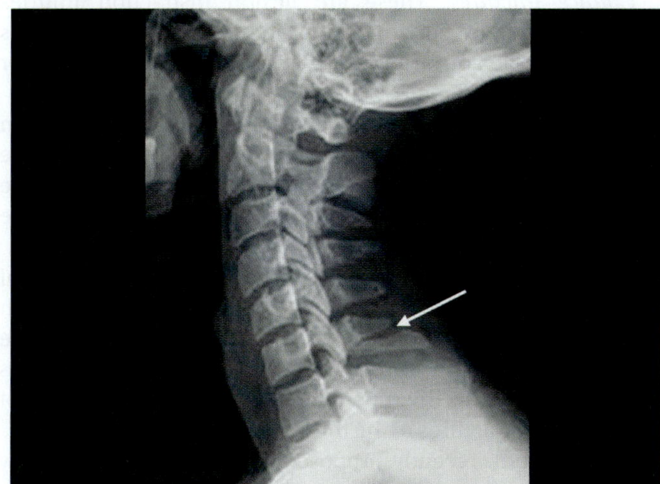

Fig. 7.35: Clay-shoveler's fracture (arrow)

- The cervical spine is the most common site of spinal cord injury.
- The most common site of cervical spine fracture is atlantoaxial junction (or C2 vertebra), but the most common site of subaxial cervical spine fracture is C5–C6.
- Flexion distraction is the most common type of injury mechanism in cervical spine injury.
- Commonly missed fractures in cervical spine injury on plain X-ray include odontoid fracture, tear drop fracture, facet injury and Hangman's fracture.

THORACOLUMBAR FRACTURES

Relevant Anatomy

In the thoracic spine the vertebrae are linked to each other via disks and facet joints and also linked to the ribs via costo-transverse joints and costovertebral joints. The thoracic spine, protected by the rib cage, is thus the least mobile spine. A transition comes at transitional area D12–L2, where a rigid thoracic spine meets the relatively flexible lumbar spine. The majority of the fractures in this area, thus tend to involve this transitional segment D12–L2 (D12 >L1). The spinal canal in this area is relatively narrow and, therefore, cord damage is not uncommon in these fractures. The cord ends at the lower border of L1 and injuries distal to this level involve the nerve roots. Very commonly these fractures are also associated with injuries in the chest and abdomen.

The treatment of unstable fractures and fracture dislocations of the thoracic and lumbar spine has long been controversial. The classifications of thoracolumbar injuries have evolved over many years. McAfee classification divides these injuries in six types:

1. *Wedge compression fracture*: There is isolated failure of anterior column due to compression. Usually it is not associated with neurological impairment.

2. *Stable burst fracture*: It is characterized by failure of the anterior and middle column and intact posterior column.
3. *Unstable burst fracture*: It is characterized by failure of the anterior and middle columns in compression and also the failure of posterior column in distraction. It is an unstable injury with high chances of kyphotic deformity and neural compression due to retropulsion of bony fragments into the canal.
4. *Chance fractures*: These are flexion distraction injuries characterized by horizontal avulsion of the vertebral bodies caused by flexion around an axis anterior to the anterior longitudinal ligament.
5. *Flexion-compression injuries*: In these injuries, the flexion axis is posterior to the anterior longitudinal ligament. The anterior column fails in compression, whereas the middle and posterior columns fail in tension. This is an unstable due to disruption of the posterior ligament complex.
6. *Translational injuries*: These are characterized by failure of all three columns in shear. These are unstable injuries with a complete displacement of neural canal in the transverse plane. Although this is one of commonly used classifications of these injuries, this does not explain the mechanism of injury of all fractures of the thoracolumbar spine.

Vaccaro et al. recently proposed the thoracolumbar injury classification and severity score (TLICS) to simplify injury classification and facilitate decision making in thoracolumbar fractures **(Table 7.10)**. It evaluates fracture morphology, the posteroligamentous complex (an important component in stability) and neurologic function to aid decision making. A maximum score of 10 is possible. Surgery is indicated if the score is 5 or more and nonoperative treatment is indicated for score 3 or less. Treatment is individualized (operative or nonoperative) for a score of 4.

Table 7.10: Thoracolumbar injury classification and severity score (Vaccaro et al.)

Features	*Points*
Fracture mechanism	
Compression fracture	1
Burst fracture	1
Translation	3
Distraction	4
Neurological involvement	
Intact	0
Nerve root	2
Cord, conus medullaris, incomplete	3
Cord, conus medullaris, complete	2
Cauda equina	3
Posterior ligamentous complex	
Intact	0
Indeterminate	2
Injured	3

Source: Vaccaro AR, Zeiller SC, Hulbert RJ, et al. The thoracolumbar injury severity score: a proposed treatment algorithm. J Spinal Disord Tech. 2005;18:209.

Specific Thoracolumbar Fractures

Wedge Compression Fractures

These are the most common thoracolumbar fracture type and result due to a combination of flexion and compression forces resulting in failure through the anterior column. The posterior column is usually not involved. Being mostly stable, these fractures are often managed on a hyperextension brace (ASHE brace). Surgical stabilization may be considered when there is significant traumatic kyphosis (> 30°) or when vertebral body height loss is larger than 40%, which indicates setting in of posterior ligamentous complex compromise due to distraction posteriorly.

Burst Fractures

Burst fractures are caused by pure axial compression through the vertebral body. In severe injuries, retropulsion of the fractured middle column fragments into the spinal canal is the hallmark of a burst fracture **(Figs 7.36A and B)**. The generally accepted differentiation between wedge compression fractures and burst fractures occurs in the middle column, which is spared in compression fractures and involved with burst fractures. The identification is relatively simple on radiographs. Loss of vertebral body height with splaying of pedicles (increased interpedicular distance) is characteristic of burst fractures.

Stable burst fractures can be treated with bracing while unstable burst fractures (loss of vertebral height more than 50%, posterior column disrupted or neurological deficit present) should be managed with surgery. Direct decompression (corpectomy) via an anterior approach is preferred, but it can also be performed via a posterior transpedicular approach, followed by instrumented fusion of the spine (with pedicle screws). Posterior pedicle screw fixation and fusion restore the posterior ligament tension-band effect and is the instrument of choice (*see* **Figs 7.25A and B**).

Chance Fractures (Seat Belt Injury/Jack Knife Injury)

These are typically seen in head on collision of vehicles when the passengers are wearing seat belts. The mechanism involved is flexion distraction **(Figs 7.37A to C)**.

When the collision occurs, the body is thrown forward and the seat belt restrains the lap. The combined flexion and posterior

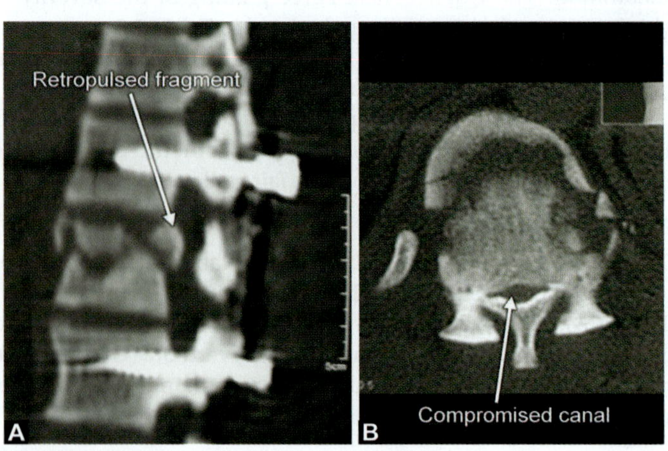

Figs 7.36A and B: Intraoperative images of burst fracture being fixed with pedicle screws showing a retropulsed fragment. (A) Sagittal view; (B) Axial view

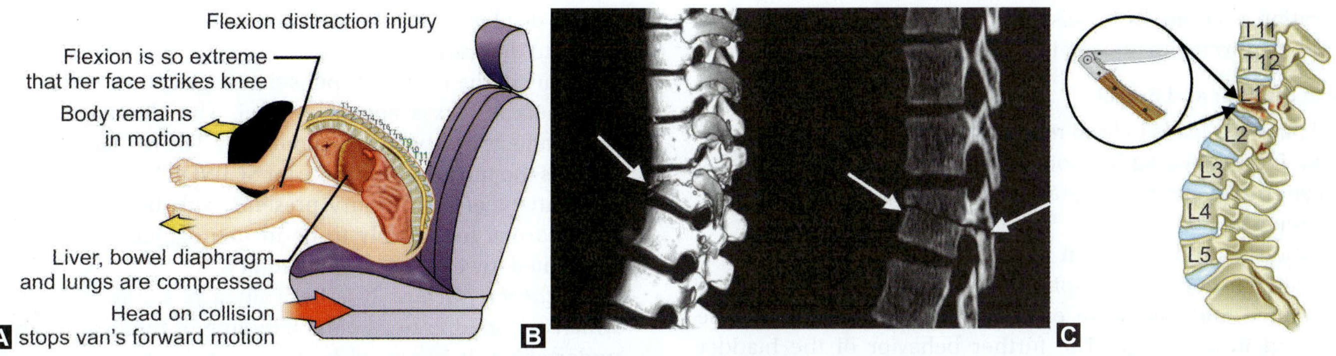

Figs 7.37A to C: (A) Flexion distraction injury mechanism; (B) 3D-CT scan image showing chance fracture (arrow); (C) Injury pattern of chance fracture simulating opening of jack knife

Courtesy: LearningRadiology.com (for Figure 7.37B).

distraction causes the lumbar spine to jack knife around an axis placed anterior to the vertebral column. Although there is no crushing of the vertebral body, but the posterior and middle column fail in distraction. The classical injury described by *chance* (Chance fracture, GQ chance, 1948) was purely an osseous lesion with a fracture line traversing the vertebral body as well as the posterior elements from front to back. However, the injury may be entirely diskoligamentous in nature (Chance variant-transaction being thorough the disk and ligaments only, with no bony involvement) or a combination of osseous and ligamentous disruption. D12–L2 is the segment mostly involved. In almost 50% cases, these fractures are associated with a concomitant intra-abdominal injury.

The incidence of neurologic deficit in flexion-distraction injuries is relatively low. Brace treatment (hyperextension braces) therefore is more likely to be successful in stable bony injuries. Unstable injuries of both the bony and ligamentous types are best treated surgically.

Fracture Dislocations

Fracture-dislocations are highly unstable injuries with high chances of neural compression owing to the translation of one vertebral body over another. All three columns fail under compression, tension, rotation or shear. Three combinations are mostly involved—(1) shear, (2) flexion-rotation, and (3) flexion distraction. The most dangerous mechanism is shear force which causes translational injuries with complete neurological deficits in all cases. Next most dangerous mechanism is flexion-rotation followed by flexion distraction. The hallmark is anterior, posterior, or lateral translation of the cephalad vertebral body on the adjacent caudal vertebral body **(Figs 7.38A and B)**. There is no role for bracing. Surgical treatment should proceed as soon as possible. Posterior pedicle screw instrumentation and fusion can usually be limited to two levels above and below the injury, though longer constructs may be required. Anterior procedures are usually not necessary.

MANAGEMENT OF TRAUMATIC PARAPLEGIA AND QUADRIPLEGIA

Paraplegia is a devastating complication of SCI and needs a team effort to rehabilitate the patient to nearly normal life. Care of a paraplegic can be divided into following parts:

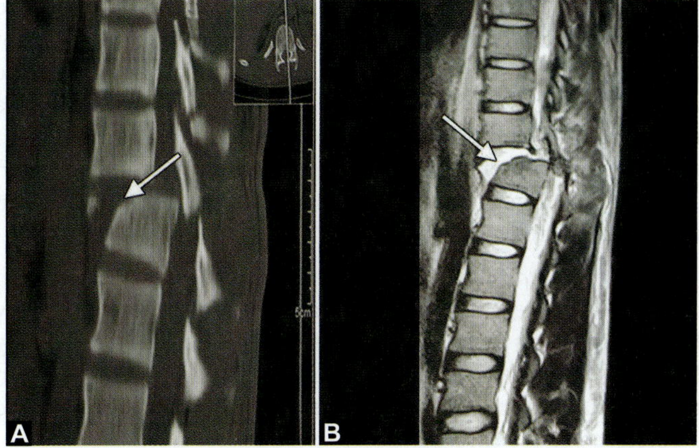

Figs 7.38A and B: CT and MRI showing a fracture dislocation (arrows) of the thoracic spine

Table 7.11: Grading of bed sores
1. *Grade 1:* Intact skin, but nonblanchable erythema present
2. *Grade 2:* Loss of tissue till dermis
3. *Grade 3:* Penetration through the whole of dermis, going into subcutaneous tissue
4. *Grade 4:* Full thickness tissue loss with exposed bone, tendon or muscle

Care of Skin

Anesthetic skin is extremely prone to develop pressure sores (**Table 7.11** for classification) and needs meticulous care. Crumples in the bed sheets must be avoided. Postural turning is advised every 2 hours. Use of air beds/water beds may assist in preventing sores. If sores have developed they need periodic debridement and if needed a surgical closure, else they never heal on their own.

Care of Muscles and Joints

Paraplegics are prone to land up with joint contractures, which may limit their functional capability further. Moreover, it restricts the possibility of undertaking them for some suitable tendon transfers to upgrade their functional capability. A good physiotherapy is must to ensure supple joints. Heterotopic ossification is common in this setting and if it occurs, excision must be performed to prevent its hazards.

Care of Bladder and Bowel

Bowel paralysis leads to fecal retention. Measures are directed to achieve fecal softening by modification is diet, use of laxatives, suppositories or enemas. Digital evacuation may be performed as and when needed.

Bladder care depends on the stage of injury the patient is in. Initially in the stage of spinal shock, the paralyzed bladder is distended and unable to empty. Catheterization should be performed in this stage. The further behavior of the bladder depends on the disruption of the pathways.

Autonomous bladder (LMN bladder) occurs when the injury involves S2 level or below. The detrusor tone is flaccid and large residual urine collects and patients tend to have stress incontinence. Periodic emptying in these patients should be assisted by manual pressure to prevent bed wetting or the patient can be taught to apply suprapubic compression. Automatic bladder (UMN bladder) occurs when there is a transection of the cord above S2 level. The detrusor is spastic and patient tends to have urge incontinence with involuntary dribbling of urine with reflex activity. Such patients can be managed with a condom catheter until recovery occurs.

Retraining of bladder function: Recovery of bladder function may take a few weeks. When the signs of sensory/motor recovery appear, retraining of the bladder function should also be taken by clamping the catheter and encouraging reflex emptying. Once an autonomous/automatic bladder is established, measures can be directed as per the case.

Psychological Care

Depression is a major and hidden ailment in these patients. Appropriate occupational, vocational and sexual rehabilitation must be ensured to deal with the same.

HIGH-YIELD POINTS

- The most common site of a spinal fracture overall is D12 followed by L1 vertebra.
- The most common site for compression fractures in spine is also D12 followed by L1.
- Vertebral fractures (of dorsal spine) are the most common fractures in elderly and the most common underlying cause is "osteoporosis".
- Most common site of fracture after fall from height is D12 vertebra, although pelvis and calcaneum are other commonly injured areas.
- Most common spinal injury mechanism overall is flexion (flexion rotation >flexion distraction specifically).
- Most dangerous spinal injury mechanism overall is translation injury followed by flexion-rotation and then flexion distraction. All these injuries cause fracture dislocations.
- *Spinal cord injury without radiological abnormality (SCIWORA):* This is a special pattern of injury seen in pediatric patients (mostly less than 8 years of age) where the patients present with a neurological deficit but a normal X-ray. Since children tend to have lax ligaments, injury often causes displacement of vertebral column resulting in traction injury to the spinal cord.

Elasticity of the ligaments pulls the displaced vertebrae back and thereby X-rays appear normal. The characteristic age group affected is the infant population. The pediatric cervical spine is the most common site for SCIWORA.

- If a patient of head injury presents with hypotension and bradycardia, he is likely to be in neurogenic shock due to associated lower cervical spine injury.
- *Undertaker's fracture:* It is basically a postmortem fracture which occurs due to careless handling of the dead body by undertakers. It is caused by falling of the head backwards forcibly, causing tearing of the intervertebral disk and subluxation of cervical spine most commonly at C6–C7 level.
- *Chalk stick fractures:* In these fractures, the fracture line is transverse to the long-axis of the bone, like a broken stick of chalk. They are seen mostly in long bones in Paget's disease and osteopetrosis. Similar transverse fractures may be seen in the spine in patients with ankylosing spondylitis and are highly unstable lesions.

SPONDYLOLISTHESIS

INTRODUCTION

Forward slip of the upper vertebra over the adjoining lower vertebra is called as "spondylolisthesis". The most common site of affection is L5 over S1 followed by L4 over L5 and the most common root irritated is L5.

Based upon the cause of the slip, there are five types described:

1. *Isthmic/Lytic:* This is the most common subtype.

   The basic lesion in this category is a defect/fracture in the "pars interarticularis" of the neural arch. Pars interarticularis **(Fig. 7.39)** is the part of the vertebrae that lies between the superior articular facets and lamina. A fracture in the pars on both sides causes the upper vertebrae (along with the whole spinal column above) to slide forward on the lower vertebrae. This lesion likely occurs in a congenitally weak pars that sustains a fatigue fracture in people involved in sports activities like weight lifting or those who sustain extensional stresses of gymnastics or wrestling. The neural arch defect appears mostly between the ages of 5 years and 7 years.

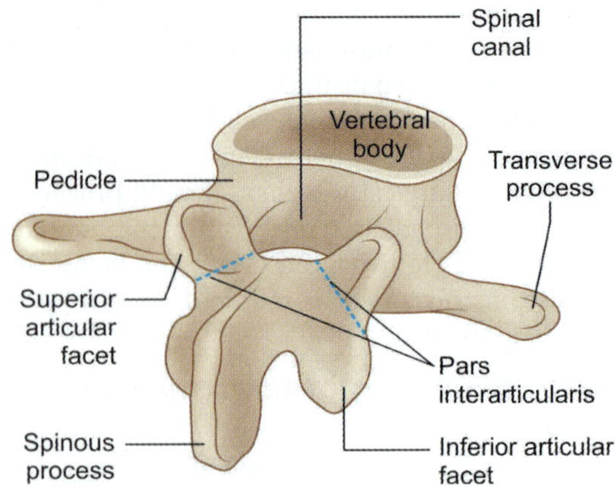

Fig. 7.39: Diagram showing pars interarticularis

Forward slipping of the vertebral body occurs most frequently between the ages of 10 years and 15 years and rarely increases after age of 20 years.

2. *Dysplastic*: This is the rare congenital variety due to either a defect in the formation of the first sacral arch and superior facets of S1 or due to attenuation and elongation of pars. There is no defect/fracture in the pars.

 In this variety the chances of developing a neurologic deficit are more than in the isthmic variety. The average age of symptom onset is usually near the final growth spurt age (14 years in girls and 16 years in boys). The onset may be quite sudden and dramatic and is aptly termed as "listhetic crisis". The patient experiences a sudden onset of backache, and on examination, characteristically, presents with a rigid lumbar spine that is commonly associated with a spastic or functional scoliosis (list).

3. *Degenerative*: This is the second most common variety. The only variety which is more common at L4–L5 level and more common in females especially with age more than 50 years. The L4–L5 segment of the lumbar spine is normally the site of the greatest mobility. The primary pathology is degeneration of the disk followed by facet joint degeneration and secondary osteoarthritis of these joints. This makes them unstable and the vertebrae slips. The neural arch, however, is intact. Usually, the slip is of low grade.

4. *Traumatic*: This is a rare variety where there is a fracture in an area other than pars causes the slip.

5. *Pathologic*: In this subtype the pars is broken secondary to a localized or a generalized bone disease.

Spondylolysis

This is a condition in which there is a defect/fracture in the pars but no obvious slipping of the vertebrae. The majority of spondylolytic lesions occur at L5, but a few will be present at higher lumbar levels. Remember that 5% of the general population walks around with a spondylolysis that is completely asymptomatic. Spondylolysis may be unilateral in up to one-third of these patients.

Retrolisthesis

A condition in which the cephalad vertebra goes posterior to the caudal vertebra. It is a sign of stability and happens in patients with degeneration who have crossed the stage of instability to enter into the stage of stability.

CLINICAL PRESENTATION

- Most of the patients are asymptomatic and the finding is incidental.
- Back pain is the presenting symptom in others and varies from severe acute low back pain to low back discomfort only on doing certain activities.
- There is hamstring stretch on raising the leg passively.
- In rare situations where the degree of slip increases, the disk may retropulse and the canal may become stenotic producing symptoms of neurological claudication, i.e. radicular pain (*see* Spinal Canal stenosis). Further compression may produce a neurological deficit.

RADIOGRAPHY

- *Plain radiographs*: Oblique radiographs **(Figs 7.40A to C)** of the lumbosacral spine may show a break in the pars interarticularis, which appears as a break in the neck of the "Scotty Terrier Dog" shadow. Scotty terrier dog shadow is a normal appearance on the oblique view of lumbosacral spine but a break in neck due to spondylolisthesis (or spondylolysis) is labeled as Beheaded Scotty terrier sign or Scotty dog wearing a collar sign. An AP X-ray shows "Inverted Napoleon Hat sign" which occurs due to superimposition of sacrum and L5 and indicates marked anterolisthesis of L5 over S1 **(Fig. 7.41)**.
- *Dynamic X-rays (Flexion and extension views)*: May be done to assess the instability in spine.
- *CT scan and single photon emission computed tomography (SPECT)*: They are useful in detecting "spondylolysis".

GRADING OF SPONDYLOLISTHESIS

In Meyerding's method the AP diameter of the superior surface of the lower vertebral body is divided into quarters and a grade of I–IV is assigned to slips of one, two, three or four quarters of the superior vertebra, respectively. Taillard method expresses the degree of slip as a percentage of the AP diameter of the top of the lower vertebra. A complete dislocation of L5 on S1 is called a "spondyloptosis".

TREATMENT

Spondylolysis

The rule of thumb here is that if the patient is asymptomatic, let him play regardless of the investigation results. If the patient is symptomatic, restrict strenuous activities until the lesion heals.

Spondylolisthesis

Low-grade slips (I and II) behave as degenerative disk disease and can mostly be managed conservatively while high-grade slips (III and IV) behave as adult deformity and when causing canal stenosis, mostly need surgery.

Conservative Treatment

Conservative treatment is the initial treatment of choice for most cases of spondylolisthesis, with or without neurologic symptoms. Mostly treatment consists of 1–2 day period of rest and anti-inflammatory medications. Physical therapy is also often prescribed in addition and includes bracing, exercise, ultrasound, electrical stimulation, and therapeutic exercise (core strengthening exercises, postural instruction, lumbopelvic mobilization exercises, and a flexion-based exercise program). Stationary bicycling is an excellent exercise as it promotes spine flexion and deconstriction of the thecal sac.

Surgical Treatment

Surgery is advocated in high grade slips where dynamic X-rays demonstrate features suggestive of spinal instability or in cases with features of canal stenosis (*see* Page 241) not responding to conservative treatment. Decompression of the neural structures by removal of the protruding disk and lamina (diskectomy and

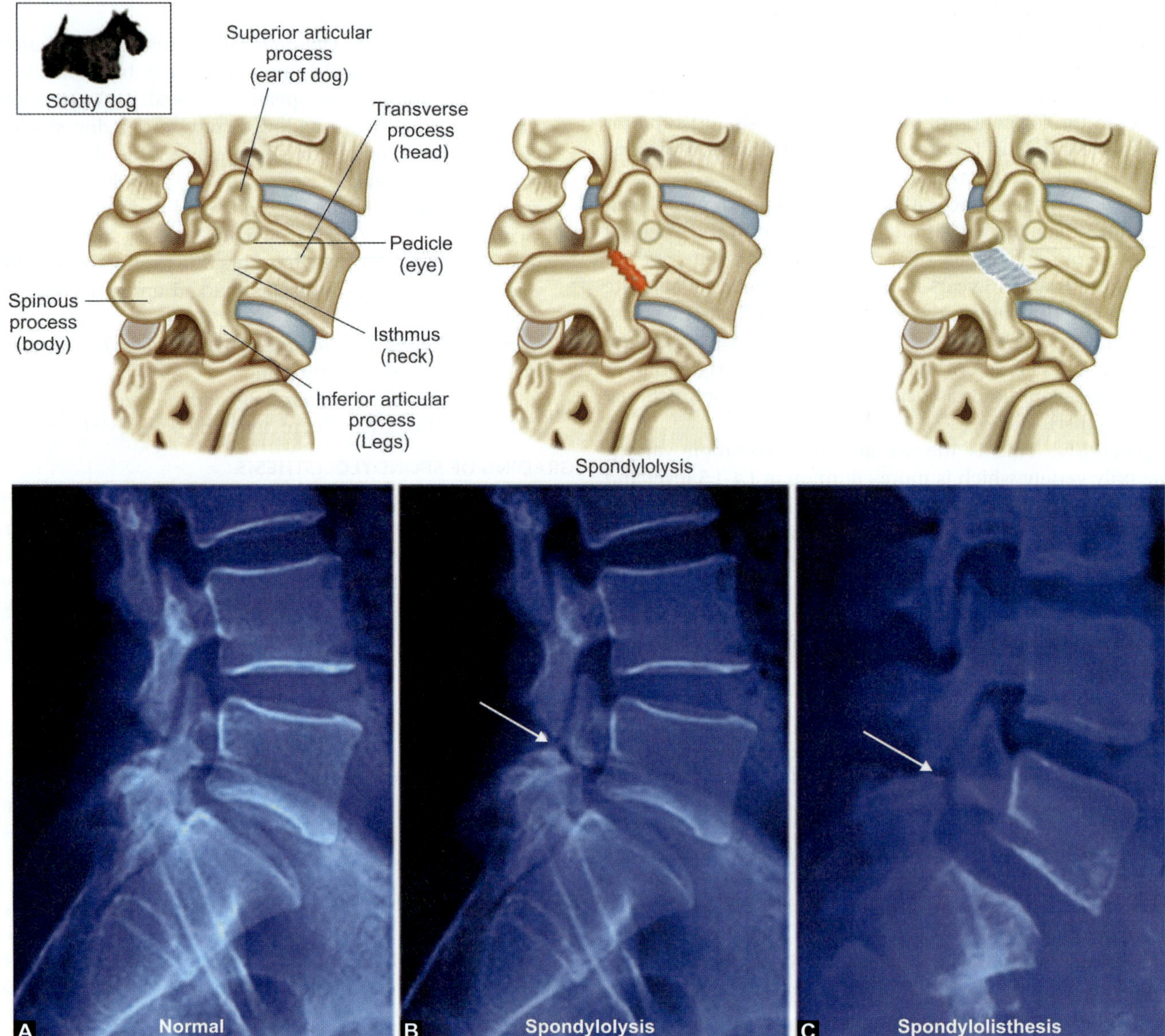

Figs 7.40A to C: (A) Diagrammatic presentation and X-ray lateral view of LS spine showing normal scotty dog shadow; (B) Diagrammatic presentation and X-ray showing spondylolysis with broken neck of scotty dog (arrow); (C) Diagrammatic presentation and X-ray showing spondylolisthesis with broken neck (arrow) and in addition forward slip of L5 vertebra over S1

laminectomy) and fusion of the adjacent vertebrae (transforaminal lumbar interbody fusion) with or without instrumentation (i.e. fixation with instruments like pedicle screws), to achieve spinal stability is the preferred procedure.

Treatment principles should actually be individualized to specific types:

1. *Isthmic*: Unlike dysplastic spondylolisthesis, further slipping is unlikely to occur in the older age group, and surgery, therefore, is not indicated to prevent further forward displacement. Continuing disabling pain constitutes the sole indication for surgery in this group of patients. A progressive neurological deficit that might end up with "cauda equina syndrome" constitutes other indications for a surgical intervention.

2. *Dysplastic*: The management here is usually surgical if the lesion is symptomatic before the age of 21 years.

3. *Degenerative*: Depending on the symptoms, decompression alone or decompression with spinal fusion may be offered to the patients.

4. *Pathologic*: The management depends on the nature of the pathology. The instance is, however, very rare.

HIGH-YIELD POINT

- An oblique X-ray gives the maximum information in spondylolisthesis while the AP view gives least.

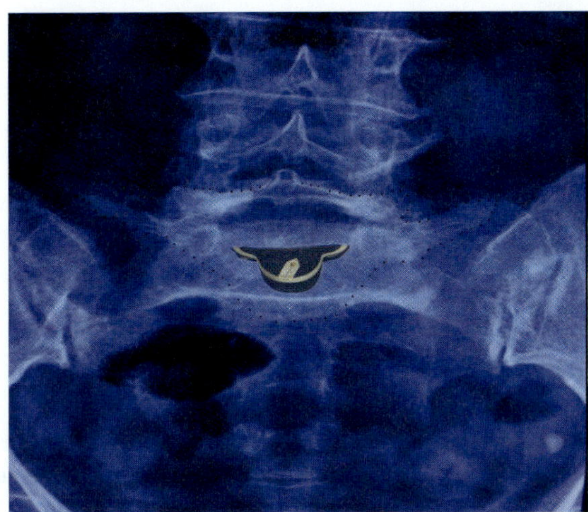

Fig. 7.41: Inverted Napoleon hat sign

INTERVERTEBRAL DISK DEGENERATION

INTRODUCTION

Degeneration of the intervertebral disks is an inevitable age-related phenomenon that occurs in almost all people who live longer than 50 years. Although in most cases it is asymptomatic, the remaining individuals develop a varied set of symptoms apart from chronic backache, depending upon the stage of degeneration their spine is in.

RELEVANT ANATOMY

The movements of the spine involve 97 diarthroses (i.e. synovial joints, having substantial motion) and an even greater number of amphiarthroses (i.e. fibrocartilaginous joints, having less motion). A spinal motion segment in the vertebral column can best be understood by the "three joint complex" model **(Fig. 7.42A)**—one intervertebral disk between the vertebrae and two articulating zygapophyseal (facet) joints.

Structure of the Intervertebral Disk

An intervertebral disk comprises of two cartilaginous end plates (made of hyaline cartilage) on either side—caudad and cephalad **(Fig. 7.42A)**, a nucleus pulposus in the center and an annulus fibrosus encircling the nucleus **(Fig. 7.42B)**. Nucleus pulposus, a remnant of notochord, is a gelatinous material, rich in type II collagen, lying slightly posterior to central axis of vertebrae that comprises almost two-thirds of the surface area of the disk. Since the nucleus is continuously under considerable pressure, to restrain it in place there is a lamellar structure the annulus, rich in type I collagen, composed of concentric fibrocartilage rings, that encircles it all around. Collagen fibers' concentration is highest in the outer annulus and it continues from the annulus to the surrounding tissues, tying it to the anterior and posterior longitudinal ligaments and the hyaline cartilage end plates superiorly and inferiorly.

The disk primarily receives its nutrition from the vascular vertebral bodies by diffusion via the endplates, although the outer third of the annulus receives blood supply from the epidural space. Motion and weight bearing are supposed to be helpful in maintain

the diffusion process. Nerve supply is predominantly from a special branch of ventral ramus of the corresponding spinal nerve, called as the "sinu-vertebral nerve".

The function of the disks primarily depends on the properties of the extracellular matrix (ECM) present in the disk. The macromolecules that form this ECM are collagen and proteoglycans, i.e. a molecule with a protein core and negatively charged Glycosaminoglycan (GAG) side chains. These macromolecules that comprise the ECM are synthesized by the small population of cells occupying less than 1% of the disk volume. The major component of the disks, however, is water and its concentration is regulated by GAGs. The concentration varies with age, location within the disk and body position. The nucleus pulposus is most highly hydrated (80–90% water), while water content of the annulus is lower than the nucleus, declining to 65% in the outer annulus in adult disks. Water content varies with load, leading to diurnal changes in disk hydration. During the diurnal cycle almost 25% of the disk's water can be lost and regained. Water is expressed from the disk during the day because of the increased forces of body weight and muscle contractions, and it is reimbibed at night when the compressive forces are removed. This diurnal cycle results in changes in disk height and affects the disk's mechanical properties.

NATURAL HISTORY OF DISK DEGENERATION

The degenerative process is divided into three separate but overlapping stages, each with its distinctive findings.

1. *Stage of dysfunction (15–45 years)*: With normal aging the disk gradually dries out with the nucleus pulposus changing from a turgid gelatinous bulb to a desiccated structure. This causes the annulus to develop circumferential and radial tears, mainly in the posterior part, where small herniations of the nuclear material may squeeze out slightly beyond the margins of the vertebral bodies. Presence of some predisposing factors like lifting a heavy weight, etc. may render these herniations symptomatic in certain predisposed individuals leading to a condition called acute posterior intervertebral disk (PIVD) prolapse, discussed subsequently in the chapter.

2. *Stage of segmental instability (35–70 years)*: Disruption of the internal structure of the disk leads to progressive disk resorption. Normally disks transmit up to 80% of the load while rest is shared by posterior structures (viz. facet joints and posterior ligaments). Loss of elasticity of disks or their resorption transfers load to facet joints (synovial joints) increasing stress in them, leading to facet joint synovitis followed by arthritis. The resultant capsular laxity and joint erosions may make these joints unstable causing a "segmental instability", which means a segment of spine is rendered malfunctional (as facet joints are integral component of spinal motion segment). Displacement of the facets may result in forward or backward shifts in the vertebral bodies. In an attempt to attain stability, the body responds by progressive development of hypertrophic bone around disks and facets, the bony ridges being erroneously called as "osteophytes" **(Fig. 7.43)**.

Radiographs may well demonstrate these signs of aging. Schmorl's nodes **(Fig. 7.44A)**, i.e. upward and downward

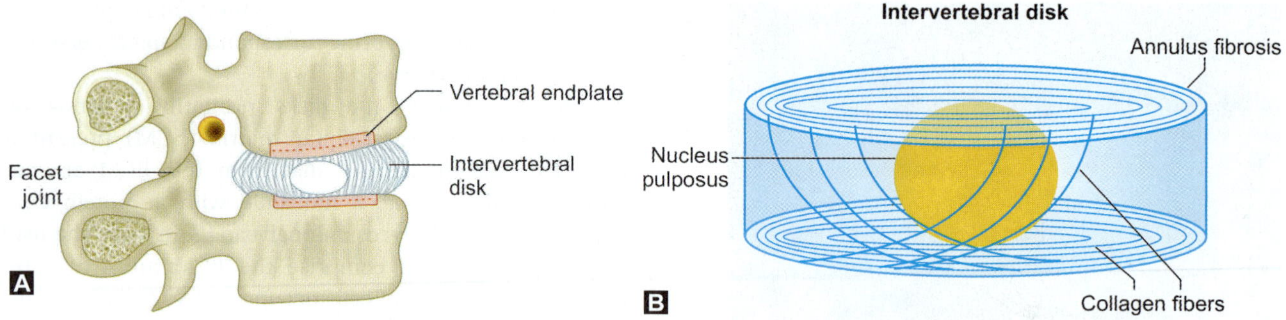

Figs 7.42A and B: (A) Vertebral motion segment; (B) Structure of intervertebral disk

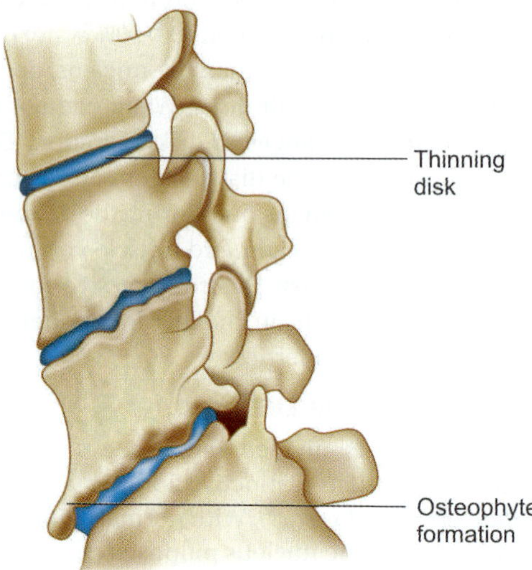

Fig. 7.43: Schematic depiction of effects of disk degeneration

protrusions of a spinal disk's tissue into the bone of the adjacent vertebrae, and vacuum phenomenon **(Fig. 7.44B)**, i.e. accumulation of gas, principally nitrogen, within the crevices of the intervertebral disks or adjacent vertebrae can be seen. As changes advance one may find reduced disk space with marginal osteophytes (typically along anterior vertebral margins) with or without small amounts of vertebral displacement (retrolisthesis >anterolisthesis), an X-ray picture vaguely termed as spondylosis* **(Figs 7.44C and D)**. Symptomatic patients with these changes are labeled as cases of "degenerative disk disease" (DDD) and present with recurrent episodes of low backache interspersed with periods of significant relief. Pain may be localized to back (axial) or at times may radiate into posterior hip or thigh (referred from malfunctional spinal motion segment).

3. *Stage of stabilization (>60 years)*: Instability is met with bony overgrowth in an attempt to attain stability. A subset of patients fails to adequately mount stabilization response ending up with degenerative spondylolisthesis (*see* Page 229). In few others, hypertrophic bone (osteophytes) and ligamentum flavum may compromise neural tissue due to stenosis of the spinal canal (central canal stenosis) or intervertebral foramina (root canal stenosis). While in former case the patients present classically with spinal claudication (pain on walking a certain distance and relieved with rest or bending forward), latter cases tend to present with a radicular pain (pain radiating to affected dermatome) due to compression of nerve root in intervertebral foramina. Spinal canal stenosis has been discussed in detail subsequently in the chapter.

HIGH-YIELD POINTS

- *Internal disk derangement:* The use of this term has recently come into practice to denote a very special category of patients who have axial spine pain likely secondary to a primary disk-related pathology. It has been postulated that disk degeneration leads to tears in annulus and cartilaginous endplates which allows foreign vertebral material or contents of spinal canal to come in contact with the degenerating disks. This may set in an autoimmune response from the body targeted against the disk. As inflammatory cascade irritates the sinu-vertebral nerves, the patient experiences diskogenic pain with no radicular symptoms. No radiographic investigation exists to date to confirm this diagnosis although magnetic resonance imaging (MRI) may show desiccated disks. It's a clinical suspicion where examination points towards disk being likely cause of pain. Confirmation can only be achieved by discography, an investigation which involves injection of an agent in disk of concern and monitoring response to the injected agent.
- *Facet joint dysfunction:* Sometimes the clinical examination may localize the source of pain to the facet joints (palpated approximately 2 cm laterally from the tip of spinous processes). Although facets may become painful due to secondary effects of disk degeneration, anatomical variations and developmental abnormalities of the facets have also been cited as a cause of this clinical situation. In case of such a diagnosis, one must consider the role of facet joint steroid and local anesthetic injections to effect remedy.

POSTERIOR INTERVERTEBRAL DISK PROLAPSE

INTRODUCTION

A disk prolapse (slipped disk) is a condition in which there is a tear in the annulus fibrosus (usually an endplate rupture) through

---

*Spondylosis is a vague term, mostly used to refer to X-ray changes of disk degeneration, although at times such patients may be clinically asymptomatic. The term is not to be confused with spondylitis which means inflammation of vertebra (e.g. tubercular spondylitis, ankylosing spondylitis, etc).

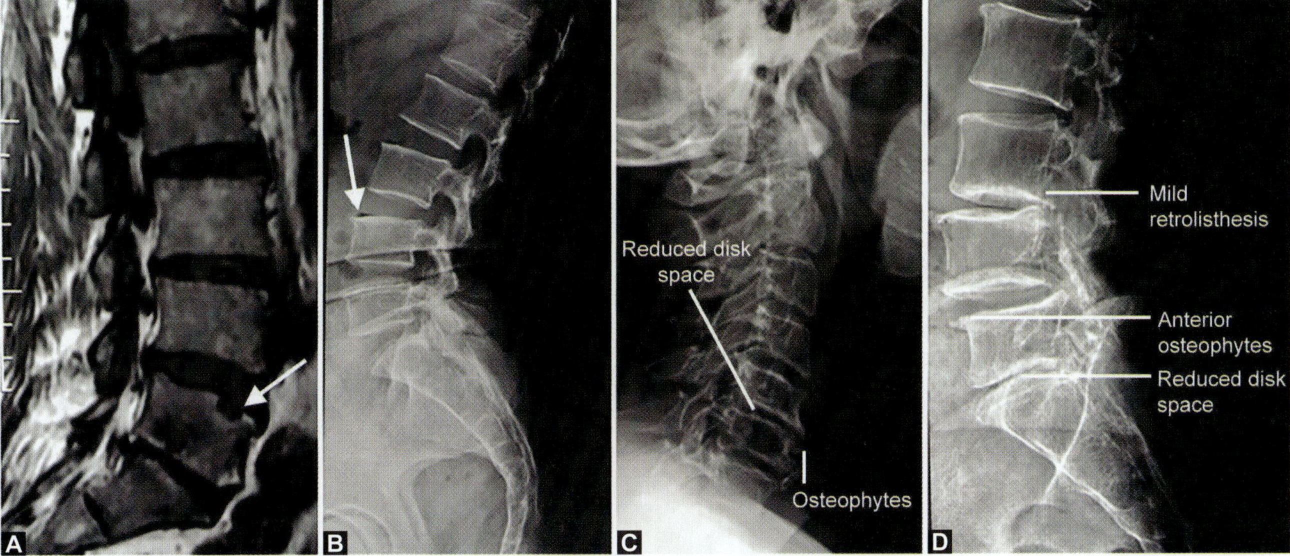

Figs 7.44A to D: Signs of disk degeneration on imaging. (A) Magnetic resonance imaging (MRI) of lumbosacral (LS) spine with visible Schmorl's nodes (arrow); (B) The vacuum phenomena (arrow) in a lateral X-ray of LS spine; (C and D) Changes of disk degeneration on lateral views of cervical and lumbar spine, respectively, a picture often vaguely labeled as spondylosis

which the gelatinous nucleus herniates out, thereby compressing the neural elements in the spinal canal. From youth into the 3rd decade the nucleus comprises of approximately 90% water by weight. Gradually over the next 4 decades the water content decreases to approximately 60%. The resultant desiccated disks are not that flexible and strong and tend to give way and herniate especially in presence of predisposing factors which include smoking, obesity, sedentary lifestyle, lifting of a heavy weight, squatting, too much of bending forward, involvement in contact sports and driving on bumpy roads. Failure generally tends to begin at the cartilaginous end plates.

The most common site for a disk prolapse is the lumbar spine (L4–L5 >L5–S1). Next in frequency comes the cervical spine (C5–C6 >C6–C7). Thoracic disks seldom prolapse due to the extrastability provided by the presence of strong rib cage in the region.

STAGES OF DISK PROLAPSE

The pathological process of disk prolapse is divided into the following stages **(Fig. 7.45)** for understanding:

- *Nuclear degeneration*: Desiccation causes degeneration and fragmentation of the nuclear material which herniates through the end plates into the vertebral body producing the characteristic "Schmorl's nodes".
- *Stage of protrusion*: The annulus becomes weak due to constant pressure by the degenerated nucleus and gives way in its weakest part, i.e. the posterolateral area thereby allowing the nuclear fragments to bulge through annulus. This is called "disk protrusion".
- *Stage of extrusion*: More bulging in the nucleus causes it to herniate through the annulus and lies underneath the posterior longitudinal ligament while still maintaining contact with the parent disk. This is called as "disk extrusion".
- *Stage of sequestration*: Once the extruded disk loses contact with the parent disk, it is called a "sequestrated disk". Now, it lies as a free fragment in the canal.

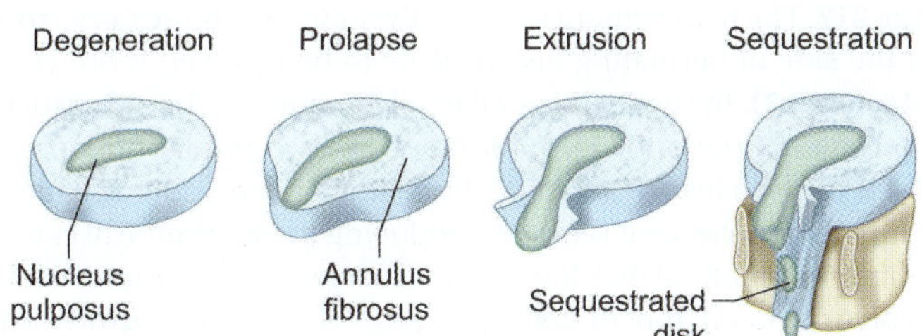

Fig. 7.45: Stages of disk degeneration

- *Stage of fibrosis and repair*: The sequestrated disk eventually becomes fibrosed and undergoes calcification. New bone forms at areas where posterior longitudinal ligament has been stripped from vertebral margins leading to osteophyte formation that adds to neural compression.
- *Secondary effects of disk prolapse*: As the disk degenerates, there is increased motion between adjacent vertebral segments which produces vertebral instability. Instability leads to more motion at facet joints which causes thickening of their capsule and induces osteoarthritis leading to osteophyte formation. All these changes further aggravate the already narrowed diameter of the spinal canal by the herniated disk, causing spinal canal stenosis eventually in chronic cases.

TYPES OF DISK HERNIATIONS

Degenerated disk is extruded posteriorly in three patterns **(Fig. 7.46)**:

1. Central herniation
2. Paracentral/paramedian type
3. Far lateral disk herniation.

Since annulus is weakest in the posterolateral part, most of the herniations are paracentral in nature and tend to involve the traversing (lower level) nerve roots, as already explained on

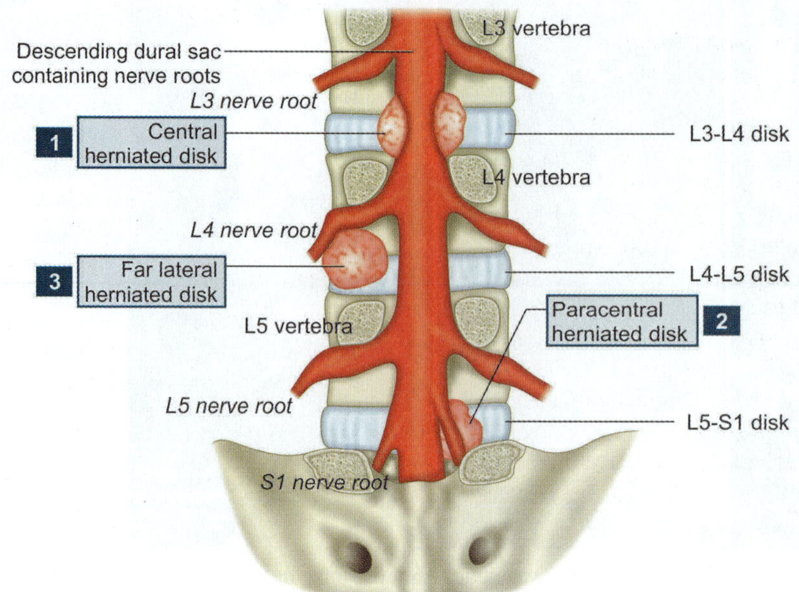

Fig. 7.46: Types of disk herniations

Page 212. The involvement is generally unilateral as the nerve root on the side of herniating disk is likely to be involved more **(Fig. 7.46, label 2)**. In case of bilateral involvement one should suspect a central herniation **(Fig. 7.46, label 1)**, as centrally prolapsing disk is likely to involve bilateral descending nerve roots and more commonly multiple nerve roots producing the syndrome of cauda equina. A far lateral disk herniation is known for its propensity to involve the nerve root of same level (viz. L4 nerve root involved in L4-L5 disk prolapse), as depicted in **Figure 7.46 (label 3)**.

PRESENTATIONS OF DISK PROLAPSE

When the disk herniates back, the herniated material may come to lie either superolateral to the affected nerve root (shoulder presentation) or inferomedial to the affected nerve root (axillary presentation). The type of presentation determines the sciatic list. List is one-plane sideways tilt of trunk without an actual structural deformity in the spine **(Fig. 7.47A)**. Patients with axillary presence of disk material bend to same side to keep the disk material away from contacting the nerve roots while those with shoulder presentations behave the opposite **(Fig. 7.47B)**.

CLINICAL FEATURES

Many patients who present with a disk prolapse tend to give a history of lifting of heavy weight in the recent past. The most common presenting symptom is acute low back pain. Often the pain radiates down the back of thigh and leg when the condition is referred to as "sciatica". The pattern of radiation depends upon the nerve root that has been compressed (remember, spinal cord terminates at lower border of L1, so the disk compresses the hanging nerve roots in the canal). In L5 root compression the pain radiates to the anterolateral aspect of leg and ankle while in S1 nerve root compression the radiation is along the posterolateral calf and heel. Sometimes, the patient may even complain of numbness or paresthesias (pins and needles like sensation) in the dermatome that corresponds to the compressed nerve root. And at times, when the disk material is large and predominantly

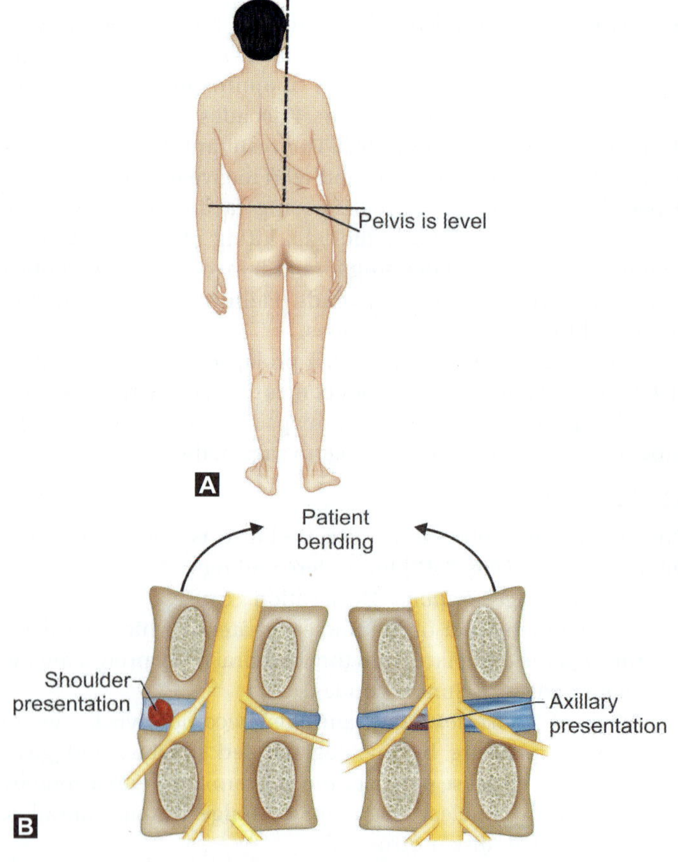

Figs 7.47A and B: (A) Shoulder and axillary presentation in disk prolapse. The disk bulge in shoulder presentation produces a list to the opposite side while a disk bulge in the axillary presentation will produce a list to the same side (mnemonic: psoas); (B) Diagrammatic depiction of a sciatic list

central, it can cause a significant compression of multiple nerve roots, a condition called cauda equina syndrome (*see* Page 213).

EXAMINATION

Patient is undressed and local examination of back is done followed by a thorough neurological examination.

Local Examination

Local examination includes assessment of the following:

- *Posture*: When the patient is observed from the back, the central furrow becomes more prominent due to paraspinal (erector spinae) muscle spasm. The spasm obliterates the normal lumbar lordotic curve and the patient's back goes flat. The trunk may be tilted to one side owing to sciatic list, the side of list being dependent on whether disk presentation is shoulder or axillary as already explained.
- *Spinal tenderness*: In the midline, the tips of spinous processes should be palpated for any localized tenderness if present, to correlate the level of lesion. Generally, most patients tend to have a diffuse tenderness in lower back owing to the paraspinal muscle spasm in the region.
- *Movements*: Spinal movements become painful. Flexion, i.e. forward bending is relatively more difficult in patients with this condition.

Neurological Examination

A thorough neurological examination is important to localize the site of spinal lesion **(Table 7.12)**. One must be meticulous in testing reflexes as the search is for a missing reflex since nerve root compressions are lower motor lesions. For motor function assessment, examination of the foot is particularly useful in this setting as one can assess L4, L5 and S1 nerve roots, all at once. L4 supplies tibialis anterior, the dorsiflexor of foot while S1 supplies the gastroc-soleus, the plantar flexor of foot and L5 brings about the contraction of the extensor hallucis longus, the extensor of the great toe. So the patient can be asked to walk on heels (dorsiflexion), that assesses L4, then on toes (plantar flexion) to assess S1 and finally to extend the great toe to assess L5. If motor power in all three activities is normal then good chances are there that no neurological deficit exists. Similarly, abductor weakness or lurch and a positive Trendelenburg test are suggestive of L5 weakness and hip extensor weakness or gluteal lurch is found in S1 weakness. But to make the inference, sensory examination of the concerned dermatomes is as important because at times, the deficit is not complete but just in form of a hypesthesic patch. In every patient with disk disease, especially with bladder or bowel dysfunction,

Table 7.12: Nerve root involved with resulting deficit

Nerve root compression	Sensory deficit	Motor weakness	Reflex change
C5	Upper lateral arm and elbow	Deltoid, Biceps (C5, C6)	Biceps (variable)
C6	Lateral forearm, thumb, index finger	Biceps (C5, C6), ECRL, ECRB	Biceps, brachioradialis (supinator)
C7	Middle finger (variable because of overlap)	Triceps, wrist flexors (FCR), finger extensors (variable)	Triceps
C8	Ring and little finger, ulnar border of palm	Interossei, finger flexors (variable), FCU	
T1	Medial aspect of elbow	Interossei	
T2		Medial upper arm and adjacent chest (intercostobrachial)	
T4		Nipple line	
T10	Umbilicus	Trunk flexion (Beevor sign)	Abdominal reflex
L1	Anterior proximal thigh near inguinal ligament	Iliopsoas (seated hip flexion)	
L2	Anteromedial thigh midway between inguinal ligament and patella	Iliopsoas (seated hip flexion)	
L3	Skin just proximal or medial to patella	Quadriceps (L3, L4)	Knee reflex (L3, L4)
L4	Posterolateral thigh, anterior knee, medial leg	Quadriceps (L2, L3, L4), hip adductors, tibialis anterior (heel walking)	Knee reflex (L3—secondary, L4)
L5	Anterolateral leg, dorsum of foot, great toe (autonomous zone is dorsal first web space and dorsum of third toe)	EHL, gluteus medius, extensor digitorum longus and brevis	Tibialis posterior reflex, medial hamstring reflex
S1	Lateral malleolus, lateral foot, heel, plantar surface of foot, web of fourth and fifth toe (autonomous zone is dorsum of fifth toe)	Peroneus longus and brevis, gastro-soleus S1—toe walking, Gluteus maximus	Ankle (L5, secondary—S1)
S2		Center of popliteal fossa (best to evaluate) supplies posterior thigh and proximal calf	
S3, S4, S5		Perianal area (arranged in concentric rings around anus) S5—central, S3—most peripheral	

Abbreviations: ECRL, extensor carpi radialis longus; ECRB, extensor carpi radialis brevis; FCR, flexor carpi radialis; FCU, flexor carpi ulnaris; EHL, extensor hallucis longus.

perianal sensations and voluntary anal contraction must be looked for to rule out "cauda equina syndrome".

Localizing the nerve root involved: As a rule, most disk prolapses are central or paracentral and it is usually the traversing root (lower level nerve root) which gets affected in "lumbar disk diseases". Details have already been explained on Page 212. *Exception*: in far lateral disk herniations, it is the exiting root which gets compressed (*see* **Fig. 7.46**).

Important Clinical Tests

The important clinical tests signifying nerve root compression that become positive before a detectable neurological deficit develops include the conventional straight leg raising test (SLRT) and its modifications as discussed below:

- *Straight leg raising test* (**Fig. 7.48**): The patient lies supine on the table. The affected leg is lifted up by flexing the hip with the knee straight. The angle between the back of the leg and the couch is noted when the patient complains of pain radiating down the limb. Test is considered to be indicative of disk pathology when the leg symptoms are reproduced at an angle between 30° and 70° (Mechanism of SLRT: sciatic nerve is tethered at the sciatic notch up and the fibular neck below, so when the leg is elevated the nerve at the back of thigh is stretched and the symptoms become apparent).
- *Bragard's sign* (**Fig. 7.49**): Straight leg raising test is performed as described. Just when the patient experiences the radicular symptoms, the leg is just lowered a little. Now, the ankle of the patient is dorsiflexed and if this reproduces the leg symptoms, it further strengthens the diagnosis (mechanism same as SLRT, ankle dorsiflexion stretches the nerve).
- *Lasegue test* (**Fig. 7.50**): Lasegue test is performed in two steps. In first step SLR test is done as described. This produces pain of nerve root compression. Now in second step knee is bent. This relaxes the nerve and pain disappears if it is due to nerve root compression. This further confirms the presence of sciatic pain and helps to differentiate sciatic pain from pain arising due to hip pathology. SLRT will be painful in both conditions but knee flexion in Lasegue test will relieve only sciatic pain and not the hip pain.

- *Well leg SLRT/contralateral SLRT*: When the patient reports sciatic pain in the affected leg upon lifting the limb that does not have the symptoms, this test is said to be positive. It basically signifies a large central type of disk herniation indenting the thecal sac.
- *Bowstring sign of McNab* (**Fig. 7.51**): Straight leg raising test is done as described. The angle at which the pain starts in the leg, the knee is flexed so that the symptoms disappear. Now the tibial nerve is palpated and compressed in the popliteal fossa to replicate the symptoms. This further helps in confirmation of the disease.

INVESTIGATIONS

- *X-ray* is generally the first investigation that is ordered. In acute cases the findings are subtle except for loss of the normal lordotic curvature of the lumbar spine. In chronic

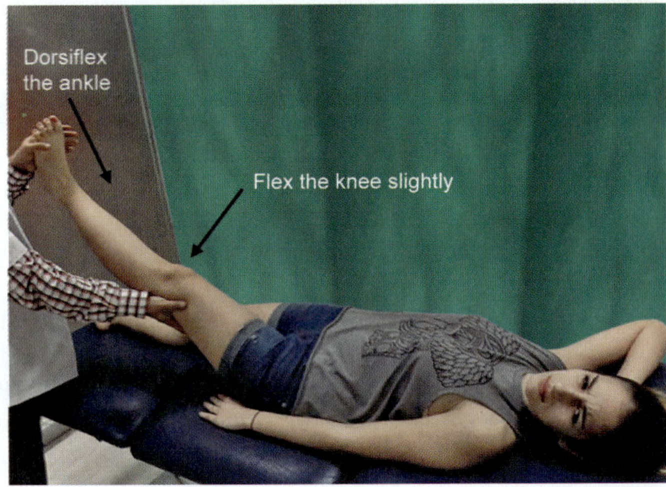

Fig. 7.49: Bragard's sign (ankle dorsiflexion produces pain while doing straight leg raising test)

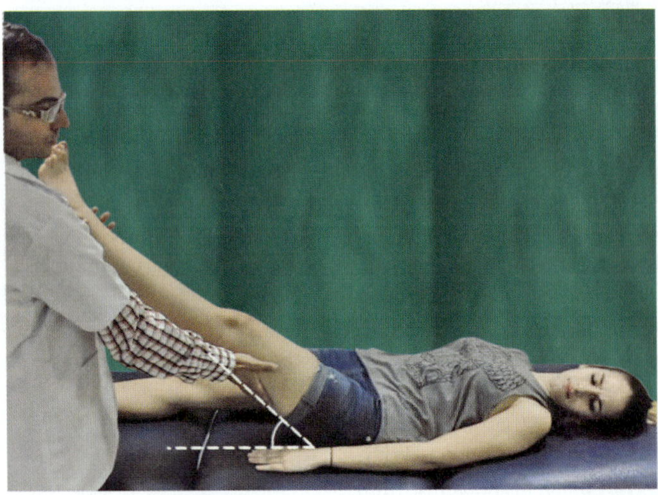

Fig. 7.48: Straight leg raising test

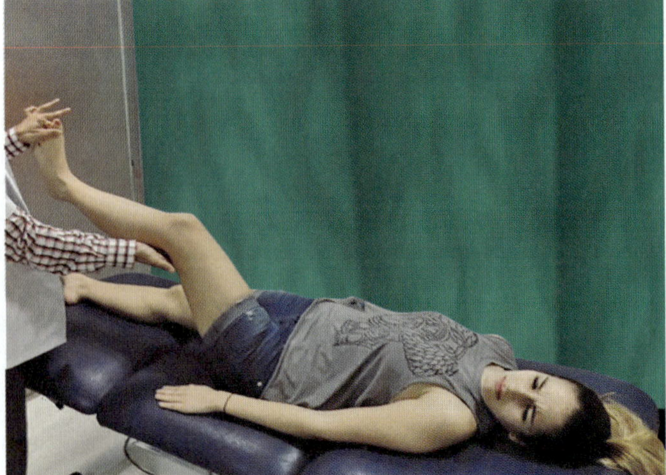

Fig. 7.50: Lasegue test

cases, the disk space may be narrowed and there may be lipping of the vertebral margins or signs of facet joint arthritis **(Fig. 7.52)**, similar to cases with DDD.

- *Magnetic resonance imaging* **(Figs 7.53A and B)** is the investigation of choice. It can document compression over the thecal sac as well as the nerve roots. It also helps in identifying the location of the disk (central, paracentral or far lateral) and to locate any sequestrated fragment.
- *Myelography* involves injecting a radiopaque dye in the cerebrospinal fluid (CSF) and then taking an X-ray. In case there is disk herniation, there may be an indentation in the thecal sac visible on X-ray. In cases where the disk is lateral and compressing on the nerve root, there may be abrupt blunting of the dye column as it fills the nerve root sheath (the root cut off sign). Myelography has largely been overtaken by MRI.

TREATMENT

Conservative Treatment

Most patients with slip disk are initially given a trial of conservative treatment which includes bed rest for 2–4 days nonsteroidal anti-inflammatory drugs (NSAIDs), muscle relaxants and spinal exercises.

- *Intermittent lumbar traction* **(Fig. 7.54A)** can be used in cases which are not responding wherein a traction belt is used to apply distraction force to the vertebrae to create space for prolapsed disk to retreat and widen the intervertebral foramina. A pull of 30–40 kg is generally needed. The procedure can at times increase the pain. So, it has a little role as per the current evidence.
- *Electrotherapy:* Local electrotherapy modalities may be added for additional benefit. These deliver heat to the body tissues thereby increasing local blood flow, washing off the inflammatory mediators. Superficial heat modalities (effective up to 0.5 cm from surface) include hot packs, infrared therapy, etc. while short wave diathermy and ultrasound are deep heat therapies (effective to depth of 3–5 cm from surface). However, the ideal therapy for radicular

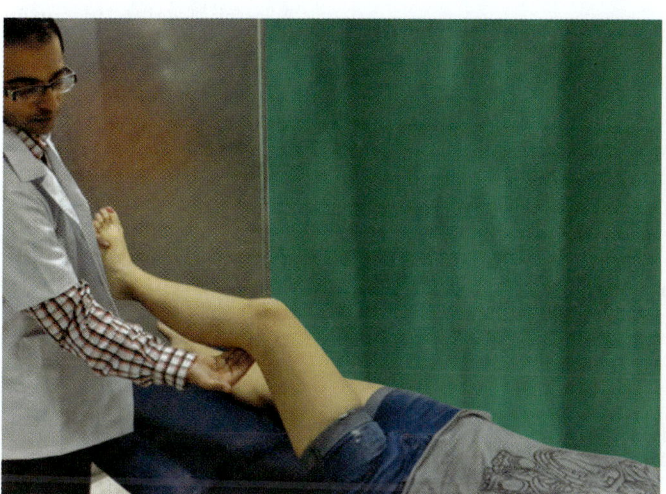

Fig. 7.51: Bowstring sign of McNab

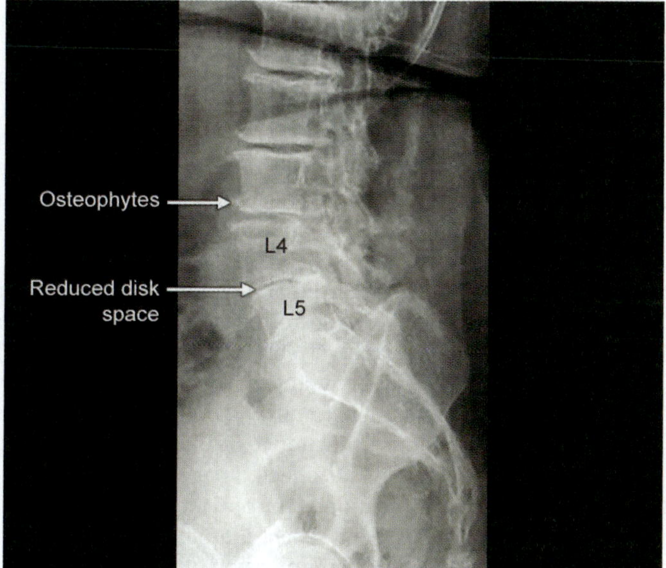

Fig. 7.52: X-ray lumbosacral spine lateral view showing signs of chronic posterior intervertebral disk prolapse

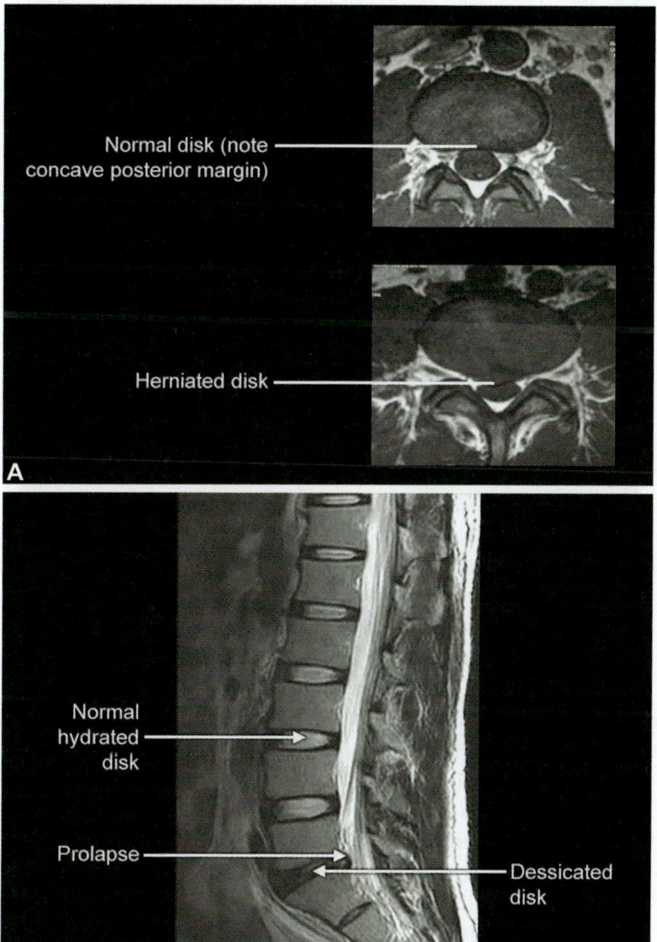

Figs 7.53A and B: Magnetic resonance imaging of lumbosacral spine. (A) Sagittal cut; and (B) Axial cut showing disk prolapse

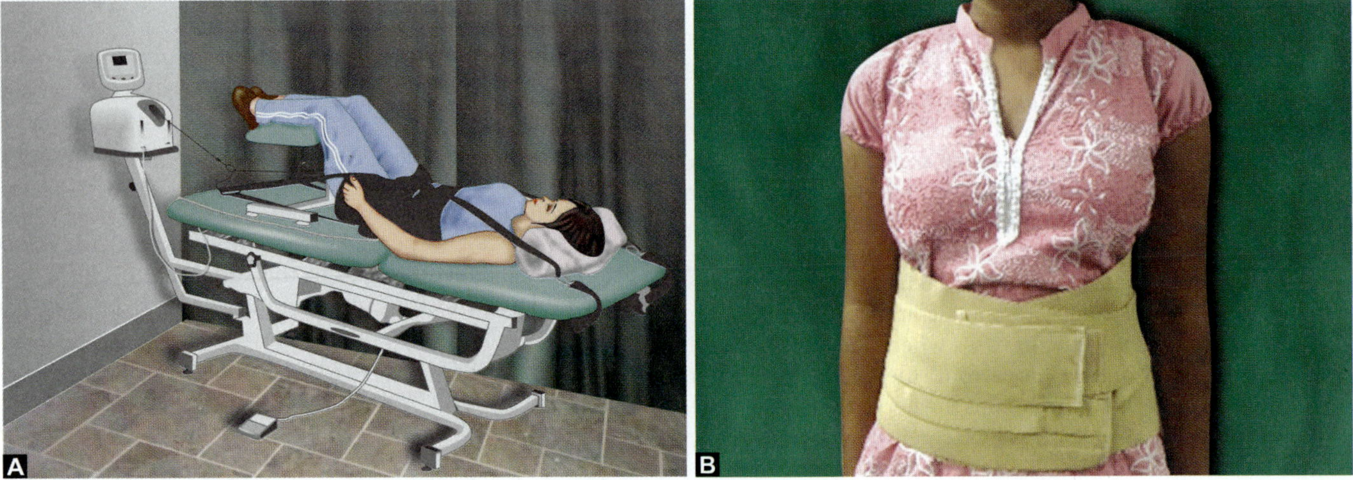

Figs 7.54A and B: (A) Intermittent lumbar traction; (B) Lumbosacral corset belt

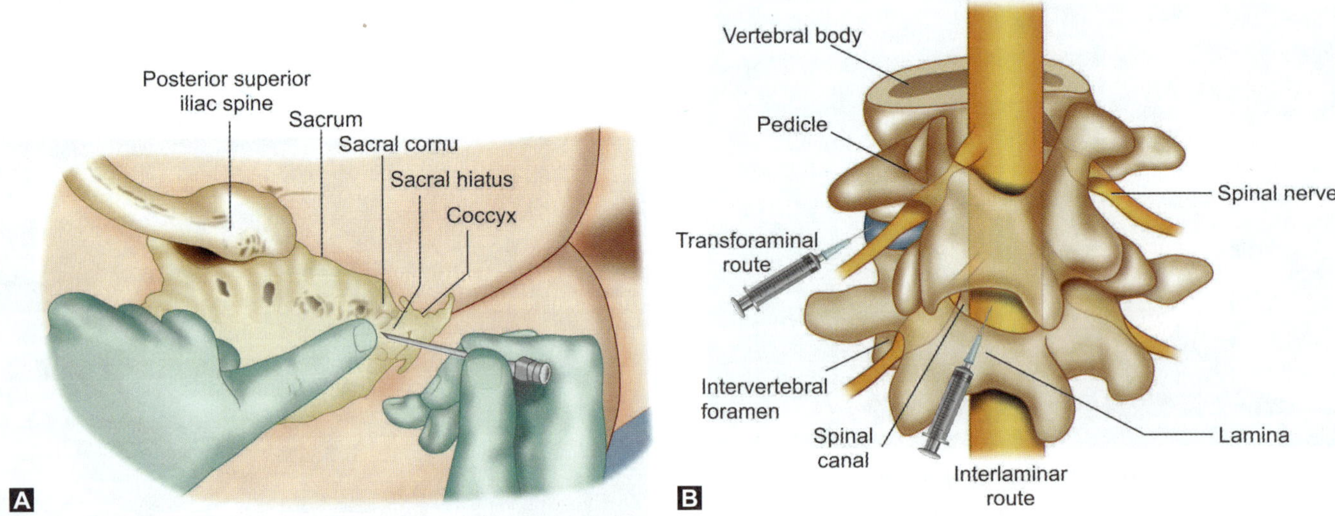

Figs 7.55A and B: (A) Caudal epidural injection being given; (B) Transforaminal and interlaminar routes for spinal epidural injections

symptoms is electrical stimulation called as transcutaneous electrical nerve stimulation (TENS).

- *Braces:* A lumbosacral corset belt **(Fig. 7.54B)** may be advised for pain relief during the acute stage. Belts increase the intra-abdominal pressure and create the spine and abdomen into a stable cylinder. Current evidence is against prolonged rest and lumbar corsets as they both gradually weaken the muscles and prolong the duration of illness.
- *Spinal manipulation techniques* (chiropractic medicine) are also described that alter the neurophysiological activity and decrease pain by release of beta endorphins and releasing the muscle spasm. However, it is only recommended in the hands of trained chiropractitioners.
- *Epidural steroid injections* are another treatment methods for diskogenic and radicular pain emanating from the herniated disks. The procedure consists of injecting into the dural sac or around the nerve root, a long acting steroid (for decreasing disk edema and local inflammation) along with a local anesthetic (for acute pain relief).

Injections can be given under fluoroscopic control via either of three routes:

1. *Caudal:* Injection is given into epidural space reached via the sacral hiatus **(Fig. 7.55A)**. Since site of inflammation is remote, relatively large amounts of drug need to be administered. The route is preferred in cases where localization of pathological disk is relatively uncertain.
2. *Transforaminal route:* Preferred mode of injection in lumbar disk pathology. Injection is introduced at site of nerve root compression via the intervertebral foramen **(Fig. 7.55B)**. Since one can inject directly anterior to compressed nerve root, expected benefit is maximum with relatively lesser doses of drug. However, for the injection to be effective, appropriate localization of pathology (i.e. affected nerve root) is must.
3. *Interlaminar route:* Injection is introduced into the epidural space from direct posterior aspect piercing the ligamentum flavum **(Fig. 7.54B)**. Since compression of nerve occurs from disk herniation from anterior side, drug delivery at targeted area is difficult to achieve and hence is not as preferred

mode as transforaminal injections. However, transforaminal injections have been met with catastrophic neurological complications owing to intra-arterial injections in cervical spine, hence, interlaminar is the preferred mode here.

Surgical Treatment

Indications for surgery include:

Absolute Indications

- Progressively increasing neurological deficit despite conservative treatment
- Cauda equina syndrome (orthopedic emergency).

Relative Indications

- Severe sciatic pain persisting despite 6 weeks of conservative treatment
- Recurrent incapacitating sciatica attacks (more than three in 1 year).

Surgery: Since a prolapsed disk compresses the neural elements in the spinal canal, surgery involves decompressing the canal by removing a piece of its wall (i.e. the lamina) apart from removal of the herniated disk (discectomy); the surgery being called decompression with discectomy.

*Methods of Spinal Decompression **(Fig. 7.56)***

- *Fenestration:* This involves creating hole in the ligamentum flavum that connects the adjacent laminas, thereby opening up the spinal canal.

- *Laminotomy:* In addition to fenestration, a part of lamina is excised to widen the hole and create wider space for decompressing the canal.
- *Hemilaminectomy:* This involves removing whole of lamina but only on one side.
- *Laminectomy:* The lamina on both the sides is removed along with the spinous process. This is generally required for large central disks and patients with cauda equina syndrome.

Methods of Disk Excision

- *Open disk excision:* Disk is reached and excised after decompressing the wall by either of the method mentioned earlier.
- *Microdiscectomy:* This involves a minimal incision where under microscopic view the herniated disk is excised after creating a fenestration in ligamentum flavum to reach the disk. It is a day care procedure and currently, the method of choice.
- *Endoscopic disk excision:* Fine instruments (camera, probes and other endoscopic instruments) are inserted via stab incisions and disk is excised in a percutaneous manner. It is a day care surgery that is recently coming up in big way.
- *Chemonucleolysis:* In this an enzyme chymopapain (derived from papaya) is injected into the herniated disk under X-ray control. The enzyme hydrolyses proteoglycans (noncollagenous proteins) which reduces water-holding capacity of nucleus pulposus. This decreases the intradiskal tension and reduces the disk bulge. Since the enzyme has no effect on collagen; tendons, bones and ligaments are

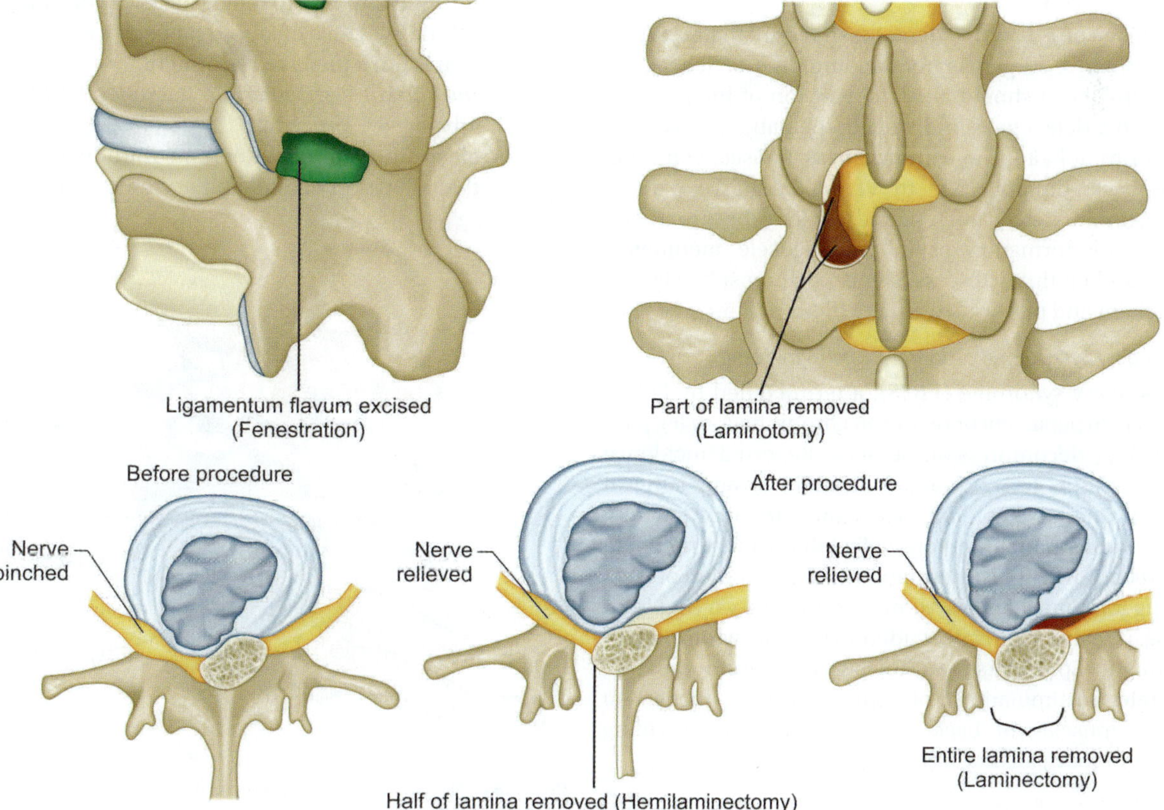

Fig. 7.56: Methods of spinal decompression

not affected. An important side effect is hemorrhage since the enzyme can erode glycosaminoglycans present in the capillary walls. Repeated use of enzyme is to be avoided due to chances of sensitization.

Complications of Invasive Disk Herniation Treatment Procedures

Some important complications that can follow disk surgery, epidural injections, chemonucleolysis or myelography, that merit a special mention are discitis and arachnoiditis.

Discitis

The term literally meaning infection limited to disk space in isolation is rare. Inoculation mostly occurs following invasive disk herniation treatment procedures. The vertebral end plates are rapidly attacked and infection spreads into the vertebral bodies. Patients classically develop severe acute back pain, muscle spasm and high-grade fever following the procedure. MRI provides the diagnosis. Treatment involves antibiotics as first line but nonresolving cases need surgical evacuation of pus.

Arachnoiditis

This is a rare diagnosis made mostly after myelography as a complication of oil-based contrast media used. Patients present with diffuse back pain, vague lower limb symptoms and at times with sphincter disturbances. MRI may demonstrate obliteration of subarachnoid space. Steroid injections may give temporary relief else surgical neurolysis may be needed. Treatment is generally unrewarding so many surgeons follow palliative measures only.

Dural Rupture (Durotomy)

With an incidence of 1–17%, incidental tear of dura mater during spinal decompressive surgery is not uncommon. CSF leakage in the intraoperative field should alert the surgeon of the possible complication. If a defect goes undetected, the patient is likely to experience postural headache with dizziness, nausea, vomiting, pain in the back, diplopia due to VI cranial nerve paresis, photophobia, tinnitus, etc. If not repaired properly these tears can lead to CSF fistula formation, pseudomeningocele, meningitis, arachnoiditis and epidural abscess. Hence, one must be vigilant in detecting them and performing a meticulous repair.

Failed Back Surgery Syndrome/Postlaminectomy Syndrome

Failed back surgery syndrome (FBSS), a term coined by Follett and Dirks, refers to persistent or recurrent chronic back or leg pain even after spinal decompression surgery. Reported incidence varies from 20% to 40%. Wrong indication, wrong surgical technique (postoperative epidural scar tissue formation), wrong level surgery, wrong patient (emotionally labile) and wrong fate of surgeon (recurrence of disk herniation or degeneration of facet joints altering joint mechanics), all may contribute varying from case to case. Treatment involves identifying the wrong factor and correcting it. Epidural steroid injections, neuromodulation therapies (electrostimulation of spinal cord), focus on strengthening muscles of back and core (trunk), providing psychological support, all may have a role.

CERVICAL DISK PROLAPSE

After the lumbar spine cervical spine is the next most common site for disk prolapse. The most common level involved is C5–C6

followed by C6–C7. Identification of nerve root involvement needs understanding of the anatomy of the area. The spinal canal here is occupied by spinal cord. Hence, not uncommon is compression of the cord in this region which leads to upper motor features. Nerve roots branching from the cord in this area exit above the corresponding vertebrae **(Fig. 7.57)**. Unlike in lumbar spine, there are no traveling or descending roots in this area, only exiting nerve roots are there. Hence, it is the exiting root which gets involved (*see* **Fig. 7.57** for explanation) so the most common roots irritated are C6 followed by C7. Diagnosis rests on meticulous examination aided by the same investigations as already mentioned. Management principles are also nearly the same. However, as far as surgery is concerned, preferred modality of treatment is removal of the disk via anterior approach (anterior cervical discectomy) with or without spinal fusion with bone graft to achieve stability.

HIGH-YIELD POINTS

- Intervertebral disk is the largest avascular structure in the body and constitutes 33% of the vertebral height.
- In total there are 23 disks in the spine. No disk exists between C1 and C2.
- The most damaging motion for the disk is axial rotation.
- Brachialgia (pain radiating from the neck down the upper limb) is the upper limb counter part of sciatica.
- Some newer modalities that have recently been introduced for disk treatment include:
  - *Ozone therapy*: It is a recently introduced minimally invasive modality where ozone-oxygen mixture is injected into disk to reduce disk volume. Presently, there is little evidence of any advantage over other procedures so it is not a preferred treatment.
  - *Intradiskal electrothermic therapy (IDET)*: It is a fairly advanced procedure wherein specially designed electrothermal catheters are introduced into the disk that allows for careful and accurate temperature control

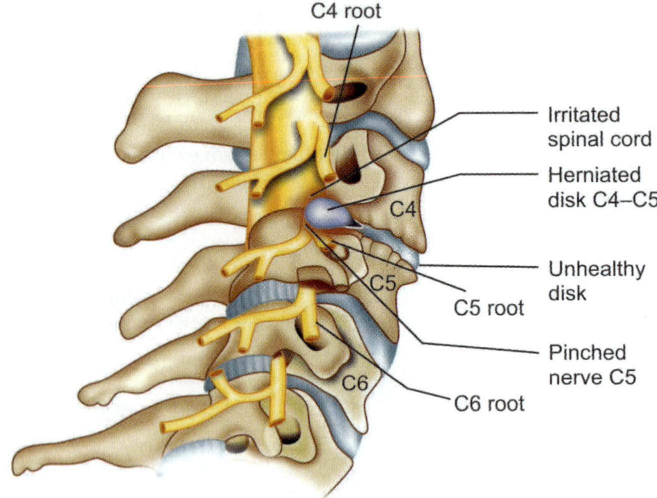

Fig. 7.57: Nerve root involvement in herniated cervical disk. With cord present in spinal canal and nerve roots exiting above corresponding vertebrae, C4–C5 disk herniates as shown to involve the cord behind it and the C5 nerve root

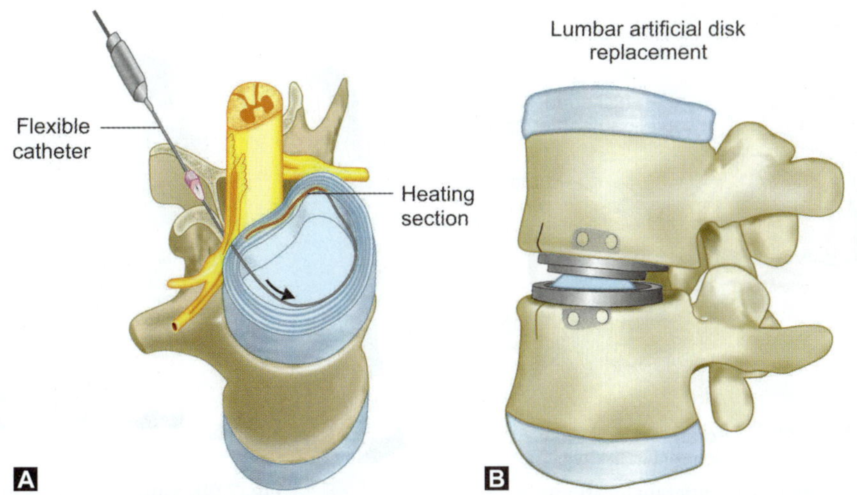

Figs 7.58A and B: (A) Diagrammatic representation of intradiskal electrothermic therapy;
(B) Diagrammatic representation of artificial disk replacement

(Fig. 7.58A). The procedure works by cauterizing the nerve endings within the disk wall to help block the pain signals. This minimally invasive outpatient surgical procedure has been developed over the last few years to treat patients with chronic low back pain caused by small herniations of their lumbar disks.

– *Artificial disk replacement*: It is an upcoming surgical procedure (similar to joint arthroplasty) in which the degenerated intervertebral disk is replaced with artificial device **(Fig. 7.58B)**, employed primarily in cases of cervical disk herniation.

SPINAL CANAL STENOSIS

SPINAL CANAL STENOSIS

INTRODUCTION

Spinal canal stenosis is a disabling disorder that generally occurs in the elderly in 6th or 7th decade of life. In this disorder diameter of spinal canal is compromised thus causing neural compression and producing symptoms. Lumbar canal that is normally round, oval or trefoil-shaped in cross section, is most commonly involved followed by cervical canal.

CAUSES

Spinal canal stenosis can result from congenital (achondroplasia, scoliosis, kyphosis, etc.) or more commonly acquired causes with the most common being DDD. Paget's disease, hyperparathyroidism, fluorosis, spinal tumors, infection such as TB, surgery and trauma remain some rare causes in the list.

PATHOPHYSIOLOGY

Degenerative lumbar canal stenosis (LCS) is the most common form of spinal canal stenosis. Degenerative LCS anatomically can involve the central canal, lateral recess, intervertebral foramina (root canal stenosis) or any combination of these locations **(Fig. 7.59)**. Degenerative changes in the intervertebral disk result in microinstability at the facet joints causing weakening of the joint capsule, hypertrophy of facet joints, hypertrophy and calcification of ligamentum flavum, formation of vertebral body osteophytes (in attempt to attain stability) and eventually subluxation of the vertebral joints. These pathological changes ultimately lead to stenosis of the spinal canal. Chronic compression of nerve roots in LCS leads to congestion and ischemia of nerves. Neurogenic claudication results, i.e. patient develops pain on walking a fixed distance as increased metabolic demands of nerves are not met due to vascular compromise.

CLINICAL PRESENTATION

Clinical presentation depends on the site of involvement. In the most common LCS neurogenic claudication pain is the hallmark (i.e. pain arising in the lower back radiating down the buttock, thigh, leg to the foot on prolonged physical activity like walking a fixed distance). Pain worsens on standing or walking but is generally relieved by either bending forward (trunk flexion) or sitting. Posture-related pain in LCS is due to the fact that the available space in the central canal decreases in axial loading and extension and increases in axial distraction and flexion. This also explains that why do patients get more relief in lying on the side (allowing flexion posture) than lying flat. For the same reason patients find walking uphill easier and pushing a shopping cart gives them relief (positive shopping cart sign) **(Fig. 7.60)**. Since they mostly remain stooped forward to relieve pressure on their neural structures, their posture is said to be ape-like. Symptoms may be unilateral in root canal stenosis.

DIAGNOSIS

The classical clinical signs point well towards the diagnosis. On examination, straight leg raising test and neurological examination tests are usually normal unless the patient is made to get up and walk for 5–10 minutes. Diagnosis can be confirmed on computed tomography (CT) scan by measuring the canal diameter. Two measurements are used: the mid-sagittal [anteroposterior (AP)] diameter and the interpedicular (transverse) diameter of the spinal canal. Values less than 11 mm for AP and 16 mm for transverse diameter are considered abnormal.

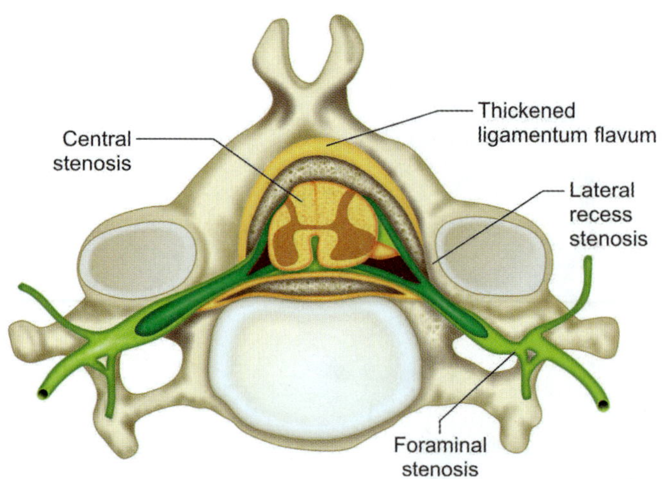

Fig. 7.59: Spinal canal stenosis at different locations

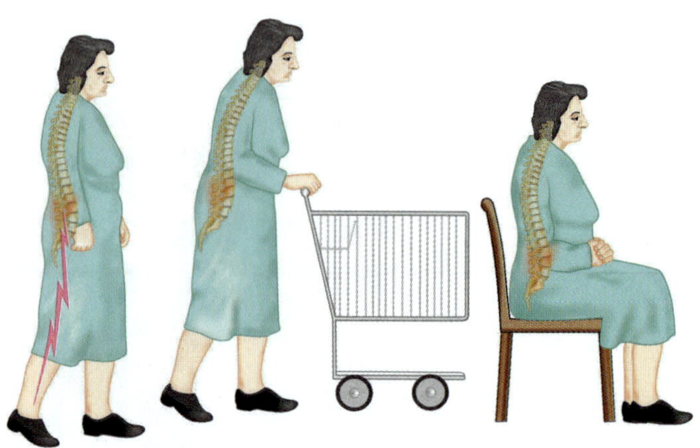

Fig. 7.60: Symptomatology in canal stenosis

Table 7.13: Differences between neurogenic and vascular claudications

Features	Neurogenic claudication	Vascular claudication
Claudication distance	Variable	Fixed
Provoking factors	Walking, standing	Walking
Relieving factors	Sitting, bending forward	Sitting, standing
Daily activities	Walking uphill, bicycling, pushing a shopping cart relieve the pain due to flexed lumbar posture	These activities provoke pain
Pulses and skin	Normal	Pulses are feeble or absent. Skin changes (loss of hair, skin atrophy) may be present
Back pain, back motion	Back pain is usually present and back motion may be limited	No back pain, back movements are normal
Neurological deficit	May be present	Absent
Time to get relief	Slow (few minutes)	Quick

Differentials (Table 7.13)

An important differential is vascular claudication pain (i.e. pain due to a peripheral artery disease). Pain on standing alone is the most sensitive symptom to differentiate neurogenic claudication from vascular claudication.

TREATMENT

Conservative treatment includes rest, NSAIDs and a spinal rehabilitation program consisting of spinal flexion exercises, electrotherapy, intermittent traction and epidural injections. In not responding cases, surgical decompression (laminectomy) of affected segments sometimes combined with spinal fusion is required. Laminoplasty is a method of spinal decompression mainly used in canal stenosis in cervical spine (use of laminoplasty for disk removal is not advocated). Here the lamina is not removed. Rather bone is cut and swung open to decompress the cord and then repositioned **(Figs 7.61A to C)**.

HIGH-YIELD POINT

- *Baastrup's disease (kissing spines):* This is degenerative disease characterized by hypertrophy and enlargement of adjacent spinous processes in lumbar spine of elderly leading to focal midline back pain which worsens in extension. Most common level involved is L4-L5. Disk height and neural foramina are normal. Treatment is mostly conservative, rarely surgical excision of bursa or osteotomy may be needed.

APPROACH TO A PATIENT WITH BACK PAIN

INTRODUCTION

Low backache (LBA), vaguely called as lumbago, is the most common cause of chronic disability in modern society with almost 80% of people experiencing it at some point of their lives. It is the second most common symptom seen in general practitioners' clinic, first being common cold. Almost in 10% of cases the complaint is chronic.

CLASSIFICATION

Broadly, back pain is categorized into two types: acute (symptoms with duration of less than 3 months) and chronic (symptoms persisting for more than 3 months). Acute backache in young is mostly due to a postural cause or a muscular strain, a prolapsed disk or a spondylolisthesis lesion, elderly with this condition must be evaluated for an osteoporotic compression fracture, metastatic disease or myeloma. Although in most cases acute backache is

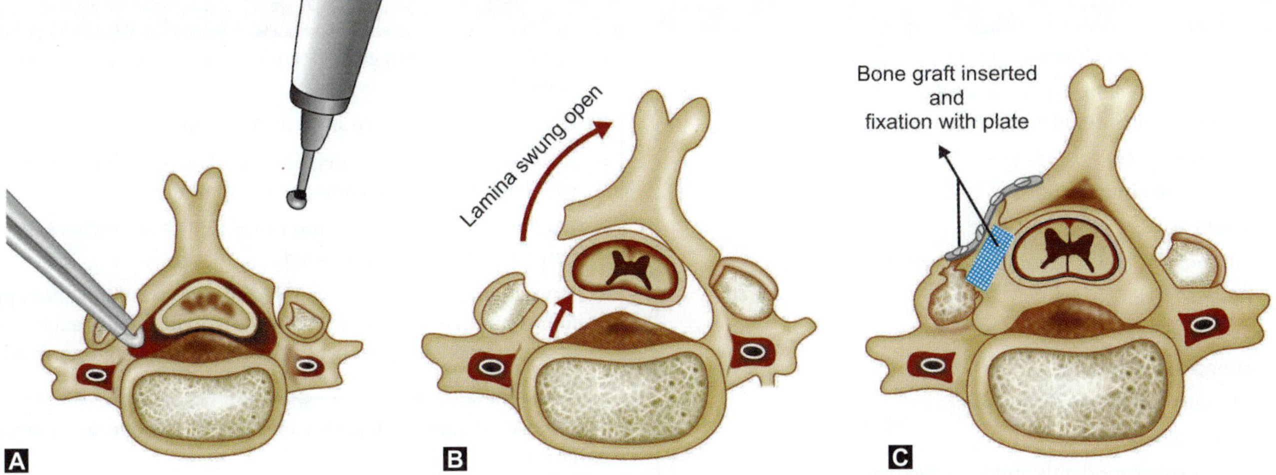

Figs 7.61A to C: Schematic depiction of laminoplasty

transient and investigations (X–ray, etc.) serve no purpose in treatment, work-up for the complaint should focus on ruling out a serious pathology by screening for "Red Flag Signs" **(Table 7.14)**. Presence of red flags suggests presence of a serious underlying pathology as the genesis factor for LBA and must be thoroughly investigated. Evolution of chronic LBA is rather complex, with physiological, psychological and psychosocial influences. In no way should it be viewed as just an extension of acute back pain. Work-up for chronic back pain (and acute LBA) should include a screen for "Yellow Flag Signs" that indicate risk for problem ending up in long-term disability.

CAUSES

Although most pains tend to be secondary to postural problems or muscular strains, a number of causes can be listed **(Box 7.1)** that need to be ruled out especially in patients with chronic symptoms. Despite making use of all modern day investigations, in almost 85% of cases, no cause is usually identified.

HISTORY AND EXAMINATION

Careful history taking and a thorough examination are cornerstones to reach the appropriate diagnosis in patients with back pain.

History Taking

It is essential to correlate factors like age, sex, occupation, etc. to genesis of pain. For example, almost 70% of pregnant females can complaint of LBA, during their course of pregnancy. In chronic cases it is often useful to inquire about the nature of pain as to whether it is mechanical or inflammatory. Mechanical back pain, more common type encountered, worsens with activity, improves with rest and is associated with acute or cumulative trauma to the spinal joints, disks, vertebrae or soft tissues of the back. Inflammatory type of back pain (seen in conditions like seronegative spondyloarthropathies) is generally worsened by rest, rather improves with activity and is associated with an element of morning stiffness.

Examination

Clinical examination must always include checking local area for tenderness and muscle spasm, detailed neurological evaluation,

Table 7.14: The red flags and yellow flags of back pain	
Red flags	*Yellow flags*
• Age <20 years or >50 years	• A belief that back pain is severely disabling
• History of significant trauma	
• The pain is constant, at night and getting worse	• Fear-avoidance behavior (avoiding activity due to anticipation of pain
• History of cancer, steroid use, IV drug use	• Tendency to low mood
• Unexplained fever and/or weight loss	• Expectation of help from passive treatment(s)
• Neurological deficit detectable	• Poor job satisfaction
	• Lack of family support

SLRT and Schober's test (*see* Page 428) for inflammatory LBA. Since at times back pain may be referred from nearby viscera (e.g. pain referred to back in pancreatitis), it is also advisable to do abdominal, rectal and per-vaginal examinations.

An important part of examination in such patients is to identify those with functional pain, i.e. malingerers. Waddell's signs **(Box 7.2)** are useful in such a scenario and must be elicited to avoid a wrong surgery and hence, the FBSS (*see* Page 240).

INVESTIGATIONS

Acute back pain is mostly self-limiting and needs no investigations (as almost 30% of asymptomatic people can have MRI abnormalities) but those with red flag signs should be subjected to imaging. CT/MRI of the lumbosacral (LS) spine is mandatory in LBA with neurological deficit. Blood investigations like hemoglobin (IIb), complete blood count (CBC), erythrocyte sedimentation rate (ESR), C-reactive protein (CRP) and human leukocyte antigen B27 (HLA-B27) should be done in the evaluation of inflammatory LBA. Calcium, phosphorus, alkaline phosphatase and vitamin D levels are estimated in the evaluation of suspected metabolic bone disease patients. Although LBA in elderly is mostly secondary to disk degeneration, serum protein electrophoresis and urinary Bence Jones proteins should be done in the work-up of elderly suspected to have multiple myeloma. Bone scan may be warranted in cases of spinal metastasis.

Box 7.1: Causes of back pain

- Congenital and developmental causes
  - Vertebral developmental anomalies (e.g. Spina bifida, block vertebra, transitional vertebra, etc.)
  - Kyphoscoliosis
  - Facet joint abnormalities
- Traumatic causes
  - Lumbosacral muscle strain (most common)
  - Prolapsed disk
  - Vertebral fractures
  - Spondylolisthesis
- Inflammatory and infective causes
  - Tuberculosis
  - Ankylosing spondylitis and seronegative spondyloarthropathies
- Degenerative
  - Degenerative disk disease and its sequel
- Neoplastic
  - Benign (most common benign tumor of spine is osteoid osteoma)
  - Malignant
    - *Primary:* Multiple myeloma is the most common primary malignant tumor of spine
    - Metastasis from other sites (breast is the most common source)
- Metabolic causes
  - Osteoporosis
  - Osteomalacia
- Iatrogenic
  - Failed back surgery syndrome
  - Discitis/arachnoiditis
- Postural back pain
  - Protuberant abdomen
  - Occupational or habitual bad posture
  - Pregnancy
- Miscellaneous
  - Functional pain syndromes and adjustment disorders (e.g. fibromyalgia)
- Referred pain from genitourinary and gynecological diseases.

Box 7.2: Signs of Waddell (for identifying those with functional pain)

- *Tenderness tests:* Superficial tenderness or nonanatomic location of tenderness
- *Overreaction:* Excessive show of emotions
- *Regional disturbances:* Regional weakness or sensory changes which deviate from accepted neuroanatomy
- *Distraction tests:* Positive tests (e.g. SLRT) are rechecked while patient's attention is distracted
- *Simulation tests:* Patient is subjected to movements that appear to be painful but actually do not cause pain such as axial loading of spine by pressing on head or rotating body holding shoulders and hips in one plane

Note: Three or more categories of signs if positive are considered significant.

relieving muscle spasm although evidence citing their benefit is insufficient. There are conflicting results on the benefits of using antidepressants and gabapentin to treat chronic pain. Electrotherapeutic modalities may have a role although it is yet to be proven by randomized controlled trials. Physiotherapy should be instituted once pain has settled and should focus on strengthening of spinal musculature (especially multifidus and transversus abdominis) and muscles of the core (trunk). Weight reduction should be encouraged and postural advice on maintaining correct postures while prolonged sitting or standing should be given to all.

Surgical intervention should be reserved for those who are not responding to conservative measures, barring some patients who present with orthopedic emergencies (e.g. cauda equina syndrome). The type of surgery should be individualized depending on the diagnosed cause.

An important treatment goal for both acute and chronic back pain is for the patient to be active as soon as possible, hence, patient education and psychological support are equally important aspects, especially in those with yellow flag signs.

HIGH-YIELD POINT

- *Transitional vertebra:* Transitional vertebrae are those that have the characteristics of two types of vertebra. They can occur at the cervicothoracic, thoracolumbar or lumbosacral junction. Sacralization of the fifth lumbar vertebra and lumbarization of the first sacral segment are classic examples. For instance, in the former condition **(Fig. 7.62)**, L5 is found fused with sacrum either partially or completely, altering mechanics of the region, likely causing lumbar back pain (association with back pain is still debatable). Treatment mostly is conservative only.

TREATMENT

Since back pain can result from a diverse category of causes, no single management approach can suffice treatment in all cases. Rather, investigative and management approach **(Flow chart 7.1)** should be tailored on individual basis depending on suspected cause.

Bed rest should be limited to 1–3 days. Patients should be advised to use firm mattresses for sleeping. Paracetamol and tramadol can be used as preferred analgesics and even NSAIDs (oral or transdermal patches) can be safely administered for a short duration of 4–6 weeks. Muscle relaxants can be added for

SCOLIOSIS

INTRODUCTION

Scoliosis refers to deviation of the normal vertical line of the spine that when measured on a radiograph is deviated for more than 10° **(Fig. 7.63)**.

Flow chart 7.1: Algorithmic approach to low backache

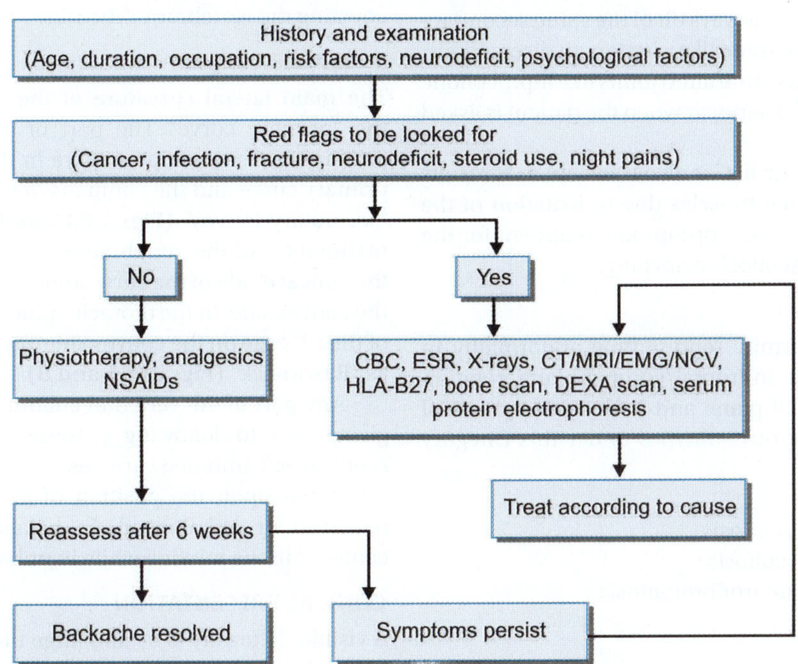

Abbreviations: CBC, complete blood count; ESR, erythrocyte sedimentation rate; CT, computed tomography; MRI, magnetic resonance imaging; EMG, electromyogram; NCV, nerve conduction velocity; HLA-B27, human leukocyte antigen B27; NSAIDs, nonsteroidal anti-inflammatory drugs; DEXA, dual-energy X-ray absorptiometry.
Source: By courtesy of Vikram A Londhey.

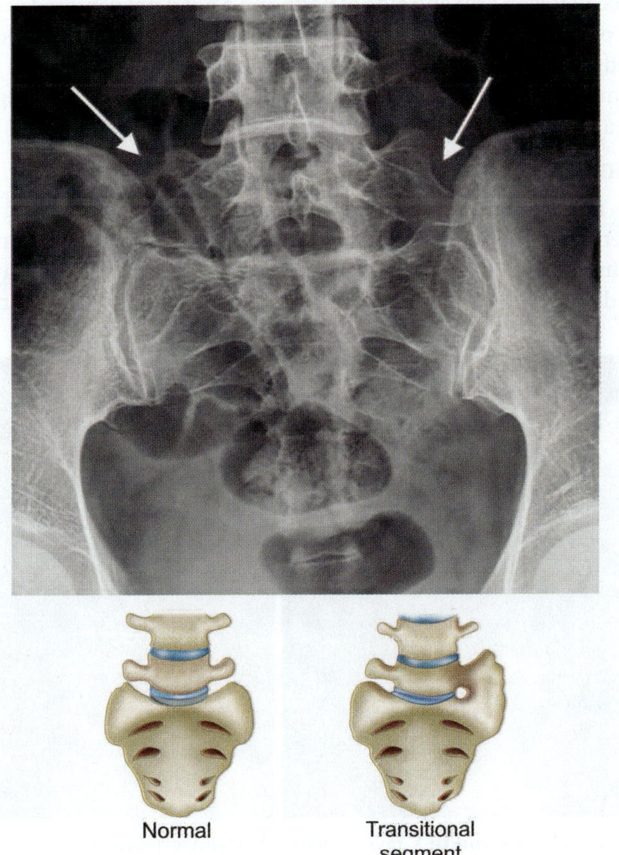

Fig. 7.62: X-ray showing sacralization of fifth lumbar vertebra (arrows)

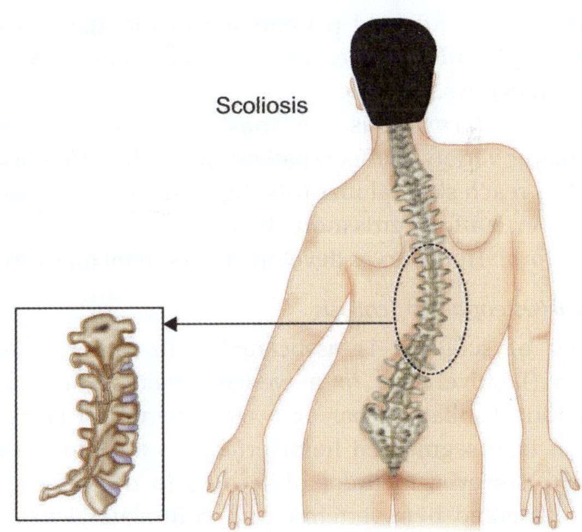

Fig. 7.63: Diagrammatic depiction of scoliosis

CLASSIFICATION OF SCOLIOSIS

It can be either nonstructural (mostly transient) or structural (permanent and fixed) deformity.

Nonstructural

This type includes postural scoliosis and compensatory scoliosis.

Postural Scoliosis

This is the most common nonstructural variety of scoliosis. The curves in postural scoliosis generally disappear when the patient bends forward while in the structural variety on forward bending the tilt becomes more prominent (Adam's Test).

Compensatory Scoliosis

In this type there is a transient sideways tilt of the spine secondary to some conditions outside the spine like a leg length discrepancy, a tilted fixed pelvis or a contracture around joints like hip. Scoliotic curve in these patients would disappear when the patient is asked to sit.

A "sciatic scoliosis or sciatic list" is also transient as it results due to spasm of the paraspinal muscles due to irritation of the nerve roots by the prolapsed disk. Appropriate treatment for the disk prolapse eliminates the scoliotic deformity.

Structural/Fixed Scoliosis

This type is a complex deformity representing abnormality in three planes—lateral bending in frontal/coronal plane, rotation of vertebral body around axial plane and lordosis of the spinal column in sagittal plane. Various subtypes under this category include:
- Idiopathic scoliosis
- Congenital (osteopathic) scoliosis
- Neuropathic/myopathic scoliosis
- Scoliosis associated with neurofibromatosis.

Idiopathic Scoliosis

This is overall the most common variety (almost 80% cases of scoliosis). It is further subdivided as follows:
- *Infantile form*: It affects children in 0–3 years of age group. Left-sided curves are more common. It affects boys more than girls.
- *Juvenile form*: Affected patients are in the age group 3–10 years. Right-sided curves are more common. Affects girls more than boys.
- *Adolescent form*: It is the most common amongst the idiopathic variety. It affects patients more than 10 years of age till they reach skeletal maturity. Right-sided curves are more common. It affects girls more than boys.
- *Adult form*: Here curves develop after skeletal maturity.

Congenital (Osteopathic) Scoliosis

This kind of scoliosis is associated with either defects of formation (hemivertebra or a wedge vertebra) or defects of segmentation (unilateral bar or a block vertebra) **(Figs 7.64A and B)**. A fully segmented hemivertebra is the most common pathology. However, in order of severity in descending order, a fully segmented hemivertebra with contralateral bar causes the maximum deformity followed by a unilateral bar, and then a fully segmented hemivertebra. Progression of the deformity is minimum with a block vertebra as it has lowest growth potential.

Neuropathic/Myopathic Scoliosis

Scoliosis may be associated with neuromuscular conditions like poliomyelitis (the most common cause in India), cerebral palsy, syringomyelia, etc. which cause an unbalanced trunk muscle paralysis. The curve in these patients is long C-shaped with the convex side towards the weaker muscles.

Scoliosis Associated with Neurofibromatosis

Almost one-third patients with neurofibromatosis tend to have some degree of scoliosis. The curves in these patients are classically short and sharp and are due to bony dystrophy affecting the vertebrae or the ribs.

SCOLIOTIC CURVES

The main lateral curvature of the spine to one side is called the "primary curve". The part of spine above and below the primary curve develops a curve in the direction opposite to the primary curve and the compensatory curves being referred to as "secondary curves" **(Figs 7.65A and B)**. The prime problem is malrotation of the vertebrae with spinous processes tilting into the concave side of the curve and transverse processes occupying the convex side. In the thoracic spine this leads to the prominence of the rib cage on the convex side, giving rise to a rib hump called as "Razorback" **(Figs 7.66A and B)**.

Any part of the vertebral column can be affected commonly giving rise to following patterns—thoracic scoliosis, lumbar scoliosis or combined varieties.

Based upon the position of the head, the curves may be balanced or unbalanced. In balanced curves the occiput is centered in the midline while in unbalanced curves it is not.

CLINICAL PRESENTATION

A visible deformity is by and large the most common complaint, otherwise most patients tend to be asymptomatic. Back pain is generally there in long-standing cases only.

On examining, these patients one may observe an asymmetry of shoulders, unequal scapular prominence (more on convex side), elevated or prominent hip (on the concave side), increased space between arm and side of body and a head not centered over the pelvis **(Fig. 7.67)**. All these findings can be used to screen children for the condition. In deformities that have progressed to advanced levels, one may detect a neurological deficit, although it is a relatively uncommon presentation.

DIAGNOSIS

For a thorough assessment of the deformity a full length anteroposterior (AP) view of spine **(Fig. 7.65B)** in standing and supine positions along with a lateral view is obtained. Sideways bending of the vertebral column can be clearly appreciated and

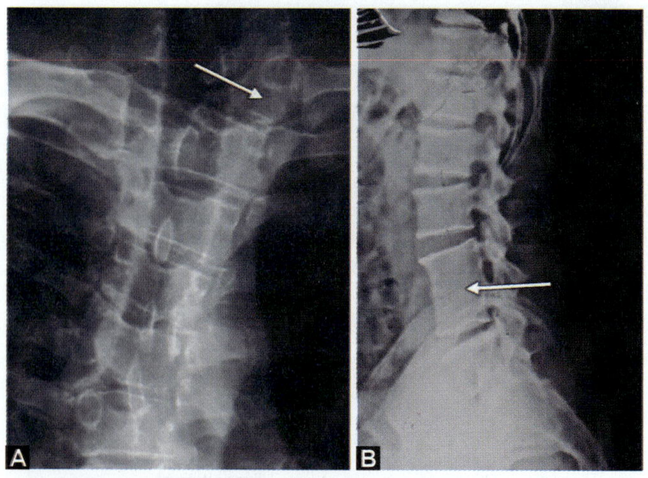

Figs 7.64A and B: X-rays showing (A) Hemivertebra (arrow); and (B) Block vertebra (arrow)

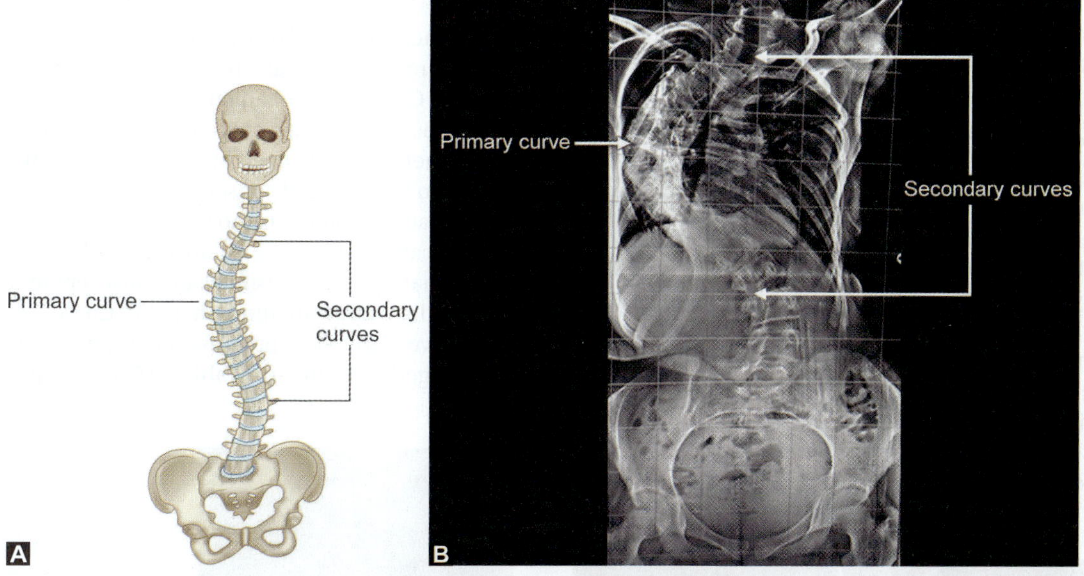

Figs 7.65A and B: Scoliotic curves

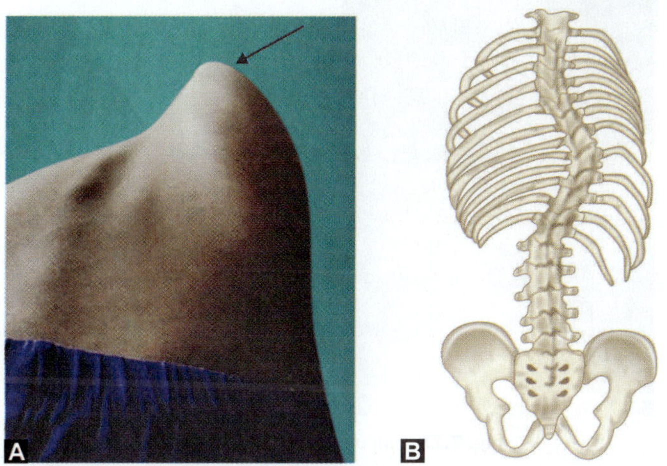

Figs 7.66A and B: Rib hump (arrow)

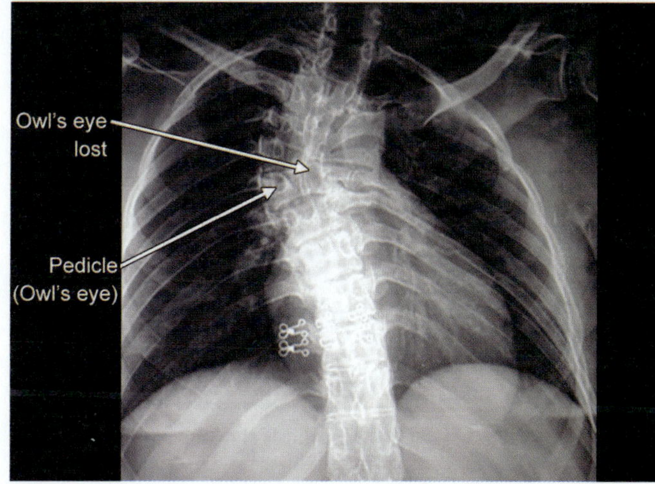

Fig. 7.68: X-ray of scoliotic spine showing loss of owl's eye appearance

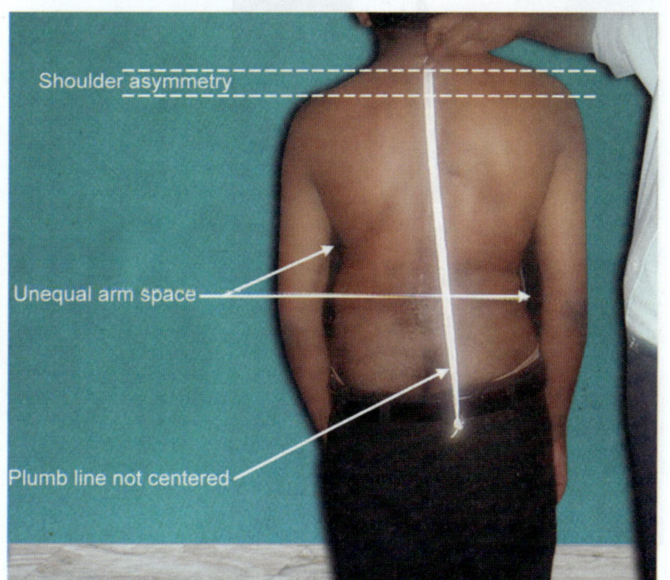

Fig. 7.67: Clinical findings on examination in scoliosis

the primary as well as the secondary curves can be documented. Abnormal rotation of the vertebrae can be appreciated by identifying the spinous processes and the pedicles. The spinous processes shift to one side and the pedicles of two sides loose the normal classical owl's eye appearance **(Fig. 7.68)**. In congenital scoliosis one may find a vertebral anomaly **(Figs 7.64A and B)**.

A lateral view in idiopathic scoliosis generally shows lordosis of the affected part **(Fig. 7.69)** and traction or bending X-rays **(Figs 7.70A and B)** are needed to see if the deformity is correctable or fixed.

Grading the Severity

The full length AP radiographs are used. The vertebra exactly in the middle of the primary curve is called the "Apical vertebra". To assess the severity, vertebrae at the upper and lower ends of the primary curve are identified. A line is drawn along the superior margin of the topmost vertebra and another line is drawn along the lower margin of the bottom vertebra. The two lines are allowed to meet to form an angle called as "the Cobb's angle" **(Fig. 7.71)**. The greater angle, the more severe the deformity is.

Vertebral rotation can be estimated by placing special calibrated instruments on radiographs called as "torsionometers (Perdriolle method)". Else a computed tomography (CT) scan is a more sensitive method.

Predicting Progression of the Deformity

Scoliotic curves tend to worsen up with skeletal growth. A clinical way of estimating progression is by using the Tanner's index (based on assessment of breasts and genitalia) as the growth potentially slows down after skeletal maturity. A radiological assessment can be made by observing the appearance of iliac apophysis on a pelvis AP X-ray. If the iliac apophysis has fused with the iliac bone, it indicates completion of the growth and hence no likelihood of curve worsening any further. This is called as "Risser's sign". Five grades of the sign are described that start with the appearance of iliac apophysis till it fuses with the iliac bone (**Figs 7.72A and B**). Lesser the Risser's grade, more are the chances of progression.

MANAGEMENT

Management is guided by the type of scoliosis.

Postural curves can be well managed by conservative methods. Curves in congenital scoliosis, myopathic scoliosis and scoliosis associated with neurofibromatosis tend to progress very fast and hence mostly need operative management. Only milder curves can be managed conservatively.

Idiopathic scoliosis is mostly treated by conservative means. The indications to operate are cases where the deformity is greater than 30° and cosmetically unacceptable to the patient or when the curves are more than 45°. Curves in young patients which have high risk of progression (as per Risser's grading) also are managed with surgery (**Table 7.15** for synopsis of treatment).

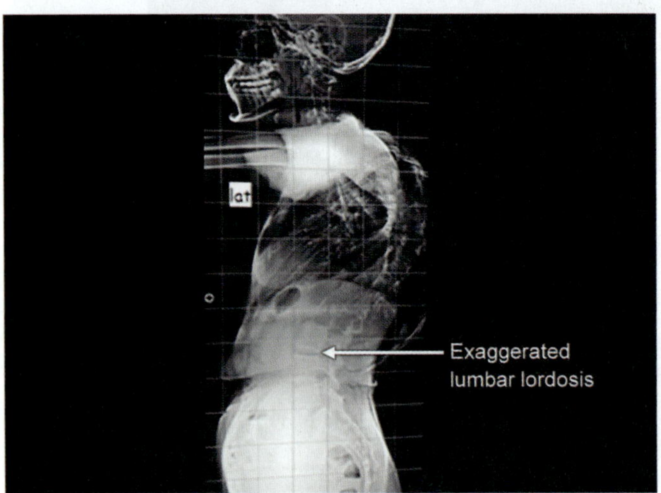

Fig. 7.69: Lateral film of scoliosis showing lordosis

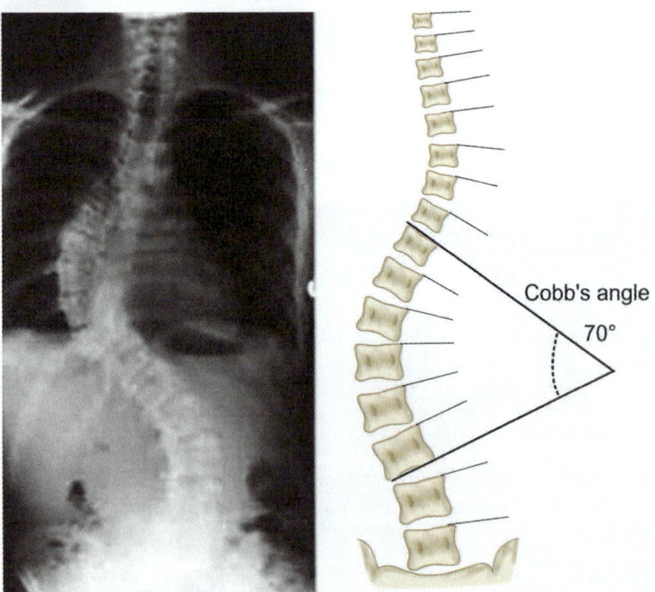

Fig. 7.71: Calculation of Cobb's angle

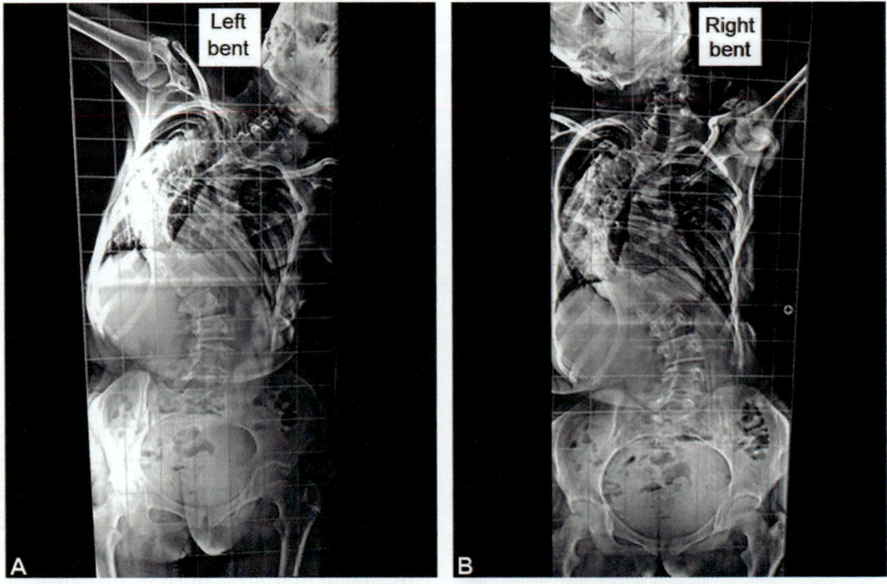

Figs 7.70A and B: Bent films in patient with scoliosis

Conservative Treatment

This involves physiotherapy to tone up the spinal and trunk muscles and thereby strengthen the spinal support and use spinal braces to prevent progression and hasten correction of the deformity.

- *Braces*: Thoracolumbar spinal orthoses (TLSOAs) **(Figs 7.73A to C)** are mostly used. They are useful only when the apex of deformity is below T7 vertebra. Patient's compliance is very important as brace wear time is 20 hours/day. Some commonly used braces are as follows:
    - *Milwaukee brace (named after the city where it was designed):* Only brace that can be used with a higher apex.
    - *Boston brace (most commonly used):* Cosmetically more acceptable. It is made from a negative mold of a patient's X-ray.
    - *Reisser's turn buckle cast:* Body cast with a buckle fitted on the concave side. Turning the buckle stretches the concave side.
    - *Charleston's night time bending brace:* To be worn only during the night time.
    - *Minerva jacket* **(Figs 7.74A and B):** Old method for correction with casting.

Contraindications to brace wear: These are only prescribed in idiopathic varieties. Congenital and neuromuscular scoliosis can worsen while waiting to see the result of brace treatment.

Operative Treatment

The surgery for scoliosis involves correction of the deformity by some forms of instrumentation and then fusion of the spine in

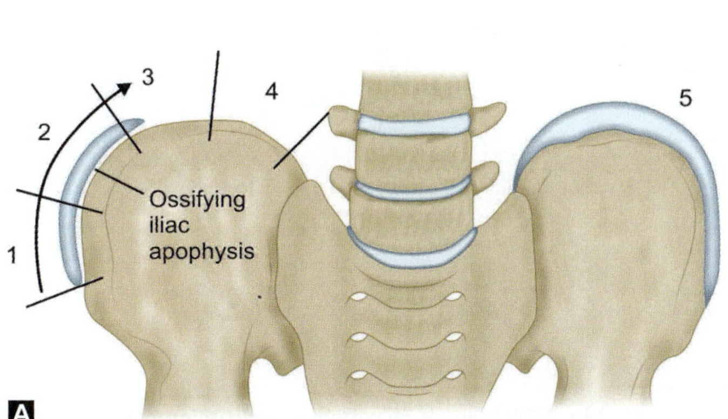

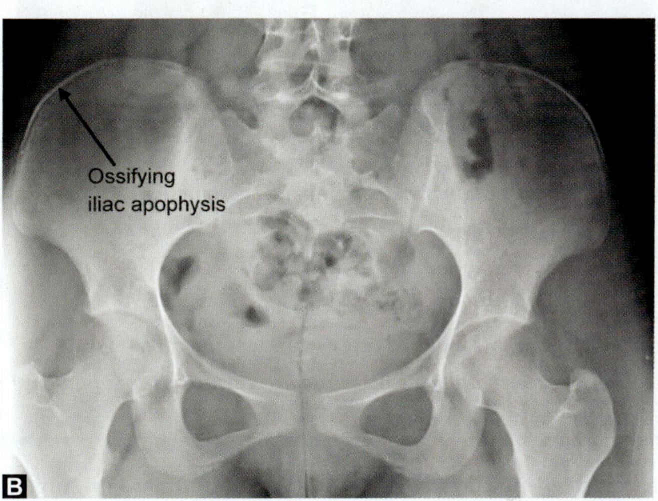

Figs 7.72A and B: (A) Pictorial representation; and (B) X-ray pelvis with both hips anteroposterior views showing ossifying iliac apophysis

Table 7.15: Management of idiopathic scoliosis

Curve magnitude (degrees)	Risser's grade 0/Premenarchal	Risser's grade 1/2	Risser's grade 3, 4, 5
<25	Observation	Observation	Observation
25–45	Brace	Brace	Observation
>45	Surgery	Surgery	Surgery (>50°)

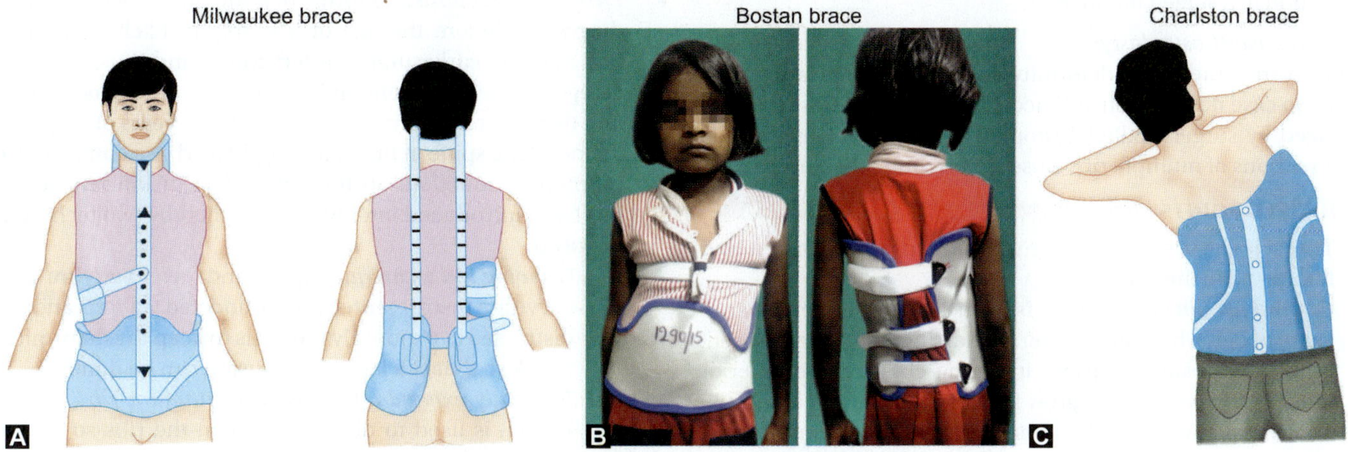

Figs 7.73A to C: Thoracolumbar spinal orthoses used in scoliosis

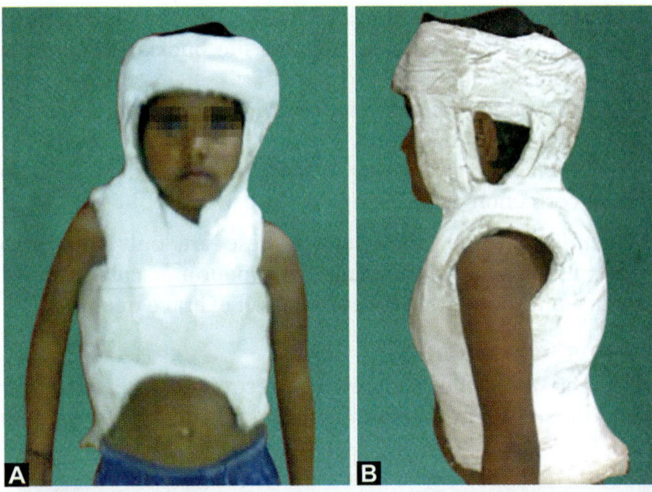

Figs 7.74A and B: Minerva jacket

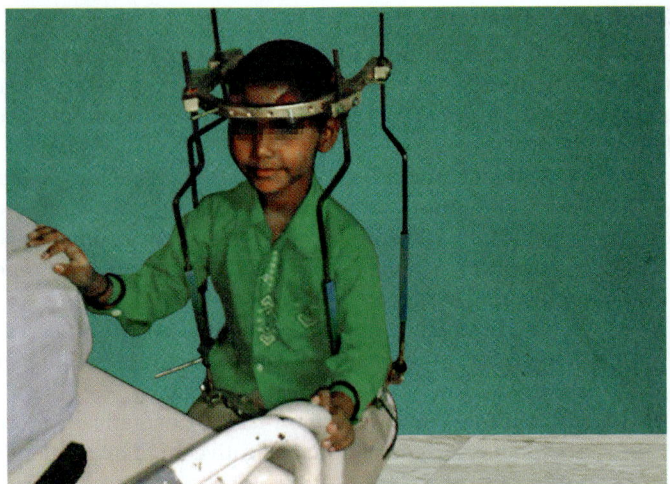

Fig. 7.75: Halo-pelvic distraction system

> **Box 7.3:** Various forms of instrumentation used for spinal fixation in scoliosis
>
> *Posterior instrumentation methods (applied via a posterior approach)*
> - Hartshill rectangles
> - Harrington rod system
> - Luque rods and sublaminar wire fixation
> - Pedicle screws (modern day preferred instrumentation)
>
> *Anterior instrumentation methods (applied via an anterior approach)*
> - Dwyer Zielke instrumentation

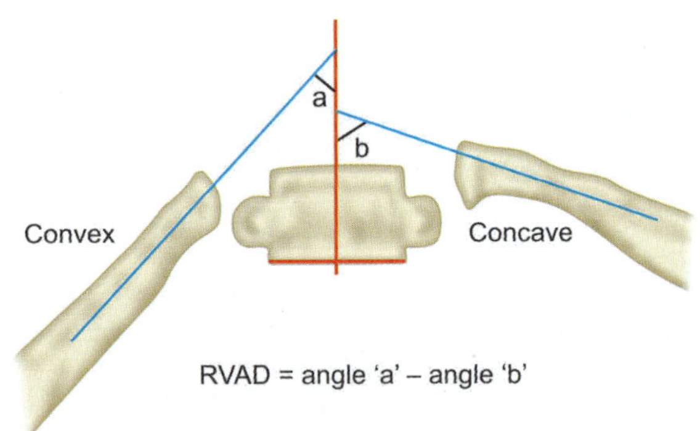

Fig. 7.76: Mehta's rib vertebral angle difference

the corrected position by means of bone grafting. For surgery the spine can be approached from either posterior aspect (more preferred and more surgeon friendly) or anterior aspect (via the transthoracic or transabdominal route). Once approached some forms of instrumentation **(Box 7.3)** can be applied to distract the spine and to bring it in a corrected position for fusion.

Note: In case deformity is very severe to be corrected on the table, then preoperatively the spine can be stretched to lessen the deformity by using the Halo-pelvic distraction system **(Fig. 7.75)** or a halo femoral traction and thereafter fused after adequate distraction in a staged manner.

Thoracoplasty/Costoplasty: The surgical methods discussed earlier correct the spinal deformity, but may not alleviate the rib hump. In case it is cosmetically acceptable, then the same can be managed by surgery called costoplasty which involves excising short sections of multiple ribs close to vertebral articulation.

HIGH-YIELD POINTS

- Thoracic curves have maximum propensity to worsen and lumber have the least.
- *Crankshaft phenomenon:* It is seen in children less than 8 years of age when only posterior Harrington system is used. With only posterior fusion, in young children the anterior body would continue to grow leading to increased deformity known as crankshaft phenomenon. It is not seen nowadays due to use of the pedicle screw system that fixes all the three columns of the vertebra.

- *Mehta's rib vertebral angle difference* **(Fig. 7.76)**: This is a trustable method of predicting curve progression in infantile idiopathic scoliosis. It is an angle between the end plate of vertebra at the apex of the curve and ribs attached to it on either side of the curve. A difference more than 20° is linked to high chance of curve progression. Difference less than 20° indicates likelihood of spontaneous recovery.
- *Early onset scoliosis:* All forms of structural scoliosis that are diagnosed before the age of 5 years are likely to progress and need an early surgical intervention and thus, fall in this category. The management in such cases differs as the lungs and thoracic cavity are not developed till 5 years of age and so fusion of the spine at this stage would lead to a compromised pulmonary function. So the concept of fusion-less surgery has been introduced into this group whereby two techniques are used:
  - *Growing rod technique:* Upper and lower vertebra of the curve are instrumented and connected via rods and then distracted at 6 monthly intervals to keep the deformity in check so that at a later stage, fusion can be done.
  - *Vertically expandable prosthetic titanium rib (VEPTR):* VEPTR is used to distract between the ribs so that the chest and spine keep growing till the age lungs get mature and allow a fusion.

INTRODUCTION

Kyphosis refers to excessive forward bending of the vertebral column. Normally also the thoracic vertebral column has a forward bend around 20–45°. When the bend is exaggerated the deformity appears at the back **(Fig. 7.77)**.

Some common terms used for description of deformity are:
- *Knuckle kyphus*: Involving one vertebra
- *Angular kyphus*: Involving two to three vertebrae
- *Rounded kyphus*: Involving more than three vertebrae.
  (Note: Gibbus is an old term not used these days more or less equivalent to angular kyphus).

TYPES OF KYPHOSIS

Nonstructural Kyphosis (Correctable)

Postural kyphosis is a non-progressive condition that is due to flexibility of spine in adolescents. It appears when the child stands and resolves in supine position. It is a self-limiting condition with no vertebral abnormality and postural training and exercises are all that is required.

Compensatory kyphosis occurs in compensation to some other deformity in the spine, usually increased lumbar lordosis.

Structural Kyphosis (Noncorrectable)

In contrast to nonstructural kyphosis, structural kyphosis is associated with vertebral structural abnormality.

Different conditions that lead to structured or fixed kyphosis in different age groups:
- *In infants and children*: Congenital kyphosis is due to either failure of formation defect or failure of segmentation defect of vertebrae. Failure of formation defect may present at birth as kyphotic deformity and worsen with growth. Failure of segmentation defect is slow to grow and usually become apparent when the child starts walking. For progressive deformity fusion of deformed vertebrae may be required. Braces have no role in congenital kyphosis. Skeletal dysplasia like spondyloepiphyseal dysplasia congenita, spondylometaphyseal dysplasia, Morquio's disease, pseudoachondroplasia, etc.
- *In adolescents*: Scheuermann's disease (see later) is the most common cause of fixed kyphosis in adolescents. Tuberculosis can also lead to the problem.
- *In adults*: Traumatic kyphosis (due to spinal trauma), tuberculosis and ankylosing spondylitis are common causes in this group. Traumatic kyphosis mainly involves the thoracolumbar or lumbar regions and usually associated with paraplegia.
- *Elderly*: Osteoporosis resulting in multiple compression factors is the main culprit for kyphosis in the elderly although, metastatic vertebral tumors or TB spine can be other causes leading to vertebral collapse.

SCHEUERMANN'S DISEASE (ADOLESCENT IDIOPATHIC KYPHOSIS)

Scheuermann described this disease in 1920 as juvenile dorsal kyphosis. The exact etiology of Scheuermann's disease is not clear. Radiological findings suggest it to be osteochondritis of the ring epiphyses of the vertebra. Defective endochondral ossification in the vertebral end plates is also a consistent pathological finding. After idiopathic scoliosis, it is the second most common spinal deformity.

Clinical Presentation

It affects adolescents (usually between 13 years and 17 years of age). Painless kyphotic deformity of the thoracic spine (apex between D7 and D9) is the most common presenting symptom **(Fig. 7.78A)**. Back pain may be there with a tendency to aggravate on exertion. Compensatory lumbar and cervical lordosis, cutaneous pigmentation at the apex of deformity due to continuous friction on the back of the chair are other associated signs, flexion contractures of hip and shoulder joints and hamstring spasm are the other common findings. It mainly involves the thoracic spine but can also affect thoracolumbar and lumbar regions. Lumbar Scheuermann's disease does not produce typical kyphosis but have similar radiological changes. Neurological deficits are rare.

X-ray findings **(Fig. 7.78B)**: Sorenson criteria are used to diagnose Scheuermann's kyphosis.
- Anterior wedging of more than 5° of three consecutive adjacent vertebrae at the apex of deformity.
- Irregular vertebral apophyseal lines.
- Presence of Schmorl nodes
- Narrowing of intervertebral disk spaces.

Differential Diagnosis

Condition has to be differentiated from other causes of kyphosis in this age group.

Treatment

Natural history is benign. So majority of patients are managed conservatively.

Conservative Management
- Postural training and back exercises.
- Serial cast treatment
- *Brace therapy*: Only brace available is a Milwaukee brace.

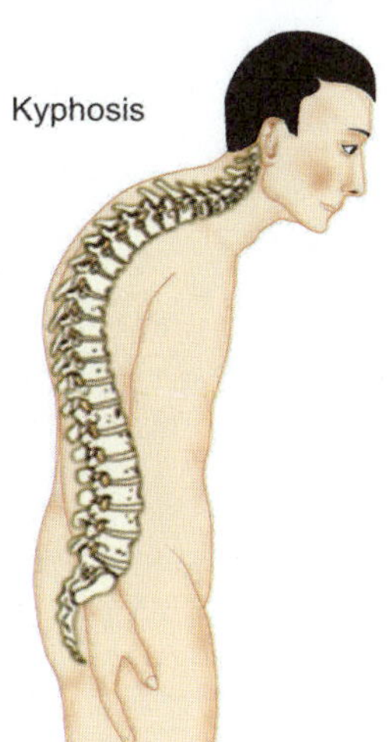

Fig. 7.77: Diagrammatic representation of kyphosis

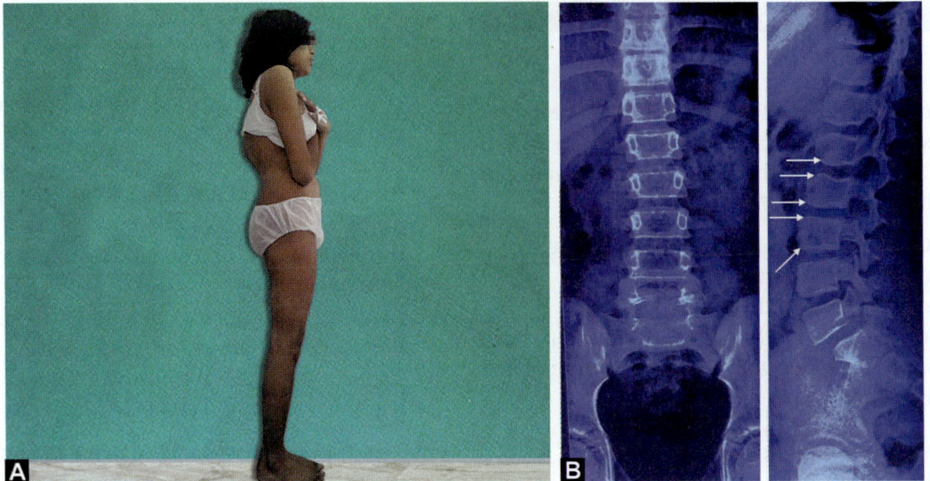

Figs 7.78A and B: (A) Clinical presentation (thoracic kyphosis) in a young patient with Scheuermann's disease; and (B) X-ray lateral view of dorsal spine showing irregular vertebral end plates with anterior wedging of vertebrae (arrows)

Surgery

It is reserved for patients with pain, a rigid deformity, a curve of more than 70–75° and an unacceptable cosmetic appearance. Anterior release and fusion followed by posterior instrumentation and fusion is the accepted standard of care. *Rule of thumb*: Never correct more than 50% of the deformity as it can cause neurological deficits.

HIGH-YIELD POINTS

- Osteoporotic fractures of the vertebrae are the most common causes of kyphosis in adults.
- Scheuermann's disease is the most common form of fixed kyphosis in adolescents.

Peripheral Nerve Injuries

PERIPHERAL NERVE INJURY: ANATOMY, CLASSIFICATION AND DIAGNOSIS

GROSS ANATOMY

Four different regions of spinal cord namely the cervical, thoracic, lumbar and sacral are organized into segments. Each segment gives rise to one pair of spinal nerve. Spinal nerves are mixed nerves, arising one on each side of the cord in pairs (total being 31 pairs). Each spinal nerve is formed by convergence of dorsal (sensory) and ventral (motor) roots **(Fig. 8.1A)**. Now for supplying the trunk, these spinal nerves divide into ventral and dorsal rami, which further subdivide into motor and sensory branches, which finally supply the targeted trunk areas. However, the supply to limbs is very different and peculiar. For the upper limb, the spinal nerves C5-T1 join in front of the scapula and form the brachial plexus (cf. lumbosacral plexus for lower limb). From this plexus, the nerves that sprout are the peripheral nerves (viz. median, ulnar, radial, etc.) **(Fig. 8.1B)** again each being a mixed nerve. So, these peripheral nerves are basically distributing the fibers of spinal nerves to the skin and musculature of the limb. By the same token, one can well imagine that one peripheral nerve may contain fibers from several spinal nerves or the fibers of single spinal nerve may get divided amongst several peripheral nerves.

MICROSCOPIC ANATOMY (FIG. 8.2)

Nerve fibers can be myelinated or unmyelinated. In the peripheral nervous system, the Schwann cells form a multilaminated myelin sheath around the myelinated nerve fibers. Each nerve fiber is enclosed by endoneurium. A few nerve fibers together make a fascicle, which is enclosed by perineurium. All fascicles of a nerve are bundled by epineurium to make a nerve. Myelin sheath is an insulating membrane and interrupted by nodal gaps or nodes of Ranvier where myelin sheath is deficient. Nodal gaps are rich in ion channels and action potential jumps from one node to another node of Ranvier (saltatory conduction) during nerve conduction. Vessels supplying nerves are called vasa nervorum. These are tiny vessels running in the loose connective tissues, mesoneurium surrounding the nerves. Mesoneurium also helps in gliding of nerves during joint motion.

NEURONAL DEGENERATION AND REGENERATION

When an axon is detached from its cell body degeneration begins in both the distal (Wallerian degeneration) and the proximal (Retrograde degeneration) segments. However, detached axon remains excitable and can transmit nerve signal for several days following injury. Depending upon the site of injury (proximity to cell body) and severity of injury degeneration in the proximal

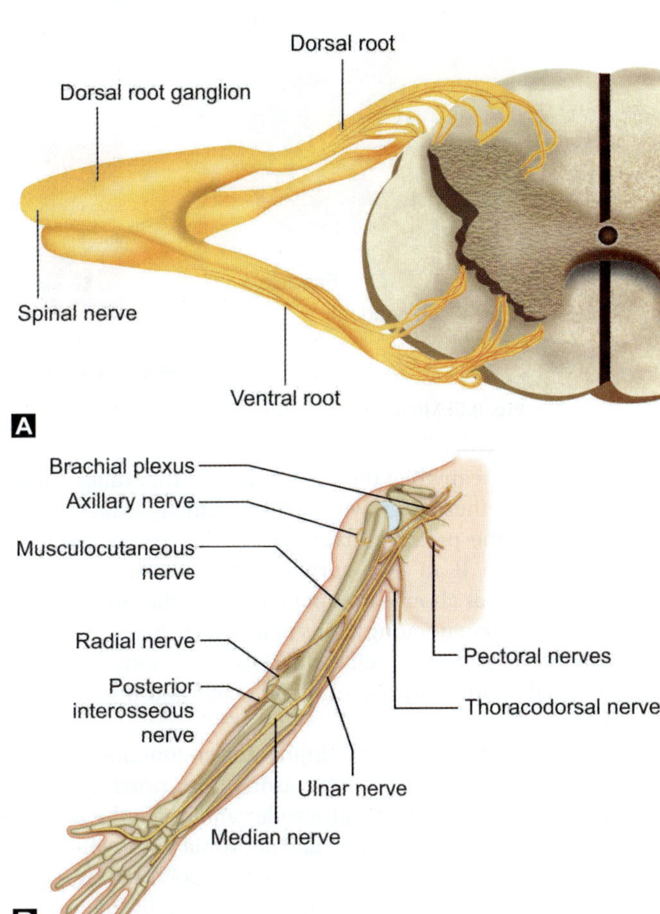

Figs 8.1A and B: Spinal nerve diagrammatic depiction and the peripheral nerves of upper limb

segment can be minimal and limited to next node of Ranvier or extensive involving the entire segment up to the cell body. Approximately 72 hours after nerve injury calcium influx initiates cytoskeletal degradation of axon by activating a protease calpain. Axonal disintegration is also accompanied by increase in astrocytes, macrophages and Schwann cells to clear axonal debris and help regenerative attempts by the proximal axon. The axon's neurilemma (the outermost layer of Schwann cells) does not degenerate and remains as a hollow tube encircling the debris. Between 4 and 30 days macrophages clear the axonal and myelin debris. Wallerian degeneration is also seen in several degenerative neurological diseases like Parkinson's disease, Alzheimer's disease and amyotrophic lateral sclerosis.

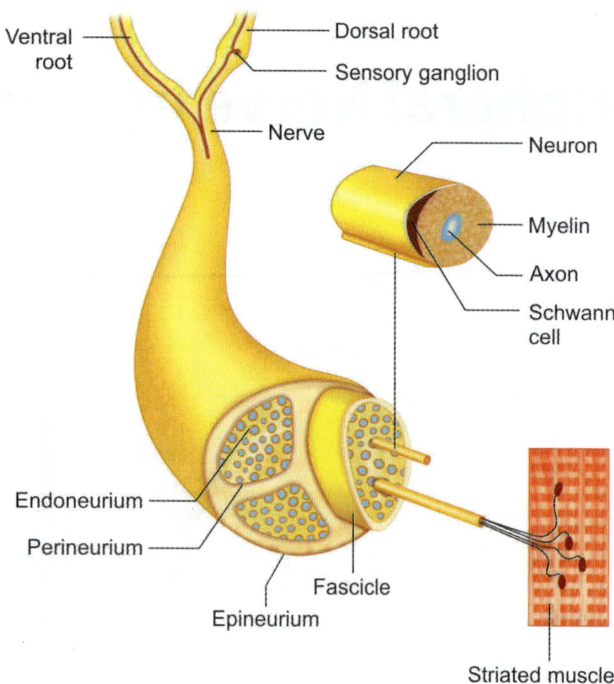

Fig. 8.2: Microscopic anatomy of a nerve

After injury meanwhile the Schwann cells that make up the hollow tube, synthesize growth factors, which attract axonal sprouting from the proximal axon stump that try to reach the distal axon stump. If an axon sprout reaches the tube, it grows into it and advances about 1 mm per day. The tubes thus provide pathways for the regenerating axons to follow to their innervation of muscles and skin. The Schwann cells then remyelinate the newly formed axons, which eventually reach and innervate the target tissue.

In some severe cases of nerve injury, the endoneural tube also gets damaged. Then the sprouting axons from proximal stump fail to enter the guiding tube and wander aimless in the adjacent tissues and form an end neuroma. End neuroma forms when there is complete cut of the peripheral nerve with widely separated ends while a partial cut with a similar situation ends up in "neuroma in continuity". Full functional return would not be possible in these situations. As the reinnervation proceeds, the muscles nearest to the site of injury are reinnervated first, followed by others. This phenomenon of reinnervation of muscles from proximal to distal is referred to as motor march, and is an evidence of recovery.

Tinel's sign (Hoffman's sign): When regenerating axonal sprouts progress along the endoneurial tubes, slight percussion along the course of the injured nerve produces sensation of tingling along the cutaneous distribution of the nerve. Tingling sensation is hardly perceived at the site of percussion and radiates, and felt only distally along the course of the nerve. A positive Tinel's sign indicates axonal regeneration. With progressive regeneration, Tinel's sign moves distally and it is a favorable sign. Presence of Tinel's sign indicates sensory recovery (cutaneous distribution) and with progressive axonal regeneration, Tinel's sign fades proximally and moves distally.

MECHANISMS OF NERVE INJURIES

Although the most common cause of nerve injuries remain fracture dislocations, a number of other mechanisms may be involved which include a cut/laceration, crushing, thermal injury (frost bite/electrical shock), ischemia to nerve (*see* Volkmann's ischemia), radiation exposure and iatrogenic causes such as accidental drug injections into the nerves.

CLASSIFICATION OF NERVE INJURIES

Seddon's Classification (1943)

Neurapraxia

It designates a situation where transmission of impulses is physiologically interrupted for a time but there is no cut in the nerve (generally, only compression of the nerve is there). Recovery is complete in a few days or maximum by 6 weeks and no Wallerian degeneration occurs. Recovery is complete all at once and all groups of muscles recover at the same time so no motor march or no advancing Tinel's sign are seen.

Axonotmesis

It designates more significant injury with damage to the axon but with preservation of the Schwann cell and endoneurial tubes. Distal Wallerian degeneration is present and spontaneous regeneration (motor march and progressive Tinel's sign) occurs with reasonably good functional recovery.

Neurotmesis

It is a more severe injury with complete anatomical severance of the nerve. The axon, the Schwann cell and endoneurial tubes are completely disrupted. The perineurium and epineurium also are disrupted to varying degrees. Significant spontaneous recovery cannot be expected unless nerve is surgically repaired.

Sunderland Classification

In 1951, Sunderland expanded Seddon's classification to five degrees of peripheral nerve injuries (PNIs):

First degree (Class I): Same as Seddon's neurapraxia.

Second degree (Class II): Same as Seddon's axonotmesis.

Third degree (Class II): The endoneurium is disrupted but the perineurium and epineurium remain intact. Chances of recovery are fair but surgical intervention may be required.

Fourth degree (Class II): In fourth-degree injury, perineurium is also disrupted and only the epineurium remains intact. In this case, surgical repair is required.

Fifth degree (Class III): This refers to complete transection of the nerve. Recovery is not possible without surgical intervention.

High versus Low Nerve Palsy

By convention, the major nerve injuries of upper limb are divided into high and low types depending on whether the injury site is proximal to elbow (high injury) or distal to elbow (low injury).

DIAGNOSIS OF A NERVE INJURY

A thorough history and a meticulous examination forms the cornerstone of making diagnosis of any nerve injury and localizing the site of affection.

Examination in a Case of Nerve Injury

Look (observing the attitude of the limb): The moment patient enters the room, observing the specific attitude of the limb or a specific gait (wrist drop in radial nerve palsy or high stepping gait in common peroneal nerve palsy) may suggest diagnosis. Wasting of the innervated muscles is evident in long-standing cases of nerve injury that provide clue to diagnosis.

Feel (sensory examination): For performing a thorough sensory examination, one needs to confront with the concept of maximal, submaximal and autonomous zones. Every nerve supplies a large area of skin often overlapped by adjacent nerves, referred to as its maximal zone while the area that is exclusively supplied by each nerve is called its autonomic zone **(Fig. 8.3)**. Interruption of a nerve causes complete insensibility in the autonomic zone while only a decreased sensibility in the maximal zone.

Move (motor examination including reflexes): Functional tests are described for all nerves, which basically work on the same underlying principle, i.e. making the innervated muscle contract and preferably testing it against resistance to grade strength.

Checking for reflexes: Since injury to a nerve is a lower motor neuron type of lesion, the reflexes are absent in the area of nerve distribution.

Examination of autonomic function: The sympathetic nerve fibers are generally considered to be the most resistant. They can be tested by the conventional sweat test (iodine starch test). An intact sympathetic function may reassure the surgeon that the injury to the nerve is not complete.

SPECIAL INVESTIGATIONS

Electrodiagnostic Studies

These are sequential studies, complementary to each other, performed in cases with a PNI that provide the clinician with a base of knowledge as follows:

1. Confirmation of diagnosis
2. Locating the site of injury
3. Estimating the extent of injury
4. Determining chances of recovery
5. Documenting recovery, if any
6. Selection of suitable donor nerves for reconstruction of lost function.

Electrodiagnostic studies (EDS) include the following:

Nerve Conduction Studies

Stimulation of a peripheral nerve by an electrode placed on the skin overlying the nerve readily evokes a response from the muscle innervated by that nerve. This response can be picked up either from surface electrode placed into the innervated muscle or even from a distant area of the nerve trunk itself. The measurements that are of interest include the latency, the amplitude and the conduction velocity. Latency is the time (in milliseconds) taken by the impulse to reach the muscle and amplitude is the magnitude of response obtained from the muscle stimulated, measured in millivolts. The velocity of conduction can also be calculated by estimating the distance between the measuring electrodes and noting the time taken by impulse to travel the distance.

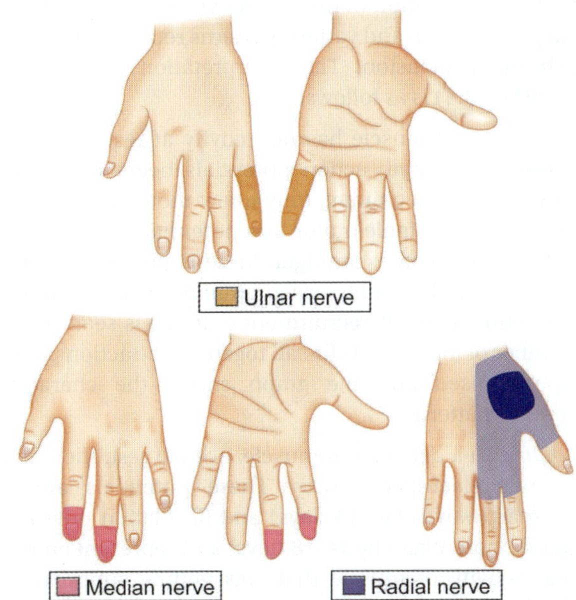

Fig. 8.3: Autonomic zones of major peripheral nerves of upper limb

When a sensory nerve is stimulated at the skin surface action potential recorded distally (antidromic response) are called sensory nerve action potential (SNAP). SNAP can also be recorded proximally (orthodromic response) with a stimulus applied distally. Stimulation of a motor or a mixed nerve generates compound muscle action potential (CMAP) amplitude of which is directly proportional to the number of motor units stimulated, e.g. the amplitude of the compound muscle action potential will be reduced by 50% compared to normal side if 50% of the nerve fibers are cut.

Interpretation of nerve conduction studies: Within first few days (7–10 days) after nerve transaction, stimulation distal to the site of injury may evoke normal response, as the distal axonal fragment remains electrically excitable. So, despite severe nerve injury proximally, normal response may be recorded. One can have an idea of site of injury as both sensory and motor responses will be absent in case the stimulation is done proximal to the site of injury. After 10–12 days, in axonotmesis/neurotmesis, due to Wallerian degeneration the distal axon will degenerate. Hence, there will be no sensory and motor response on stimulation distal to injury site. However, in neurapraxia (focal demyelination of the nerve) distal responses will be preserved because of the underlying intact axons. In neurapraxia decrease in the amplitude or conduction velocity may be noted, due to loss of, rapidly conducting large diameter myelinated axons (conduction block).

Therefore, if an acute nerve injury is suspected, best time to perform nerve conduction studies is 10–14 days after the injury as at this time the studies will reveal the severity of injury (demyelination or partial or complete cut) that can be correlated with the prognosis.

Electromyography

Electromyography (EMG) is a graphical recording of the muscle activity observed with a needle electrode placed in muscle. The test involves observation of muscle activity at rest and then with voluntary contraction and various patterns recorded are analyzed to reach the conclusion. The interpretation of the patterns observed **(Fig. 8.4)** is as follows:

Normal: A normal muscle has no activity at rest. As voluntary contraction is initiated, action potentials begin to develop in the muscle. In the beginning, only a few motor units are firing, so recordings show single motor unit potentials on the graph. As the contraction becomes stronger, there is progressive increase in the number and then increased amplitude of the motor unit action potential (MUAP, recruitment pattern) is seen. Finally, a large number of motor units fire all together, the action potentials get superimposed and the graph shows the characteristic "interference pattern".

Nerve injury: In a denervated muscle, even at rest, there is some spontaneous electrical activity. These potentials are called positive sharp waves (10–14 days) and fibrillation potentials or denervation potentials (by 14–18 days) and represent embryonic electrical activity of muscle that was getting suppressed due to inhibition by the stronger nerve action potential. At times, these fibrillations are so strong that they can be seen and are then called fasciculations. However, one must remember that these potentials develop by about 2 weeks after the injury. So, absence of these potentials by about 3 weeks would signify a good prognosis as the muscle in that case would not be denervated. In case, these potentials develop, then they last indefinitely until the muscle is reinnervated or becomes fibrotic. Analysis of MUAP morphology and recruitment pattern is the key element of needle EMG to diagnose myopathy. Small, polyphasic MUAPs (due to dysfunctional muscle fibers) is a characteristic finding of myopathy. Other commonly seen findings of myopathies in needle EMG are fibrillations and positive sharp waves, which are waxing and waning action potentials in both frequency and amplitude. Occasionally, in chronic myopathies, complex repetitive discharges (CRDs) may be seen.

Application: The clinical value of an EMG test lies in that it can determine whether the nerve injury is complete or an incomplete one. If the injury would be incomplete, there will be evidence of reinnervation that appears much before visible muscle contraction. EMG also differentiates a myopathy from a neuropathy (*see* **Fig. 8.4**). By performing an EMG of all the muscle supplied by a nerve, it is even possible to decide the possible site of injury, as only those muscles will be paralyzed, which are being supplied distal to the site of lesion.

*Strength Duration Curve **(Fig. 8.5)***

This is a graphical method of quantifying the excitable property of the nerve and the muscle under consideration and thereby quantifying the amount of recovery that has taken place.

Underlying principle: A normal muscle can be excited by a small amount of current if the stimulation reaches the muscle via the neuromuscular junction. A denervated muscle would thus need a higher strength of current.

Procedure: A low strength current is given to excite the muscle contraction, for a fixed duration for example say 300 milliseconds. The minimum current required to elicit muscle contraction is

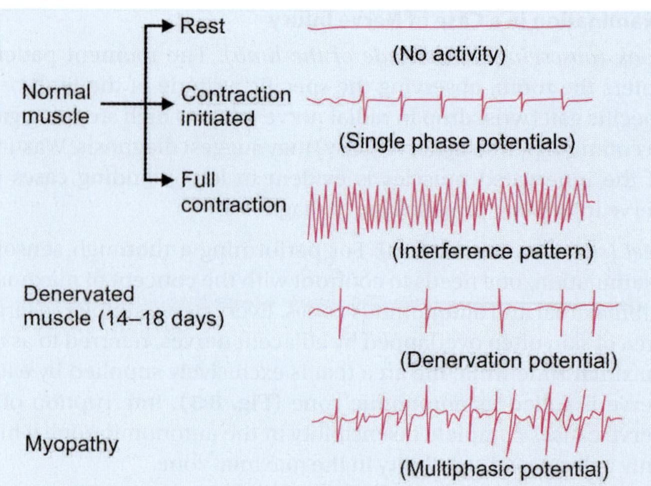

Fig. 8.4: Electromyographic record interpretation

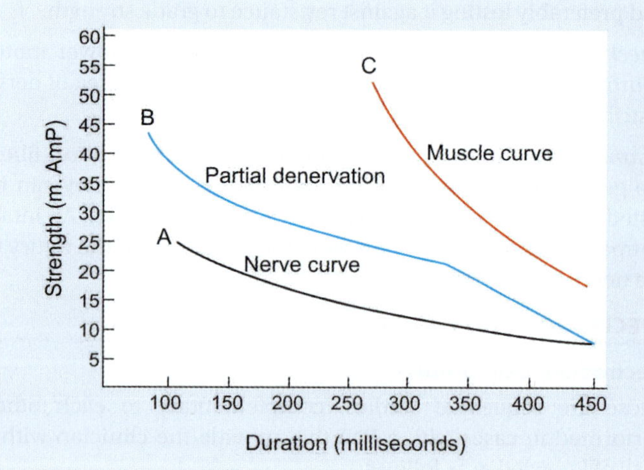

Fig. 8.5: Strength duration curve

noted and is called rheobase for that muscle. As the duration is decreased, the amount of current needed to elicit the contraction proportionally increases and the recording follows the pattern shown in curve A, in the **Figure 8.5**. Next, a double the rheobase current is given, and the time interval is gradually reduced, carefully noting the minimum time for which a double rheobase current needs to be given to elicit the muscle contraction. This minimum time period required to elicit contraction (at double rheobase current) is called chronaxie.

Interpretation: A normal pattern curve is called nerve curve (curve A). If the muscle is denervated, then for eliciting contraction, a greater amount of current would be needed at every time duration, and hence the curve would shift to right (curve C). Such a curve is called as muscle curve. In cases of partial denervation, the curve of the recovering muscle lies between the nerve and muscle curves and is characterized by a kink at some point as shown (curve B). Thus, strength duration (SD) curve can differentiate a completely and a partially denervated muscle and also quantify the rate of recovery, as with recovery, the curve will shift from right to left (curve C–curve A).

HIGH-YIELD POINTS

- Loss of SNAP indicates a disease distal to spinal foramen (peripheral nerve entrapment) and intact SNAP indicates a proximal disease differentiating it from peripheral entrapment neuropathy.
- *Late potentials (H reflex and F-wave)*: Late potentials take substantially longer time (more than 10–20 ms) than direct responses to appear after stimulation of motor nerves. Two distinct types of late responses are the H-reflex and the F-wave. F-waves are smaller responses seen after CMAP when a motor or mixed nerve is stimulated. H reflex is a monosynaptic reflex, which can be elicited by stimulating the tibial nerve submaximally and then recording potentials from the calf muscle (gastrosoleus). Late responses are useful to evaluate nerve conduction (in radiculopathies, and peripheral polyneuropathies) in the portion of the nerve that is relatively near the spine, and therefore, inaccessible to conventional techniques.

PERIPHERAL NERVE INJURIES OF UPPER LIMB

RELEVANT ANATOMY

The musculature of the arm is divided into an anterior, medial and a posterior compartment. Medial compartment is largely rudimentary and in it lies the coracobrachialis, originating from coracoid process of scapula. Although vestigial, the muscle is incredibly important landmark as all peripheral nerves change their compartments just distal to the place where this muscle is inserted into the medial aspect of middle humerus. The main bulk of anterior compartment is composed of the biceps (supplied by musculocutaneous nerve) and the brachialis (motor supply by musculocutaneous and sensory fibers by radial nerve). The posterior compartment mainly comprises of the triceps with its three heads, supplied by the radial nerve. So, no muscle in the arm is supplied by the median and ulnar nerves.

The forearm has the flexors on the anterior aspect and the extensors on the dorsal aspect.

The forearm flexor muscles are classified as superficial, intermediate and deep. The superficial group includes those muscle tendons that are visible under the skin **(Fig. 8.6)**, viz. palmaris longus (PL), flexor carpi radialis (FCR), flexor carpi ulnaris (FCU) and pronator teres (PT). Underneath it lies the intermediate group [flexor digitorum superficialis (FDS)] while the deep group comprises of the flexor digitorum profundus (FDP) and flexor pollicis longus (FPL) tendons. All these flexors have a common origin, the medial epicondyle of humerus but varying insertions. The superficial group inserts onto the corresponding carpal bones just as the tendons cross the wrist. The intermediate and deep groups extend beyond and play a role in the flexion of the digits. FDS splits in front of proximal phalanx and the two slips insert onto the sides of the middle phalanx. The FDP and for thumb the FPL, are the only tendons that reach till the distal phalanges inserting at its base, and thereby acting as sole flexors of the distal interphalangeal (DIP) joints. All flexors of forearm are supplied by median nerve except one and a half flexors (the FCU and the medial tendons of FDP), that are supplied by ulnar nerve.

The extensor side of the forearm comprises of six compartments as shown in **Figures 8.7A and B**. The extensor carpi radialis longus (ECRL) and extensor carpi radialis brevis (ECRB) are primary extensors of the wrist while the extensor indicis (EI) and extensor digitorum communis (EDC) are primarily finger extensors. All these extensor muscles have a common origin from the lateral condyle of humerus and are supplied by posterior interosseous branch of radial nerve.

The palmar aspect of the hand comprises of the thenar and the complimentary hypothenar muscles. The thenar muscles are short muscles that guide the movements of the thumb **(Fig. 8.8)**. There are four thenar muscles, namely flexor pollicis brevis (FPB), adductor pollicis, abductor pollicis brevis and opponens pollicis (no extensor pollicis as it is an extensor compartment muscle). Just like all flexors, all thenar muscles are also supplied by median nerve except one and a half muscles (deep head of FPB and adductor pollicis), that are supplied by the ulnar nerve.

The peripheral nerves that supply the skin and musculature of the upper limb arise from the brachial plexus. The plexus finally ends as three cords: lateral, middle and posterior. The cords are named so because of their relation to the axillary artery in the axilla and the upper arm. The medial cord continues as the ulnar nerve, the posterior as the radial nerve and the lateral cord is joined by a twig from medial cord to continue as the median nerve.

ULNAR NERVE PALSY (C8–T1)

Course (Fig. 8.9)

Arm

Ulnar nerve (Musician's nerve) is a continuation of the medial cord of brachial plexus. Hence, in the upper arm, it lies medial to the axillary artery. At the junction of middle and distal thirds of humerus, just distal to the insertion of coracobrachialis, the ulnar nerve pierces the medial intermuscular septum to enter the posterior compartment. At the elbow, the nerve lies behind the medial epicondyle, almost superficially palpable in a bony tunnel called the cubital tunnel.

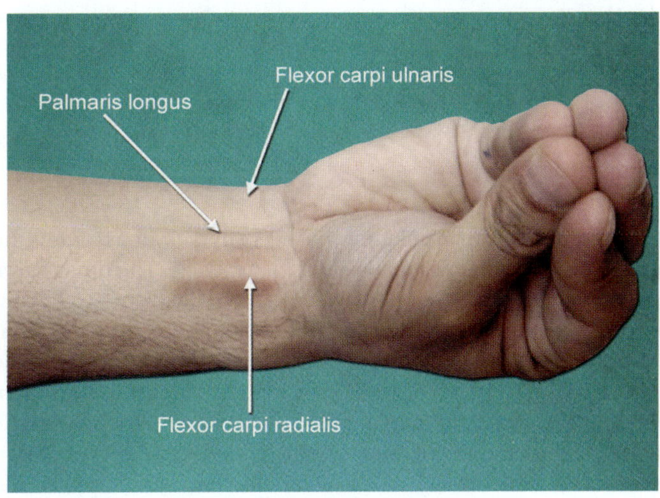

Fig. 8.6: Superficial flexors of forearm

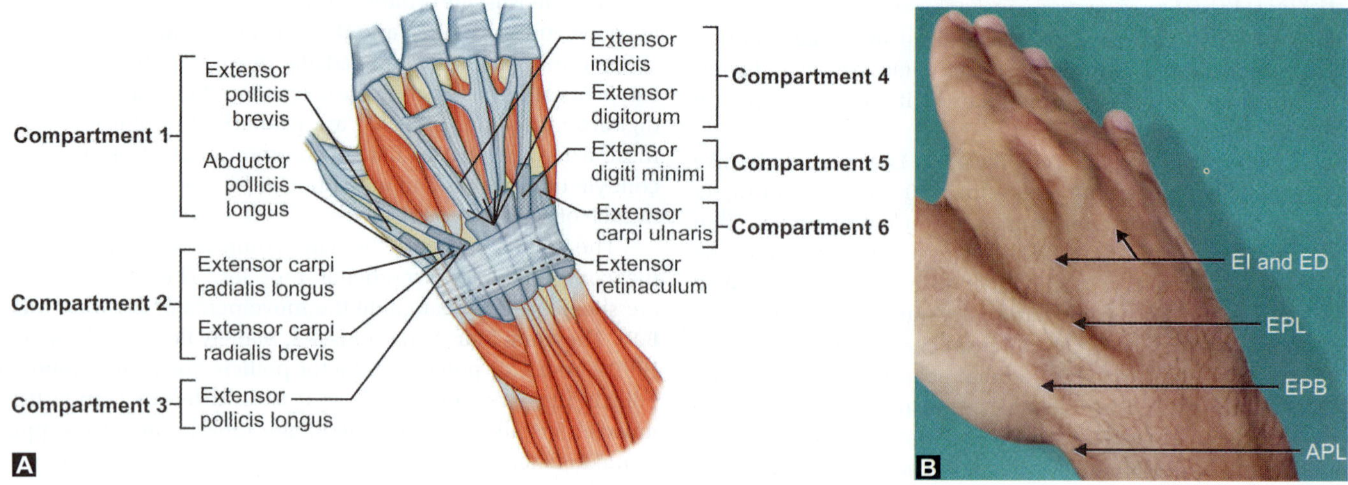

Figs 8.7A and B: Extensor compartment of wrist

Abbreviations: EI, extensor indicis; ED, extensor digitorum; EPL, extensor pollicis longus; EPB, extensor pollicis brevis; APL, abductor pollicis longus.

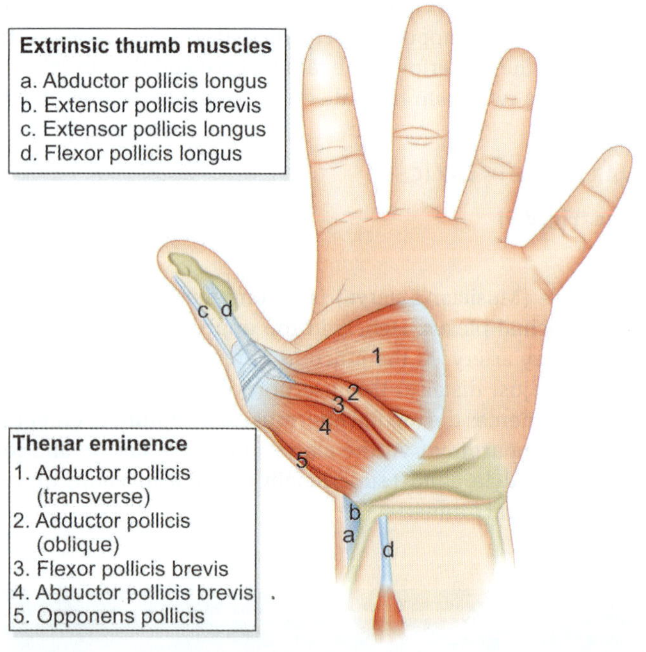

Fig. 8.8: Thenar muscles

Forearm

It is a general dictum in anatomy that every nerve when it enters the forearm, it enters between two heads of a muscle. The ulnar nerve enters the forearm passing between the two heads of FCU. From here, the nerve travels under the FCU, accompanied by the ulnar artery (the neurovascular bundles generally travel together), to lie at the wrist just underneath the fleshy tendon of this muscle. Before entering the hand, the nerve gives two sensory branches for the hand: (1) the palmar cutaneous branch (supplies the hypothenar eminence), and the (2) dorsal cutaneous branch (supplies the medial dorsum of hand and the proximal parts of dorsum of 2 and a 1/2 digits).

Hand

The ulnar nerve enters the hand by passing superficial to flexor retinaculum lying between the pisiform bone medially and the ulnar vessels laterally.

The FCU tendon that was overlying the ulnar nerve in forearm also enters the hand. Although the tendon is inserted into pisiform, which is a sesamoid in the tendon, the true insertion of FCU is the hook of hamate, the terminal part being called as the pisohamate ligament. The ulnar nerve courses under this pisohamate ligament (an area called Guyon's canal). Here the nerve divides into superficial terminal branch, which is primarily a sensory branch (Palmaris brevis in only muscle supplied) and supplies the skin of medial one and a half digits with their nail beds. The deep branch is primarily motor and ends by supplying muscles of the hand.

Muscles Innervated (Fig. 8.9)

Arm

No muscle is supplied by the ulnar nerve in arm.

Forearm

Since the nerve enters the forearm between two heads of FCU, it is the first muscle to be supplied. Now, all flexors of forearm are supplied by median nerve except one and a half flexors supplied by ulnar nerve—the one flexor is FCU, the half flexor is medial half of the FDP.

Hand

Deep branch supplies three hypothenar muscles—the abductor digiti minimi, flexor digiti minimi, and opponens digiti minimi (palmaris brevis the fourth hypothenar muscle is supplied by the superficial branch).

Amongst the thenar muscles, it again supplies one and a half muscles—the adductor pollicis and deep head of FPB.

It innervates all the interossei muscles. The interossei bring about adduction and abduction of the fingers (PAD, palmar interossei are adductors and DAB, dorsal interossei are

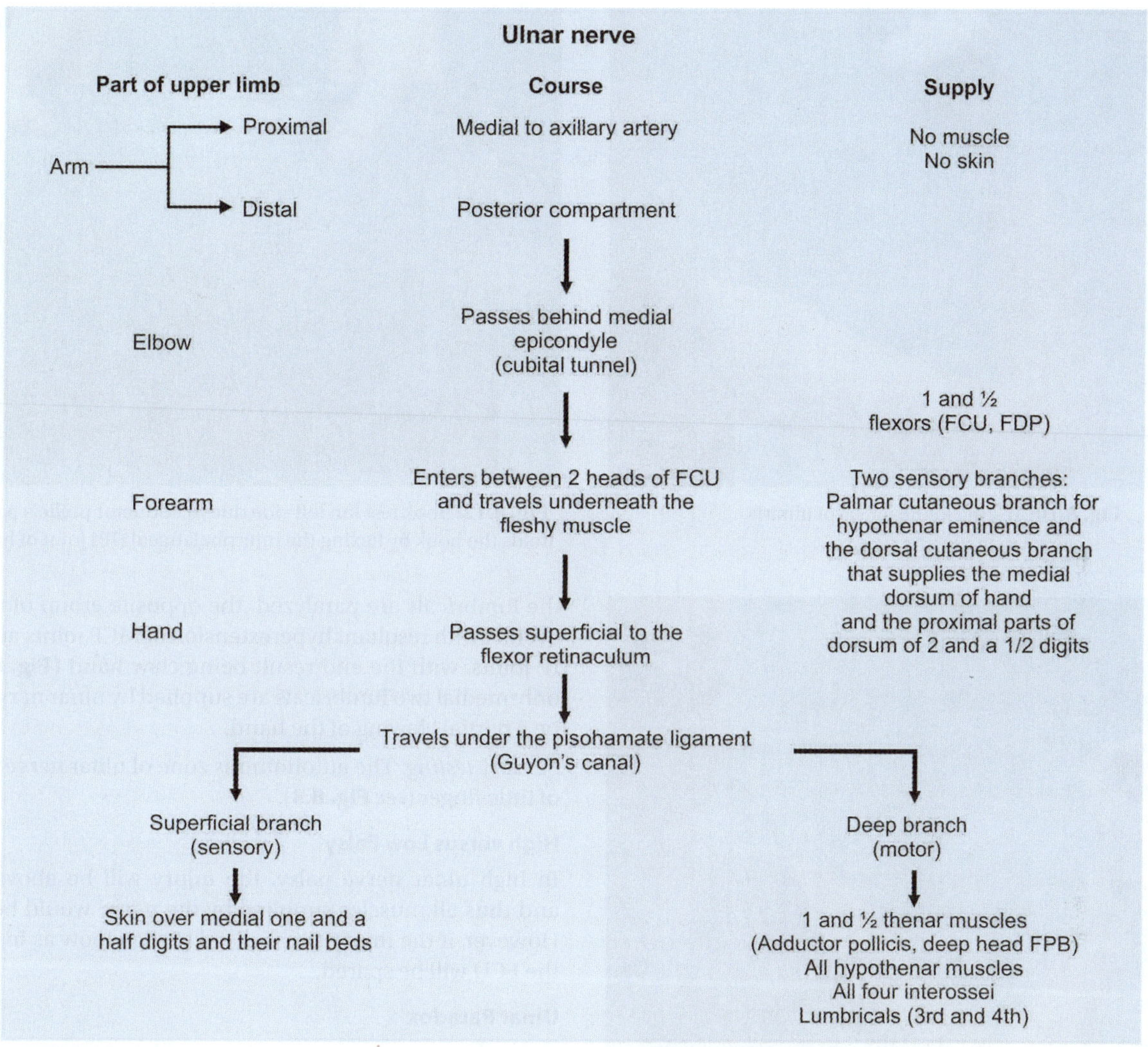

Fig. 8.9: Ulnar nerve course and distribution

abductors), and hence this movement is brought about by the ulnar nerve. One can well imagine the importance of adduction and abduction of fingers for playing a piano and thereby the use of the term musician's nerve.

Lumbricals originate from the tendons of FDP only, so just like FDP, they have a dual nerve supply. So, only the medial two lumbricals get supplied by ulnar nerve.

Important Sites of Compression

Arm

Arcade of Struthers (the arcade is a thin aponeurotic band lying approximately 8 cm above medial epicondyle, extending from medial head of triceps to the medial intermuscular septum) may be a compression site in cases where a transposition of ulnar nerve has been done as a surgical treatment (not a site in ordinary cases).

Elbow

Behind medial epicondyle: Cubitus valgus deformity (tardy ulnar nerve palsy) or compression in the cubital tunnel (most common site) when the nerve passes between two heads of FCU.

Hand

Guyon's canal (area under the pisohamate ligament).

Clinical Testing

Forearm

Flexor carpi ulnaris: The muscle is tested by asking the patient to flex the wrist. If the FCU is paralyzed, the wrist deviates toward radial side **(Fig. 8.10)** due to pull by FCR (supplied by median nerve).

Flexor digitorum profundus (medial half): This is the sole flexor of the DIP joints and is tested by asking the patient to make a fist. While all fingers close, the DIP joints of the medial two digits remain extended **(Fig. 8.11)**.

Hand

In chronic cases, there may be atrophy of the hypothenar eminence and hollowing of intermetatarsal spaces due to atrophy of the interossei.

Adductor pollicis: The muscle is tested by the book test. The patient is asked to hold a book by the side of thumb and medial

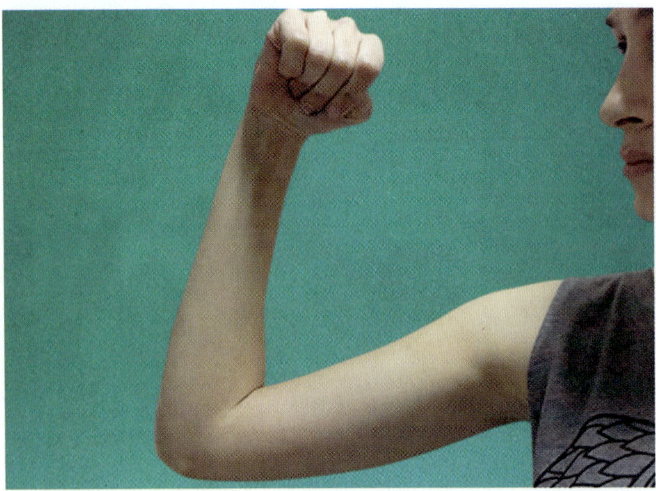

Fig. 8.10: Testing for flexor carpi ulnaris

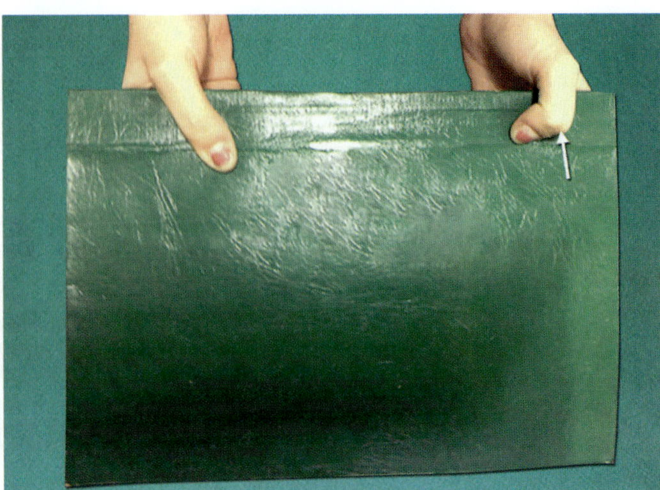

Fig. 8.12: Book test [on left side due to adductor pollicis palsy patients holds the book by flexing the interphalangeal (IP) joint of hand (arrow)]

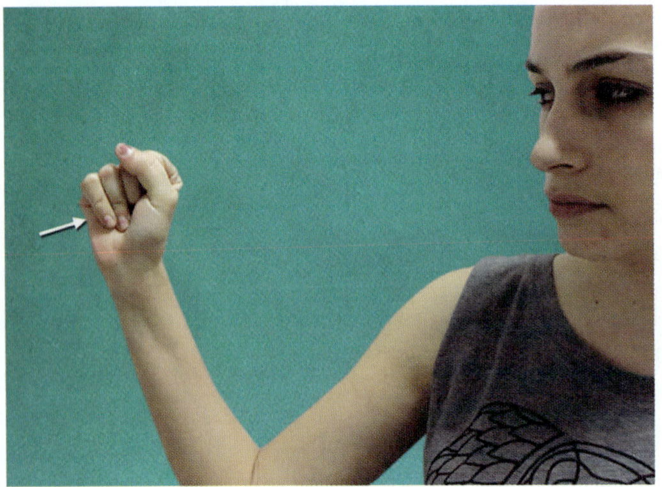

Fig. 8.11: Testing for flexor digitorum profundus of medial two digits

border of palm by just adducting the thumb. When this muscle is paralyzed, the patient holds the book by flexing the thumb at the interphalangeal joint, due to action of FPL (which is supplied by median nerve). The test is called book test and the sign is called Froment's sign **(Fig. 8.12)**.

Interossei: Both dorsal and palmar interossei are tested. Dorsal interossei are abductors of fingers and are tested by the Egawa's test **(Fig. 8.13A)**. The patient is asked to place his hand on the table and fan all the fingers. The palmar interossei are adductors of fingers and are tested by the card test **(Fig. 8.13B)**. The patient is asked to hold a card by adducting the fingers while the examiner tries to pull the card away.

Since all interossei are supplied by ulnar nerve, it controls adduction-abduction of fingers, a movement unique for playing a piano. Hence, it is called the Musician's nerve.

Lumbricals: The function of the lumbricals is flexion of the metacarpophalangeal (MCP) joints and extension of the IP joints (or simply they make an "L" shape of the hand). When the lumbricals are paralyzed, the opposite group of muscles will overact with resultant hyperextension at MCP joints and flexion at IP joints, with the end result being claw hand **(Fig. 8.14)**. Since only medial two lumbricals are supplied by ulnar nerve, there will be a partial clawing of the hand.

Sensory testing: The autonomous zone of ulnar nerve includes tip of little finger (*see* **Fig. 8.3**).

High versus Low Palsy

In high ulnar nerve palsy, the injury will be above the elbow and thus all muscles supplied by the nerve would be paralyzed. However, if the injury site is distal to the elbow as in a low palsy, the FCU will be spared.

Ulnar Paradox

Going by common sense, one would expect that high palsy is associated with greater paralysis and hence should have more clawing while the reverse should be expected in low palsy. However, what is seen is absolutely opposite. In high lesions since the FDP gets paralyzed, the IP joints of fingers extend masking the clawing. This is called ulnar paradox.

MEDIAN NERVE PALSY (C5–8, T1)

Course (Fig. 8.15)

Median nerve (Laborer's nerve) is formed by joining of medial and lateral (main contribution) cords of brachial plexus.

Arm

In the upper arm, it runs around the lateral side of the axillary/brachial artery till middle of arm where it crosses medial to the artery just distal to coracobrachialis insertion, lying in the anterior compartment. Thereafter, the nerve runs along the medial side of the brachial artery occupying the cubital fossa at the elbow. The nerve enters the forearm passing between two heads of PT.

Forearm

Just on entering the forearm, it passes under the fibrous arch of the FDS. It travels in the forearm (giving anterior interosseous branch in proximal forearm) lying deep to FDS and over the surface of

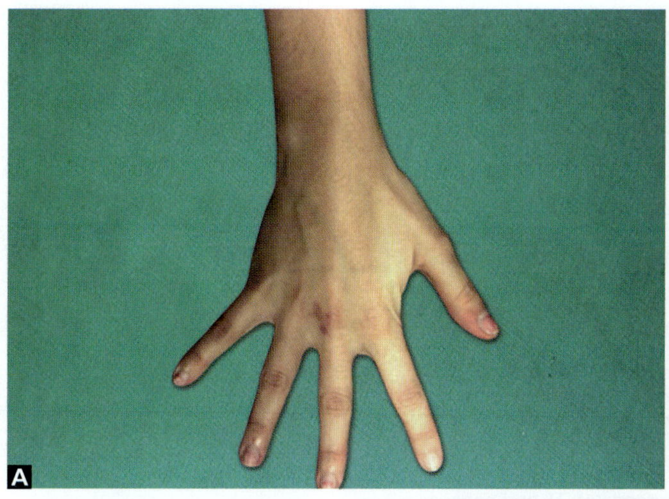
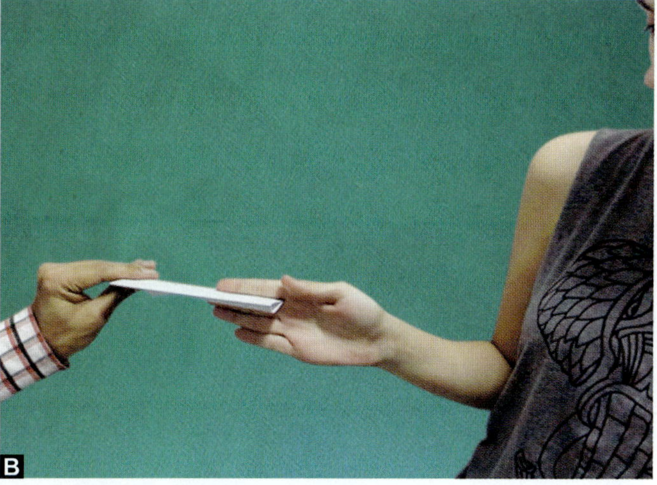

Figs 8.13A and B: Egawa's test and card test

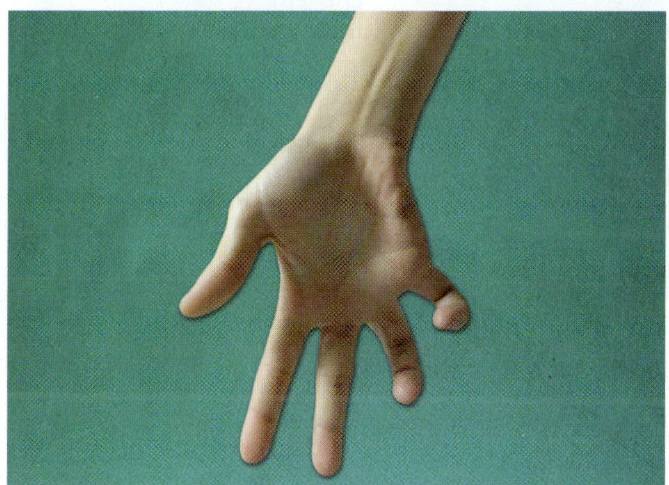

Fig. 8.14: Clawing of medial two digits in ulnar nerve palsy

FDP, to reach near the wrist **(Fig. 8.16)**. About 5 cm proximal to the flexor retinaculum (wrist), the nerve comes toward the lateral side of FDS tendons, becomes a bit superficial and can be traced between the tendons of FCR (lying laterally) and FDS (lying medially) with tendon of PL almost overlapping the nerve **(Fig. 8.17)**. Just before entering the hand (a short distance above flexor retinaculum), the nerve gives the palmar cutaneous branch that supplies the skin over the thenar eminence.

Hand

The nerve enters the hand deep to the flexor retinaculum (area called the Carpal tunnel). Immediately below the retinaculum the nerve divides into lateral (stouter branch) and medial divisions. The lateral division primarily supplies the two and a half thenar muscles and first lumbrical (sensory supply is only to thumb and lateral border of index finger) while the medial division is primarily sensory (supplies the left over index, middle and half of ring finger to complete up the sensory supply— the lateral three and a half fingers; it also supplies second lumbrical).

Muscles Innervated (Fig. 8.15)

Arm

No muscle in the arm is supplied by median nerve.

Forearm

The nerve passes between two heads of PT and thus it is the first muscle to be supplied. Then it supplies all (but one and a half) flexors of the forearm. These include the superficial flexors, viz. PL, FCR and the intermediate group, viz. FDS and the deep flexors (more specifically, these are supplied by the anterior interosseous branch given off in the proximal forearm), viz. FPL, pronator quadratus and the lateral two tendons of FDP.

Since finger flexors (FDS and FDP) get predominantly supplied by median nerve, the nerve is also called Laborer's nerve owing to the strong gripping action, it provides to the hand.

Hand

The lateral division supplies all (but one and a half) thenar muscles, viz. FPB (superficial head), abductor pollicis and opponens pollicis. The lateral two lumbricals are the only other muscle group in hand supplied by the median nerve (first lumbrical by lateral and second by medial division).

Important Sites of Compression

Distal Arm

Supracondylar humerus fracture is an important cause of median nerve injury.

Proximal Forearm

The nerve may be compressed as it passes between two heads of PT (pronator syndrome). The anterior interosseous branch (AIN) may be compressed by the deep head of pronator teres, edge of laceratus fibrosus or by the tendinous FDS arch (*see* AIN syndrome/Kiloh-Nevin syndrome later).

Wrist (Most Common Site)

Compression may be there in the carpal tunnel (*see* carpal tunnel syndrome), fracture of distal end radius, lunate dislocations.

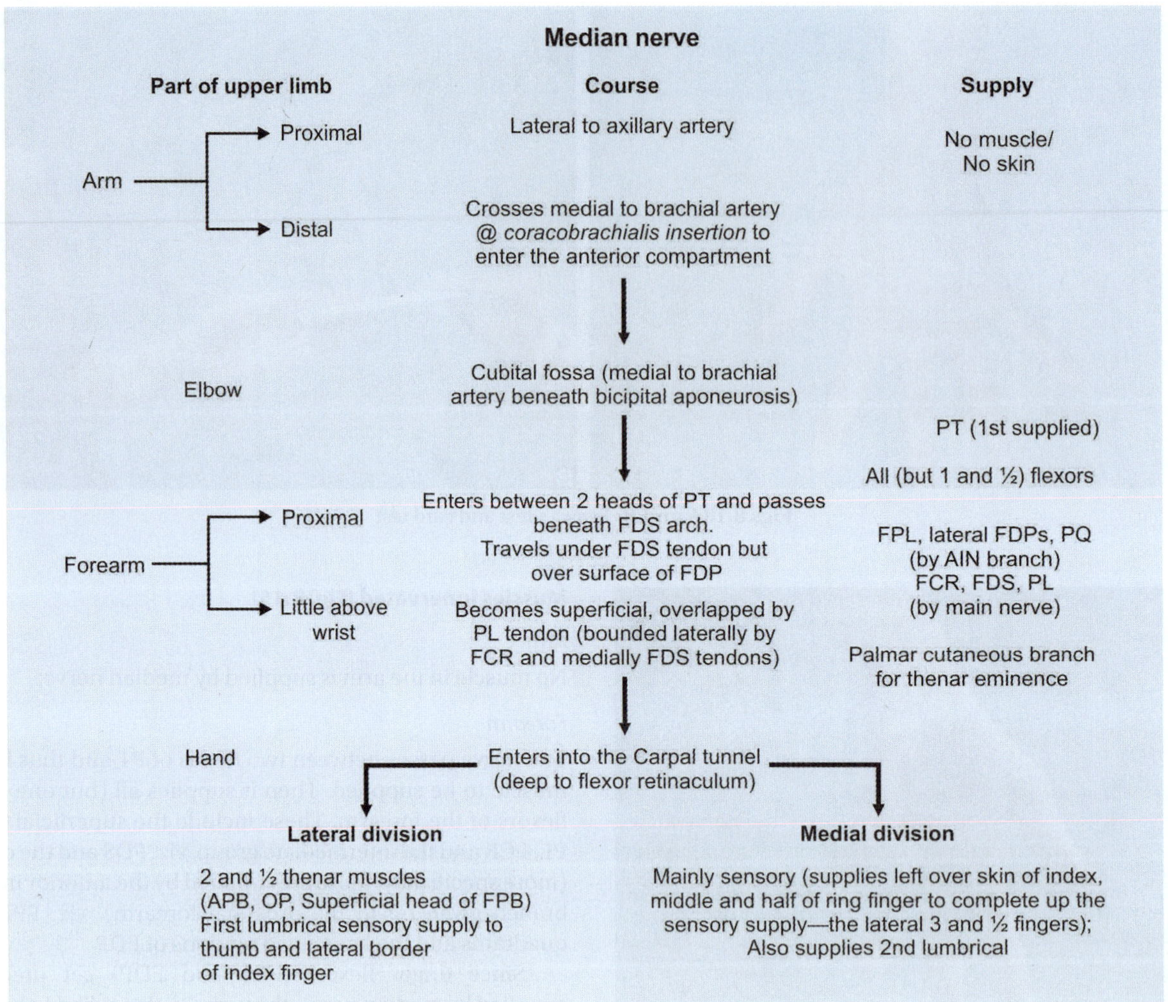

Fig. 8.15: Median nerve course and distribution

Clinical Testing

Forearm

Flexor carpi radialis: Ask the patient to flex the wrist. The wrist deviates to ulnar side **(Fig. 8.18)** if the FCR is paralyzed (due to unopposed action of the FCU supplied by the ulnar nerve).

Flexor pollicis longus: This muscle is inserted onto the base of distal phalanx of thumb and is the sole flexor of the IP joint of thumb (FPB inserts at base of proximal phalanx and flexes MCP joint of thumb). So, FPL is tested by checking flexion of the thumb IP joint **(Fig. 8.19)**.

Flexor digitorum superficialis and lateral FDPs: These are tested together by eliciting the pointing sign. When a patient with median nerve palsy is asked to close the hand and make a fist, he closes the ring and little fingers as these fingers have intact FDPs (supplied by ulnar nerve). The middle finger also partially closes (as all FDPs are partially interlinked) but the index finger remains open and gives the pointing sign **(Fig. 8.20A)**. The other ways of eliciting this test are the Benediction/Pope's hand or the Ochsner's clasping sign **(Fig. 8.20B)**.

Hand

Abductor pollicis brevis: It can be tested by the pen test **(Fig. 8.21)**. The patient places his hand flat on the table. Examiner brings a pen in front of the palm and the patient is instructed to abduct the thumb and touch the pen with the tip of the thumb.

Opponens pollicis: Tested by asking the patient to touch the little finger with the pulp of the thumb by swinging the thumb across the palm **(Fig. 8.22)**. A rather simpler way is to observe the attitude of the thumb. When opponens (and abductor) pollicis is paralyzed, with adductor pollicis (supplied by ulnar nerve) still intact, the thumb goes into adduction, and hence these patients land up with ape thumb deformity (thumb in the same plane as the palm).

Lumbricals: Ideally, the paralysis of the lateral two lumbricals should cause clawing of the lateral two digits. However, due to complex cross connections between the lumbricals (just like the FDPs), clawing gets masked in isolated median nerve palsy. Clawing gets manifested either in ulnar nerve palsy where only the medial two digits show clawing or in combined median and ulnar nerve injuries where all the four digits show clawing.

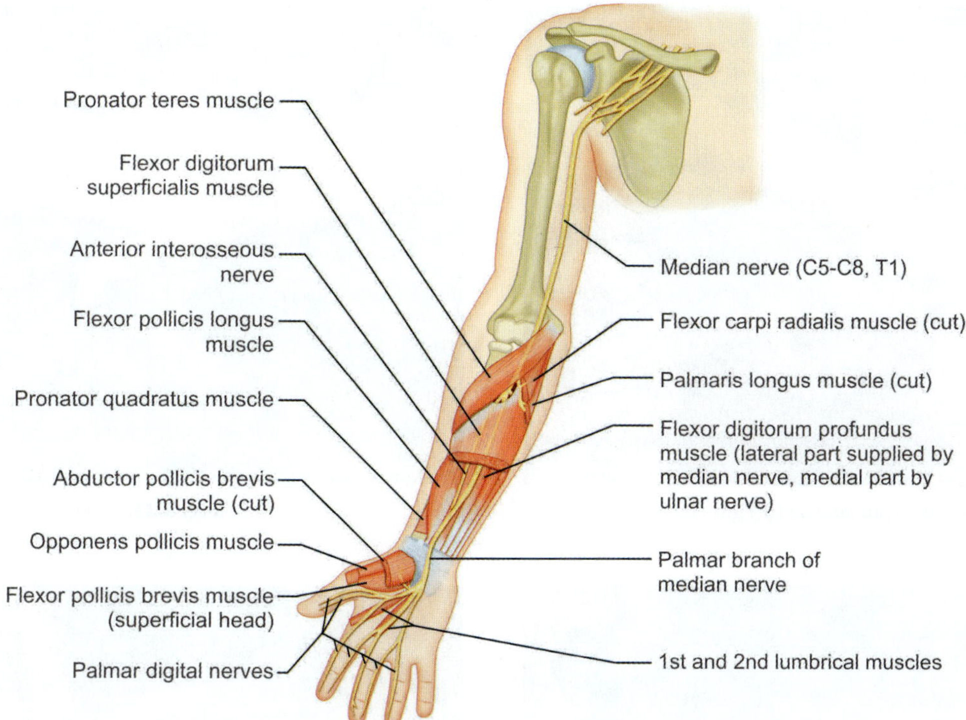

Fig. 8.16: Median nerve in forearm

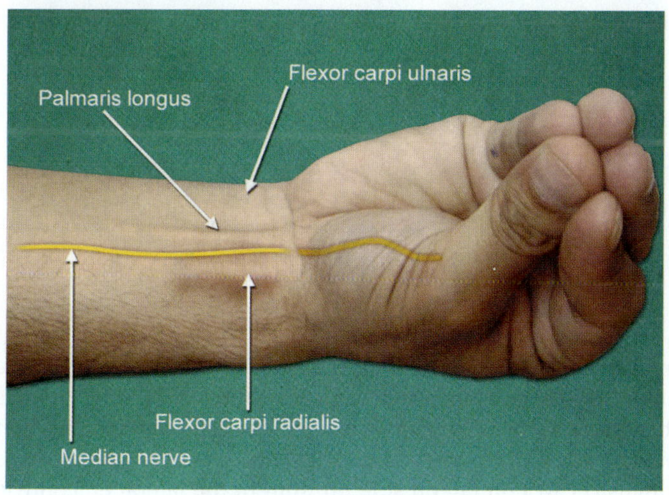

Fig. 8.17: Median nerve at wrist

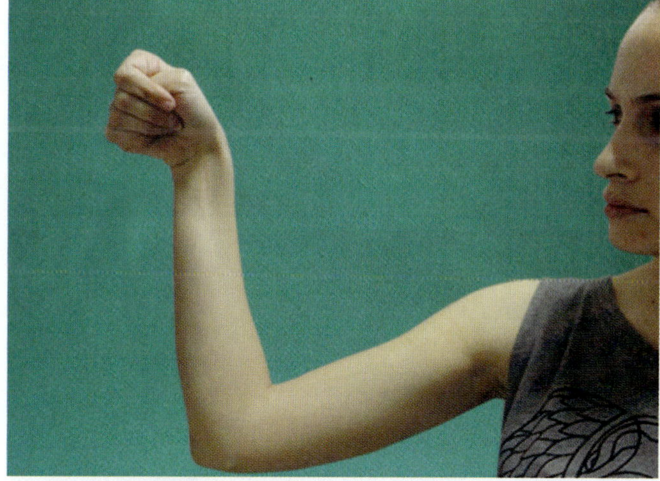

Fig. 8.18: Testing for flexor carpi radialis

Sensory testing: Tips of index and middle finger form the autonomous zone (*see* **Fig. 8.3**). Since these finger tips are at times used by people in sensing surfaces, median nerve has been equated to an 'eye' of the hand.

High versus Low Palsy

Median nerve injuries are classified as "high" or "low," specifically depending on whether the lesion is proximal or distal to the origin of the anterior interosseous nerve in the proximal forearm but grossly that simulates with the lesion being proximal or distal to the elbow as with the ulnar nerve. In high lesions, all muscles supplied by the nerve would be paralyzed, but in low lesions classically only the hand function is affected.

RADIAL NERVE PALSY (C5–8, T1)

Course (Fig. 8.23)

The radial nerve is the largest branch the posterior cord and is primarily its continuation.

Arm (Fig. 8.24)

In the upper arm, it lies posterior to the artery and travels into the lower triangular space. Then the nerve enters into the radial groove

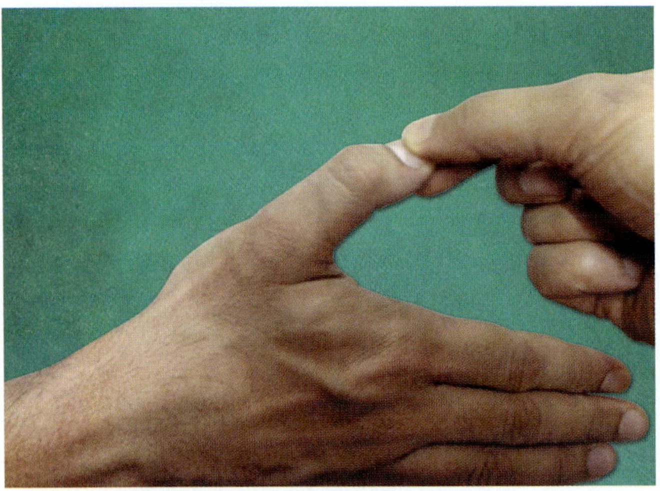

Fig. 8.19: Testing for interphalangeal (IP) joint flexion thumb

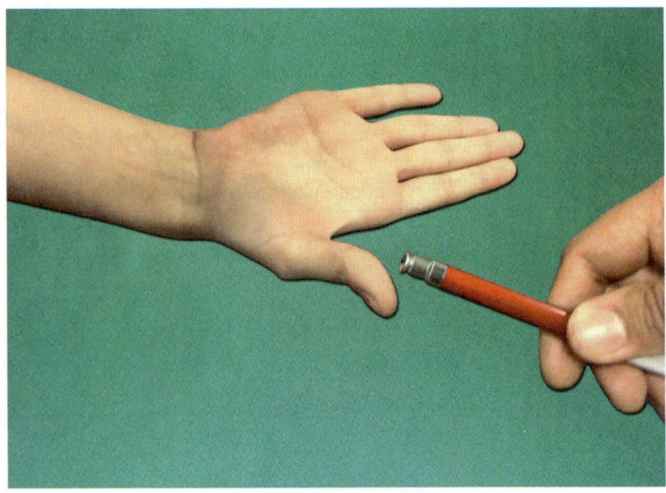

Fig. 8.21: Pen test

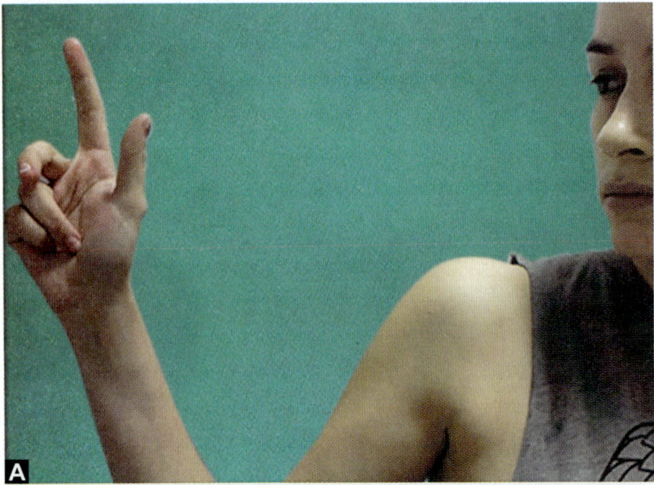

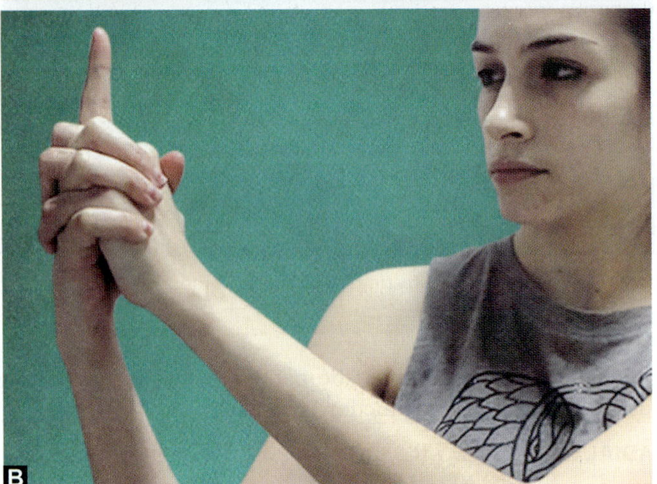

Figs 8.20A and B: Pointing sign or Ochsner's clasping sign

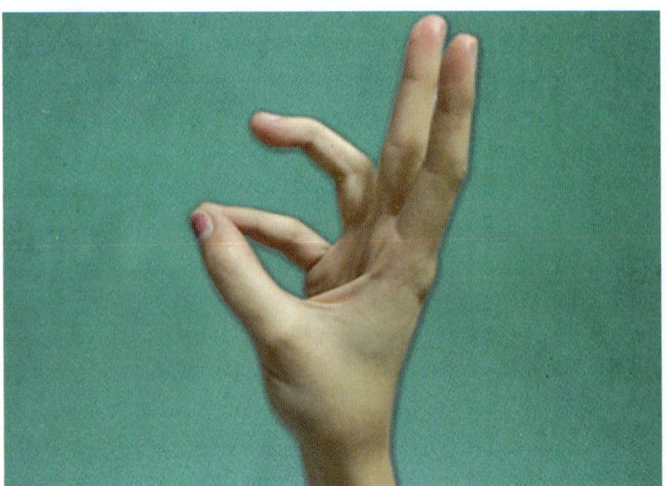

Fig. 8.22: Testing for opponens pollicis

intermuscular septum to enter the anterior compartment. At the elbow, it is sandwiched between two muscles (cf. other nerves that pass between two heads of same muscles) the brachialis on medial side and brachioradialis (BR) and extensor carpi radialis longus (ECRL) on lateral side. In front of the lateral epicondyle of humerus (cf. ulnar nerve is behind medial epicondyle), the nerve divides into a superficial sensory branch and a deep motor branch, the posterior interosseous nerve (PIN).

Forearm

The sensory branch travels alongside the radial artery, going underneath the brachioradialis and gives sensory supply to lateral part of dorsal aspect of hand and dorsal aspect of lateral two and a half fingers (*see* **Fig. 8.3**). The PIN is a pure motor nerve. It pierces the supinator in the proximal forearm and comes to lie on the extensor side of forearm (about 8 cm below the elbow joint). Here, it travels a very short distance before dividing into terminal branches that supply all the six extensor compartments of the forearm (PIN itself is part of fourth extensor compartment).

on the posterior aspect of humerus, traveling between medial and lateral heads of triceps. Here, it crosses from medial to lateral aspect. At the junction of middle and distal third of humerus (bit distal to coracobrachialis insertion), the nerve pierces the lateral

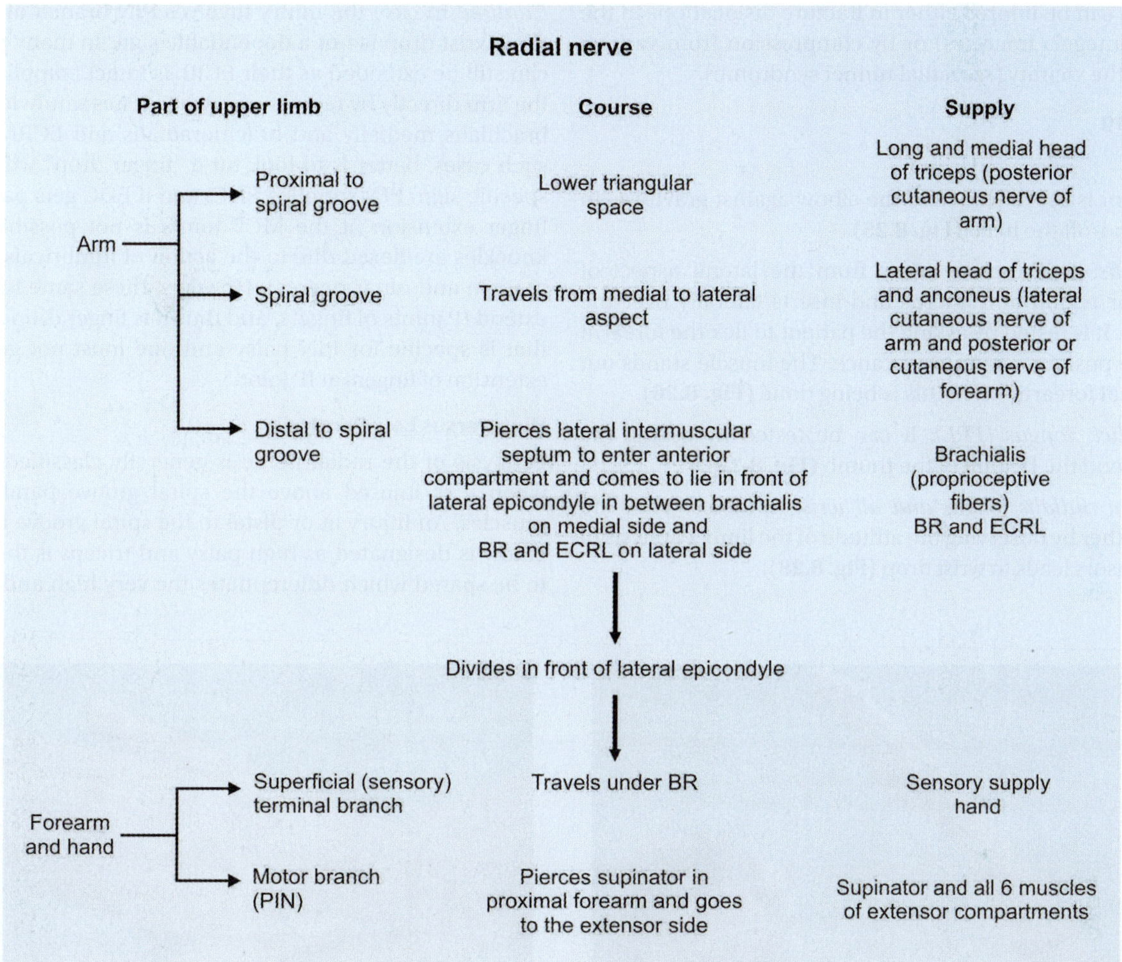

Fig. 8.23: Radial nerve course and distribution

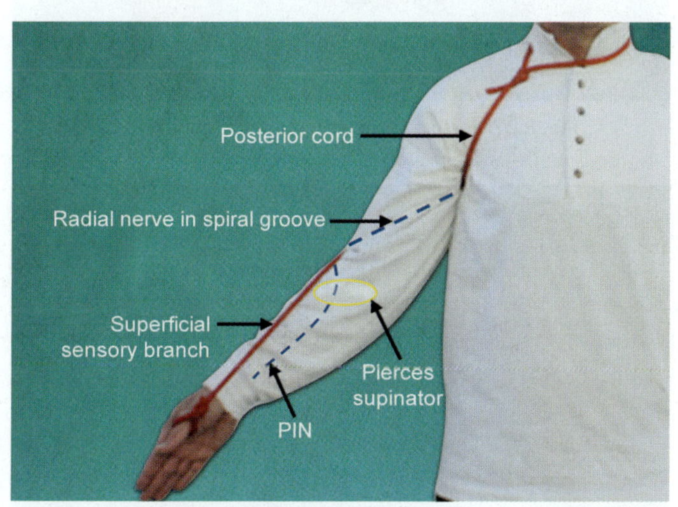

Fig. 8.24: Diagrammatic representation of radial nerve course in arm and forearm

Muscles Innervated (Fig. 8.23)

Arm

Before spiral groove: Triceps (long and medial head)

In the spiral groove: Lateral heads of triceps, anconeus

Below the spiral groove: Brachialis (only sensory supply, motor supply is from musculocutaneous nerve), BR and ECRL.

Forearm

The PIN supplies supinator and all six extensor compartment muscles on the dorsal aspect of forearm, viz. abductor pollicis longus (APL), extensor pollicis brevis (EPB), extensor carpi radialis brevis (ECRB), extensor indicis proprius (EIP), EDC, extensor digiti minimi (EDM) and extensor carpi ulnaris (ECU).

Sensory Supply

Posterior cutaneous nerve of the arm (given off above spiral groove), the lateral cutaneous nerve of arm and posterior cutaneous nerve of forearm (given in the spiral groove). The autonomous zone of the radial nerve is the dorsal aspect of the first webspace, through the superficial terminal branch (*see* **Fig. 8.3**).

Important Sites of Compression

Common sites of compression of radial nerve include:

Arm (most common site): Compression high up in axilla above the spiral groove by an axillary crutch (crutch palsy), in the spiral groove (Saturday night palsy) or in or below the groove as in injury during fractures of the shaft humerus (most common cause) and elbow region and intramuscular injections of the arm.

Forearm: PIN can be injured either in fracture dislocations in the area (e.g. Monteggia fractures) or by compression from various structures in the vicinity (*see* radial tunnel syndrome).

Clinical Testing

Arm

Triceps: Patient is asked to extend the elbow against gravity as in lifting the hand-off the head **(Fig. 8.25)**.

Brachioradialis: This muscle arises from the lateral aspect of supracondylar region of humerus and inserts laterally over the radial styloid. It is tested by asking the patient to flex the forearm in mid-prone position against resistance. The muscle stands out in the proximal forearm when this is being done **(Fig. 8.26)**.

Extensor pollicis longus (EPL): It can be tested by asking the patient to extend the IP joint of the thumb **(Fig. 8.27)**.

Extensor carpi radialis longus and all wrist extensors: They are checked together by observing the attitude of the limb. Paralysis of all wrist extensors leads to wrist drop **(Fig. 8.28)**.

Caution: In case the injury involves PIN branch of radial nerve, then wrist drop is not a dependable sign. In many patients wrist can still be extended as their ECRL is intact (supplied high up in the arm directly by radial nerve when it lies sandwiched between brachialis medially and brachioradialis and ECRL laterally). In such cases, better is to look for a "finger drop", which is a more specific sign. PIN supplies EDC, and if EDC gets paralyzed, then finger extension at the MCP joints is not possible, rather the knuckles are flexed due to the action of lumbricals (supplied by median and ulnar nerves). However, these same lumbricals can extend IP joints of fingers, and thus it is finger drop at MCP joints that is specific for PIN palsy and one must not get mislead by extension of fingers at IP joint.

High versus Low Paralysis

Paralysis of the radial nerve is generally classified as very high when it is injured above the spiral groove paralyzing all the muscles. An injury at or distal to the spiral groove but above the elbow is designated as high palsy and triceps is the first muscle to be spared which differentiates the very high and high lesions.

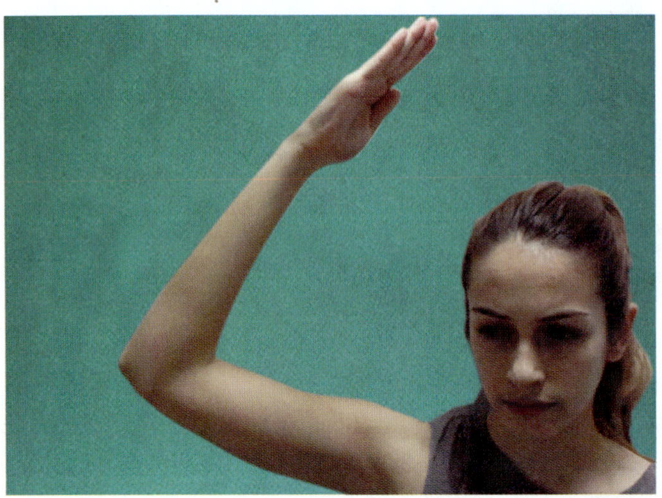

Fig. 8.25: Testing for triceps

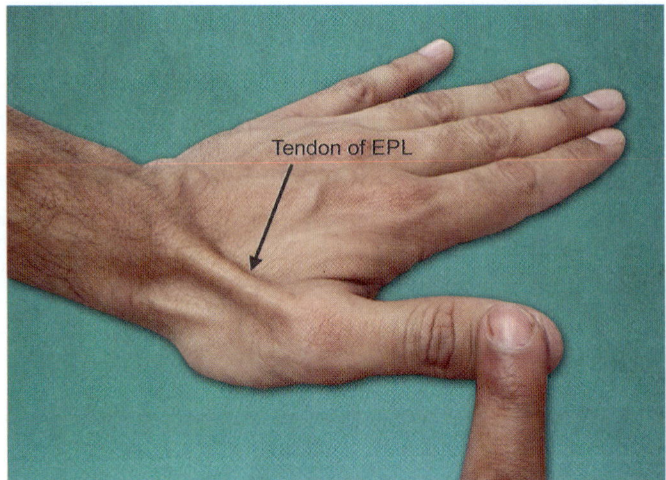

Fig. 8.27: Testing for extensor pollicis longus (EPL)

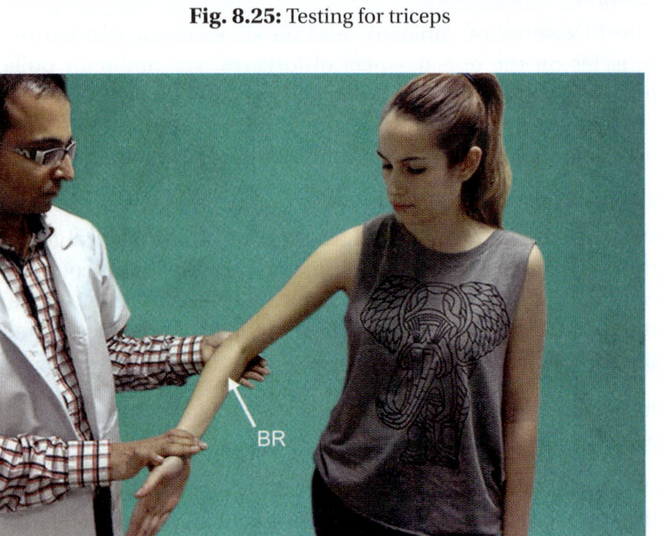

Fig. 8.26: Testing for brachioradialis (BR)

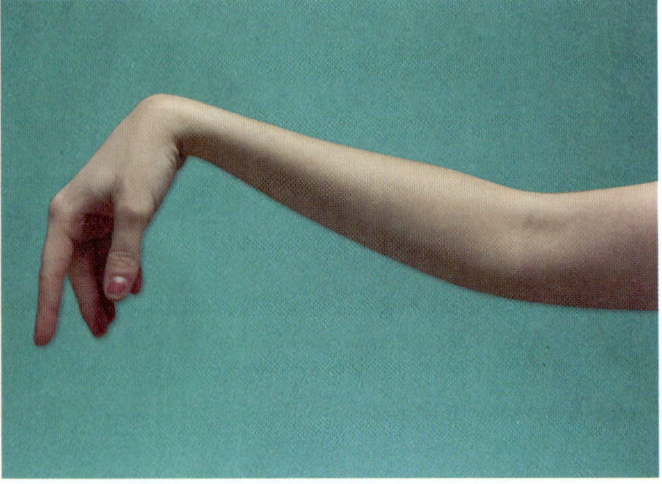

Fig. 8.28: Wrist drop after radial nerve palsy

The low lesions involve injury of the PIN mostly below the elbow and in these injuries, testing for intact brachioradialis is used as a distinguishing factor. Also since it is entirely a motor nerve, the sensations in the autonomous zone are intact.

AXILLARY NERVE PALSY (C5–6)

Course

It is a branch of the posterior cord of the brachial plexus. It winds around the neck of humerus (around 4–5 cm distal to acromion) to pass through the quadrangular space **(Figs 8.29A and B)** and supplies the deltoid and the teres minor muscle (nerve to teres minor bears a pseudoganglion). The nerve gives sensory innervation to lateral aspect of lower deltoid (regimental badge area).

Muscles Innervated

Deltoid and Teres minor.

Sensory supply: Regimental badge area (lateral aspect of shoulder and upper arm).

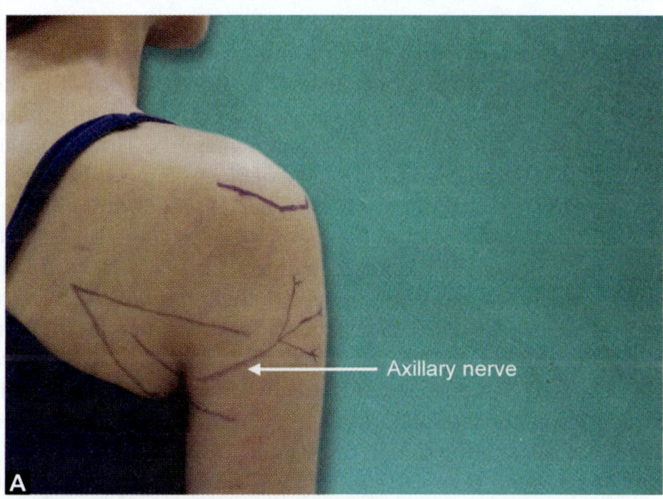

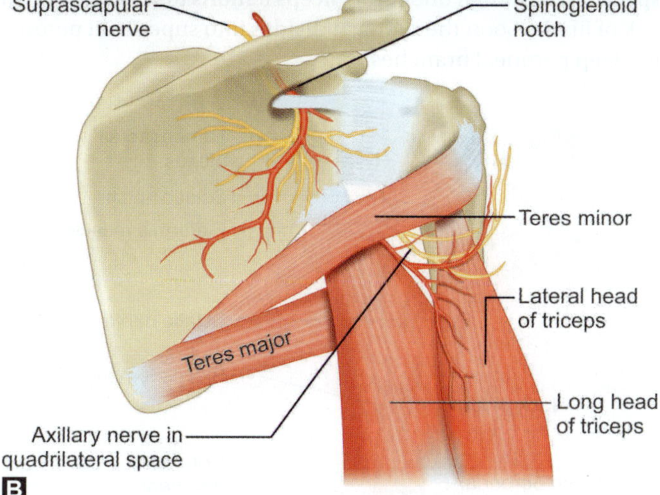

Figs 8.29A and B: (A) Surface anatomy of axillary nerve; (B) Axillary nerve in quadrangular space

Injury Sites

It is commonly injured in fractures of the surgical neck of humerus and shoulder dislocation. Other important causes are iatrogenic injury during lateral approach to shoulder and shoulder arthroscopy.

Most common site of injury is just proximal to quadrangular space.

Clinical Testing

Examination reveals loss of contour of affected shoulder and weakness of abduction from 15 to 90 degrees. Sensations are lost in the regimental badge area (regiment badge sign) **(Fig. 8.30)**.

SUPRASCAPULAR NERVE PALSY (C5–6)

Course (Figs 8.29A and B)

Arises from upper trunk of brachial plexus and lies in the posterior triangle of neck. Passing under the belly of omohyoid muscle, the nerve enters the suprascapular notch of scapula. The notch is bridged on top by the transverse scapular ligament. The nerve passes beneath the ligament and travels the supraspinatus fossa where it supplies the supraspinatus. Then it arches around the lateral border of the spine of the scapula (area called spinoglenoid notch) to enter the infraspinatus fossa, where it sends a muscular branch to the infraspinatus muscle.

Muscles Innervated

- Supraspinatus (before entering the spinoglenoid notch)
- Infraspinatus (after crossing the spinoglenoid notch).

Sites of Injury

- *Posterior triangle of neck*: Penetrating trauma, cancer surgery
- *Suprascapular fossa*: Fractures of scapula involving suprascapular notch, entrapment in the notch due to thickened transverse scapular ligament and rarely anterior dislocation of shoulder
- *Spinoglenoid notch*: Commonly compressed by a space occupying lesion like a ganglion in the notch.

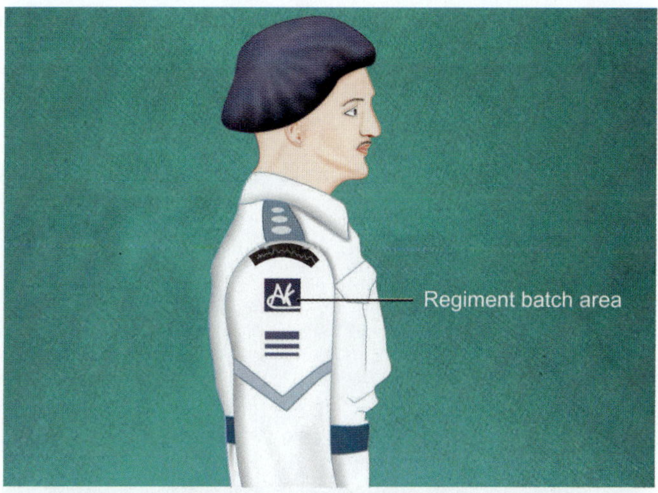

Fig. 8.30: Diagrammatic depiction of regiment badge sign

Clinical Presentation

If the nerve is compressed proximal to spinoglenoid notch (usually in the suprascapular fossa), both the supraspinatus and the infraspinatus show atrophy.

A compression in the spinoglenoid notch (distal to the suprascapular fossa) manifests only with atrophy of the infraspinatus.

LONG THORACIC NERVE PALSY (C5–7) (NERVE OF BELL)

It arises from the ventral rami of C5–7 and descends behind the brachial plexus to supply the serratus anterior muscle. This muscle works in conjunction with the trapezius in aiding overhead abduction. This nerve is generally injured in traction injuries to the shoulder while few other causes may include exposure to cold, viral infections, and placing patients in the Trendelenburg position with shoulder braces that compress the supraclavicular areas.

Paralysis of the nerve makes it difficult for the patient to flex the arm above shoulder level. When these patients attempt forward pushing movements pressing hands against a wall, "winging" of the scapula occurs **(Fig. 8.31)** and its vertebral border and inferior angle become unduly prominent.

SPINAL ACCESSORY NERVE PALSY

The spinal accessory nerve supplies the trapezius. It is susceptible to damage from penetrating injuries or during operations such as lymph node biopsy or radical neck dissection that involve the posterior triangle of neck. The patient reports generalized weakness in the affected shoulder girdle and arm, inability to abduct the shoulder more than 90 degrees. On examination, one may find winging of the scapula, but it is bit different from classical winging. Here, the scapula rotates laterally such that the superior angle moves away from midline while the inferior angle moves toward midline. In such a position, the medial flare of scapula is accentuated when the arm is abducted but the same disappears when the arm is flexed forward (unlike classical winging seen in serratus anterior palsy).

MUSCULOCUTANEOUS NERVE PALSY (C5–6)

The nerve is a branch of lateral cord of brachial plexus. It is mostly injured by penetrating injuries but seldom in anterior dislocation shoulder or fracture of humerus neck. The nerve supplies coracobrachialis (vestigial), brachialis and biceps brachii. This nerve palsy is generally overlooked as it hardly causes any problems. Sensory loss is ill-defined and even though biceps and brachialis are paralyzed, elbow can still be flexed by a strong brachioradialis.

PERIPHERAL NERVE INJURIES OF LOWER LIMB

RELEVANT ANATOMY (FIGS 8.32A AND B)

Sciatic Nerve (L4–S3)

Sciatic nerve is the continuation of the sacral plexus and main contribution to the nerve supply of the lower limb. It is composed of two parts, outer common peroneal arising from dorsal division of anterior rami of L4–S3 and inner tibial part arising from ventral divisions of anterior primary rami of L4–S3. After formation, nerve passes below the piriformis and leaves the pelvis by passing through the sciatic notch. After leaving the pelvis, it enters the gluteal region. Here it passes beneath the gluteus maximus midway between the greater trochanter and ischial tuberosity to enter the back of the thigh and finally terminates at the apex of popliteal fossa by dividing into the common peroneal (aka. lateral popliteal) and tibial branches. The tibial part supplies the hamstrings, viz. semimembranosus, semitendinosus, long head of biceps and ischial head of adductor magnus. The common peroneal part supplies the short head of biceps femoris.

The *tibial nerve* descends at the back of the leg and supplies the calf muscle (soleus) and the plantar flexors of the foot [flexor digitorum longus (FDL), flexor hallucis longus (FHL), tibialis posterior (TP)]. Sensory supply covers the region of the back of the leg and the sole of the foot (latter is the autonomous zone). In the popliteal fossa, it gives off a sensory branch, the sural nerve (L5, S1-2) that descends between the two heads of gastrocnemius passing across the lateral border of the foot to end at the tip of the little toe supplying the skin in these areas.

The *common peroneal nerve* (CPN) descends on the lateral aspect of lower thigh under the biceps femoris to wind around the neck of fibula. Soon thereafter, it divides into superficial peroneal and deep peroneal branches.

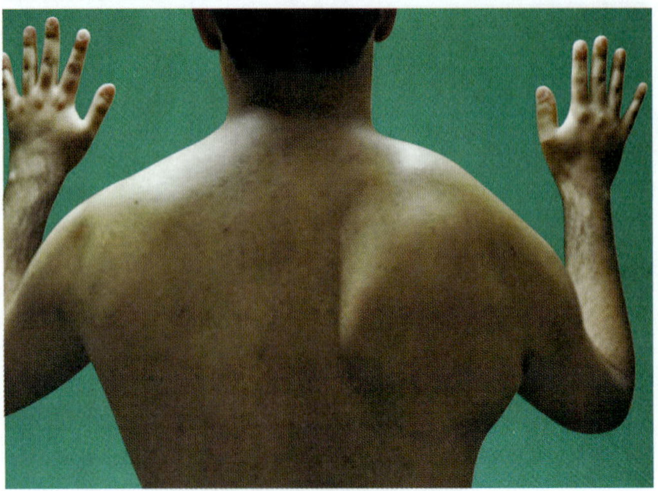

Fig. 8.31: Winging of scapula

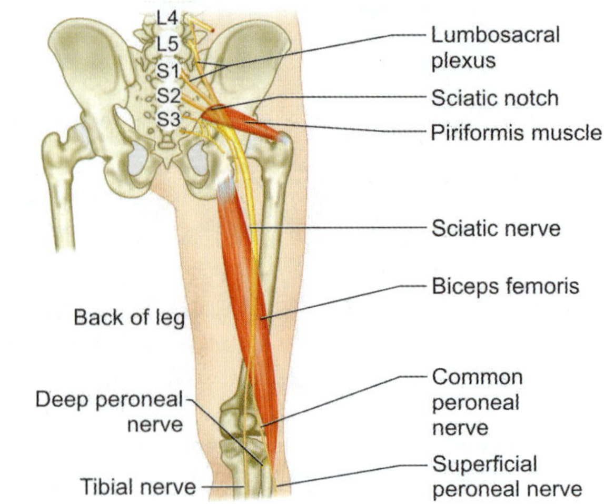

Fig. 8.32A: Course of sciatic nerve (diagrammatic representation)

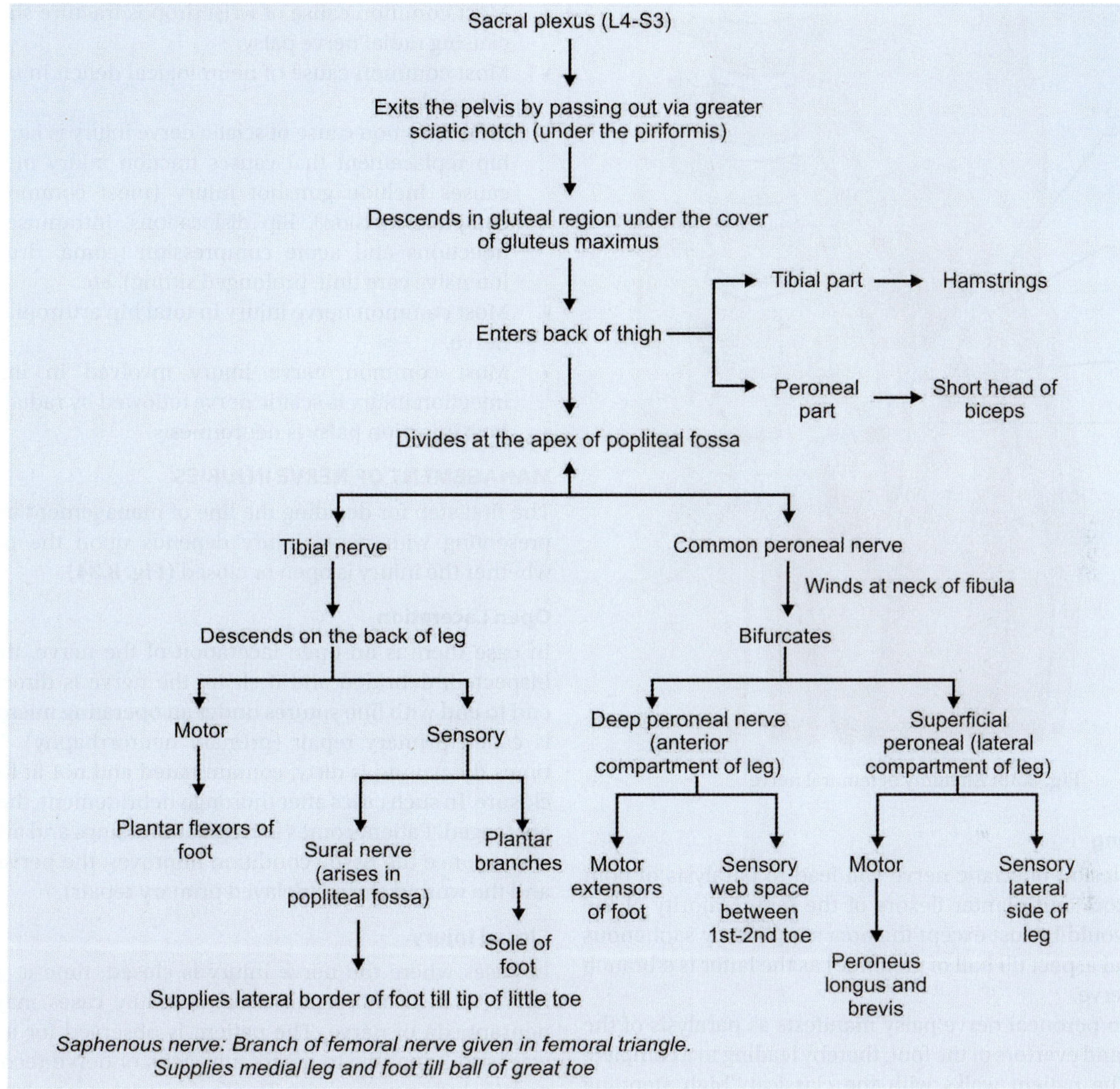

Fig. 8.32B: Sciatic nerve course and distribution

The *superficial peroneal* supplies the peroneus longus and brevis and terminates by supplying the skin over the lateral aspect of leg and majority of the dorsum of the foot.

The *deep peroneal nerve* (counterpart of PIN in forearm) pierces the anterior intermuscular septum, to enter the anterior compartment of leg. It is the main nerve of this extensor compartment of leg and foot and supplies the dorsiflexors of the foot [tibialis anterior, extensor digitorum longus (EDL), extensor digitorum brevis (EDB), extensor hallucis longus (EHL) and peroneus tertius]. It also gives sensory supply to the skin of the first web space between the first and second toes (autonomous zone).

Femoral Nerve (L2, L3, L4)

The main nerve on the front of the thigh is the femoral nerve. This is a relatively rarely injured nerve as it lies quite near to the femoral artery and the arterial injury takes precedence in these patients. The nerve travels across the femoral triangle lying 1–2 cm lateral to the femoral artery and supplies the quadriceps **(Fig. 8.33)**. In the triangle, it gives a saphenous branch (L3–4) (arising from posterior division) that supplies the skin over the medial leg and medial foot till ball of great toe.

SCIATIC NERVE PALSY

Traumatic injury is the most common cause (gunshot/fracture dislocations) followed by iatrogenic injury due to intramuscular injections and surgery around hip. However, complete lesions of sciatic nerve are rare. Most lesions injure the common peroneal part as these are the outermost fibers. Moreover, CPN is relatively a fixed nerve as it winds around the neck of fibula and is hence more amenable to injury. CPN may also be injured in fracture dislocations around the knee, especially fibular neck fractures and knee dislocation, iatrogenic injuries by insertion of pins for skeletal traction, compression by tumors and leprosy are other rare causes of CPN palsy.

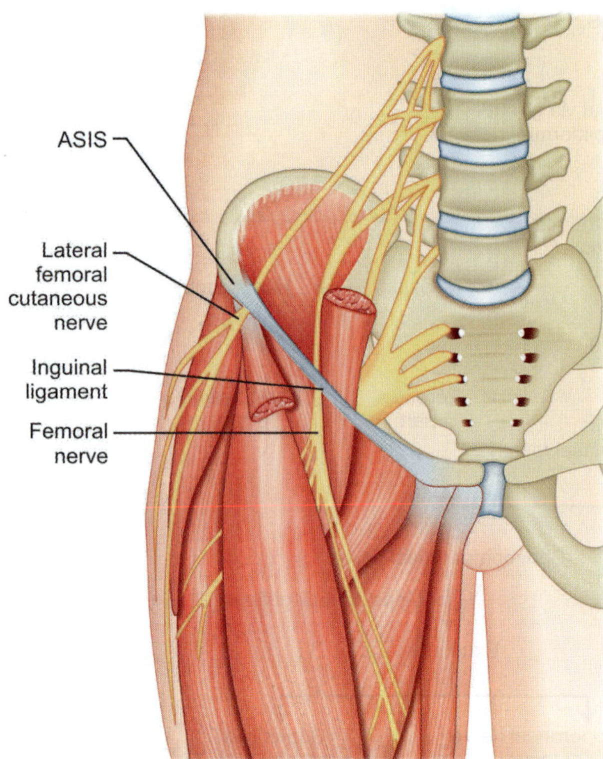

Fig. 8.33: Anatomy of femoral nerve

Clinical Testing

A complete lesion of sciatic nerve will lead to paralysis of both the dorsiflexors and plantar flexors of the foot. Majority of the sensations would be lost except the area supplied by saphenous nerve (medial aspect till ball of great toe) as the latter is a branch of femoral nerve.

Common peroneal nerve palsy manifests as paralysis of the dorsiflexors and evertors of the foot, thereby leading to a complete foot drop. The patient walks with the classical "high stepping gait". The plantar flexors on examination are normal (as they are supplied by tibial nerve).

At times only the *deep peroneal nerve* may be injured. It supplies the dorsiflexors of foot. Injury would lead to foot drop but since peronei escape (supplied by superficial peroneal) the drop is not complete as eversion masks the drop to some extent. One can detect good power in the peronei (evertors) in such cases and finding sensory loss in the autonomous zone (first web space), with intact sensation over lateral leg (from superficial peroneal) further strengthens the diagnosis.

In injuries of the *tibial nerve*, the plantar flexors are paralyzed and can be evaluated by asking the person to plantar flex the foot against resistance. Moreover, sensations on the sole of the foot may also be lost.

HIGH-YIELD POINTS

- Most common PNI is radial nerve. Most common nerve injury in athletes is stingers (*see* Page 277). Most common combined nerve injury is median plus ulnar nerve.
- Least common nerve involved in entrapment is femoral nerve.

- Most common cause of wrist drop is fracture shaft humerus causing radial nerve palsy.
- Most common cause of neurological deficit in upper limb is Erb's palsy.
- Most common cause of sciatic nerve injury is iatrogenic (total hip replacement that causes traction injury mostly). Other causes include gunshot injury (most common cause for complete division), hip dislocations, intramuscular gluteal injections and acute compression (coma, drug overdose, intensive care unit, prolonged sitting), etc.
- Most common nerve injury in total hip arthroplasty is sciatic nerve.
- Most common nerve injury involved in intramuscular injection injury is sciatic nerve followed by radial nerve.
- Post injection palsy is neurotmesis.

MANAGEMENT OF NERVE INJURIES

The first step for deciding the line of management in the patient presenting with nerve injury depends upon the presentation, whether the injury is open or closed **(Fig. 8.34)**.

Open Laceration

In case there is an open laceration of the nerve, the wound is inspected, debrided and if clean, the nerve is directly repaired end to end with fine sutures under an operating microscope. This is called primary repair (primary neurorrhaphy). However, at times the wound is dirty, contaminated and not fit for a primary closure. In such cases after thorough debridement, the nerve ends are tagged. Patient comes for regular dressings and after around 2 weeks, once the tissue condition improves, the nerve is repaired and the wound closed (delayed primary repair).

Closed Injury

In cases where the nerve injury is closed, time is given to the nerve to heal and repair itself, as many cases may be only a neurapraxia of nerve. The patient is observed for a period of 6 weeks to 3 months to assess any signs of nerve recovery, which may include a progressive Tinel's sign, motor march or sequential electrodiagnostic study (EDS) analysis indicating nerve regeneration.

If there is positive evidence of regeneration, conservative treatment is continued. But if there are no signs of recovery by 3 months or a maximum by 6 months, the patient is planned for a nerve exploration procedure. The nerve is explored and the further treatment decided by the results of exploration.

Two situations are possible on exploring the nerve:

1. *Nerve is found intact but engulfed in scar tissue, as would be the scenario in cases with partial cuts/axonotmesis*: In such cases, the appropriate management is neurolysis. This procedure involves relieving the nerve from the enveloping scar when it is called external neurolysis or splitting the nerve sheath and then longitudinally dissecting the nerve to relieve pressure from the fibrous tissue inside, called internal neurolysis.

2. *Nerve if found to be completely transacted*: In these cases, a nerve repair is planned (called secondary repair or secondary neurorrhaphy as it is being done after few weeks or months). If the two ends of the nerve can be brought together without any tension on the suture line, the nerve is repaired end to

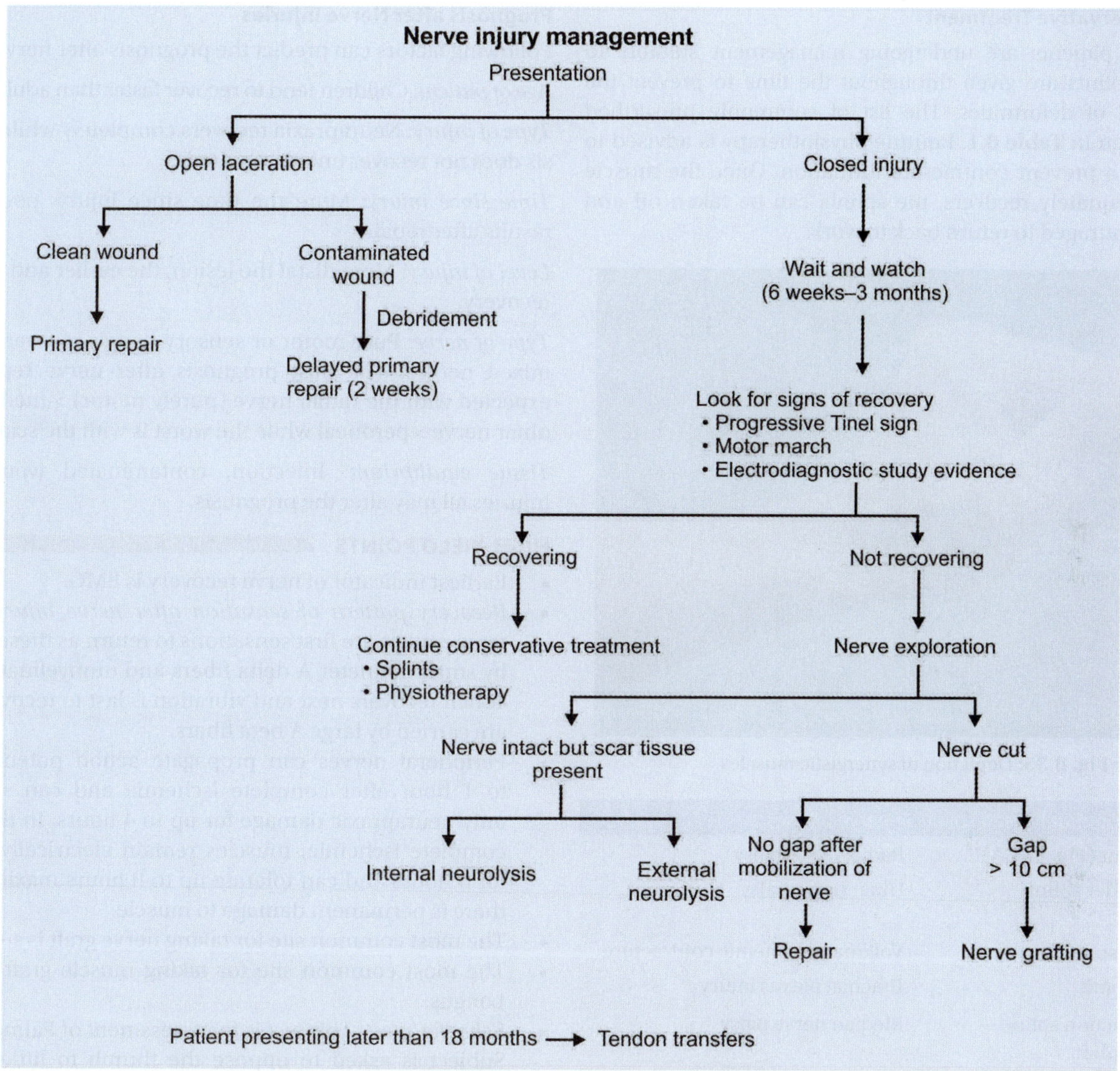

Fig. 8.34: Protocol for management of nerve injuries

end. In cases where there is an anticipation of tension on the stitches, a nerve grafting procedure is generally opted for.

Important sites of harvesting nerve grafts include:
Sural nerve (most common and largest donor graft of approximately 10 cm), superficial radial nerve, cutaneous nerve grafts.

However, before deciding to opt for nerve grafting, one must adequately mobilize the nerve trunk to ensure easy approximation of nerve ends. There are various methods of mobilizing a nerve, which include mobilization of the nerve, positioning of the limbs, transposition, bone resection, nerve stretching and bulb suture, nerve grafting and nerve crossing.

Nerve repairs can have good results up to a year after injury. At times the patient may present even late. If the time since injury has been more than 18 months to 2 years, then repairing the nerve is generally of no use as the neuromuscular junctions have already degenerated by this time. The treatment under such circumstances is tendon transfers.

Tendon Transfers

These are reconstructive surgical procedures where the lost function of a denervated muscle/tendon is reconstructed by using an expendable/extra donor tendon.

Important principles of tendon transfers to decide appropriate donor include:
- The donor muscle should be expendable, powerful enough (more than grade 4 power) and be an agonist or synergist. Synergist muscles are those that simultaneously contract during single movement, e.g. in gripping an object, wrist dorsiflexes while fingers flex (**Fig. 8.35**). So, wrist dorsiflexors and finger flexors are synergistic muscles and can be used to replace each other.
- The recipient site must have supple and mobile joints.
- The transferred tendon should be routed subcutaneously and placed in straight line of pull.
- The patient should be motivated and cooperative enough to attend physiotherapy and rehabilitation clinics.

Role of Conservative Treatment

While these patients are undergoing management suitable to the injury, splints are given throughout the time to prevent the development of deformities. The list of commonly prescribed splints is given in **Table 8.1**. Routine physiotherapy is advised to all patients to prevent contracture formation. Once the muscle function adequately recovers, the splints can be taken off and patients encouraged to return back to work.

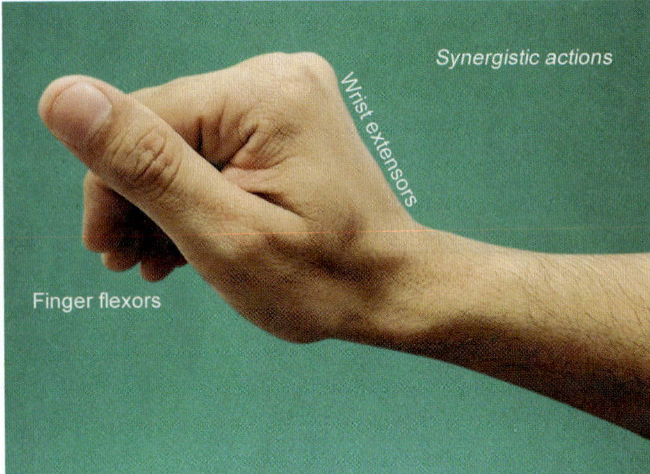

Fig. 8.35: Depiction of synergistic muscles

Table 8.1: Commonly used splints in nerve injuries	
Cock up splint **(Fig. 8.36A)**	Radial nerve palsy
Knuckle bender splint **(Fig. 8.36B)**	Ulnar nerve palsy
Turn buckle splint	Volkmann ischemic contracture
Aeroplane splint	Brachial plexus injury
Thumb abduction splint, opposition splint	Median nerve palsy
Ankle foot orthosis (foot drop splint)	Common peroneal nerve palsy

Prognosis after Nerve Injuries

Following factors can predict the prognosis after nerve repair:

Age of patient: Children tend to recover faster than adults.

Type of injury: Neurapraxia recovers completely while neurotmesis does not recover unless repaired.

Time since injury: More the time since injury, poorer are the results after repair.

Level of injury: More distal the lesion, the earlier and better is the recovery.

Type of nerve: Pure motor or sensory nerves recover better than mixed nerves. The best prognosis after nerve repair can be expected with the radial nerve (purely motor) > median nerve > ulnar nerve > peroneal while the worst is with the sciatic nerve.

Tissue equilibrium: Infection, contaminated wounds, crush injuries all may alter the prognosis.

HIGH-YIELD POINTS

- Earliest indicator of nerve recovery is EMG.
- *Recovery pattern of sensation after nerve injury:* Pain and temperature are first sensations to return as these are carried by small diameter A delta fibers and unmyelinated C fibers. Touch recovers next and vibration is last to recovers as these are carried by large A beta fibers.
- Peripheral nerves can propagate action potentials for up to 1 hour after complete ischemia and can survive with only neurapraxic damage for up to 4 hours. In the setting of complete ischemia, muscles remain electrically responsive for 3 hours and can tolerate up to 8 hours maximum before there is permanent damage to muscle.
- The most common site for taking nerve graft is sural nerve.
- The most common site for taking muscle graft is Palmaris Longus.
- *Schaefer's test:* This test is for assessment of Palmaris Longus. Subject is asked to oppose the thumb to little finger and then flex the wrist which makes the tendon prominent (*see* **Fig. 8.17**).

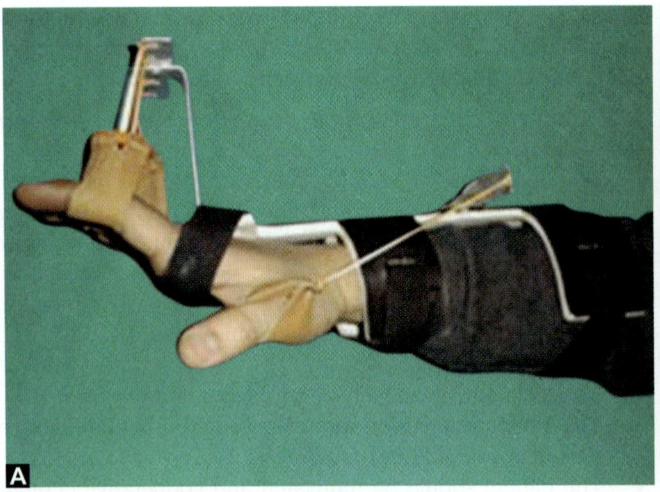

A

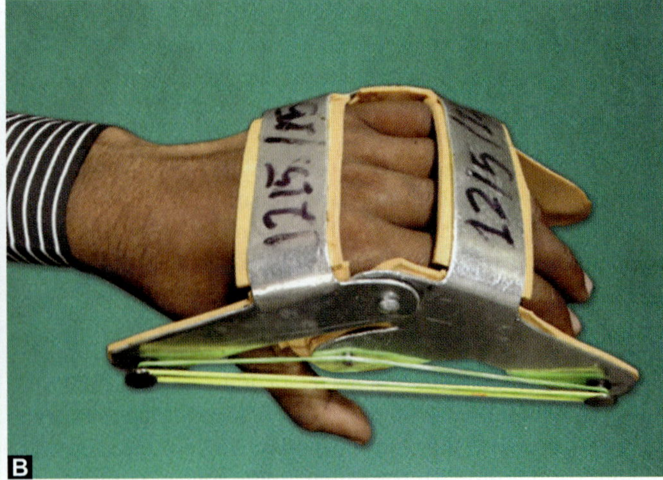

B

Figs 8.36A and B: (A) Cock up splint for wrist drop in radial nerve palsy; (B) Knuckle bender splint for neutralizing clawing in ulnar nerve palsy

NERVE ENTRAPMENT SYNDROMES (COMPRESSION NEUROPATHIES)

Few nerves have some part in their course when they have to travel in a confined space. In such areas, these nerves or their branches are highly susceptible to compression **(Table 8.2)**. Some important compression neuropathies include the following.

Carpal Tunnel Syndrome

Definition

It is the compression neuropathy of the median nerve below the flexor retinaculum. It is the most common compression neuropathy.

Etiology

This entity is common in middle-aged females and is associated with rheumatoid arthritis, hypothyroidism (second most common cause), pregnancy, acromegaly, diabetes, amyloidosis and hyperparathyroidism. However, the most common cause is idiopathic.

Clinical Features

The patient usually presents with pain, paresthesias in the wrist and hand and sensory motor weakness in the median nerve distribution. Pain characteristically occurs at night awakening the patient from bed and increases on activity.

Examination

Examination reveals a positive Phalen's test (symptoms reproduced when wrist is kept in flexion for a minute; **Fig. 8.37A**), Durkan's test (compression over the flexor retinaculum reproduces symptoms) and a positive Tinel's sign. Symptoms are reproduced when a tourniquet is applied and inflated. Positive hand diagram and Semmes-Weinstein monofilament testing are other tests of less practical utility. Durkan's test is best out of these.

Investigations

Diagnosis is usually confirmed by delay in conduction velocity on NCV. A distal motor latency of more than 8.5 ms and distal sensory latency of more than 3.5 ms is considered positive.

Treatment

Management involves treatment of the underlying condition. Nonsteroidal anti-inflammatory drugs (NSAIDs) and steroid injections are useful in selected patients while nonresponders need surgical decompression of the nerve.

Cubital Tunnel Syndrome

Cubital tunnel syndrome involves compression of ulnar nerve in the cubital tunnel under Osborne's ligament. It is the second most common compression neuropathy after carpal tunnel syndrome. Causes of ulnar nerve compression in cubital tunnel may be primary (idiopathic) or secondary (following trauma, arthritis, lipoma, ganglion, etc.)

Clinical Features

Patients present with forearm pain and numbness and paresthesia in of the 4th and 5th fingers. Examination may reveal typical features of ulnar nerve involvement (i.e. positive book test, card test, etc.). Atrophy of the intrinsic muscles of the hand and clawing is seen in long standing cases.

Table 8.2: Compression neuropathies	
Carpal tunnel syndrome	Median nerve at wrist
Pronator syndrome	Median nerve between two heads of pronator teres
Kiloh-Nevin syndrome	AIN branch of median nerve
Radial tunnel syndrome	PIN branch of radial nerve
Cubital tunnel syndrome	Ulnar nerve behind the medial epicondyle
Guyon's canal	Ulnar nerve at wrist below pisohamate ligament
Piriformis syndrome	Sciatic nerve compression
Meralgia paresthetica	Lateral cutaneous nerve of thigh (branch of femoral nerve)
Cheralgia paresthetica	Superficial sensory branch of radial nerve
Tarsal tunnel syndrome	Posterior tibial nerve
Morton's metatarsalgia	Interdigital nerve compression

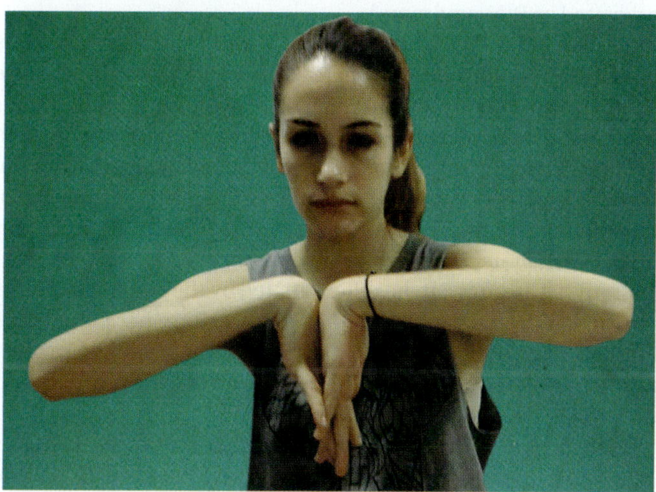

Fig. 8.37A: Phalen's test

Management

Diagnosis is mainly clinical and can be confirmed by positive electrodiagnostic studies. Mild cases with a recent history are observed with physiotherapy and nocturnal elbow splinting. In nonresponding cases cubital tunnel decompression (either open or endoscopically assisted) is done.

Tarsal Tunnel Syndrome

It is analogous to carpal tunnel syndrome in the upper limb. The nerve involved is the tibial nerve at the flexor retinaculum or the laciniate ligament.

Etiology

It is usually idiopathic in nature but may occur in association with rheumatoid arthritis (next common cause), ankylosing spondylitis, ganglion or tumors encroaching the tarsal tunnel or in talar and calcaneal fractures.

Clinical Features

The patient presents with burning pain or paresthesias over plantar aspect of the foot more at night and on bearing weight.

Examination

Positive Tinel's sign is evident. Muscle weakness may not be severe and sensory signs predominate. Diagnosis is confirmed by increased difference of the conduction velocities between lateral and medial plantar nerves.

Management

Treatment by release of tarsal tunnel is not as satisfactory as carpal tunnel syndrome.

Radial Tunnel Syndrome

Radial tunnel is approximately 5 cm long space in front of elbow extending from the radiocapitellar joint to proximal margin of supinator. The term radial tunnel syndrome (RTS) indicates compression of PIN in radial tunnel by fibrofascial bands coursing superficial to the radial head, the radial recurrent artery, the fibrous edge of the extensor carpi radialis brevis (ECRB), the proximal and distal edges of the supinator. The most common point of compression is the arcade of Fröhse (free aponeurotic proximal margin of supinator, in which case the condition is specifically designated as PIN syndrome).

Radial tunnel syndrome and posterior interosseous nerve (PIN) syndrome (supinator syndrome) both are cause of intractable lateral elbow pain and can present with similar symptoms. The clinical presentation includes pain 5 cm distal to the lateral epicondyle over the course of the radial nerve down the forearm. Typically, patients have pain with resisted extension of the long finger with the elbow in extension, forearm in pronation and the wrist in neutral.

Both syndromes can be differentiated by the fact that patients with PIN syndrome have a loss of motor function whereas patients with RTS have only lateral forearm pain without motor involvement. The difference in clinical presentation may be due to differences in the degree of compression.

Nonsurgical treatment of radial tunnel syndrome includes rest, NSAID and steroid injection if associated with lateral epicondylitis. Surgical decompression provides excellent result in most of patients.

Anterior Interosseous Syndrome (Kiloh-Nevin Syndrome)

It refers to compression of the AIN branch of Median nerve usually by the deep head of Pronator teres, FDS arch, edge of lacertus fibrosus or Gantzer's muscle (accessory head of FPL). Typically, these patients have only motor deficits) and they fail to make an "O.K." sign (Kiloh-Nevin sign, **Fig. 8.37B**), as flexion of the interphalangeal joint of the thumb (FPL) and the distal interphalangeal joint of the index finger (FDP) is impaired. Parsonage-Turner syndrome is a variant where there are bilateral AIN signs caused by viral induced brachial plexus neuritis.

Nonsurgical treatment is same as above but surgical decompression may be needed in nonresponding cases.

Morton's Neuroma/Morton's Metatarsalgia

It is a benign neuroma of an intermetatarsal plantar nerve, most commonly of the second and third intermetatarsal spaces. It presents with pain and numbness or paresthesias, particularly on weight bearing. On examination, one may find Mudler's click (a click on squeezing the two metatarsal heads). Ultrasound

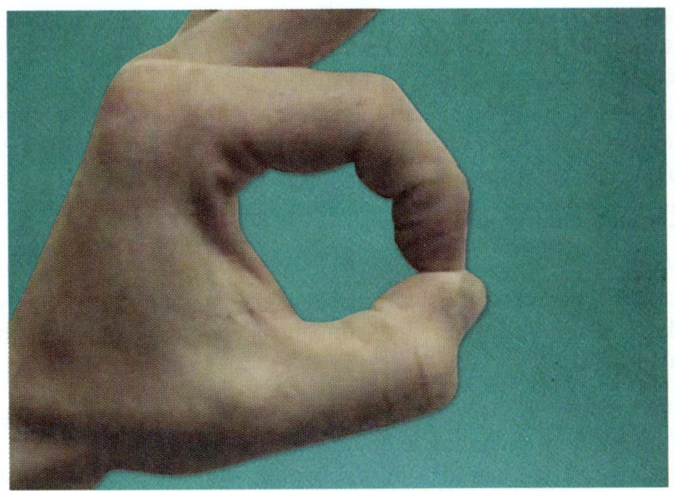

Fig. 8.37B: Kiloh-Nevin sign in anterior interosseous nerve (AIN) syndrome

accurately demonstrates thickening of the interdigital nerve within the web space of greater than 3 mm, diagnostic of a Morton's neuroma. Biopsy reveals that the affected nerve is markedly distorted, with extensive concentric perineural fibrosis. Orthotics, steroid injections and neurectomy are methods of management. Radiofrequency and cryoablation is upcoming treatment modality.

Meralgia Paresthetica

This chronic neurological disorder involves entrapment or compression of the lateral cutaneous nerve of thigh where it passes between the iliac crest and the inguinal ligament near the attachment at the anterior superior iliac spine. Injury to the nerve can also occur after performing McRobert's maneuver for delivering a child. Pain on the lateral side of the thigh radiating to the groin or outer side of the knee is the usual presenting complaint in the adult. It may be associated with a burning sensation, tingling and numbness in the same area. EMG, nerve conduction studies may help in the diagnosis. NSAIDs and heat therapy may help initially. Refractory cases respond to surgical decompression of the nerve.

HIGH-YIELD POINTS

- The growth potential of adult nervous system is limited. The lack of axonal growth after injury is due to several factors:
  - Due to formation of glial scar (formed by astrocytes and acts as a physical barrier to growth)
  - Intrinsic growth state of neuron
  - Absence of neurotrophic growth factors
  - Presence of myelin associated growth inhibitory molecules i.e. myelin associated glycoproteins (MAG), oligodendrocyte myelin glycoprotein (Omgp) and Nogo-A (an integral membrane protein predominantly expressed by oligodendrocytes).
- Anomalous connections between median and ulnar nerves
  - Martin-Gruber anastomoses can occur when branches of the median nerve cross over in the forearm and merge with the ulnar nerve to innervate portions of the ulnar supply in the hand.

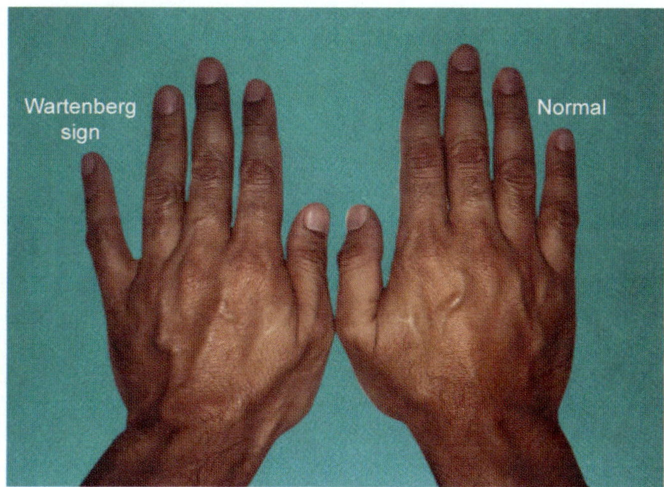

Fig. 8.37C: Wartenberg sign. Note greater abduction of little finger on side of ulnar nerve palsy as the finger is extended and kept flat on table

- – Riche-Cannieu anastomoses can occur when there is connection between recurrent branch of the median nerve and deep branch of the ulnar nerve of the hand.
- *Mobile wad of Henry:* It consists of three forearm muscles— brachioradialis, extensor carpi radialis longus and brevis. It presents in dorsolateral aspect of forearm and is important landmark for surgical approaches in this area.
- *Wartenberg sign:* This is a neurological sign seen in ulnar nerve neuropathy. Since the palmar interossei (adductor) of the 5th digit is paralyzed in ulnar nerve palsy, one may notice little finger resting in slightly greater abduction as it is extended by the radial nerve innervated extensor digiti mini muscle **(Fig. 8.37C)**. This should not be confused with Wartenberg's syndrome, which is also called cheiralgia paresthetica. It is a rare condition in which compression of the superficial branch of the radial nerve causes pain and paresthesiae on the radial side of the dorsum of the hand, and in the thumb.
- Even though there is more clawing in low ulnar nerve palsy (ulnar paradox), the sensory loss in hand is same in both high and low palsies.
- *Double-crush phenomena:* The double-crush syndrome was initially described by Upton and McComas in 1973. They postulated that nonsymptomatic impairment of axoplasmic flow at more than one site along a nerve might summate to cause a symptomatic neuropathy. The hypothesis was postulated to explain the frequent association of a proximal and distal nerve compression syndrome, including carpal tunnel syndrome associated with cervical radiculopathy, brachial plexus compression with diabetic neuropathy.
- *Causes of winging of scapula:* Serratus anterior (true winging), trapezius paralysis and paralysis of rhomboides.
- Vasa nervorum are small blood vessels that supply the peripheral nerves. Sciatic nerve vasa nervorum is a branch of inferior gluteal artery.

BRACHIAL PLEXUS PALSY

INTRODUCTION

The brachial plexus is formed by the union of the anterior rami of C5, C6, C7, C8 and T1. Just distal to the scalene muscles, the C5 and C6 roots unite to form the upper trunk, the C7 root continues alone to form the middle trunk, and the C8 and T1 roots unite to form the lower trunk. The three trunks formed proceed inferolaterally behind the clavicle, and each divides into anterior and posterior divisions. The three posterior divisions unite to form the posterior cord, the anterior divisions of the upper and middle trunks unite to form the lateral cord, and the anterior division of the lower trunk continues alone to form the medial cord. These three cords embrace the axillary artery in the relationships that their names imply. A diagrammatic description of the plexus and its branches is shown in **Figure 8.38**.

Common causes of injury to the brachial plexus include traction injuries to the nerves during birth (most common cause) or during an accident and rarely fractures and dislocations around the shoulder or penetrating injuries of the axilla.

Injuries of the plexus can be either preganglionic or postganglionic. Avulsion of the nerve root from the spinal cord is a preganglionic lesion, i.e. disruption proximal to dorsal root ganglion. Rupture of a nerve root distal to ganglion or of a trunk or peripheral nerve is a postganglionic lesion. It is important to differentiate the two lesions **(Table 8.3)** as they have prognostic significance with preganglionic lesions seldom showing recovery.

Based upon the location of injury, the lesions can be classified into upper plexus injuries (almost 90% cases), lower plexus injuries and pan plexus lesions.

The upper plexus lesions tend to have a very good prognosis while the lower and pan plexus lesions have a poor prognosis.

Important features of the upper and lower plexus injuries are as follows.

UPPER PLEXUS INJURY (ERB'S PALSY)

It is the most common plexus injury causing neurological deficit in the upper limb. The injury occurs due to undue traction to the plexus when the shoulder is pulled to one side and head bends on to the opposite side as may occur during a difficult delivery or at times during anesthesia. Rarely, the cause may be a direct blow to the shoulder.

The lesion involves injury to upper trunk of brachial plexus (mainly C5 and partly C6) at the Erb's point, which is meeting point for six nerves.

The nerves involved and the muscles thus paralyzed are as under:

Musculocutaneous: Biceps, brachialis, coracobrachialis

Axillary: Deltoid, teres minor

Nerve to subclavius: Subclavius

Suprascapular nerve: Supraspinatus, infraspinatus.

Clinical Presentation

These patients present with the characteristic policeman tip hand/ porter's hand **(Fig. 8.39)**. The arm is adducted and internally rotated, elbow is extended and forearm is pronated. The opposite movements are lost, i.e. there is loss of abduction and external rotation of arm, loss of flexion of elbow, loss of supination of forearm and loss of supinator and biceps reflexes. Sensations may be lost over the regimental badge area (lateral aspect of upper arm).

LOWER PLEXUS INJURY (KLUMPKE'S PARALYSIS)

This type of lesion generally is caused by hyperabduction of the arm as in catching hold of a support while falling from height. The

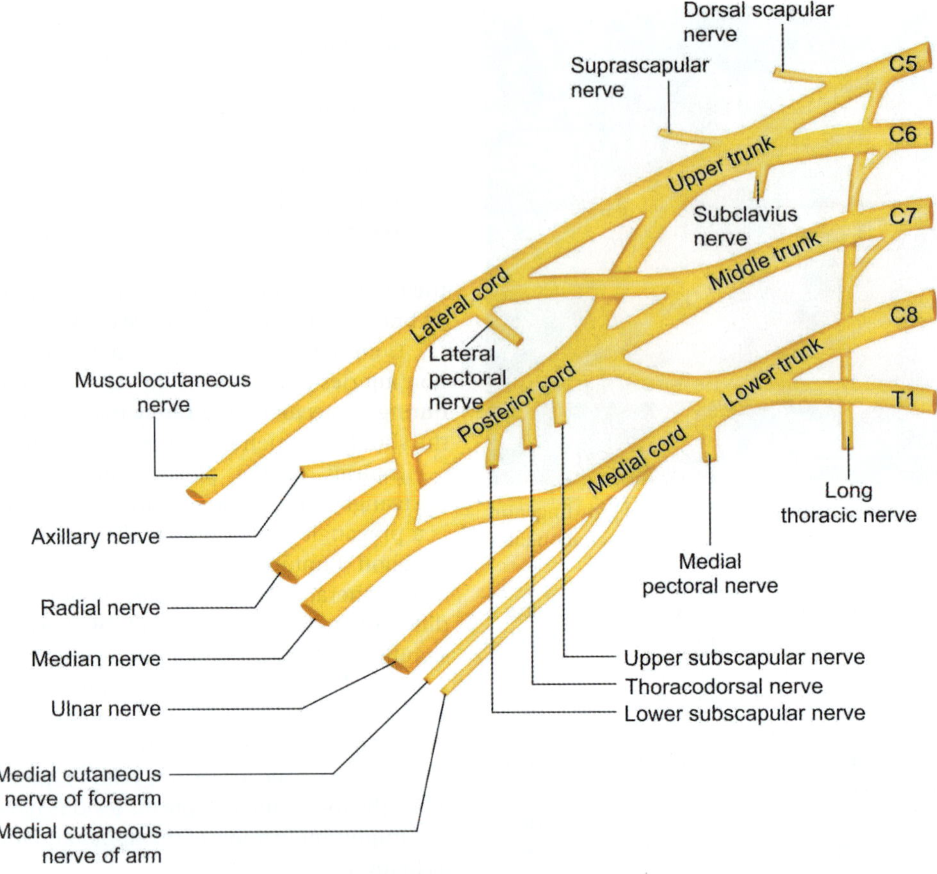

Fig. 8.38: Diagrammatic representation of brachial plexus

Table 8.3: Preganglionic versus postganglionic lesions

	Preganglionic lesion	Postganglionic lesion
Site	Proximal to the dorsal root ganglion (avulsion of root from cord)	Distal to dorsal root ganglion (disruption of peripheral nerve)
Histamine test	Intact (Put histamine on skin. There is cutaneous vasodilatation followed by wheal and then flare response.)	Flare response is absent
MRI	Pseudomeningomyeloceles are produced due to root avulsion	—
Nerve conduction study	Intact somatosensory conduction with absent somatosensory evoked potentials	—
Recovery	Poor	Potentially capable of recovering
Horner's syndrome	Present	Not seen

injury tears the lower trunk of the brachial plexus (mainly T1 and partly C8).

Muscles Paralyzed

- Intrinsic muscles of the hand (lumbricals and interossei) due to T1 involvement
- Ulnar flexors of the wrist due to C8 involvement.

Clinical Presentation

Paralysis of the intrinsic muscles of the hand causes the claw hand deformity. Horner's syndrome may be associated due to injury to sympathetic fibers to head and neck that leave the spinal cord through T1. The sensations in a narrow zone on the medial side of the forearm and hand may be diminished.

MANAGEMENT

Most injuries initially are managed conservatively with appropriate physiotherapy to prevent contractures. An aeroplane splint **(Fig. 8.40)** is given to keep shoulder abducted. Patient is observed for recovery of biceps function. If no recovery in the muscle is documented by 3 months, then the patient is advised a microsurgical exploration of the plexus and surgical repair of the lesion. Late cases present often with a deformity that may need appropriate release operations.

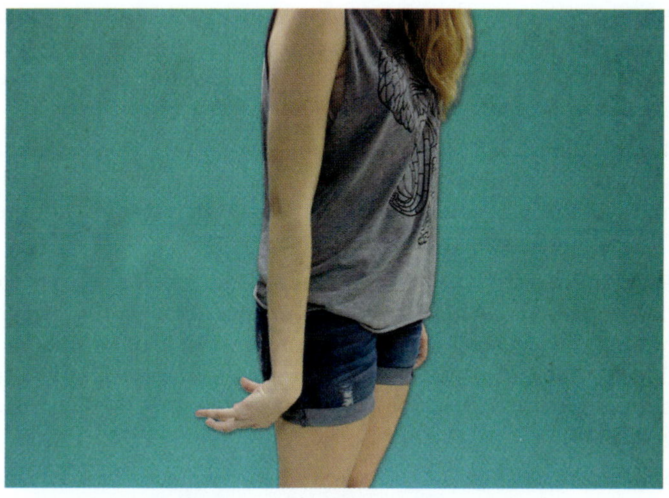

Fig. 8.39: Policeman tip/Porter's hand

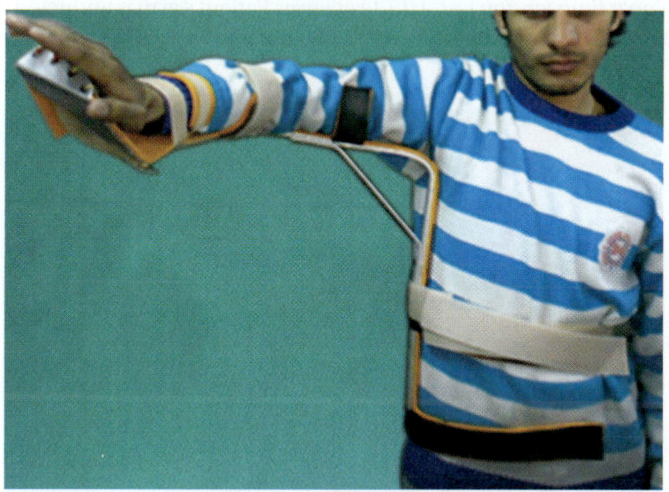

Fig. 8.40: Aeroplane splint

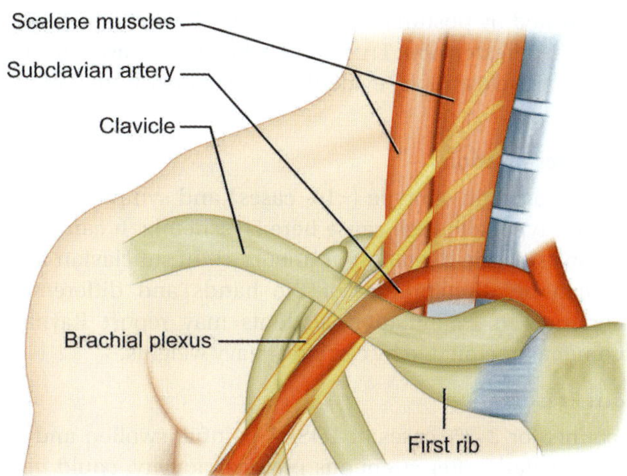

Fig. 8.41: Diagrammatic depiction of thoracic outlet

HIGH-YIELD POINTS

- In preganglionic lesions, repair is not possible and these avulsion injuries are managed by special procedures called neurotization, which involve nerve transfers like suprascapular to spinal accessory or intercostal nerves to musculocutaneous.
- *Burners/stingers*: These are mild traction injuries of brachial plexus in sports persons.

THORACIC OUTLET SYNDROME

INTRODUCTION

The thoracic outlet syndrome (TOS) describes a constellation of symptoms that arise from compression of the neurovascular structures as they course through the axilla to pass from base of neck to the arm. The outlet is basically bounded by the clavicle above, the first rib below, the scalenus anterior in front and scalenus medius behind **(Fig. 8.41)**. The structures mainly involved are the brachial plexus, the subclavian vein, and rarely, the subclavian artery. The outlet comprises of three narrow passages:

1. *Interscalene triangle*: Its boundaries are the scalenus anterior anteriorly, the scalenus medius muscle posteriorly and the medial surface of the first rib inferiorly. The triangle becomes even narrower with certain provocative maneuvers. Important pathologies causing constriction in this area are fibrous bands, cervical ribs and anomalous muscles.
2. *Costoclavicular triangle*: It is bounded by the clavicle anteriorly, the first rib posteromedially and the upper border of scapula posterolaterally.
3. *Subcoracoid space:* It lies beneath the coracoid process deep to the pectoralis minor tendon.

ETIOLOGY

The most common cause of TOS is physical trauma from probably nonergonomic postures and sports-related activities (repetitive stress injury). TOS results due to decreased outlet space due to abnormal posturing, hypertrophy of scalenus muscles (scalenus anticus syndrome), by compression from the cervical rib (fibrous/bony) or fractures/anomalies of nearby bones and shoulder girdle on arm movement. A pancoast tumor (superior sulcus pulmonary tumor) can also lead to TOS. Pregnancy can predispose to development of TOS as well. Rib exostosis and osteomyelitis in the area are few rarer causes.

CLINICAL PRESENTATION

Thoracic outlet syndrome manifests with signs and symptoms involving the arms and hands. Involvement may be unilateral or bilateral. The manifestations depend upon which structure (isolated or combinations) is compressed in the area of thoracic outlet: axillary/subclavian artery, subclavian vein or neurological structures (brachial plexus or the sympathetic nerves). Pain and paresthesia in ulnar nerve distribution are the most common symptoms.

Neurological Presentation

This is the most common presentation and account for more than 95% cases of TOS. Most patients complain of pain and paresthesias travelling down the arm from base of the neck that are aggravated by postural changes especially abduction of arm and neck hyperextension. True motor weakness is rare but can be there with muscle atrophy evident mostly in distribution of ulnar nerve (C8, T1).

Arterial Presentation

It is least common subtype (<1% cases) and symptoms mimic neurologic type, although cause here is ischemia. It can present with a poststenotic dilatation or aneurysm of subclavian artery. There can be discoloration of the hands and difference in temperature on examination. Patients may report Raynaud's phenomena precipitated by carrying heavy weights.

Venous Presentation

It accounts for 2–3% cases of TOS. A painful, swollen and blue arm, particularly after strenuous physical activity, could be the first sign of a subclavian vein compression. This rare entity and is known as Paget-Schroetter syndrome (PSS) or effort-induced thrombosis syndrome. The main pathophysiology of PSS involves congenital aberration of the costoclavicular ligament, which inserts far lateral to its usual insertion on the first rib. In the presence of hypertrophied scalenus anticus muscle vein is compressed and occluded.

ORTHOPEDIC CLINICAL TESTING MANEUVERS

*Adson's test (**Fig. 8.42**)*: Radial pulse is palpated with the arm by the side of the body. Now patient's arm is slightly abducted and extended. Patient is asked to turn the head to the side of symptomatic arm. A decreased pulse volume indicates positive compression. However, the sensitivity and positive predictive value of Adson's test is low and some surgeons have modified this test by tilting neck to opposite side or by looking for aggravation of symptoms rather than an absent pulse.

*Wright's test (**Fig. 8.43**) (also called hyperabduction maneuver)*: Palpate the radial pulse of the patient when the arms are by the side of the body. Now examiner places the patient's shoulder into hyperabduction above the head and holds this position for 1–2 minutes. Positive test is indicated by diminution of radial pulse and/or symptom reproduction.

*Halstead's test (**Fig. 8.44**)*: The examiner palpates the radial pulse and applies downward traction on the test extremity. The patient's neck is hyperextended and rotated to the opposite side. Disappearance of the radial pulse indicates a positive test.

*Military posturing/costoclavicular maneuver (**Fig. 8.45**)*: Patient stands in "attention position" with shoulders drawn posteriorly and inferiorly. Patient holds this position for one minute. Diminution of radial pulse constitutes a positive test.

Roos stress test/EAST test (Elevate abduct stress test: test for intermittent claudication): With the arms abducted, externally rotated and elevated overhead, patient is asked to open and close fingers, time and again for 1–3 minutes. A positive test is indicated by reproduction of symptoms (pain, numbness, tingling, etc.) (**Fig. 8.46**).

*Spurling's test (**Fig. 8.47**)*: Patient's head is placed in extension and lateral flexion and axial compression applied to the patient's head in an effort to simulate radicular pain.

Upper limb tension test (ULTT) of Elvey: Patient's arm is abducted to 90° with elbows extended now wrist is dorsiflexed. These maneuvers

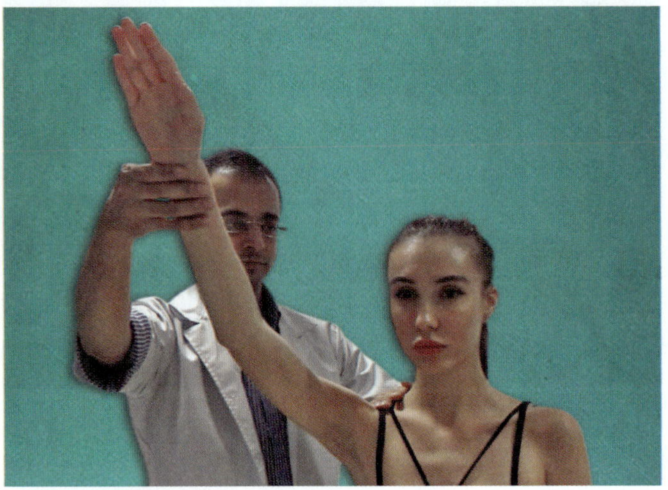

Fig. 8.43: Hyperabduction maneuver (Wright's test)

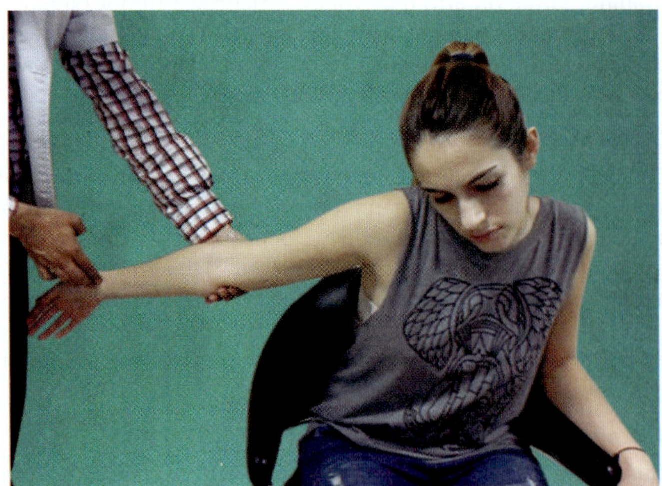

Fig. 8.42: Adson's test

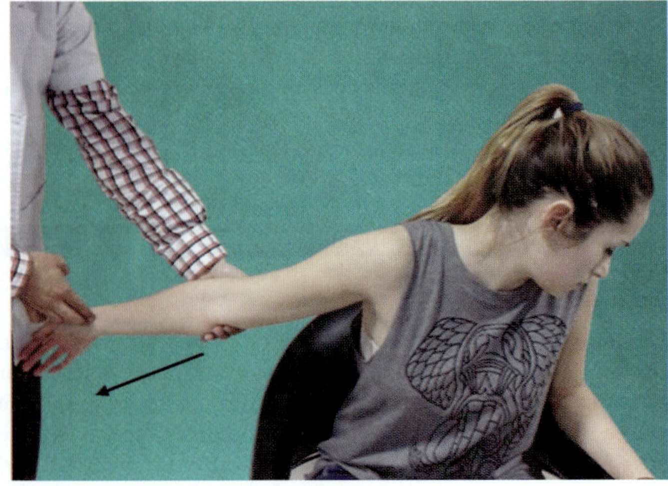

Fig. 8.44: Halstead's maneuver

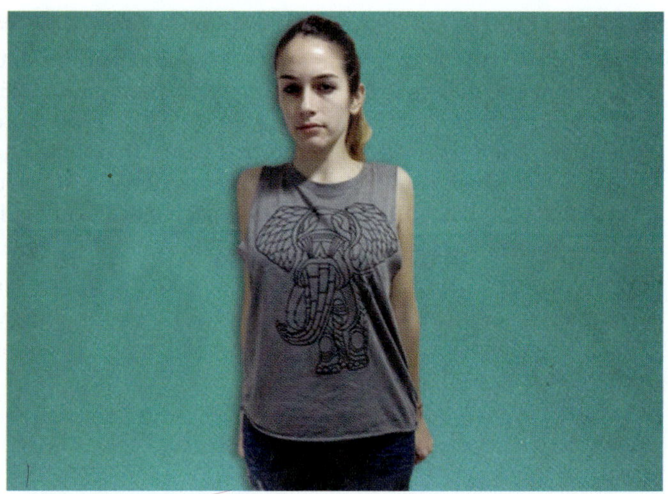

Fig. 8.45: Military posture

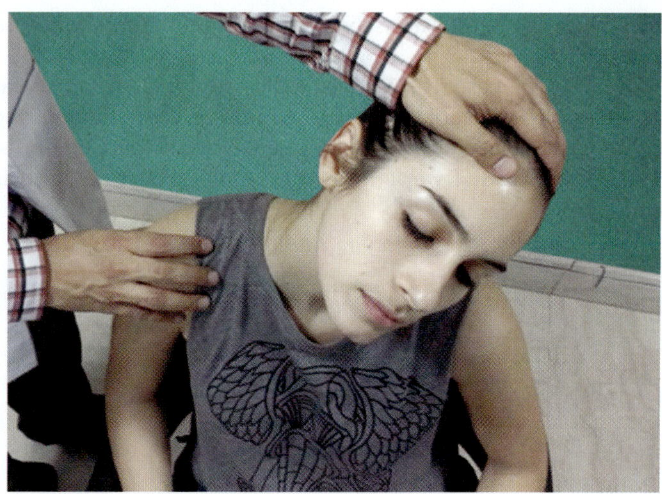

Fig. 8.47: Spurling's test

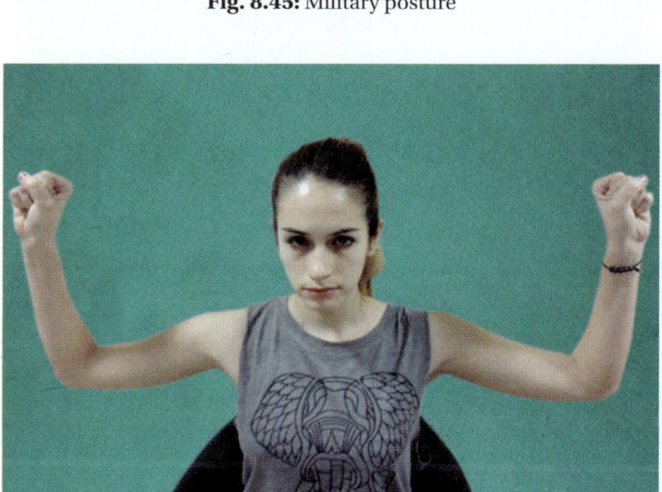

Fig. 8.46: Roos test

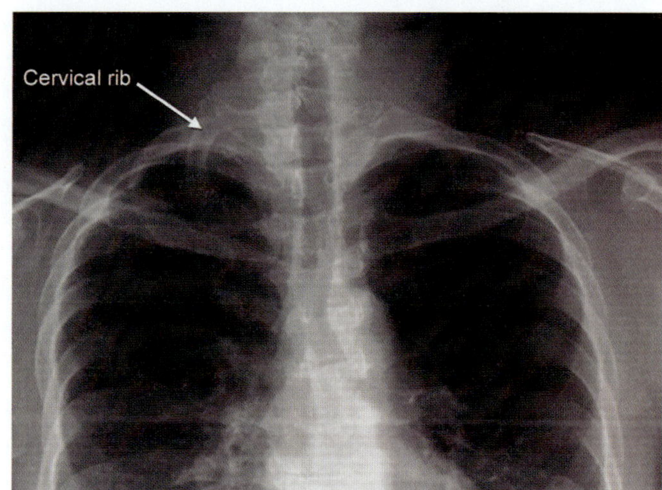

Fig. 8.48: X-ray showing cervical rib on right side

progressively stretch the brachial plexus and cause symptoms on ipsilateral side. Now patient is instructed to tilt the head to contralateral side, ear to shoulder. This will further increase the stretch on the brachial plexus. Reproduction of nerve compression signs and symptoms (pain, paresthesia and numbness) indicate neurogenic TOS. This test can be done simultaneously for both sides.

Gilliatt-Sumner hand: Atrophied abductor pollicis brevis, interossei, hypothenar muscles (ulnar distribution) can point toward the diagnosis.

ESTABLISHING THE DIAGNOSIS

Although a number of cardiac, pulmonary and esophageal disorders may mimic the presentation, the prime conditions to be ruled out include:

- Cervical discogenic pain
- Peripheral neuropathies (like carpal tunnel syndrome)
- Shoulder impingement syndrome.

Careful examination and serial X-rays **(Fig. 8.48)** are required to differentially diagnose between the positional/static and dynamic etiologies like first rib anomalies, scalene muscle spasm, and a cervical rib or fibrous band. Computed tomography (CT) scan and magnetic resonance (MR) scan may be helpful in dubious situations. Adson's test, Wright's test and costoclavicular maneuver are vascular tests they are of little value in diagnosis of much more common neurological TOS. Provocative clinical testing for TOS has been reported to display high rates of false positive findings. Diagnosis can be supported by vascular and electrodiagnostic studies. Venous ultrasound studies, venous scintillation scans and venography for venous TOS and Doppler ultrasound and angiography for arterial TOS can establish the diagnosis. Similarly, nerve conduction velocities and EMG of the medial antebrachial cutaneous nerve for the true neurogenic TOS are helpful investigations. Although these tests can support the diagnosis but diagnosis is mainly based on clinical findings as negative tests do not rule out the disease.

TREATMENT

All other patients should receive nonoperative treatment that includes adequate rest, NSAIDs, cervicoscapular strengthening exercises and modalities to counter pain and muscle spasm such as ultrasound, transcutaneous nerve stimulation and biofeedback.

Surgery in cases of TOS is indicated for acute vascular insufficiency (arterial/venous), progressively increasing neurological deficit and intractable pain for more than 3 months. Postoperative use of warfarin/low-molecular-weight heparin is mandatory.

HIGH-YIELD POINT

- *Allen's test*: This is a test for patency of ulnar artery and collateral circulation of the hand. Here, the ulnar and radial arteries are occluded and hand is exercised. The pressure on ulnar artery is released. In normal cases, the blanching completely disappears and this test is considered *positive* in such a case. If blanching persists in a specific distribution, it indicates absence of normal collateral supply–*negative test*.

Bone and Joint Infections

OSTEOMYELITIS

INTRODUCTION

Osteomyelitis (term coined by Nelaton) refers to inflammation of the bone and the marrow caused by an infective organism.

CLASSIFICATION

Osteomyelitis can be classified in a number of ways based on different criteria:

- *Waldvogel classification (modified):* Osteomyelitis is first described based on duration of symptoms as acute (<2 weeks), subacute (2–4 weeks) or chronic (>4 weeks), the time limits are though arbitrary. Second, it is further classified based on mode of spread of infection, which can be either hematogenous spread from a distant infective focus (commoner) or contiguous/direct spread from a nearby focus (open fractures, surgical wound) or infection occurring in an area of vascular insufficiency (usually seen in diabetes mellitus patients).

- *Cierny-Mader classification:* This system classifies osteo-myelitis based on the local environment (status of the affected bone/tissue) and adds a second dimension in the form of the physiological status of the host. While the status of affected bone/tissue is depicted as one of the four anatomical stages **(Fig. 9.1)**, a host is classified into either of three types: (1) Type A—normal, (2) Type B—immunocompromised, or (3) Type C—prohibitive (where the morbidity of treatment may be more than the expected benefits), allowing a total of 12 possible categories. The major advantage of this system is that the classification lends itself to guiding treatment and prognosis of the disease. Stage I may be managed only with conservative measures while higher stages may require aggressive debridement or even limb reconstructive procedures. The classification does not make use of the words "acute" or "chronic", rather, a peculiarity of the classification system is its dynamic nature, where the stages can change with time with treatment.

PATHOGENESIS

The infection usually starts in the metaphysis of long because of vascular stasis due to the "hair pin" like arrangement of metaphyseal blood vessels. As shown in **Figure 9.2**, as the arteries take a U-turn at the growth plate and return to become venous channels, there occurs stasis of blood flow which leads to accumulation of bacteria that overpower host's immunity.

Bacterial seeding in the metaphysis leads to inflammatory reaction, which causes local tissue necrosis and thus metaphyseal abscess formation. As the abscess enlarges, intramedullary pressure rises and pus escapes through the Volkmann's canal into the subperiosteal space. The periosteum is lifted from the bone and new bone formation occurs (it is an innate response in bone that whenever periosteum is lifted, there occurs new bone formation), which is referred to as periosteal reaction. This periosteal reaction is seen after 7–10 days of onset of symptoms **(Fig. 9.3A)**.

Now, after 2 weeks, acute osteomyelitis starts entering into a chronic phase. As periosteum is lifted, blood supply to underlying bone is damaged, so a part of the bone is rendered avascular. This avascular segment becomes dead, gets surrounded by infected granulation tissue and segregates from viable parent bone to form "sequestrum" (sequestrum means separated). Sequestrum formation generally takes around 3 months postinfection. Lack of blood supply to involved area makes it difficult for body to halt infection, so the body tries to wall off sequestrum by forming reactive new bone around it, which is referred to as "involucrum". But the organisms in the sequestrum have proteolytic enzymes and create openings in the involucrum that are called *cloaca*.

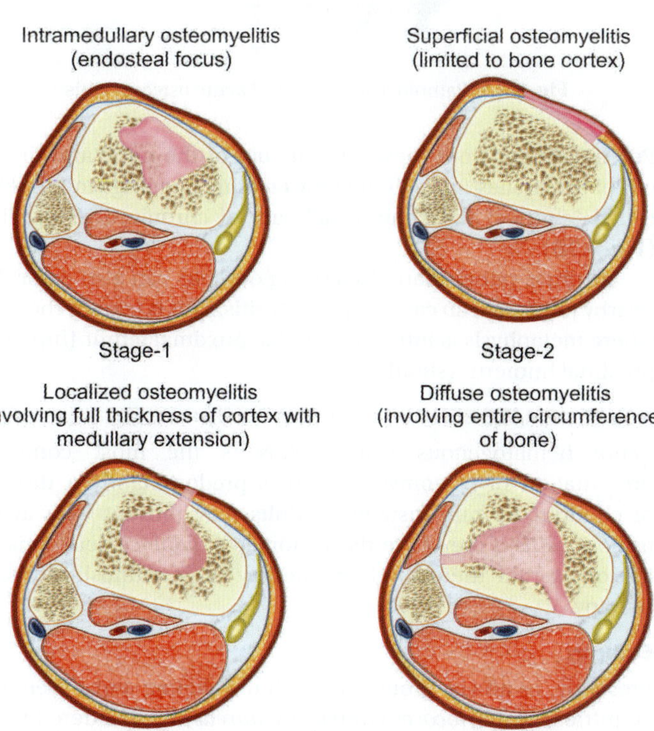

Fig. 9.1: Cierny-Mader classification of osteomyelitis depicting four stages (1–4)

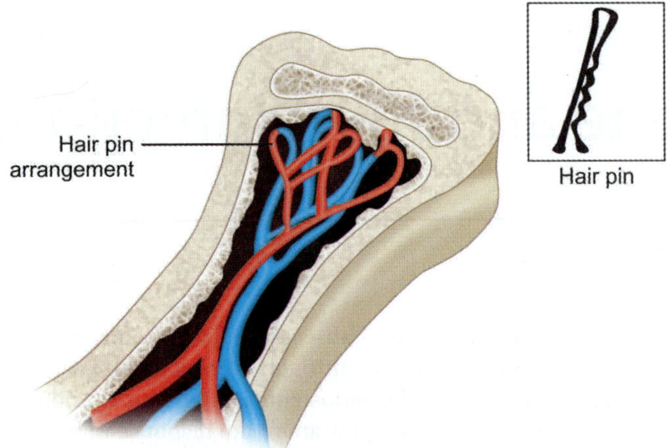

Fig. 9.2: Hair pin arrangement of vessels at metaphysis

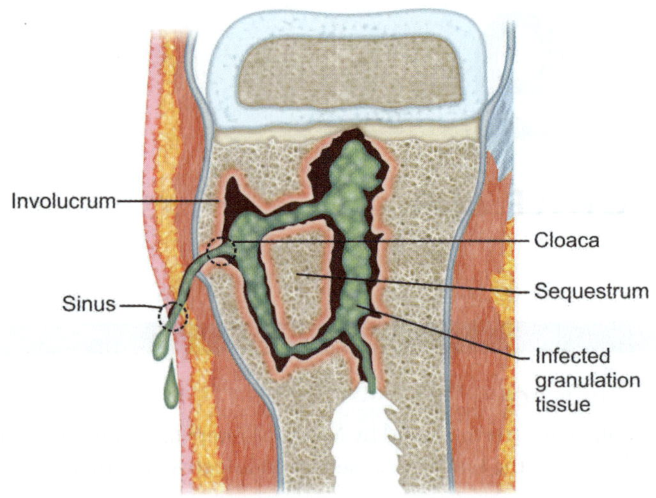

Fig. 9.3B: Pathological changes of chronic osteomyelitis

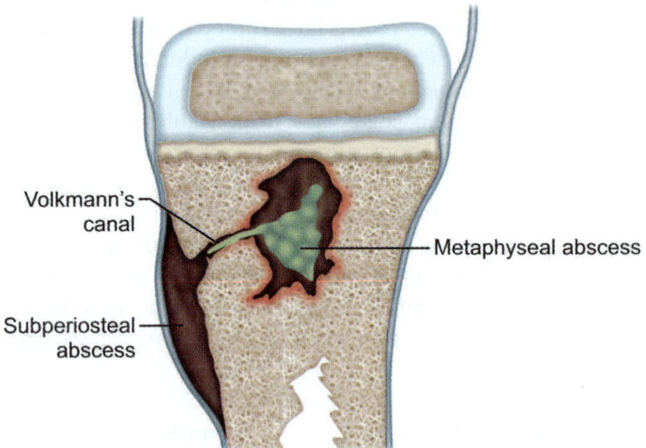

Fig. 9.3A: Pathological changes of acute osteomyelitis

> **Box 9.1:** Most common causative organisms of acute hematogenous osteomyelitis
>
> - In sickle cell disease patients—*Salmonella*
> - In IV drug abusers—*Pseudomonas*
> - In HIV and immunocompromised patients—*Staphylococcus aureus*
> - After an animal bite—*Pasteurella multocida*
> - After human bite—*Eikenella corrodens*
> - Diabetic foot ulcers—*Staphylococcus aureus*
> - In open fractures and post-traumatic cases—*Staphylococcus aureus*
> - In postsurgery cases—*Staphylococcus aureus*

Abbreviations: IV, intravenous; HIV, human immunodeficiency syndrome.

Pus travels out from these cloacae, out of the bone and finally out of the tissues and skin thereby creating openings in the skin, called "sinuses", the clinical hallmark of chronic osteomyelitis **(Fig. 9.3B)**.

At times rather than discharging out, pus can also enter the nearby joint and can cause septic arthritis. This is usually the case where metaphysis is intracapsular like proximal femur (hip) and proximal humerus (shoulder).

ACUTE HEMATOGENOUS OSTEOMYELITIS

Acute hematogenous osteomyelitis is the most common presentation of osteomyelitis and is predominantly a disease of children. In rare instances, adults may present with acute osteomyelitis if they have risk factors like diabetes, leukemia or are on steroid therapy, chemotherapy or immunosuppressive therapy.

Etiology

Presently, in all age groups (in both developing and developed countries) *Staphylococcus aureus (S. aureus)* is considered to be the most common causative organism, seen in 80–90% culture positive cases. Group B *Streptococci* are commonly (but not most common) seen in 0–6 months old infants. *Haemophilus*

influenzae infections were once very common in 6 months to 4 years aged children, the number having gone down significantly after introduction of Hib vaccine. **Box 9.1** shows the common etiological agents in some special categories of patients.

Clinical Features

The child classically presents with acute febrile illness with pain and swelling in the involved area (lower end of femur more than upper end of the tibia are the most common sites of affection in acute osteomyelitis). A history of injury may coincidentally be obtained. The cause is often difficult to trace unless the clinician has a high index of suspicion. The only clinical sign that may suggest the diagnosis is tenderness on pressing the metaphysis (metaphyseal tenderness).

Investigations

The diagnosis of acute osteomyelitis is by and large clinical, supplemented by following investigations **(Box 9.2)**:

Blood investigations: The white blood cell (WBC) count, erythrocyte sedimentation rate (ESR) and C-reactive protein (CRP) are elevated. Blood culture is positive in 50% of cases. Serum procalcitonin (> 0.4 ng/mL) is a sensitive and specific marker for acute osteomyelitis (and also septic arthritis).

X-ray: Haziness/soft tissue shadow due to increased blood flow is the earliest sign seen on X-ray within 48 hours of infection.

Box 9.2: Differential diagnosis of acute osteomyelitis

- *Acute septic arthritis:* In these patients, movements at the involved joint are extremely painful and aspiration of the joint would reveal pus
- *Scurvy:* Bone pain due to subperiosteal hemorrhages (pseudoparalysis of parrot) simulates acute osteomyelitis. Look for other features of malnutrition
- *Ewing sarcoma:* Ewing sarcoma patients may have a very similar clinical presentation as acute osteomyelitis. The two, however, can easily be differentiated from magnetic resonance imaging (MRI) and biopsy
- *Osteosarcoma:* Dilated veins in osteosarcoma (*see* **Figs 11.32A and B**, Page 326) arouse the suspicion. Classical X-ray signs, MRI and biopsy findings can help in cases with doubtful diagnosis
- *Acute rheumatic arthritis and juvenile rheumatoid arthritis (JRA):* Usually multiple joints are involved. Rheumatic arthritis has the characteristic fleeting (transient) and flitting (migratory from one joint to another joint) nature of joint pains
- *Sickle cell crises:* These are acute painful episodes occurring in patients with sickle cell anemia when sickled red blood cells get entrapped in the microvasculature. Patients may experience excruciating bone pain, however, blood smears can easily resolve the diagnostic dilemma

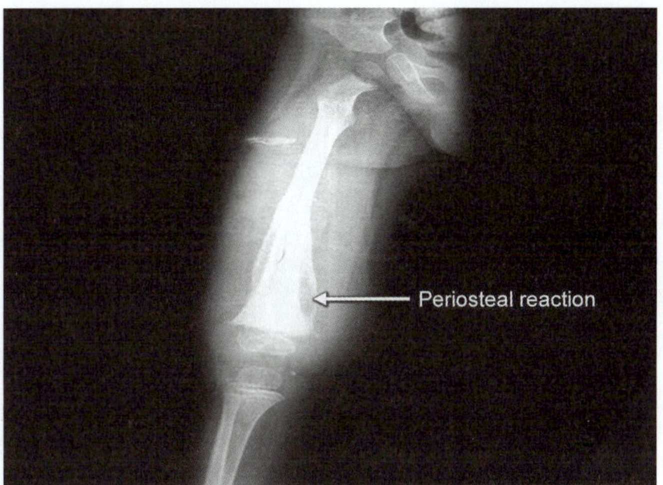

Fig. 9.4: X-ray of thigh with knee and hip joint showing periosteal reaction in acute osteomyelitis

However, the classical sign, easier to recognize, is the periosteal new bone formation evident at around 7–10 days postinfection **(Fig. 9.4)**.

Bone scan: It (Indium-111 labeled leukocytes preferred over Ga-67 or Technetium Tc-99m MDP) is useful in early stages where radiographs may be negative. It shows an area of increased uptake in the affected region within 24–48 hours and gives an early diagnosis. However, its nonspecific.

Magnetic resonance imaging (MRI): It provides the earliest diagnosis and it is the investigation of choice for acute osteomyelitis.

Bone aspiration of pus, gram stain and culture sensitivity: It is considered the gold standard for confirming diagnosis.

As per Morrey and Peterson criteria, definite diagnosis of osteomyelitis should be made only when histological evidence or organism can be recovered from bone tissue. They suggested osteomyelitis to be labeled 'probable' when X-ray findings, clinical features and blood cultures are positive but histological evidence is not obtained. And when blood cultures are also negative then osteomyelitis is 'likely' only if patient is responding to antibiotics.

Differential Diagnosis

The important conditions to exclude before finalizing the diagnosis of osteomyelitis have been tabulated in **Box 9.2**. If any doubt in diagnosis remains, Peltola and Vahvanen criteria may be used to establish the diagnosis of osteomyelitis. As per the criteria osteomyelitis exists when two out of following four factors are identified:

1. Pus aspirated from bone
2. Positive bone/blood culture
3. Clinical features present
4. Radiographic features present.

Management

Acute osteomyelitis is an emergency. The key to management is an early diagnosis.

General principles: General supportive care is given to the patient consisting of splintage and rest to the affected limb, elevation of the extremity, intravenous (IV) fluids and analgesics.

Antibiotics: Empirical broad spectrum antibiotics (cephalosporins to cover gram-positive and fluoroquinolones for gram negative coverage) are started and are changed to definitive on the basis of culture and sensitivity report. The antibiotics are given via IV route for first 2 weeks and oral for the next 4 weeks (total 6 weeks). But the antibiotic therapy is effective only before pus formation.

Surgery: Pus formation occurs by 2–3 days and hence if there is failure to improve despite appropriate antibiotic therapy for 72 hours, the patient is undertaken for urgent surgery. Incision and drainage of pus are the mainstay of surgical treatment. If no pus is found in soft tissue planes, drill holes are made in the metaphyseal area of bone and still if no pus comes out, one can go on to make a small metaphyseal bone window to drain out the pus.

Complications

- *Chronic osteomyelitis*: It is the most common complication. It is almost the outcome in immunocompromised patients
- Metastatic abscesses
- Septicemia in untreated cases
- Septic arthritis usually at joints where metaphysis is intra-articular
- Pathological fractures
- Growth plate disturbances ending up in limb length discrepancy.

BRODIE'S ABSCESS

This is a long standing localized form of osteomyelitis seen in cases where either the virulence of the infective organism is low or the immunity of the host is good, such that the host is able to localize the infection within the metaphysis. Proximal tibia is the

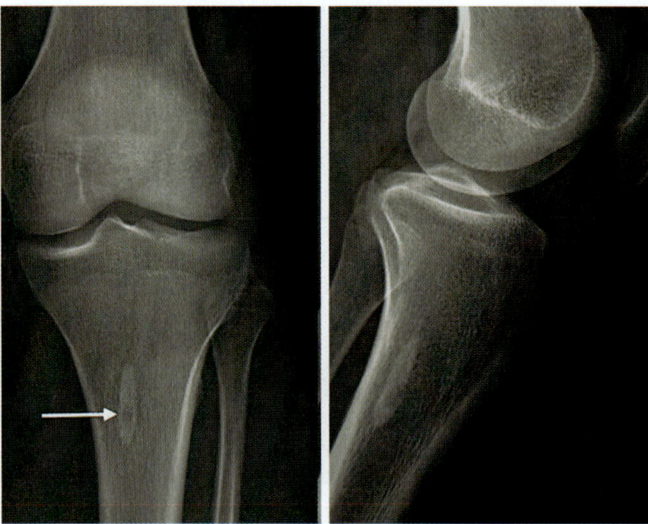

Fig. 9.5: X-ray, anteroposterior (AP) and lateral views of knee joint showing Brodie's abscess (arrow) in proximal tibia

most common site of affection and most affected patients are 10–20 years old (slightly older as compared to patients with acute osteomyelitis). A label "subacute osteomyelitis" was added to the entity by Billroth based on the classical clinical presentation. The condition typically has an indolent course and severity of symptoms is limited as compared to acute osteomyelitis. Most patients present with mild to moderate localized tenderness and intermittent pain that is worse at night and has persisted for more than 2 weeks.

Blood investigations (WBC counts, ESR, CRP) are usually within normal limits or mildly elevated. X-ray **(Fig. 9.5)** shows cavity at metaphyseal-epiphyseal junction with a rim of reactive new bone. Diagnosis can be confirmed by bone biopsy. *S. aureus* is the most common organism isolated. Treatment is curettage and bone grafting under an antistaphylococcal antibiotic cover.

CHRONIC OSTEOMYELITIS

Chronic osteomyelitis is defined as the presence of ongoing bone infection for longer than 1 month in the presence of devitalized/necrotic bone. It can simply be considered as a consequence of acute osteomyelitis that may lead to extensive bone necrosis, formation of sequestra and ultimately, segmental bone defects.

Etiology

Chronic osteomyelitis occurs as a sequel of acute osteomyelitis because of delay in its diagnosis or when acute osteomyelitis is inadequately treated. Open fractures, prolonged surgery (especially involving implant placement) and impaired host immunity are other important factors that lead to persistence of infection. Most common causative organism again is *S. aureus* and the most common bone involved is tibia followed by the femur and humerus.

Clinical Features

There are usually no systemic symptoms. Discharging sinus (especially with history of discharge of bony chips) is the clinical hallmark and the most common presenting symptom. On examination, the discharging sinus is generally fixed to the underlying bone and at times multiple puckered scar marks of healed sinuses may be visible **(Figs 9.6A to C)**. The surface of bone becomes irregular due to periosteal reaction and new bone formation and hence, irregular bony thickening and tenderness on deep palpation can be appreciated.

Diagnosis

The diagnosis is based on a combination of the clinical picture (presence of sinus) and laboratory (elevated ESR, CRP in all and raised WBC levels in 35% cases) and imaging studies.

X-rays: Sequestrum, the radiological hallmark of chronic osteomyelitis may indicate the diagnosis in some cases **(Fig. 9.7)**.

Sequestrum appears more radiodense than adjacent bone because of its avascularity as calcium is not resorbed from dead bone. Different etiologies may present with different types of sequestra **(Box 9.3)**. Involucrum (also radiodense) is the reactive new bone present outside the infected granulation tissue. In late cases, X-ray classically shows the typical appearance of multiple lytic and sclerotic areas which is called honeycombed pattern/moth-eaten appearance **(Fig. 9.9)**.

Other investigations: The valuable information provided by X-rays can be supplemented by MRI. MRI **(Fig. 9.6C)** may reveal a well-defined rim of high signal intensity surrounding the focus of active disease (Penumbra/Rim sign). A bone scan is mainly useful in acute cases not much in chronic as the former often has negative plain films. The gold standard for diagnosis remains a biopsy and preferably the sample should also be cultured to isolate the organism and guide antibiotics. A sinogram (injecting a radiopaque dye in the sinus to delineate it) should be done to localize the source of pus.

Treatment

Surgery is the mainstay of treatment. Since the source of persistent infection is sequestrum, surgery involves sequestrectomy (removal of the sequestrum), curettage of the walls of the cavity, creating the cavity into shape of a saucer (saucerization) and filling the cavity with antibiotic impregnated bone cement [polymethylmethacrylate (PMMA)] beads or bone grafts to eliminate dead space **(Fig. 9.10)**. Excision of sinus tract should follow to complete all the steps. After the surgery wound is usually closed over a continuous suction and irrigation system (Willenger's closed instillation suction technique) wherein irrigating fluid goes in via an inlet tube into the medullary cavity of bone and the same drains out after flushing the cavity via an outlet tube connected to a suction source. Amputation may rarely be done in cases with chronic discharging sinuses with malignant change or infected nonunion with failed multiple previous surgeries.

An antibiotic cover is always added to surgery. Rifampin is favored as a supplement to first-line antistaphylococcal antibiotics in chronic infection because it achieves intraleukocytic bactericidal concentration. Treatment involves IV antibiotics for 6 weeks and then oral antibiotics for another 6 weeks. However, depending upon response, medications for up to 6–9 months may be necessary.

Complications

- *Acute on chronic osteomyelitis:* Acute exacerbation is the most common complication of chronic osteomyelitis

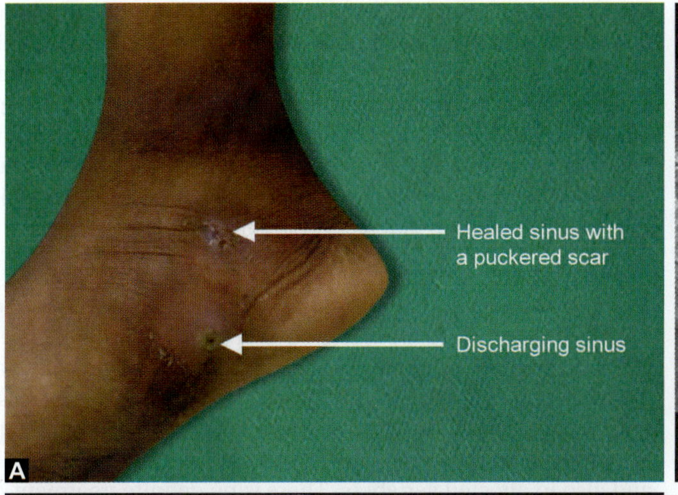

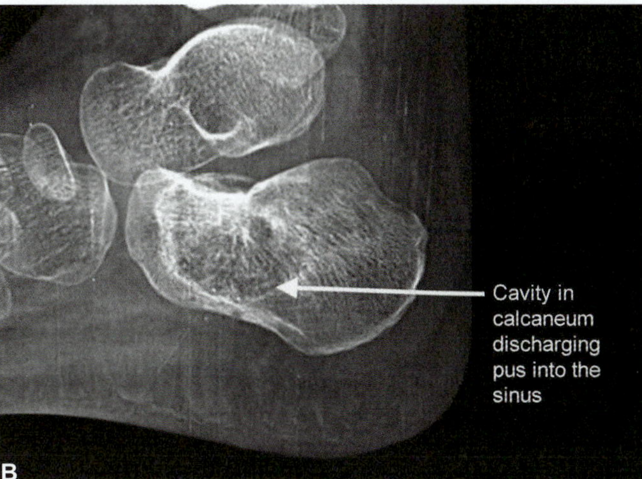

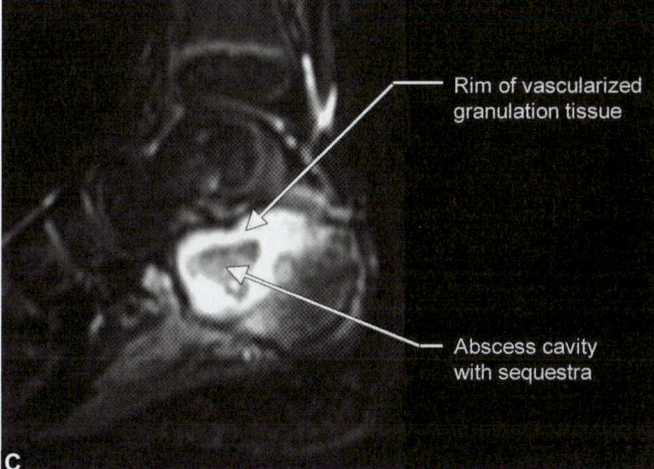

Figs 9.6A to C: (A) Sinus in the foot of a child, discharging pus with chronic osteomyelitis; (B) Lesion in the calcaneum on X-ray; and (C) An MRI showing the Rim (Penumbra) sign

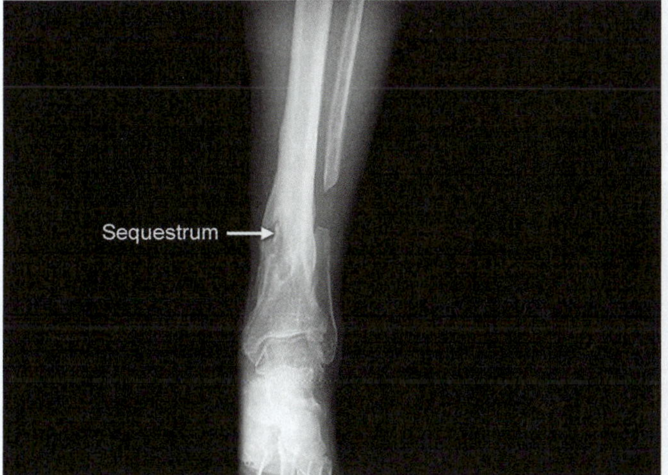

Fig. 9.7: X-ray, anteroposterior (AP) view of the ankle with leg showing sequestrum in the distal third of the tibia

> **Box 9.3:** Types of sequestrum in osteomyelitis
>
> - *Tubular sequestrum* **(Fig. 9.8D)**: Pyogenic osteomyelitis, infants
> - *Pencil like sequestrum*: Infants
> - *Ring sequestrum*: At the end of amputation stumps, around Steinman pins or pin tracts of external fixator **(Fig. 9.8C)**
> - *Conical/Annular sequestrum*: Amputation stumps
> - *Ivory sequestrum*: Syphilis
> - *Feathery sequestrum*: Tuberculosis (in cavity) **(Figs 9.8A and B)**, syphilis
> - *Coarse sandy sequestrum*: Tuberculosis (outside cavity)
> - *Rice grain sequestrum*: Tuberculosis
> - *Fine sandy sequestrum*: Viral osteomyelitis, in metaphyseal lesions of tuberculous osteomyelitis
> - *Kissing sequestrum*: Paradiscal tuberculosis spine
> - *Black sequestrum*: Actinomycosis, fungal osteomyelitis
> - *Colored sequestrum*: Fungal osteomyelitis
> - *Coralliform sequestrum*: Perthes disease
> - *Bombay sequestrum*: On the exposed surface of bone due to hydrogen sulfide deposition

- *Growth disturbances and limb deformities*: Both shortening (more common) and limb lengthening (due to increased blood flow) may result
- Pathological fractures
- Restricted joint movements leading to joint stiffness
- Amyloidosis
- Marjolin's ulcer, i.e. squamous cell carcinoma in the sinus tract (rarely sarcoma of bone).

SCLEROSING OSTEOMYELITIS OF GARRE

This is a nonsuppurative (i.e. no pus formation) chronic osteomyelitis characterized by marked bony sclerosis (whitening of bone) and cortical thickening **(Fig. 9.11)** and absence of sequestra. It is thought to be caused due to low grade possibly anaerobic bacteria. The mandible is most commonly affected site followed by diaphysis of a tubular bone (mostly tibia). Involved patients are mostly children and young adults (0–20 years). Clinically, patients may present with fever and pain worse at night, but unlike chronic osteomyelitis there are no discharging sinuses. The bone is tender to deep palpation. The ESR may be slightly elevated. Due to a fusiform osseous enlargement it is often confused with a bone tumor, but the classical age and the X-ray picture are diagnostic. Treatment is largely supportive and broad spectrum antibiotics may be given.

CHRONIC RECURRENT MULTIFOCAL OSTEOMYELITIS

This is a diagnosis that comprises of several different syndromes with features of an inflammatory bone disorder occurring in association with chronic skin lesions, viz. pustular lesions of palms and soles (palmar-plantar pustulosis) and pustular psoriasis. In 1972, the term "CRMO (chronic recurrent multifocal osteomyelitis)" was initially used to describe this condition as few cases were identified but as association with dermatological lesions was observed, and in 1987, the term "SAPHO (synovitis, acne, pustulosis, hyperostosis and osteitis)" was coined. Despite "osteomyelitis" in the name, there is no microorganism which has been isolated and neither is a discharge present. An autoimmune cause can be likely. Histology shows signs of chronic inflammation, but the exact etiology still remains to be elucidated.

Few of the clinical syndromes included in this spectrum are:

Sternocostoclavicular hyperostosis: This presentation is seen mostly in men aged between 40 years and 50 years. Disease affection is predominantly in sternum and adjacent bones and the vertebral column. X-rays classically depict hyperostosis of the medial ends of the clavicles and sternum. Radioscintigraphy also depicts increased activity around the sternoclavicular joints and also in affected vertebrae. There is no definite treatment, but symptoms tend to fade away in long-term follow-up. Recurrent flares are common and eventually lead to ankylosis of the affected joints in some patients.

Subacute recurrent multifocal osteomyelitis: This presentation is seen mainly in children and adolescents. There are recurrent

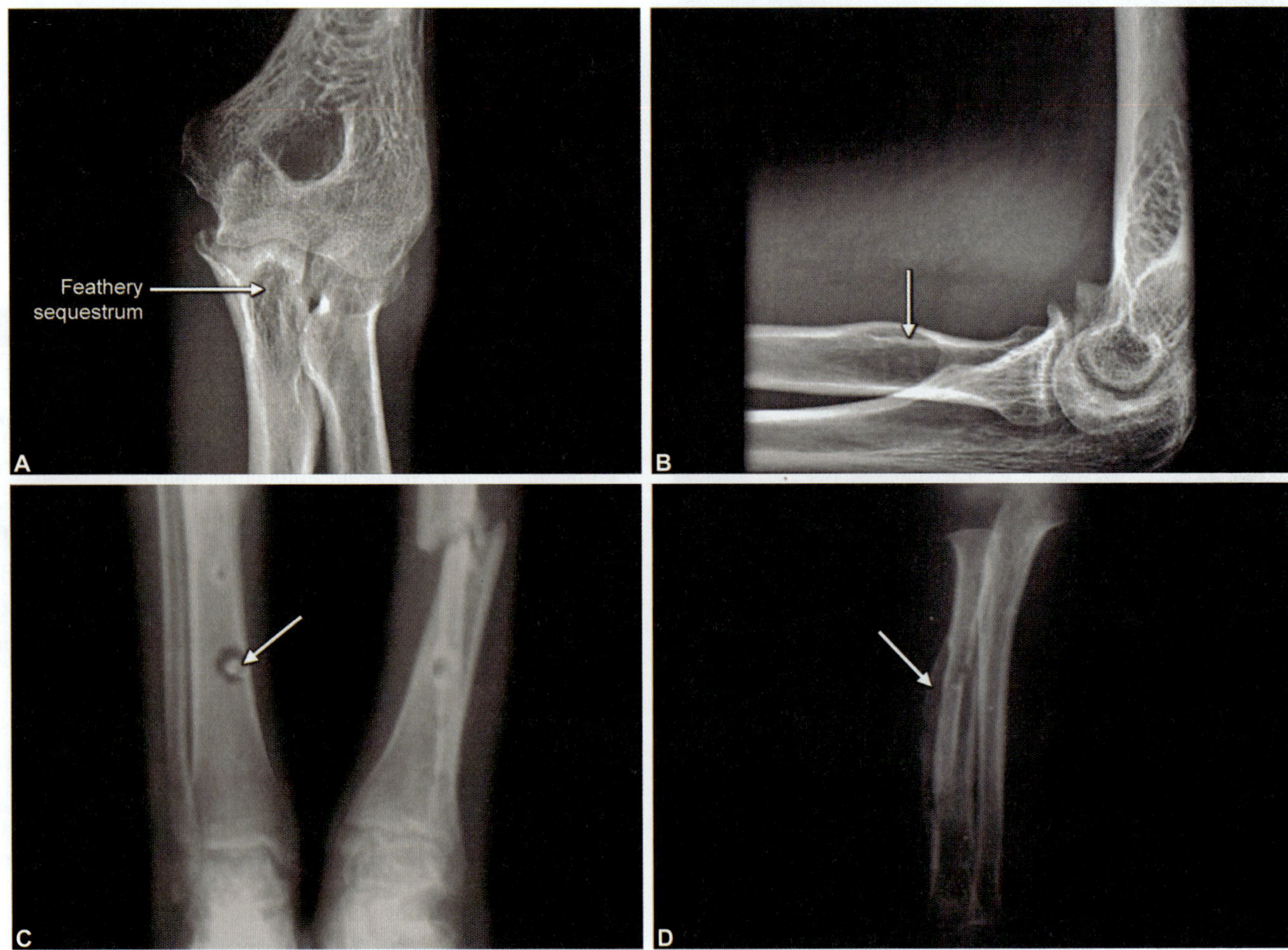

Figs 9.8A to D: (A and B) Feathery sequestrum of tuberculosis (arrows); (C) X-ray showing ring sequestrum (arrow) at the site of insertion of external fixator pin in the bone; (D) X-ray forearm anteroposterior (AP) view showing tubular sequestrum (arrow) in radius

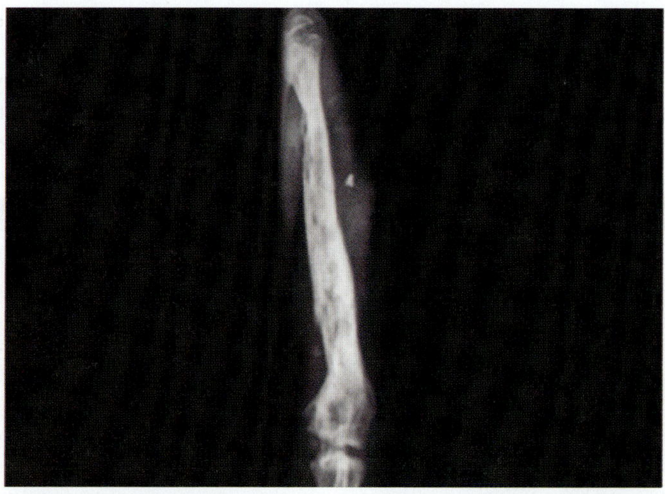

Fig. 9.9: Moth-eaten appearance in chronic osteomyelitis of humerus

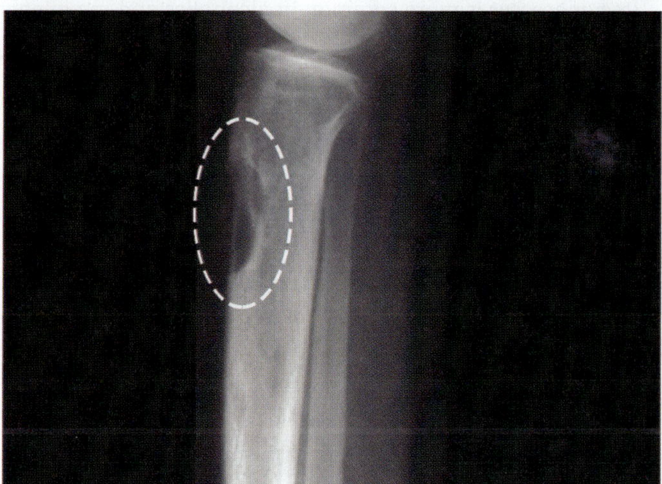

Fig. 9.10: X-ray of tibia lateral view showing saucer-shaped cavity (saucerization) after sequestrectomy and curettage in chronic osteomyelitis

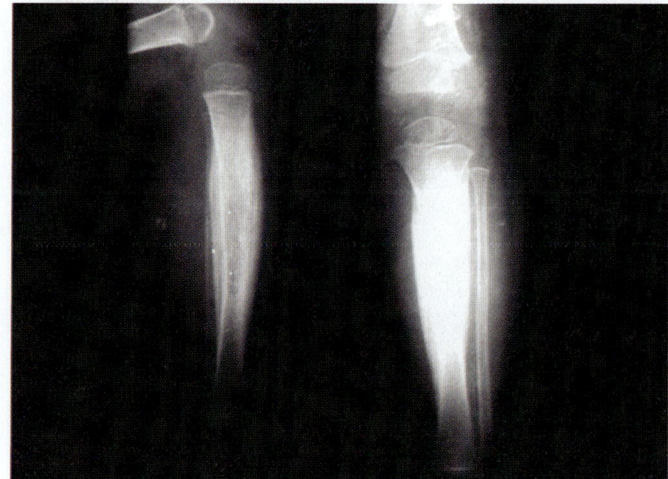

Fig. 9.11: X-ray of leg, anteroposterior (AP) and lateral views showing marked sclerosis and cortical thickening in Garre's osteomyelitis

episodes of pain, swelling and tenderness around long bone metaphysis (most common sites are the distal femur and the proximal/distal tibia), medial ends of clavicles or a vertebral segment. The involvement is mostly multifocal but may or may not be symmetrical. Radiographic changes include small, lytic lesions in the metaphysis with surrounding sclerosis. The clavicle is markedly thickened. Radioscintigraphy shows increased activity around these lesions. Antibiotics have no role and treatment is generally palliative. Although the disease runs a protracted course, prognosis is good, as lesions heal well without any sequelae.

HIGH-YIELD POINTS

- The most common site of osteomyelitis (both acute and chronic) in adults is vertebral bodies.
- Sequestrum usually takes 2–3 months to separate from parent bone. It has an inner smooth surface and an outer rough surface. The outer surface is rough as the latter is being continually eroded by infected granulation tissue. Another feature is that if this piece is placed in water, it sinks and if it is examined on histopathology, one finds a closed haversian system.
- Sequestra may not be seen in children (particularly infants) as they have loose periosteum that gets easily lifted and whole bone becomes sequestrum. In case small sequestra have formed, then they get rapidly absorbed over time.
- Ideal timing of sequestrectomy is when three out of four cortices (two cortices each in AP and lateral X-ray views) of involucrum are well formed.
- *Osteomyelitis in HIV patients*: After septic arthritis the next most prevalent musculoskeletal infection in HIV infected patients is osteomyelitis. The disease in HIV patients also is mostly caused by *S. aureus*, although in one-third cases the infection is polymicrobial. The pathology is absolutely similar with necrosis of bone and a periosteal reaction. However, involvement may at times be bilateral. The bone most commonly involved is tibia.
- *Salmonella osteomyelitis*: Salmonella infection is mostly seen in children with sickle cell disease. It occurs during the convalescent phase of the disease. Usual sites of involvement are diaphysis of long bones (most commonly tibia and forearm bones). Sometimes involvement may be multifocal or bilaterally symmetrical. The radiological hallmark is marked diaphyseal sclerosis.

SEPTIC ARTHRITIS

INTRODUCTION

The term septic arthritis refers to infection of the joint caused by pyogenic bacteria with the exception of tuberculosis. Knee is the most common joint involved, followed by the hip (most common in infants) and shoulder.

PATHOGENESIS

Septic arthritis is more common in children, with males more commonly affected than females. The possible routes of infections are hematogenous (most common), open injuries or infection through contiguous sites like a nearby site of osteomyelitis (the hip is commonly involved by this mode from a focus in proximal femur). Not uncommonly, in infants, the umbilical cord sepsis travels to the joint.

Infection begins mostly with systemic bacteremia and once the bacteria invade the joint, the synovium gets involved triggering an inflammatory cascade. Lysosomal enzymes are released by the macrophages that destroy the articular cartilage. Gradually the whole joint gets destroyed and bony trabeculae form that run across the articulating surfaces as the lesion heals, leading to the bony ankylosis as an end result.

ETIOLOGY

S. aureus is the most common causative organism in all age groups except in healthy, sexually active young adults where *Neisseria gonorrhoeae (N. gonorrhoeae)* is isolated in 75% of cases. *Streptococcus pyogenes* and *Pneumococcus* are others in the list. **Box 9.4** shows some important etiologies to consider in some special situations.

CLINICAL PRESENTATION

The child is toxic with high-grade fever and presents with sudden onset pain, swelling and erythema around the affected joint. There is severe limitation of joint movements in all directions; a reliable way to differentiate the condition from acute osteomyelitis where the restriction of nearby joint movement is relatively milder. The child keeps the joint in the position of the maximum capacity of joint also known as "position of ease", which is flexion, abduction and external rotation for hip, flexion for knee and elbow and palmar flexion for the wrist. If at all patient attempts to walk, there is a painful limp.

An important condition to rule out before moving to management is Psoas abscess. A bacterial infection (either primary or secondary to appendicitis or inflammatory bowel disease) can result in pus formation within or on the surface of the iliopsoas muscle. Differentiation of a psoas abscess from septic arthritis of the hip can be a diagnostic challenge. Patients with a psoas abscess present with a pseudo hip flexion deformity (due to spasm of iliopsoas, not due to hip involvement). The Psoas sign (Cope's Psoas Test) has been described as being useful in differentiating it from septic arthritis. It is performed by determining hip pain during hip movements when the hip is in a flexed versus an extended position. When the hip is flexed, tension on the psoas is relaxed, and the patient with a psoas abscess may have minimal pain with hip rotations, whereas the patient with septic arthritis will have significant pain with the same motion. Extending the hip places the psoas muscle and the hip capsule under tension, resulting in severe pain with internal and external rotation in both patient groups.

INVESTIGATIONS

Blood investigations reveal increased WBC counts with predominant neutrophilia.

Blood cultures may show causative organism in 60% cases.

X-rays in early stages are usually normal. At times, due to joint effusion one might appreciate an increased joint space on the affected side in comparison to normal side **(Fig. 9.12)**. As the infection progresses, there is joint space narrowing due to

destruction of cartilage and in the end stage bony ankylosis of the joint may be seen **(Fig. 9.13)**.

Ultrasonography (USG) is a useful investigation, especially in the deep seated joints like the hip, as it can detect even small amount of collections. Fluid can be aspirated under ultrasound

Box 9.4: Common organisms isolated in some special situations

- In patients with prosthetic joints *Coagulase negative staphylococci (S. epidermidis) closely followed by S. aureus and Propionibacterium acnes* are the common isolates
- Patients with systemic lupus erythematosus have increased risk of infection with *Salmonella*
- *Group A (beta hemolytic) streptococci* are the most common infecting organisms after varicella infection
- Intravenous drug abusers have increased likelihood of *Pseudomonas* infection
- Patients on TNF inhibitors (e.g. RA patients) have increased risk of *Mycobacterial* infections
- *Pneumococcus* is more common in alcoholics and in patients with hemoglobinopathies

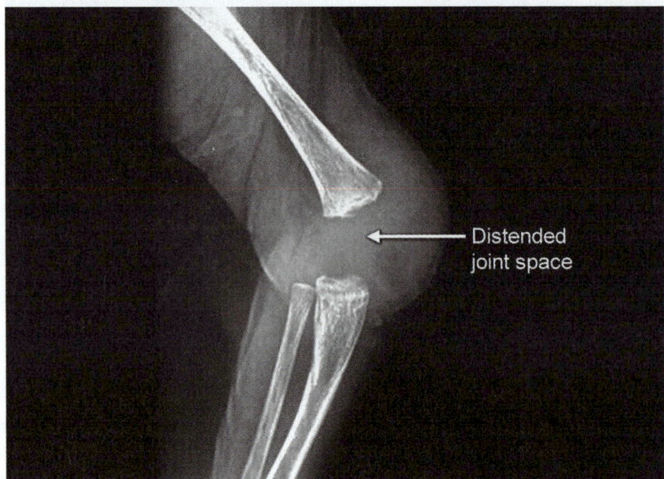

Fig. 9.12: X-ray of septic knee in acute stage showing increased joint space

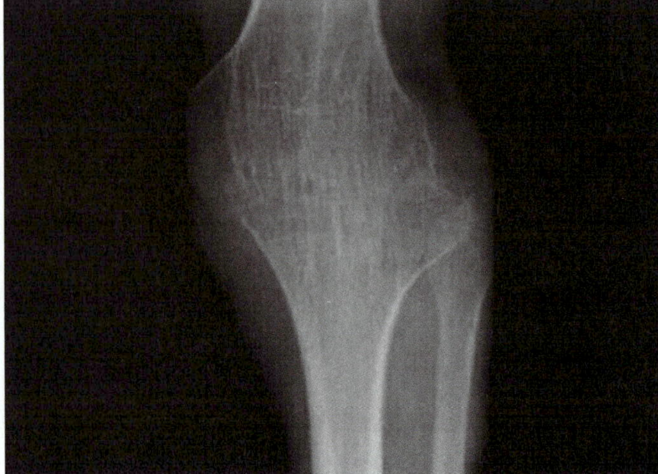

Fig. 9.13: X-ray showing bony ankylosis postseptic arthritis of knee

guidance and the aspirate analysis remains the most accurate diagnostic tool for concluding the diagnosis. If infected, total leukocyte count (TLC) is increased with neutrophilic leukocytosis while proteins increase and glucose level reduces in synovial fluid. Gram staining with culture sensitivity isolates the causative organism confirms the diagnosis and guides the antibiotic treatment.

In cases where cultures are negative, Morrey et al. suggested to label the diagnosis if five out of following six factors are present:
1. Temperature > 38.3°C
2. Painful joint range of motion
3. Swelling of affected joint
4. Systemic symptoms present
5. Absence of other pathological process that could be attributed
6. Satisfactory response to antibiotic therapy.

Differential Diagnosis

Acute osteomyelitis, psoas abscess, rheumatic arthritis, hemophilic arthritis and tubercular arthritis.

TREATMENT

Adequate drainage of pus from the joint (arthrotomy), IV antibiotic cover for 6 weeks and immobilization in functional position are the main principles in the management of septic arthritis. If the aspirate is pus, arthrotomy is done as an emergency procedure and wound closed over a negative suction. Empirical antibiotics are started and tailored after the culture sensitivity report is received. In case there has already been significant destruction of the articular cartilage or a pathological dislocation, a thorough debridement of infected tissue is done and the joint is immobilized in optimum position to ensure maximum function in case the bony ankylosis is the end result.

COMPLICATIONS

- Septicemia in untreated cases
- Stiffness and deformity
- Secondary osteoarthritis
- Pathological dislocation.

TOM SMITH ARTHRITIS (THOMAS SMITH, 1874)

Tom Smith arthritis is the septic arthritis of the hip in infants. It occurs mostly secondary to generalized bacteremia or as an extension of a metaphyseal focus from proximal femur, but can occur in the neonatal period as a spread from umbilical sepsis. Peculiarly of this condition is that in a child of less than 1 year of age, the head of the femur is largely cartilaginous, which gets easily and rapidly destroyed by the bacteria.

Presentation is acute with rapid destruction of the head of femur, however, localization of pathology is challenging owing to the classical age group involved. In the infant, particularly the neonate, the major features of infective process are those of septicemia, viz. irritability, muscular spasms, failure to thrive, fever, tachycardia, etc. Involvement of the hip joint must be suspected if there is an abnormal posture of the leg, swelling in buttock or the genitalia region or pain on palpation or movement of the hip. An older child walks in with a painful limp. There is shortening of the affected limb with attitude of external rotation and range of motion of the hip is increased in all the directions. Telescopy (*see* Pages 124, 125) at the joint is positive. Many a times the initial diagnosis is missed and the child comes months or years later with a painless limp. The gait is unstable, Trendelenburg type (*see* Page 121) and affected leg is shorter.

Ultrasonography-guided aspiration remains the mainstay of diagnosis in suspected cases, especially the neonates. X-ray may be done in relatively older child and may show complete absence of head and neck of the femur (**Figs 9.14A and B**). One needs to differentiate it from developmental dysplasia of the hip (DDH). In Tom Smith arthritis, the acetabulum is well developed while in DDH, the acetabulum is additionally abnormal.

Management in an infant is aggressive same as in septic arthritis. Older children/adults with sequel develop rotational and angular deformities (increased anteversion, coxa vara or valga) around the proximal femur and depending upon the amount of remnant of head or neck present, need appropriate osteotomies or reconstructive procedures.

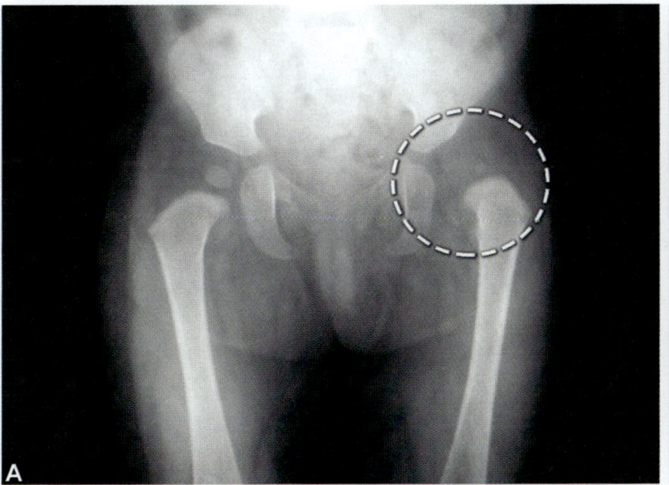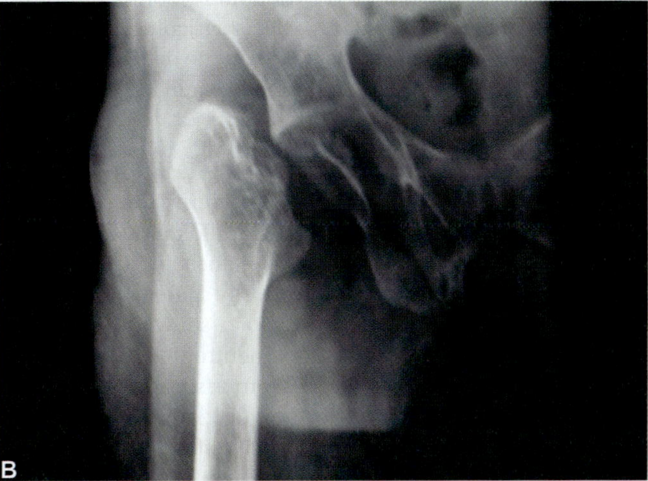

Figs 9.14A and B: (A) Tom Smith arthritis with destruction of head but normal looking acetabulum; (B) Sequel of Tom Smith arthritis in an adult (*see* well-developed acetabulum)

HIGH-YIELD POINTS

- Septic arthritis is the most common cause of bony ankylosis.
- *Gonococcal arthritis: N. gonorrhoeae* is the most common cause of septic arthritis in healthy, sexually active adults, although a septic joint develops in even less than 3% of cases infected with *N. gonorrhoeae*. Joint infection generally manifests within 2 weeks of urethral discharge. Inflammation as a rule is restricted to subsynovial layers. Involvement can be polyarticular (although the knee is the most common joint involved) and associated with papular rash. Joint cultures are usually negative, but cultures from pharynx and urethra may be positive. Gonococcal arthritis has generally good prognosis if treated with appropriate antibiotics (drug of choice is penicillin) and drainage is usually not necessary.
- Recently, there have been upcoming reports on septic arthritis occurring in people involved with agricultural occupations, secondary to Brucella infections (zoonosis transmitted to man from farm animals). The most common joint affected in Brucellosis is Hip joint.
- Spread of infection from a metaphyseal focus of osteomyelitis is different in children of different age groups. In children above the age of 2 years, the growth plate (physis) acts as a barrier and prevents the spread towards the epiphysis and into the joint. Rather, the abscess tracks towards the diaphysis commonly producing a diaphyseal involvement. However, in children below the age of 2 years, there are vessels that travel from the metaphysis across the growth plate into the epiphysis. Hence, infection easily spreads across the physis and epiphyseal and joint involvement is relatively common.

MADURA FOOT

INTRODUCTION

Mycetoma (Madura foot) is a chronic granulomatous infection of skin and subcutaneous tissues caused by fungi (eumycetomas) or bacteria (actinomycetes). Bacteria account for about 60% of cases. It is mainly a disease of tropical countries namely Africa, Mexico and India. In India, maximum cases are found in Rajasthan and Tamil Nadu. It was first reported in Madurai (South India) in 1942 and hence the name. It mainly affects agricultural workers, herdsmen and farmers who walk barefoot in the field. The foot is the most commonly affected site followed by hand.

PATHOPHYSIOLOGY

Causative organism enters through the minor cut or splinters on the skin of the foot and the hand. A neutrophilic response initially occurs, which is followed by a granulomatous reaction. The infection spreads through the facial planes and can lead to osteomyelitis. Nerves and tendons are mostly spared.

Hematoxylin and eosin (H and E) stain shows suppurative granulomas, which are composed of neutrophils, histiocytes and a mixed inflammatory infiltrate comprising lymphocytes, macrophages, plasma cells, and eosinophils. These granulomas surround characteristic granules. Granules of actinomycetoma consist of fine, branching filaments, whereas in eumycetomas the granules are composed of septate hyphae. H and E staining and Gram staining of the histological slides show club shaped fungi in eumycetoma infection and filamentous bacteria in case of actinomycetoma infection. Common organisms causing Madura foot are as follows:

Actinomycetes:
- *Actinomadura madurae*
- *Actinomadura pelletieri*
- *Streptomyces somaliensis*
- *Nocardia* species

Eumycetes:
- *Pseudallescheria boydii*
- *Madurella mycetomatis.*

CLINICAL FEATURES (FIG. 9.15)

The disease is commonly seen in young and middle aged men. The disease is characterized by the triad of tumor like swelling, discharging sinuses and granules in the discharge. Pathogenic organism (e.g. fungal spore) enters the skin through the minor breaks in the skin. After an incubation period of several weeks or months the disease usually begins as a painless swelling or thickening of the skin and subcutaneous tissue. As the disease progresses nodules develop which suppurate to form discharging sinuses. The overlying skin is often depigmented. Sinus tracts discharge serosanguinous fluid which may contain grossly visible granules of various colors and size depending upon the organism involved. Granules are firm 0.2–5 mm aggregates of organized vegetative septate hyphae/branching filaments, which often are embedded in a matrix substance that contains sulfur. The color of these granules is specific for a particular species **(Box 9.5)**. Regional lymphadenitis secondary to bacterial superinfection of the lesion may be present.

INVESTIGATIONS

Plain X-ray may show calcification, obliteration of fascial planes and in advanced cases, bone scalloping and periosteal reaction may be seen. USG can help to differentiate between eumycetoma, actinomycetoma and nonmycetoma lesions. MRI scans can provide a better assessment of the degree of bone and soft tissue involvement, and may be useful in evaluating the differential

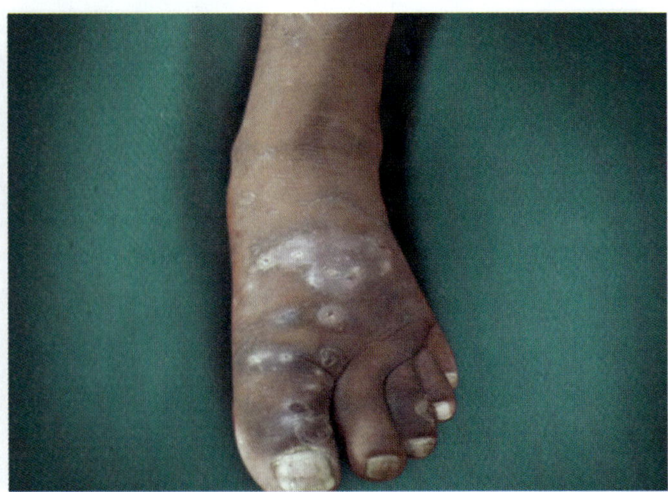

Fig. 9.15: Mycetoma foot
Courtesy: Dr. Rajendra Jangir, Ganganagar (India).

diagnosis of the swelling. Histopathological examination and culture of exudate and grains can reliably establish the diagnosis.

MANAGEMENT

Eumycetoma is usually refractory to medical treatment. Few reports of successful treatment with prolonged chemotherapy (many years) with antifungal agents like ketoconazole and itraconazole have been reported. Surgery is required in most of the cases which include wide local excision, repetitive debridement excisions and amputations in refractory cases. Actinomycetoma is often amenable to medical treatment. Combination chemotherapy is often required and cotrimoxazole plus streptomycin/dapsone are first-line drugs.

HIGH-YIELD POINTS

- Most commonly actinomycosis involves orocervicofacial region.
- Overall, the most common site of actinomycosis is mandible.

SYPHILIS AND ORTHOPEDICS

INTRODUCTION

Syphilis is a sexually transmitted infection where the causative agent is a spirochaete, *Treponema pallidum*. The disease manifests not only in the host to which the organism is transmitted (acquired syphilis) but also in the fetus in case the transmission has occurred (congenital syphilis). However, the manifestations are unique to each type.

ACQUIRED SYPHILIS

The course of disease passes through four phases:

1. *Primary stage*: 2–10 weeks after transmission a painless oval chancre develops at the site where the bacteria have entered the body (usually penis/vagina). The lesion mostly heals within 6 weeks without treatment.
2. *Secondary stage*: After around 3 months, disease enters the secondary stage and the nonitching rashes develop over the palms and soles that usually heal in about another 6 weeks. During this stage the organism spreads through the tissues of the host and the patient is highly contagious.
3. *Latent stage*: Duration varies from a few years to decades. The patient is noninfectious with the bacteria lying inactive in lymph nodes and spleen. From here the disease may or may not progress to tertiary stage.
4. *Tertiary stage (Late syphilis)*: One-third of patients generally progress to this stage. The patient is noncontagious but the organism produces damage to various tissues of the body. Invasion of the neural tissue is characteristic and referred to as "Tabes Dorsalis (neurosyphilis)".

Orthopedic Manifestations in Acquired Syphilis

Joints may be affected in secondary or tertiary stage of the disease. In secondary stage, there are transient polyarthralgias that generally involve large joints. In the tertiary stage, gummatous arthritis (synovial and osseous forms) is the characteristic manifestation. An indirect consequence that may occur in the tertiary stage (Tabes Dorsalis) is Charcot's arthropathy (*see* Page 440).

CONGENITAL SYPHILIS

Transmission across the placenta causes syphilis in the fetus and the newborn, that presents as chronic osteitis, periostitis and osteochondritis. The tibia is the most commonly affected bone.

Orthopedic Manifestations in Congenital Syphilis

- Frontal bossing/Olympian brow.
- *Higoumenakis sign*: Bilateral enlargement of the sternal end of clavicle due to periostitis.
- *Saber shin*: Anterior bowing of mid-portion of the tibia.
- *Parrot joints*: Syphilitic osteochondritis in children.
- *Clutton joints*: Painless, symmetrical synovitis most commonly involving knee in children near puberty.
- Bilateral symmetrical metaphyseal erosions most commonly seen in the tibia.

LEPROSY AND ORTHOPEDICS (HANSEN'S DISEASE, 1873)

INTRODUCTION

Leprosy is a chronic granulomatous infection affecting multiple tissues like skin, peripheral nerves, testes, eyes, and upper respiratory tract mucosa. It is caused by acid fast bacillus *Mycobacterium leprae,* an obligate intracellular parasite confined to humans and armadillos. The disease is only mildly contagious with infection being usually acquired by inhaling airborne droplets contaminated with bacteria on coming in close contact with affected untreated individuals. Once the organism enters the body from the nasal mucosa, it spreads by the hematogenous route to skin, peripheral nerves and other areas. As the bacilli are very slow dividing, it may take 3–5 years for the symptoms to appear, although an incubation period of even up to 20 years has been reported.

PREVALENCE

Leprosy is one of the oldest known diseases of the mankind, earliest described in India-China (mentioned as *Kushta Roga* in Sanskrit by Sushruta Samhita) around the 6th century BC. Although elimination of leprosy (i.e. a prevalence rate of leprosy less than 1 case per 100,00 persons at global level) was achieved in the year 2000, pockets of high endemicity still remain in some areas of countries like Bangladesh, Brazil, China, Ethiopia, India, Indonesia, Myanmar, Nepal, Nigeria, Philippines, Sri Lanka, etc. Countrywise, India accounts for the maximum number of cases (approximately 58% of the total cases) worldwide (as in 2011).

PATHOLOGY

Most people who are infected with the organism get rid of the infection by virtue of their immunity. However, in those where the immunity level is not appropriate, the organism produces the manifestations. Based upon the immune response mounted by the host, Ridley and Jopling classified the disease into "indeterminate", "tuberculoid", "borderline" and "lepromatous" subtypes.

The "indeterminate" type, an early form of the disease, consists of the first type of skin lesions (hypopigmented macules) that mostly heal spontaneously.

The "tuberculoid" form occurs in those who are able to mount up a reasonably good delayed type hypersensitivity (DTH) response. The granulomas are circumscribed, focal and have few scattered giant cells and lymphocytes. The disease in these cases is paucibacillary.

The "lepromatous" form is seen in those who are unable to mount effective cell-mediated immunity (CMI) against the infecting organism. Here the granulomas are diffuse and extensive and are loaded with bacilli (multibacillary).

The "borderline" types are intermediate forms that show some features of each of the above two forms.

ORTHOPEDIC MANIFESTATIONS

The orthopedic manifestations of the disease primarily span the following areas:

Skin Involvement

Hypopigmented skin patches with impaired sensibility are seen in all forms of "leprosy". Skin lesions in tuberculoid leprosy are well demarcated, few, hypopigmented, anesthetic macules while in lepromatous leprosy, skin lesions are extensive, multiple, symmetrical with only some sensory impairment. Nodules may develop in advanced stage. Coarsening of facial skin and loss of eyebrow hair may produce the classical "leonine facies". Nasal muscosal involvement may lead to destruction of nasal septum producing a nasal deformity.

Nerve Involvement

The nerve involvement is extensive in "lepromatous leprosy" while in "tuberculoid" it is focal in distribution. However, clinical defects in nerve function appear early in tuberculoid leprosy while they are much later seen in lepromatous type.

Pattern of Nerve Involvement

Nerve trunks of the upper limb are involved more commonly than the nerves of lower limb. Overall, the ulnar nerve is the most common nerve involved, followed by common peroneal nerve. Most common cranial nerve involved is facial nerve (VII) closely followed by the trigeminal (V).

Nerve involvement in leprosy occurs in the following forms:

- *Nerve thickening*: Peripheral nerve involvement is almost always a rule in leprosy. The affected nerves become chronically thickened due to hypertrophy of epineurium and perineurium, granuloma formation and endoneural fibrosis. A thickened nerve may be strangulated by its own sheath or by the walls of a narrow passage that may be there in its course producing symptoms of nerve ischemia and compression.
- *Acute neuritis*: The chronic course is often punctuated by acute episodes of neuritis due to the classic "lepra" reactions that greatly increase the nerve damage. While Type I reactions (erythema nodosum leprosum) are due to deposition of immune complexes, the Type II (reversal reactions) reactions are due to increase in CMI (delayed type hypersensitivity). The reactions occur in 30–50% of patients with leprosy either before, or more often, after the start of treatment and are induced by medicines, stress and surgical procedures.

- *Nerve abscesses*: Occasionally nerve lesions in tuberculoid leprosy undergo caseation and liquefaction to form "cold abscess" that may break through the epineurium to present as a chronic collar stud abscess.

Clinical Presentation

The end result of nerve damage may bring the patient to the doctor with the following problems:

- *Muscle paralysis and joint deformities*: Damage to the affected nerves leads to paralysis and atrophy of the muscles supplied. The end result may be joint deformities **(Box 9.6)** and contractures depending upon the nerve involved. For example, peroneal nerve involvement may end up in foot drop while ulnar nerve involvement may lead to claw-hand deformity in hand.
- *Trophic ulceration*: Insensibility in area of affected nerve distribution predisposes to abnormal stresses of pressure especially on hands and feet. Thereby heads of first and fifth metatarsals, heel and sometimes the distal phalanges tend to develop trophic ulcers that are chronic in nature, resistant to healing and that progressively increase in size. Not uncommonly do these ulcers get secondarily infected.
- *Mutilations*: Neglect in treatment leads to the mutilations of terminal extremities caused by recurrent trophic ulcers and sequestration of bone.

DIAGNOSIS

Diagnosis of leprosy is established on detection of at least two of the following features:

1. Characteristic skin lesions
2. Thickened peripheral nerves
3. Areas of sensory loss
4. Demonstration of Acid Fast Bacilli (*M. leprae*) in skin or nasal smear biopsy.

RLEP real-time polymerase chain reaction (PCR) is coming up as a useful tool for an early diagnosis in cases where skin smears are negative or a skin biopsy is not feasible. However, the role of Lepromin test (intradermal injection of inactivated *M. leprae* antigen) in primary diagnosis is limited. It is more useful in determining the type of leprosy (tuberculoid or lepromatous) that the patient has.

TREATMENT

Multidrug Therapy

Drugs used to cure the condition include rifampicin, dapsone and clofazimine. The course and dosages depend upon whether leprosy is paucibacillary or multibacillary. Acute lepra reactions are generally managed with a course of steroids and thalidomide. Kindly refer to medicine textbook for more information.

Box 9.6: World Health Organization (WHO) grading for orthopedic deformities in leprosy

- *Grade I*: No sensory impairment/no visible deformity
- *Grade II*: Sensory impairment present, but no visible deformity
- *Grade III*: Both sensory impairment and visible deformity (e.g. claw hand) are present

Surgical Treatment

Indicated in following conditions:

- *Compression neuropathies*: Nerve decompression may be required in cases not responding to conservative treatment. The procedure involves tunnel release from which nerve is passing and incising epineurium over an affected segment of nerve.
- *Nerve abscesses*: Abscesses likely to burst or those causing neurological deficit need to be drained.
- *Managing residual paralysis and trophic ulcerations*: These conditions are best prevented by early treatment. Insensate areas must be offered extraprotection. Proper physiotherapy is must to prevent deformities. In case deformities result, then they can be managed by appropriate release operations and tendon transfers **(Box 9.7)**.

HIGH-YIELD POINTS

- The first sign of the disease is the feeling of numbness or loss of sensation for temperature (heat) followed by touch and pain which usually begins in the extremities.
- Patients undergoing surgery should not have had acute neuritis for at least 6 months prior to surgery.
- Lucio phenomenon is a cutaneous vasculitis in patients with lepromatous leprosy and tends to affect people who have not taken their medication regularly.
- Fluorescent leprosy antibody absorption test (FLA-ABS) is a highly sensitive technique in detecting antibodies against *M. leprae* antigen by immunofluorescent technique. It is useful in identifying the contacts of leprosy patients who can be at risk of developing the disease.

HAND INFECTIONS

INFECTIONS AROUND NAIL

Acute Paronychia

Paronychia is the infection of soft tissue fold around the fingernail (eponychium) most commonly caused by *S. aureus* associated with poor nail hygiene. The patient presents with pain, redness and swelling around the nail fold. Nail fold is extremely tender. Risk factors include diabetes, steroid therapy, chemotherapy, immunocompromised individuals, manual laborers and farmers.

Treatment

When there is no pus point visible, infection is controlled by oral or IV antibiotics. In late stages when there is abscess only on one side of the nail, incision and drainage are done **(Fig. 9.16)**. If pus is extended to opposite side and under the nail, a second incision is made and proximal third of the nail is removed.

Chronic Paronychia

Seen in patients whose hands have prolonged exposure to water, which causes thickening of eponychium due to chronic

inflammation and recurring infection. The organisms responsible are *S. pyogenes*, *S. epidermidis* and *C. albicans*.

Treatment

Eponychial marsupialization is to be done.

INFECTIONS IN THE HAND

Relevant Anatomy

Spaces of the Hand

The fascia and fascial septae in the hand form many spaces. The anatomy of these spaces is important because these spaces may get infected and infection from one space may reach the other space. The important spaces of hand are:

- *Palmar spaces*:
  - Pulp space of fingers
  - Web space
  - *Deep palmar spaces*:
    - Mid-palmar space
    - Thenar space
- *Dorsal spaces*:
  - Dorsal subcutaneous space
  - Dorsal subaponeurotic space
- The forearm space of Parona.

Pulp Space Infections

Felon: A felon is the infection of the subcutaneous tissue of the distal pulp of a digit, the most common site being thumb followed by the index finger. The distal pulp is divided into tiny compartments by strong fibrous septae that traverse from skin to bone, because of these septae any swelling in this space causes very pain due to increased pressure within the pulp **(Fig. 9.17)**. Infection is generally caused by penetrating foreign body or pinprick for medical reasons (hematocrit or blood glucose estimation). *S. aureus* is the most common causative organism. Throbbing pain, swelling and redness of the terminal pulp are the presenting symptoms. Abscess formation may follow rapidly. An abscess can extend into underlying bone and may cause osteomyelitis of the distal phalanx. Treatment consists of antibiotics after incision and drainage.

Whitlow: Whitlow is an infection of the pulp space of digit usually caused by Herpes simplex type I virus. The distinction between "felon" and "whitlow" is made primarily on the basis of history. Herpetic whitlow usually presents with a prodromal phase of

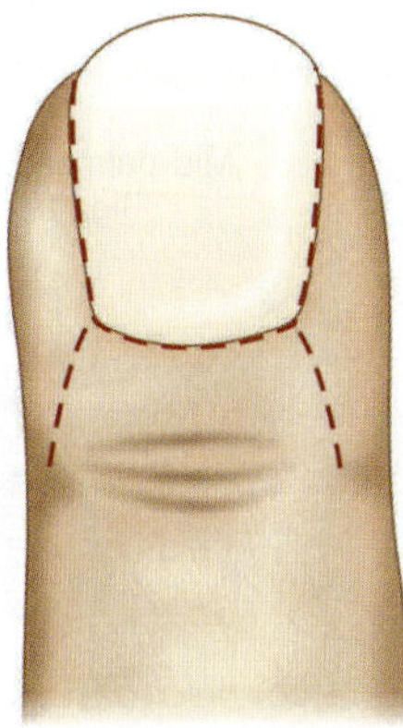

Fig. 9.16: Incision for draining a paronychium

24–72 hours of burning pain prior to the development of the classical skin changes. First, there is erythema and swelling, then the formation of clear vesicles. The vesicles coalesce, often around the nail folds. The fluid within the vesicles is turbid, but not frankly purulent. The pulp of the affected digit is not tense as in a felon. The disease persists over approximately 2 weeks and then resolves over the next 1 week.

Web Space Infection (Collar Button Abscess)

Web space is a fat-filled triangular interdigital space at the level of the metacarpophalangeal (MCP) joints. This infection usually seen in laborers, begins beneath palmar creases. The patient presents with redness, swelling and tenderness over the web space **(Fig. 9.18A)**. Abscess, if undrained may spread through the lumbrical canal into the mid-palmar space. Treatment involves incision and drainage **(Fig. 9.18B)**.

Deep Palmar Space (Mid-palmar and Thenar Space) Infections

Deep palmar space lies deep to the flexor tendons and their synovial sheaths. This space is divided into a mid-palmar space (medially) and a thenar space (laterally) by a fascial membrane that passes obliquely from third metacarpal to fascia, dorsal to flexor tendons of the index finger **(Figs 9.19A and B)**. Lateral to the thenar space lies thenar muscles and medial to mid-palmar space lies hypothenar muscles.

Mid-palmar Space

Triangular space is present under ulnar half of the hollow of the hand. Proximally, it extends up to the distal margin of flexor retinaculum and communicates with forearm space. Distally it extends up to the distal palmar crease and communicates with fascial sheaths of third and fourth lumbrical muscles.

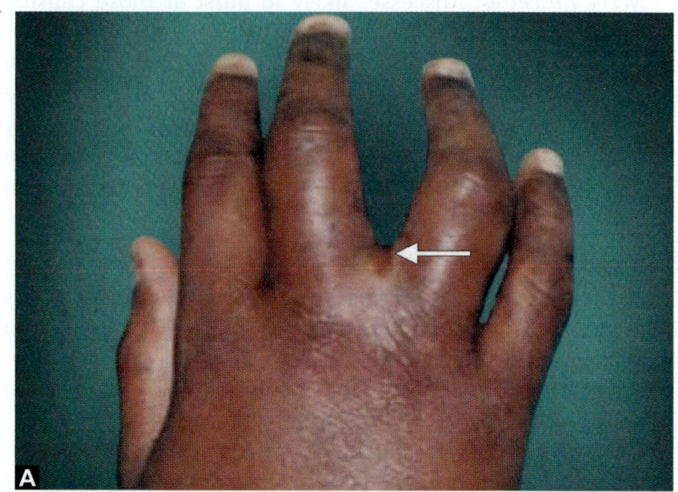
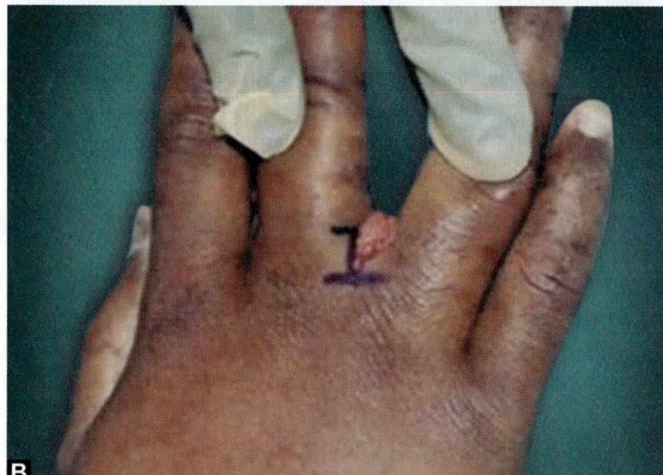

Figs 9.18A and B: (A) Collar button abscess (arrow) being taken up for incision; and (B) Drainage

Courtesy: Kyle J. Jeray, MD, Greenville Hospital System, USA.

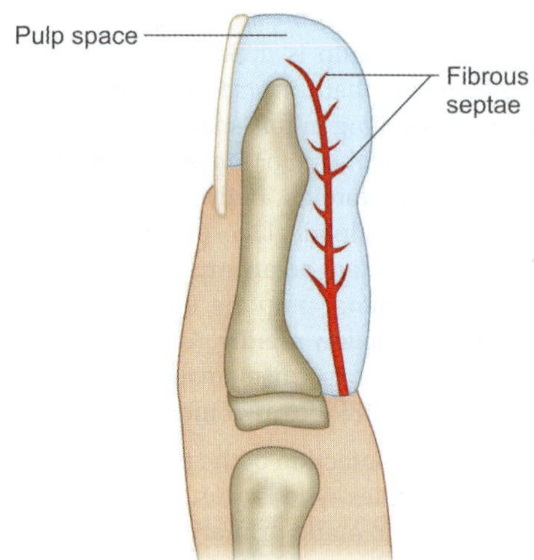

Fig. 9.17: Pulp space of digit

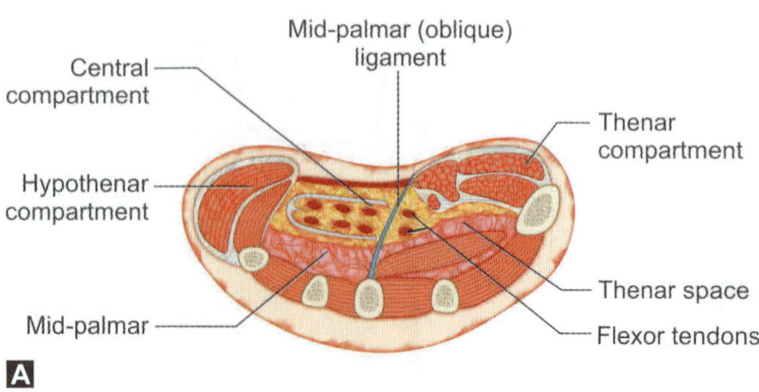

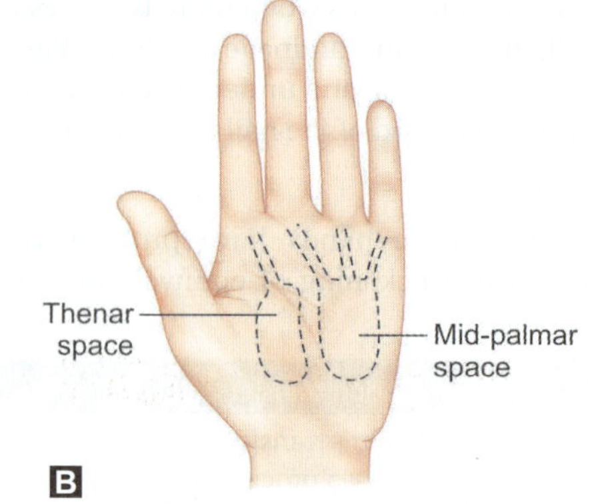

Figs 9.19A and B: Deep palmar spaces of hand

The space is bounded anteriorly by palmar aponeurosis and flexor tendons of third, fourth and fifth fingers and posteriorly by third, fourth and fifth metacarpals, medially by hypothenar septum and laterally by mid-palmar (oblique) septum.

Thenar Space

Triangular space is present under radial half of the hollow of the hand. Proximally, it extends up to the distal margin of flexor retinaculum and communicates with forearm space. Distally, it extends up to the proximal transverse palmar crease and communicates with the subcutaneous web of the thumb. It is bounded anteriorly by palmar aponeurosis and posteriorly by first dorsal interosseous muscle, medially by a mid-palmar septum and laterally by a lateral palmar septum.

The infection in these spaces can be reached by penetrating wound, hematogenous route or infection from a nearby site like web space infection or flexor tenosynovitis. There is pain, swelling and tenderness on the volar aspect of the hand. A mid-palmar abscess can cause a systemic reaction, pain, tenderness, inability to move the long and ring fingers actively and swelling of hand and fingers. A thenar abscess causes similar symptoms, but thumb web is more swollen.

Treatment: Incision and drainage under antibiotic cover. A transverse palmar incision is given between the two parallel flexion palmar creases for mid-palmar abscess. A thenar crease incision is given for thenar abscess **(Fig. 9.20)**.

Dorsal Space Infections

Dorsal spaces include the *dorsal subcutaneous space* that lies deep to the loose skin of the dorsum of the hand and the *dorsal subaponeurotic space* that lies deep to the dorsal aponeurosis of the hand. Infection of the subaponeurotic space needs more attention. These are usually caused by penetrating injuries to the dorsum of the hand or local spread from another infection. Swelling, redness, and warmth over dorsum of hand, tenderness, painful finger extension and draining sinuses are usually seen.

Treatment

Incision and drainage along with antibiotics are the mainstay of the treatment. Most dorsal abscesses are drained through a single longitudinal incision centered over the abscess. A large abscess may require two parallel incisions, one over second metacarpal and another between fourth and fifth metacarpals.

Infections of the Forearm Space of Parona

Rectangular space situated deep to the lower part of the forearm just above the wrist. It is bordered by the pronator quadratus dorsally, flexor pollicis longus laterally, flexor carpi ulnaris medially and long flexor tendons on the palmar aspect. Inferiorly, it extends up to flexor retinaculum and communicates with the mid-palmar space and superiorly it may extend up to the oblique origin of flexor digitorum superficialis. Infections in this space generally are related to infections of the digital synovial sheaths, especially the ulnar bursa (*see* later).

ACUTE SUPPURATIVE TENOSYNOVITIS

Relevant Anatomy

The flexor tendons of the fingers are surrounded by their own synovial sheaths. The digital synovial sheaths of the second, third and fourth digits are independent and terminate proximally at the level of the MCP joints. The digital synovial sheath of the little finger continues proximally in the palm as the ulnar bursa while that of the thumb as radial bursa **(Fig. 9.21)**. The two bursas extend proximally for 2–3 cm above the wrist and communicate with each other and may communicate with the forearm space of "parona".

Acute suppurative tenosynovitis is a purulent infection of the digital tendon sheaths. Although rare, this is the most serious hand infections as if left untreated, this infection can lead to the destruction of the gliding surfaces in the sheath, necrosis of tendons, osteomyelitis and even amputation. Most commonly affected are the ring, middle and index fingers and *S. aureus* is the most common infective organism. A history of penetrating injury is typical, by a sharp object like a needle, however, a few cases can occur as a result of hematogenous spread, usually caused by gonococci.

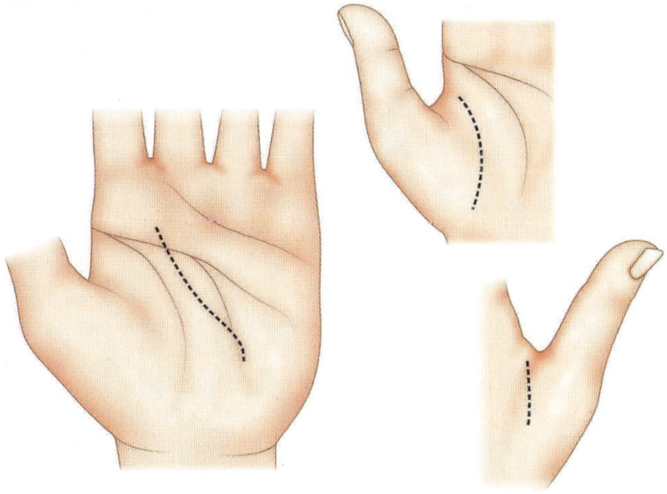

Fig. 9.20: Drainage of deep palmar abscesses

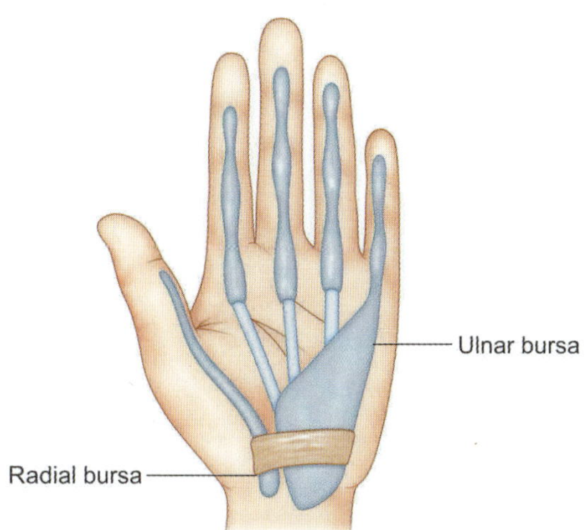

Fig. 9.21: Digital synovial sheaths

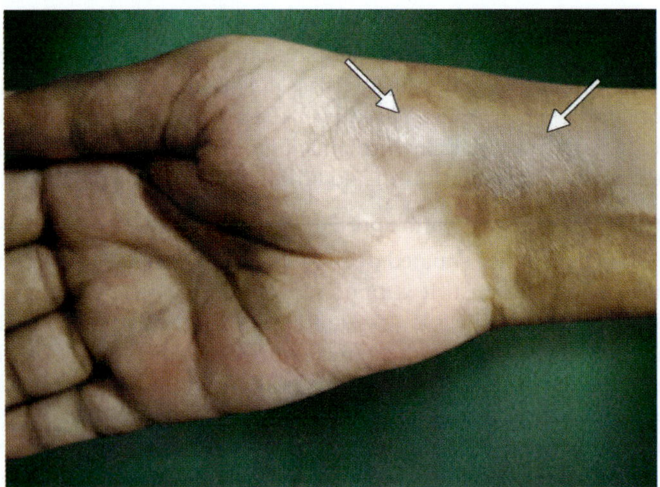

Fig. 9.22: Compound palmar ganglion (arrows)
Courtesy: Dr. Navdeep Gupta, FNB Sports Medicine, Sports Injury Center, Safdarjung Hospital, New Delhi.

Clinical Features

The affected finger is grossly swollen and tender. Kanavel described the four cardinal signs of flexor tenosynovitis: (1) fusiform swelling of the finger, (2) partially flexed posture of the digit, (3) tenderness over the entire flexor tendon sheath, and (4) disproportionate pain on passive extension. The last sign is the most constant and typically the first being present in early cases.

Spread

Infections of the thumb can spread to radial and then to ulnar bursa while the infections of the little finger spread to involve the ulnar bursa primarily and then the forearm space of "parona". This results in an hour glass swelling both proximal and distal to the wrist (flexor retinaculum) producing the "compound palmar ganglion" **(Fig. 9.22)**, a clinical picture more commonly seen in patients with rheumatoid arthritis and tuberculosis.

Treatment

An aggressive treatment is needed. Infections of the digital synovial sheaths are drained by two transverse incisions, one in the DIP joint crease and the other in distal palmar crease. Ulnar bursa is approached by an incision along the lateral margin of the hypothenar eminence while the radial bursa is approached via an incision along the medial margin of thenar eminence. A good antibiotic cover is added.

HIGH-YIELD POINTS

Spread of infections in hand:
- *Thenar space infection:* It results from index finger or thumb.
- *Mid-palmar space infection:* It results from middle and ring fingers.
- Infection of the thumb spreads to radial bursa.
- Infection of little finger spreads to ulnar bursa.

Skeletal Tuberculosis

INTRODUCTION

The tubercle bacillus has coexisted with Homo sapiens since time immemorial. The Vedas (3000–1800 BC) and Samhita of Charaka and Sushruta (1000 & 600 BC) recognized the disease as "Yakshma". Tuberculous lesions have even been found in Egyptian mummies (3400 BC) and mentions about the disease have been made in the Greek-Roman civilization literature.

Although the osteoarticular tuberculosis (TB) is disappearing in western countries but in developing countries it is still a major public health problem. After the lungs and lymph nodes, the bones and joints are the third most common site of TB. Amongst skeletal system, spine is the most common site of involvement, followed by the hip, knee, foot, elbow, hand and shoulder in order of frequency. The least common bone or joint to be involved are the mandible and the temporomandibular joint. However, the least common orthopedic site for TB is a bursa (out of which the trochanteric bursa is most commonly involved).

ETIOLOGY

The causative organism is *Mycobacterium tuberculosis*. Although the tuberculous bacilli are omnipresent, the disease manifests in those, in whom the load of infecting bacilli trip over the amount of immune response the host can mount. Hence, malnutrition, environmental conditions and living standards such as poor sanitation, overcrowded housing and slum dwellings, serve as important predisposing factors. Diabetes mellitus, acquired immunodeficiency syndrome (AIDS) (30 times greater risk), repeated pregnancies and lactation in women are also predisposing conditions. Trauma as a causative factor is debatable.

PATHOGENESIS

Infection is paucibacillary (bacterial load in skeletal lesion is 10^5 as compared to pulmonary lesion where it is 10^7–10^9) and is always secondary to lung infection (50–75% patients have concomitant pulmonary lesion). Bacilli reach the bone via hematogenous route (more common) or by direct extension from a neighboring focus. Lesion starts in the metaphysis in children and in the epiphysis in adults. The organism on reaching the bone switches on body's cell-mediated immunity, whereby, body self-destructs via the delayed type hypersensitivity reaction. This chronic granulomatous inflammatory response produces the classical lesions with central caseous necrosis. On the basis of pathology, actually the lesion may be either of the two types. The caseous exudative type (more common in children) has more exudate and is more destructive with sinus and abscess formation. The granular dry type (more common in adults) is less destructive and abscess formation is rare (e.g. caries sicca). In clinical practice, both types coexist with one predominating over the other.

CLINICAL FEATURES

The disease is more common during the first three decades of life although all age groups can be involved. The disease is equally distributed amongst both sexes. Patients usually present with monoarticular or mono-osseous involvement with insidious onset dull aching pain and often night cries (relaxation of muscles at night removes their splinting effect on involved joints, permitting movements between inflamed surfaces). Constitutional symptoms like low-grade fever, evening rise of temperature, weight loss, anorexia, etc. are present in 20–30% of patients. On examination, tenderness, muscle spasms, painful restriction of movements and regional lymph node enlargement may be seen.

INVESTIGATIONS

Hemoglobin level is low (normocytic normochromic anemia of chronic disease). Total leukocyte count (TLC) increases with lymphocytosis in differential count. Erythrocyte sedimentation rate (ESR) is elevated. Conventional methods like Ziehl-Neelsen (ZN) staining and culture on solid Lowenstein-Jensen medium or an automated liquid culture system (e.g. BACTEC MGIT 960) may be done to confirm the diagnosis. However, the sensitivity and specificity of staining and culture is low apart from fact that culture may take 6–8 weeks to show growth. Nucleic acid amplification from synovial fluid, synovium, pus, etc. and histopathological examination of diseased tissue are highly specific tests for TB. Nucleic acid amplification tests (NAAT) are Polymerase Chain Reaction (PCR) based assays that amplify target nucleic acid regions unique to mycobacterium tuberculosis complex. They can detect as low as 10–50 bacilli from the clinical sample with sensitivity and specificity near to 90%. The results can be obtained within hours from the receipt of the specimen and drug resistant strains (e.g. rifampicin resistance) can be identified as well. Commercially available NAAT kits for TB include GeneProbe Amplified Mycobacterium Tuberculosis Direct [(AMTD), San Diego, CA, USA] and the Roche Amplicor MTB and Cobas Amplicor tests (Roche molecular diagnostics, CA, USA). The QuantiFERON-TB Gold assay (sensitivity 84% and specificity 95%) is a recently introduced blood test to detect a latent or active TB infection. It detects cell-mediated inflammatory responses to TB infection by measuring interferon-gamma levels in patient's plasma sample, which has been exposed to *M. tuberculosis* antigens in vitro. Considering the fact that India is a high burden country, the interpretation remains questionable and use of the test has not been recommended in the 2016 RNTCP guidelines.

X-RAY FEATURES

In tuberculous arthritis, localized osteoporosis is the first radiological sign of active disease. The articular margins and bony cortices become irregular and hazy with no periosteal reaction or new bone formation. Bony destruction in the absence of periosteal new bone formation is pathognomonic of TB. The synovial fluid, thickened synovium and pericapsular tissues may cause a soft tissue swelling. With the destruction of articular cartilage, the joint space is reduced. In later stages, there is bone destruction with collapse, subluxation or dislocation and deformity of the joint. Features of spinal TB on radiographs have been discussed on Page 301.

PRINCIPLES OF TREATMENT

Various principles of treatment include:

- *Chemotherapy*: Anti-tubercular therapy (ATT) is the mainstay of treatment. Same drugs, as per the WHO's directly observed treatment, short (DOTS) regimen are used. However, duration and regimens remain debatable. Authors prefer daily dose therapy (cf alternate regimen in DOTS), owing to presence of dead bone and poor bone penetration of these drugs. The duration preferred ranges from 9 months to 12 months with intensive phase (all four drugs) for 2 months followed by maintenance phase (isoniazid and rifampicin). ATT is stopped once the ESR of patient returns to normal, radiograph shows signs of healing and clinically tenderness in affected area disappears.
- *Nutrition*: High-protein diet and exposure to fresh air and sunlight provide good resistance to fight with infection.
- *Rest and traction*: The affected extremity should be kept in functional position during the period of pain, to decrease pain and to avoid the deformity or contractors.
- *Physiotherapy*: With the start of ATT, the disease activity and pain is reduced, gradual mobilization exercises are started followed by strengthening exercises.
- *Surgical management*: Following surgeries may be required in different patients depending upon the clinical situation:
  - *Aspiration of cold abscess*: Resolve with chemotherapy only. For those that are peripherally palpable and for those that are causing symptoms (like a psoas abscess causing pseudoflexion deformity of the hip), aspiration (by antigravity method*) and instillation of streptomycin injection in the cavity is needed.
  - *Curettage of lesion*: For tubercular osteomyelitis, lytic lesion in the bone is curetted and the sample is sent for biopsy.
  - *Joint debridement*: For tubercular arthritis, joint debridement is done and material is sent for biopsy. This is also known as "joint clearance surgery".
  - *Synovectomy*: In case of primarily synovial involvement (e.g. in knee), synovectomy is done, partial or total, depending on the extent of involvement.
- *Chemoprophylaxis:* Close contacts of infectious cases (e.g. infants staying in contact with infected mothers) should be administered with chemoprophylaxis for the disease. The

recommended dose is isoniazid 5 mg/kg/day for at least 6 months.

HIGH-YIELD POINTS

- The basic microscopic lesion of TB, "the tubercle", was discovered by Laennec (inventor of stethoscope), in the beginning of 19th century. It was an irony of fate that he himself scummed to the disease at an early age of 45 years.
- The most common chronic vertebral infection worldwide is TB.
- The most common opportunistic infection in human immunodeficiency virus (HIV) infected individuals is TB. Treatment of TB in patients with HIV follows the same principles as treatment of uninfected patients. However, it is important to consider the potential for drug interactions particularly between rifampicin and anti-retroviral agents.
- *ATT in pregnancy*: All drugs, i.e. isoniazid, rifampicin, ethambutol and pyrazinamide (except Streptomycin that is ototoxic to fetus, hence avoided during pregnancy), can be given to pregnant and lactating mothers. Prophylactic pyridoxine (10 mg/day) must be added along with ATT.

TUBERCULOSIS OF SPINE

*Also known as "Pott's Disease", named after Percival Pott (1779)***

INTRODUCTION

The spine is the most common site of skeletal TB and accounts for nearly half of the cases of musculoskeletal TB. 50% of these cases of spinal TB involve dorsal region (specifically lower dorsal) followed by lumbar and then dorsolumbar (D12-L1) region, with lumbosacral being the least common. 7% cases may have skipped lesions (i.e. involvement of more than one noncontiguous level). Although people across all age groups are involved, most commonly the disease affects people in their most productive ages (10–30 years). Children also constitute a high-risk group for acquiring the disease.

PATHOLOGY

Tuberculosis of spine is always secondary to lung lesion. Bacilli reach the spine via the hematogenous route through arteries or Batson paravertebral plexus of veins (Batson's paravertebral venous plexus in the vertebra is a valveless system that allows free flow of blood in both directions depending upon the pressure generated by the intra-abdominal and intrathoracic cavities following strenuous activities like coughing). Upon reaching the spine, bacilli establish either of the four types of anatomical lesion **(Fig. 10.1)**:

1. *Paradiskal*: This is the most common type. Contiguous areas of two adjacent vertebrae along with the intervening disk are affected **(Fig. 10.2)**. The classical patter results because, the lower half of one vertebra and the upper half of one vertebra below it with the intervening disk, develop from the same pair of sclerotome and thus have a common blood supply **(Fig. 10.2)**. Strictly speaking the infection initially starts in the anterior inferior portion of the vertebral body. Later on it spreads into the disk, once the vertebral end plates are eroded.

---

*Antigravity aspiration is done to minimize the chances of sinus formation.
**Currently, the term "Pott's Disease/Pott's spine/Caries spine" describes tuberculous infection of the spine and the term "Pott's paraplegia" describes paraplegia resulting from TB of the spine.

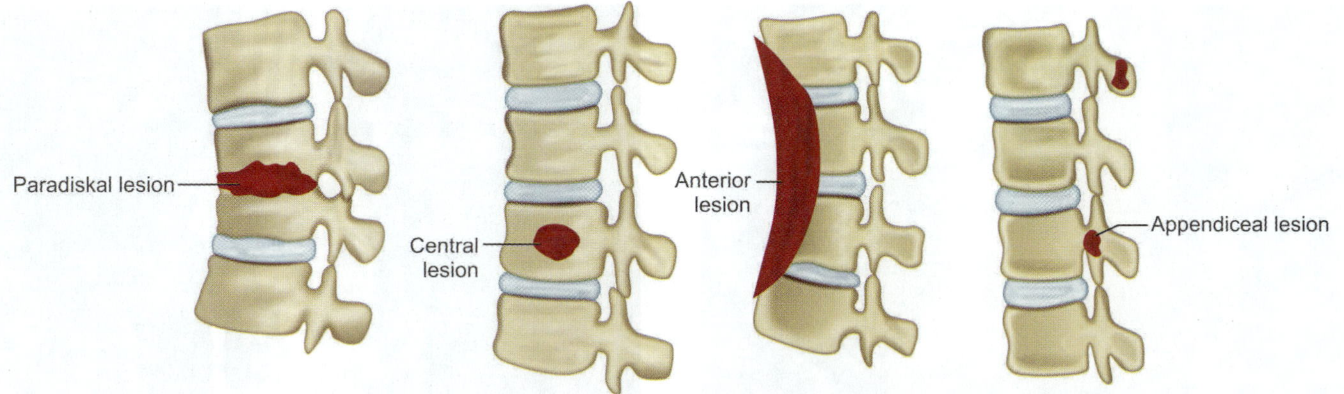

Fig. 10.1: Anatomical types of spinal lesions in tuberculosis spine

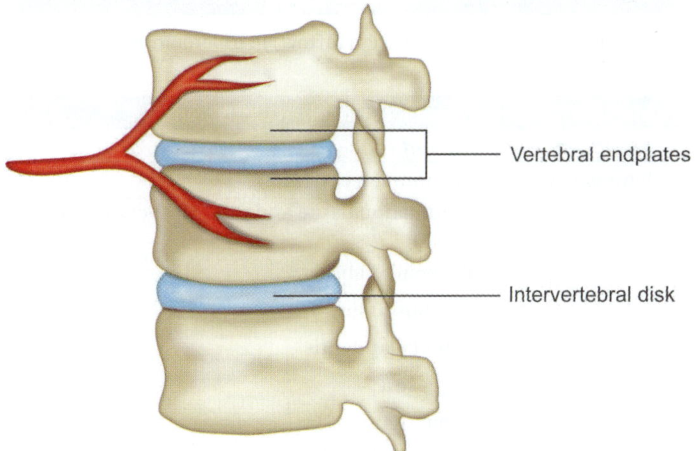

Fig. 10.2: Pattern of blood supply of a vertebra

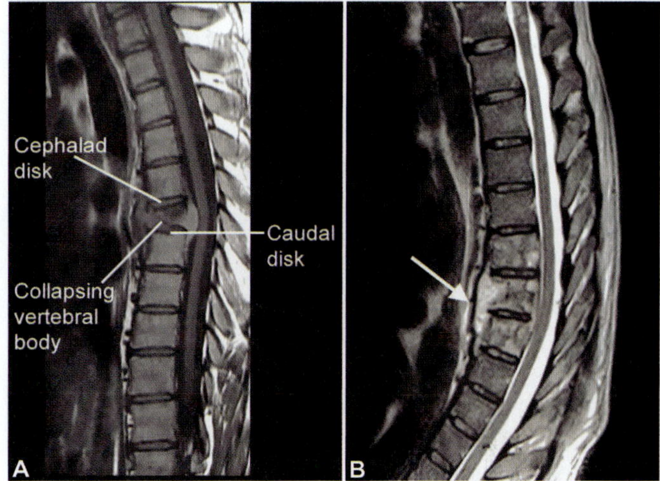

Figs 10.3A and B: (A) Magnetic resonance imaging (MRI) (sagittal section) of dorsal spine showing involvement of vertebral body with preserved disk space [central tuberculosis (TB)]; (B) MRI (sagittal section) of dorsal spine showing involvement of anterior margins of vertebral body with pus collection (arrow) under the anterior longitudinal ligament (anterior TB)

2. *Central*: Central lesions result when infection spreads by intraosseous venous systems (not Batson's plexus). Here body of a vertebra is affected, but, the disk space is preserved **(Fig. 10.3A)**. The whole vertebra collapses in later stages leading to a "concertina collapse", resulting in formation of vertebra plana (a flat vertebra that results from complete compression of a vertebral body).

3. *Anterior*: Infection starts beneath the anterior longitudinal ligament (ALL) and involves anterior margin of the vertebral body **(Fig. 10.3B)**. Relative lack of proteolytic enzymes in mycobacteria (compared with pyogenic bacteria) prevents vertebral erosions but promotes a subligamentous spread with infection spreading up and down under the ALL. The pus that accumulates in this area often on an X-ray gives an appearance of an aneurysm of the aorta, hence called the "Aneurysmal phenomena".

4. *Posterior (Appendiceal)*: Posterior involvement is very rare and involves the posterior elements (pedicles, laminae, transverse process, facet joints and spinous process). Facet joints followed by spinous processes are the least commonly involved structures in posterior type.

CLINICAL FEATURES

Many patients who come with the disease have a past history or family history of TB. Back pain is the earliest and most common symptom, they present with. Associated with pain in mid back, patient may complain of stiffness, swelling (cold abscess), deformity, and/or paraparesis with constitutional symptoms like low-grade fever with evening rise of temperature, malaise, anorexia and weight loss. Pain is insidious in onset, diffuse and dull aching in character. It may be radiating in nature, if the disease process involves a nerve root.

On examination, the spine is stiff and painful on movement. In fact, the first clinical sign is paraspinal muscle spasm. The collapse of vertebral bodies leads to localized kyphotic deformity on the back, causing prominent spinous process, which is tender to palpation **(Fig. 10.4)**. Kyphus can be of three types: (1) knuckle (single vertebra involved) kyphus, (2) angular kyphus (two or three vertebrae involved, gibbus was an older term for the same) or (3) rounded kyphus (more than three vertebrae involved).

A cold abscess may be present far away from vertebral column along the fascial planes or course of neurovascular bundle. The usual sites are anterior or posterior triangles of the neck, paraspinal region of back, along the brachial plexus in axilla, along intercostal nerves in the lateral or anterior chest wall,

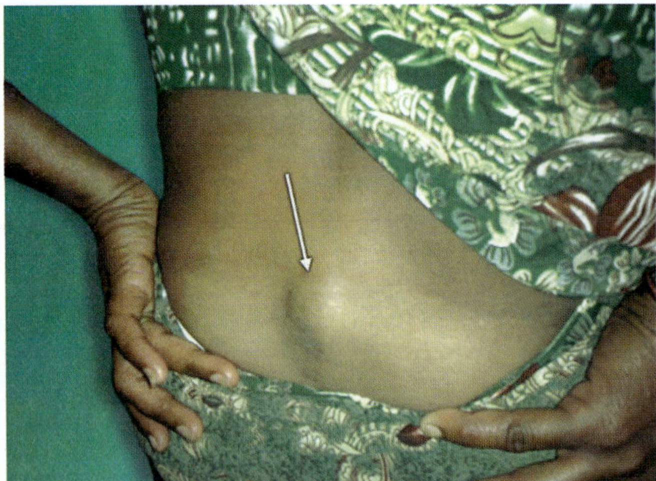

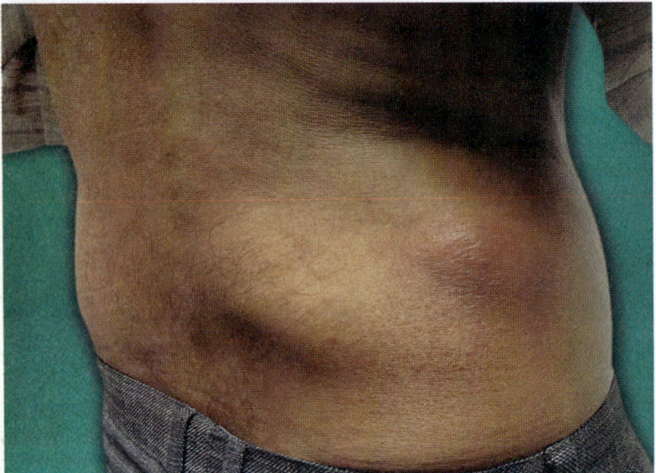

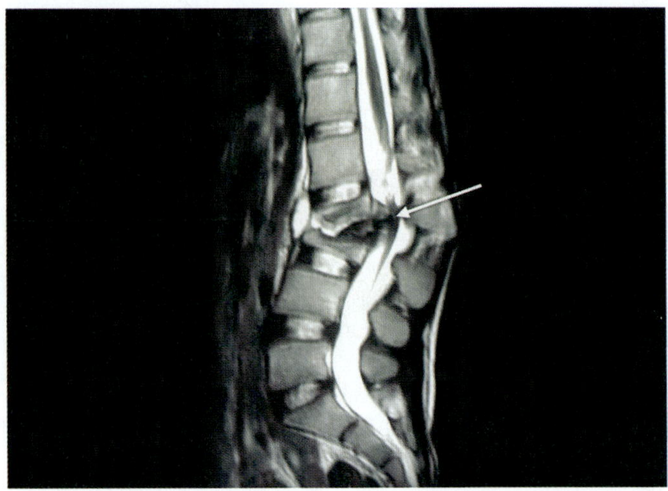

Fig. 10.4: Prominent spinous process at back (Knuckle, arrow)
Courtesy: Dr Matad Lokeshwaraiah Chetan.

Fig. 10.5: Clinical picture showing cold abscess in tuberculosis tracked to the lumbar triangle at the back

Fig. 10.6: Cord compression (arrow) in tuberculosis spine

Table 10.1: Causes of paraplegia in tuberculosis spine	
Extrinsic compression of cord	
Inflammatory	Inflammatory edema
	Granulation tissue and pus (Most common cause)
	Tubercular abscess
	Caseous tissue
Mechanical	Tubercular debris
	Sequestra
	Canal stenosis
	Internal gibbus*
	Pathological dislocation of spine
Intrinsic pathology in cord	
Vascular	Thrombosis or endarteritis of spinal vessels
Degenerative	Myelitis
	Syringomyelic changes
	Cord stretching due to severe deformity
Atypical causes	Spinal tumor syndrome[†]

* Internal Gibbus: *See* **Figure 10.7**.
[†] Spinal tumor syndrome: *See* "differential diagnosis".

iliac fossa, along psoas muscle (psoas abscess), lumbar triangle **(Fig. 10.5)** and in the upper part of the thigh. Patients with psoas abscess may present with a pseudoflexion deformity of the hip (*see* Page 288).

NEUROLOGICAL COMPLICATIONS (POTT'S PARAPLEGIA)

If TB spine is neglected, more and more vertebral body collapses and the necrotic caseous material herniates back and compresses the neural structures, the patient then may present with paraparesis **(Fig. 10.6)**. The incidence of Pott's paraplegia is 10–30% and is commonly seen in disease of the upper thoracic spine because of narrow canal space. Causes of paraplegia can be grouped as shown in **Table 10.1**. Although the most common cause is compression by pus and tubercular granulation tissue, sudden onset paraplegia may result from ischemia of the cord due to thromboembolic phenomena, or cord transection due to pathological dislocation or a rapidly accumulated epidural abscess.

Order of Neurological Involvement

Rarely is paraplegia the presenting symptom. However, when it develops, the motor system is almost always affected before the sensory system because the diseased area in the spine (i.e. vertebral body) lies anterior to the cord near the motor tracts **(Fig. 10.7)**. As motor tracts are compressed, the first neurological sign that appears is ankle clonus followed by plantar extensor. Thereafter, the patient develops mild spastic motor weakness manifesting as clumsiness or incoordination of gait which ends in severe weakness to the extent where the patient is unable to stand and is bedridden. The sensations carried by lateral spinothalamic tract—pain, crude touch and temperature are affected first, followed by sensations carried by dorsal column—vibration and proprioception. Lastly, there is paralysis of the anal sphincter and bladder. In extremely severe cases, spasticity disappears and paralysis becomes flaccid **(Box 10.1)**.

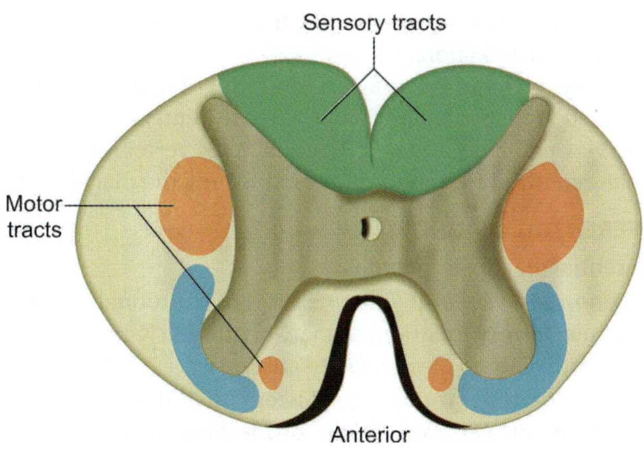

Fig. 10.7: Compression of cord from anterior

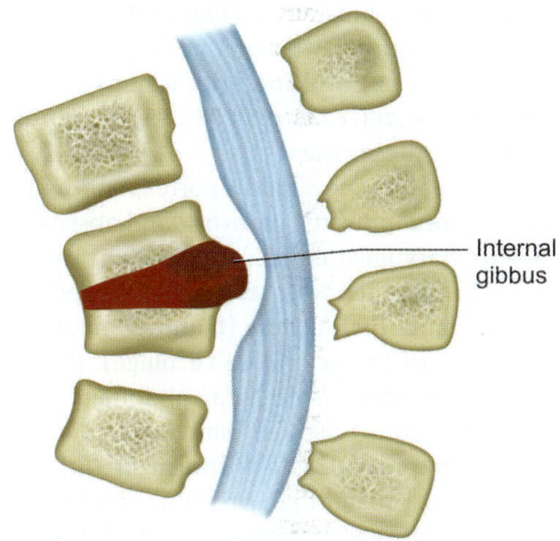

Fig. 10.8: Diagrammatic representation of internal gibbus. (Collapse of vertebral body causes angulation of the spine that leads to the formation of a bony spur that may press on the anterior aspect of the spinal cord)

Box 10.1: Stages of tubercular paraplegia

- *Stage 1*: Patient is unaware of neural deficit, physician detects plantar extensor and/or clonus

- *Stage 2*: Patient is aware of neural deficit, presents with complaints of clumsiness or incoordination while walking, but is able to manage to walk with or without support

- *Stage 3*: Nonambulatory patient due to paraplegia in extension; sensory loss is less than 50%

- *Stage 4*: Stage 3 plus flexor spasms/paraplegia in flexion/flaccid paraplegia/sensory loss more than 50%/bladder-bowel involvement

---

Classification of Paraplegia in TB Spine (Griffith's Classification)

Griffith classified paraplegia into early and late onset types, to highlight the different pathological processes involved in two different situations:

1. *Early onset paraplegia*: It occurs during the active phase of the disease usually within 2 years of onset. It is caused due to inflammatory edema, granulation tissue, abscess, caseous tissue or ischemic lesion of cord.

2. *Late onset paraplegia*: It occurs after 2 years of the persistence of disease. It may be associated with recrudescence of the disease or due to mechanical pressure on the cord. It is caused due to caseous tissue, tubercular debris, sequestra, internal gibbus **(Fig. 10.8)**, canal stenosis or severe kyphotic deformity.

DIAGNOSIS

Blood investigations show low hemoglobin, increased TLC and elevated ESR. QuantiFERON-TB Gold assay yields positive results.

Radiological Features

The classic radiographic triad of TB spine is disk space reduction, lysis of the vertebra and paravertebral soft tissue abscesses **(Fig. 10.9A)**. Loss of definition of paradiskal margins (due to erosion of endplates and prolapse of the nucleus pulposus into the soft cancellous diseased body) followed by disk space reduction are the earliest findings, seen in the more common paradiskal type of TB. Thereafter, the contiguous parts of the affected vertebrae get eroded and osseous destruction becomes evident. However, it's not until 2–4 months that osteopenia manifests, as 30–40% of

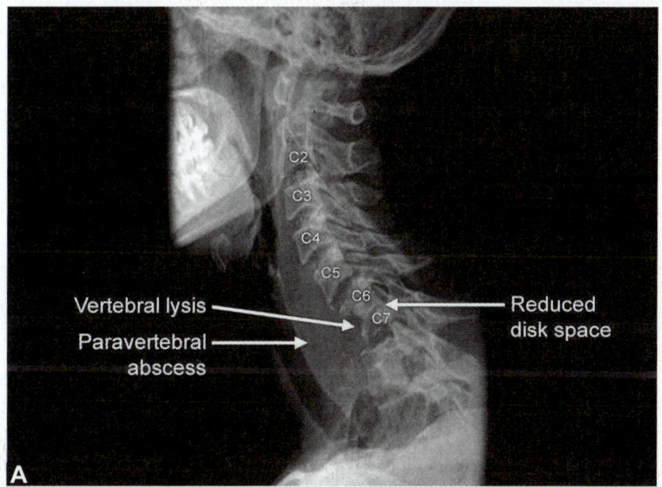

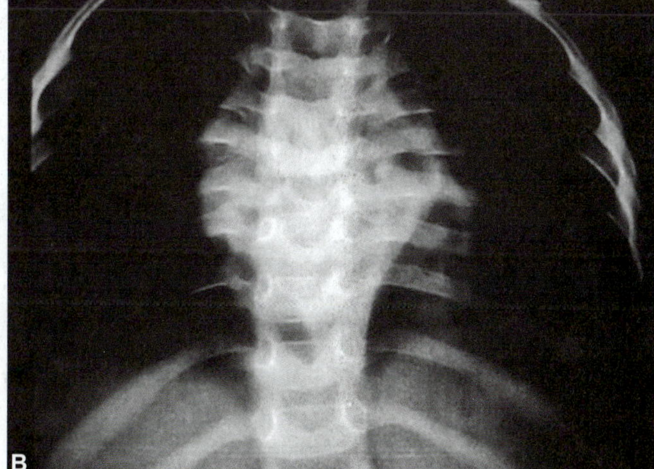

Figs 10.9A and B: (A) X-ray of cervical spine lateral view showing the classic triad of tuberculosis (TB); (B) Paravertebral abscess in TB thoracic spine

calcium must be lost from any bone to show up as radiolucent area on X-ray. As destruction of the vertebral bodies continues, there is anterior wedging of vertebra leading to kyphotic deformity [classified based on kyphus angle **(Fig. 10.10 and Table 10.2)**]. On the contrary, central TB lesions present with a concertina collapse (vertebra plana) while anterior lesions can be identified by the aneurysmal sign (*see* Pages 298-299). Diminution of disk space is minimal in these cases.

Paravertebral soft tissue shadow corresponding to the site of the affected vertebra indicates paravertebral abscess. In cervical spine TB, a retropharyngeal abscess may be seen on the lateral view **(Fig. 10.9A)**. It is identified when the space between the pharynx and the spine is more than 0.5 cm (if above cricoid cartilage) or more than 1.5 cm (if below cricoid cartilage). Psoas abscess is seen as a soft tissue shadow on X-ray abdomen as widening of psoas shadow. In thoracic spine, paravertebral collection **(Fig. 10.9B)** may either present as a fusiform or bird nest abscess (abscess with length greater than breadth) or a tense or globular abscess (abscess with width greater than length indicating pus under pressure). An abscess in upper dorsal spine may lead to a widened superior mediastinum on an anteroposterior film.

Computed tomography (CT) scan is a useful tool in assessing the extent of destruction of the vertebral body. Shape, extent and route of spread of cold abscess can be very well visualized on CT scan.

Magnetic resonance imaging (MRI) provides earliest diagnosis and is the investigation of choice as it can additionally evaluate the status of spinal cord **(Fig. 10.11A)**. It is extremely useful in diagnosis of difficult and rare sites like craniovertebral or cervicodorsal region. It also shows the type and extent of

paravertebral abscess. Use of contrast (Gadolinium) may enhance areas of active infection.

Biopsy is required only in doubtful diagnosis. However, CT-guided transpedicular (biopsy needle enters into vertebral body via pedicle, under CT guidance) vertebral biopsy is considered the gold standard for establishing the diagnosis.

DIFFERENTIAL DIAGNOSIS

Differential diagnosis includes:

- *Traumatic vertebral fracture*: No constitutional symptoms, rather history of trauma may be there. X-ray shows the fracture with no paravertebral abscess.
- *Disk prolapse*: Young age, history of lifting heavy weight and intact vertebral body on radiography with absent paravertebral shadow clinch the diagnosis.
- *Tumor* **(Fig. 10.11B)**: It is the most important differential, especially in older individuals where the metastasis is to be ruled out. Preservation of disk space and absence of paravertebral shadow provide the diagnosis. Mostly tumors tend to involve pedicles, an infrequently involved area in TB.
- *Ankylosing spondylitis*: Patients may present with chronic back pain, however, absence of constitutional symptoms, characteristic age, presence of sacroiliitis on X-ray and reduced chest expansion provide the diagnosis.
- *Spinal tumor syndrome* **(Figs 10.12A and B)**: The name is a misnomer as it is not a tumor of the spine. It refers to a condition when an extradural mass (a granuloma over dura mater/tuberculoma) compresses the cord. On X-ray, there are no osseous changes, but the patient may present with neurological deficit. MRI is the investigation of choice. Since vertebra is not eroded, surgical management involves decompression via laminectomy unlike Pott's spine where laminectomy is contraindicated and anterolateral decompression (ALD) is the treatment of choice (*see* later).
- *Hydatid disease of bone*: Although liver followed by lung are the most common sites of hydatid cysts, *Echinococcus granulosus* (dog tapeworm) produces cystic lesions in bone in only 0.5–4% of cases. Spine followed by femur is the most common site of affection. MRI provides a reliable tool of establishing the diagnosis in this rare condition. Treatment is largely surgical with removal of the cyst and surrounding

Table 10.2: Clinicoradiological classification of spinal tuberculosis (grading of kyphosis based on K angle, **Fig. 10.10**)

Stage	Clinicoradiological features
I (Predestructive stage)	Straightening of spine on X-ray; No kyphus
II (Early destructive stage)	Disk space reduced on X-ray; K angle <10°
III (Mild kyphus)	2–3 vertebrae collapse; K angle 10–30°
IV (Moderate kyphus)	>3 vertebrae collapse; K angle 30–60°
V (Severe kyphus)	>3 vertebrae collapse; K angle > 60°

Note: Patients having stage I disease have healing with no defects; stages II–IV may heal with progressive kyphotic deformity; in stage V patients' chances of complete neural recovery are remote.

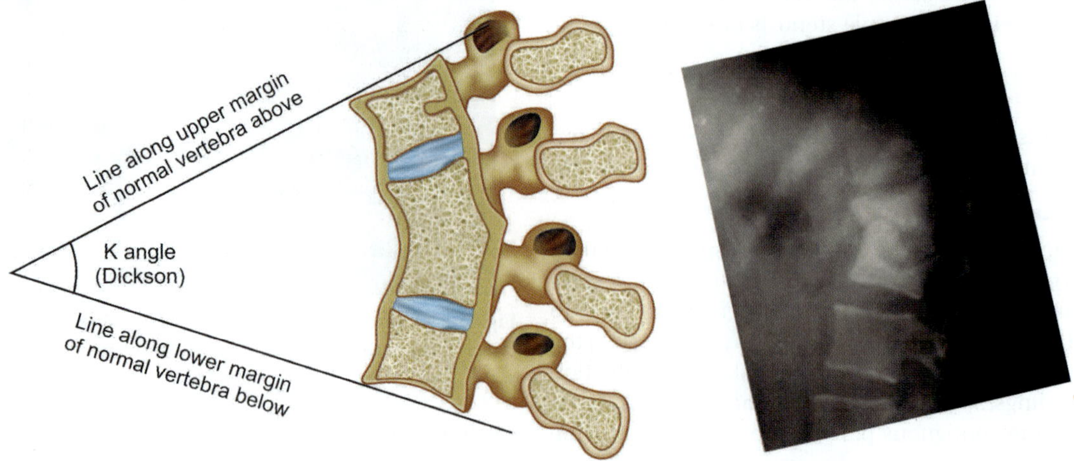

Fig. 10.10: Kyphus angle (Dickson) measurement being depicted in caries spine L1-L2

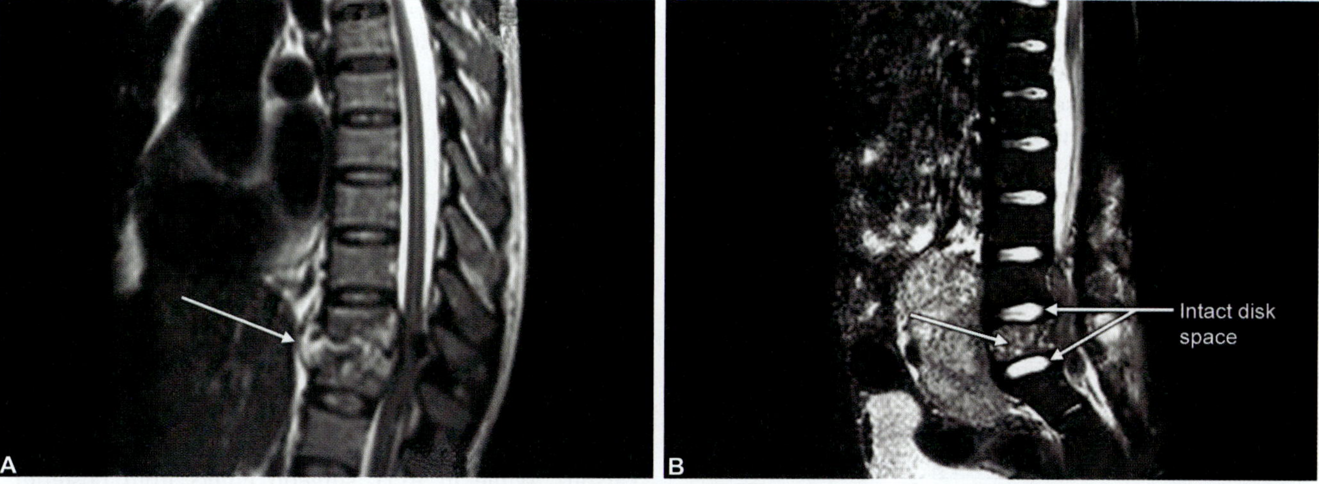

Figs 10.11A and B: (A) Magnetic resonance imaging of the thoracic spine (sagittal section) showing loss of disk space and compression of spinal cord in the tubercular affection of thoracic spine; (B) Tumor (Ewing sarcoma, arrow) of L5 vertebrae

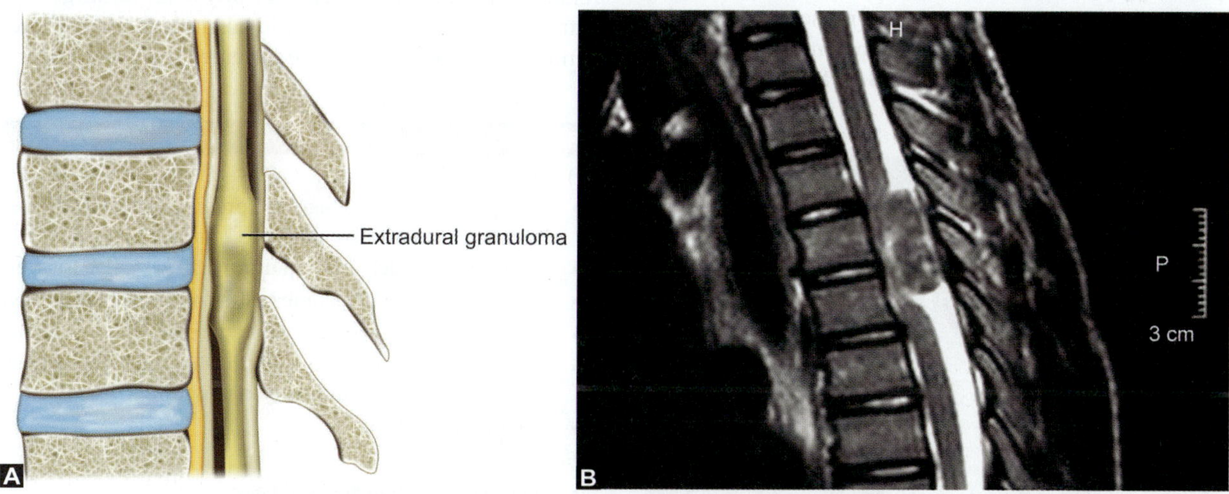

Figs 10.12A and B: Spinal tumor syndrome. (A) Pictorial description; (B) Magnetic resonance imaging of thoracic spine (sagittal section) showing extradural granuloma

bone and replacement of bone defects with bone grafts under cover of Benzimidazoles (Albendazole).

TREATMENT

Various options of treatment include:

- *Chemotherapy:* ATT is administered to all cases (with or without neurological deficit).
- *Bed rest and traction*: Absolute bed rest is required for pain relief and to prevent further collapse of the vertebra, pathological dislocation and neurological complications. In the treatment of cervical spine TB (if lesion seems unstable), skeletal traction by Crutchfield tongs is used to put the diseased part at rest.
- *Mobilization*: Gradual mobilization is encouraged with help of spinal brace as soon as the patient is comfortable **(Fig. 10.13)**.
- *Treatment of abscess*: Aspirated when palpable or symptomatic and 1 g of streptomycin is instilled.

Treatment of a Case with Paraplegia

All patients are initially started on ATT as soon as the diagnosis is made and put on absolute bed rest.

- *Paraplegic care*: A paraplegic patient is bedridden and is vulnerable to numerous complications associated with recumbency. These complications are bed sores (decubitus ulcer), hypostatic pneumonia, deep venous thrombosis, constipation, urinary tract infection due to Foley's catheter, joint stiffness, osteoporosis, muscle atrophy and depression. To prevent these complications, the patient is encouraged to take frequent turns in bed specially 2-hour log rolling and application of talcum powder over the back to avoid bed sores. Air mattress is also used. Incentive spirometer and chest thumping (chest physiotherapy) are done to avoid chest complications. High-fiber diet and bulk laxatives for constipation and bladder wash to prevent urinary tract infection are prescribed.

- *Operative treatment*: Operative treatment is needed for those who do not respond to minimum 3 weeks of ATT. The principle behind surgery is to decompress the spinal cord by removing the diseased portion of vertebral body and the tuberculous pus, caseous matter and granulation tissue. The operative procedures used vary with part of vertebral column involved and have been listed below. The indications for surgery are given in **Box 10.2**.

Operative Procedures

Anterior decompression: It refers to going via anterior approach and removing the diseased vertebral body and caseous tissue to decompress the cord. Theoretically, it is the best surgical procedure, but most orthopedic surgeons are unfamiliar with this approach as in thoracic or lumbar spine, it involves going via pleural or peritoneal cavities. Hence, it is generally not the preferred approach. It is mostly advocated in cases of cervical spine TB.

Capener's lateral rachiotomy (modified costotransversectomy): This is a posterior approach (incision is on posterior side of spinal column) to vertebral column via paraspinal muscles and involves removal of transverse processes and 6–8 cm of medial end of ribs attaching to diseased vertebrae **(Fig. 10.14A)**. Minimum two and maximum four ribs can be removed.

Anterolateral decompression: It is most commonly performed procedure. Going with a posterior incision, dividing paraspinal muscles, along with costotransversectomy, the diseased part of vertebra lying anterior and lateral to the spinal cord is debrided and the cord is decompressed from its anterolateral aspect **(Fig. 10.14B)**. In ALD, the structures removed are ribs, transverse process, pedicle and posterolateral part of the vertebral body. Spinous process and lamina are not removed as damaging these intact posterior structures may risk the stability of the spine. The main drawback of this approach is that if surgeon plans to fix spinal column (with instruments, e.g. pedicle screws) for immediate postoperative stability to ensure early mobilization of patient, the same can be very difficult.

Lateral extracavitary approach (LECA): A procedure that is increasingly being used in recent times is the LECA (Stanford Larson). While in ALD, surgeon enters from posterior side dividing paraspinal muscles, in LECA **(Fig. 10.14C)**, the trajectory is ventrolateral to paraspinal muscles (as paraspinal muscles are reflected medially). Going posteriorly it allows surgeon to remain extrapleural and/or extraperitoneal but at the same time entering ventral to spinal musculature provides relatively better access to

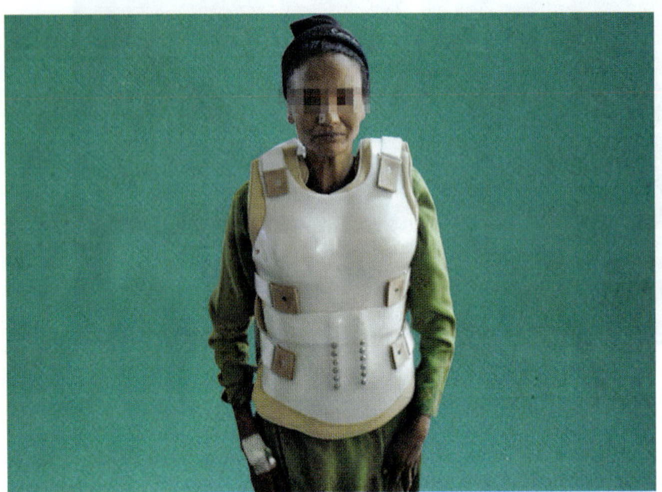

Fig. 10.13: Mobilization in brace

Box 10.2: Indications of surgery

Absolute indications

- Paraparesis with no signs of progressive recovery on at least 3 weeks of conservative therapy
- Paraparesis which develop during conservative treatment
- Paraparesis which becomes worse on conservative therapy
- Patients with recurrence of paraparesis
- Patients of cervical spine TB, having large prevertebral abscess causing dyspnea or difficulty in deglutition
- Grade 4 paraplegia

Relative indications

- Paraplegia with onset in old age
- Painful paraplegia

Rare indications

- Spinal tumor syndrome
- Cauda equina syndrome
- Posterior spinal disease

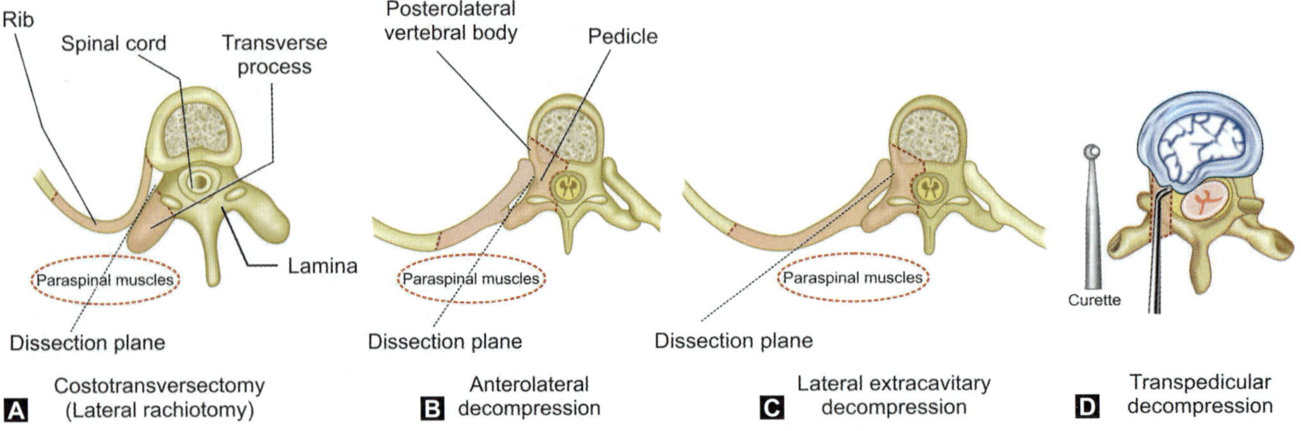

Figs 10.14A to D: Posterior surgical approaches for Pott's paraplegia

anterior, middle and posterior aspects of spinal column and also offers direct visualization of the dural sac and neural elements for decompression (somewhat comparable to what an anterior approach would offer). Additionally if surgeon plans to fix spinal column with instrumentation (e.g. with pedicle screws) for immediate postoperative stability to ensure early mobilization, the same is much easier via the LECA, where one can reflect paraspinal muscles laterally (rather than medially as initially done) to expose the pedicles and go ahead with pedicle screw fixation (*see* Page 220).

Posterior transpedicular decompression: This is another variation of posterior approach to spinal column. The surgeon uses special currents to scoop out diseases portion of vertebra, entering the body via the pedicle of vertebra **(Fig. 10.14D)**. However, the amount of decompression that can be performed is limited, so the procedure is mainly used for those with early stage of disease (minimal vertebral destruction or incomplete paraplegia).

Laminectomy: Removal of the lamina in TB spine is contraindicated because TB usually involves anterior structures and removal of posterior structures (i.e. lamina) will further jeopardize stability of the spine. However, laminectomy is indicated in cases of spinal tumor syndrome and posterior spinal disease.

Spinal fusion: If the patient being operated has severe kyphotic deformity (K angle > 60°), it is preferable to add a posterior spinal fusion (*see* Page 220) after decompression surgery and deformity correction, as such a large deformity is invariably associated with delayed neurological complications, 10–15 years later. Else patient will have to be taken up later for removal of the internal gibbus deformity.

HEALING OF DISEASE

As the disease heals, lytic focus gets surrounded by sclerotic bone. Even the whole of the vertebral body may become sclerotic (ivory vertebra). Earliest radiological sign of healing is sharpening of fuzzy paradiskal margins. However, one should remember that radiological as well as MRI evidence of healing, lags behind the biological process in spinal TB. Prognostic factors for spinal TB are given in **Table 10.3**.

End result: Even though infection may be eliminated by chemotherapy, when several vertebrae have been damaged and disk space destroyed, the adjacent vertebrae undergo fusion resulting in bony ankylosis or bone block formation **(Fig. 10.15)**. This is in contrast to other joints where TB leads to fibrous ankylosis, as in the spine the area of contact between cancellous vertebral surfaces is high and in addition weight-bearing induces bone formation.

HIGH-YIELD POINTS

- Tuberculosis is the most common cause of kyphosis in India.
- Cold abscesses in TB may track along psoas muscle producing psoas abscess. Psoas abscess as a rule is associated with a detectable tuberculous disease of vertebral column from D10 vertebra to sacrum, or a disease of sacroiliac joint, pelvis or hip.
- *"Spine at Risk" signs:* Prof Rajasekaran (India) described "spine at risk signs" (X-ray signs) in TB to caution against a progression of the tuberculous deformity. These include:
    - Subluxation of the facet joint at the apex of the kyphus deformity
    - Presence of retropulsion (posterior displacement) of the vertebra
    - Posterior toppling of the vertebra
    - Lateral translation of the vertebra.
- *Middle path regime*: It is a general guide for treatment of TB spine *advocated by Dr SM Tuli, Delhi, a pioneer in the field.* It simply refers to "nonoperative treatment for all cases of caries spine and operative treatment in cases of failure of conservative therapy and development of complications".
- *Anterolateral decompression surgery:* ALD is the traditional approach for posterior decompression in Pott's paraplegia. Although the procedure was originally described by Griffith and Seddon (1956) with patient in prone position, a modification of patient positioning has been advocated by Dr SM Tuli. He recommends performing it in right lateral position (right side of patient down) and approach the spine from left side via a semicircular incision centered over the diseased vertebra **(Fig. 10.16)**. The proposed

Table 10.3: Prognostic factors in tuberculosis (TB) spine*

Factors	Good	Bad
Age	Young	Old
Onset	Early onset	Late onset
Duration	Shorter	Longer
Progression	Slow	Rapid
Lesion type	Wet (Exudative)	Dry
Severity	Stages 1 and 2	Stages 3 and 4
General condition	Good	Poor
Vertebral disease	Active	Healed
Kyphosis	<60°	>60°
Cord status on MRI	Normal	Myelomalacic changes

*Tuberculosis of the skeletal system by Dr SM Tuli.

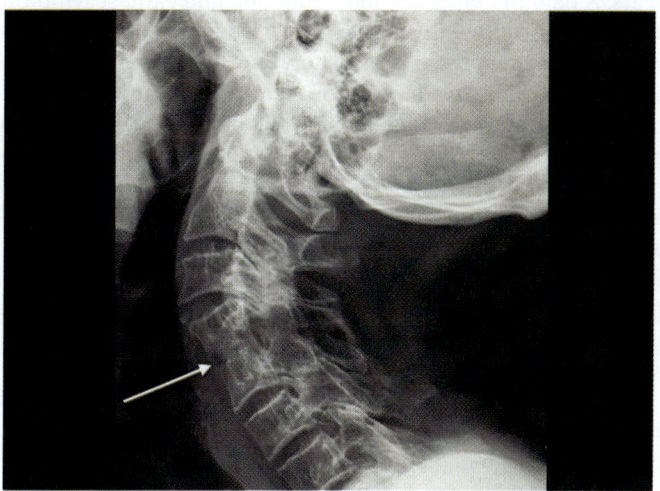

Fig. 10.15: Bony ankylosis (arrow) between C4 and C5 vertebrae

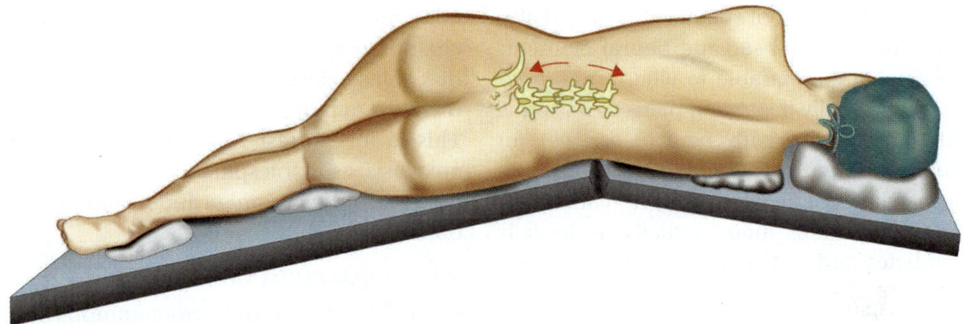

Fig. 10.16: Patient positioned in right lateral position for anterolateral decompression (as recommended by Dr SM Tuli, Delhi). A semicircular incision centered over the diseased vertebra (marked with arrows) is used for the surgery and spine is approached from left side

advantages of this modification are: avoidance of venous congestion and excessive bleeding, freer respiration as lung and mediastinal contents fall anteriorly and a better look at lesion.

- *Hong Kong procedure (radical anterior decompression and spinal fusion)*: If surgical decompression is to be performed in patients with cervical spine TB, an anterior approach is preferred. Hong Kong procedure involves a radical anterior debridement of spine followed by removal of diseased vertebral body and bone grafting in the area of the removed body. It helps in early healing of the disease and prevents also a deformity in a better way, but needs appropriate facilities.

TUBERCULOSIS OF THE HIP JOINT

INTRODUCTION

The most common site of extraspinal TB is the hip joint (15% of skeletal TB cases). The initial focus may start in the acetabular roof (most common), epiphysis, metaphysis (an area of watershed between obturator and femoral circulation called as Babcock's triangle) or greater trochanter. If the disease starts in acetabulum, the joint involvement is late and mild in severity. Rarely the disease may start in synovium and involve the bones later.

CLINICAL FEATURES

Mostly affected are children between the age of 5 years and 15 years. A painful limp is the most common and earliest symptom. The patient walks with an antalgic gait (decreased stance phase by putting a little pressure for a short time on affected limb). Pain around the hip is insidious in onset, gradually progressive and may be referred to the medial aspect of the knee. Muscle wasting of anterior thigh and gluteus maximus is seen. Additionally child may present with deformity, stiffness, shortening and fullness around the hip. Constitutional symptoms like fever, weight loss and loss of appetite are usually present. A child may wake up from sleep due to night cries. Rarely the patient may present with palpable cold abscess (in femoral triangle, over medial, lateral or posterior part of the thigh, ischiorectal fossa, etc.), discharging sinuses or pathological dislocation of hip, if neglected.

On examination, tenderness may be present over anterior hip joint elicited 1–1.5 cm down and lateral to mid-inguinal point. In the sagittal plane, flexion deformity is present (detected by Thomas Test), which is compensated by exaggerated lumbar lordosis (up to 30° of flexion deformity can be compensated). In the coronal plane, any of adduction or abduction deformity may be seen. There may be a global restriction of movements in all directions. In late stages, there is just a jog of movement possible (fibrous ankylosis).

STAGES OF TUBERCULOSIS HIP

The disease process progresses through the following clinical stages:

- *Stage 1 (Stage of tubercular synovitis)*: Due to synovitis, there is joint effusion and the joint is held in position of maximum capacity, i.e. flexion, abduction and external rotation causing apparent lengthening. On X-ray, all that is visible is a widened joint space due to effusion and generalized osteopenia.
- *Stage 2 (Stage of early arthritis)*: With the advancement of the disease process, there is destruction of articular cartilage. With spasms of the flexors and adductors of the hip, there is flexion, adduction and internal rotation deformity with apparent shortening.* True shortening* is also present due to damage to articular cartilage, but is less than 1 cm. X-ray shows decrease in joint space and osteopenia.
- *Stage 3 (Stage of late arthritis)*: With further destruction, clinical signs of flexion, adduction, internal rotation deformities and apparent shortening are exaggerated. True shortening is more than 1 cm. There is gross restriction of movements and muscle wasting. X-rays may show complete loss of joint space with destruction of the head or acetabulum.
- *Stage 4 (Late arthritis with subluxation/dislocation)*: There are flexion, adduction and internal rotation deformities with gross shortening. With the destruction of acetabulum, femur head and ligaments, the upper end of the femur may displace upwards and dorsally leaving the lower part of acetabulum empty but forming a false acetabulum higher up (wandering acetabulum, **Fig. 10.17A**). In some cases, the head and neck of femur get smaller in size and contained in an enlarged acetabulum (mortar and pestle appearance, **Fig. 10.17B**). Severe destruction of the capsule and acetabulum may eventually lead to pathological dislocation of femur head.

RADIOLOGICAL FEATURES

X-ray pelvis with bilateral hip, anteroposterior (AP) view and a hip lateral view is required. Radiographs with tubercular arthritis

---

*See Examination of Hip (Chapter 5).

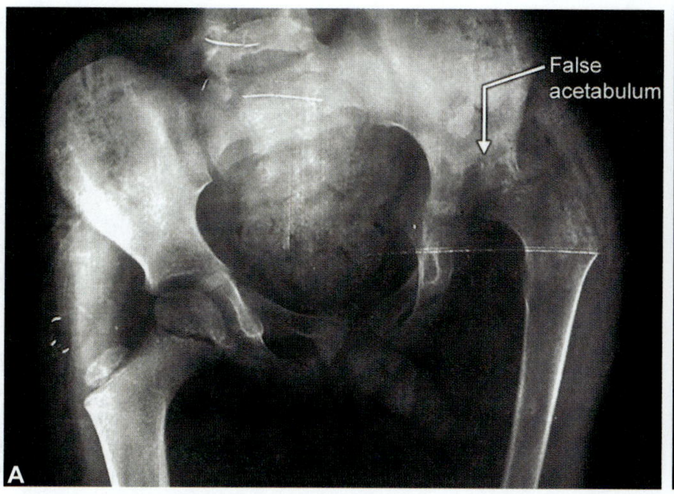

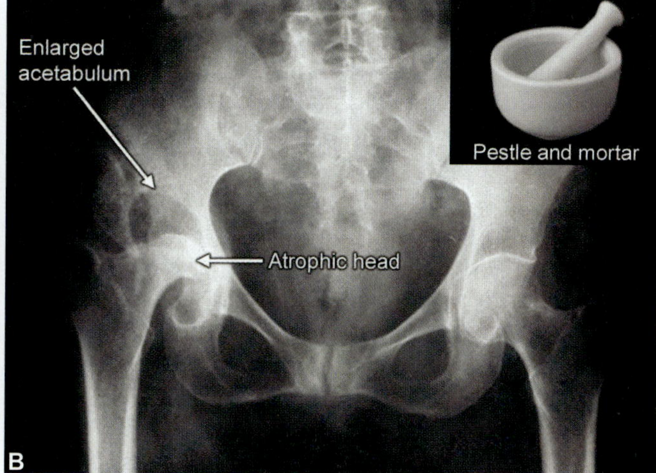

Figs 10.17A and B: Tuberculosis of the hip joint. (A) Wandering acetabulum; and (B) Pestle and mortar appearance

Courtesy: Dr Gaurav Gupta.

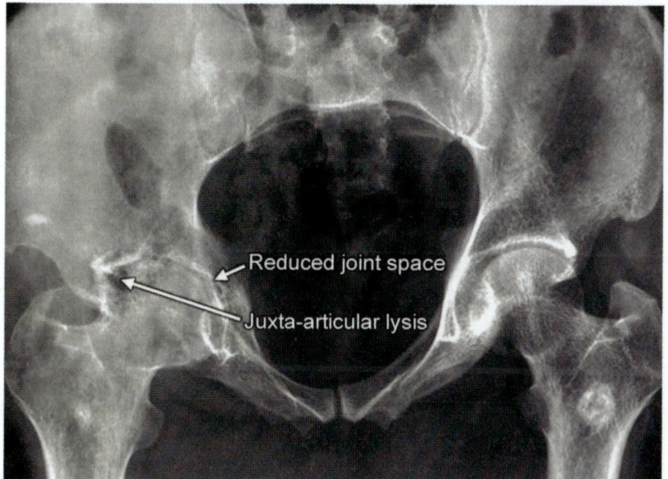

Fig. 10.18: X-ray pelvis with both hips anteroposterior views of patient with tuberculosis right hip joint

exhibit the classical Phemister's triad consisting of juxta-articular osteopenia, periarticular erosions and reduced joint space **(Fig. 10.18)**. Although the classic feature is reduction of joint space that occurs because of destruction of cartilage, haziness of articular margins (due to juxta-articular osteopenia) is the earliest radiological sign. Lytic lesions (periarticular erosion) develop as disease advances and may be seen in acetabular roof or femoral head. In even later stages, a wandering acetabulum or a pestle and mortar appearance may develop.

DIFFERENTIAL DIAGNOSIS

In Children

Perthes disease: It is the closest differential. It affects classically children in the age group of 4–8 years. Symptoms are intermittent and child may present with painful limp. Clinically, these patients have limited abduction and internal rotation while in TB, all range of motions are painful. MRI may be done where TB may show destruction of both acetabulum and femoral head while in Perthes disease only the head is destroyed and there is no evidence of any collection.

Low-grade septic arthritis: Aspiration of pus and Gram stain and culture solve the query.

Developmental dysplasia of the hip (DDH): Limp is painless, so is the range of movements. Also, telescopy is positive.

Congenital coxa vara: Children with this condition present with painless limp and restricted abduction and internal rotation. Fairbank's triangle may be visible in the neck (*see* Page 375).

In Adults

Monoarticular rheumatoid arthritis: Rare disease. The joint space is uniformly narrowed. A positive rheumatoid factor or anti-cyclic citrullinated peptide antibody test may aid the diagnosis.

Osteoarthritis: Pain along with crepitus may be present. Rather than osteopenia, on X-ray there is subchondral sclerosis. Constitutional symptoms are absent, so is the collection on MRI.

MANAGEMENT

Active Stage

Tuberculosis hip is said to be active when the hip is extremely painful with presence of constitutional symptoms. On examination, there is rise in local temperature, hip is tender, and range of motion is painful.

- *Nonoperative treatment:* Patient is admitted and ATT is started. The affected hip is put to rest by using skin or skeletal traction. Traction relieves spasm, reduces pain, prevent or correct deformity and prevent subluxation of the hip. Abscess if present, is aspirated. When pain subsides, active-assisted range of motion exercises are started.
- *Operative treatment:* If there is no adequate response to conservative therapy, joint debridement (Wilkinson's joint clearance surgery) is done. In this, the joint is opened and pus, necrotic caseous tissue, debris, inflamed synovium, and other dead tissues are removed, joint is curetted and washed. Synovium and tissues are sent for histopathological examination.

Healed Stage

When a patient presents in healing or healed stage, the disease has already eaten up the normal bone and patient presents mainly with deformity, instability and shortening with minimal pain. In such cases, the main aim is to provide painless hip with maximum useful functions.

Four options are there to tackle such a situation:

1. *Corrective osteotomy*: Cases where the hip is ankylosed in an unacceptable position, a subtrochanteric osteotomy will be helpful to correct the deformity.
2. *Girdlestone excisional arthroplasty* **(Fig. 10.19)**: In this procedure, the head and neck of the femur are excised. The dead necrotic tissues and granulation tissues are removed. Postoperatively, skeletal traction is given for 3 weeks, followed by range of motion exercises of the hip is started. It provides painless, mobile but unstable joint. Advantages are ability to squat and sit cross legged. Drawbacks are instability and shortening.
3. *Arthrodesis*: Classically, this operation is indicated in an adult presenting with unsound or painful ankylosis. In this procedure, the hip joint is fused in functional position to provide painless, stable but fixed joint **(Fig. 10.20)**. The patient is unable to squat after arthrodesis. With advent of modern joint replacement surgery, this option has relatively fallen out of favor.
4. *Total hip replacement (THR)*: Joint replacement after TB of the hip is still a debate. Despite the best of selection, reactivation of the disease may occur. THR should be done after a long quiescent period of maintaining healed status under perioperative antitubercular treatment cover.

HIGH-YIELD POINTS

- In certain cases of tubercular arthritis (stages II–IV), the hip may not have the classical deformities pertaining to that stage. This may be either due to the effect of traction used or due to continuous adoption of a specific posture that is offering the patient pain relief or because of destruction of the iliofemoral ligament by the disease process unrestraining the stability of the joint.
- *Shanmugasundaram classification*: This is a radiological classification of TB hip that classifies the disease into seven types: (1) normal, (2) traveling acetabulum, (3) dislocation hip, (4) Perthes type, (5) protrusio type, (6) atrophic type and (7) pestle and mortar type. There is a relationship between these types and functional outcome.
- While the end result of TB spine is bony ankylosis (i.e. osseous tissue fuses two bones together), osteoarticular TB (TB hip, knee, etc.) ends in false ankylosis or fibrous ankylosis (i.e. fibrous connective tissue or contracture of capsule and surrounding structures fuse the joint).

TUBERCULOSIS OF THE KNEE JOINT

INTRODUCTION

The knee is the third most common site for skeletal TB. Commonly affected patients are relatively older children and young adults.

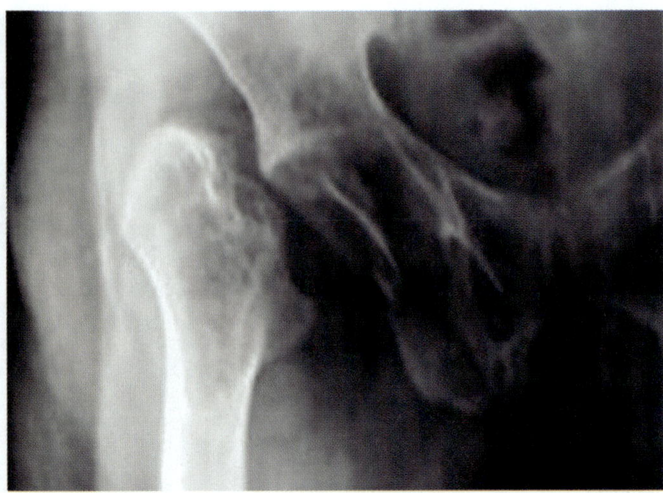

Fig. 10.19: X-ray pelvis with both hip joints anteroposterior views showing Girdlestone arthroplasty on right side

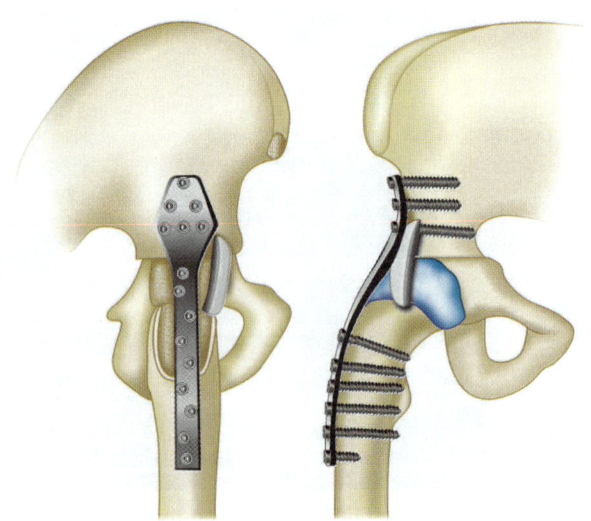

Fig. 10.20: A schematic diagram to show fusion of hip (arthrodesis) using a specially designed "cobra plate"

PATHOLOGY

The origin of TB in the knee can be:

- Synovial
- Osseous, involving articular surfaces
- Osseous but involving nonarticular parts of the tibia or femur.

Somehow, most cases of TB knee start in synovium and tend to remain purely so for a long time. The infection then spreads as a pannus under the articular cartilage, denuding the same and leading to reduction of joint space and arthritis. Eventually cold abscess may form that may track out as discharging sinuses. The end result generally is a fibrous ankylosis.

CLINICAL FEATURES

Most patients tend to present with pain and swelling in the knee that is of long duration. There may be grossly visible muscle wasting in quadriceps muscle (especially vastus medialis).

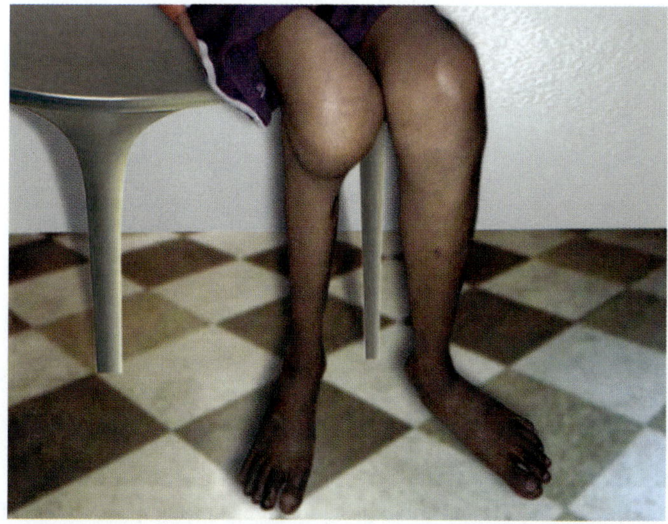

Fig. 10.21: Patient with "triple deformity" right knee secondary to TB knee. Note the flexion, external rotation and posterior subluxation of right tibia (relative to femur)

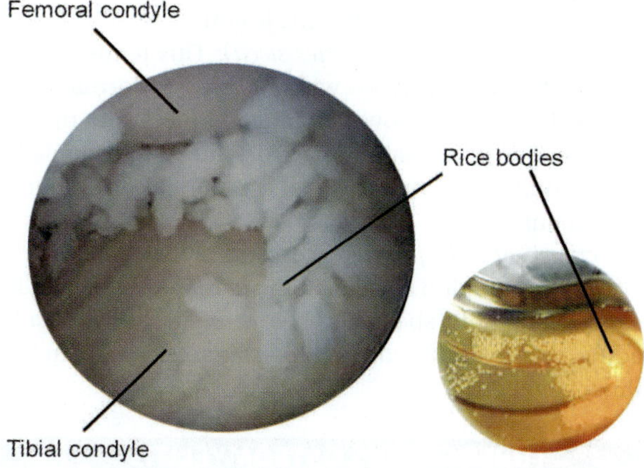

Fig. 10.22: Rice bodies as visible on arthroscopic examination and gross examination

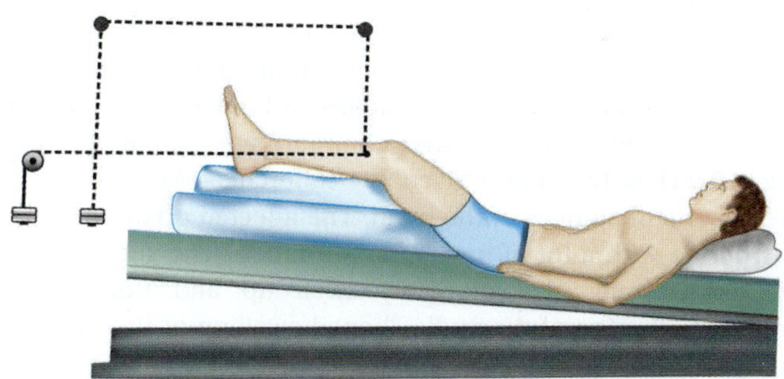

Fig. 10.23: Double traction being used to neutralize a triple deformity of knee

Sinuses either discharging or healed with puckering of skin may be noticed.

On examination, doughy or boggy thickening may be palpable in the suprapatellar region owing to synovial thickening. It is best felt on the medial side of the knee as vastus medialis remains muscular till its insertion onto the patella and is wasted early in the disease. On the contrary, muscles on the lateral side are aponeurotic and covered by thick iliotibial band that relatively masks the feeling. There is generally painful limitation of both flexion and extension. In advanced stages, triple deformity results (due to spasm of iliotibial band, biceps femoris and hamstrings) where there is flexion, external rotation and posterior subluxation of tibia on femur **(Fig. 10.21)**.

DIAGNOSIS

Diagnosis includes:

- *Radiography*: In initial stages radiographs shows juxta-articular osteopenia, reduction of joint space and articular erosions. Late cases show the classical triple deformity.
- *Magnetic resonance imaging*: It is needed in cases where radiographic findings are uncertain. MRI can demonstrate the pus collection, synovial thickening as well as osseous destruction.
- *Joint aspiration*: It forms the cornerstone in cases where the diagnosis remains a dilemma. Aspirated fluid can be sent for ZN staining, culture and PCR for *M. tuberculosis* DNA.
- *Biopsy*: It remains the gold standard. Arthroscopic biopsy is generally preferred nowadays. Additionally one can find typical "rice bodies" that are accumulations of fibrin and articular cartilage inside the joint on arthroscopic examination **(Fig. 10.22)**.

DIFFERENTIAL DIAGNOSIS

Important differentials include:

- Chronic recurrent traumatic synovitis
- Monoarticular rheumatoid arthritis
- Subacute septic arthritis
- Pigmented villonodular synovitis.

MANAGEMENT

The management is on the same lines as TB hip. ATT is started in all patients. Gentle traction is applied and the joint is immobilized in Thomas splint. Triple deformity can be reduced by using a "double traction" **(Fig. 10.23)**. As the deformity reduces and lesion enters healing phase, traction is removed and a plaster cast is given and once the lesion seems quiescent, range of motion is instituted. Initially weight-bearing is protective (using walkers or crutches) for 18–24 months, later unprotected weight-bearing is allowed. Surgical management in the form of synovectomy or an arthrodesis is generally required in nonresponders.

HIGH-YIELD POINT

- Tuberculosis is the most common cause of monoarthritis in children.

TUBERCULOSIS OF OTHER JOINTS

INTRODUCTION

Almost any joint may be affected with TB, including elbow, shoulder, ankle and wrist. Clinical features, diagnostic aspects and management principles remain the same as discussed earlier. Of particular interest are the following lesions:

- *Tuberculosis of shoulder (Caries sicca):* This tends to be the granular dry type of lesion without any pus formation and osseous destruction. However, range of motion is markedly restricted. The presentation is almost indistinguishable from frozen shoulder and must be kept as a possible differential in such patients.
- *Tuberculosis of wrist joint:* Abscess formation at this site may involve flexor tendon sheaths in the palm producing an hour glass swelling both above and below the flexor retinaculum, leading to the formation of the characteristic compound palmar ganglion.

TUBERCULOUS OSTEOMYELITIS

Although TB mostly involves the epiphyseal area and joints, rarely shafts of long bones may be involved leading to tubercular osteomyelitis. Lesions are mostly multifocal and there is shear lysis without any attempt at new bone formation.

More common is rather a tuberculous affection of short bones of hand and feet. The phalanges and metacarpals may be involved. Calcaneum is another common site. "spina ventosa" **(Fig. 10.24)** is the name given to "tubercular dactylitis" that involves the phalanges of the hand. The affected phalanx shows destruction with a lot of new bone formation. The surrounding soft tissues may also markedly swell up and the patient presents with a painful spindle-shaped swelling of the affected finger.

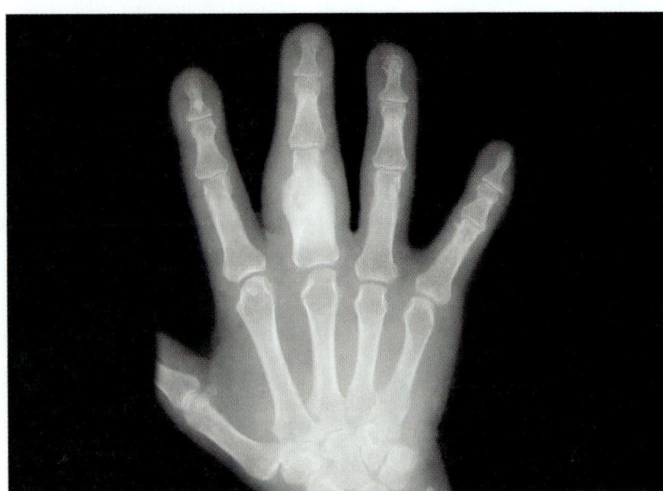

Fig. 10.24: X-ray of hand anteroposterior view showing spina ventosa of proximal phalanx of the middle finger

HIGH-YIELD POINTS

- *Poncet's disease (tubercular rheumatism):* It describes a polyarthritis resembling rheumatoid arthritis occurring in patients with TB. On treating TB, polyarthritis also disappears.
- *Bacille Calmette-Guérin (BCG) osteomyelitis:* It is a rare complication (occurs in approximately 1 in 10,000 vaccinations) that has been reported to occur a few months to 5 years after BCG vaccine administration in children. Mostly involved are long tubular bones. The course is benign and fortunately patients respond favorably to ATT.

Orthopedic Oncology

GENERAL PRINCIPLES

Although bone malignancies form a small spectrum (approximately 1%) of all malignancies in the body, their clinical significance cannot be underrated. The diagnosis and management aspect can be badly challenging unless one has a meticulous knowledge on the subject.

CLASSIFICATION

Broadly speaking, the bone tumors are divided into tumor-like lesions [fibrous dysplasia, fibrous cortical defect (FCD), bone cysts, etc.], osteochondroma/exostosis (a lesion in between the tumor-like lesions and true tumors) and the true tumors of the bone. The last ones are further subclassified into benign and malignant subtypes.

World Health Organization (WHO) has provided a relatively simple way of classifying the true bone malignancies based on their origin, as shown in **Table 11.1**. However, the greatest majority of bone malignancies is actually formed by the metastasis that arise from other sites, the most common source being the breast in females and prostate in males (overall breast being the most common).

DIAGNOSTIC FUNDAMENTALS

Thorough history and good clinical examination are essentially the first step while imaging and biopsy complement.

Imaging in Bone Tumors

On plain radiography one must note:
- *The anatomical location*: Epiphysis, metaphysis or diaphysis **(Fig. 11.1)**.
- *The margins:* Well-defined with a surrounding zone of reactive sclerosis in benign lesions, while the same are ill-defined in malignant lesions.
- *The pattern of bone destruction*
  - *Geographic:* Seen in slow-growing tumors where there is a narrow zone of transition between the normal and abnormal bone as seen in most benign lesions **(Fig. 11.2A)**.
  - *Moth eaten:* Where there are multiple scattered lytic areas in bone like in Ewings and osteosarcoma **(Fig. 11.2B)**.
  - *Permeative:* Seen in poorly demarcated lesions with a wide zone of transition, as in high-grade Ewings and chondrosarcomas **(Fig. 11.2C)**.
- *Types of Periosteal Reaction*
  - *Solid:* Cortical thickening as in osteoid osteoma
  - *Lamellated:* As in Ewing's sarcoma (onion skinning)
  - *Complex:* As in osteosarcoma (sunburst pattern).

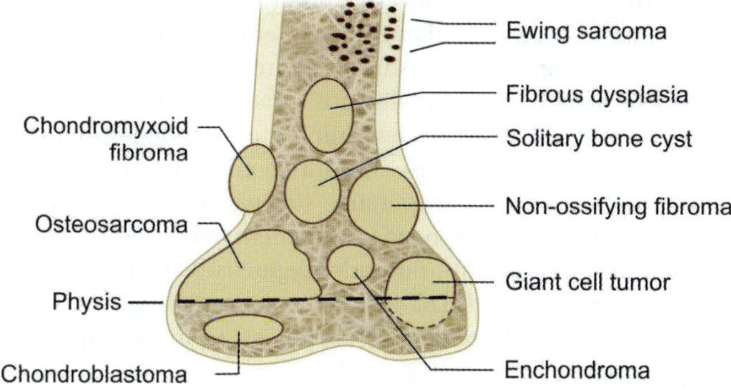

Fig. 11.1: Anatomical distribution of various bone tumors

Table 11.1: Origin-based classification of true bone tumors (simplified WHO classification)		
Types	*Benign*	*Malignant*
Bone-forming tumors (arising from osteoblasts)	Osteoma Osteoid osteoma Osteoblastoma	Osteosarcoma
Cartilage-forming tumors (arising from chondroblasts)	Enchondroma Chondroblastoma Chondromyxoid fibroma	Chondrosarcoma
Giant cell tumor (has osteoclast-like cells, origin uncertain, likely from mononuclear cell)	Osteoclastoma (locally aggressive tumor)	
Marrow tumors		Ewing sarcoma, Multiple myeloma (plasma cells)
Vascular tumors	Hemangioma	Angiosarcoma
Other tumors		Chordoma Adamantinoma

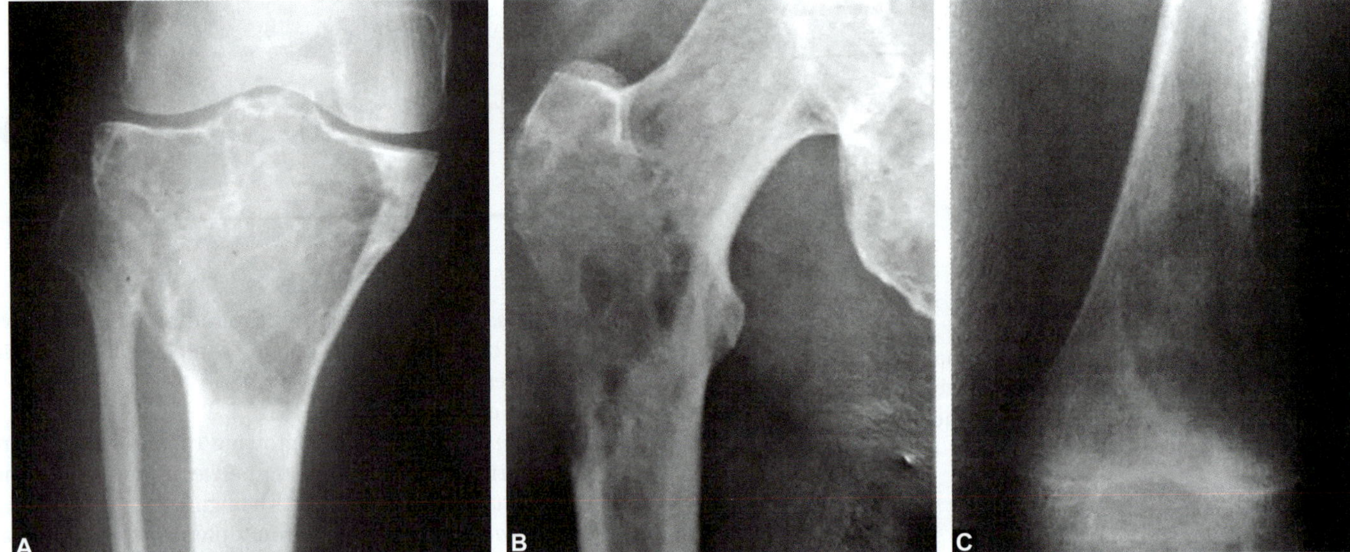

Figs 11.2A to C: Pattern of bone destruction. (A) Geographic; (B) Moth-eaten; and (C) Permeative

Magnetic resonance imaging (MRI), computed tomography (CT) scan and bone scan are vital add on investigations in indicated situations. The gold standard in making diagnosis of bone tumors is a biopsy (best taken from the peripheral margins as the center of the tumor often is necrotic). Most surgeons today recommend MRI as a precursor investigation (investigation of choice) to determine the size, extent of intramedullary and extraosseous disease and the relationship to neurovascular structures in suspected aggressive and malignant tumors. Technetium bone scans are primarily used to determine the presence of multiple lesions or skeletal metastases. Positron emission tomography (PET scan) is useful in preoperative staging, planning the treatment, to evaluate the response to treatment and to detect recurrences. Fluorine-18 (18F)-fluorodeoxyglucose-labeled positron emission tomography (FDG-PET) in conjunction with CT and MRI is used to differentiate recurrences from postoperative changes.

Biopsy of a Suspected Musculoskeletal Tumor

A biopsy is the gold standard in making the diagnosis of a musculoskeletal tumor. It can be a needle biopsy, where a special needle is inserted into the tumor and fluid and cells are drawn out or an open biopsy where tissue is obtained after giving incision. A biopsy should be well planned and carefully performed. Recommendations regarding biopsy of a musculoskeletal tumor are given in **Box 11.1**.

STAGING OF BONE TUMORS

Enneking, the father of "Orthopedic Oncology", developed a rational system for staging the bone tumors that serves as a protocol for deciding surgical management and assessing prognosis **(Table 11.2)**. The system is based on the histological grade (low or high), anatomical location (T1: intracompartmental and T2: extracompartmental) and the presence of secondary metastasis (M). Recently, American Joint Committee on cancer system has also provided a classification system for bone sarcomas

Box 11.1: Recommendations for a biopsy of musculoskeletal tumor

- All imaging studies including magnetic resonance imaging (MRI) should be performed before biopsy. It helps in planning biopsy incision and avoids possible artifacts in imaging studies
- A biopsy track should be so planned that it can be included into future incisions of the surgery
- It is best to perform biopsy by the same surgeon who is going to perform surgery later on
- If tourniquet is used, exsanguination should be avoided to prevent squeezing of tumor cells into the normal tissues
- Incisions should be given through the single muscle and intermuscular plane and neurovascular bundles should be avoided
- Sampling should include peripheral extension (soft tissue extension) of the bone tumor. Peripheral growing edge of the tumor or the soft tissue extension contains most viable tumor cells to make the diagnosis. Biopsy from the center of the tumor should be avoided
- If a tourniquet is used it should be deflated before closure and adequate hemostasis should be achieved and wound should be tightly closed in layers
- A frozen section should be sent intraoperatively to ensure that adequate diagnostic tissue has been obtained

that depends on grade, size (<8 cm or >8 cm) and presence of metastasis **(Table 11.3)**.

OPERATIVE MANAGEMENT

The operative management depends on the type of lesion—benign or malignant. Benign lesions are adequately treated with excision of the tumor, curettage of walls to remove any leftover tumor tissue, followed by filling the defect with bone graft or bone cement. Aggressive lesions generally need an extended curettage where an additional agent (adjuvant) like phenol, hydrogen peroxide, liquid nitrogen or bone cement is used to promote killing of tumor cells. Frankly malignant lesions mostly need adequate surgical

Table 11.2: Enneking staging system for benign and malignant bone tumors

Staging of benign musculoskeletal tumors (Enneking system)		Staging of malignant musculoskeletal tumors (Enneking system)			
		Stage	Grade	Site	Metastasis
Stage 1: Latent lesion	• Intracapsular usually asymptomatic, incidental finding • *Radiological features:* A well-defined margin with a thick rim of reactive bone	IA	Low	Intracompartment (T1)	No
Stage 2: Active lesion	• Intracapsular, actively growing • *Radiological features:* Well-defined margins with only a thin rim of reactive bone	IB IIA	Low High	Extracompartment (T2) Intracompartment (T1)	No No
Stage 3: Aggressive lesion	• Extracapsular, aggressive nature • *Radiological features:* The tumor has broken through the reactive bone and possibly the cortex	IIB III	High Low/high	Extracompartment (T2) Any	No Present (regional/distant)

Table 11.3: American Joint Committee on Cancer System for staging bone sarcomas

Stage	Grade	Site	Metastasis
IA	Low	≤8 cm	None
IB	Low	>8 cm	None
IIA	High	≤8 cm	None
IIB	High	>8 cm	None
III	Any	Any	Skip metastasis
IVA	Any	Any	Pulmonary metastasis
IVB	Any	Any	Nonpulmonary metastasis

clearance. Based on the amount of tumor removed, the surgical margins can be classified as:

- *Intralesional*: The plane of dissection lies within the tumor tissue.
- *Marginal excision*: Plane of excision is through the pseudocapsule.
- *Wide excision*: Plane of excision includes a cuff on normal tissue.
- *Radical excision*: Involves removing the entire compartment containing the tumor.

HIGH-YIELD POINTS

- Cryotherapy is a type of extended curettage where liquid nitrogen is used to kill the leftover tumor cells by freezing effect. Liquid nitrogen has been postulated to give least recurrence rate, although it is debatable. Cryotherapy also increases risk of fracture due to necrosis of surrounding tissues (side effect of freezing).
- Bone cement and bone graft both are popular options for filling bone defects left after excisional curettage. While bone graft offers the most rapid and reliable healing rate, it may at times not be available in sufficient quantities. Harvesting autogenous grafts may additionally add on problems of donor site morbidity. Bone cement on the other hand not only avoids donor site morbidity, but also acts as an adjuvant by providing heat of polymerization that additionally kills the tumor cells. Moreover, it provides an immediate stability and hence speeds up rehabilitation. Tumor recurrences are also easier to detect with cement. However, the choice of agent to use is largely surgeon dependent.

- In the following tumors or conditions multiple lesions are seen in bone:
  Histiocytosis, enchondroma, osteochondroma, fibrous dysplasia, multiple myeloma, metastases, hemangioma, hyperparathyroidism (Brown's tumors).

TUMOR-LIKE LESIONS

FIBROUS DYSPLASIA

The term "fibrous dysplasia" refers to a benign nonfamilial disorder caused by mutations of the gene (GNAS1) that encodes the α subunit of stimulatory G protein (Gsα). This results in inhibition of the differentiation and proliferation of bone forming stromal cells and leads to the replacement of normal bone and marrow by fibrous tissue and woven bone. Affected individuals are generally in the age group of 5–30 years. It is generally a metaphyseal lesion that extends into the diaphysis. The most common sites of affection are the proximal femur (overall the most common site), tibia, humerus, ribs and craniofacial bones (zygomatic-maxillary complex is the most common site in craniofacial area).

The disease may be monostotic when affecting a single bone or may be polyostotic when a number of bones are affected. Monostotic form is six times more common than polyostotic form. Patients generally present with pain, deformity or a pathological fracture. A majority of the monostotic cases does not progress, and the long-term outcome is usually satisfactory. Deformities in patients with polyostotic disease may continue to progress after skeletal maturity. Generalized fibrous dysplasia involving the face and skull is called "leontiasis ossea".

Radiographs in fibrous dysplasia show a multiloculated translucent lesion expanding the cortex of the bone, classically demonstrating the so called "ground glass appearance" (a shadow similar to the density of a cancellous bone, but with absence of normal trabecular pattern due to replacement of bony tissue by solid fibro-osseous mass that gives a more homogenous appearance, **Fig. 11.3**). In some cases, the lesion is surrounded by a sclerotic rim. This is referred to as the Rind sign (**Fig. 11.4**). In neglected cases, the proximal femoral lesion develops microfractures as the patient continues to bear weight, leading

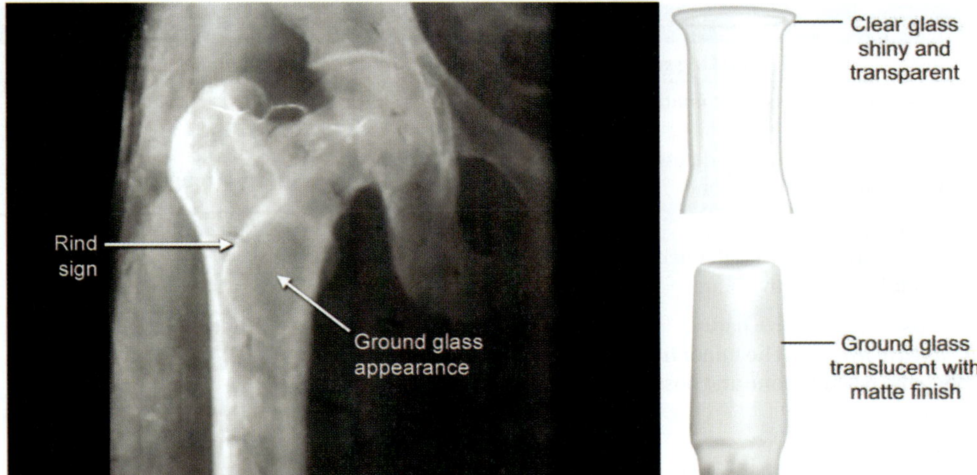

Fig. 11.3: Fibrous dysplasia of neck of femur showing the ground glass appearance

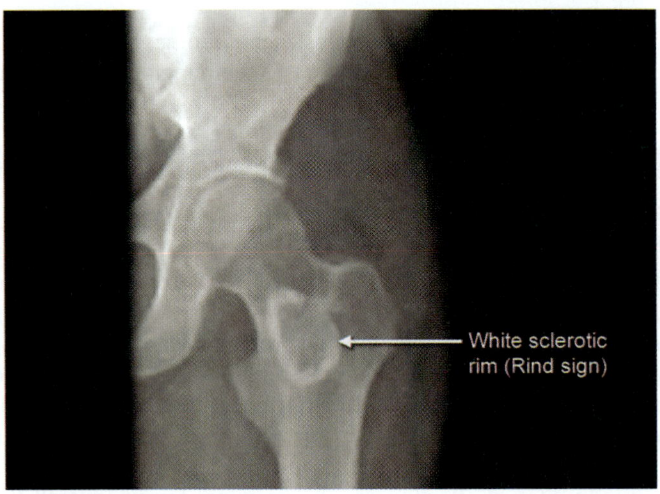

Fig. 11.4: Rind sign in fibrous dysplasia of neck of femur

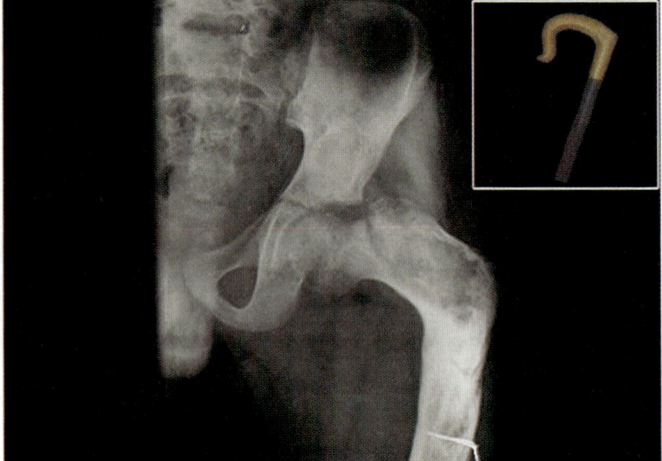

Fig. 11.5: Shepherd crook deformity (a crook is a curved stick used by shepherds to control their sheep when they are grazing, see inset image)

to the medial wall collapse, eventually ending up with a femur that becomes hook shaped—The shepherd crook deformity **(Fig. 11.5)**. Diagnosis is confirmed on biopsy that shows the well-recognized "Chinese letter pattern" **(Fig. 11.6)**.

Treatment generally involves excisional curettage with bone grafting, as in most benign lesions. Medical treatment (bisphosphonate therapy to decrease pain and lower fracture risk) may be offered to appropriately selected patients with fibrous dysplasia.

HIGH-YIELD POINTS

- Fibrous dysplasia may also have nonskeletal manifestations in certain patients. Most common nonskeleton manifestation of fibrous dysplasia is café-au-lait spots.
- *McCune Albright syndrome*: It refers to the triad of polyostotic fibrous dysplasia, precocious puberty and skin pigmentation in the form of café-au-lait spots. These spots are hallmarks of neurofibromatosis, but in neurofibromatosis these are smoothly marginated (Coast of California) in contrast to the irregular margins (Coast of Maine) these spots have when

found in McCune Albright syndrome. 90% of patients with McCune Albright syndrome have craniofacial involvement.
- *Mazabraud syndrome*: It includes polyostotic fibrous dysplasia with intramural myxomas.

FIBROUS CORTICAL DEFECT OR NONOSSIFYING FIBROMA

Most authors consider it to be a smaller version of fibrous dysplasia only. FCD is a small eccentric metaphyseal lytic lesion with sclerotic margins **(Fig. 11.7)**, most commonly found in the lower femur, where a nest of fibrous tissue persists in the bone for a variable time before finally ossifying. Nonossifying fibroma (NOF) is larger, lobulated, well-circumscribed geographic lesion with sclerotic margins **(Fig. 11.8)**.

People generally affected with FCD are in the age group of 2–20 years; it is rare outside this age group. In fact, it is estimated to occur in approximately 35% of children. Mostly, it is an incidental finding and as it ossifies, it disappears with age. The importance of this condition lies in the fact, that it is the most common reported lesion (not a tumor) of the bones.

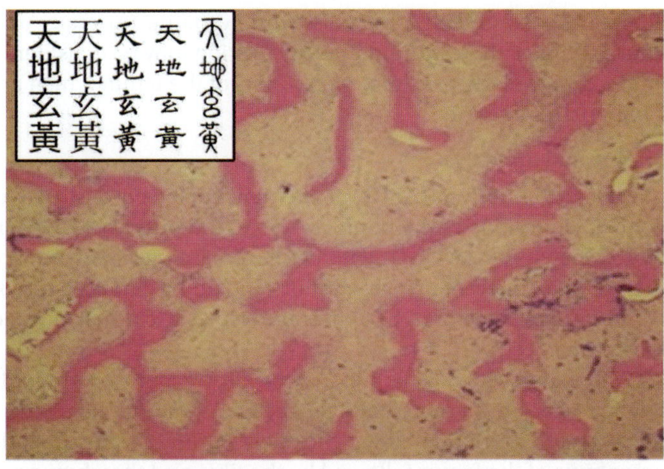

Fig. 11.6: Histology of fibrous dysplasia, see Chinese letter pattern appearance

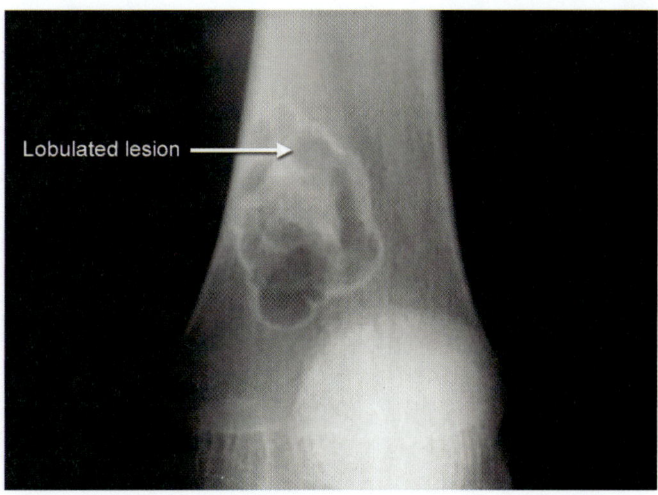

Fig. 11.8: Nonossifying fibroma of distal femur

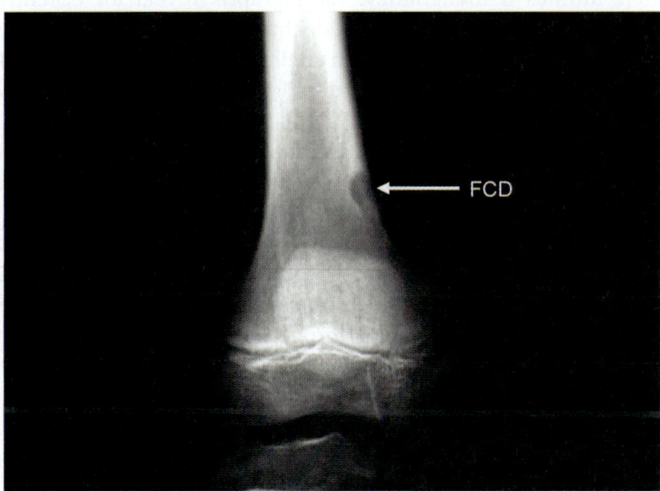

Fig. 11.7: Fibrous cortical defect (FCD)

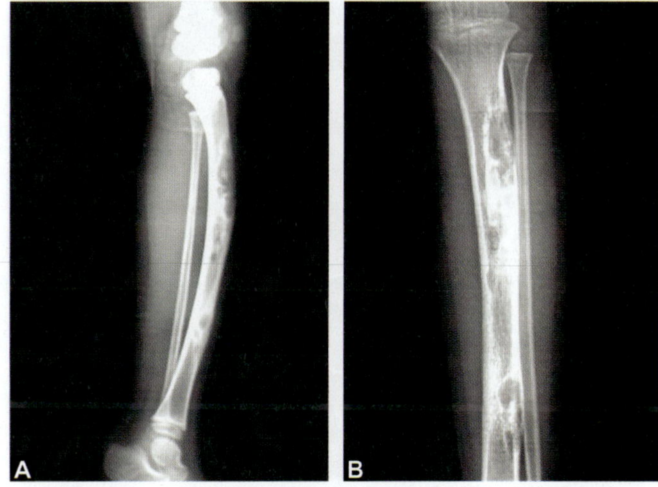

Figs 11.9A and B: X-ray leg anteroposterior and lateral views showing osteofibrous dysplasia

OSTEOFIBROUS DYSPLASIA

Osteofibrous dysplasia (ossifying fibroma of long bones, also known as Campanacci disease) usually affects patients in their first two decades of life. The diaphysis of the tibia followed by fibula is the most frequently affected location. Tibia is often bowed anterolaterally and the radiographs show eccentric, intracortical osteolysis with the expansion of the cortex **(Figs 11.9A and B)**. Management involves observation as some lesions regress spontaneously while most do not progress after puberty. Surgical management is aimed at preventing pathological fracture and/or correcting deformity.

BONE CYST

A bone cyst refers to a cavity in the bones. Two varieties of cysts may be encountered as described.

Simple or Unicameral Bone Cyst

It is the only "true" cyst of the bones as most other lesions that appear cystic are actually osteolytic. Although the exact pathogenesis is unclear, some believe it as a defect of growth plate development, while others suggest it is due to venous obstruction to the drainage of interstitial fluid. The resulting pressure changes due to blockage of interstitial fluid drainage lead to cyst formation within the bone. Pathologically, the cyst wall is generally lined by a thin fibrous membrane (<1 mm thick) and the contents comprise of yellowish or straw-colored serous fluid. It usually occurs during the first two decades of life (more in 4–10 years of age group) with a 2:1 male-to-female preponderance.

Most commonly affected site includes the metaphysis of proximal humerus followed by the distal femur and the proximal tibia. Although initially they start as metaphyseal lesions, with time they move closer to the diaphysis. Unicameral cyst is classified as active when it is within 1 cm of the physis and latent when it is closer towards the diaphysis. The cyst generally is asymptomatic but as many as two-thirds of patients may present with a pathological fracture after a trivial trauma.

X-ray would usually show up an aseptate lytic lesion in the metaphyseal area of a long bone. The lesion is centrally placed and symmetrically expansile, but almost never penetrates the

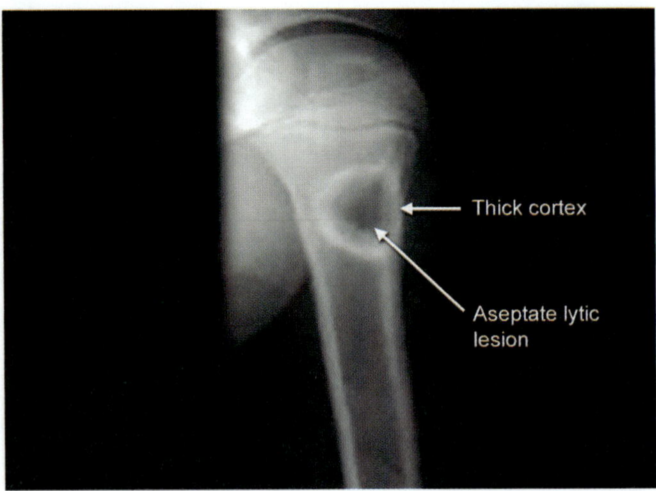

Fig. 11.10: Simple bone cyst (SBC) of proximal humerus metaphysis

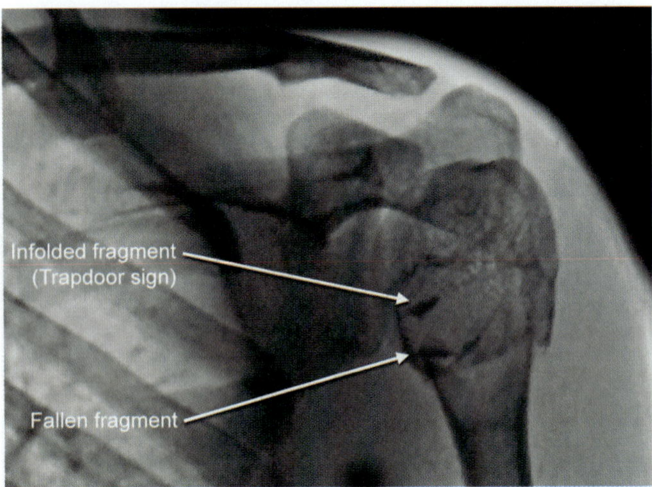

Fig. 11.11: Simple bone cyst (SBC) of proximal humerus showing fallen fragments in cyst cavity and an infolded fragment (trapdoor)

cortex. The width of the simple bone cyst (SBC) usually does not exceed the width of the neighboring growth plate **(Fig. 11.10)**. Diagnostic of the SBC is the "fallen fragment/leaf sign" **(Fig. 11.11)**. A small fragment of cortex, sometimes breaks and the piece settles to the most dependent part of the cyst, confirming its empty cystic nature. However, in some cases the broken fragment does not fall as it remains attached to the periosteum but it folds inwards. This is called as "trapdoor sign" **(Fig. 11.11)**.

Treatment is individualized to the patient. Small asymptomatic lesions in the upper extremities require only periodic observation and restriction of activities. Larger cysts in the lower limbs or symptomatic cysts are treated with aspiration and injection of corticosteroid (one or two injections of 80–200 mg methylprednisolone). Injection may be repeated after 2 months if no evidence of healing is seen. Corticosteroid injection has replaced curettage and bone grafting as a first-line of treatment because of high success rate. Other materials used for percutaneous treatment of unicameral bone cysts include autogenous bone marrow mixed with demineralized bone matrix, injectable bioresorbable calcium phosphate paste and high-porosity hydroxyapatite. Curettage and bone grafting with or without internal fixation may be considered for large cysts of the proximal metaphysis of the femur which are at high risk of fracture.

Aneurysmal Bone Cyst

Aneurysmal bone cysts (ABCs) are benign, but locally destructive, blood-filled lesions of the bone. ABCs are the primary lesions in approximately 70% of cases, whereas in remaining cases, they are secondary to different primary tumors, including giant cell tumor (GCT), chondroblastoma, SBC, fibrous dysplasia, chondromyxoid fibroma, etc.

Although a wider age group may be affected, most commonly they are seen in patients younger than 20 years of age, with a slight female preponderance. The most common sites include metaphysis of the femur followed by the tibia and then humerus. Vertebral lesions involving the posterior elements are common (approximately 20%). The clinical course is much rapid and often mimics a malignancy. Radiographs reveal an eccentric lytic lesion, often multiloculated, that elevates the periosteum but remains contained by a thin shell of cortical bone, signifying its asymmetrical expansion and ballooning nature **(Figs 11.12A and B)**.

Differentiating it from SBC is important **(Table 11.4)** and MRI often helps. MRI in ABC classically shows intralesional septations and double-density fluid levels.

Treatment has to be more aggressive and involves an extended curettage and bone (or bone graft substitute) grafting where after the curettage tumor cavity is treated with agents like liquid nitrogen, phenol, hydrogen peroxide or bone cement to kill the leftover tumor cells. Recently, many studies have shown high healing rate and good functional outcome with intralesional calcitonin and methylprednisolone injection in ABC. Embolization is useful in treating aneurysmal cysts located in areas of limited access, such as the spine and pelvis.

After treatment, the recurrence rate is high (approximately 10–20%) especially in patients younger than 15 years, centrally located lesions and in cases where there is incomplete removal of cyst contents. Recurrences can be treated in the same way as primary lesions, but with greater care.

HIGH-YIELD POINT

- A solid variant of ABC is often referred to as a giant cell reparative granuloma.

OSTEOCHONDROMA OR EXOSTOSIS

Osteochondroma (also called as exostosis) is an aberration at the growth plate where a few cells at the periphery of the plate rather than growing up and down, start growing centrifugally to form a separate lump on one side. It originates at the physis or growth plate, but with bone growth the tumor gets "left behind" and comes to lie at the metaphysis and sometimes even diaphysis. Even though it is the most common benign tumor of bone, it is generally not considered to be a true neoplasm as the growth often ceases once the skeletal maturity is reached. Being developmental lesions, they generally become evident before the individual reaches 20 years of age, with most lesions found near the rapid skeletal growth. Although they can involve any

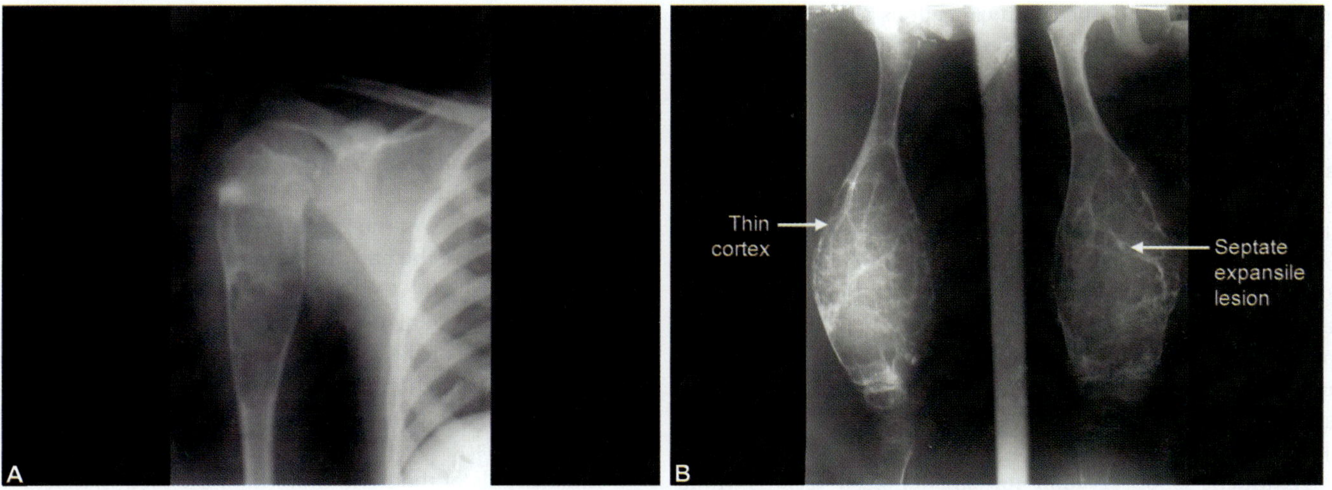

Figs 11.12A and B: (A) Aneurysmal bone cyst (ABC) of proximal humerus; (B) A large ABC of distal femur

Table 11.4: Simple bone cyst (SBC) versus aneurysmal bone cyst (ABC)

Features	SBC	ABC
Sex	Male preponderance	Slight female preponderance
Location	Central to start	Eccentric lesion initially
Most common site	Proximal humerus	Distal femur
X-ray appearance	Centrally located, purely lytic, metaphyseal lesion with a well-marginated outline. No periosteal new bone formation is present, unless there has been a fracture. No periosteal elevation is seen "Fallen fragment" sign is pathognomonic of a unicameral bone cyst Cortical thinning without disruption may be seen	Eccentrically located, metaphyseal, expansile lytic lesion that elevates the periosteum. Cyst expands eccentrically and expands cortex. Typically described as "blow out" or ballooned-out lesion that is outlined by a thinned-out cortex A thin shell of subperiosteal new bone formation is seen surrounding the lesion
Magnetic resonance imaging (MRI) appearance	MRI will demonstrate a low-signal intensity on T1-weighted images and high-signal intensity on T2-weighted images in the typical SBC. Usually aseptate appearance, but osseous ridges on the inner cortical wall may give it a multiloculated appearance	MRI shows characteristic fluid-fluid levels (double-density fluid levels) due to blood sedimentation, septations (multiloculated) and high-signal intensity (T1- and T2-weighted) of the upper fluid layer. Sclerotic rim is often seen surrounding the lesion
Expansion	Symmetrically expansile	Asymmetrical/ballooning expansion
Aspiration	Straw-colored fluid	Hemorrhagic fluid
Treatment	Aspiration and intralesional corticosteroid injection. In non-healing cases, curettage with bone grafting	Extended curettage with bone grafting

bone developed by endochondral ossification, the most common site includes distal femur followed by proximal tibia and then proximal humerus, which show that the lesion is common around the metaphysis of long bones.

The lesion usually comprises of a pedunculated bony mass **(Fig. 11.13A)**, often in the form of a stalk (can rarely be sessile, **Fig. 11.13B**), produced by progressive endochondral ossification of a growing cartilaginous cap. Although most lesions are solitary, multiple lesions (approximately 5%) do occur. In fact, "hereditary multiple exostosis (HME)" (synonym diaphyseal aclasis, **Fig. 11.14A**) is an autosomal dominant condition with variable penetrance. These patients have mutations in one of the two genes: *EXT1* (chromosome 8) or *EXT2* (chromosome 11). The striking feature of the disease apart from the presence of multiple

osteochondromas is the presence of growth anomalies such as abnormal tubulation of bones producing broad metaphysis and sometimes causing bowing of radius and shortening of ulna (Masada syndrome, **Fig. 11.14B**).

Clinically, most lesions are asymptomatic and discovered incidentally. Sometimes they cause mechanical symptoms by irritating the surrounding structures (e.g. bursitis over the tip of osteochondroma) or rarely become painful due to a pathological fracture of the osteochondroma itself (not of bone). False aneurysms of the neighboring vessels and neuropathies also have been reported.

Plain radiographs are generally sufficient to make the diagnosis. Important differentials to rule out in exostosis are Trevor's disease (*see* Page 392) and myositis ossificans. In exostosis, the projecting part of the lesion has cortical and cancellous components, both of which are continuous with the corresponding components of the parent bone (cf myositis ossificans where this continuation is absent). The lesion is covered with a cartilaginous cap that is often not visible on an X-ray, unless calcification in the cap may be seen. CT is sometimes needed to confirm the diagnosis. Thickness of the cartilage cap more than 2 cm **(Fig. 11.15)** is often indicative of malignancy (mostly chondrosarcoma arises). However, malignant degeneration is exceedingly rare (only 1% for solitary osteochondroma but 5% for HME). If at all it occurs, the previously quiescent lesion in the adult may show signs of rapid growth, causing mechanical symptoms or the patient may start complaining of pain in a previously painless swelling or one may find ulceration of the overlying skin or involvement of the adjacent lymph nodes.

Treatment is observation for smaller-sized lesions while problematic lesions should undergo an extraperiosteal excision (excising overlying periosteum to avoid leaving any abnormal cartilage cells). If a chondrosarcoma occurs in exostosis, a wider excision is needed, however, the prognosis after excision of chondrosarcoma is excellent.

HIGH-YIELD POINTS

- *Subungual osteochondroma **(Figs 11.16A and B)**:* A variant of osteochondroma that generally involves the distal phalanx, most commonly of the great toe. Excision is indicated when the elevation of the nail produces pain.
- *Bizarre parosteal osteochondromatous proliferation (Nora's lesion):* It is a benign lesion affecting patients in second or third decade of life. The lesion is an exophytic outgrowth similar to osteochondroma arising from the cortical surface of bone **(Fig. 11.17)**, consisting of elements of bone, cartilage and fibrous tissue. It is mostly seen in the phalanges and metacarpals of the hand more than the feet. Classical X-ray picture and biopsy may provide the diagnosis. Excision is needed, but the recurrence rate is high.

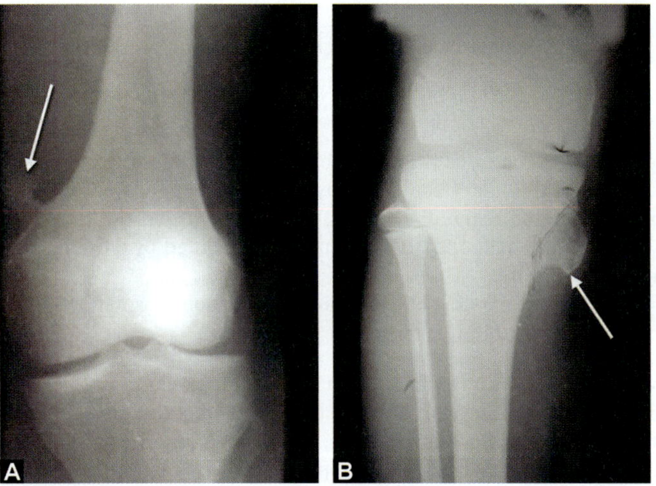

Figs 11.13A and B: X-ray knee anteroposterior (AP) and lateral views showing pedunculated and sessile osteochondromas (arrows)

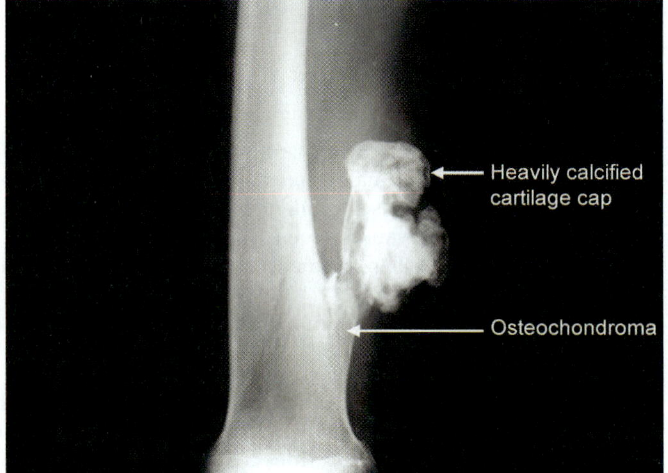

Fig. 11.15: Chondrosarcomatous change in osteochondroma

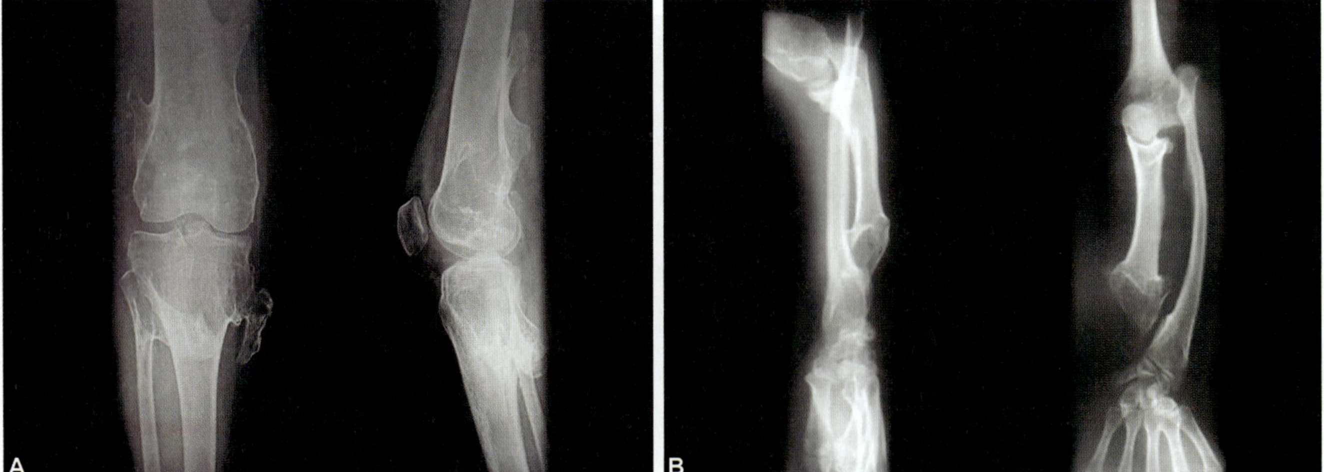

Figs 11.14A and B: (A) X-ray knee anteroposterior and lateral views showing multiple exostosis; (B) Forearm deformities of hereditary multiple exostosis—metaphyseal broadening and shortening of ulna with radial bowing and radial head dislocation

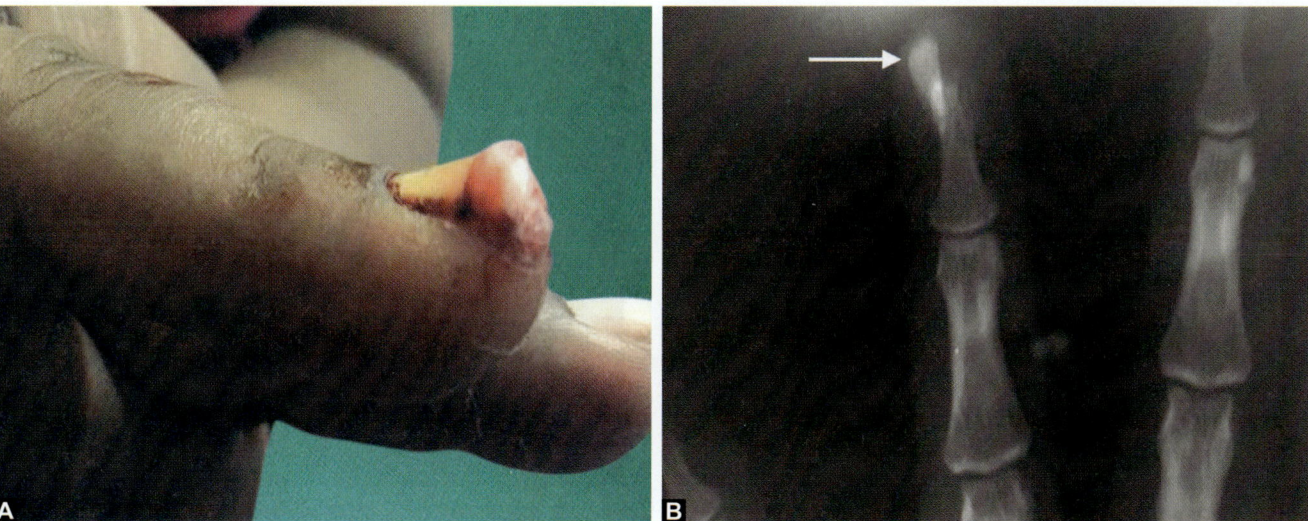

Figs 11.16A and B: Subungual osteochondroma. (A) Clinical picture; and (B) X-ray showing growth below nail due to subungual osteochondroma (arrow)

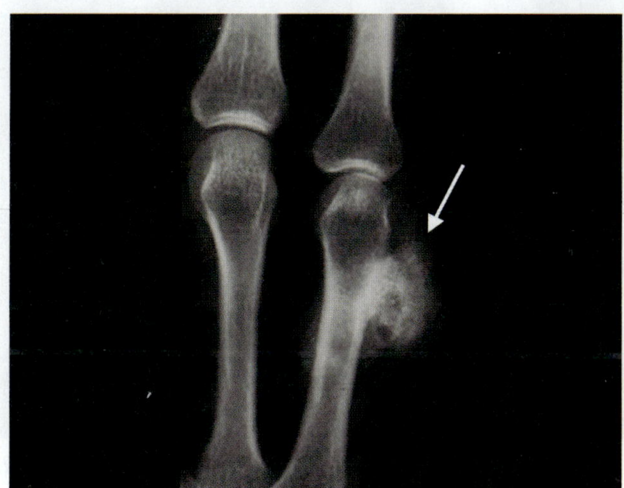

Fig. 11.17: Nora's lesion in the metacarpal neck (arrow)

BENIGN BONE TUMORS

OSTEOMA

Osteoma is a benign slow-growing osteogenic lesion, characterized by the proliferation of compact or cancellous bone, almost exclusively found in the head and neck regions (skull being the most common site). Central, peripheral and extraskeletal are the three variants of osteoma. Paranasal sinuses are the favorite locations of peripheral osteoma of the craniofacial region; frontal and ethmoidal sinuses being the common ones. Although, peripheral osteomas are usually benign, innocuous lesions, their size and prominent location on the visible parts of the face makes the surgical intervention necessary.

OSTEOID OSTEOMA

It is a benign bone forming lesion considered to be the most common true benign tumor of the bone. With a slight male preponderance, it is usually seen in second or third decade of life. The lesion is diaphyseal generally, sometimes metaphyseal, with most lesions affecting the femur greater than the tibia. It is also known to occur in the vertebrae (7–20% incidence) where it mostly affects the posterior elements. Osteoid osteoma is usually cortical lesion but can be intramedullary, subperiosteal and intra-articular.

Clinically, patients typically present with pain that is worse at night. Possible cause seems to be the elevated levels of prostaglandins and cyclooxygenase that have been demonstrated in the lesions. This fact explains the dramatic and diagnostic relief provided by aspirin (nonsteroidal anti-inflammatory drugs) in patients with this tumor.

X-ray is usually diagnostic **(Figs 11.18A and B)**. Typical lesion consists of a radiolucent nidus surrounded by a thick rim of dense sclerotic bone. Nidus (made up of a fibrovascular stroma and elements of woven bone) may have a central region of mineralization. CT scan is the investigation of choice to identify the nidus, the size of which is generally less than 1.5 cm. Biopsy is not needed, but may show immature bony trabeculae with a fibrovascular stroma that is rimmed by prominent osteoblasts.

The malignant potential of the lesion is almost nil, so most patients are given a trial of anti-inflammatory medications initially. If the symptoms are controlled, the treatment is continued and most lesions show spontaneous healing in 3–4 years. Surgical management involves removal of the entire nidus mostly done by a special technique called as "burr down technique". In this manner, a minimal amount of surrounding sclerotic bone is removed, thereby minimizing the subsequent risk of pathological fracture. A more popular method is a percutaneous CT guided radiofrequency ablation of the lesion. Here under CT guidance a needle is inserted into the nidus which is then burnt down by radiofrequency waves.

HIGH-YIELD POINTS

- Osteoid osteoma is the most common primary benign tumor of the spine.

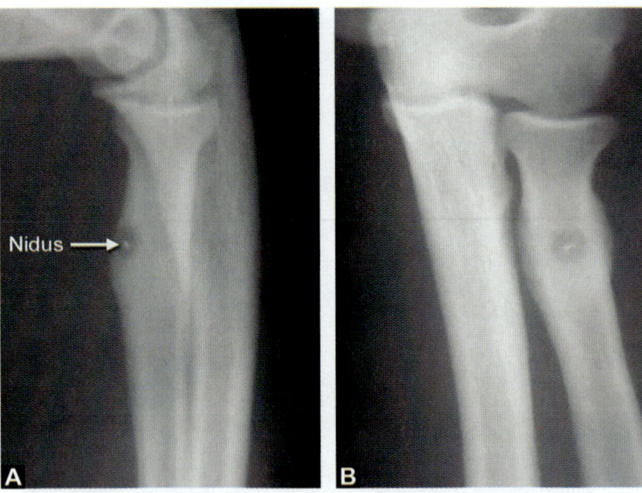

Figs 11.18A and B: Osteoid osteoma of the radial tuberosity (with mineralized dot in the center of the radiolucent nidus)

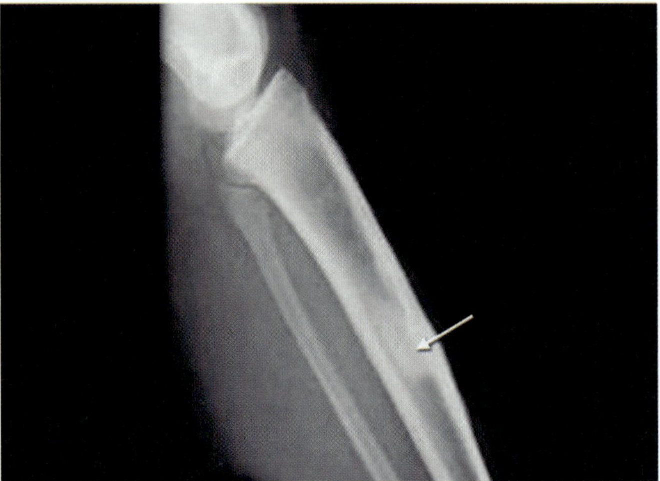

Fig. 11.19: Osteoblastoma in tibial diaphysis (arrow)

- Technetium-99m scintigraphy in osteoid osteoma reveals increased uptake in the nidus and may be used to confirm the diagnosis.

OSTEOBLASTOMA

It is a rare bone-forming benign neoplasm that occurs in 10–30 years old individuals with a 3:1 male preponderance. About 30–50% of the lesions are located in the spine with most involving the posterior elements of the vertebrae. In the long bones, the lesion is mostly in the diaphysis, can be in metaphysis but is never in the epiphysis. It can be intramedullary or intracortical (intramedullary location is more common). Pain is the most common symptom and may be similar in nature to osteoid osteoma.

Unlike osteoid osteoma, X-rays usually reveal a mineralized sclerotic focus surrounded by a radiolucent halo (nidus) with hardly any rim of reactive sclerosis **(Fig. 11.19)**. If sclerosis occurs, then one has to differentiate it from osteoid osteoma by going for a CT scan. The differentiation is then based on the size of the nidus which in these cases is usually larger than 1.5 cm.

Microscopically the lesion resembles osteoid osteoma but as far as the clinical behavior is concerned, the lesion is much more aggressive than osteoid osteoma. Treatment consists of extended curettage with bone grafting.

CHONDROMA (ENCHONDROMA)

They are benign neoplasms of hyaline cartilage. Since they usually lie inside the medullary canal, they are often referred to as "enchondromas". Very rarely they arise from the surface of the bone in which cases they are referred to as "juxtacortical chondromas". Any age group can be involved (more so in second decade). The most common site is the hand and foot bones (particularly phalanges), although any bone formed in cartilage can be involved. Radiographs classically show an expansile radiolucent lesion in the metaphysis of bone with wisps of calcification (stippled calcification) giving a septate appearance **(Fig. 11.20)**. One has to differentiate it from the ABC or tubercular dactylitis (spina ventosa, i.e. tuberculosis of phalanges).

Most lesions are solitary but at times can be multiple. Multiple enchondromatosis (nonhereditary disorder) is referred

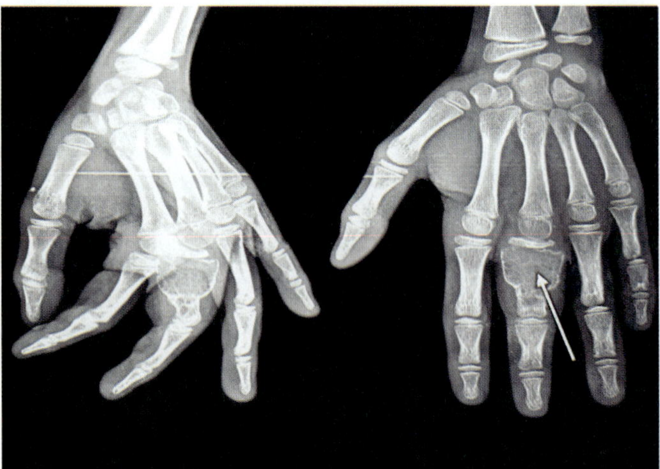

Fig. 11.20: Enchondroma in metaphysis of proximal phalanx middle finger (arrow)

to as Ollier's disease **(Fig. 11.21)** and if along with multiple enchondromas there are multiple cavernous hemangiomas and phleboliths, then the condition is called as Maffucci syndrome (hereditary disorder).

Treatment is generally advised for enlarging lesions and consists of excisional curettage and bone grafting.

HIGH-YIELD POINTS

- Enchondromas are the most common bone tumors and, most commonly benign bone tumors of the hand bones.
- Most common malignant bone tumor of the hand is chondrosarcoma.
- Most common malignant tumor of hand is squamous cell carcinoma.
- Most common soft tissue mass in the hand is a ganglion (*see* Page 452).
- Malignant transformation to chondrosarcoma occurs in less than 2% of solitary cases of enchondroma, 25% cases in Ollier's disease (by the age of 40 years) and in almost 100% cases in Maffucci syndrome.

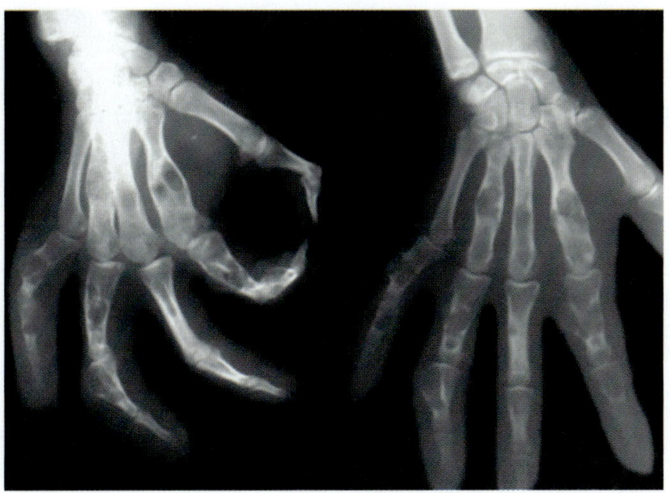

Fig. 11.21: X-ray hand anteroposterior and oblique views showing multiple enchondromatosis

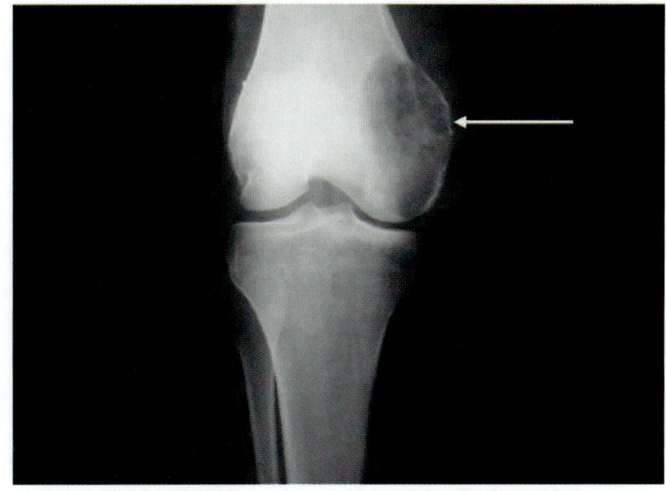

Fig. 11.22: Chondroblastoma (arrow) of distal femur

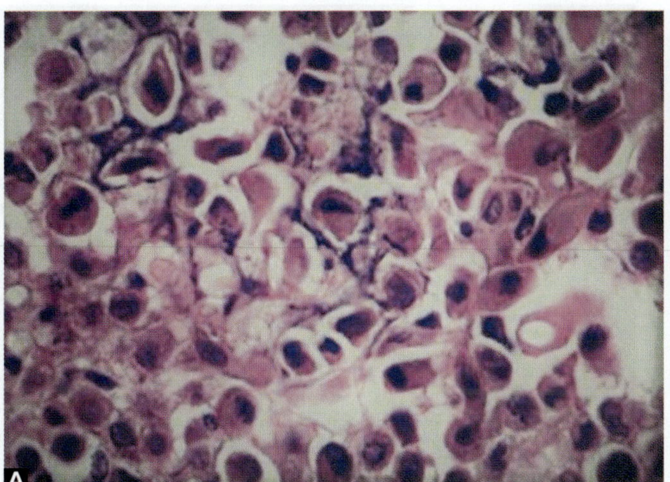

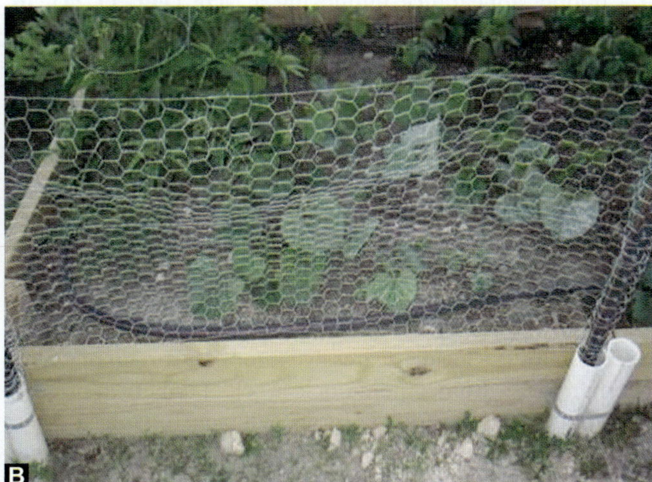

Figs 11.23A and B: (A) Chicken wire fence appearance of chondroblastoma cells due to dystrophic calcification that may surround individual cells; (B) A chicken wire fence

- Computed tomography is the best investigation to evaluate endosteal erosion that can signify a chondrosarcoma.

CHONDROBLASTOMA

Chondroblastoma is an epiphyseal lesion mainly seen in the distal femur followed by proximal humerus and then proximal tibia, in 10–25 years of age group with a 2:1 male preponderance. At times, the lesion may be seen in an apophysis like greater tuberosity or greater trochanter. Since they are epiphyseal lesions, most patients complain of progressive pain that often mimics an intra-articular pathology like chronic synovitis.

Radiological findings are characteristic with the X-ray showing a well-circumscribed eccentric epiphyseal lytic lesion with a rim of sclerosis **(Fig. 11.22)**. About 30–50% exhibit matrix calcification on CT evaluation.

The differential is a GCT in older individuals. GCT would not have a rim of sclerosis or intralesional calcification and might have a soft tissue component. Biopsy confirms the diagnosis and demonstrates dystrophic calcification surrounding individual cells the so called "chicken wire fence appearance" **(Figs 11.23A and B)**. Multinucleate giant cells are abundant. Treatment is excisional curettage with bone grafting.

HIGH-YIELD POINTS

- Since this lesion was described by the famous scientist Codman (in 1931), chondroblastoma is also sometimes called as Codman's tumor.
- Histological grading is of no prognostic significance in chondroblastoma.

CHONDROMYXOID FIBROMA

Chondromyxoid fibroma is a benign cartilage tumor that also has myxoid and fibrous elements. Most lesions occur in patients 10–30 years old. Chondromyxoid fibroma rarely is included in the differential diagnosis of a lesion, unless the lesion is in the proximal tibial metaphysis, which remains its most common location.

Radiographically, it is usually a well-circumscribed lesion with a rim of sclerosis in the metaphysis of a long bone and may

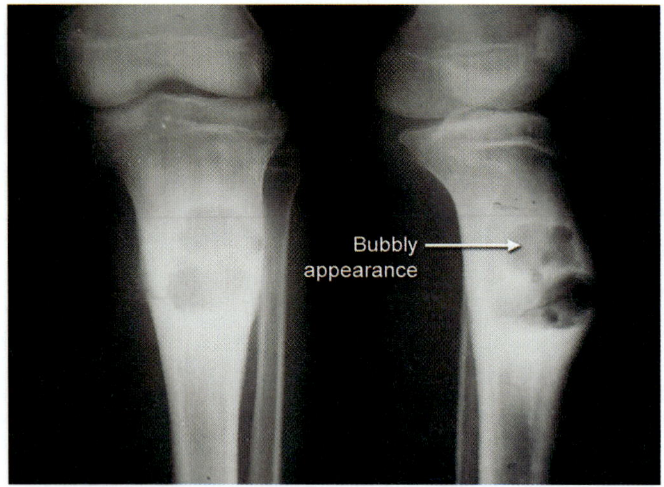

Fig. 11.24: Chondromyxoid fibroma of proximal tibia

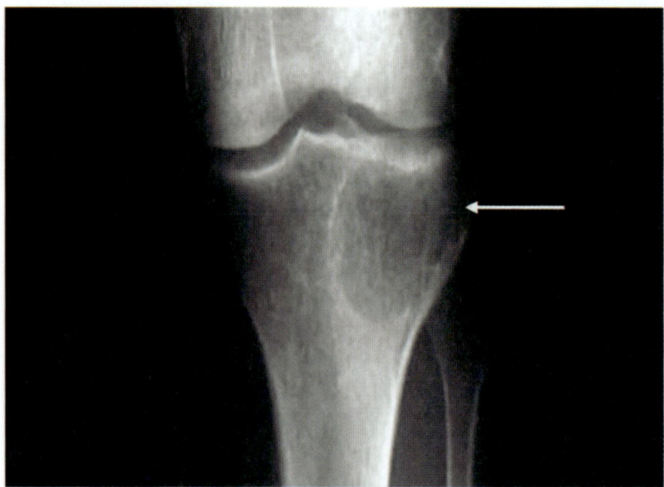

Fig. 11.25: Giant cell tumor (arrow) of proximal tibia

have a bubbly appearance mimicking a NOF **(Fig. 11.24)**. In contrast to other cartilaginous lesions, radiographic evidence of intralesional calcification usually is absent.

Microscopically, chondromyxoid fibroma appears lobulated. The center of the lobules contains loose myxoid tissue and the periphery contains a more cellular fibrous tissue. The background often appears chondroid, although distinct areas of hyaline cartilage are rare. Microscopic calcification may be present.

Treatment consists of resection or extended curettage with bone grafting. Sarcomatous change is rare.

GIANT CELL TUMOR (OSTEOCLASTOMA)

Giant cell tumor is a locally aggressive tumor, the origin of which is uncertain (likely from a mononuclear cell of unknown origin). Since it is composed of giant cells (non-malignant) on microscopy, mistaken as osteoclasts, it is also referred to as osteoclastoma. The characteristic age group of affection is 20–40 years with a slight female preponderance. Although classically categorized as an epiphyseal lesion, in adults, it spans across both the epiphysis and metaphysis. However, in adolescents it is primarily limited to metaphysis being confined proximally by the growth plate. One theory suggests that these lesions originate in the metaphysis and later extend into the epiphysis on closure of the growth plate. The most common sites of occurrence include the distal femur followed by proximal tibia and then distal radius.

Clinically, patients usually present with progressive pain. In 10–30% cases pathological fractures are evident at presentation. On examination, the clinician can elicit "egg shell cracking" sound on tapping the lesion.

Radiographic appearance is characteristic **(Fig. 11.25)**. An eccentric expansile lytic lesion is located in the epiphyseal-metaphyseal area usually abutting the subchondral bone (the so called "soap bubble appearance", **Fig. 11.26**). Initially GCT is covered by a thin shell of reactive bone, but with expansion it may break through the cortex; however, intra-articular extension following a break in subchondral bone is very rare. Matrix calcification is not seen in GCT. MRI clearly defines the extent of the lesion within bone and in soft tissue. The lesion is dark on T1-weighted images and bright on T2-weighted images.

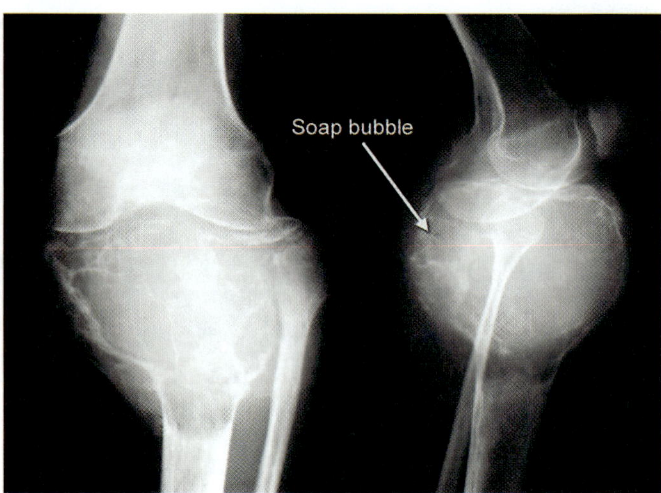

Fig. 11.26: X-ray knee anteroposterior and lateral views showing the classical soap bubble appearance of expanding giant cell tumor (GCT)

Microscopically, the tumor is composed of many multi-nucleated (having 40–60 nuclei per cell) giant cells lying in a sea of mononuclear stromal cells **(Fig. 11.27)**. The nuclei of mononuclear cells are identical to the nuclei of the giant cells, a feature that helps to distinguish GCT from other tumors that may contain giant cells. It should be noted that these osteoclast-like giant cells are reactive and benign in nature. Mononuclear mesenchymal stromal cells having mitotic activity are the real neoplastic component of the tumor.

Campanacci grading system for GCTs is based on the radiographic appearance of the tumors.

- A grade 1 lesion (latent) has a well-defined margin and an intact cortex.
- A grade 2 lesion (active) has a relatively well-defined margin, but no radiopaque rim, and the cortex is thinned and moderately expanded.
- A grade 3 lesion (aggressive) has indistinct borders and cortical destruction.

Treatment is extended curettage with bone grafting or bone cement. Cementing is generally preferred as cement provides immediate stability aiding quicker rehabilitation and allows easier detection of recurrence than a bone graft. The lesions around the knee that abut the subchondral bone sometimes require excision with reconstruction or arthrodesis of the joint. Excision of the tumor and reconstruction arthroplasty is preferred over arthrodesis nowadays. For aggressive Campanacci grade III GCT with extensive tumor wide excision and joint reconstruction using megaprosthesis are done **(Figs 11.28A to C)**. For GCT of distal end radius treatment of choice is excision of tumor and reconstruction with fibular grafting. Chemotherapy has limited success and irradiation should be reserved for symptomatic inoperable cases. Denosumab (*see* Page 403 and 412), monolonal antibody against RANK receptors (expressed by osteoclasts in GCT) may offer symptom and disease control in patients with unresectable lesions. However, the optimal indications and long-term side effects remain to be defined. Recently bisphosphonates have been postulated to delay tumor progression in aggressive lesions and prevent recurrence. Reported recurrence rate is 5–15%. Treatment of recurrent lesions is same as primary lesions provided biopsy demonstrates them to be benign.

Although these tumors typically are benign or more appropriately locally aggressive, pulmonary metastasis can occur in approximately 3% of patients. Both recurrence and pulmonary metastases usually occur within 3 years, but have been reported even after 20 years. Most common malignancies in the GCT are osteosarcoma followed by malignant fibrous histiocytoma and fibrosarcoma.

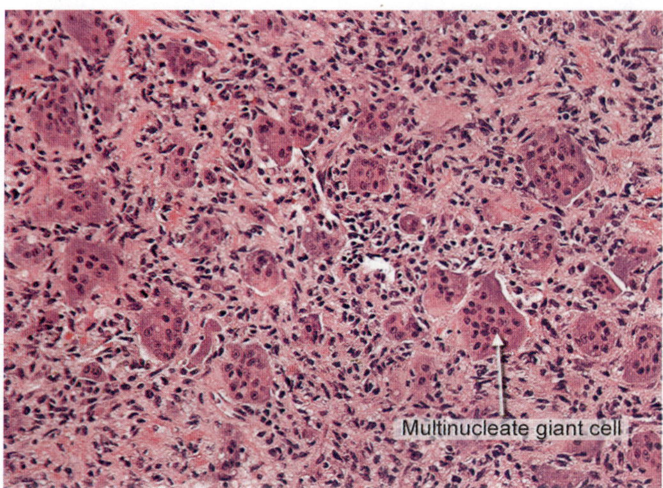

Fig. 11.27: Microscopic picture of giant cell tumor

HIGH-YIELD POINTS

- Giant cell tumors represent less than 5% of neoplasms of bone. Less than 5% are multicentric and less than 5% show pulmonary metastasis.
- The "Es" of GCT:
    - E—Occurs during epiphyseal closure (20–40 years)
    - E—Epiphyseal eccentric lytic lesion (distal femur > proximal tibia > distal end of radius)
    - E—Expansile lesion (causes expansion of the overlying cortex, giving the soap bubble appearance on X-ray)
    - E—Egg shell cracking sound on tapping the lesion is heard
    - E—Extended curettage with bone grafting is the treatment.
- In spine most commonly GCT occurs in the vertebral body of sacrum followed by lumbar and then thoracic vertebrae.
- Giant cell tumor is a pulsatile bone tumor. Other pulsatile bone tumors include telangiectatic variant of osteosarcoma, ABC and metastasis from follicular carcinoma thyroid and renal cell carcinoma.

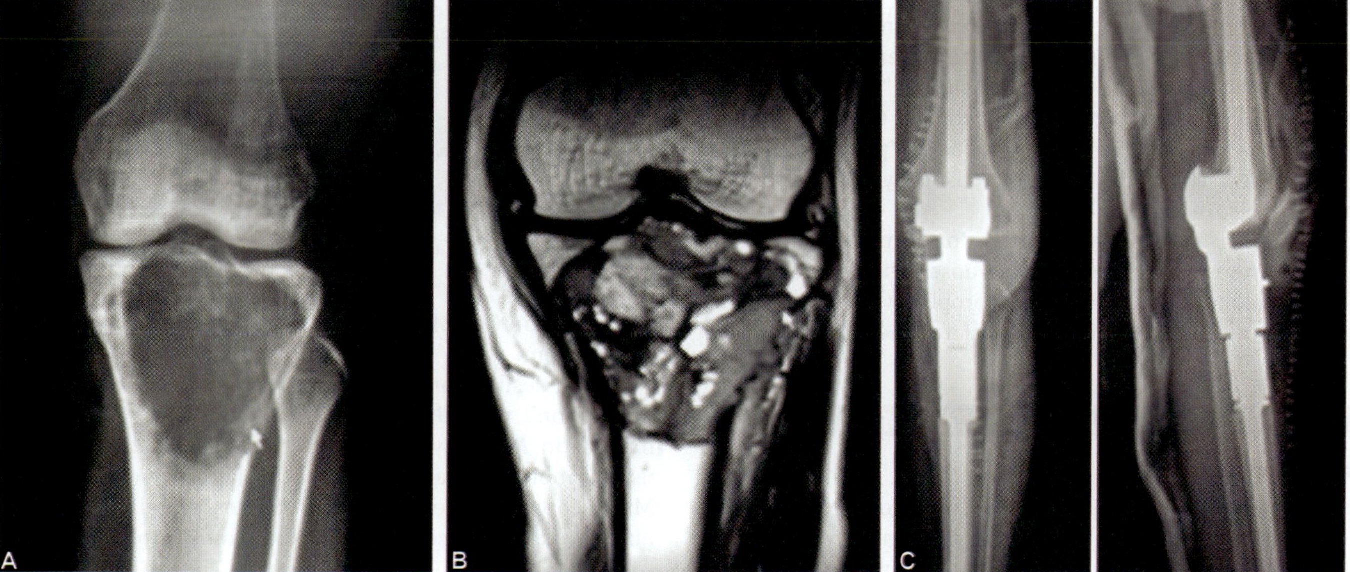

Figs 11.28A to C: (A) Aggressive giant cell tumor of proximal tibia; (B) Magnetic resonance imaging showing intra-articular extension; and (C) Joint reconstruction after excision of tumor using megaprosthesis
Courtesy: Dr Shailendra Singh Thakur. Custom prosthetic reconstruction of proximal tibial GCT. J Mahatma Gandhi Inst Med Sc. 2014;19(2).

- *Giant cell tumor variants*: These are those lesions which resemble GCT on microscopic examination because of the presence of giant cells on microscopy. The lesions include:
  - A—ABC and SBC
  - B—Brown's tumor of hyperparathyroidism
  - C—Chondroblastoma and chondromyxoid fibroma
  - D—Desmoplastic fibroma
  - E—Epulis (giant cell reparative granuloma), epithelioid cell variant of osteoblastoma
  - F—Fibrous dysplasia and nonossifying fibroma
  - G—Giant cell rich osteosarcoma, giant osteoid osteoma
  - H—Benign fibrous histiocytoma.
- Aneurysmal bone cyst is the closest GCT variant and nonossifying fibroma is the most common GCT variant.
- Mostly malignancies appearing in GCTs are secondary malignancies following radiation and primary malignant transformation is rare.
- Giant cell tumor of tendon sheath or giant cell synovioma or localized nodular tenosynovitis, is a firm lesion, measuring 1–3 cm in diameter, and is most commonly attached to the tendons of the hands and wrist, with a predilection for the flexor surfaces. These tumors (mostly seen in 20–30 years of age) are typically painless but can cause cortical erosion. Surgical excision is commonly needed, but the tumors tend to recur.

HEMANGIOMA

This common benign lesion is appropriately a hamartoma in bone being composed of masses of vascular channels (capillary, venous, cavernous, etc.). The most common age group is fifth decade of life with a female preponderance. Hemangioma is the most common benign neoplasm of the spine. The most common sites of occurrence are vertebrae (T4–L4) followed by the skull. In fact, it is estimated to be present in approximately 10% of the population in the form of asymptomatic spinal lesions that at times are discovered incidentally.

Radiographic features are characteristic and biopsy is almost never required. On X-ray **(Figs 11.29A to C)** vertebra shows vertically oriented trabeculae giving the classic "Jailhouse appearance" or the so called "corduroy appearance". On cross-sectional images on CT scan, the pattern is called as "polka dot pattern" **(Fig. 11.30)**. The lesions are characteristically bright in both T1 and T2 images of MRI.

Treatment is necessary mostly for symptomatic lesions. Selective arterial embolization or low-dose radiation are generally the preferred modes. Recently, vertebroplasty (*see* Page 403) has been advocated as another modality of treatment with promising results.

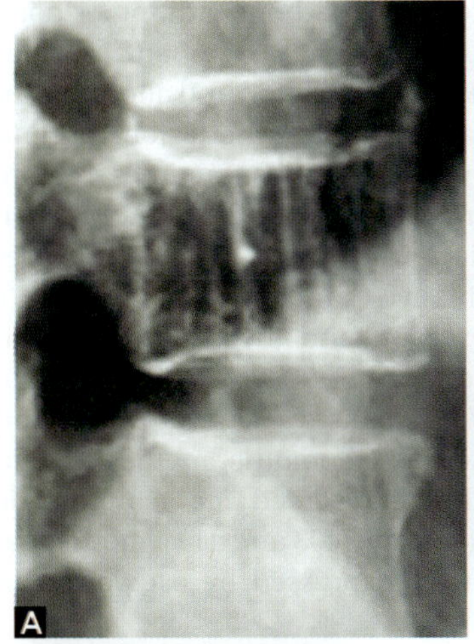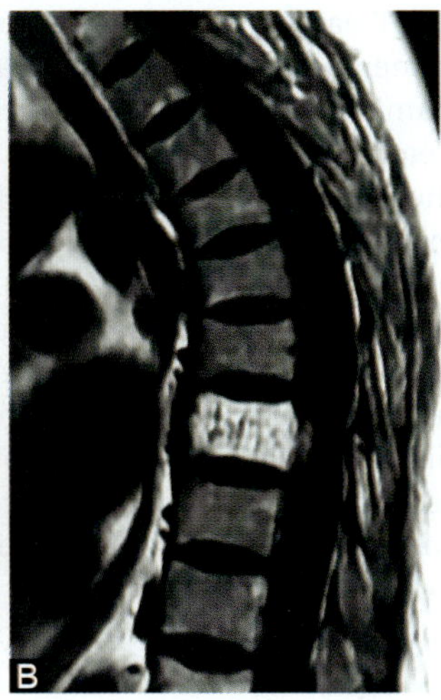

Figs 11.29A to C: (A) X-ray; and (B) MRI of thoracic spine showing the classical corduroy appearance of vertebral hemangioma; (C) Corduroy cloth: a thick cotton fabric showing the characteristic velvety ridges running in parallel fashion

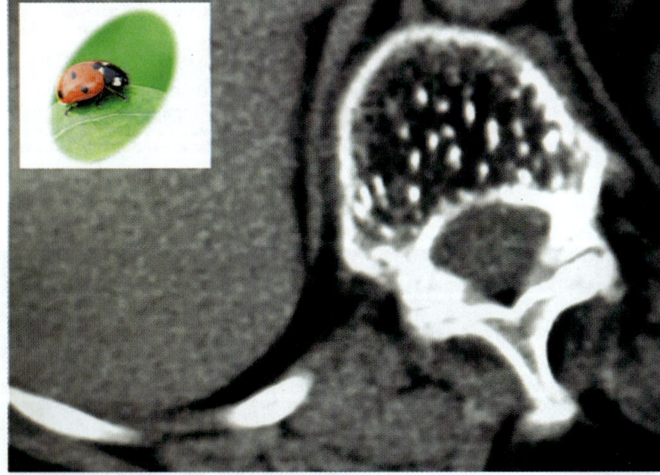

Fig. 11.30: Axial CT scan cut showing the characteristic Polka dot pattern

MALIGNANT BONE TUMORS

CHORDOMA

This rare malignant neoplasm arises from notochord remnant. It is the second most common primary malignancy in the spine (after MM) and is the most common primary malignancy of the sacrum with a peak incidence in fifth to seventh decades of life. Greater than 50% arise in the sacrococcygeal area (below S3 level) while more than 30% arise at the base of the skull. The most common presenting complaint for sacrococcygeal tumors is low back pain while larger masses may present with neurological involvement.

Bone destruction is the radiographic hallmark of the lesion. The lesions virtually arise from the midline. Often they are missed on AP X-rays due to overlying gas shadows. They are usually more easily appreciated on the lateral view of the sacrum. Microscopically, they consist of lobules of cells separated by fibrous bands. The cells contain abundant vacuolated cytoplasm (physaliferous cells—pathognomonic). The primary treatment is surgical resection with wide margins even if it creates a neurological deficit. Effort should be to protect S2, S3 nerve roots to avoid bladder, bowel function. Radiation may benefit nonresectable cases. Chemotherapy is of no proven benefit.

HIGH-YIELD POINTS

- In adults, remnant of the notochord is nucleus pulposus.
- A more distal location for sacral lesions is associated with a better prognosis.

CHONDROSARCOMA

This malignant bone tumor arising from the cartilage cells is the third most common primary malignant bone tumor (most common—multiple myeloma, second most common—osteosarcoma) or the second most common primary nonhematological malignancy of the bone. Peak incidence occurs in fourth to sixth decades of life. In fact, it is the most common primary malignant tumor of the bone in people above 40 years of age, with a slight male preponderance. Lesions may arise de novo or in a pre-existing tumor like an enchondroma or osteochondroma. The tumor has a predilection for flat bones and the most common sites are pelvis followed by proximal femur. It is also most common malignant chest wall tumor. Although malignant, patients generally present with a slowly enlarging mass and a dull aching pain.

Radiographically, the tumors are characterized by metaphyseal radiolucent lesions with cortical erosions and rarely a soft tissue mass. There is abundant matrix calcification, the so called "mottled/popcorn like/comma-shaped calcification" **(Figs 11.31A and B)**. Biopsy demonstrates malignant cells with abundant cartilaginous matrix.

Treatment in most cases is wide or radical excision (excision of whole compartment that contains the tumor) or at times an amputation is needed. There is no role of chemotherapy and radiotherapy is only palliative. Since cartilage is avascular, it survives transplantation easily and hence recurrences are common. Metastasis is mostly hematogenous and most frequently to the lungs. The prognosis for patients with chondrosarcoma depends mostly on the size, grade and location of the lesion.

HIGH-YIELD POINTS

- There is no osteoid production in chondrosarcoma. If at all, even minimal amounts of osteoid are found, then the diagnosis is chondroblastic osteosarcoma (a variant of osteosarcoma)—a tumor with a different prognosis and treatment.
- Less common histological subtypes of conventional chondrosarcoma include dedifferentiated chondrosarcoma, clear cell chondrosarcoma and mesenchymal chondrosarcoma. Clear cell type (low grade) has tendency to occur in epiphysis and can have giant cells on biopsy (giant cell variant). Mesenchymal variety (high-grade variant) has cellular portions that often have a hemangiopericytomatous pattern of growth with "stag-horn-like" vessels.

OSTEOSARCOMA

Osteosarcoma is a highly malignant tumor characterized by the production of osteoid by the tumor cells. It is the second most common primary malignancy of bone, but the most common nonhematological primary malignancy of bone. Areas with high rate of bone growth are more commonly affected and most common sites being metaphyseal areas of distal femur followed by proximal tibia and then proximal humerus. Classically, it has a bimodal age distribution with a primary variety (conventional osteosarcoma) that arises de novo and predominates in second decade of life and a secondary variety that arises in premalignant lesions **(Box 11.2)** and spans the 40–60 years of age group. Overall, males are more commonly affected than females. Although the tumor is present in association with hereditary forms of retinoblastoma, Rothmund-Thomson syndrome and Li-Fraumeni syndrome, genetic factors rarely have been shown to play a role.

Clinically, patients mostly report progressive pain as a first symptom that results from microinfarctions as the invasive tumor

> **Box 11.2:** Premalignant lesions associated with secondary osteosarcoma
>
> - Fibrous dysplasia
> - Paget's disease
> - Post-irradiation
> - Osteochondromatosis (multiple)
> - Bone infarction

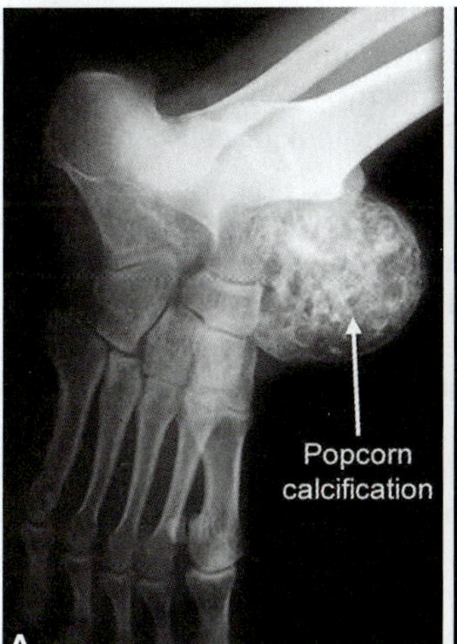

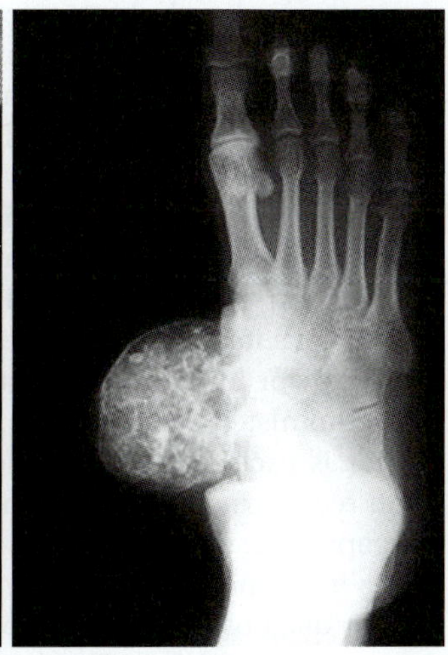

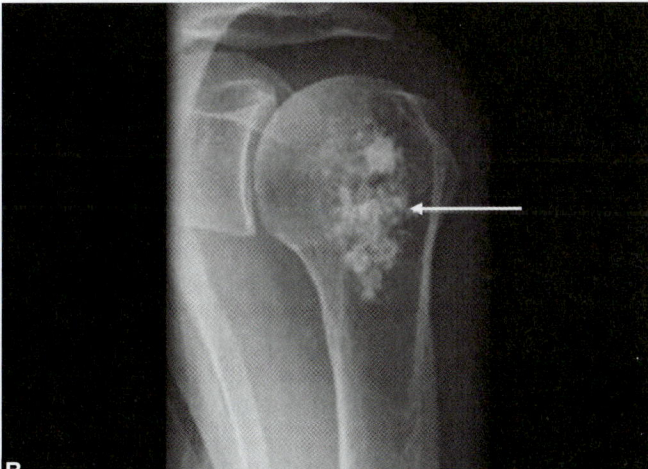

Figs 11.31A and B: Chondrosarcoma of (A) Talus and (B) Proximal humerus showing popcorn calcification (arrow)
Source: Figure 11.31B is reproduced with permission from "The Radiology assistant".

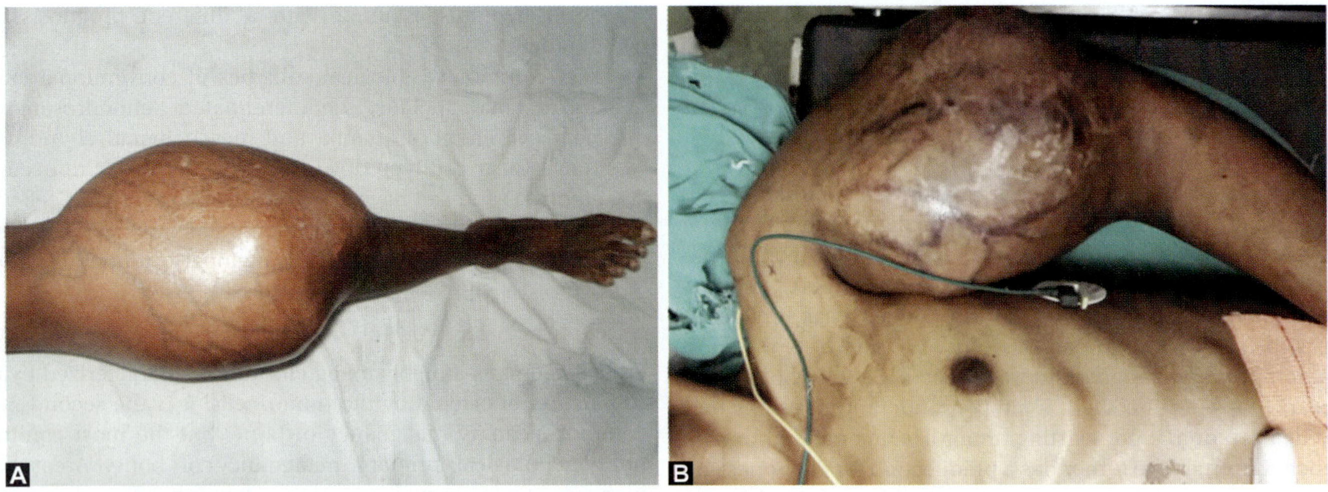

Figs 11.32A and B: Massive swelling and dilated veins due to osteosarcoma of (A) distal femur and (B) distal humerus

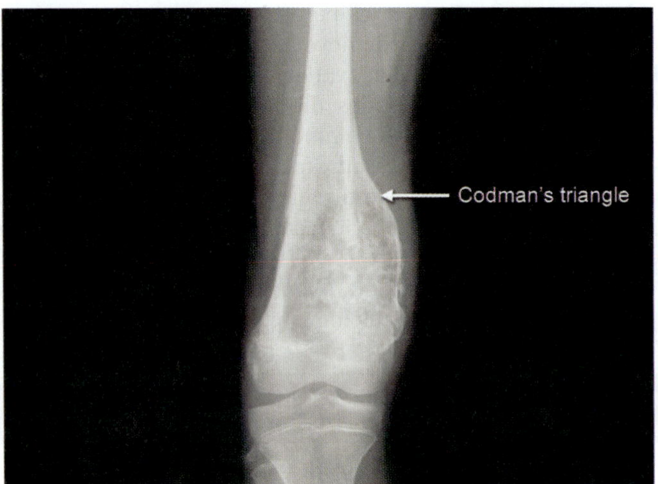

Fig. 11.33: Codman's triangle in osteosarcoma distal femur

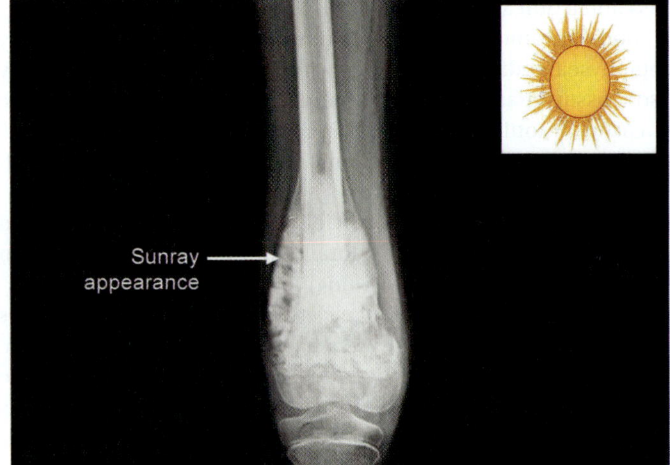

Fig. 11.34: Sunray appearance in osteosarcoma distal femur

Courtesy: Dr Gaurav Gupta, JN MCH, Aligarh.

cells weaken the involved bone. Night pains may be present in 25% of these people. Later on, swelling may be evident with overlying skin appearing warm and tender and dilated veins crossing the swelling **(Figs 11.32A and B)**.

Plain radiographs are valuable to make the diagnosis. Primary or conventional osteosarcoma is characterized by a permeative lytic lesion with ill-defined borders with evidence of bone formation. Periosteal reaction may take the form of Codman's triangle **(Fig. 11.33)**, a triangular area of subperiosteal new bone at the tumor host cortex junction at the ends of the tumor or may appear as the classical sunray appearance **(Fig. 11.34)**, which is due to calcification along the Sharpey's fibers that attach the periosteum to the bone cortex. Often the tumor breaks through the cortex and forms a soft tissue mass. MRI is best to know the soft tissue extent, but to detect "skip lesions", a bone scan is the preferred investigation.

Microscopically, the lesion is characterized by variable amount of osteoid production by the atypical spindle-shaped tumor cells. Based on the amount of osteoid production, the tumors are subclassified as being osteoblastic (lot of new bone formation), chondroblastic (cartilage formation predominates), fibroblastic (where fibroblasts predominate) and telangiectatic/osteolytic (with areas of tumor necrosis and blood-filled spaces) types. The latter has highly malignant-looking cells and resembles an ABC to a great extent.

Treatment of osteosarcoma has evolved considerably over the past few years. In older times, radical excision or mostly an amputation was the preferred treatment modality, but with the advent of effective chemotherapy regimens the current trend is to go for "limb salvage surgery". Chemotherapeutic drugs are administered as per the "T10" protocol **(Box 11.3)** and tumor is excised taking a safe margin (preferably >1 cm) and limb reconstruction done either with massive allografts or with megaprosthesis (*see* Chapter 19, Page 481). In the majority of cases micrometastasis already would have occurred by the time of the diagnosis and adjuvant chemotherapy is even effective in controlling them. The lung is the most common site for metastasis that generally reaches the organ via hematogenous

Box 11.3: T10 protocol for osteosarcoma

- High-dose methotrexate
- Vincristine
- BCD: Bleomycin, cyclophosphamide, dactinomycin
- Doxorubicin

Note: In patients not responding to methotrexate, cisplatin is used as a substitute.

route (lymphatic spread is extremely rare). Radiotherapy has no role as it is a highly radio-resistant tumor. However, Extracorporeal irradiation is an upcoming treatment modality. It consists of en block removal of the bone segment that has the tumor, it's irradiation and then it's reimplantation back into the body. Immunotherapy is another recently introduced treatment modality where a portion of the tumor is implanted into a sarcoma survivor and is removed after a few days. The sensitized lymphocytes from the survivors are then infused into the patient and these lymphocytes then selectively destroy the tumor cells.

With today's multiple-agent chemotherapy regimens and appropriate surgical treatment, most series report long-term survival of 60–75%. The most important prognostic factor at the time of diagnosis is the tumor stage. Patients with pulmonary metastasis at diagnosis have a poorer prognosis as do patients with skip lesions. The next most important prognostic feature is the grade of the lesion. Size and location are also important variables; most proximal tumors are larger at the time of diagnosis than distal tumors and have a bad prognosis. Paget's osteosarcomas continue to have a poor prognosis, with less than 15% long-term survival. Radiation-associated osteosarcomas also have been regarded as having a poor prognosis. Age and gender are not associated with prognosis.

Parosteal/Juxtacortical Osteosarcoma

This is a slow-growing variant (a less common variant of conventional osteosarcoma), that arises in the region of periosteum, in relation to the cortex of the bone, usually the distal femur. People in the age group of 20–35 years are generally affected. Treatment is wide excision with reconstruction using a prosthesis. The overall prognosis is much better than conventional osteosarcoma.

HIGH-YIELD POINTS

- Osteosarcoma is the most common primary tumor of bone, causing pulmonary metastasis (micrometastasis being present in 90% of cases and detectable in 15–20%).
- The most common factors associated with secondary osteosarcomas include Paget's disease and previous radiation therapy. The incidence of osteosarcoma in Paget's disease is approximately 1% and higher (5–10%) for patients with advanced polyostotic disease.
- Osteosarcoma is the most radio-resistant tumor and the most common radiation-induced tumor. Radiation-associated osteosarcoma occurs in approximately 1% of patients who have been treated with greater than 2,500 cGy and can occur in unusual locations, such as the skull, spine, clavicle, ribs, scapula and pelvis. The time to onset of the secondary osteosarcoma averages 10–15 years after radiation exposure, but may occur 3 years to several decades after treatment.

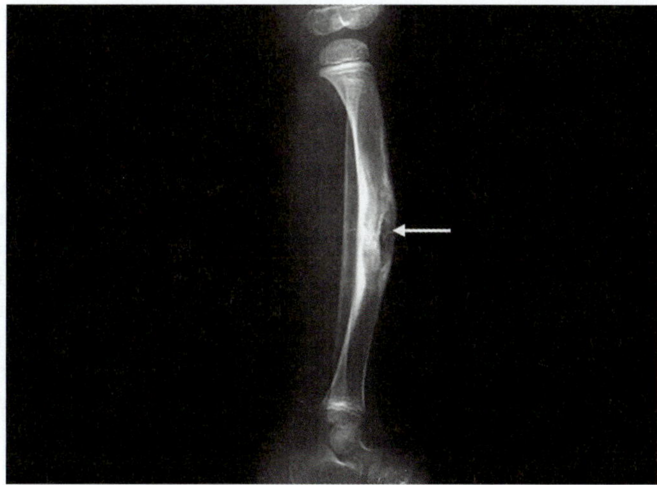

Fig. 11.35: X-ray leg lateral view showing adamantinoma (arrow)

- Serum alkaline phosphatase levels in this tumor are often raised, but rather than diagnostic significance, they are important to monitor follow-up or recurrence.
- Recently, Finkel-Biskis-Jinkins (FBJ) murine virus has been implicated in the pathogenesis of osteosarcoma.

ADAMANTINOMA

Adamantinoma is a low-grade malignant tumor that arises from an aberrant nest of specialized cells similar in histology to ameloblasts (enamel-forming cells in the mandible) that are present under the skin over bones in subcutaneous location, giving rise to adamantinoma of long bones. Tibia (85% cases) followed by fibula is the most common site. The tumor generally affects individuals in their second to third decades of life. Pain is the most common symptom with which most patients report to the clinician. The tumor is typically slow-growing in nature.

X-ray classically shows multiple demarcated radiolucent lesions in tibial diaphysis, separated by areas of dense sclerotic bone **(Fig. 11.35)**. The picture is quite similar to osteofibrous dysplasia (Campanacci disease) and some workers consider adamantinoma to be a malignant variant of the same.

Microscopic examination shows islands of epithelial cells in a fibrous stroma. Nuclear atypia is minimal. Immunohistochemical stains, viz. cytokeratins and vimentins stain positive in adamantinoma.

Treatment is wide resection with adequate margins. The tumor is chemo-resistant and radio-resistant. Local recurrences may occur in up to 25% cases and may need an amputation. Due to slow-growing nature, recurrences have been reported to occur quite late (some up to 20 years). Metastasis generally goes to the lungs and inguinal lymph nodes.

HIGH-YIELD POINTS

- Ameloblastoma, a term at times misused for adamantinoma, is an entirely separate entity. It is a benign tumor that arises from ameloblasts which are enamel-forming cells present in the mandible. Posterior part of the mandible (in the area of the molar teeth) is the most common site of ameloblastoma.

- Most common tumor of the jaw is squamous cell carcinoma of the oral mucosa. Ameloblastoma is the most common bone tumor of the jaw.

EWING SARCOMA

Ewing sarcoma (named after James Ewing, who first described it in 1921), is the third most common nonhematologic primary malignancy of the bone, but it is the second most common (after osteosarcoma) in patients younger than 30 years of age and most common in patients younger than 10 years of age. Classically it affects children in the age group of 5–15 years with those in their second decade being more commonly affected. There is a slight male preponderance. Most common bones affected include the femur (diaphysis) and pelvis. The tumor is also commonly found in the diaphysis (often extending into metaphysis) of humerus, tibia and the flat bones like the vertebrae, ribs and scapula. Multicentric lesions have also been reported.

Pain is the universal complaint, but often there is a delay in diagnosis as the clinical picture may closely resemble acute osteomyelitis with the child having complaints of intermittent fever with the raised leukocyte count, erythrocyte sedimentation rate (ESR), C-reactive protein (CRP) and anemia. Often a needle aspirate of Ewing sarcoma may grossly resemble pus further complicating the matter.

X-ray in acute osteomyelitis would show a metaphyseal lesion with well-defined cloacae and a relatively smooth periosteal reaction and may reveal a sequestrum. However, in Ewing sarcoma, X-ray classically shows a permeative lytic lesion (moth-eaten appearance) in the diaphysis of a long bone surrounded by a lamellated periosteal reaction (onion peel appearance, **Fig. 11.36**). In 80% cases extension of the tumor into adjacent soft tissues is there. Skip lesions are not reported, but at times almost the entire bone may be involved. MRI is generally required to know the full extent of the lesion.

Microscopic picture is classical with multiple small round blue cells with very scanty intercellular matrix, at times showing pseudorosette formations, a pattern attributed to the group of primitive neuroectodermal tumors (PNET) **(Fig. 11.37)**. In fact, the cells stain positive for S-100 and neuron-specific enolase, show neural elements on electron microscopy, are positive for *MIC2* gene and also demonstrate the trl (11;22) seen in the PNET group. One has to opt for tumor markers to reach the specific diagnosis. Ewing sarcoma is CD99 positive and usually is periodic acid-schiff (PAS) positive (owing to intracellular glycogen) but reticulin negative. In contrast, lymphomas (another PNET group tumor) are PAS negative and reticulin positive; additionally they stain positive for leukocyte common antigen (CD45).

Treatment concepts of Ewing sarcoma have immensely changed over the past few years. The success of chemotherapy (VDCA regime—vincristine, doxorubicin, cyclophosphamide and actinomycin D) has emerged as a game changer and both adjuvant and neoadjuvant chemotherapies are extensively used to treat the lesion as well as the distant metastasis that might have been undetectable. Also, this tumor is very radiosensitive. In fact, the tumor is said to melt on radiotherapy. So the patients who have a resectable lesion, where resection with wide margins would not cause a functional deficit are offered surgery followed by radiotherapy (60 Gy) while for most other lesions the multiagent

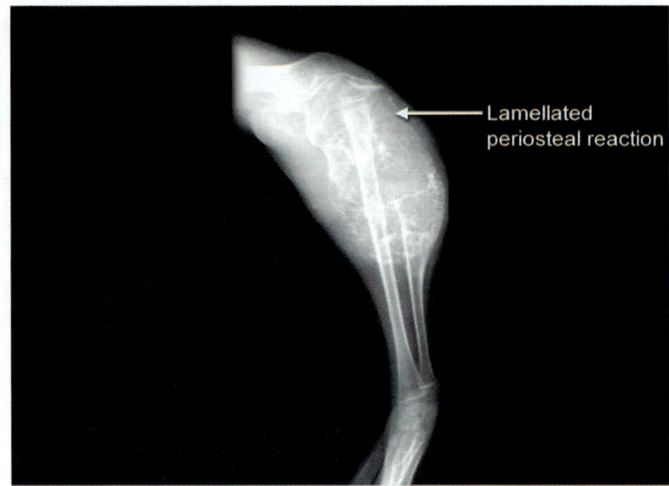

Fig. 11.36: Ewing sarcoma of proximal ulna showing lamellated periosteal reaction

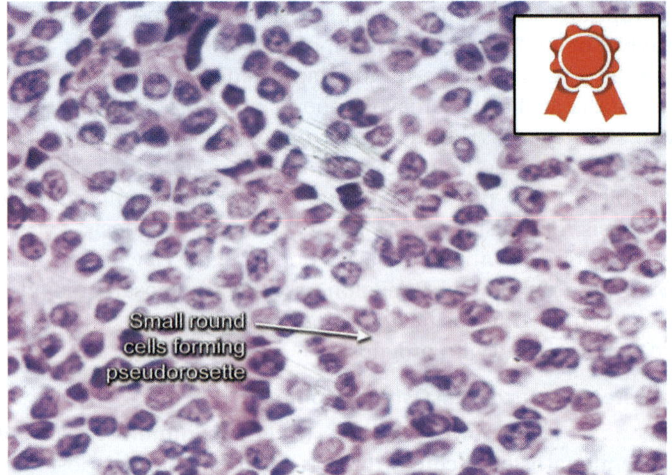

Fig. 11.37: Microscopic picture of Ewing sarcoma with pseudorosette formation ("Rosette" is a decoration typically made from ribbon that resembles a rose, see inset image)

chemotherapy remains the mainstay. Extracorporeal irradiation may be opted where lesion is huge and limb salvage is to be considered.

Metastatic deposits are not uncommon and occur primarily to the lungs (50%) and to bones (25%). Prognosis depends on a number of factors. The most unfavorable prognostic factor in Ewing's sarcoma is the presence of distant metastasis at diagnosis. Other unfavorable prognostic factors include an age older than 10 years, a size larger than 8 cm, more central lesions (as in the pelvis or spine) and poor response to chemotherapy. The histological grade is of no prognostic significance, as all Ewing's sarcomas are of high grade. Fever, anemia, and elevated white blood cell (WBC) count, ESR, and lactate dehydrogenase (LDH) values have been reported to indicate more extensive disease and a poorer prognosis. The presence of trl (11;22), which is present in 90% cases of Ewing sarcoma, however, does not seem to affect the clinical course.

HIGH-YIELD POINTS

- Ewing sarcoma is the most chemosensitive and most radiosensitive malignant bone tumor.
- Ewing sarcoma (>osteosarcoma) is the most common tumor showing bone-to-bone metastasis, hence mandating a bone scan to detect the metastasis.
- The *MIC2* gene detection (by monoclonal antibodies) is significant for the screening purposes while the most specific diagnostic measure involves the demonstration of trl (11;22) by a reverse transcription polymerase chain reaction (RT-PCR) method.
- Although classified under the PNET group, as per the latest hypothesis, the tumor actually has a mesenchymal origin. The sarcoma arises from the medullary cavity (marrow) but the trl (11;22) (*EWSR1-ETS* family gene fusions) changes the developmental pattern of these cells and makes the tumor express the ectodermal markers.

MULTIPLE MYELOMA (KAHLER'S DISEASE)

Plasma cell dyscrasias comprise a group of disorders characterized by neoplastic proliferation of a single clone of plasma cells in the bone marrow, which then produces excess of monoclonal immunoglobulins leading to a constellation of clinical signs and symptoms. The presentation is most commonly a multisystem disorder called Multiple Myeloma (MM), but in about 5% cases, they may present as an isolated bony lesion termed as solitary plasmacytoma. A third rare form of presentation is an osteosclerotic myeloma.

Epidemiology

Multiple myeloma is the most common primary malignancy of the bone. It is diagnosed in adults over 40 years of age (median age at diagnosis is 65 years). It is nearly twice as common in males as in females.

Etiology

Exact etiology is still to be elucidated. Mutations of chromosome 14 and deletions on chromosome 13 are found in many cases and portend a poor prognosis. Few other factors that have been purported to play a role in causation are radiation exposure, pesticide (dioxin) exposure and infection with human herpesvirus 8 (HHV-8) and human immunodeficiency virus (HIV). Why some patients develop MM and others plasmacytoma is also not completely understood. It might be related to differences in cellular adhesion molecules or chemokine receptor expression profiles of the malignant plasma cells.

Pathogenesis

The proliferation of abnormal plasma cells results in overproduction of heavy chains in the form of monoclonal immunoglobulin G (IgG) (most common), IgA or IgM and light chains (kappa and lambda—commonly called the Bence Jones proteins). These proteins aggregate to increase viscosity of blood or overload the renal tubules culminating in renal failure or over a longer period lead to amyloidosis. Additionally, the abnormal plasma cells lead to bone destruction by humoral mechanisms [overproduction of receptor activator of nuclear factor-kB ligand (RANKL), interleukin-6 (IL-6) and macrophage inflammatory protein 1 (MIP 1) alpha].

Clinical Features

The most common presentation of MM is generalized bone pain in an elderly patient. Pathological fractures are common and may be the presenting feature in other patients. Features indicating end-organ damage may include anemia (due to replacement of the marrow by abnormal plasma cells) or hypercalcemia and uremia due to renal failure. Hyperviscosity may lead to neural ischemia manifesting as paresthesias and areas of sensory loss. Amyloidosis may develop in some patients, causing macroglossia, skin lesions and palpebral purpuras.

Radiographic Features

Punched out lesions without a reactive zone or sclerotic zone with a sharp zone of transition to normal bone, are found throughout the skeleton **(Figs 11.38A and B)**. Common sites of involvement (in order of frequency) are spine (most common), pelvis, ribs, upper extremities, face, skull, femur and sternum.

A bone scan is usually negative (cold spot) because of lack of osteoblastic overactivity. The screening tool of choice is a skeletal survey (X-ray). MRI and CT are not routinely done but may be helpful tools in defining skeletal lesions or when a decompression of a spinal lesion is to be planned.

Diagnosis

In the majority of cases the diagnosis is self-evident from the classical clinical picture and the radiological findings. However, considering the elderly age group, metastasis to bone remains an important differential to exclude. The same can be easily excluded by a blood or urine analysis. Patients with suspected MM should be investigated with screening tests which include paraproteins in serum and Bence Jones proteins in urine.

In MM, on blood examination one would find low hemoglobin, raised serum calcium (due to the marked osteolytic action of myeloma cells), increased uric acid (due to increased cell breakdown), elevated urea (in patients with renal failure), markedly increased ESR and a high total protein value but with reversal of A:G (albumin:globulin) ratio (due to increase in the globulin fraction of proteins). Electrophoresis shows an increase in gamma fraction of globulin called the M-spike detectable in both blood and urine. Serum β2-microglobulin is a tumor marker, increase of which is a poor prognostic sign. On urine examination one can also detect the presence of Bence Jones proteins by the heating method or by immunoelectrophoresis (more sensitive method).

On histological examination, the tumor cells have an eccentric nucleus with clumped nuclear chromatin arranged in a clock face pattern (cartwheel appearance) and stain positive for CD56 and CD38 (while normal plasma cells do not). Hoffa's clear zone (clear zone near the nucleus representing Golgi apparatus) is characteristic in these cells. Amyloid collection on bone marrow biopsy in an old patient who is not on long-term hemodialysis is a very strong indicator of underlying MM.

Criteria for the diagnosis of MM have recently been changed by International Myeloma Working Group **(Box 11.4)**. Solitary plasmacytoma occurs as a single skeletal (or extraskeletal) lesion without fulfilling the above criteria and in the absence of other features of MM (i.e. anemia, hypercalcemia, renal insufficiency or multiple lytic bone lesions). It progresses to classic systemic

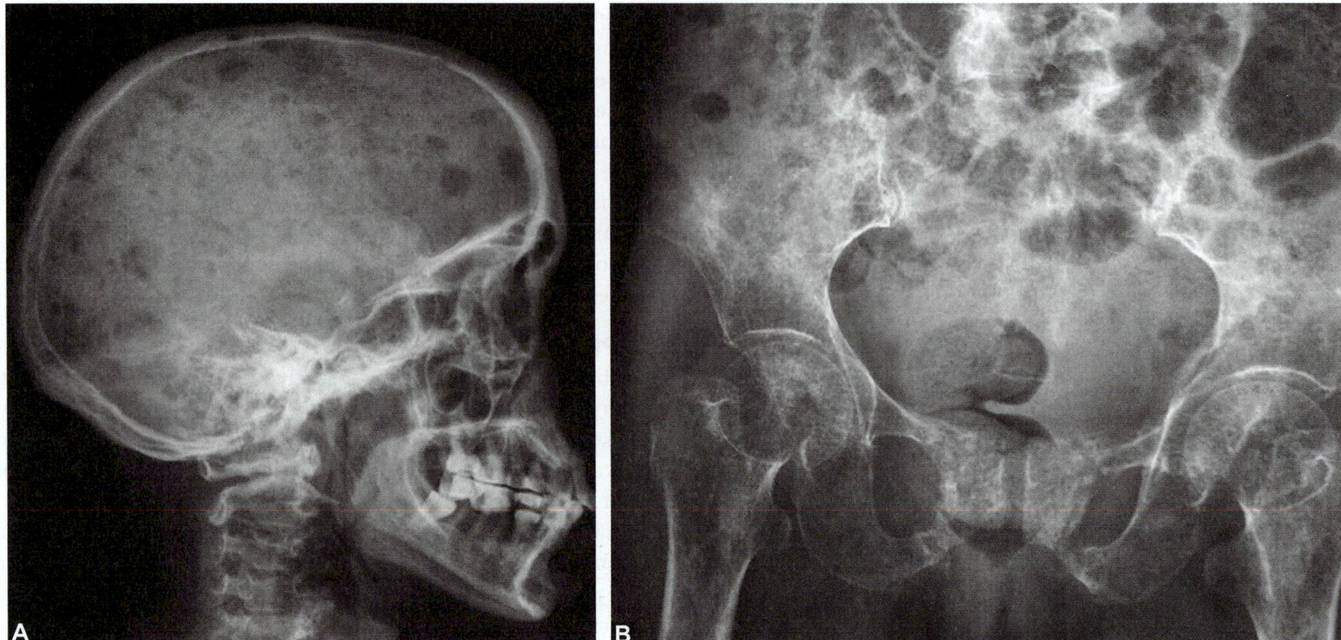

Figs 11.38A and B: X-rays showing the classical lytic lesions of multiple myeloma (mm) in the skull and pelvis

Box 11.4: International Myeloma Working Group (IMWG) criteria for the diagnosis of multiple myeloma (2015)

Diagnosis is MM when clonal bone marrow plasma cells >10% or there is biopsy-proven bony or extramedullary plasmacytoma plus any one or more of CRAB (raised calcium, renal insufficiency, anemia, bone lesion) feature or myeloma-defining event

CRAB features (markers of end organ damage)

- *Hypercalcemia*: Serum calcium >0.25 mmol/L (>1 mg/dL) higher than the upper limit of normal or >2.75 mmol/L (>11 mg/dL)

- *Renal insufficiency*: Creatinine clearance <40 mL per minute or serum creatinine >177 μmol/L (>2 mg/dL)

- *Anemia*: Hemoglobin value of >2 g/dL below the lower limit of normal, or a hemoglobin value <10 g/dL

- *Bone lesions*: One or more osteolytic lesion on skeletal radiography, CT, or PET/CT. If bone marrow has <10% clonal plasma cells, more than one bone lesion is required to distinguish from solitary plasmacytoma with minimal marrow involvement

Myeloma defining events (Biomarkers of malignancy)

- 60% or greater clonal plasma cells on bone marrow examination

- Serum involved/uninvolved free light chain ratio of 100 or greater, provided the absolute level of the involved light chain is at least 100 mg/L (a patient's "involved" free light chain—either kappa or lambda—is the one that is above the normal reference range; the "uninvolved" free light chain is the one that is typically in, or below, the normal range)

- More than one focal lesion on MRI that is at least 5 mm or greater in size

endocrinopathy, M spike, skin changes). International Myeloma Working Group diagnostic criteria of solitary plasmacytoma of bone, extramedullary plasmacytoma, monoclonal gammopathy of undetermined significance and smoldering multiple myeloma (SMM) have been summarized in **Table 11.5**.

Management

Chemotherapy is the mainstay of treatment. Drugs used are melphalan in combination with prednisolone. Other agents which may be used are cyclophosphamide, doxorubicin and thalidomide. Bisphosphonates are used to decrease bone pain and control hypercalcemia.

Autologous stem cell transplantation, although not curative (i.e. does not cause remission) improves overall survival by 2–3 years. It is an option in relatively young (<65 years) patients without comorbidities.

Orthopedic Management

Impending (Mirel score > 8, *see* Page 41) or actual pathological fractures may require long bone stabilization with intramedullary implants (to splint the entire length of the bone). Periarticular fractures are managed with joint replacements or megaprostheses. The tumor is radiosensitive so 3 weeks after surgery, radiation is also added to the treatment regimen. Kyphoplasty or vertebroplasty is used for painful vertebral compression fractures.

Solitary plasmacytoma is treated mainly with radiotherapy only, with operative stabilization employed generally in cases of actual or impending pathological fracture.

Prognosis

The overall prognosis for MM is bad, however, patients with solitary plasmacytomas tend to have a better prognosis.

form in more than 50% patients. Osteosclerotic myeloma is rare and is characterized by POEMS (polyneuropathy, organomegaly,

Table 11.5: Definitions of related plasma cell proliferative disorders

Plasma cell disorder	*Definition*
Smoldering multiple myeloma	Both criteria must be met: 1. Serum monoclonal protein (IgG or IgA) ≥30g/L or urinary monoclonal protein ≥500 mg per 24 h and/or clonal bone marrow plasma cells 10–60% 2. Absence of myeloma-defining events or amyloidosis
Non-IgM monoclonal gammopathy of undetermined significance (MGUS)	Serum monoclonal protein <30 g/L Clonal bone marrow plasma cells <10% Absence of end-organ damage such as hypercalcemia, renal insufficiency, anemia, and bone lesions (CRAB) or amyloidosis that can be attributed to the plasma cell proliferative disorder
IgM MGUS	Serum IgM monoclonal protein <30 g/L No evidence of anemia, constitutional symptoms, hyperviscosity, lymphadenopathy, hepatosplenomegaly, or other end-organ damage that can be attributed to the plasma cell proliferative disorder
Light chain MGUS	Abnormal free light chain (FLC) ratio (<0.26 or >1.65) Increased levels of the appropriate free light chain (increased κ FLC in patients with ratio >1.65 and increased λ FLC in patients with ratio <0.26) No immunoglobulin heavy chain expression on immunofixation Absence of end-organ damage such as hypercalcemia, renal insufficiency, anemia, and bone lesions (CRAB) or amyloidosis that can be attributed to the plasma cell proliferative disorder Clonal bone marrow plasma cells <10% Urinary monoclonal protein <500 mg/24 h
Solitary plasmacytoma	Biopsy-proven solitary lesion of bone or soft tissue with evidence of clonal plasma cells Normal bone marrow with no evidence of clonal plasma cells Normal skeletal survey and MRI (or CT) of spine and pelvis (except for the primary solitary lesion) Absence of end-organ damage such as hypercalcemia, renal insufficiency, anemia, and bone lesions (CRAB) or amyloidosis that can be attributed to the plasma cell proliferative disorder
Solitary plasmacytoma with minimal marrow involvement	Biopsy-proven solitary lesion of bone or soft tissue with evidence of clonal plasma cells Clonal bone marrow plasma cells <10% Normal skeletal survey and MRI (or CT) of spine and pelvis (except for the primary solitary lesion) Absence of end-organ damage such as hypercalcemia, renal insufficiency, anemia, and bone lesions (CRAB) or amyloidosis that can be attributed to the plasma cell proliferative disorder
POEMS syndrome	Polyneuropathy Monoclonal plasma cell proliferative disorder Any one of the 3 other major criteria: sclerotic bone lesions, Castleman's disease, elevated levels of vascular endothelial growth factor (VEGF) Any one of the following 6 minor criteria: 1. Organomegaly (splenomegaly, hepatomegaly, or lymphadenopathy) 2. Extravascular volume overload (edema, pleural effusion, or ascites) 3. Endocrinopathy (adrenal, thyroid, pituitary, gonadal, parathyroid, pancreatic) 4. Skin changes (hyperpigmentation, hypertrichosis, glomeruloid hemangiomata, plethora, acrocyanosis, flushing, white nails) 5. Papilloedema 6. Thrombocytosis/polycythemia
Systemic AL amyloidosis	Presence of an amyloid-related systemic syndrome (e.g., renal, liver, heart, gastrointestinal tract, or peripheral nerve involvement) Positive amyloid staining by Congo red in any tissue (e.g., fat aspirate, bone marrow, or organ biopsy) Evidence that amyloid is light-chain-related established by direct examination of the amyloid using mass spectrometry-based proteomic analysis or immunoelectron microscopy Evidence of a monoclonal plasma cell proliferative disorder (serum monoclonal protein, abnormal free light chain ratio, or clonal plasma cells in the bone marrow)

Abbreviations: IgM, immunoglobulin M; MGUS, monoclonal gammopathy of undetermined significance; FLC, free light chain; CRAB, raised calcium, renal insufficiency, anemia and bone lesions; POEMS, polyneuropathy, organomegaly, endocrinopathy, M spike, skin changes; VEGF, vascular endothelial growth factor.

HIGH-YIELD POINTS

- The levels of alkaline phosphatase are not raised in MM.
- Bence Jones proteins may be identifiable in urine in almost 50% of MM patients. These proteins precipitate when the sample is heated to 50°C and again dissolve when the sample is heated to 100°C.
- Unlike MM, solitary bone plasmacytoma does not include the presence of abnormal plasma cells throughout the bone marrow.
- The most common site for an extramedullary myeloma is skin and subcutaneous tissues followed by the liver. Over 80% of these arise in the region of head and neck, especially the upper respiratory tract.
- The most common site for a solitary plasmacytoma is the spine.
- Multiple myeloma is one tumor which can have dural deposits without bone lesions.

MISCELLANEOUS CONDITIONS OF CLINICAL INTEREST

BONE ISLAND

Bone island **(Fig. 11.39)** is an unossified piece of cartilage in the bone. At times a person may have multiple bone islands scattered in whole body, a condition called as "osteopoikilosis" (*see* Page 393).

PIGMENTED VILLONODULAR SYNOVITIS

Pigmented villonodular synovitis (PVNS) is a rare benign disease of the synovial membrane which is characterized by hypervascular neoplastic proliferation of the synovium with deposition of macrophages, multinucleated giant cells and hemosiderin. The knee joint is most commonly involved joint. On arthroscopy typical brownish pigmentation of synovium **(Fig. 11.40)** is seen due to deposition of hemosiderin pigment. On knee aspiration, the finding of blood-tinged synovial fluid is highly suggestive, although not pathognomonic, of pigmented villonodular synovitis. Two varieties have been described, diffuse variety and localized nodular variety. Chances of recurrence are higher in diffuse variety. Low-dose external beam radiotherapy and arthroscopic or open synovectomy have been tried with varying success for the treatment. Malignant transformation has been reported, but very rare.

GORHAM'S DISEASE

Gorham's disease/disappearing bones/massive osteolysis is a disorder of unknown etiology characterized by the progressive disappearance of bones in the body **(Fig. 11.41)**. Shoulder and pelvis are the most common sites, although any bone may be affected. The medical treatment includes radiation therapy, bisphosphonates (inhibit osteoclastic function) and α-2b interferon. Surgical options include resection of the lesion and reconstruction using bone grafts or prostheses. In most cases, bone grafts tend to undergo resorption and are hardly helpful.

CORTICAL DESMOID

A cortical desmoid is an irregularity in the posteromedial aspect of the distal femoral metaphysic **(Figs 11.42A and B)** that occurs as a reaction to muscle stress exerted by the adductor magnus, mostly in 10–15 years old boys. Clinical symptoms include soft tissue swelling and pain. Radiographs and MRI reveal erosion

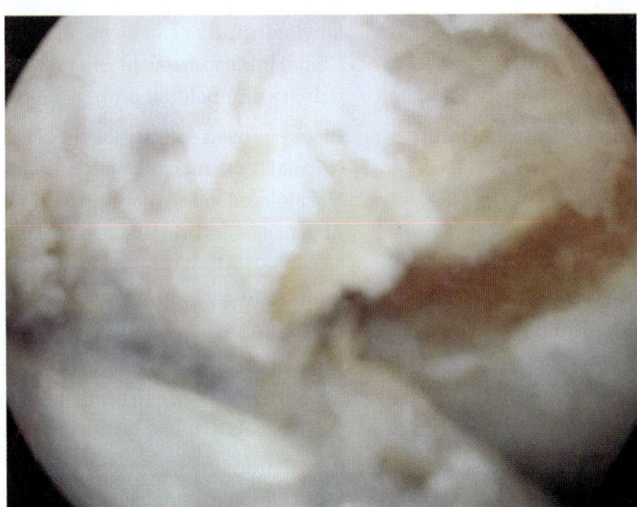

Fig. 11.40: Brownish pigmentation of synovium in pigmented villonodular synovitis (arthroscopic view)

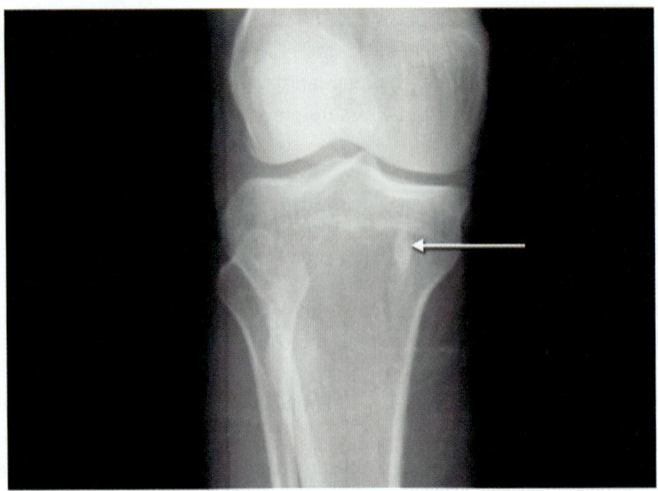

Fig. 11.39: Bone island in the proximal tibia (calcified)

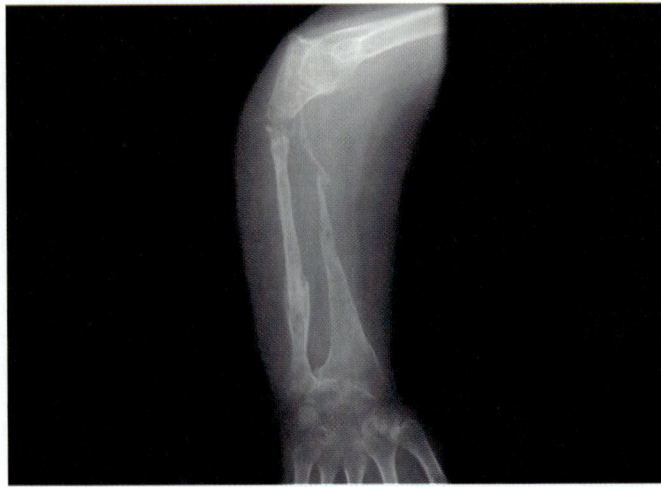

Fig. 11.41: X-ray of a patient with Gorham's disease showing disappearing forearm bones

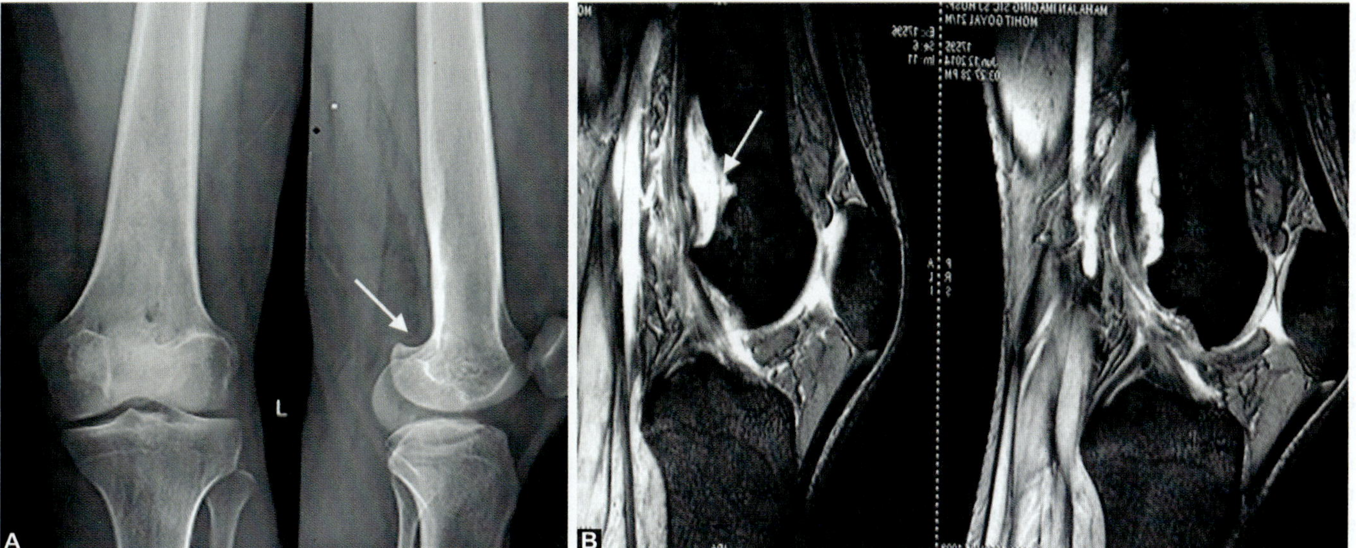

Figs 11.42A and B: Cortical desmoids. (A) X-ray knee with thigh anteroposterior and lateral views, see scalloping at the posteromedial cortex of the distal femoral metaphysis in lateral view (arrow); (B) In MRI, high signal intensity (arrow) is seen at the posteromedial aspect of the distal femoral metaphysis

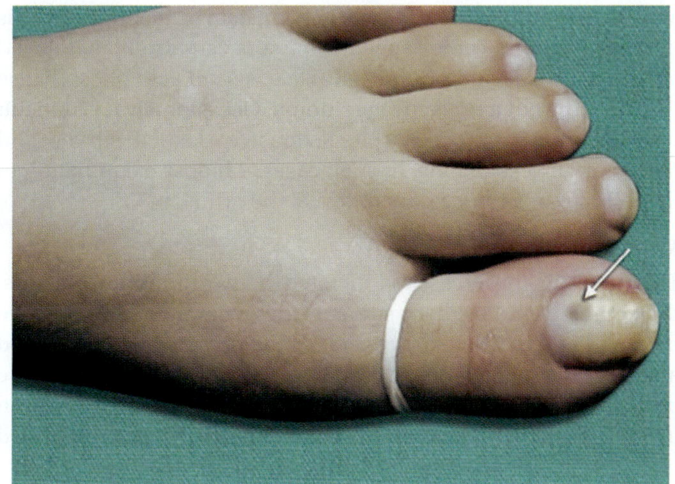

Fig. 11.43: Glomus tumor (arrow) of toe nail showing bluish discoloration

of the cortex with a sclerotic base. A biopsy is not warranted. Treatment usually consists of observation only.

GLOMUS TUMOR

Glomus tumor is a benign neoplasm, seen mostly in 30–50 years old women, arising from a neuromyoarterial apparatus called the glomus body. Glomus bodies are arteriovenous shunts located in the dermis throughout the body but concentrated densely in the apical skin areas (primarily the fingertips). They are involved in thermoregulation of extremity, a function they perform by regulating blood flow to the extremity. The most common site of occurrence of this tumor is the subungual area of the fingers, although any area may be affected. Classical triad of the tumor is intense paroxysmal pain, pin point tenderness on touching the lesion and cold hypersensitivity. The lesion often produces a bluish discoloration below the nail **(Fig. 11.43)**. Love's test, i.e. pain when applying pressure, has a high sensitivity while the

Hildreth test is more specific. It is based on the vascular nature of this tumor and consists of applying a tourniquet above the systolic pressure; if the pain disappears, it indicates glomus tumor. MRI provides the diagnosis in doubtful cases. Treatment involves complete surgical excision.

After lung and liver, skeletal system is the third most common site to receive secondary metastatic deposits from a primary site. In fact, metastasis to bone is so common that metastatic carcinomas not only constitute the most common cause of destructive bone lesion in adults, they also are the most common tumors of the bone.

Sites

Metastasis can reach the bone from a number of primary sites that include the breast, lung, prostate, kidney, thyroid, etc. **Box 11.5** summarizes common sites for primary, in case of bony metastasis in different situations. Overall, the most common site for a primary tumor that metastasizes to the bone is the breast carcinoma. These metastatic deposits preferably go to the thoracic region of spine because the venous drainage of the breast through the azygos communicates with the plexus of Batson in the thoracic region. Not uncommon is the involvement of the proximal ends of the humerus and femur, due to the predominance of the red bone marrow. However, metastases distal to the knee and elbow are very rare and generally tend to arise from lung (most common) and tibia is the most commonly affected bone in these cases.

Mode of Spread

Hematogenous spread has been documented as the most common mode of bone involvement. Vertebra is a cancellous bone highly rich in red marrow and hence the most common site of affection.

Pathophysiology of Bone Metastasis

Once the metastatic deposits reach the bone, they can produce either an osteoblastic or an osteolytic lesion **(Box 11.6)**. Tumor cells in some cancers (prostate) produce some signaling molecules that stimulate bone formation by increasing osteoblast activity. They include transforming growth factor-β (TGF-β), bone morphogenetic proteins (BMPs) and endothelin-1. Whereas in other metastatic cancers like breast cancer, tumor cells secrete parathyroid hormone-related protein (PTHrP) and IL-6, which are powerful mediators of osteoclast activation and participate in osteolysis by stimulating the production of RANKL by osteoblasts and stromal cells.

Clinical Presentation and Diagnosis

Mostly these patients are old aged and present to the orthopedic surgeon with a clinically silent primary site, but with either bone pain or a pathological fracture. In all elderly patients presenting with generalized bone pain, a detailed skeletal survey with radiographs of all suspected areas is of utmost importance to prevent missing a metastasis. Radiographs must be ordered keeping in mind that metastasis that reaches the bone, most commonly involve the axial skeleton (spine followed by the pelvis, then the ribs and then skull) and the thoracic segment of the spine is the most commonly involved site. In the spine, the vertebral body is involved before the pedicles, although

destruction of the pedicles is the most common finding initially appreciable on plain films.

In case where radiographs fail to detect the lesions, bone scan is a useful tool and it can especially pick up skip lesions. It is the investigation of choice for detecting osteoblastic metastasis while for osteolytic lesions FDG-PET scan can be employed. In fact, PET-CT can detect any tumor cell activity. MRI is more useful in primary bone tumors to find their soft tissue extent.

Not uncommon for these patients is to present with a pathological fracture. Femoral neck is the most common site of pathological fracture in such patients and these pathological fractures classically tend to produce transverse fracture lines on radiographs.

Locating the Primary Site

A challenge in these patients is to locate the primary site. A detailed history, meticulous general physical examination and a case-tailored investigation profile are necessary to appropriately locate the primary site from where the secondary deposits originated. Serum alkaline phosphatase levels may be elevated in cases with bone destruction, but attempted reparative osteoblastic reaction while in cases of massive destruction, the urine hydroxyproline levels may go up. Thus, evaluation of markers of bone formation and resorption (*see* **Box 2.6**, Page 17), can help in making diagnosis in these patients. Tumor-specific markers can also be employed to rule out suspected primary sites, e.g. serum acid phosphatase levels to rule out a prostatic carcinoma. Occasionally it is difficult to detect the primary despite extensive skeletal survey and laboratory investigations. In such cases, a biopsy examination of the lesion may be necessary to reveal the primary.

Management

Treatment in these cases is dictated by two important factors: the source of the primary site and the general condition of the patient. In cases where the general condition of the patient is good and there is a solitary metastatic deposit with a located primary, the primary lesion is treated first and the metastatic area excised. In inaccessible areas, radiotherapy or chemotherapy may be employed

---

Box 11.5: Common primary sites for bone metastasis

- *In males:* Prostate followed by lung
- *In females:* Breast followed by lung
- *In children:* Neuroblastoma
- *Overall:* Breast followed by prostate and then lung

Box 11.6: Primaries causing osteoblastic (sclerotic) and osteolytic bone metastasis

- Osteoblastic **(Fig. 11.44A)**—prostate, seminoma, carcinoids, medulloblastoma
- Osteolytic **(Fig. 11.44B)**—kidney, thyroid, lung
- Mixed—breast (more commonly lytic)

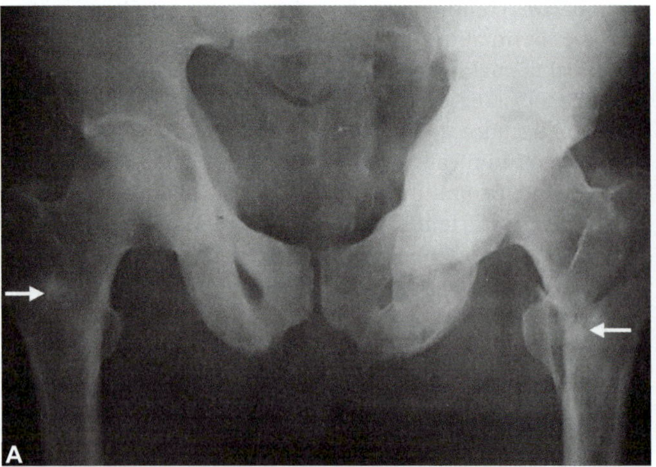

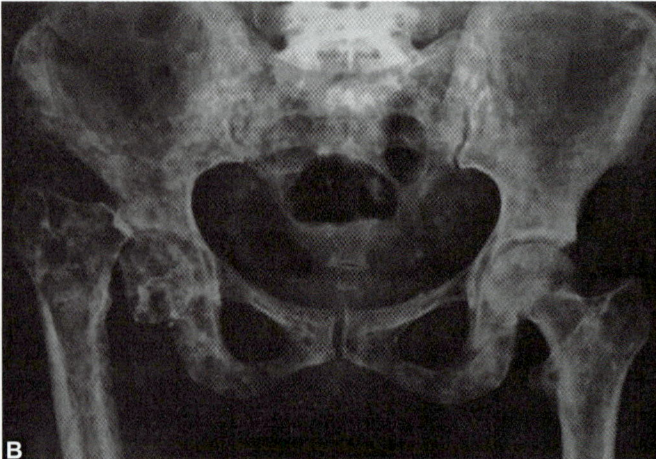

Figs 11.44A and B: (A) X-ray pelvis with both hips anteroposterior (AP) views showing osteoblastic metastasis (arrows) from carcinoma prostate and pathological intertrochanteric fracture left femur; (B) X-ray pelvis with both hips AP views showing osteolytic metastasis from lung carcinoma with a pathological fracture neck of right femur

depending on the source of metastasis. Multiple secondaries with an unknown or even a known primary are better managed with palliative chemotherapy or radiotherapy to provide some pain relief. Impending pathological fractures (*see* Mirel score > 8, Page 41) are managed with prophylactic internal fixation, before the fracture occurs and troubles the patient. Metastatic pathological fractures if result, often fail to unite and require internal fixation with intramedullary rod or long plate with the addition of bone cement to fill the defect. Joint arthroplasty is a favorable option for lesions near the joint. For the involvement of larger areas of bone, often replacement of whole bone with a tumor prosthesis (megaprosthesis) may be required.

Bisphosphonates inhibit the osteoclast-mediated bone resorption by inducing osteoclast apoptosis, inhibiting osteoclast maturation and decreasing their activity and hold an important place in the medicinal treatment of bony metastasis. Both bisphosphonates and radiotherapy are especially useful in affecting pain relief and halting the progression of bone destruction in metastatic bone cancer.

HIGH-YIELD POINTS

- Most common site for metastasis to bone is the breast, but from primary bone tumors metastasis most commonly go to the lungs.
- Bone is the primary site of metastasis in 40–75% cases of breast cancer.
- Bone-to-bone metastasis is seen in Ewing sarcoma and osteosarcoma (Ewing sarcoma is more than osteosarcoma).
- About 70% of cases with bony metastases are detected radiographically and 85% of them show lytic changes.
- Metastasis from follicular carcinoma thyroid and renal cell carcinoma are pulsatile. Most pulsatile tumors are metastasis followed by ABC and GCT.
- Radionuclide therapy is a recent addition in the treatment for palliative pain relief from metastatic bone disease. Commonly used agents are phosphorus-32 orthophosphate and strontium-89 chloride.

SOFT TISSUE SARCOMAS

INTRODUCTION

Soft tissue sarcomas are rare tumors. They account for nearly 1% of all malignancies. Based on the location and tissue of origin, following types are recognized:
- Smooth muscle: Leiomyosarcoma
- Skeletal muscle: Rhabdomyosarcoma
- Fat: Liposarcoma
- Blood vessels: Angiosarcoma
- Fibrous tissue: Fibrosarcoma
- Fibrohistiocytic: Malignant fibrous histiocytoma (MFH)
- Lymph vessels: Lymphosarcoma
- Uncertain origin: Synovial sarcoma, epithelioid sarcoma.

Soft tissue sarcomas overall are more common in males, and mostly occur in the adult population. These most commonly arise in the extremities (60%), with lower extremities being involved three times as often as upper extremity. Staging criteria for soft tissue sarcomas depends on the histologic grade, the tumor size and depth, and the presence of distant or nodal metastases.

The most important prognostic factor is the histologic grade. General indicators of poor prognosis include size greater than 5 cm, location below deep fascia, and high-grade lesions, proximal extremity location (as opposed to distal extremity). Soft tissue sarcomas most commonly metastasize to the lungs. Diagnosis is confirmed on biopsy.

MALIGNANT FIBROUS HISTIOCYTOMA

It is the most common soft tissue sarcoma in adults. It is interesting to note that the most common radiation-induced soft tissue sarcoma is also MFH (whereas osteosarcoma is overall the most common radiation-induced sarcoma).

Its most common location is thigh where it commonly presents as a deep-seated painless mass, gradually increasing in size. Rarely, it may arise from the bone also. Occasional systemic features include fever and hypoglycemia. Lesions appear hypointense on T1 and hyperintense on T2-weighted MRI. Tumor pathology is heterogeneous with predominantly storiform or cartwheel arrangement (irregular whorled pattern) of histiocytic cells (**Fig. 11.45**) with occasional giant cells. Due to its pleomorphic nature, it has been recently reclassified as pleomorphic undifferentiated sarcoma.

Management includes wide resection and radiation (preoperative or postoperative). Tumors not amenable to resection demand a more aggressive surgery in the form of amputation. Chemotherapy may also be added, but its role is not clear at present. Metastasis to the lungs and lymph nodes is common. Prognosis mainly depends on the histological grade of tumor (atypia, mitotic figures, etc.).

LIPOSARCOMA

It is the second most common soft tissue sarcoma in adults. Presentation is similar to MFH. The behavior depends on histological type. Well-differentiated type occurs in the limbs. It rarely metastasizes and has an excellent survival rate, whereas the dedifferentiated type is more aggressive and commonly occurs in the abdomen or groin region. Another rare type is myxoid type,

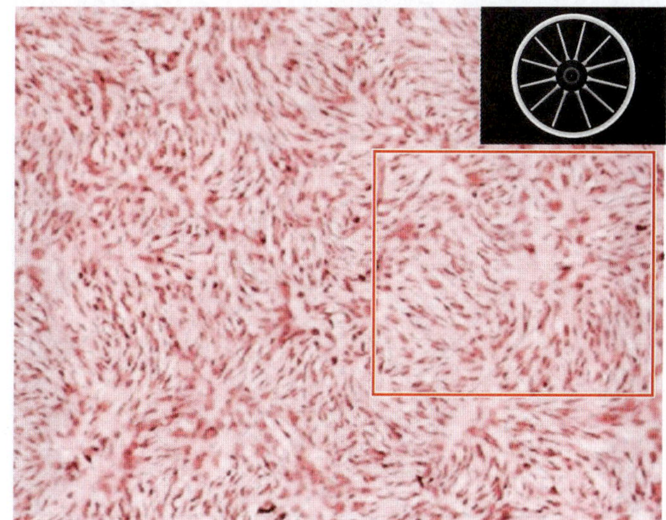

Fig. 11.45: Storiform or irregular whorled appearance of histiocytic cells of malignant fibrous histiocytoma simulating a cartwheel make cartwheel as inset

which tends to occur in relatively younger age group and has a predilection for the retroperitoneum. Well-differentiated type is treated with resection alone, whereas other types require surgery, radiotherapy and occasionally chemotherapy.

SYNOVIAL CELL SARCOMA

Synovial cell sarcoma is a soft tissue tumor that does not have a synovial origin despite its name. Occurring mostly in adolescents and young patients, it is a rare but aggressive tumor that arises in the vicinity of a bursa, tendon sheaths or joint capsules where there are multipotent stem cell rests that differentiate into mesenchymal as well as epithelial structures, hence a "biphasic tumor". Although the tumor is most commonly located around the knee, it is also the most common soft tissue sarcoma of the foot. It is characterized by trl (X;18). Wide excision is the treatment of choice and radiotherapy also is effective.

FIBROSARCOMA

Very rare entity; in fact, it has become a diagnosis of exclusion. The characteristic microscopic appearance of fibrosarcoma consists of spindle cells arranged in a herringbone pattern **(Figs 11.46A and B)**. The typical presentation is a 5–10-cm, slow-growing, painless mass in the deep soft tissues of the lower extremity in adults aged 30–50 years old.

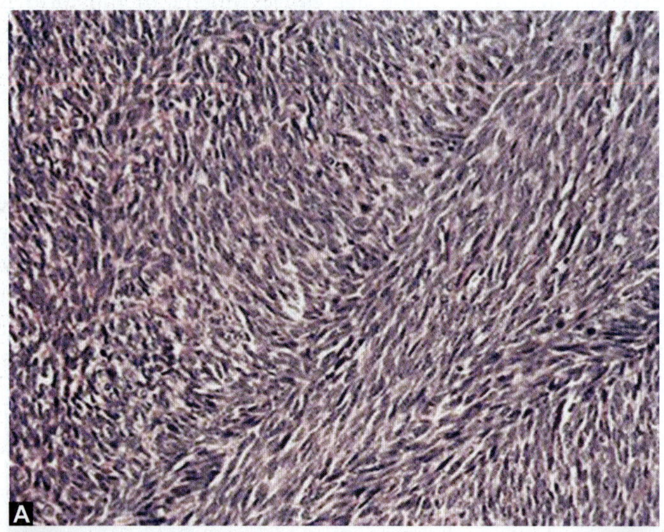

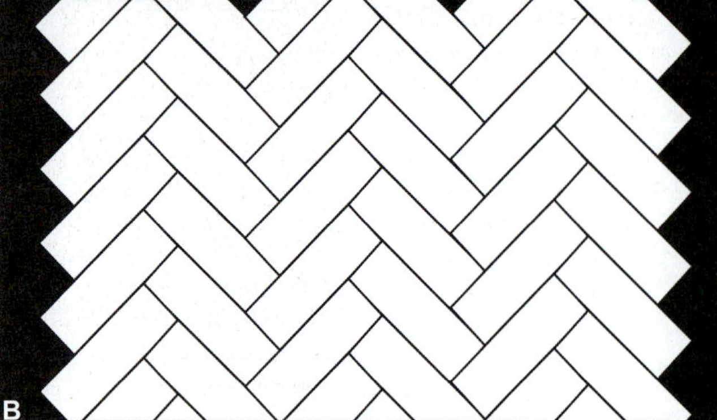

Figs 11.46A and B: Herringbone pattern in fibrosarcoma. Herringbone pattern refers to the arrangement of rectangles used in floor tiling

EPITHELIOID SARCOMA

It is the most common soft tissue sarcoma of hand. It may be confused with a benign granuloma clinically and histologically. Metastasis to lymph nodes is relatively common. Treatment is by wide resection or amputation (if nonresectable).

RHABDOMYOSARCOMA

It is the most common soft tissue sarcoma in children. The most common locations are head and neck, genitourinary and retroperitoneum. Only 15% occurs in extremities.
Histologically, three types are there:
1. Embryonal type is the most common and consists of round and spindle cells in a myxoid stroma. Visible cross-striations may be seen. Sarcoma botryoides is its variant, which occurs in hollow mucosa-lined organs (vagina, bladder, etc.).
2. Alveolar rhabdomyosarcoma commonly occurs in the extremities. It consists of septa which divide clusters of cells (similar to alveolar architecture of the lung).
3. Pleomorphic rhabdomyosarcoma is rare and consists of large eosinophilic polygonal cells. Multinucleated giant cells are prominent and the typical strap-shaped and racket-shaped cells are also seen.

Rhabdomyosarcoma frequently has a rapid and aggressive clinical course. Metastasis occurs to the lungs, lymph nodes and bone marrow. Treatment consists of wide resection and multiagent chemotherapy.

HIGH-YIELD POINTS

- Most common soft tissue sarcoma in adults—malignant fibrous histiocytoma followed by liposarcoma
- Most common soft tissue sarcoma in young adults— synovial cell sarcoma
- Most common soft tissue sarcoma in children— rhabdomyosarcoma
- Most common site of rhabdomyosarcoma—head and neck
- Most common soft tissue sarcoma of the foot—synovial cell sarcoma
- Most common soft tissue sarcoma of the upper extremity/ hand—epithelioid sarcoma
- Most important prognostic factor in soft tissue sarcomas— histological grade
- Most common radiation-induced soft tissue sarcoma is malignant fibrous histiocytoma. Otherwise, most common radiation-induced sarcoma is osteosarcoma
- Sarcomas of soft tissue origin rarely metastasize to bone, however, the following ones may metastasize to bone— angiosarcoma, liposarcoma, rhabdomyosarcoma and synovial cell sarcoma
- Sarcomas metastasizing via the lymphatic system (mnemonic "ME Loves CARS"):
  - M: Malignant fibrous histiocytoma
  - E: Epithelial sarcoma
  - L: Lymphosarcoma
  - C: Clear cell sarcoma
  - A: Angiosarcoma
  - R: Rhabdomyosarcoma
  - S: Synovial cell sarcoma.

EOSINOPHILIC GRANULOMA AND LANGERHANS CELL HISTIOCYTOSIS

Eosinophilic granuloma (EG) is a part of the spectrum of disease Langerhans cell histiocytosis, formerly called as histiocytosis X.

Langerhans cell histiocytosis is a disease of unknown etiology characterized by accumulation in body of a large number of abnormal histiocytes that actually start damaging the body itself. It can be present in three forms:

1. Letterer-Siwe disease (10% cases)—a fulminant systemic disease that occurs in children under 3 years of age and is rapidly fatal.
2. Hand-Schuller-Christian disease (10–20% cases)—a chronic disseminated that occurs in older patients and exhibits the well-known triad of diabetes insipidus, exophthalmos and skull lesions.
3. Eosinophilic granuloma or pulmonary histiocytosis-X (60–80% of all cases)—the most benign form of the three clinical variants. It is basically a solitary non-neoplastic proliferation of histiocytes that mostly produces a lesion in the lungs or bones. It is seen mostly in 5–10 years old children and sometimes in young adults, with a male-to-female ratio of 2:1.

EOSINOPHILIC GRANULOMA OF BONE

Eosinophilic granuloma may occur in the bone as either a solitary lesion of bone destruction (more common) or as multiple lesions in the skeleton. Although any bone can be involved; the more common sites include the skull (most common site), mandible, spine, ribs and the long bones. The patients are usually children that present with localized pain, tenderness, swelling, fever, elevated ESR and leukocytosis. The radiographic picture is nonspecific and varies with the site of involvement. The skull may have a lesion with a sharp, punched out borders that are uneven across the inner and outer table (affects outer table more than the inner table), causing a "beveled edge" that gives them the characteristic double contour **(Fig. 11.47)**. In spine lesions appear in the vertebral body and bone destruction may lead to collapse of the whole vertebra leading to the classical picture of vertebra plana **(Fig. 11.48)**. In long bones, EG is found in the diaphysis or metaphysis mostly in the center of the medullary cavity. The lesion is generally surrounded by a good periosteal reaction and may expand to cause endosteal scalloping. A bone scan is not much useful in delineating these lesions and MRI is more commonly employed. Biopsy remains the gold standard for confirmation. Under the microscope, EG consists of sheets of Langerhans cells that are derived from the mononuclear cells and dendritic line precursors found in the bone marrow. These cells when seen under the electron microscope demonstrate racket-shaped cytoplasmic inclusion bodies called Birbeck's granules. Additionally, on immunohistochemistry, the cells stain positive for S-100, CD-1a and neuron-specific enolase.

Although almost always symptomatic, the lesions mostly regress spontaneously in about 6 months to 2 years. At times, the biopsy may incite the regression. So treatment is mostly not required. The lesions are also highly radiosensitive and excision and curettage are employed only in resistant cases. Chemotherapy is limited to systemic form of the disease. Overall prognosis is very good.

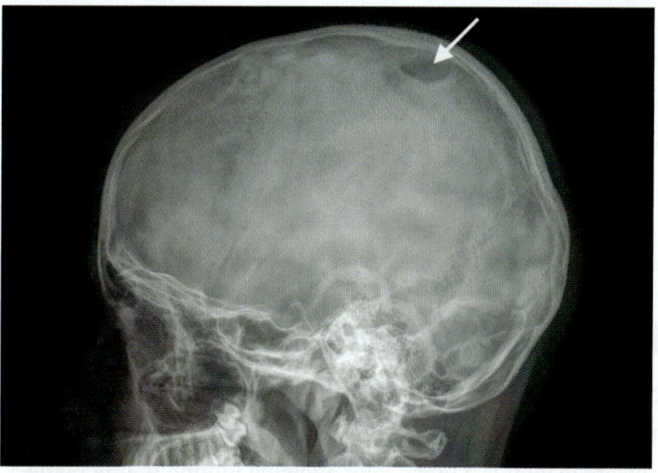

Fig. 11.47: Eosinophilic granuloma lesion in the parietal bone (arrow) of the skull depicting the classical double contour pattern
Courtesy: Radiopedia.org.

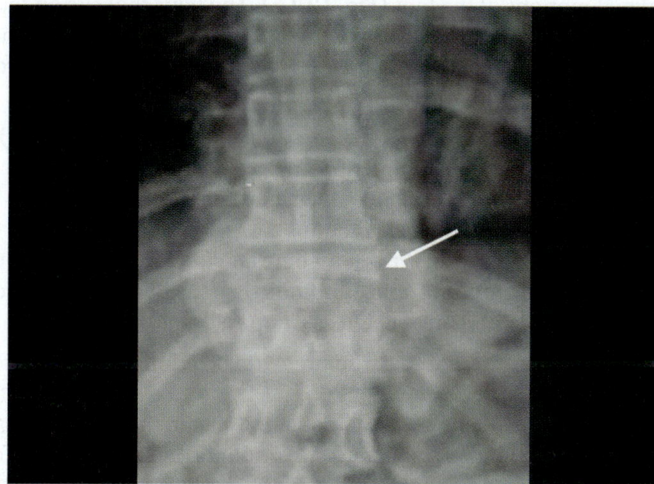

Fig. 11.48: X-ray of spine anteroposterior view showing vertebra plana, i.e. flat vertebra (arrow) at T10 level

HIGH-YIELD POINTS

- Lung involvement occurs in 20% of the patients with EG and in an older group (age, 20–40 years).
- In 50–75% of the patients, the disease is monostotic and skull involvement is seen in 50% of these patients.
- Punched out lesions in the skull may be seen in MM as well as EG. They can be differentiated by the fact that in EG, the lesions have a double contour (due to beveled edge) as there is uneven destruction of the inner and outer table of the skull.
- Important causes of vertebra plana:
    - Eosinophilic granuloma (most common cause of vertebra plana)
    - Ewing sarcoma
    - Lymphoma/leukemia
    - Gaucher's disease
    - Aneurysmal bone cyst
    - Infection—tubercular or pyogenic spondylitis.

12

CHAPTER

Pediatric Orthopedics

FOOT DEFORMITIES

CONGENITAL TALIPES EQUINOVARUS OR CLUBFOOT

Relevant Anatomy

The ankle joint is a hinge joint allowing motion in one plane, i.e. plantar flexion and dorsiflexion. This joint is formed by tibia on top and dome of talus below. Now, the talus rests on top of calcaneum and the two tarsals articulate at the subtalar (talocalcaneal joint), which accounts for the inversion (syn. varus) and eversion (syn. valgus) motions of the foot **(Fig. 12.1A)**. The talus that sits on top of calcaneus is rotated inward or medially and articulates in front with navicular while the calcaneum is rotated laterally or outward and articulates with the cuboid **(Fig. 12.1B)**.

For descriptive purposes, foot is divided into three parts (Fig. 12.1B):
1. *Forefoot*: Metatarsals and phalanges
2. *Midfoot*: Cuboid, navicular and three cuneiforms
3. *Hindfoot*: Talus and calcaneum.

While Lisfranc joint is the joint between forefoot and midfoot, joints between midfoot and hindfoot (i.e. calcaneocuboid and talonavicular joints) are labeled as Chopart or midtarsal joints.

Important ligamentous structures involved in CTEV are **(Fig 12.2A and B)**:
- *Deltoid ligament*: Medial collateral ligament of the foot attaching medial malleolus to multiple tarsals (navicular, calcaneum and talus). It consists of superficial and deep parts (*see* Chapter 6).
- *Spring ligament*: Plantar calcaneonavicular ligament, which is a thick band of fibers connecting sustentaculum tali of calcaneum to the plantar aspect of navicular. It supports the head of talus.
- *Bifurcate Y ligament*: Originates from calcaneum and then divides distally in a Y-shaped manner to give two slips, medially to navicular and laterally to cuboid.
- *Interosseous talocalcaneal ligaments*: Thick and strong ligament binding the talus and calcaneum together.
- *Plantar fascia*: Thick aponeurosis, which originates at the calcaneal tuberosity and runs toward heads of metatarsals covering the short and long plantar ligaments.

Ossification of Foot Bones

At birth talus, calcaneum and cuboid are ossified but the navicular and cuneiforms are cartilaginous. The metatarsals and phalanges are also ossified at birth. The navicular ossifies between 2 years and 5 years and the cuneiform between 6 months and 3 years.

Understanding the Condition

Congenital talipes equinovarus (CTEV) (*Latin*: tali—ankle; pes—foot; equino—horse-like) or clubfoot is basically a deformity of the foot wherein the foot is plantar flexed and turned/rotated inward such that the patient bears weight on the lateral border of the foot **(Fig. 12.3)**. The deformity is mostly idiopathic but can result due to a number of secondary causes.

This anomaly comprises of four basic deformities in the foot **(Table 12.1)**—(1) the ankle is fixed in equinus (plantar flexion), (2) the subtalar joint in varus (inversion), (3) the midfoot has cavus (a prominent medial longitudinal arch) and (4) the metatarsals are adducted toward the midline. An additional component is internal tibia torsion (inherently internal twist) in distal tibia of

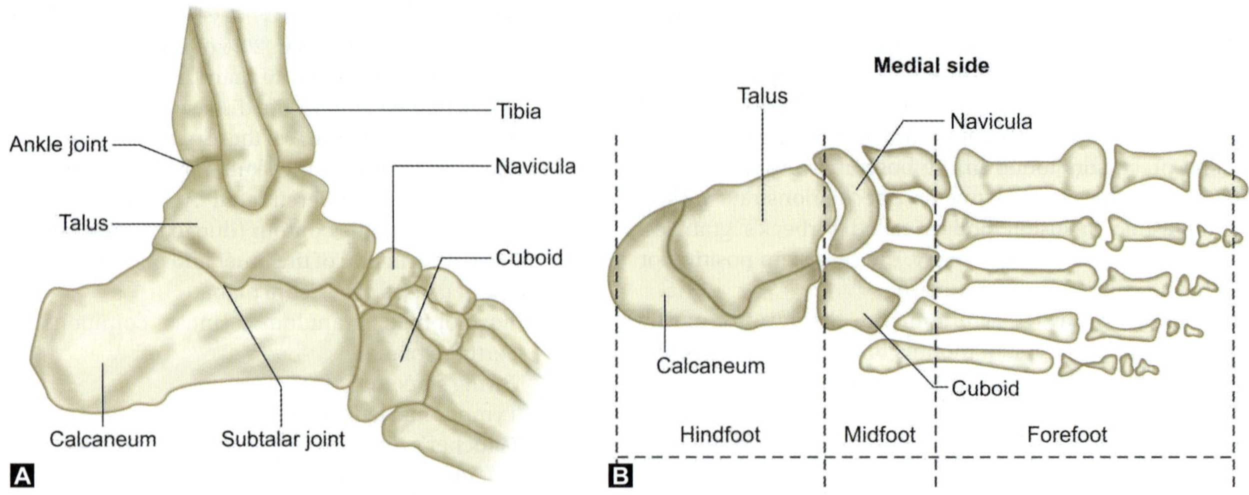

Figs 12.1A and B: Normal anatomy around foot and ankle

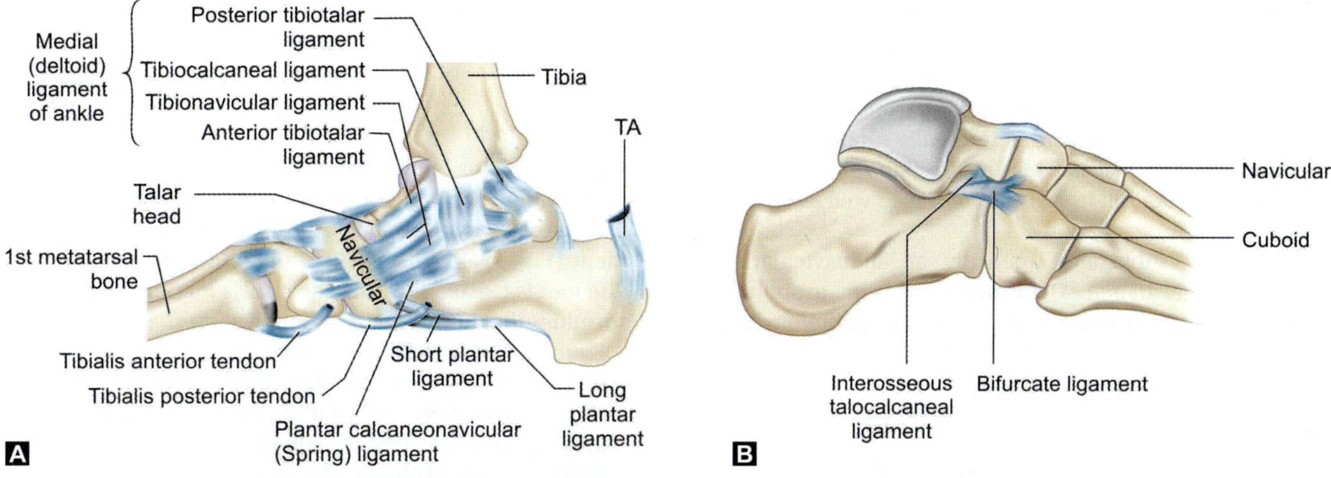

Figs 12.2A and B: Ligaments involved in CTEV. (A) Medial view and (B) Lateral view

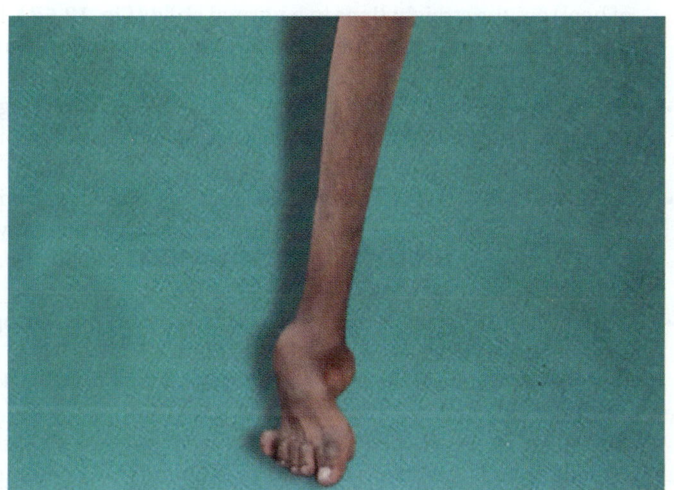

Fig. 12.3: Clinical photograph of a patient with congenital talipes equinovarus

Table 12.1: Basic deformities in the foot in congenital talipes equinovarus

Deformity	Joints affected	Zone of foot
Equinus (plantar flexion)	Ankle (tibiotalar)	Hindfoot
Varus (inversion)	Subtalar (talocalcaneal)	
Cavus	Intertarsal joints	Midfoot
Adduction	Tarsometatarsal joints	Forefoot
Internal tibia torsion	Distal tibia	Lower leg

these patients. Hence, CTEV is basically a dysplasia of the lower limb involving various joints below the level of the knee (but excluding the knee).

Incidence

- It is the most common congenital anomaly of foot affecting 1 in 1,000 live births.
- Males are affected nearly twice as often as females.
- Deformity is bilateral in nearly 50% of the cases.

- There is a high concordance rate among monozygotic twins.
- Some recent studies have implicated PITX1-TBX4 pathway (that plays critical role in lower limb development) abnormality as a key causative factor.

Pathogenesis

The primary problem in CTEV that fixes the foot in the abovementioned deformed position is the fact that all structures lying on the posteromedial side of the lower leg and foot (structures below knee level involved) are contracted. Some workers believe that these patients have genetic abnormalities and hence defective bones leading to articular malalignments that cause secondary contracture of the soft tissues while the other school of thought is that these patients may primarily have a soft tissue contracture and the bones may get secondarily deformed. Anyhow, the crux is that these patients have articular malalignments that get firmly fixed by capsular, ligamentous and musculotendinous contractures on posteromedial aspect of the foot.

Although the exact cause still remains to be elucidated, a number of theories exist that try to explain the origin of the deformity.

- *Developmental arrest theory*: Foot goes through a stage resembling clubfoot during normal development. Developmental arrest may lead to persistence of the deformity after birth.
- *Myofibroblastic theory*: Fibrotic contractile tissue present on posteromedial aspect of foot.
- *Primary germplasm defect theory*: Patients are supposed to have a genetic defect in the cartilaginous talus (bony deformity being primary cause, with soft tissue contractures occurring secondarily).
- *Multifactorial*: Most probable theory. Genetic association has been shown which accounts for familial clustering of cases. *PITX1* gene has been recently linked to CTEV.

Pathoanatomy

Following abnormalities in various structures of foot have been observed in patients who have CTEV:

- Deformities in bones of foot
- Soft tissue abnormalities.

Deformities in Bones of Foot

- Talus is the most deformed bone. Head and neck are small, plantarflexed (equinus) and medially deviated relative to body that is rather rotated outward (Herzenberg et al.).
- Calcaneum is in varus and is internally rotated. Rather the relationship between talus and calcaneum is characterized by abnormal rotation in sagittal, coronal as well as horizontal planes (McKay).
- Navicular is subluxated medially at talonavicular joint and is wedge-shaped. Deformed talus with a subluxated talonavicular joint is the most important pathology that is central to the origin of deformity in CTEV.
- Cuboid is also subluxated medially.

Soft Tissue Abnormalities

Following muscles, ligaments and capsular structures at posteromedial aspect of foot (present behind medial malleolus) are shortened and contracted:

- *Muscles/tendons*: Tibialis posterior, flexor digitorum longus (FDL), flexor hallucis longus (FHL) and tendo-Achilles (TA).
- *Capsule/ligaments*: Deltoid ligament, spring ligament, bifurcate Y ligament, interosseous ligament, posteromedial capsule of ankle, subtalar and talonavicular joints and plantar fascia.

Overall, foot size is small with absent deep creases over lateral border of foot and exaggerated deep creases over medial border of foot. Lateral border of foot is convex and long, medial border is concave and short. As these children begin to walk the weight is borne by the lateral side of the foot and callosities and bursae develop on the lateral border.

Types of Clubfoot

Based on whether the deformity was present since birth or was it acquired after birth, CTEV is divided into primary and secondary types, respectively, with syndromic type being a third but rare variant.

- *Primary (congenital clubfoot)*: Cases where clubfoot may be present since birth include:
  - Idiopathic (most common type)
  - Neurogenic—Spina bifida
  - Dysplastic—Arthrogryposis multiplex congenita (AMC)*.
- *Secondary (acquired clubfoot)*: In some diseases a muscle imbalance may result, causing contracture of the posteromedial foot structures leading to a secondary CTEV anytime during life. Secondary deformity may be seen in:
  - Paralytic (poliomyelitis)
  - Post-traumatic—contracted scar on posteromedial aspect
  - Postinfective
  - Spastic (cerebral palsy).
- *Syndromic*: Patients with following syndromes may have CTEV—AMC, Down's syndrome, Streeter's dysplasia (congenital disorder where constriction bands form around fingers), Larson syndrome, Freeman-Sheldon syndrome, Mobius syndrome, Pierre Robin syndrome, Prune belly syndrome and fetal alcohol syndrome.

Differences between primary and secondary clubfoot are given in **Table 12.2**.

Diagnosis

Clinical Assessment

Congenital talipes equinovarus is by and large a spot diagnosis, usually evident at birth. The foot is small, the calf is thin and heel is small and high lying. Deep posterior and medial creases are well evident **(Fig. 12.4A)**. The sole of the foot faces posteromedially as the foot is twisted inward. The crux is identifying the classical deformities that have been mentioned earlier.

- *Equinus*: Identified by dorsiflexing the foot. If equinus is present foot cannot be dorsiflexed beyond neutral **(Fig. 12.4A)**. Normally in a newborn, tissues are so pliable that the forefoot can be dorsiflexed to an extent to touch even the front of tibia **(Fig. 12.4B)**.
- *Varus*: Looking from behind, a line through center of calf (bisector of calf) and a line through center of heel (bisector of heel) are the straight lines in a normal child **(Fig. 12.5B)**. If there is varus present at the subtalar joint, the two bisectors will form a medially based angle **(Fig. 12.5A)**.
- *Cavus*: Exaggerated medial longitudinal arch, i.e. cavus **(Fig. 12.4A)** is easily detectable, especially in unilateral cases upon comparing to opposite side.
- *Adducted metatarsals* **(Figs 12.6A and B)**: Looking from behind normally only the great toe should be visible medially, but if forefoot is adducted, more toes are seen medially (*too many toes sign*) and none is visible laterally.
- *Internal tibial torsion*: Torsion in tibia is assessed by measuring the thigh foot angle (TFA) as shown in **Figure 12.7**.

Best views to assess these deformities are varus from back, equinus from side and forefoot adduction from front.

Once the deformities have been recognized, one can enquire if the condition is congenital (primary clubfoot) or acquired (secondary clubfoot) and then go on to look for the cause by taking appropriate history.

Table 12.2: Difference between primary and secondary clubfoot		
Feature	*Primary clubfoot*	*Secondary clubfoot*
Time of diagnosis	Presence since birth	Develops after birth
Bilaterality	More often bilateral (60%)	More often unilateral
Foot appearance and creases	Chubby short foot, posterior and medial creases present	Atrophic skin with absent creases
Heel size	Small	Relatively normal
Foot size	Clearly smaller when compared to a normal foot	Normal or somewhat small
Neurological examination	Normal	Motor/sensory loss present
Prognosis	Good	Poor

---

*Arthrogryposis multiplex congenita is a genetic disease where a group of muscles are replaced by fibrous tissue. The patients are identified by absent joint creases and presence of deformities involving multiple joints.

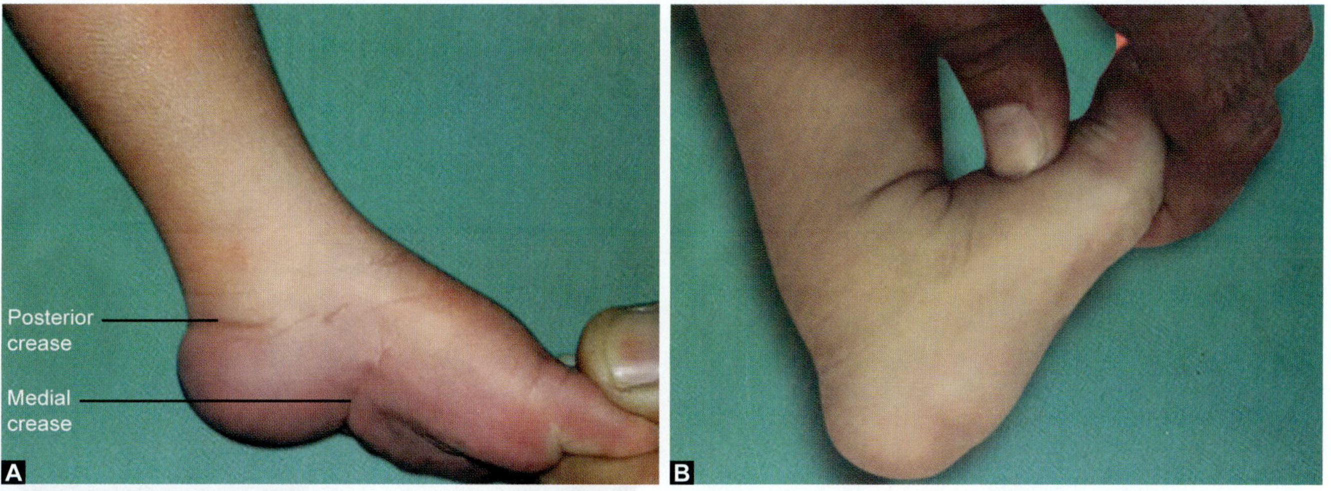

Figs 12.4A and B: (A) Equinus at ankle joint. Note presence of prominent posterior and medial creases; (B) Normal dorsiflexion at ankle joint

Courtesy: Dr Gaurav Gupta (JN Medical College, AMU).

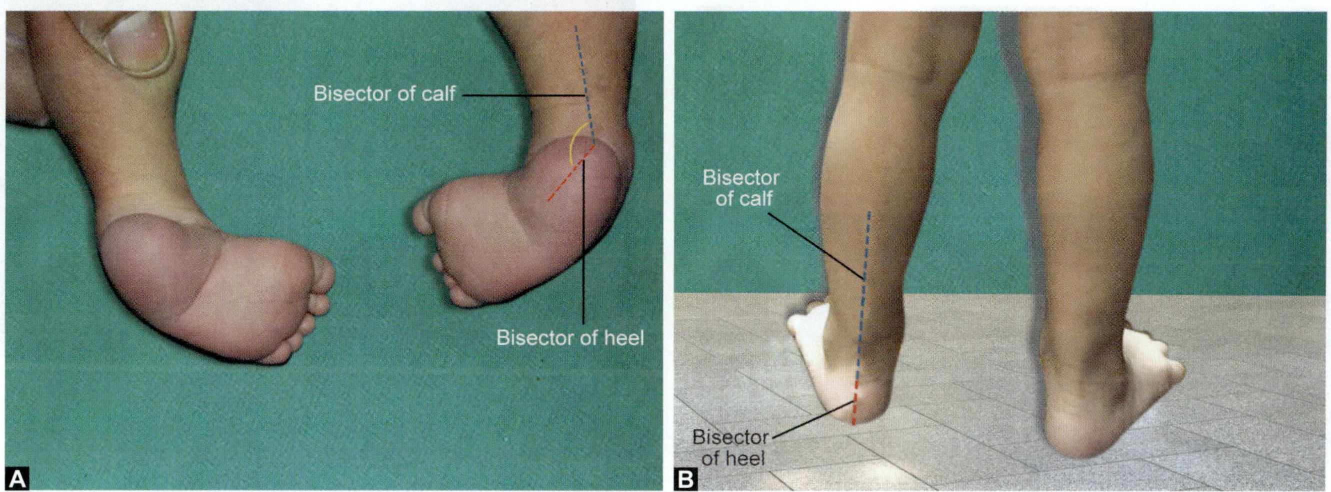

Figs 12.5A and B: (A) Varus at subtalar joint. Note bisector of calf and bisector of heel are forming a medial angle; (B) Foot of a normal child. Note bisector of calf bisecting the center of heel

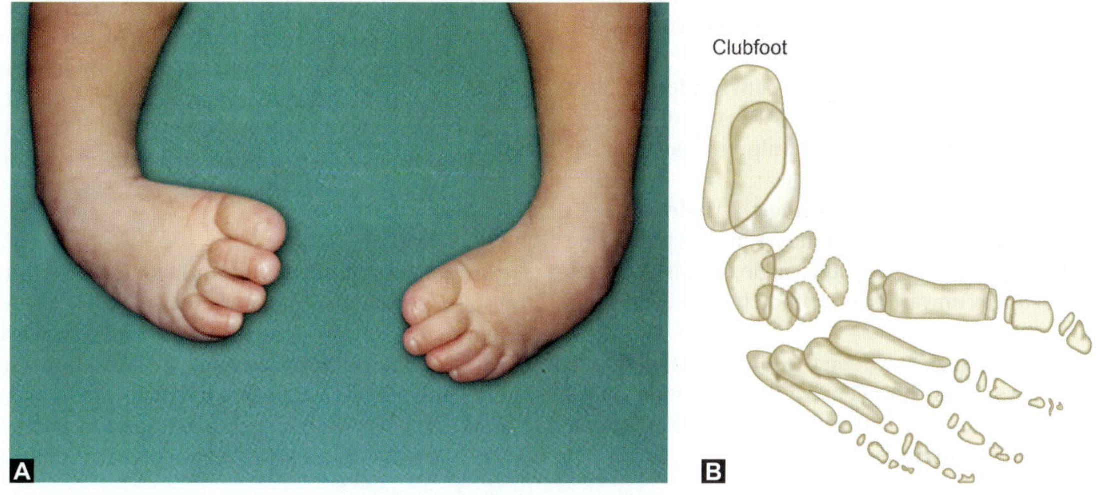

Figs 12.6A and B: Adduction of metatarsals

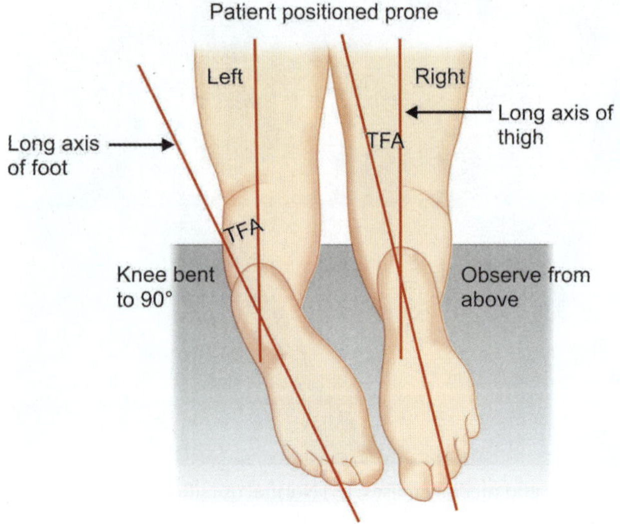

Fig. 12.7: Measurement of thigh foot angle (TFA) to detect torsion in tibia

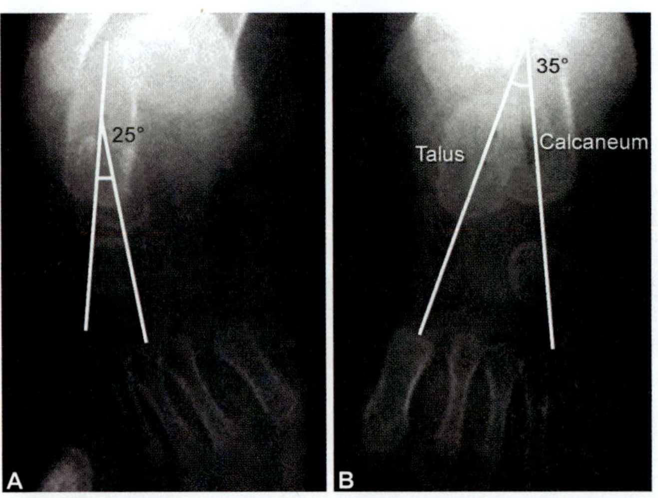

Figs 12.8A and B: Talocalcaneal (Kite's) angle in congenital talipes equinovarus and a normal patient

*Radiographic Assessment**

Routinely, radiographs are not necessary but they may be useful to confirm the diagnosis especially in relapsed or recurrent cases. Some important parameters evaluated include:

- *Talocalcaneal angle (Kite's angle)*: Angle between long axis of talus and calcaneum in anteroposterior (AP) view of the foot. Normal value is 35–55° **(Fig. 12.8B)**. A value of less than 25° **(Fig. 12.8A)** is confirmatory for clubfoot.
- *Talus first metatarsal angle (Meary's angle)*: Angle between the long axis of talus and first metatarsal in weight-bearing lateral view **(Fig. 12.9A)**. Normally, this angle is 0°. It becomes greater than 5° (convex upward) in clubfoot. It measures cavus deformity.
- *Tibiocalcaneal angle*: Angle between the long axis of tibia and calcaneum in stress lateral view **(Fig. 12.9B)**. Normal value is 10–40° in stress lateral view. The angle increases in clubfoot (>90°). It is basically a measure of heel equinus.

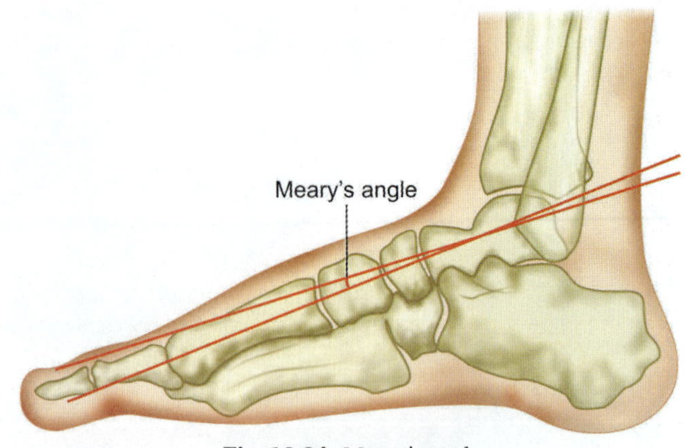

Fig. 12.9A: Meary's angle

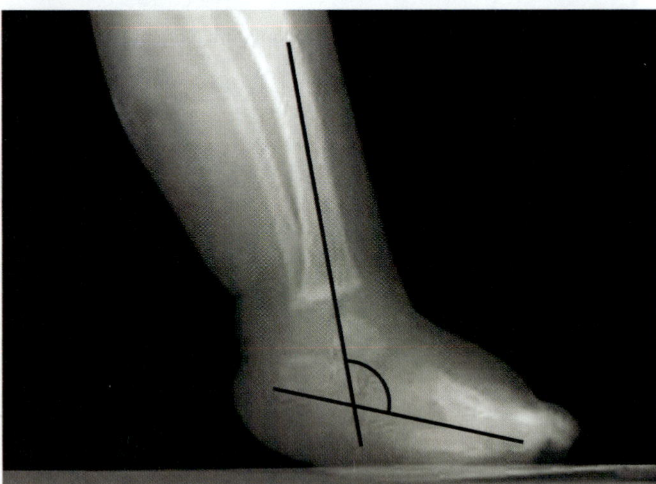

Fig. 12.9B: Tibiocalcaneal angle

Classifications (Scoring Systems)

Following scoring systems are commonly employed for grading the severity of deformity in a patient with clubfoot:

- *Dimeglio classification*: It is based on the degree of reducibility of various deformities (equinus, varus, forefoot adduction, derotation of calcaneopedal block, etc.).
- *Modified Pirani classification (more commonly used)*: Three variables for midfoot (curvature of lateral border, severity of medial crease and palpation of talar head to assess its uncovering) and three variables for hindfoot (emptiness of heel, severity of posterior crease and rigidity of equinus) are assessed. Each has score of 0, 0.5 or 1 depending on severity. Maximum score is 6 (worse).

Management

Treatment should be started immediately after birth. Early in life the soft tissues of the infant are very pliable and the deformity can be corrected by conservative means only. However, as the child grows, the deformity becomes more and more fixed and surgical management becomes necessary and more so if a particular age is crossed then even the results with surgery are not very encouraging. So, the dictum is to start the treatment just as the lanugo is shed off.

---

*While assessing X-rays, kindly note that calcaneal and talar ossification centers are present at birth but cuboid appears by 6 months and navicular will not appear until 2–4 years.

Treatment of CTEV is dictated by the age of the patient, with slight overlapping, depending on flexibility of deformity and surgeon's perception.

Age Less Than 1–2 Years

Serial manipulation and casting is the treatment of choice in this age group. It consists of manipulating the foot of the child and applying a corrective plaster every week when the child comes to attend the OPD clinic. After a few plasters the deformity is corrected in most cases, and then the correction is maintained by specific orthosis. Three philosophies of conservative gradual correction of deformity are there:

1. *Ponseti method* **(Figs 12.10A to C)** (method of choice now with a success rate of more than 95%)*: This procedure consists of manipulating the foot for 1–3 minutes into corrected position, followed by holding the correction in an above knee cast (applied with knees flexed to 90°). After 7 days, cast is removed, foot remanipulated and recast for another week in successively more corrected position. Usually five to seven casts are sufficient and deformity gets corrected. The order of correction is very important. It can be remembered by the pneumonic "CAVE". Cavus is corrected in the first cast by supinating the forefoot and dorsiflexing the first metatarsal. Forefoot must never be pronated as it will increase the cavus deformity. Adduction and varus are then corrected simultaneously in the subsequent casts by abducting the forefoot in supination with counter pressure being applied at talar head. Lastly, equinus is corrected, by dorsiflexing the fully abducted foot. The last cast is applied with foot finally in 15° dorsiflexion and 70° abduction for 3 weeks. In case dorsiflexion is difficult beyond neutral then a percutaneous tenotomy of TA is done to achieve adequate dorsiflexion.

   Caution: It is important to follow the above mentioned order. When an attempt is made to correct equinus before adduction and varus are fully corrected, the equinus gets corrected at the midfoot area (midfoot breaks) rather than at the ankle and the plantar surface of the foot becomes convex. This is referred to as Rocker bottom foot.

2. *Kite's method*: Oldest devised method, but not used nowadays. Sequence of correction was forefoot adduction, followed by heel varus, and lastly equinus. Cavus was not addressed. Kite followed a strict sequence of correction, proceeding to the next deformity only when first one is fully corrected. This is biomechanically incorrect as all joints in foot are kinematically interlinked (kinematic coupling, i.e. movement at one joint will automatically result in movement in surrounding joints also). This method is lengthy (may take up to 2 years for correction) and success rate is also around 70–75% only. The biggest mistake made by Kite (Kite's error) was that he abducted the foot by using cuboid as the fulcrum rather than talar head as in Ponseti method, which is biomechanically more sound.

3. *French physiotherapy method (functional method of Bensahel)*: This method is used mainly in Europe and involves daily corrective passive manipulations performed by an experienced physical therapist with correction being held

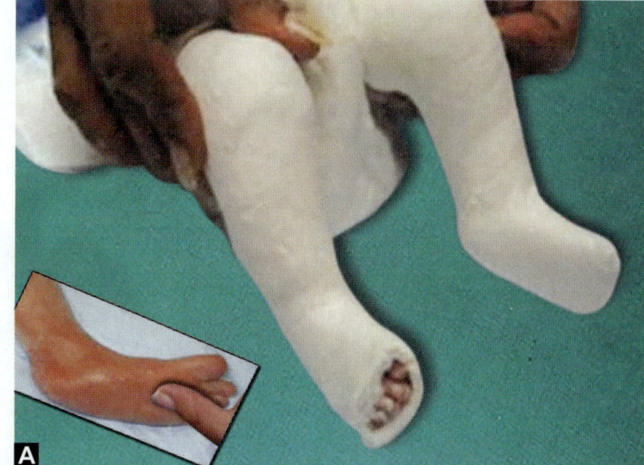
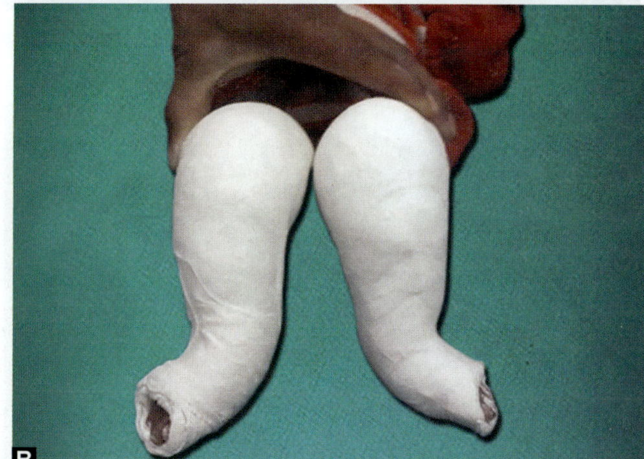
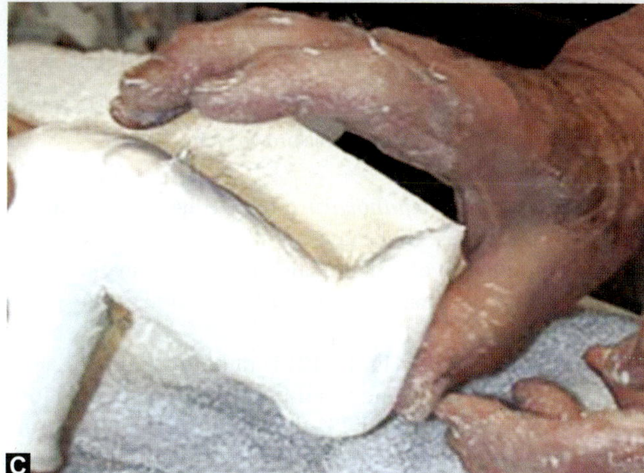

Figs 12.10A to C: Ponseti technique. (A) Cavus correction; (B) Varus and abduction corrected; and (C) Equinus correction

by special stretchable tapes in corrected foot positions and splinting (not casting) until next session.

Once the desired correction has been achieved, the same has to be maintained over next few years (2–4 years) by applying a foot abduction orthosis. Options available include Dennis brown splint or CTEV shoes.

---

*Off late there have been a number of reports of application of Ponseti casting in older children (up to 15–16 years of age) with success. However, a consensus on upper age limit still remains undefined and is limited to surgeon's choice.

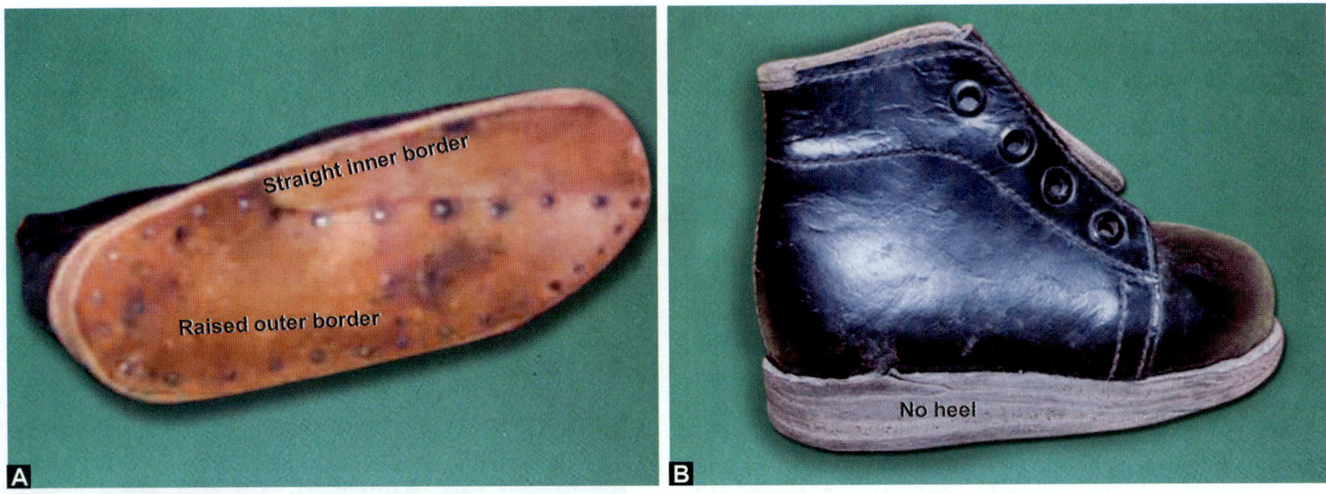

Figs 12.11A and B: Congenital talipes equinovarus shoes

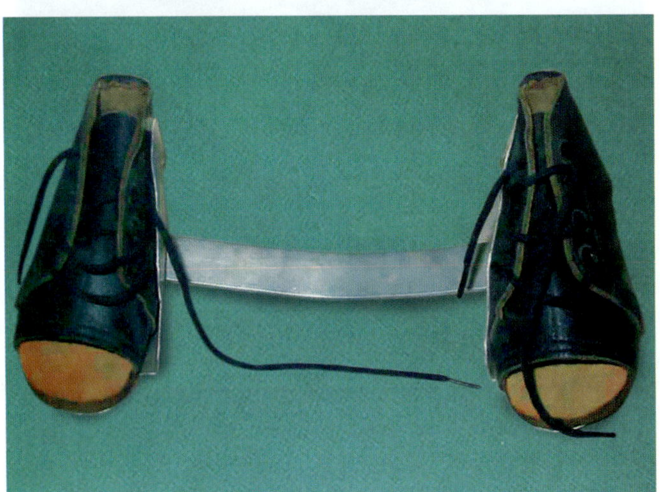

Fig. 12.12: Dennis brown splint

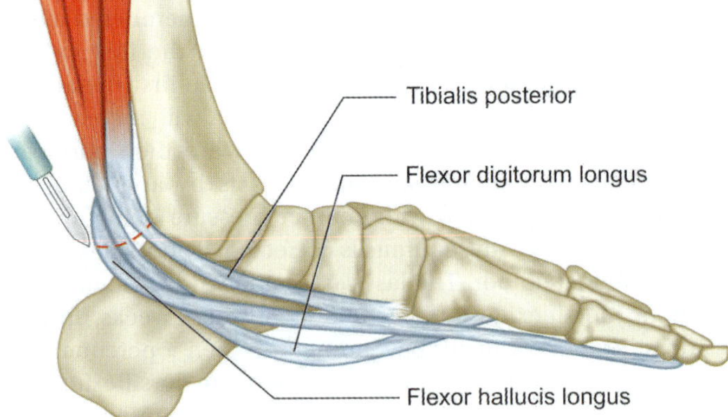

Fig. 12.13: Posteromedial soft tissue release

- *Congenital talipes equinovarus shoes* **(Figs 12.11A and B)** are special shoes that have a straight inner border (to prevent adduction of metatarsals), no heel (to avoid equinus recurrence) and raised outer border (to make foot go into eversion).
- *Dennis brown splint* **(Fig. 12.12)** is rather dynamic in action. It has a pair of shoes mounted on a steel bar in position of 70° external rotation and 15° dorsiflexion. The shoes rotate outward whenever the child kicks thereby causing more and more abduction. Mostly, a Dennis brown splint is preferred but as the child approaches the walking age, CTEV shoes are opted for. The orthosis has to be applied for 23 hours a day (i.e. full time) for 3 months and during sleep till 2–4 years of age.

Age Above 1 Year but Less Than 3–5 Years

Once the child has crossed the age of 1–2 years, the soft tissues are no longer that pliable that they can be stretched by plaster alone. Surgery is often required in these children to correct the deformity and this involves releasing the tight structures present on the posteromedial side of the foot, i.e. behind the medial malleolus, a surgery called as posteromedial soft tissue release (PMSTR). This surgery is rather best centered by most surgeons to the age group 9–12 months. Not only is the foot easier to operate upon at this age, by the time the child becomes ambulatory (usually by 1 year age), foot correction is achieved.

Posteromedial soft tissue release: Two commonly done procedures for PMSTR are Turco's release via medial hockey stick or J-shaped incision and a modified McKay extended release by a transverse incision. The structures cut in PMSTR **(Fig. 12.13)** include—tibialis posterior, FHL, FDL and TA (lengthened by "Z" plasty).

Age Above 3–5 Years but Less Than 10 Years

By the age of 5 years, isolated soft tissue release becomes ineffective and a bony osteotomy (classically Dillwyn-Evans procedure) is often required in addition to PMSTR to achieve desired correction. The principle behind bony osteotomies is to shorten the lateral column as these patients have a long lateral border and a short medial foot border. Common bony procedures performed include:

- *Dillwyn-Evans procedure (Fig. 12.14A):* It is bony procedure of choice between 4 years and 8 years of age and involves resection and fusion of calcaneocuboid joint on the lateral aspect of the foot. The growth on lateral side stops, medial side continues to grow and foot gradually corrects over time.

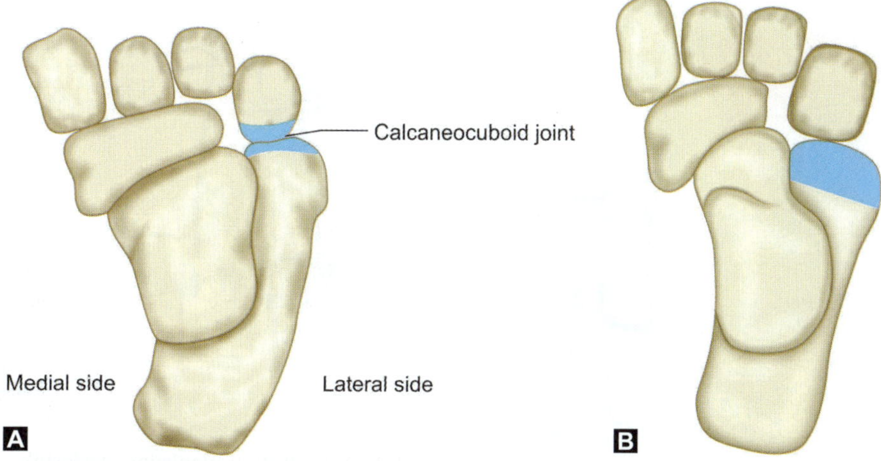

Figs 12.14A and B: (A) Dillwyn-Evans calcaneocuboid fusion; (B) Lichtblau procedure

It should never be performed in children less than 4 years of age as large amounts of cartilage between two joints make fusion difficult.

- *Lichtblau procedure (Fig. 12.14B)*: It involves lateral closing wedge osteotomy of anterior end of calcaneum. An advantage of this procedure is that it avoids hindfoot stiffness, which may occur after Dillwyn-Evans procedure. And also, the procedure can be performed in relatively younger children (3 years old) if situation or deformity demands.
- *Cuboid decancellation*: Another way of shortening the lateral column but preserving joint integrity is by decancellating cuboid on lateral aspect of foot.

Age More Than 10 Years

A neglected clubfoot by the age of 10 years becomes so rigid that it can only be salvaged by *triple arthrodesis* **(Fig. 12.15)**. The procedure involves fusion of talonavicular, talocalcaneal and calcaneocuboid joints after taking out adequate wedges to correct the deformity. It results in a stiff but cosmetically better foot. It is performed only after skeletal maturity as inadequate fusion occurs if it is performed before skeletal maturity and also growth of foot will be affected. The most common complication of this procedure is pseudoarthrosis of the talonavicular joint.

Recurrence (Box 12.1)

Failures and relapses are integral to every form of treatment and mostly occur in CTEV patients due to poor compliance with brace wear regime. Early failures can be managed with repeat manipulations and casting, while late failures (>2 years old) mostly present with fixed deformities that need operative interventions.

The most common residual deformity in clubfoot patients during early course of treatment is equinus. The deformity is generally flexible and requires TA lengthening, mostly performed adequately by a percutaneous TA tenotomy or by "Z" plasty **(Fig. 12.16A)**. If presentation is late, equinus may be fixed (not correctable passively) and then it may require a corrective Lambrinudi's arthrodesis **(Fig. 12.16B)**. Patients who present with an isolated fixed heel varus can be addressed with Dwyer's osteotomy **(Fig. 12.16C)** of calcaneum. It is calcaneal osteotomy

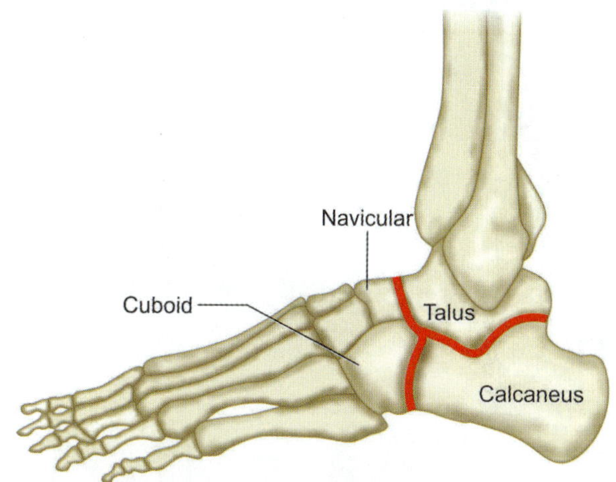

Fig. 12.15: Triple arthrodesis (Joints to be fused marked in red)

> **Box 12.1:** Important clubfoot terminologies in context of recurrence or treatment failure
>
> - *Neglected clubfoot:* Deformity that has not been treated by 2 years of age
> - *Relapsed/recurrent clubfoot:* Deformity corrected initially, but one or more components recurred
> - *Resistant clubfoot:* Not corrected or partially corrected despite correctly using the Ponseti technique

(medial opening wedge osteotomy) for correcting heel varus. An important residual deformity that needs special mention is a dynamic supination adduction that remains in some children treated with Ponseti casting. The foot twists into a supinated-adducted posture as the child swings the leg to march ahead. An overpull by tibialis anterior with a weak peroneus longus (dynamic muscle imbalance) is cited as causative factor. If the deformity interferes with gait, then it should be treated with transfer of tibialis anterior to lateral cuneiform, provided lateral cuneiform is ossified (2–3 years of age) and the child is old enough to undergo rehabilitation process for tendon transfers.

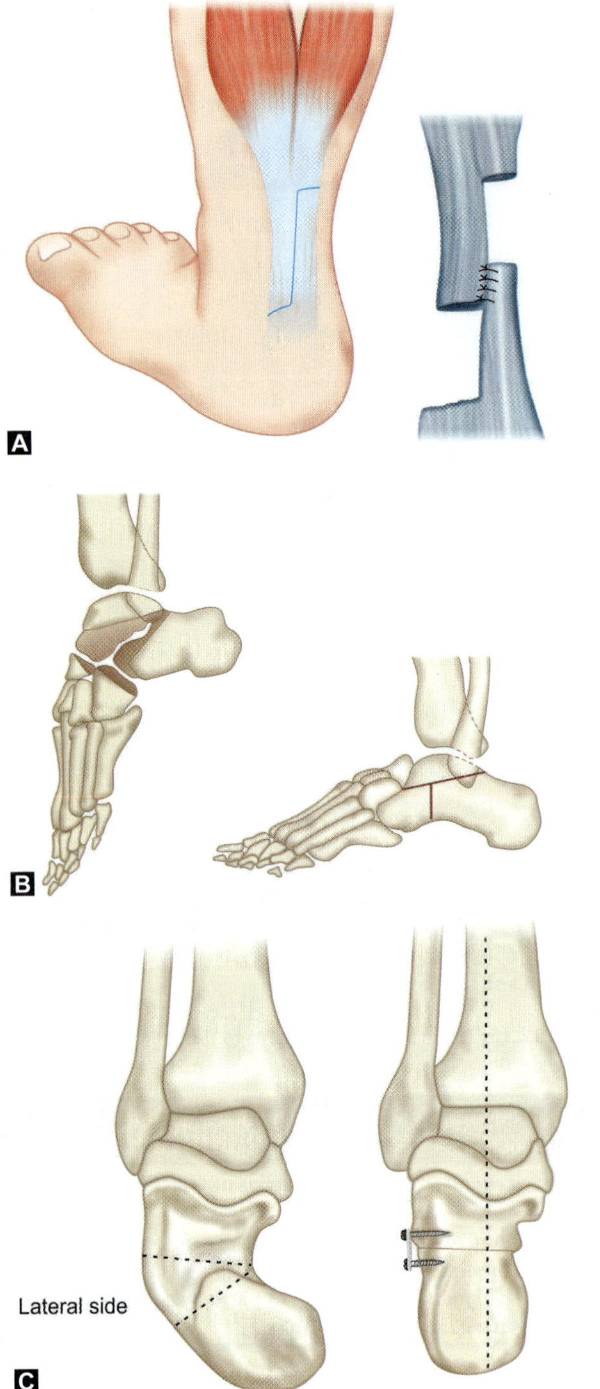

Figs 12.16A to C: (A) Tendo-Achilles lengthening by "Z" plasty; (B) Lambrinudi's arthrodesis; (C) Dwyer's osteotomy of calcaneum

Atypical or Complex Clubfoot

This term refers to a very rigid clubfoot. These feet are short and chubby with underdeveloped calf muscles and are characterized by severe cavus and marked equinus (due to hyperflexed metatarsals) that tend to produce a single deep transverse crease in the middle of the sole. Often these are not identified in the beginning of the treatment but recognized when the Ponseti casting commences. Although the medial soft tissues stretch

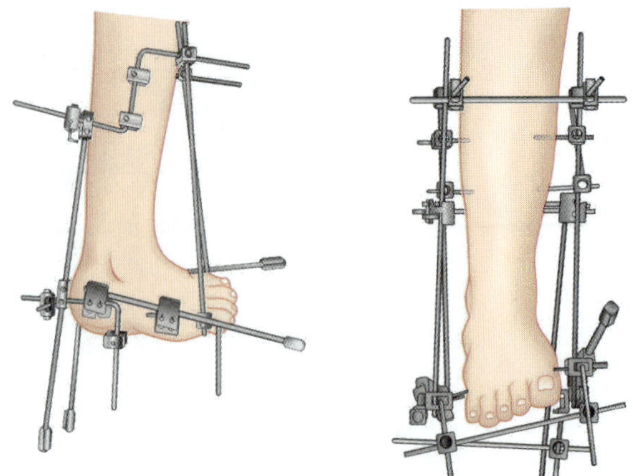

Fig. 12.17: Schematic depiction of a Joshi's external stabilization system (JESS) fixator applied on a congenital talipes equinovarus patient

up, cavus and equinus show great resistance. In such patients the Ponseti technique needs to be modified a little bit. The aim should be to achieve 20–40° of abduction (rather than routine 70° as it may lead to exaggerated flexion of metatarsals) while a dorsiflexion of 5° usually suffices as the latter spontaneously improves after a few months.

HIGH-YIELD POINTS

- Supination and pronation are complex movements. While supination at foot is a combination of varus of hindfoot, plantar flexion at ankle and adduction of forefoot; foot pronation involves a combination of valgus of hindfoot, dorsiflexion at ankle and abduction of forefoot.
- Congenital talipes equinovarus is associated with hypoplasia or absence of anterior tibial artery (dorsalis pedis) in many children.
- *Kite's index*: This refers to sum of talocalcaneal angles in AP and lateral views of foot. Normally, it is more than 40°. A decreased value indicates diagnosis of CTEV.
- *Fulcrum of correction:*
  - Kite's method—calcaneocuboid joint.
  - Ponseti method—talar head.
- The term "Rocker bottom foot" refers to convex plantar surface of the foot. Although it can result if the correct order of correction is not followed during Ponseti casting, it is also seen in congenital vertical talus (CVT) (*see* Page 349).
- *Serpentine foot/skew foot/Z foot*: A complex deformity of foot where the forefoot is adducted, navicula is subluxated dorsolaterally over the talar head and the heel (hindfoot) is in valgus.
- *Master knot of Henry*: It is a tough fibrous tissue encasing the crossings of FDL and FHL at plantar aspect of foot. It must be released during PMSTR.
- Joint not fused in triple arthrodesis—ankle (tibiotalar).
- *Joshi's external stabilization system (JESS):* Indigenous external fixation system (**Fig. 12.17**) developed by Dr BB Joshi (Mumbai) based on the principle of "fractional distraction", where the shortened posteromedial side of the foot is distracted by an external fixator to correct CTEV. The system offers a relatively less invasive correction than conventional surgical procedures for any CTEV patient, irrespective of

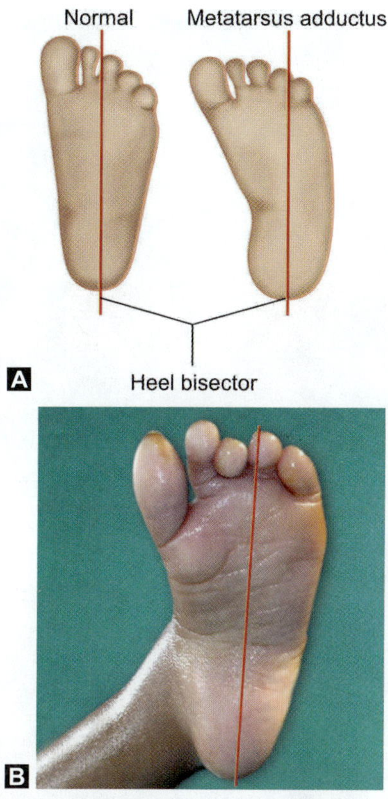

Figs 12.18A and B: Metatarsus adductus

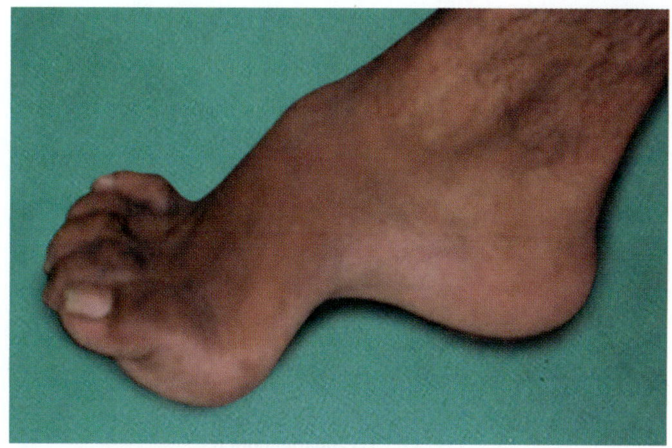

Fig. 12.19: Pes cavus

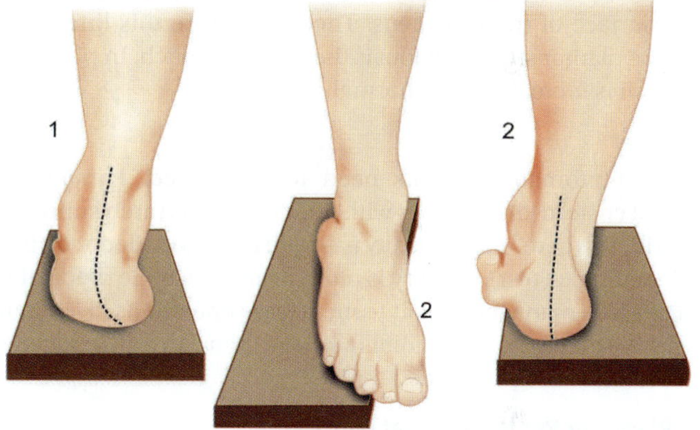

Fig. 12.20: Coleman block test—when the patient stands on the edge of a block, the hindfoot recorrects itself, if it is supple

age group. And moreover, it can be used for correction of relapsed, resistant or even a neglected clubfoot.

METATARSUS ADDUCTUS

This is a congenital foot deformity that resembles a mild form of clubfoot. These infants have isolated adduction of metatarsals such that the forefoot is curved inside **(Figs 12.18A and B)**. The anomaly has strong association with developmental dysplasia of hip (DDH) (*see* Page 363). The majority of cases improve spontaneously with growth. Mild residual deformities can be managed with serial corrective plasters plus shoe modifications while small percentage of children with severe deformities may need multiple metatarsal dome osteotomies (Berman and Gartland procedure).

PES CAVUS AND PES PLANUS

Relevant Anatomy

Since the foot has to act as a pliable platform to support body weight, it is an arched structure. There are two longitudinal (medial and lateral) and two transverse (anterior and posterior) arches. Both the longitudinal arches have distal ends formed by the corresponding metatarsal heads and the proximal limit formed by the base of calcaneum. However, out of the two, the medial longitudinal arch is higher, more pliable and a better shock absorber.

Pes Cavus (High-arched Foot)

In "Pes cavus", the medial longitudinal arch of the foot is exaggerated, and often there is also clawing of the toes **(Fig. 12.19)**. The heel is mostly inverted (in varus) and the soft tissues of the sole are tight.

Causes

All forms of this deformity generally result from some kind of muscle imbalance and hence it is seen mostly in association with neuromuscular disorders like poliomyelitis (most common cause), hereditary motor or sensory neuropathy (HMSN), cerebral palsy, diastematomyelia, tethered cord syndrome, muscular dystrophies, etc. Occasionally the deformity occurs secondary to trauma (e.g. burns contracture or compartment syndrome leading to Volkman's contracture of sole).

Clinical Presentation

Patients are generally older children or young adolescents that present with a calcaneo-cavo-varus deformity of foot. Due to associated clawing of the toes, the metatarsal heads are forced into the sole and callosities form over pressure areas that may be painful. An important aspect of examination is to check if the deformity is reversible. For this the Coleman block test is performed **(Fig. 12.20)**. A thorough neurological examination must also be done to elucidate the cause.

Diagnosis

On a lateral foot radiograph, the Meary's angle and the calcaneal pitch are useful to deduce the diagnosis.

Meary's angle is drawn **(Fig. 12.9A)** and an angle that is greater than 4° convex downward is considered "pes planus" while an angle greater than 4° convex upward is considered as "pes cavus".

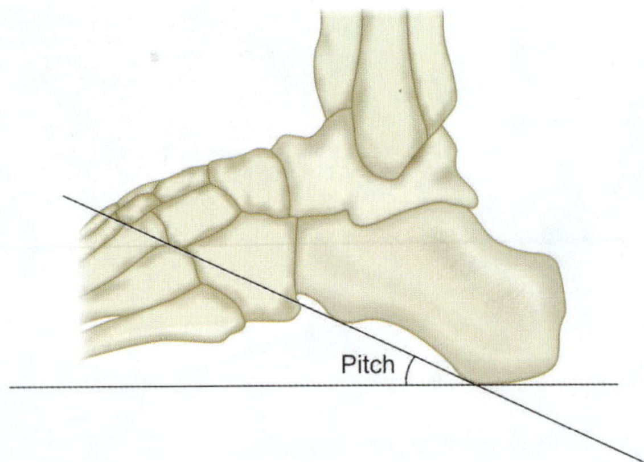

Fig. 12.21: Calcaneal pitch

Calcaneal pitch **(Fig. 12.21)**: A line is drawn from the plantar-most surface of the calcaneus. The angle made this line makes with the plantar surface of foot is the calcaneal pitch. In pes cavus, the pitch is increased than normal.

Treatment

Only symptomatic patients need to be treated. Patients are advised custom-made shoes with molded inserts (arch supports). In patients where the deformity is severe and fixed (deduced from Coleman block test), surgery is often needed. Mobile deformities can often be managed by soft tissue release operations like plantar fascia release while in case joints are fixed then corrective calcaneal osteotomies are the options.

Pes Planus or Pes Valgus (Flat Foot)

Flat foot refers to flattening of the medial longitudinal arch of the foot. In these patients the medial border of the foot touches the ground, and often the heel is in valgus (planovalgus, **Fig. 12.22A**). In these patients, an ink impression of the foot if taken will show an increased contact of the medial foot border **(Fig. 12.22B)**. On lateral foot X-ray one can confirm the diagnosis by finding a decreased Meary's angle **(Fig. 12.9A)**.

The deformity is classified into following types for a better understanding:

Compensatory Flat Foot

A compensatory flat foot deformity may be acquired at times in life to compensate for any condition that affects the posture like a genu valgum deformity of knee, spasm of peroneal muscles, malunited fracture of calcaneum, arthritis in foot joints as in rheumatoid arthritis, diseases causing flaccid paralysis and loss of foot muscle tone and sometimes even in cases with morbid obesity. Treating the causative condition treats the deformity.

Flexible (Correctable) Flat Foot

In flexible type, the deformity appears when the patient is bearing weight on the foot but once the foot is in the air, the arch reappears. Or one may be able to recreate the arch in such patients by dorsiflexing the great toe (Jack's test). This maneuver stretches the plantar fascia that makes the medial arch prominent even in normal people (Wind-lass mechanism). Most of the cases are idiopathic, however, it may appear in patients with ligament laxity and in those who have a hypermobile foot. At times the deformity is just physiological in toddlers as the intrinsic muscle

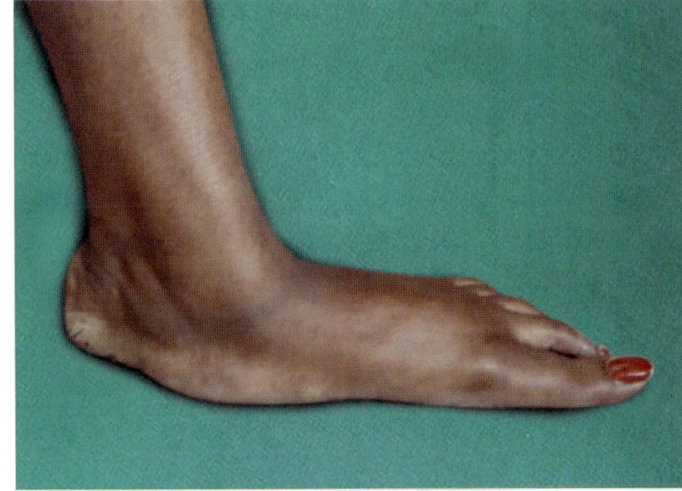

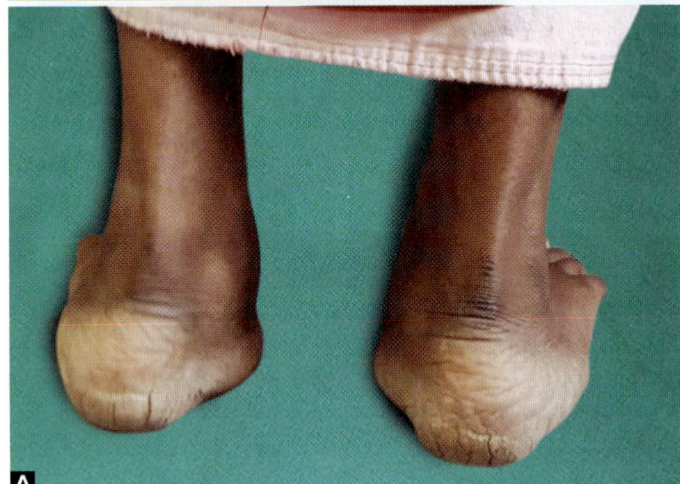

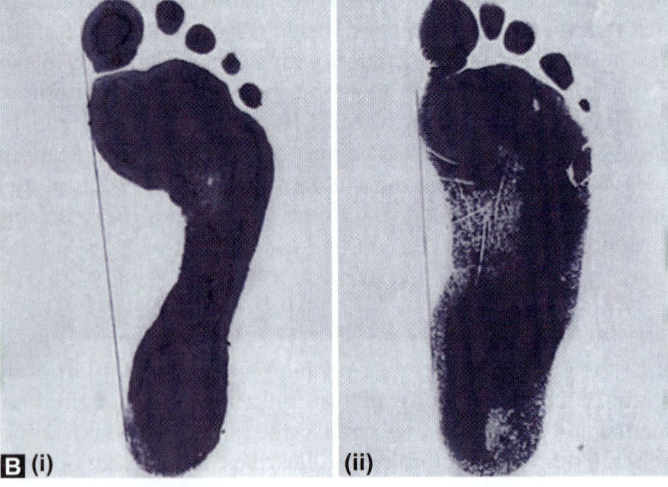

Figs 12.22A and B: (A) Flat foot (side view and view from dorsum); (B) Ink impression in a (i) normal, and (ii) a flat-foot patient. Note the medial "hollow" in normal foot due to presence of medial longitudinal arch

tone in foot takes some time to develop and the arches thus take some time to fully appear.

Treatment in most such cases is conservative. Patients are prescribed flat foot exercises (e.g. rolling the foot over a ball or clenching a towel with toes) and may be given special shoes with

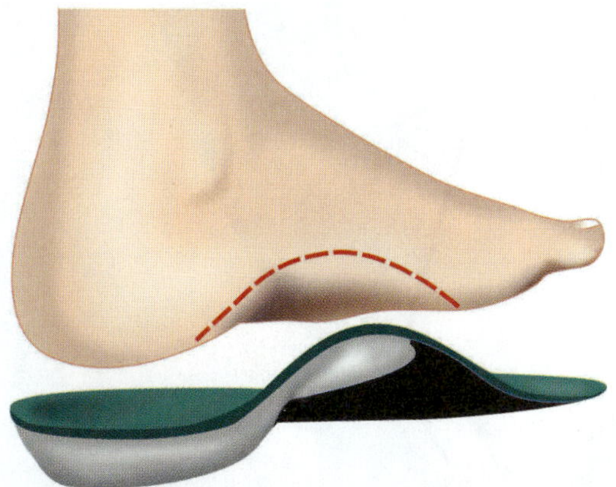

Fig. 12.23: Arch support insole for flat feet

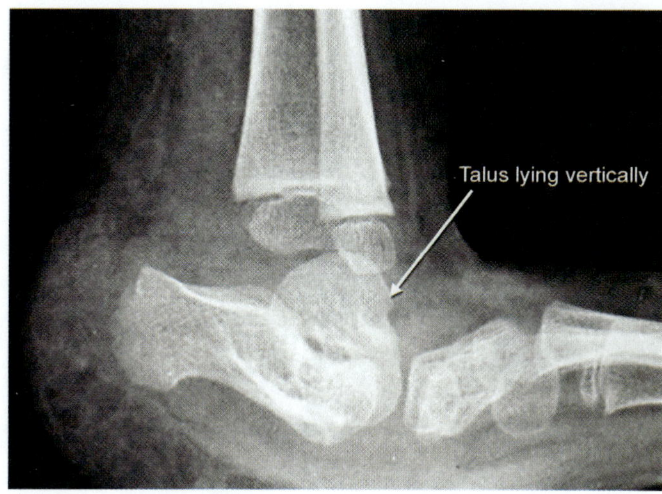

Fig. 12.24: Congenital vertical talus
Courtesy: Dr Heren Patel (BJ Medical College, Ahmedabad).

elongated and crooked heels (Thomas heel) or arch supports **(Fig. 12.23)** to tone up the arches. Although these patients are compatible for almost all normal life activities, however, they face eligibility problems at times when they apply for jobs requiring high level of fitness, so reassurance is important.

Rigid Flat Foot

This is the noncorrectable fixed variety of flat foot, the cause of which varies as per the age of presentation. When small children or infants are brought with this deformity, a condition called as "congenital vertical talus" (*discussed later*) must be considered while in the adolescents and adults the cause is generally a segmentation defect of tarsal bones, a condition called as "tarsal coalition" (*discussed later*) or presence of an "accessory navicular bone" (*discussed later*). Not uncommon cause in middle aged women is a condition called "tibialis posterior tendon dysfunction". The etiology is unknown but the tendon attrition occurs mostly in diabetic people or in those who have been injected steroids into the tendon. Since "tibialis posterior" is an inverter and plantar flexor important for maintaining medial longitudinal arch of foot, its dysfunction often ends in flat foot.

Congenital vertical talus: This is a rare congenital condition seen in infants where the medial longitudinal arch is not just flat but the undersurface of the foot is convex downward giving the appearance of rocker bottom chair (hence called rocker bottom foot). The deformity is called "congenital vertical talus" as the talus in these patients lies malpositioned vertically as opposed to normal horizontal position **(Fig. 12.24)**. X-ray clearly shows the malpositioned talus with the navicular dislocated dorsally over the talar head.

Treatment is very difficult as by the time the child is seen the dorsolateral structures are severely contracted. Hence, surgery must be done early usually before the age of 2 years. Surgery involves open reduction and realignment of talonavicular and subtalar joints (Ramsay procedure). In later stages (generally later than 4 years) the subtalar joint has to be fused (Grice Green subtalar arthrodesis).

Tarsal coalition (peroneal spastic flat foot): This is an autosomal dominant (AD) condition characterized by segmentation defect of tarsal bones. The problem although is present since birth usually becomes symptomatic during early adolescence. The patient generally presents with a painful rigid flat foot often accompanied

by the spasm of peroneal muscles. On X-ray one finds coalition (a connecting bar of bone) between talus and calcaneum (most common) and/or between calcaneum and navicular. Tarsal coalition between calcaneum and navicular typically resembles appearance of nose of the anteater (anteater nose sign, **Fig. 12.25**). Treatment is initially conservative but nonresponders usually need excision of the connecting bar.

Accessory navicular (prehallux): Some patients (with flexible flat foot mostly) have an accessory ossicle lying just medial and little proximal to the navicular bone on their X-ray **(Fig. 12.26)**. It is usually asymptomatic. This accessory navicular may be a cause of flat foot in some although the real significance is still debatable. In symptomatic cases tenderness can be elicited directly over it. Conservative treatment is usually successful. In nonresponding cases excision of accessory navicular is performed (Kinder's procedure).

HALLUX VALGUS

It refers to lateral deviation of the hallux (great toe) in relation to the first metatarsal **(Figs 12.27A and B)**. It is the most common toe deformity with females affected more often than men.

Etiology

Exact cause is unknown but contributing factors include pronated flat foot, hypermobility of foot, long first ray, etc. Other disorders which may cause hallux valgus include gout, rheumatoid arthritis, Ehler-Danlos syndrome, Marfan syndrome, Charcot-Marie-Tooth disease, etc. People who wear tight shoes may be more prone.

Pathoanatomy

On the medial side of the great toe's metatarsophalangeal (MTP) joint, there is medial joint capsule and abductor hallucis muscle while on the lateral aspect lies the lateral joint capsule and the adductor hallucis muscle. As the toe deviates toward lateral aspect, the lateral structures, viz. adductor hallucis and lateral joint capsule get contracted while the medial structures are

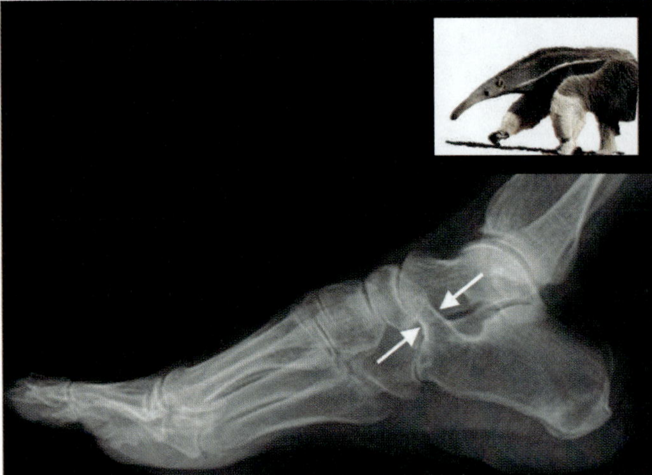

Fig. 12.25: X-ray of tarsal coalition between calcaneum and navicular showing anteater nose sign

Courtesy: Abcradiology.blogspot.com.

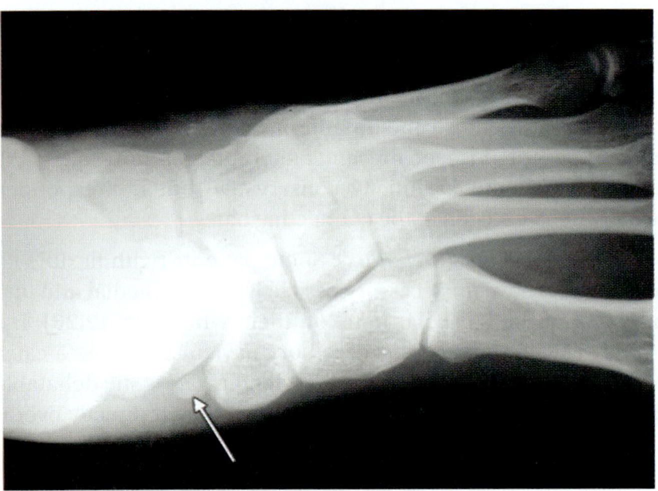

Fig. 12.26: Accessory navicular

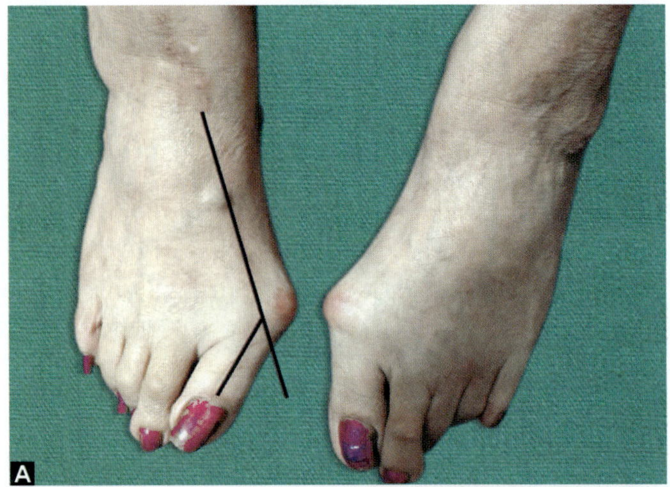

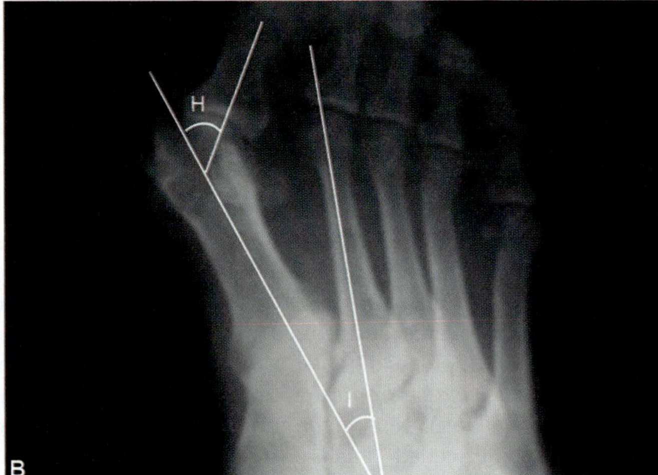

Figs 12.27A and B: (A) Bilateral hallux valgus; (B) X-ray of patient with hallux valgus depicting hallux valgus angle (H) and intermetatarsal angle (I)

long axis of first and second metatarsals) is also increased (normal is 9°).

Treatment

In initial stages joint degeneration is minimal and deformity is flexible (i.e. toe can be pulled into normal position). In such cases, treatment is nonoperative and includes prescription of shoe modifications (wide-toe box), orthotics **(Fig. 12.28)** or inserts like toe wedges or spacers that are to be worn for a long time (2–3 years). If conservative treatment fails or if deformity is fixed (i.e. toe cannot be pulled passively into correct position), then operative treatment is opted. In low-demand geriatric people, the joint would have degenerative changes. Such cases may benefit by an arthrodesis or excision arthroplasty (Keller's operation, **Fig. 12.29A**). However, in active patients and patients with minimal degenerative changes in the joint, surgery is directed to correct the hallux valgus and intermetatarsal angles. Correction of increased hallux valgus angle depends on whether the joint is congruent on X-ray or not. If joint is congruent despite a valgus deformity of great toe, it means the deformity is because of abnormality in bony structure near the joint **(Fig. 12.29B)**. Such cases would need a corrective osteotomy (Akin or Chevron) of the distal

stretched. Over time the deformity gets fixed. As subluxation of the first MTP joint occurs, the metatarsal head gets prominent medially. A bursa develops in the overlying area that together with thickened soft tissues lead to bunion formation. As the deformity increases, there occurs crowding of the lesser toes and lesser toe deformities may also result.

Clinical Features

Patient presents with unsightly deformity, difficulty in wearing shoes and pain over the bunion (most common presenting complaint). Secondary to the deformity, more weight is borne on lateral metatarsal heads, resulting in transfer of metatarsalgia, stress fractures and callosities of the lateral metatarsals. In long-standing cases, there may be osteoarthritis of MTP joint causing severe pain.

Diagnosis

An X-ray is done to measure the hallux valgus angle (angle between first metatarsal and proximal phalanx); an angle greater than 15° is diagnostic **(Fig. 12.27B)**. Intermetatarsal angle (between (neck) metatarsal. However, if joint is incongruent **(Fig. 12.29B)** that means the deformity is because of soft tissue imbalance (tight lateral structures and lax medial structures). Such cases need a soft tissue release on lateral side with medial-sided imbrication of joint capsule. And once the hallux valgus angle is corrected, a basal osteotomy of the (proximal) metatarsal may need to be added in those who have increased intermetatarsal angle **(Fig. 12.29C)**. The treatment algorithm has been summarized in **Flow chart 12.1**.

HIGH-YIELD POINT

Hallux rigidus: It refers to stiffness or rigidity of the first MTP joint. It can occur in a number of conditions such as gout, pseudogout or even osteoarthritis and mostly it is bilateral.

OTHER IMPORTANT DIGITAL DEFORMITIES

Claw toes: This is characterized by hyperextension at MTP joints and flexion at both proximal and distal interphalangeal joints **(Fig. 12.30)**. It is an intrinsic minus deformity due to paralysis of intrinsic muscles of foot, and hence is seen mostly in diseases such as peroneal muscular atrophy, poliomyelitis, peripheral neuropathies, etc. Rheumatoid arthritis is also an important cause. Surgical treatment involves rerouting the long toe extensor

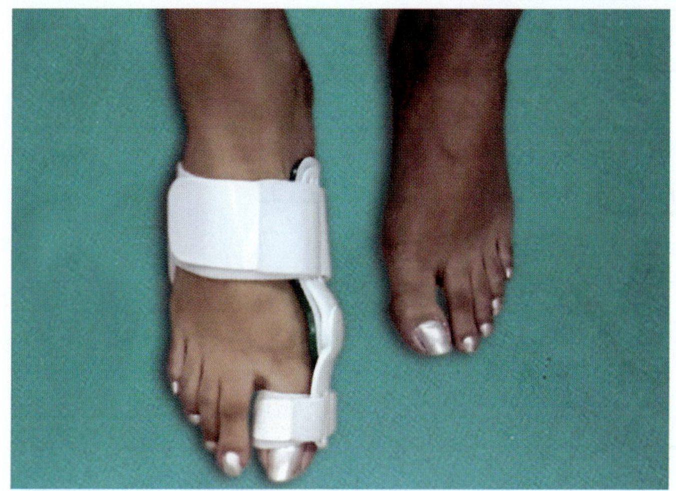

Fig. 12.28: Hallux valgus splint

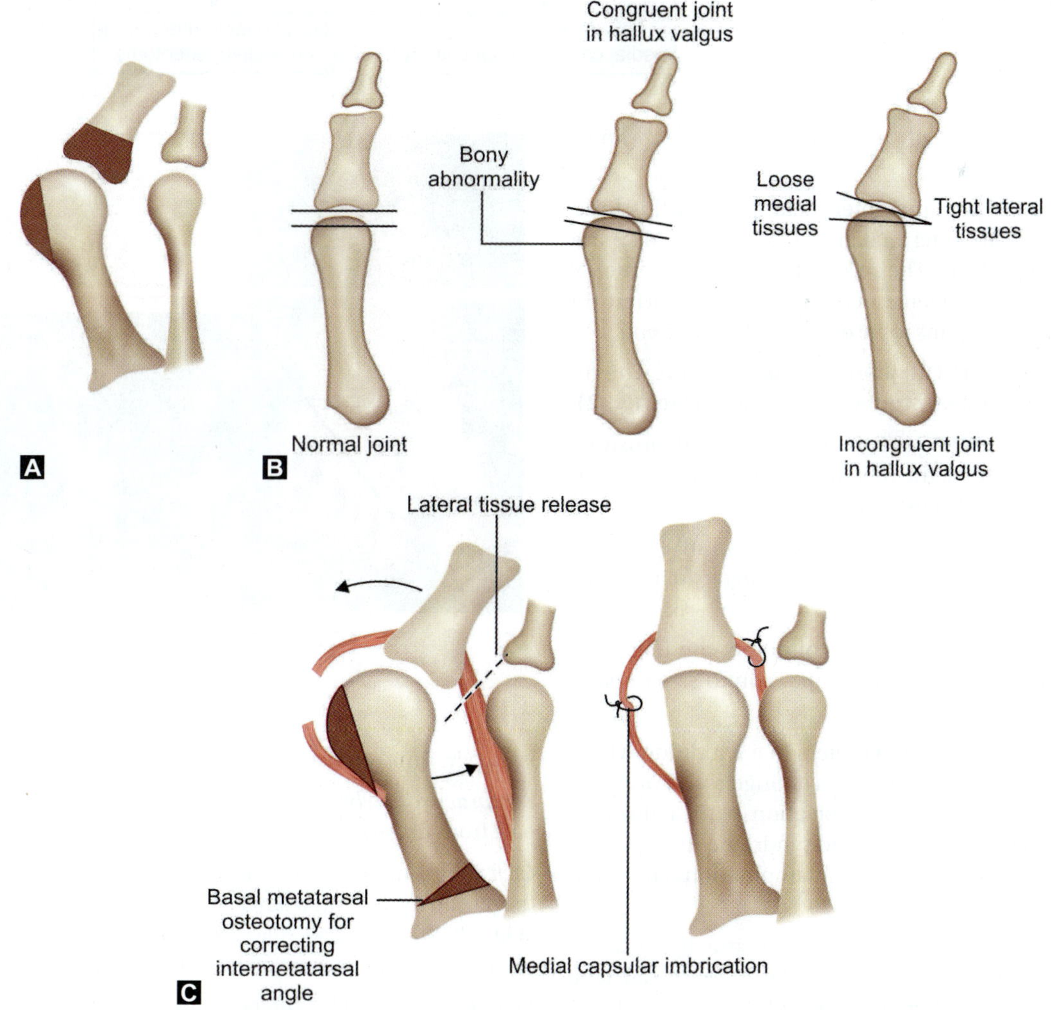

Figs 12.29A to C: (A) Keller's operation; (B) Diagram showing etiology in hallux valgus with congruent and incongruent joints; (C) Schematic depiction of treatment in a patient with hallux valgus (increased hallux valgus and intermetatarsal angles) with incongruent joint

Flow chart 12.1: Treatment algorithm in a patient with hallux valgus

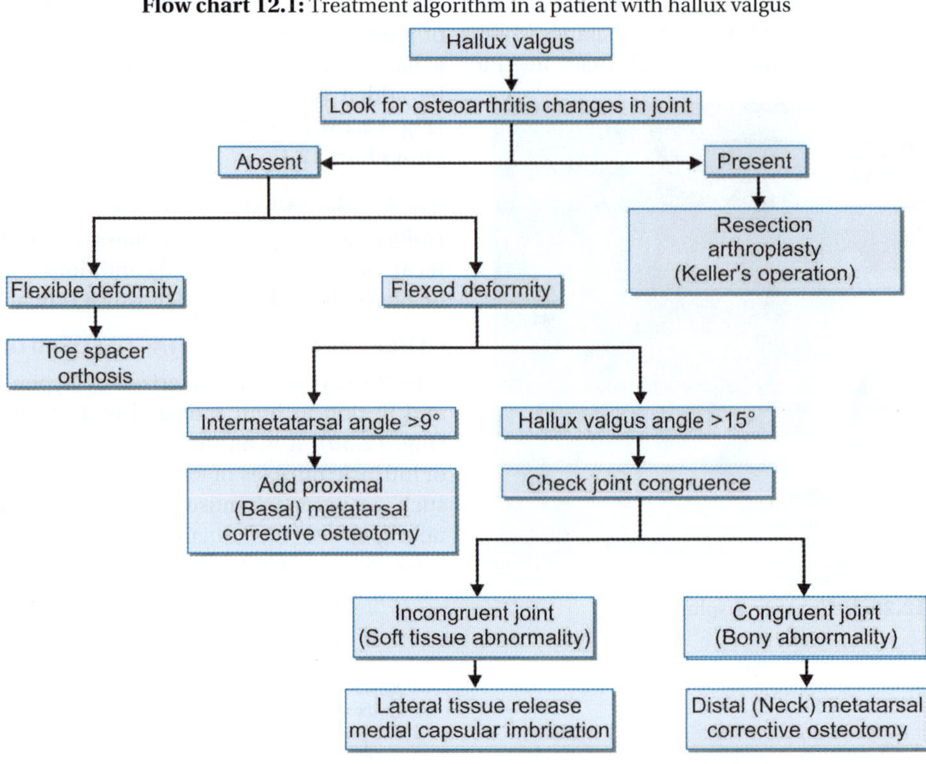

tendons through the neck of metatarsals (modified Jones operation).

Hammer toe: In this, the proximal interphalangeal (PIP) is fixed in flexion while the distal interphalangeal (DIP) and MTP are fixed in extension **(Fig. 12.31)**. The second toe is most commonly affected. The deformity is congener of Boutonniere's deformity of finger and possible cause seems to be extensor dysfunction.

Mallet toe: In Mallet toe, the DIP joint is fixed in flexion. The tip of the toe presses into the shoe producing a callosity **(Fig. 12.32)**.

Cock-up deformity: The MTP joint is dislocated and proximal phalanx sits on the dorsum of the metatarsal head **(Fig. 12.33)**. It is generally seen as a sequel of osteoarthritis.

Macrodactyly (Fig. 12.34): Refers to presence of an enlarged-sized digit. Most commonly affected is index finger followed by the long finger.

Arachnodactyly (spider fingers): In this condition, the fingers or toes are long and slender in relative comparison to size of palm or sole.

Syndactyly: Syndactyly **(Fig. 12.35A)** refers to a condition where two or more digits are fused (webbed toes or fingers). A condition called acrosyndactyly is found in association with a disorder called Streeter's dysplasia (amniotic band syndrome) where there are congenital constriction rings (or even amputations) found in the extremities of neonates **(Fig. 12.35B)**.

Polydactyly (Figs 12.36A and B): Presence of an extra digit is called "polydactyly". The deformity can be preaxial or postaxial type (Venn Watson classification, **Figs 12.37A and B**). If cosmetically unacceptable, the accessory digit can be amputated.

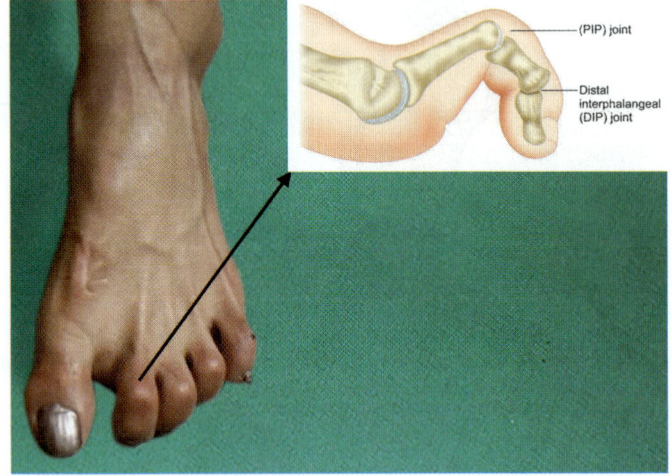

Fig. 12.30: Claw toe deformity

Adactyly: This refers to complete absence of a finger(s) or toe(s).

Symbrachydactyly: This is a condition when there is absence of a part from fingers or toes.

Cleft foot: This is an anomaly where the central rays are absent (partial adactyly) and a single cleft extends proximally into the foot **(Fig. 12.38)**. It is also called as "lobster foot". Treatment requires plastic surgery for closure of the cleft using rectangular flaps.

Symphalangism: This refers to ankylosis (fusion) of the PIP joints in either toes or fingers.

Camptodactyly: It refers to flexion deformity at PIP joint (usually seen in fingers).

Clinodactyly: In this condition, there is curving of little finger toward ring finger due to a wedge-shaped middle phalanx **(Figs 12.39A and B)**. The condition is associated with many genetic disorders but the strongest association exists with Down's syndrome, the condition being present in 60% of newborns with Down's syndrome.

Kirner's deformity: This refers to palmoradial curvature of the distal phalanx of the little finger. It is associated with Down's and

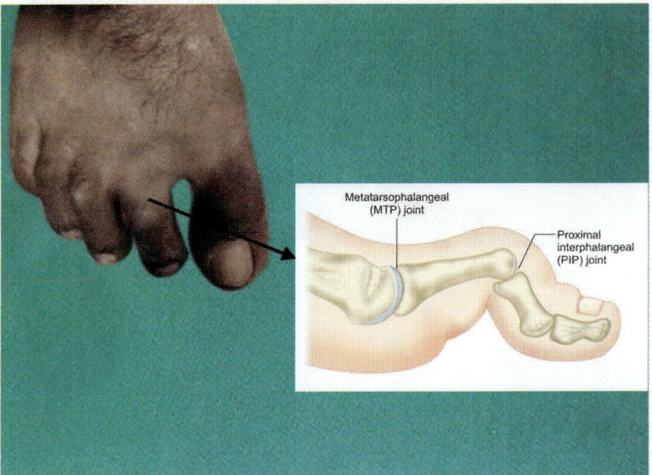

Fig. 12.31: Hammer toe

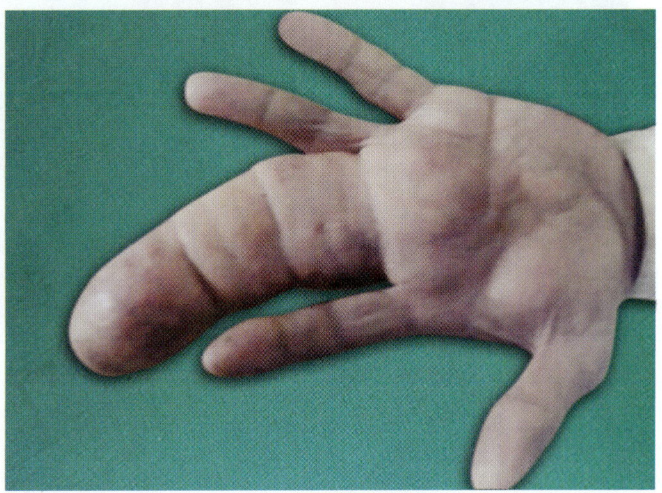

Fig. 12.34: Macrodactyly

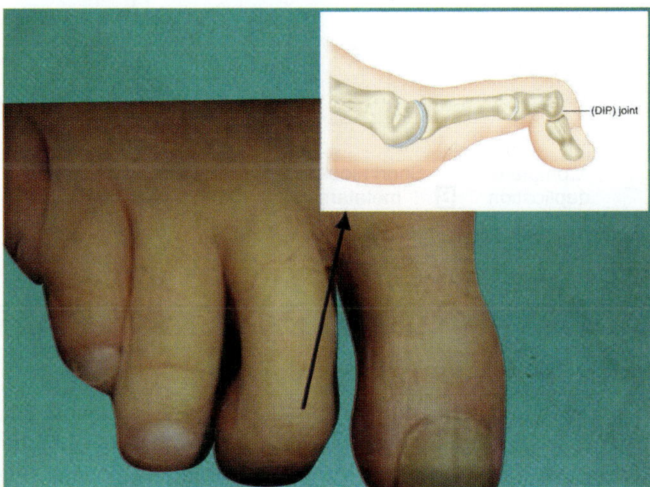

Fig. 12.32: Mallet toe

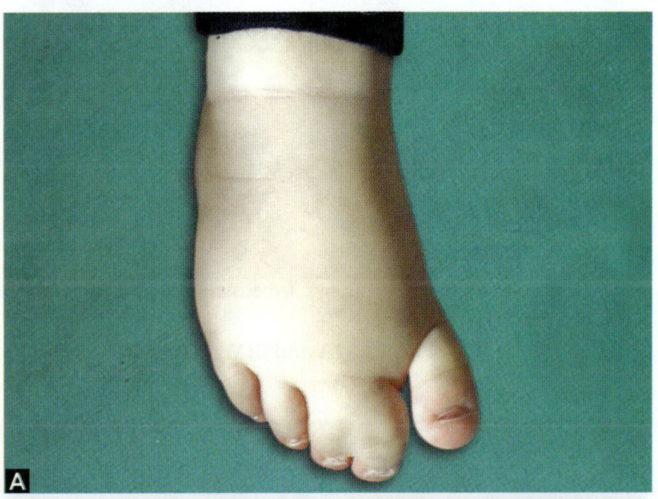

A

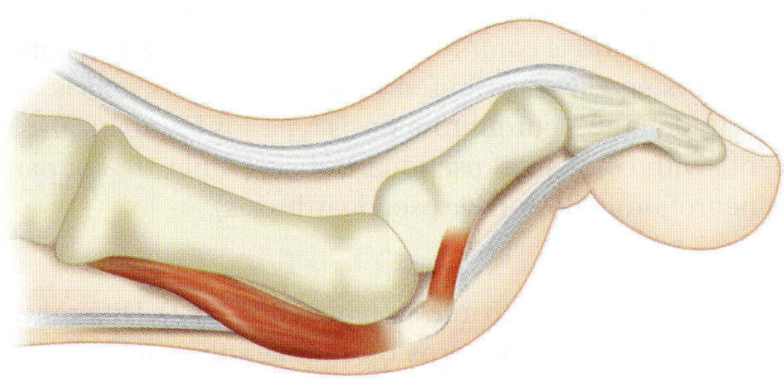

Fig. 12.33: Cock-up deformity

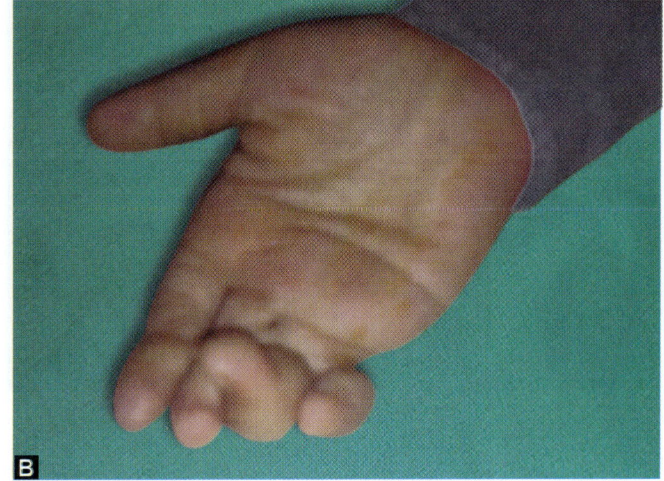

B

Figs 12.35A and B: (A) Syndactyly; (B) Acrosyndactyly

Courtesy: Chelsea Lafleur and M-cm community.

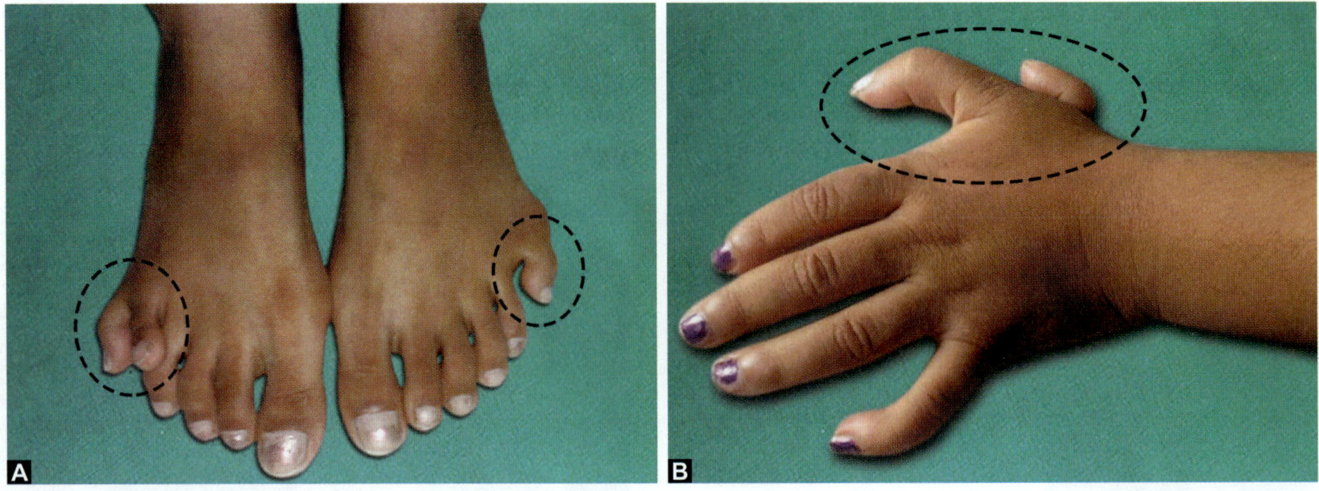

Figs 12.36A and B: Polydactyly

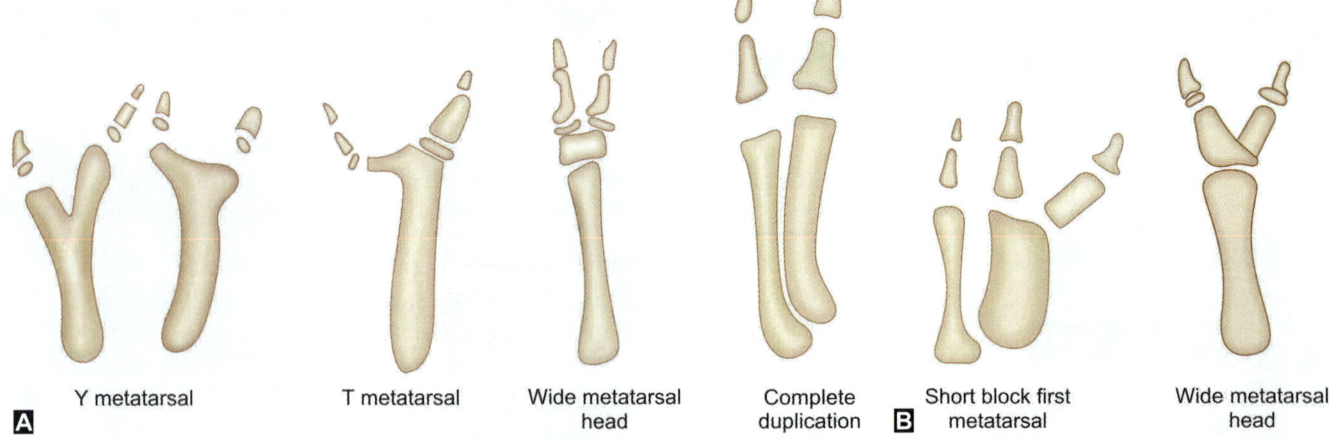

Figs 12.37A and B: Venn Watson classification of polydactyly. (A) Postaxial types; (B) Preaxial types

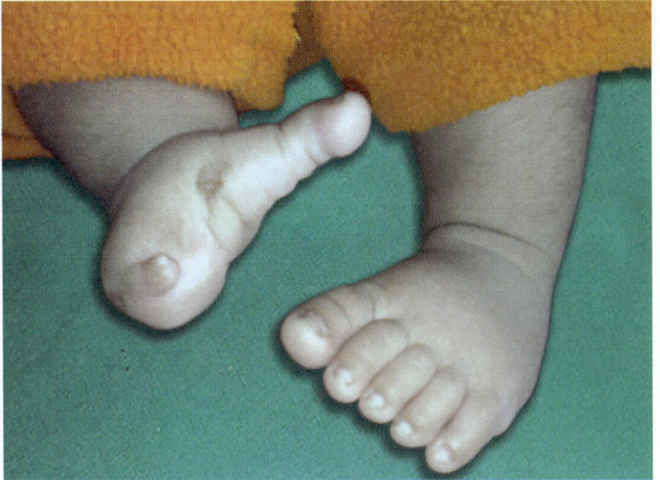

Fig. 12.38: Cleft foot

Turner's syndromes and these patients often have congenital cardiac abnormalities.

DEFORMITIES OF LEG

CONGENITAL PSEUDOARTHROSIS OF TIBIA

This is a congenital condition (disease process is present since birth) characterized by dysplasia in the distal half of tibia, that presents with tibial bowing (mostly anterolateral bowing, **Figs 12.40A and B**), generally evident within a year after birth. There is little tendency for the lesion to regress. The dysplastic tibia fractures easily through the weakened area and fractures often fail to unite, hence the term pseudoarthrosis. Refracture through the lesion is common if at all, initially union occurs. The condition is equally distributed in boys and girls and is almost always unilateral. Neurofibromatosis type 1 is found in 50–55% of patients with congenital pseudoarthrosis (while 10% of patients with neurofibromatosis have pseudoarthrosis).

Diagnosis

Boyd classified this lesion into six types **(Box 12.2)**. Different types may present different patterns on radiographs such as sclerosis of medullary canal **(Fig. 12.41)**, an hour-glass constriction of the

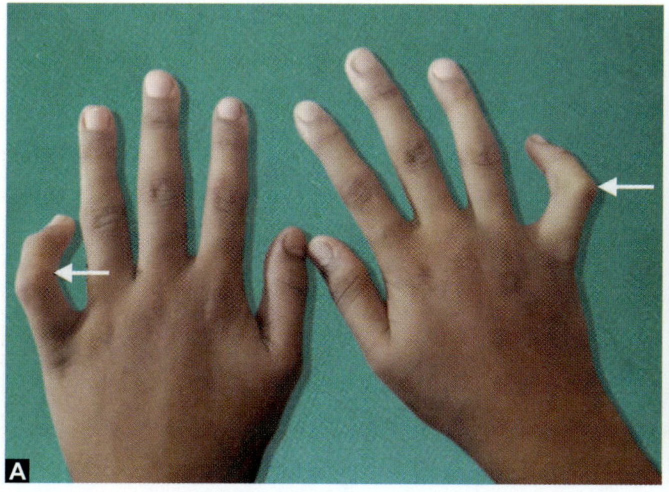

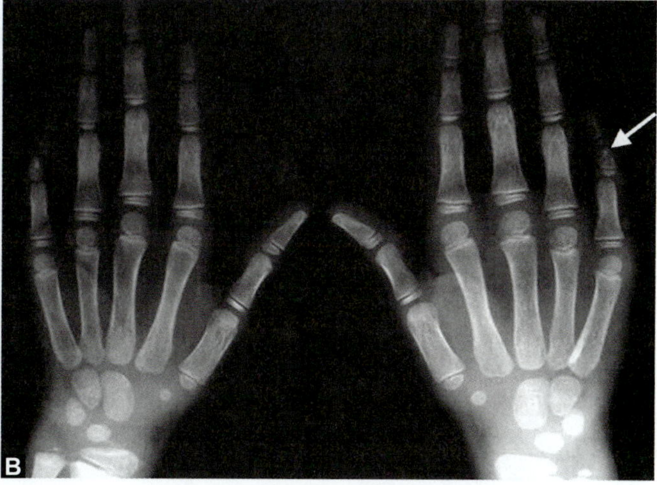

Figs 12.39A and B: Clinodactyly (arrows). (A) Clinical picture; (B) X-ray bilateral hands (anteroposterior view) of a patient with clinodactyly showing wedge-shaped middle phalanx

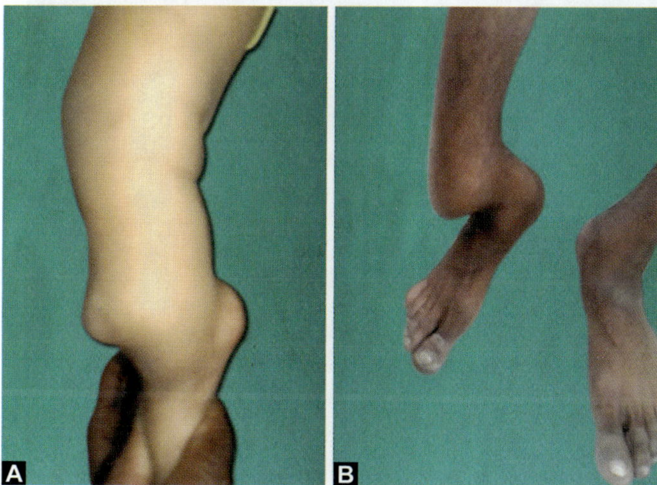

Figs 12.40A and B: (A) Child with congenital pseudoarthrosis of tibia; (B) Deformity of distal leg in neglected pseudoarthrosis of tibia

Courtesy: Dr Matad Lokeshwaraiah Chetan (SS Institute of Medical Sciences, Davangere, Karnataka).

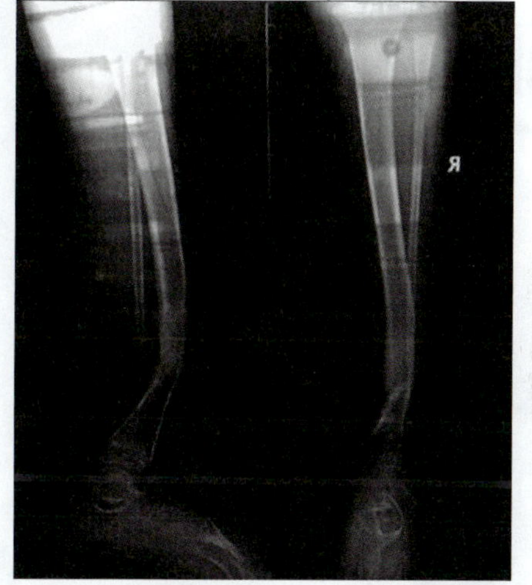

Fig. 12.41: X-ray of pseudoarthrosis of tibia showing anterolateral angulation and sclerotic segment in distal tibia

---

Box 12.2: Boyd classification of congenital pseudoarthrosis of tibia

Type I: Defect present in distal tibia

Type II (high-risk tibia): Hour-glass constriction present in distal tibia is associated with neurofibromatosis and has poorest prognosis

Type III: Congenital cyst is present

Type IV: Sclerotic segment is present at dysplasia site

Type V: Dysplastic fibula along with tibia pseudoarthrosis

Type VI: Intraosseous neurofibroma is present

---

tibia or a cystic lesion in the medullary canal of tibia. An important step is to differentiate this condition from fibular hemimelia (*read below*), that commonly has anteromedial bowing rather than anterolateral. Moreover, the latter will have an absent fibula which is identifiable in pseudoarthrosis.

Treatment

Before a fracture occurs, a total contact orthosis (providing circumferential support) is prescribed as prophylaxis. Orthotic support and weight-bearing stresses sometimes lead to union. However, if the deformity is hindering quality of life or once a fracture occurs, surgery is indicated. The procedure of choice in the first attempt is resection of pseudoarthrosis tissue, shortening of bone, fixation with intramedullary nail (William's technique) and bone grafting. If this fails to achieve union, vascularized fibular grafting may be opted. Limb length discrepancy (LLD) is an untoward event that may need external fixation with distraction osteogenesis (Ilizarov fixator). An amputation (disarticulation through ankle with motion at pseudoarthrosis site controlled with prosthetic socket) is indicated in cases with two to three failed surgical attempts, severe stiffness or shortening more than 2–3 inches.

CONGENITAL DEFICIENCIES OF LONG BONES (HEMIMELIA)

Hemimelia are a group of disorders where there are congenital deficiencies of long bones. They can be of two types: (1) terminal deficiencies where a complete body part distal to the affected site is absent **(Fig. 12.42)**, and (2) intercalary deficits where a middle

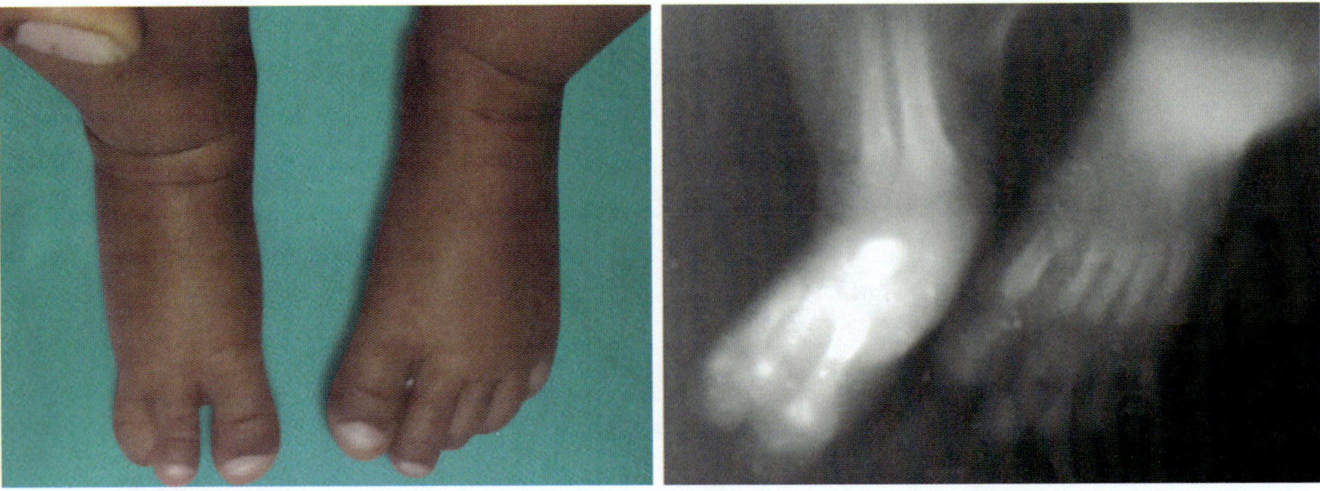

Fig. 12.42: Complete absence of fourth and fifth ray in foot (terminal hemimelia)

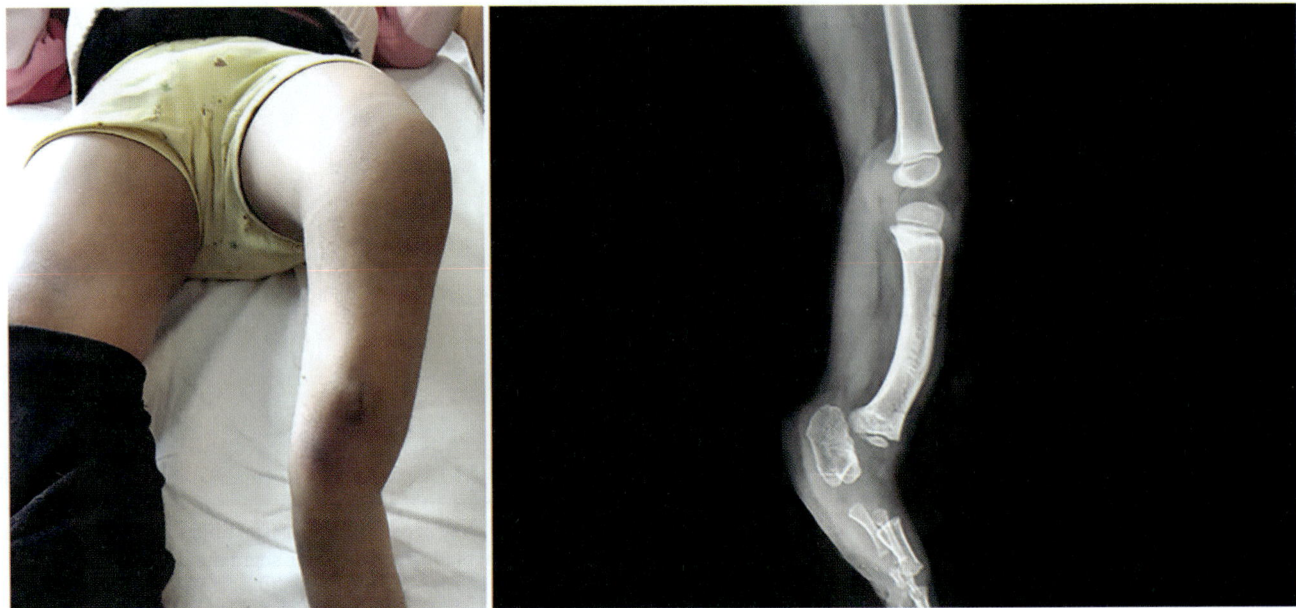

Fig. 12.43: Fibular hemimelia showing absent fibula and bent tibia (intercalary hemimelia). Note anteromedial bowing of the leg

segment of limb is missing, e.g. fibular hemimelia **(Fig. 12.43)** where fibula in leg is absent but distal structures are present. Fibula, Radius, Femur and Tibia are the common bones involved in decreasing order of frequency.

Fibular Hemimelia

This is characterized by a congenital longitudinal deficiency of fibula. It is the most common long bone deficiency reported in orthopedics. Classical presentation is a child who comes with anteromedial bowing of tibia (as opposed to anterolateral bowing which is common in congenital pseudoarthrosis of tibia) with skin dimpling over the bowed tibia **(Fig. 12.43)** and foot pushed into equinovalgus. LLD is significant as proximal femoral focal deficiency (PFFD) (*see* Page 376) and congenital coxa vara (*see* Page 375) are common associations. In fact treatment depends on amount of shortening. If limb shortening is more than 15 cm, a primary amputation followed by prosthetic fitting is the advisable treatment. However, in less severe cases, reconstructive procedures may be offered which involve corrective osteotomies for the ankle foot deformity (Wiltse varus supramalleolar osteotomy) and limb lengthening (by distraction osteogenesis).

Tibial Hemimelia

This is an AD condition where the patient has a congenital longitudinal deficiency of tibia. The extremity is shortened with anterolateral bowing of leg. Treatment depends on amount of tibial remnant present. Severe deformities with completely absent tibia need a knee disarticulation. If some proximal tibial anlage is present and quadriceps mechanism is functioning, then fibula can be surgically transferred into the intercondylar notch (Brown's procedure). However, if there is proximal tibia of varying sizes is present a proximal tibiofibular synostosis (a surgery to joint tibia-fibula) up combined with a syme's amputation at ankle below gives good functional results.

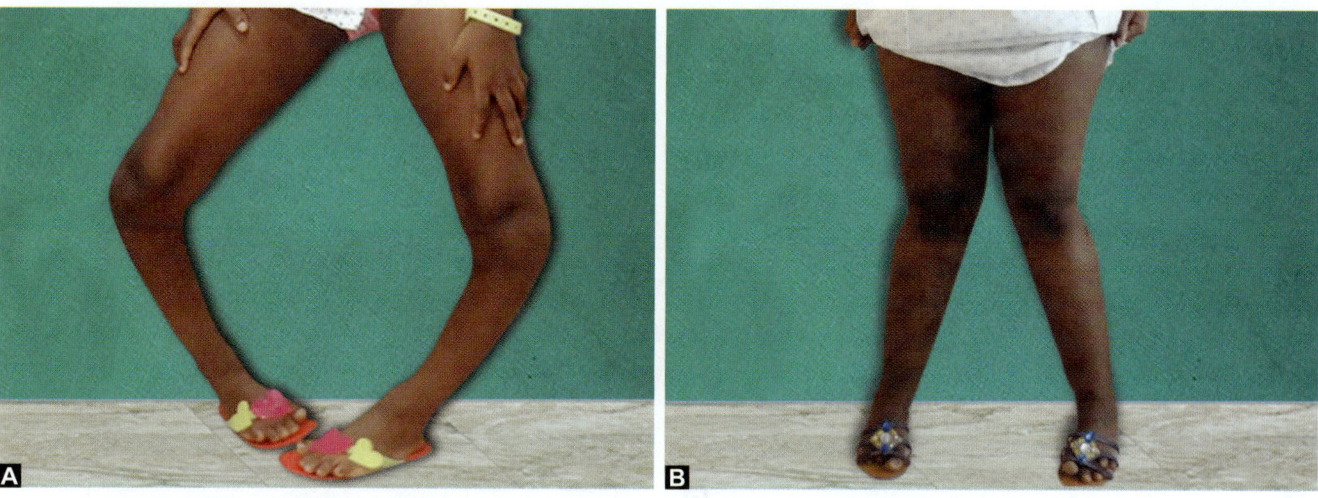

Figs 12.44A and B: (A) Child with bilateral genu varum deformity; (B) A child with bilateral genu valgum deformity

Courtesy (Fig. 12.44A): Dr RK Sharma (Indraprastha Apollo Hospital, New Delhi).

Courtesy (Fig. 12.44B): Dr Sachin Ingole (Indraprastha Apollo Hospital, New Delhi).

HIGH-YIELD POINTS

- Apart from tibia, congenital pseudoarthrosis may be seen in fibula and clavicle.
- Congenital pseudoarthrosis of fibula invariably involves the distal fourth of the bone and is rarely symptomatic unless leg is vigorously stressed so that ankle develops valgus. Such cases may need a tibiofibular synostosis (fusion).
- Congenital pseudoarthrosis of clavicle is mainly seen on right side (possibly from pressure of right subclavian artery). There occurs failure of lateral and medial ossification centers to fuse resulting in pseudoarthrosis in the middle. Spontaneous union is unknown and bone grafting is required.

DEFORMITIES AROUND THE KNEE

ANGULAR KNEE DEFORMITIES

Introduction

Genu varum* (bow legs) and genu valgum (knock knees) are very common pediatric concerns that worry many parents. In genu varum when ankles are approximated in a standing child, the knees remain divergent apart **(Fig. 12.44A)** while in genu valgum* when the knees are touching each other, the ankles tend to be divergent apart **(Fig. 12.44B)**.

To label a pathological diagnosis, one needs to have detailed knowledge of lower limb alignment axes and normal progression of lower limb alignment with age.

Lower Limb Alignment Axes

Axial alignment of the lower limb is studied by obtaining a full length standing AP radiograph from hips to ankle (scanogram). Following axis and angles are evaluated in the radiograph:

- Mechanical axis of the lower limb **(Fig. 12.45A)** on this radiograph refers to a vertical line that extends from the center of the femoral head to center of the ankle joint. Individually speaking, mechanical axis of both tibia and femur are in line with each other (i.e. make an angle of 0° with each other). In normal person, the mechanical axis of lower limb crosses the knee joint slightly medial to the tibial spine.

- The anatomical axis on this radiograph is defined as lines drawn along the intramedullary canals of the femur and tibia. While, for tibia the mechanical and anatomical axes coincide, the mechanical and anatomical axes of femur make an angle of 6° with each other. Hence, if referred from a vertical line, anatomical axis of the femur and tibia would make an angle of 9° and 3°, respectively.

- Femorotibial angle (FTA) is the angle between the anatomical axis of femur and the anatomical axis (or mechanical axis) of tibia. Since mechanical axis of tibia is same line as mechanical axis of femur, FTA is similar to angle between anatomical and mechanical axes of the femur itself. Normally, it is 6°.

Genu varum **(Fig. 12.45B)** is labeled, when on a scanogram, the mechanical axis of lower limb crosses more medial to the tibial spine than normal while genu valgum **(Fig. 12.45B)** is labeled, if it passes lateral to the tibia spine. Another way to define these deformities is by measurement of the FTA. The anatomical axis of tibia is in 6° of valgus with respect to anatomical axis of femur.

Medial proximal tibial angle (MPTA) and lateral distal femoral angle (LDFA): MPTA and LDFA are outlined in **Figure 12.46**. These angles when drawn on scanogram assist the surgeon in localizing the site of deformity in cases of varum or valgum. On most occasions, genu varum deformity is due to deformed tibia and in these patients, the MPTA (normal is 87° ± 3°) is decreased while on the contrary, most people with genu valgum have deformity contributed by malformed femur and in these people, the LDFA (normal is 88° ± 3°) is decreased.

*Lower Limb Alignment in Different Age Groups***

From birth to 1 year a physiological (natural) varum (up to 10–15°) is present at knee. After 1 year of age, varum starts to reduce. By

---

*Varum means the limb distal to a joint is deviated toward midline while valgum means the limb distal to the joint is deviated laterally, i.e. away from midline.
**Values based on femorotibial angle (FTA).

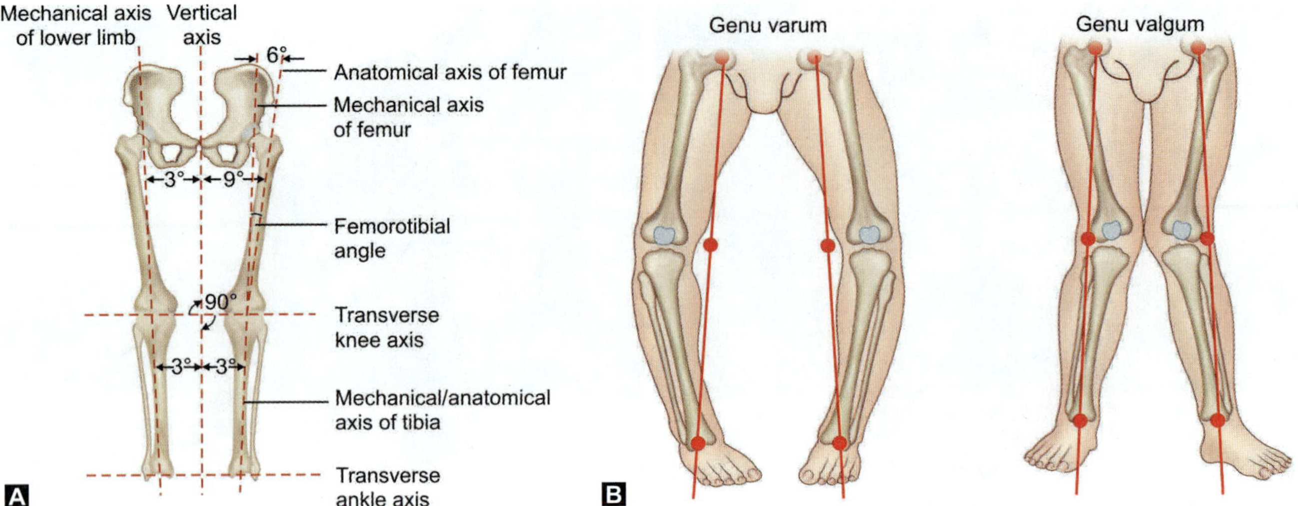

Figs 12.45A and B: (A) Lower limb alignment axes; (B) Deviation in mechanical axis in genu varum and genu valgum

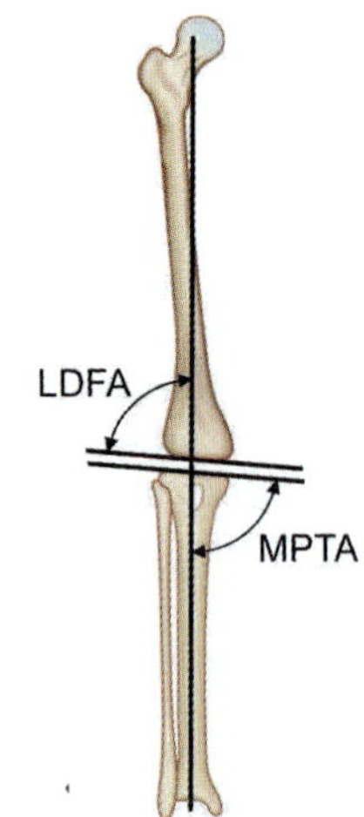

Fig. 12.46: Measurement of medial proximal tibial angle (MPTA) and lateral distal femoral angle (LDFA)

18–24 months, a neutral relationship is attained. After 2 years a rapid transition to valgum occurs that peaks at 3–4 years of age (may go up to 15–20°). Thereafter, the valgum gradually reduces such that by 5–6 years of age, valgus of about 5–6° is established, which persists into adult life.

Genu Varum

Although the deformity is generally apparent to a naked eye, it is confirmed in the clinical setting by measuring the distance between medial joint lines of both knees with ankles of the patient approximated. If genu varum is present at knee, then this distance is more than 6 cm. Important causes for the deformity have been tabulated in **Box 12.3**.

Evaluation of a Child with Bowleg Deformity

Owing to valgum being the natural alignment, the deformity is generally obvious to the naked eye. Crucial steps in evaluation are to reach the pathological cause (physiological genu varum, rickets, Blount's disease, etc.) and this should entail the assessment of site of deformity, gait analysis, limb length measurements, symmetry of involvement and the radiological assessment.

> **Box 12.3:** Common causes of genu varum deformity
>
> - Physiological genu varum (most common cause of bowlegs in a toddler)
> - Pathological genu varum
>   - Rickets (most common cause in India)
>   - Blount's disease or tibia vara (most common cause worldwide)
>   - Congenital familial form of tibia vara
>   - Physeal injury (trauma, infection, tumor involving medial side of knee, etc.)
>   - Osteogenesis imperfecta (OI)
>   - Skeletal dysplasias such as achondroplasia and metaphyseal dysplasia
>   - Focal fibrocartilaginous dysplasia

Site of deformity: This may be focal in the distal femur, knee or the tibia or it may be generalized. In physiologic genu varum and rickets, there is a gentle curve involving both the distal thigh and the proximal leg. In Blount's disease (*discussed later in detail*) an acute medial angle is seen just below the knee due to involvement of proximal medial tibial physis. In the congenital familial form of tibia vara deformity is at the lower tibia at the junction of the middle and the lower thirds.

A gross way to decipher which bone (femur or tibia) is primarily contributing to the deformity is by asking the patient to lie supine or sit on table's edge and then place both his legs parallel to each other while both knees are flexed to 90°. The clinician then observes from the foot end **(Fig. 12.47)**. If the deformity disappears, it is likely in femur and must be corrected by a procedure on femoral side else, if the deformity is in tibia, it will persist on flexion and should be addressed by procedure on tibial side.

Gait analysis: In both the physiological genu varum and Blount's disease (tibia vara), the foot progression angle (*see* Page 120) may be medial but it is more severe in tibia vara. Lateral thrust is a brief and dynamic lateral move of the femur on the medially depressed tibia during stance phase. It is characteristically seen in Blount's disease due to lateral ligamentous laxity or incompetency but absent in the physiological genu varum and rickets.

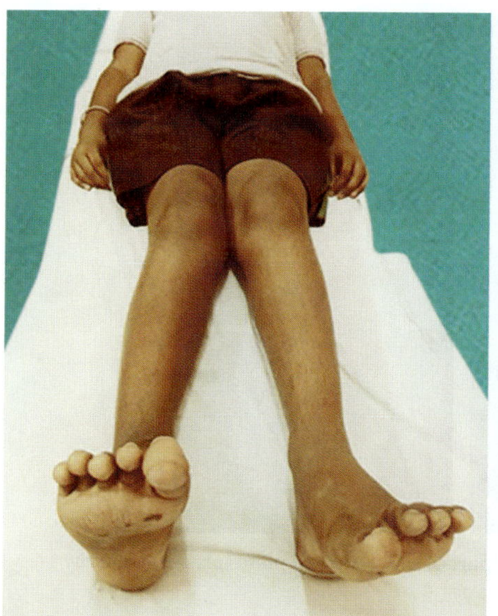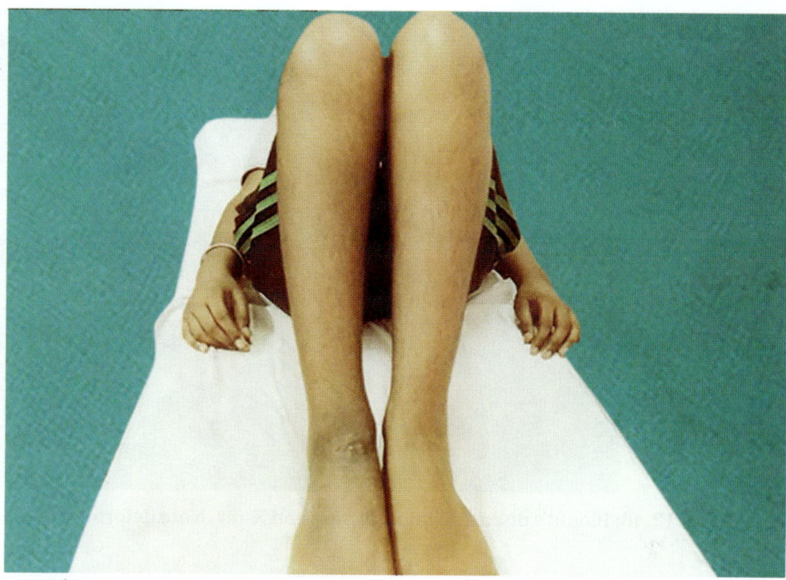

Fig. 12.47: Deciphering the site of involvement in a patient with angular deformity at knee

Symmetry of involvement and limb length: Involvement is usually bilateral in rickets and physiological genu varum but may be unilateral or bilateral in Blount's disease. Affected limb may be shorter in tibia vara but of equal length in rickets and physiological genu varum. Children of rickets may be short-statured in addition to bowlegs.

Radiological assessment: In physiological genu varum physes are normal, but distinctive radiological features are seen in rickets (*see* Page 406) and in Blount's disease.

General Principles of Management

A varus alignment in a child below 2 years is simply physiological, where the X-ray usually shows a gentle curve involving distal femur and proximal tibia with normal physes. Early walking has been postulated as causative factor for this physiological bowing. Along with this physiological genu varum an internal tibial torsion is also a common companion causing intoeing gait in these toddlers. Both physiological genu varum and internal tibial torsion correct simultaneously and just need reassurance to be given to the parents. Persistent varus after 2 years is considered pathological and should be thoroughly evaluated.

The first step is to identify the cause and see, if it has a remedy. On many occasions, correction of pathology may lead to resolution of the condition. In cases where the cause cannot be remedied (e.g. Blount's disease*) or in cases where the deformity persists beyond the age of 3–4 years, despite elimination of pathological cause (e.g. rickets†), a surgical intervention is warranted.

Type of surgery is chosen depending upon the age and remaining growth potential in the child. If there is significant growth potential remaining, i.e. boys less than 12 years and girls less than 10 years of age, hemiepiphysiodesis (surgical fusion of growth plate) that is reversible (e.g. growth plate fixed with staples that can be removed later) is done. Staples are applied on lateral side of growth plate to prevent the lateral side from growing so that only the medial side grows with age and the deformity corrects itself. Once the desired correction is achieved, staples may be removed. Otherwise, a timed permanent hemiepiphysiodesis can be done at a time when the remaining growth potential of the opposite half of the physis just corrects the deformity before naturally fusing (generally when only a year or two of growth are remaining).

In skeletally mature cases, a corrective osteotomy (achieve slight overcorrection especially in varum) is done. The bone to receive the osteotomy should be the one that harbors the deformity (*see* **Figs 12.46 and 12.47**).

Blount's Disease (Tibia vara)

This is a developmental (not a congenital) disorder characterized by progressive bowleg deformity **(Fig. 12.48)**. Exact etiology is not known but physiological bowing and Blount's disease are considered as parts of a same spectrum. Since majority of the affected kids are early walker and overweight (>95th percentile), the disease is thought to result from excessive mechanical stresses due to early weight-bearing on the growth plate. Excessive medial pressure due to weight-bearing stresses on the bowed legs causes osteochondrosis of the medial proximal tibial physis. Disturbed growth of proximal medial tibial physis leads to progressive bowing and shortening of the limb. A bony bridge (physeal bar) develops in severe cases resulting in growth arrest across the physis.

Clinical Features: Affected kids are mostly obese and have acute angular bowing just below the knees. There is associated internal tibial torsion with or without a genu recurvatum (hyperextension) deformity at the knee. On gait analysis, some children show a positive lateral thrust at the knee due to lateral ligament laxity. In other cases where the medial tibial plateau is severely deformed

---

*Treatment discussed in detail subsequently in this chapter.
†Treatment of knee deformity in patient of rickets has been discussed in detail on Page 409.

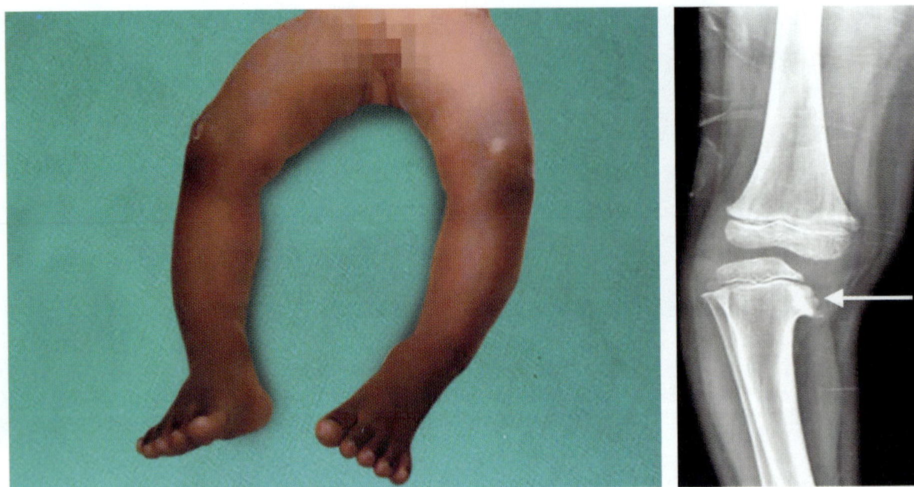

Fig. 12.48: Blount's disease; clinical picture and X-ray. Note deformed medial part of tibial growth plate (arrow) on X-ray

due to abnormal growth plate, the medial femoral condyle may be seen subluxating posteromedially into the depressed medial tibial plateau at 10–20° of knee flexion (Siffertz Katz sign). Intoeing due to internal tibial torsion is a frequent component. Distal femur is typically normal but rarely may show a compensatory valgus deformity.

Based on the time of presentation, the disease is categorized as infantile (onset up to 4 years of age, most common subtype), juvenile (4–10 years) and adolescent (after 10 years of age) forms. Late onset tibia vara (juvenile and adolescent) is more often unilateral and less severe than infantile form. These children usually have a mild pre-existing varus deformity. Adolescent tibia vara and slipped capital femoral epiphysis (SCFE) are often seen in association.

Diagnosis: Most of the cases are bilateral like physiological genu varum and unilateral cases may have concomitant physiological bowing of other leg, hence diagnosis is challenging. Moreover, acute angulation may be masked in obese children. The diagnosis hence needs to be confirmed by drawing metaphyseodiaphyseal (MD) angle of Drenan **(Figs 12.49A and B)**. It is subtended between two lines, one line is perpendicular to long axis of tibia and other is tangent to proximal tibial metaphysis. An angle more than 11° favors the diagnosis while an angle more than 16° confirms the diagnosis.

Differential Diagnosis: Physiological genu varum is the closest differential to the infantile tibia vara. These two can easily be differentiated based on X-ray features of infantile tibia vara. Characteristic X-ray features are usually seen by 2 years of age. MD angle of Drenan **(Figs 12.50A and B)** helps in differentiating the two conditions. **Table 12.3** gives a detailed account of important differentials to consider along with differentiating features to look for.

Classification: Based on X-ray features Langenskiold described six stages **(Table 12.4)** of the disease.

Treatment: Brace should be given to all children aged less than 2 years with early Blount's disease (stages I and II) and older than 2 years with persistent bowing and risk factors (MD angle 11–16°, obesity) for Blount disease. Braces (e.g. mermaid splints) have

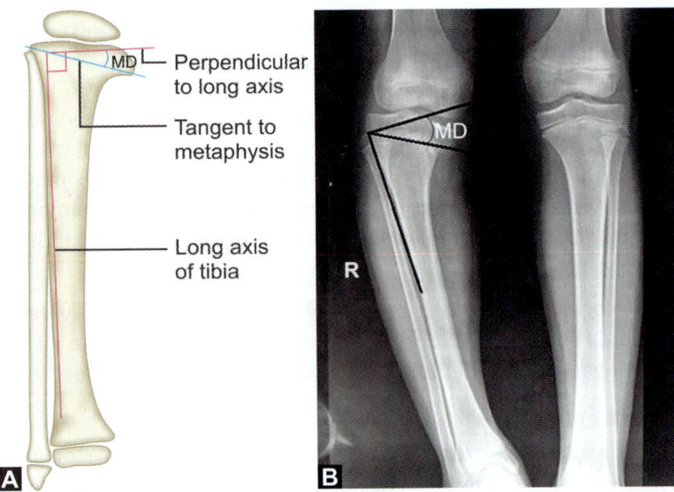

Figs 12.49A and B: Metaphysiodiaphyseal (MD) angle of Drenan

proven beneficial in Blount's disease by offloading the diseased proximal medial tibial physis. Brace treatment should be continued until the X-ray features of early Blount's disease (metaphyseal beaking and depression) resolve. This may take 1–2 years.

Operative treatment (proximal tibia fibula valgus osteotomy) is required in older children aged 3 or more with late stages of Blount's disease (stages III and IV) and who are unresponsive to braces. Early surgery prevents progression of the disease and it is recommended that the osteotomy should be done before the child is 4 years old. If physeal bar has formed it should be resected along with correcting osteotomy. Stages V and VI may have severe depression of medial tibial plateau. Medial tibial plateau elevation is required along with osteotomy in these cases. Proximal lateral tibial hemiepiphysiodesis is indicated for adolescent tibia vara, if the growth plates are still open and the varus deformity is not too severe.

Genu valgum

Genu valgum is labeled in the outpatient clinics when the distance between medial malleoli of both ankles with knees of patient approximated is greater than 8 cm.

Table 12.3: Differentiating features of some common conditions that lead to bowleg deformity

	Physiological genu varum	*Blount's disease*	*Rickets*
Site of varus angulation	A gentle curve involving distal thigh and upper half of the leg	Acute angle below knee	A gentle curve involving distal thigh and upper half of the leg
Lateral thrust (Gait)	Absent	May be present	May be present
Limb lengths	Equal	Affected limb may be shorter	Equal, but the child is relatively short (height is usually in the lower 10th percentile)
Symmetry of involvement	Usually bilateral	May be unilateral or bilateral	Usually bilateral
Radiological features	Normal physes around knee joint, some varus in both the distal femur and the proximal tibia, without an acute angular component Metaphyseodiaphyseal (MD) angle is < 10° Proximal fibular epiphysis is well inferior to the knee joint line	Medial fragmentation and beaking of the proximal tibial metaphysis (earliest radiographic finding) Physeal enlargement which occupies the space created by metaphyseal depression Cleft in the epiphysis and closure of medial physis (a physeal bar) are late features MD angle is > 11° (mostly > 16°) The proximal fibular epiphysis is nearer to the knee joint line (i.e. proximally migrated) due to relative overgrowth of the fibula	Radiographic abnormalities include widening of the physes, cupping of the physes and bowing of the long bones MD angle < 10° Proximal fibular epiphysis is well inferior to the knee joint line

Table 12.4: Langenskiold classification of Blount's disease

Stage	I	II	III	IV	V	VI
Features	Medial and distal beaking of the metaphysis	Depression/ tapering in the medial metaphysis	Deepening of the metaphyseal beak to form a sharp angular step	Ossification into the metaphyseal step causing epiphyseal enlargement	Cleft in the epiphysis (a separate medial fragment can be seen)	Closure of the medial proximal tibial physis (bony bridge formation)
Pictorial description						

Parents often become concerned for knock knees when their child is around 4 years of the age because at this age physiological valgum is maximum. This physiological genu valgum is characterized by symmetrical and bilateral deformity between 3 years and 7 years of the age. After this age, neutral to 12° of valgus may be considered normal, provided the child is asymptomatic.

Pathological causes of genu valgum have been listed in **Box 12.4**. Most cases are simply a valgus that persists into adolescence without any obvious cause (idiopathic).

Evaluation of a Child with Knock Knee Deformity

Other than obvious knock knee deformity, knee pain due to overloading of lateral compartment is a common complaint in these children. Due to lateral mechanical axis deviation, lateral recurrent subluxation of patella may occur. Knock knees are often associated with increased femoral anteversion (assessed by Craige test, Page 118) and external tibial torsion (assessed by measuring thigh foot angle, **Fig. 12.7**), both of which are assessed in prone patient. If children with knock knees have height less than the 3rd percentile they should be assessed for causative pathologic condition (e.g. skeletal dysplasia and renal osteodystrophy). Gait should be evaluated for presence of any medial thrust. Medial thrust is a brief knee joint protrusion to medial side during stance phase of the gait that indicates medial knee ligaments incompetency. A full length scanogram **(Fig. 12.50A)** from hip to ankle joint with patella facing forward should be taken for accurate assessment of the deformity and measurements of the axis and femorotibial angles **(Fig. 12.45A)**.

General Principles of Management

Physiological genu valgum (up to 7 years) requires observation and reassurance of the parents. Radiographs are warranted in only those 3–4 years old children who have excessive tibiofemoro angle falling outside the physiological range (>20° valgus at 3–4 years) or for a unilateral deformity. Surgical treatment is usually deferred until the child is 10 years of age in hope for spontaneous correction. Mostly genu valgum develops in adolescents due to a deformity in distal femur that persists without any obvious cause

Box 12.4: Common causes of pathological genu valgum deformity

- Persistent genu valgum of idiopathic nature (most common)
- Rickets (when onset is after 2 years*)
- Physeal injury (trauma, tumor, infection of lateral part of physis, etc.)
- Skeletal dysplasias (chondroectodermal dysplasia, mucopolysaccharidosis type IV, and spondyloepiphyseal dysplasia tarda)
- Multiple hereditary exostosis
- Proximal tibial metaphyseal fractures (Cozen's fracture†)

*In children < 2 years of age, there is physiological varus and soft bones in rickets dip into genu varum. However, in older children genu valgum may be seen more commonly.

†Malunion of a proximal tibial fracture commonly produces a genu valgum deformity (Cozen's fracture of proximal tibial metaphysis).

(idiopathic). In adolescents, surgical treatment of genu valgum should be considered, if

- Femorotibial angle is more than 15° or
- Intermalleolar distance is more than 10 cm or
- When mechanical axis passes lateral to lateral tibial cortex (zone 3, **Fig. 12.50B**) or
- When lateral deviation of mechanical axis (zone 2) is associated with knee pain or recurrent patellar subluxation.

Hemiepiphyseal stapling of distal medial femoral physis (and sometimes proximal medial tibial physis also) is indicated in skeletally immature children with significant remaining growth. Corrective varus osteotomy is required in skeletally mature patients with valgus deformity and in young children with severe valgus deformity when immediate correction is required.

Genu Recurvatum

Genu recurvatum refers to hyperextension at knee (extension beyond 5°). The deformity is commonly encountered in those who have ligament laxity from any cause (e.g. poliomyelitis, Larsen syndrome, Marfan syndrome, Ehlers-Danlos syndrome, etc.). However, it can also be a sequel of malunited fracture, old trauma to physis or a condition like Osgood-Schlatter disease. The posterior soft tissue structures are stretched and these patients display muscle imbalance and poor proprioceptive control during gait. Initial treatment in these patients consists of rehabilitation program in conjunction with bracing, however, resistant cases may eventually need corrective osteotomies.

In neonates most common cause of genu recurvatum deformity is congenital dislocation of the knee, which has been discussed subsequently.

Congenital Dislocation of the Knee

It is thought to result from abnormal fetal position that causes the knee to get locked in hyperextension **(Fig. 12.51)**. It is usually seen in patients with neuromuscular syndromes such as AMC, Larsen syndrome, Ehler-Danlos syndrome, etc. Classically, newborns present with hyperextension deformity of the knee **(Fig. 12.51)**. Often there is congenital absence of cruciate ligaments with fibrosis of quadriceps and hypoplastic patella. About 70% cases are associated with ipsilateral DDH and 50% with CTEV. Patients

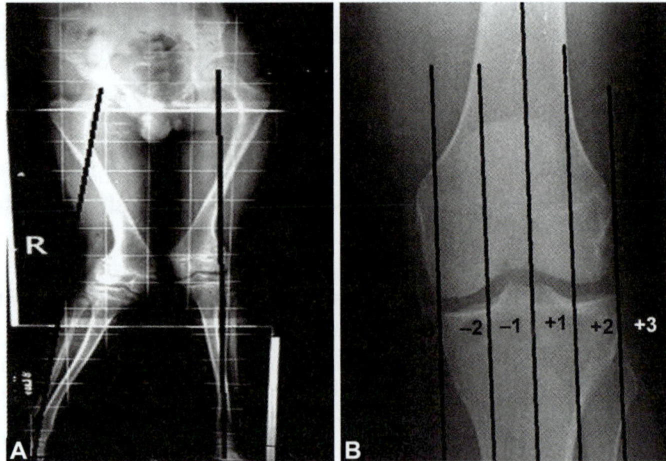

Figs 12.50A and B: (A) Mechanical axis drawing on the scanogram showing bilateral genu valgum with more severe valgus deformity (mechanical axis falling outside the lateral tibial cortex) on the right side; (B) Tibial plateau is divided into four zones. Positive values are given for valgus and negative values are given for varus deformity. Zone 1 is centered over tibial spine and mechanical axis should pass through this zone. Zone 3 is outside the tibial cortex and mechanical axis passing through this zone, always requires correction

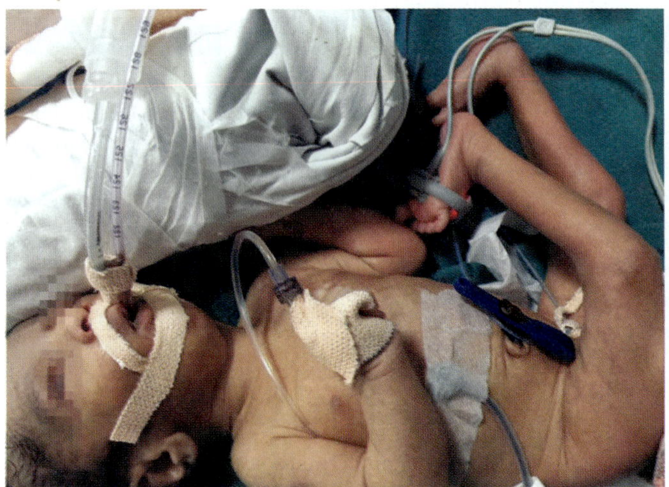

Fig. 12.51: Congenital dislocation of knee. Note hyperextension (recurvatum) deformity of bilateral knees

are managed with serial casting to achieve up to 90° flexion. If it fails surgical correction is undertaken by 6 months to 1 year.

HIGH-YIELD POINTS

- Rickets more commonly causes genu varum because the most common form of rickets is nutritional rickets which occurs during the age group of physiological varus. Hypophosphatemic rickets also causes genu varum. But renal osteodystrophy typically occurs later in life, hence it produces genu valgum.
- In reversible hemiepiphysiodesis for genu varum, staples are applied on lateral side while in genu valgum, they are applied on medial side.

DEFORMITIES AROUND THE HIP

DEVELOPMENTAL DYSPLASIA OF HIP

Introduction

Hip joint is the most stable joint in the body with a big socket, i.e. the acetabular cup and a well-sized ball, i.e. the femoral head. Also the strongest ligament in the body (iliofemoral ligament) is present around this joint to provide stability. To dislocate such a stable joint a good velocity trauma would be needed. However, the term "congenital dislocation of hip (CDH)" refers to spontaneous dislocation of hip that occurs at birth without any documented evidence of severe trauma. This clearly indicates that these patients must be having some predisposing factors that make their hip unstable so that a dislocation results spontaneously.

A better understanding of the condition was provided by Klissic. He observed that although a group of patients with this condition are born with a hip that is dislocated at birth, a subset of children exists in whom the joint spontaneously dislocates shortly after birth. Thereby, he introduced the term developmental dysplasia of hip (DDH) to signify that these patients have dysplastic hips that are the predisposing cause. Either their femoral head is small and does not ossify on time or their acetabulum is flat and shallow due to faulty development.

Technically, DDH comprises a spectrum of disorders (just hip dysplasia, subluxation, frank dislocation, teratological dysplasia, late adolescent dysplasia, etc.) with the common underlying etiology, i.e. a lax hip capsule and dysplastic hip joint resulting in failure to maintain the femoral head within the acetabular socket. In children where dislocation exists from birth, the primary cause is faulty development while in those where dislocation generally occurs bit later, ligament laxity is the more important predisposing factor.

Incidence

- Actual dislocation is reported in 1/1,000 live births (incidence of positive clinical findings, i.e. Frank dislocations and lax dislocatable hips combined, is higher).
- Male:female ratio is 1:5.
- It is bilateral in approximately one-third cases.
- Left hip involvement is more common (left > bilateral > right).

The condition is more common in *F*irst born *F*emale child with *F*air complexion (whites or Caucasians) who had a positive *F*amily history and at birth had a *F*aulty intrauterine position (breech deliveries, oligohydramnios, etc.)—"The Five F's".

It is uncommon in India because mothers carry child straddled on the side of their waist with the hips of child abducted **(Fig. 12.52)**. This tends to reduce unstable hips because when the femur goes into abduction, the head falls back into the acetabulum.

Etiology

Important factors implicated are:

- *Ligamentous laxity*: Often inherited. Maternal hormone relaxin may play a role. It is possible that the hormone crosses the placenta and if patient is a female the environment is more conducive for the hormone to relax the hip capsule and ligaments.

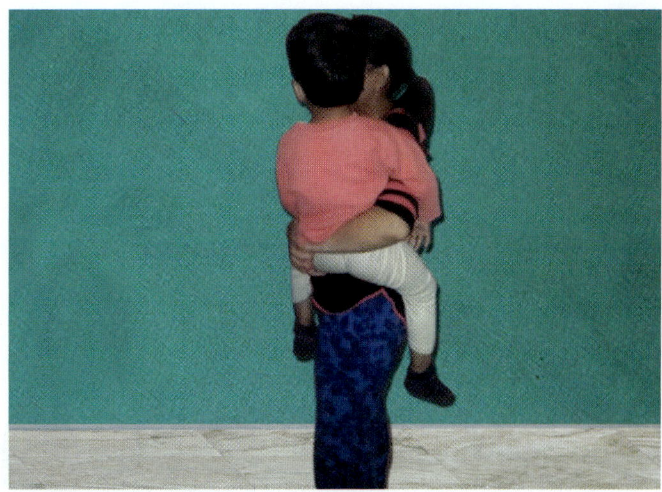

Fig. 12.52: Mother carrying baby by side causing abduction of hips

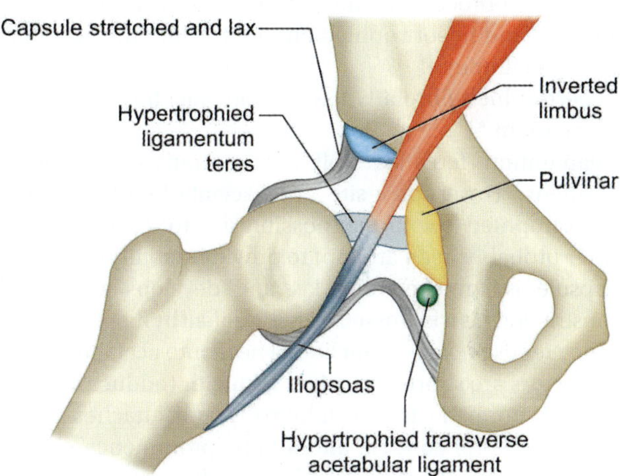

Fig. 12.53: Pathological changes in developmental dysplasia of hip

- *Breech presentation*: Unstable hip is 10 times more common.
- *Postnatal positioning of child*—wrapped up with the hips swaddled in extension predispose to easy dislocation.
- *Oligohydramnios*: Likely that this causes crowding of the fetus *in utero* and faulty presentation thereby predisposing to dislocation.
- *Packaging disorders*: The condition is thought to be associated with congenital packaging disorders viz. torticollis (strongest association, 20% cases), metatarsus adductus (10% cases) and congenital knee dislocation. No proven association with genu varum or CTEV exists.

Pathological Changes Seen in these Dysplastic Hips (Fig. 12.53)

- The femoral head epiphysis is small and ossifies late and when dislocated, the head moves upward and laterally. This is due to the upward pull of gluteal muscles that arise from pelvis and are inserted on the greater trochanter.
- The acetabulum is shallow (not cup shaped) due to faulty development. This is the most common pathology central to the pathogenesis.

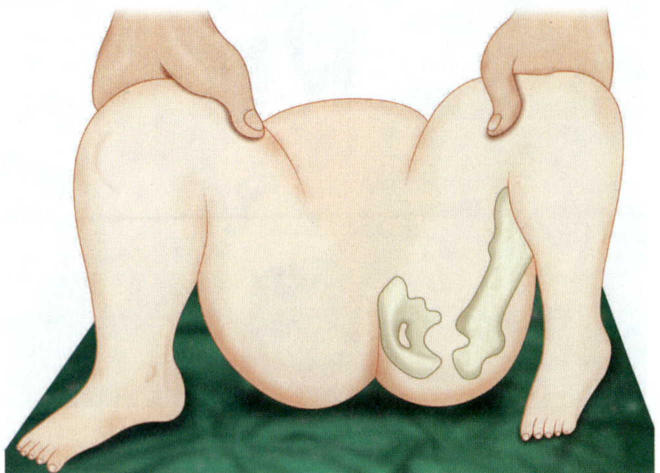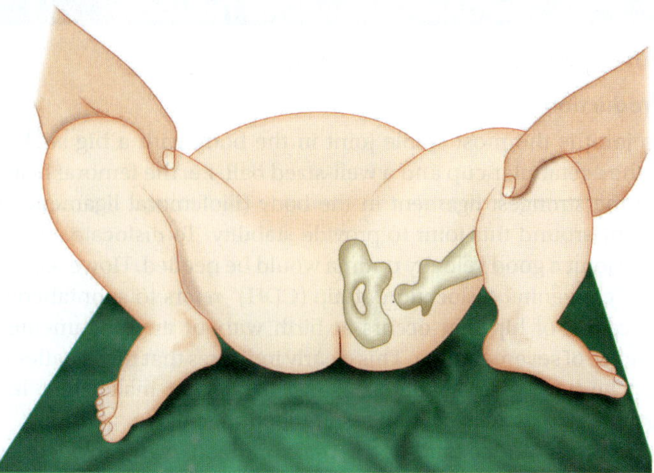

Fig. 12.54: Barlow's test

- Labrum (fibrocartilaginous rim around acetabulum) is inverted and hypertrophied and folded into the acetabulum (inverted limbus).*
- Hypertrophied fibrofatty tissue (pulvinar) fills up the empty acetabulum.*
- Ligamentum teres as well as the transverse acetabular ligament (insertion site of acetabulum labrum) is hypertrophied (the former possibly due to stretching and the latter probably in an attempt to provide stability).*
- Capsule is stretched and lax and develops an hourglass constriction (as it is crossed in its lower half by iliopsoas tendon) which tends to block reduction of head into acetabulum.*
- Adductors are shortened. Main adductor (adductor magnus) extends from the ischial tuberosity and attaches near the medial femoral condyle into a bony prominence called the adductor tubercle. When the head is dislocated, this muscle pulls the distal femur medially and over time the adductors relatively shorten up.*
- There is excessive anteversion of both femoral neck and acetabulum. Also the neck shaft angle is increased (coxa valga). These changes are ascribed to altered growth across the femoral neck and trochanteric growth plates owing to disturbed muscle forces in a dislocated hip.

Clinical Presentation

Newborn

Although no standard guidelines for screening of DDH exist, it is a general consensus that all newborns must be screened for an unstable hip. Two conventional methods in practice for this are the Ortolani and the Barlow's tests **(Fig. 12.54)**. Both the tests use a similar principle, the unstable hip is dislocated or reduced and the clunks of dislocation or reduction are appreciated.

*Barlow's test (more preferred, **Fig. 12.54**):* The test has two parts: (1) adduction and (2) abduction.

With the hips and knees flexed, grasp thighs with fingers over greater trochanter and thumb in front. Gently adduct the hip and give slight outward pressure with thumb to dislocate the hip, producing the characteristic "clunk of dislocation". This occurs in unstable dislocatable hips, which are not already dislocated. This part of test is negative in already dislocated hip.

In second part, pressure is released and hips abducted, which will relocate the hip and produce the "clunk of relocation". Clunk, and not click, is significant.

Ortolani test (Abduction test): Similar to second part of Barlow's test so can be applied only to already dislocated hips.

Older Children

Ortolani and Barlow's tests are rarely positive after 3 months of life because of soft tissue contractures. Other clinical findings that may suggest the diagnosis in older child include:
- Asymmetrical thigh folds/groin creases and a wide perineum **(Fig. 12.55A)**.
- The affected limb is shortened and externally rotated.
- Restricted abduction (especially in flexion) is one of the most sensitive sign (sensitivity—69%, specificity—54%).
- There is excessive internal and external rotation of the dislocated hip.
- *Galeazzi's sign (Allis sign):* With the child lying supine with both hips and knees flexed, the knee is lower on affected side **(Fig. 12.55B)**. It is due to shortening of the affected lower extremity.
- Telescopy (*see* Pages 124, 125) at hip is positive.
- Vascular sign of Narath (*see* Page 126) may be appreciated.
- Lumbar lordosis may be exaggerated (mostly in bilateral cases).
- In a walking child Trendelenburg's gait (abductor lurch) and Trendelenburg's test may be positive. Children with bilateral CDH walk with a waddling gait/duck gait/sailor's gait.
- *Klisic sign **(Figs. 12.56A and B)**:* In a supine child, place middle finger over greater trochanter and index finger over anterior superior iliac spine (ASIS). Normally, an imaginary line through these points crosses at umbilicus, but in

---

*These factors prevent successful closed reduction on treatment attempt.

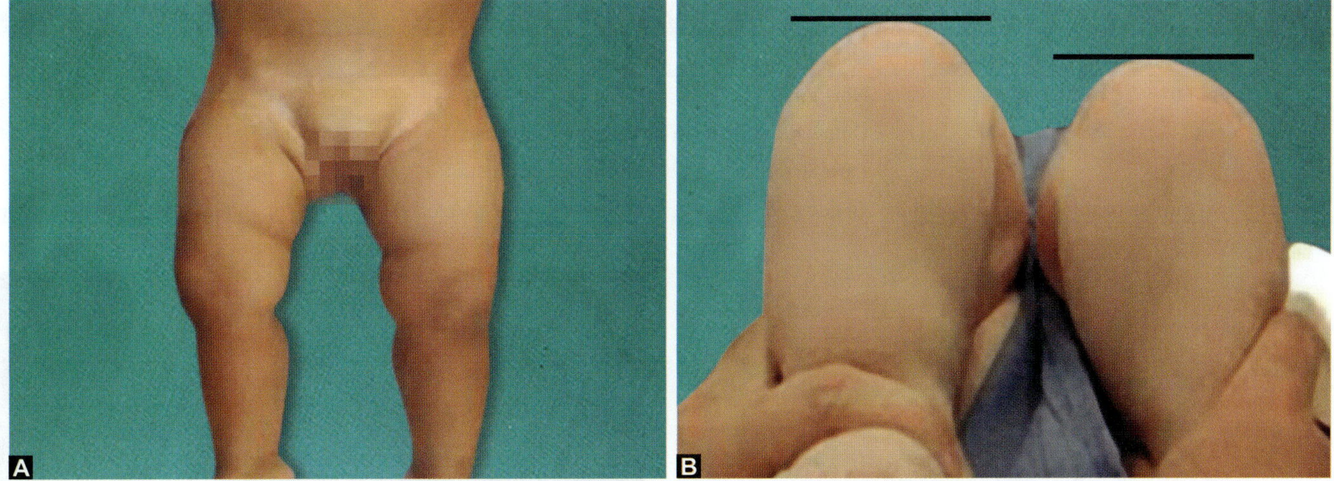

Figs 12.55A and B: (A) Asymmetrical skin folds; (B) Allis sign

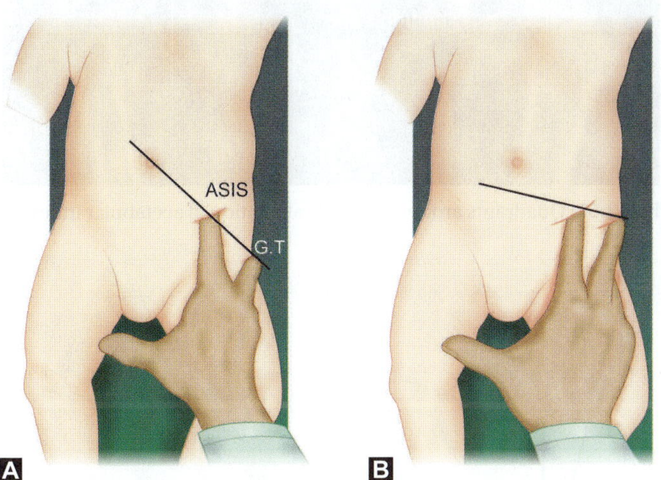

Figs 12.56A and B: Klisic sign

dislocation the line crosses below the umbilicus. The sign is positive in both unilateral and bilateral cases.

Investigations

X-ray is of little value in a child less than 6 months. This is because the proximal femoral epiphysis is not ossified at birth (ossification occurs at 4–6 months), and hence not visible on X-rays for the first 6–12 months of life. The investigation of choice (for screening as well as for diagnosis) for this age group (<6 months old) is ultrasonography (USG), although the best investigation for any age is magnetic resonance imaging (MRI) that provides the best details.

On USG, DDH is classified by Graf's method **(Table 12.5)**. The radiologist measures two angles on hip ultrasound—(1) alpha angle (between baseline of ilium and roof of bony acetabulum) and (2) beta angle (between baseline of ilium and cartilaginous acetabular roof). Normally alpha angle is more than 60° and decreases with increasing severity while beta angle is less than 55° and increases with increasing severity of DDH. Various grades are described and this grading helps in guiding treatment. However, the ultrasound findings commonly improve with age,

so the decision to treat DDH should be based on USG at 6 weeks and not at birth.

X-rays are useful in relatively older children. Delayed appearance of upper femoral epiphysis (Normally it appears at 6 months) and delayed development (smaller size), shallow acetabulum, a broken Shenton's line (line from proximal medial neck to inferior border of superior pubic rami) and lateral and upward displacement of ossific center of femoral head are some of the findings that guide the diagnosis.

Von Rosen's view may be especially useful in children under 1 year of age. The view is taken with hips abducted, internally rotated and extended. Normally, axis of the femoral shaft should intersect the acetabulum (triradiate cartilage). In dislocation, the line crosses above the acetabulum **(Fig. 12.57)**.

Another way to confirm the findings is to draw the Hilgenreiner's line (horizontal line connecting the two triradiate cartilages) and the Perkin's line (vertical line on each side passing through lateral margin of acetabulum) such that four quadrants are formed across each hip **(Fig. 12.58)**. Normal position of femoral head (proximal metaphyseal beak more specifically if head is not visible) is the inner lower quadrant whereas a dislocated head migrates into the upper outer quadrant.

Acetabular index **(Fig. 12.58)** is calculated from these radiographs to know if the acetabulum is dysplastic or not. The index is determined by measuring the angle between Hilgenreiner's line and a line connecting triradiate cartilage and lateral lip of acetabulum. Normally this angle is less than 30°. Greater values mean a more vertical, shallow and dysplastic acetabulum.

Center edge angle of Wiberg **(Fig. 12.59)** is another radiographic measurement to establish the diagnosis. The angle is formed by a line drawn from the center of femoral head to the outer edge of the acetabular roof, and a vertical line drawn through the center of femoral head. Normally this is greater than 20° and lesser values indicate dislocated hip.

Treatment

Treatment of this condition is dictated by the age at which the patient presents to the doctor. Aim is achieving concentric and stable reduction of head into acetabulum and maintaining the same. It has been seen that in young children if the head is

Table 12.5: Classification of developmental dysplasia of hip (DDH) by Graf's method

Grade (Class)	Alpha angle	Beta angle	Description (head)	Treatment
I	>60°	<55°	Normal	None
II	43–60°	55–77°	Delayed ossification	Abduction orthosis
III	<43°	>77°	Lateralization	Abduction orthosis
IV	Unmeasurable	Unmeasurable	Dislocated	Abduction orthosis/closed reduction/open reduction (age dependent)

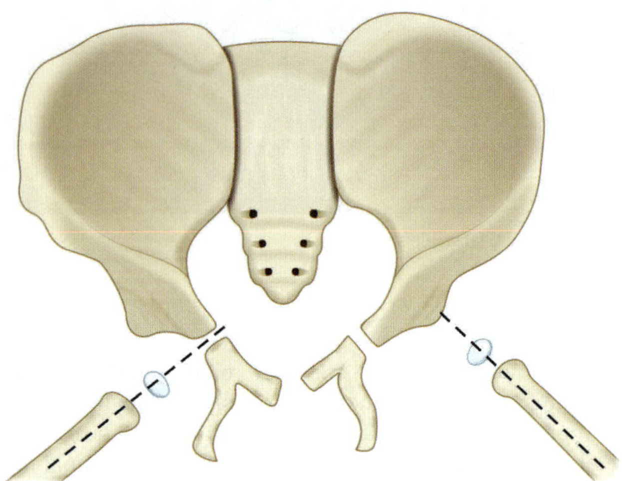

Fig. 12.57: Von Rosen view to identify dislocated hip

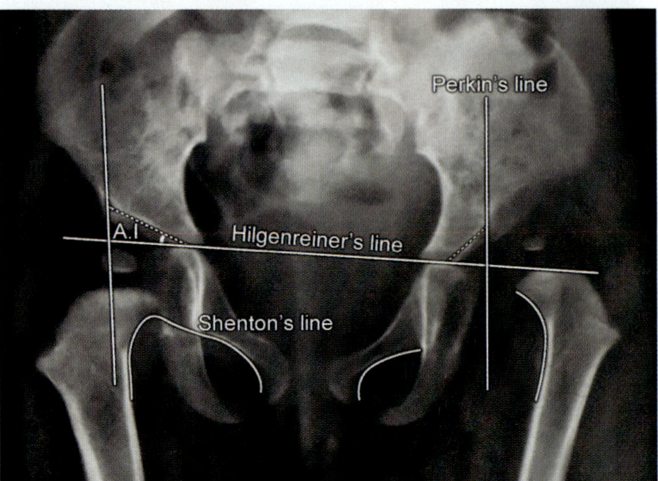

Fig. 12.58: Quadrants around hip and calculation of acetabular index (AI)

maintained inside the acetabulum for a time, under the mold-like effect of the head the acetabulum gradually develops into a cup-like shape and covers the head to full extent.

Age Less Than 6 Months

Method of reduction: Child with an unstable hip (Ortolani or Barlow test positive) but reduced by examiner (i.e. Ortolani positive) is placed in a hip abduction splint* and reduction confirmed by von Rosen X-ray view **(Fig. 12.57)**. If the hip remains dislocated despite examiner's attempt then also the child is placed in an abduction splint or orthosis but with higher degrees of hip flexion such that on von Rosen AP radiograph line along femoral shaft intersects the triradiate cartilage **(Fig. 12.57)**.

Maintenance of reduction: This is taken care by the abduction splint itself that has been applied for reduction. Pavlik harness **(Fig. 12.60A)**, a dynamic abduction splint is the most commonly used apparatus while von Rosen splint **(Fig. 12.60B)** and a Frejka pillow **(Fig. 12.60C,** not preferred due to high complication rate) are other abduction orthoses available. A recheck of reduction is performed between 3 weeks and 6 weeks by USG or arthrography (radiography after injection of a contrast agent in hip; a reduced hip shows the classical "rose thorn" appearance). Two situations may be encountered:

1. *Hip is found reduced*: Treatment is continued if findings are normal and patient may be called every 3–6 weeks for follow up. It is advised to wear the harness for 23 hours in a day. In a neonate continue it for minimum 6 weeks while in 1–6 months old continue it for 6 weeks after the hip attains

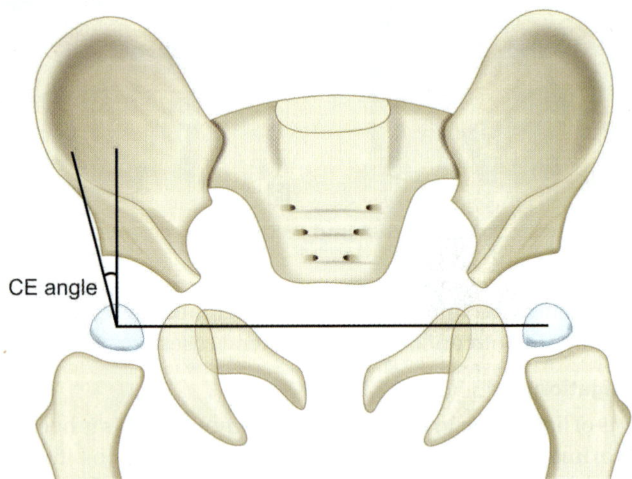

Fig. 12.59: Center edge (CE) angle of Wiberg

stability (i.e. Ortolani and Barlow tests become negative). Then wean off the infant over next 6 weeks by prescribing it for only night time wear.

2. *Hip is found dislocated*: If recheck findings suggest that reduction has not been achieved then closed reduction followed by spica casting (*read below*) is opted. If patient will be continued on Pavlik harness despite finding an unreduced hip at 3–6 weeks, "Pavlik disease" may develop (erosion of pelvis just superior to acetabulum) that interferes subsequently with closed reduction attempts.

---

*On abducting the femur, head will fall into the acetabulum achieving reduction.

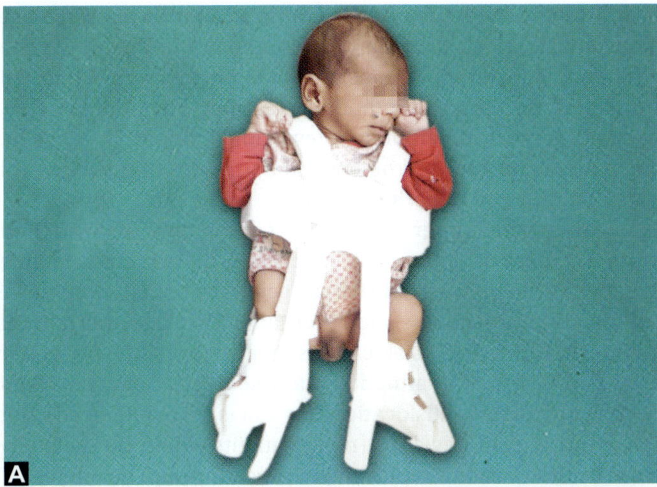

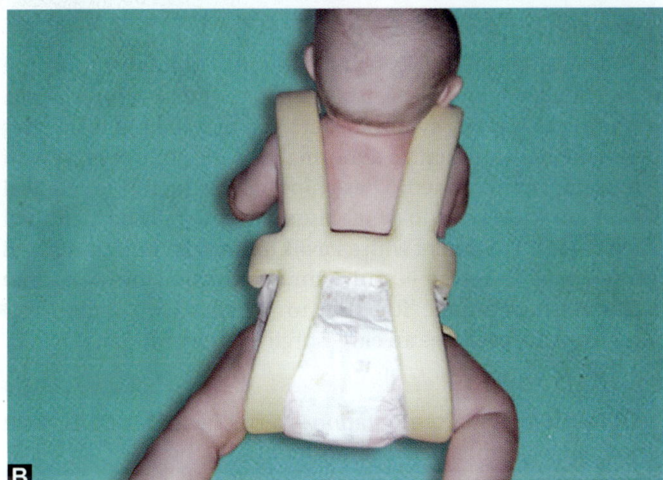

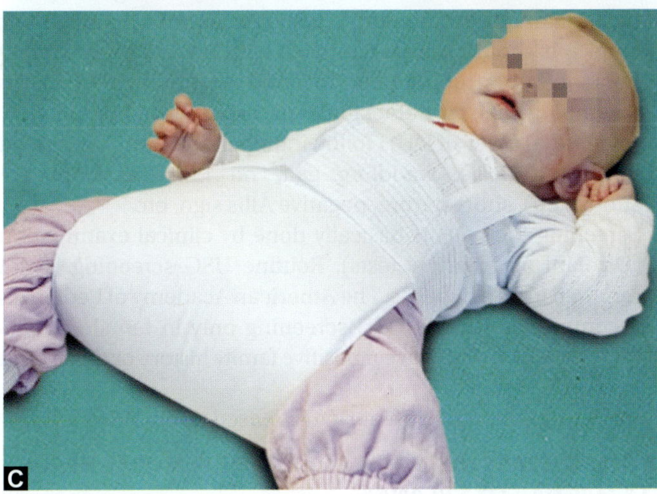

Figs 12.60A to C: (A) Pavlik harness; (B) von Rosen splint;
(C) Frejka pillow
Courtesy **(Fig. 12.60B):** Dr. Zeeshan Khan, JN Medical College, AMU.
Courtesy **(Fig. 12.60C):** John Furnes, SITZ ApS, Denmark. *www.siz.dk*).

Important complications to look for during Pavlik harness (abduction orthoses) use include:

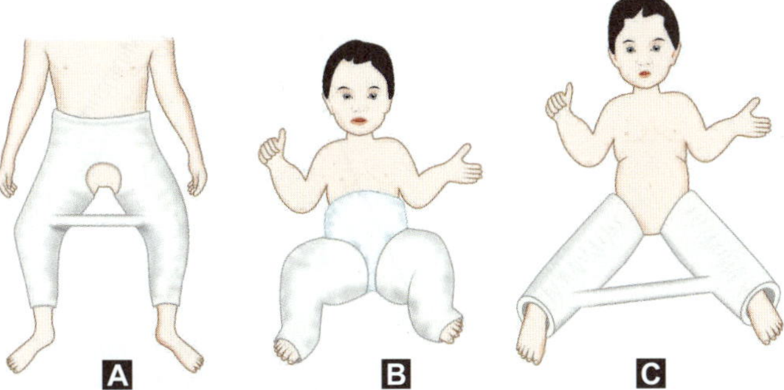

Figs 12.61A to C: (A) Hip spica; (B) Frog leg; (C) Bachelor's cast

- *Transient femoral nerve palsy*: Develops in those where excessive flexion (>110°) is needed to maintain reduction.
- *Avascular necrosis (AVN) of the femoral head*: Develops in those where excessive abduction (>50°) that compresses posterosuperior retinacular branches of medial circumflex femoral artery, is needed to maintain reduction.

Age 6–18 Months

Method of reduction: A trial of closed reduction (confirmed on table under c-arm) under anesthesia is given. However, at times closed reduction fails as the acetabulum is filled with fibrous tissue. This necessitates open reduction. Preoperatively a short period of traction (role still controversial) or an adductor tenotomy (if adduction contracture is present) performed during closed reduction, has been cited to be useful in facilitating reduction. Investigation of choice to confirm adequacy of reduction in this age and beyond (or once spica has been applied) is CT scan.

Maintenance of reduction: Pavlik harness is not effective in this age group, so a "hip spica cast" or "frog leg (Lorenz)" or "bachelor cast" for 3 months* is used **(Figs 12.61A to C)**. Reduction is deemed unacceptable and unstable in cast if with head in reduced position, the position of hip falls outside Ramsey's safe zone of abduction **(Fig. 12.62)**. Once the head is reduced (by flexing and abducting the hip) the hip is moved to maximum abduction possible. Now on adducting the hip, range at which hip dislocates is noted. A minimum safe zone more than 20° is desirable before hip dislocates when adducted. If safe zone is narrow, consider the patient for adductor tenotomy (to widen abduction and hence the safe zone). The reduced hip should ideally be maintained in cast in "human position" (90° hip flexion and 45° abduction) to minimize any complications (AVN or femoral nerve palsy).

Age 18 Months to 3 Years

The treatment in this age group is essentially the same as mentioned above except that open reduction is generally the initial treatment (closed reduction attempts have been associated with high incidence of AVN) followed by spica casting in abduction. The surgery is generally done through an anterior approach (Somervillie approach) so as to ensure least risk to the medial circumflex femoral artery (that lies posteriorly), the dominant vessel carrying blood to the femoral head. A femoral shortening should be considered if open reduction is being performed in child over 2 years of age to release any undue pressure that the head

---

*Spica should be changed once at 6 weeks.

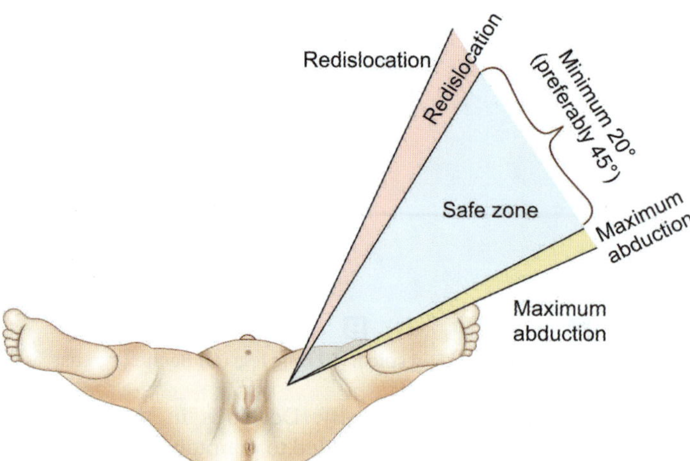

Fig. 12.62: Ramsey's safe zone concept

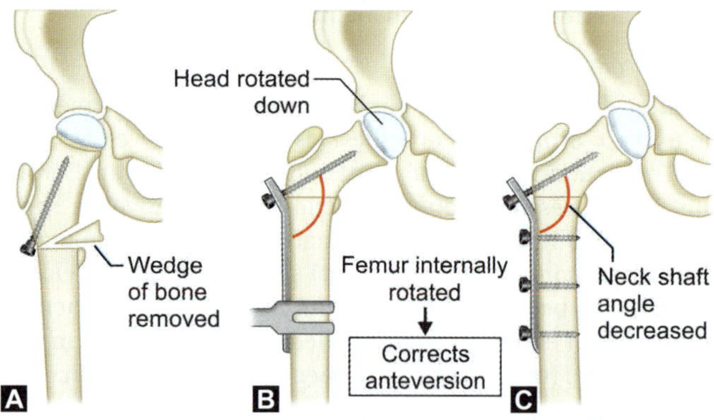

Figs 12.63A to C: Femoral derotation osteotomy

might be subjected to as it is brought down to fit the acetabulum. And once head is reduced stability should be assessed on table. If hip requires flexion and abduction for stability (i.e. anterolateral acetabular coverage is deficient), an acetabular reconstructive procedure (*read below*) should be added. On the other hand, if hip requires extreme abduction and internal rotation for stability (i.e. increased femoral neck anteversion and coxa valga are causing problem) to relocate during surgery, femoral subtrochanteric varus derotation osteotomy **(Figs 12.63A to C)** is done to provide inherent abduction-internal rotation to proximal femur to ensure head stays reduced.

Age 3 years and Above

After this age the development potential of acetabulum is no longer there. So even if the head is reduced and maintained, once the maintenance brace is removed the head would dislocate again. So children older than 3 years of age invariably need an additional bony procedure (either a femoral derotation or an acetabular reconstructive osteotomy) after open reduction to ensure head stays in the acetabulum even if further development is not there.

Choice of femoral or acetabular ostetomies is largely surgeon-dependent.* If on preoperative X-rays the acetabular index is high (i.e. acetabular coverage is deficient) an acetabular reconstructive procedure is generally chosen. These acetabular reconstructive

procedures or pelvic osteotomies **(Table 12.6)** basically decrease the acetabular index to better accommodate the head. On the other hand, if acetabular index is close to normal range, femoral subtrochanteric varus derotation osteotomy (to address coxa valga and increased femoral anteversion) should be chosen. Many patients may have problems on both sides of the joint and need a combination of both procedures.

As far as the upper age limit of reduction of head and performing these osteotomies is concerned, there is considerable debate. Children up to age of 10 years generally benefit from these reconstructive procedures, however, after that age the natural outcome of untreated dislocations might probably be better than the outcome of treatment. So a wise neglect may be opted especially for bilateral dislocations (as gait is more balanced), but when arthritis pain develops (most patients would be skeletally mature by then), a joint replacement procedure can be offered.

Teratological Dislocation of Hip

This is a severe form of DDH where the patient has a congenital neuromuscular paralytic disorder (e.g. meningomyelocele, arthrogryposis, Larsen syndrome, etc.) so that the hip dislocates in utero, the development is abnormal and the child is born with the deformity almost fixed. These hips are irreducible on clinical examination and a pseudoacetabulum can generally be identified on their X-rays. Treatment with a Pavlik harness is contraindicated in these cases (harness is a dynamic abduction orthoses that requires normal muscle function to be effective), rather, this severer form necessitates an early surgical intervention.

HIGH-YIELD POINTS

- Although fetal malpresentation is a risk factor for DDH, twin pregnancy is not a risk factor.
- *Neolimbus* refers to thickened articular cartilage over the posterolateral acetabulum (responsible for characteristic clunk). It should not be confused with inverted limbus that refers to hypertrophied and inverted labrum in DDH that is a pathological factor blocking a successful closed reduction.
- In bilateral cases of DDH following signs are seen—increased lumbar lordosis, waddling gait, no LLD (as both are shortened), short stature, negative Allis sign, etc.
- Screening for DDH is basically done by clinical examination (Ortolani and Barlow tests). Routine USG screening is not required in all newborns. The American Academy of Pediatrics recommends routine USG screening only in female infants (at 4–6 weeks) who have a positive family history or those born in breech position.
- Kashiwagi classification of DDH is based upon MRI findings.

PERTHES DISEASE (OSTEOCHONDRITIS OF FEMORAL HEAD/COXA MAGNA/COXA PLANA)

Introduction

This disorder of a growing child characterized by avascular necrosis (osteonecrosis) of the femoral head was described almost at same time (1910) by three different scientists—Legg (USA), Calve (France) and Perthes (Germany), hence better known as Legg-Calve-Perthes disease. The condition affects children in the age range of 4–10 years.

---

*Some surgeons like to go with femoral osteotomy in children below 4 years while in those who are older they prefer to choose pelvic-acetabular osteotomies.

Table 12.6: Acetabular reconstruction procedures **(Figs 12.64A to G)**

Osteotomy	Age	Procedure	Requirement
Salter's innominate osteotomy (most commonly performed procedure)	18 months to 6 years	Transiliac osteotomy (above the acetabulum) which passes through the greater sciatic notch. Acetabulum rotates hinging at the pubic symphysis (in older children pubic symphysis does not rotate well) improving coverage of the head. It requires temporary internal fixation and corrects acetabular index maximum to 15°	Concentric hip reduction* Triradiate cartilage should be open
Pemberton's acetabuloplasty	18 months to 10 years	It is curved osteotomy starting just above the anterior inferior iliac spine. It hinges at the triradiate cartilage. No internal fixation is required and >15° of acetabular index correction can be achieved. However, a demerit is that acetabular volume is decreased	Concentric hip reduction* Triradiate cartilage should be open
Dega	3–8 years	Transiliac osteotomy that hinges on an intact posteromedial iliac cortex (not sciatic notch as Salter). Intact notch allows better stability (limits internal fixation use). It is favored in neuromuscular conditions. Demerit is acetabular volume is reduced	Concentric hip reduction* Best results when triradiate cartilage is open. Can be done with fused cartilage also
Steel (Triple osteotomy)	Above 8 years	Acetabular reorientation procedure where an osteotomy of both rami is added to Salter's procedure	Concentric hip reduction* Triradiate cartilage should be open
Shelf procedure (Staheli)	Above 8 years (adolescents and skeletally mature)	Lateral acetabular augmentation is performed by adding extra-articular shelf of bone to. Fibrocartilage metaplasia occurs to provide eventual support tissue for the subluxated femoral head	Non-concentric hip Triradiate cartilage can be open or closed
Ganz (Bernese)	Above 8 years (adolescents and skeletally mature)	Triplanar periacetabular osteotomy allowing large amount of correction (3D correction) without altering shape of true pelvis. Immediate crutch walking is possible	Fused triradiate cartilage
Chiari	Above 8 years (adolescents and skeletally mature)	Salvage procedure is done when concentric reduction of head is not possible. It is transverse osteotomy just above acetabulum to greater sciatic notch, with medialization of acetabulum. Depends on fibrocartilaginous metaplasia	Non-concentric hip Fused triradiate cartilage

*Femoral head and acetabular opposing surfaces should be congruent on X-ray.

Incidence

- One in 10,000
- Boys affected five times more commonly than girls
- Bilateral in 10% cases.

Etiology

Exact cause is unknown but the common underlying feature is ischemia of the head (Caffey's hypothesis).

Factors linked to causation of this ischemia include:

- Coagulopathies (protein C and S deficiency, factor V Leiden mutation)
- Sickle cell anemia
- Hereditary (mutation in type II collagen)
- Hyperactivity (attention deficit hyperactivity disorder —ADHD)
- Passive smoking
- Trauma
- Sequelae of synovitis (controversial).

Pathogenesis

The characteristic age range (4–10 years) is related to the variation in blood supply of femoral head with age (**Fig. 12.65** and Page 119). From birth till 4 years of age supply is from retinacular (lateral epiphyseal) as well as metaphyseal vessels, after 8 years of age supply from vessels from ligamentum teres takes over. So, during the age 4–10 years, supply is mostly from retinacular vessels only. This single source during this age range renders the head susceptible to ischemia if any insult or predisposing factor comes up.

It is postulated that the inciting event may be traumatic or an episode of transient synovitis (**Flow chart 12.2**), but this remains to be proved.

Pathology

The course of the disease is divided into four stages (Waldenstrom classification):

1. *Ischemia*: Ischemia leads to necrosis of ossific nucleus, which stops growing and becomes dense.
2. *Revascularization and repair*: Dead bone is then slowly resorbed and replaced by new bone during the repair process in an attempt to restore normal shape. However, during this repair stage the soft head deforms under pressure. This stage is also known as fragmentation stage.
3. *Repair (reossification)*: If the repair is rapid head shape returns to normal. In other situations, epiphysis collapses and head becomes flattened (mushroom-shaped/coxa plana) and enlarges (coxa magna).
4. *Healed*: Gradual return to normal architecture.

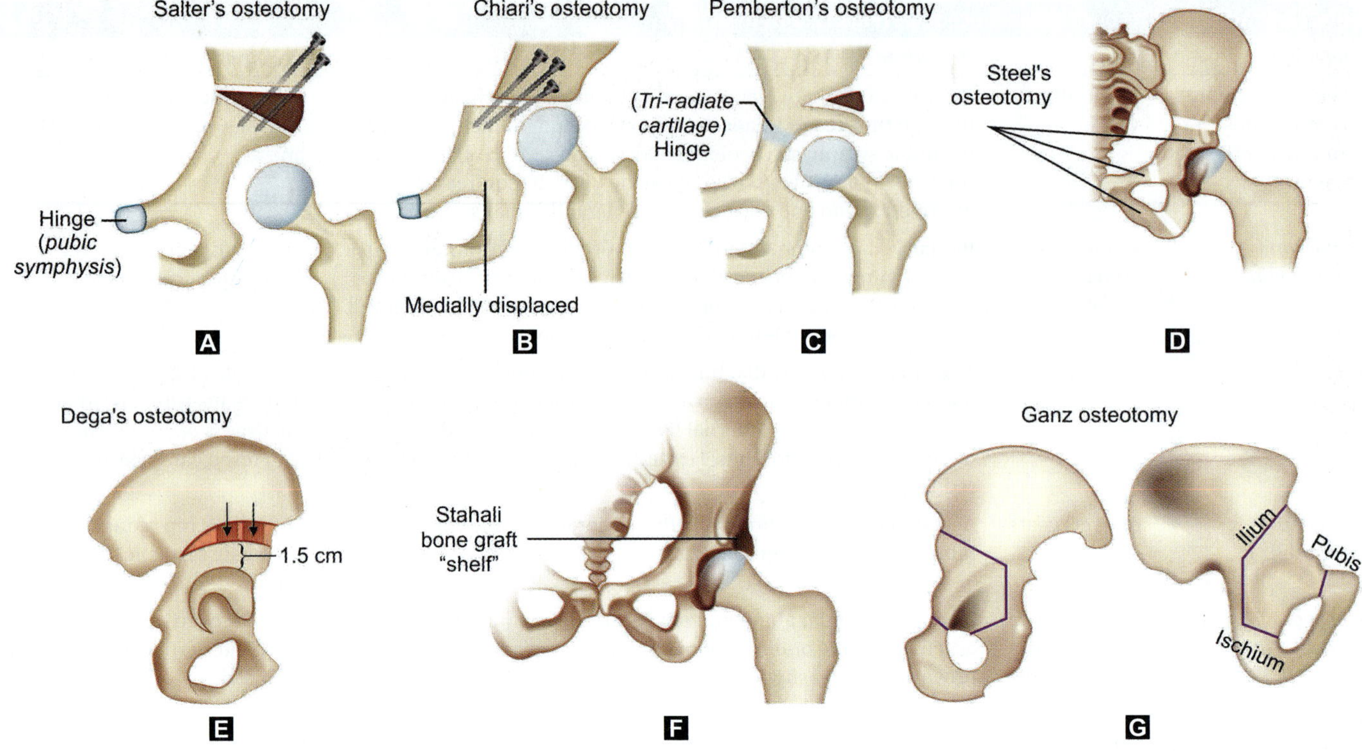

Figs 12.64A to G: Some important pelvic osteotomies (acetabular reconstruction procedures)

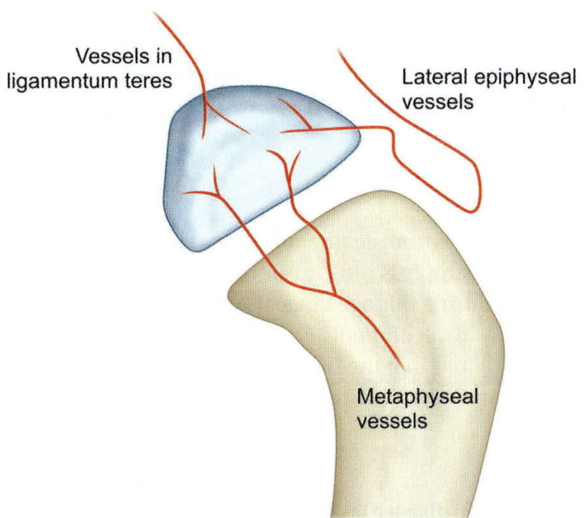

Fig. 12.65: Pathogenesis of Perthes disease (blood supply of femoral head)

Flow chart 12.2: Pathogenesis of ischemia of femoral head in Perthes disease.

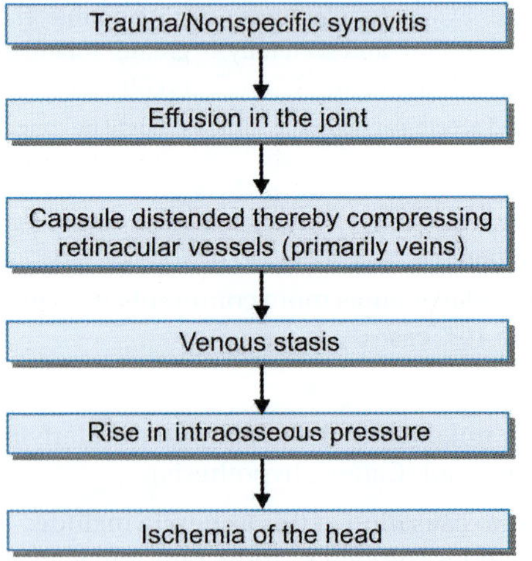

Clinical Features

This disease characteristically has a waxing and waning course, with periods of alleviation and exacerbation of symptoms. Most common presenting complaint is limp. Classically, a painless limp is present but there may be pain during the periods of exacerbation. Second most common complaint is pain in the hip (may be referred to knee). There is limitation of abduction and internal rotation in severe cases. When the hip is flexed, it may go into obligatory external rotation (Catterall sign). On examination, Trendelenburg test is positive (as the head is flattened there is upward migration of greater trochanter which slackens the gluteus medius). One may also note shortening of the affected limb.

Radiographic Features

In the early course the X-ray may be normal with only widening of the joint space appreciated. As the head undergoes ischemia and bone death, the area becomes sclerotic (appears radiodense) and starts fragmenting **(Fig. 12.66A)**. Eventually the head collapses, becomes flattened (mushroom-shaped) and enlarged (coxa magna) **(Fig. 12.66B)**. Some other X-ray signs that may aid the diagnosis include Gage sign **(Fig. 12.66A,** a radiolucent V-shaped area can be appreciated in the lateral part of femoral head epiphysis

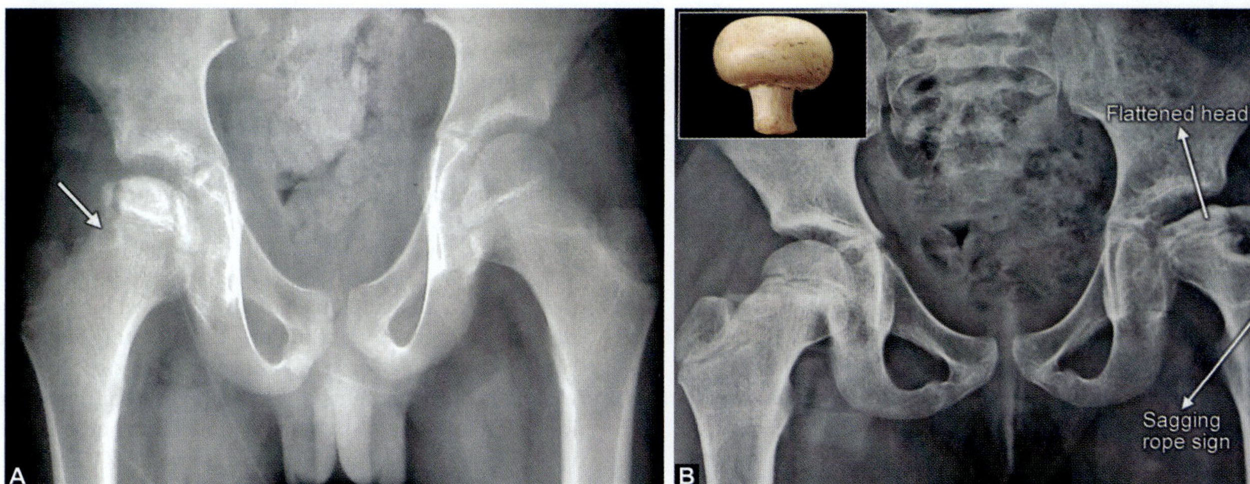

Figs 12.66A and B: Radiological signs of Perthes disease (A) fragmented head with Gage sign;
(B) Mushroom-shaped head, Gage sign and sagging rope sign

and adjacent metaphysis) and sagging rope sign (**Fig. 12.66B,** a thin radio-opaque line in upper femoral metaphysis. It indicates damage to growth plate with marked metaphyseal reaction).

Bone scan detects changes quite early in the course of disease but MRI is the investigation of choice and detects the changes at the earliest.

Classification Systems

Important classification systems are:
- *Catterall classification*: It is based on the amount of epiphysis involved. It classifies the disease in four stages ranging from stage I (only anterior part of head is involved) to stage IV (whole of the head is involved).
- *Salter Thompson classification*: It classifies into two groups based on extent of head involved in X-rays, Group A (less than half of head involved) and Group B (more than half).
- *Herring's lateral pillar classification (**Figs 12.67A to C**)*: It is most commonly used classification nowadays to guide the treatment. It is based on the height of the lateral pillar of the head (the head being divided into medial central and lateral pillars).
  - Group A—no loss of height in lateral pillar
  - Group B—more than 50% height maintained
  - Group C—less than 50% height maintained.
- *Stulberg classification*: It is a prognostic classification based on the final appearance of head and its relation to acetabulum (roundness of head and its congruency in relation to acetabulum) in the healed stage. Spherical congruent head has best outcome and aspherical noncongruent head has poorest outcome.

Differential Diagnosis

The most important differentials to consider are tuberculosis (TB) of hip and multiple epiphyseal dysplasia (MED). While early acetabular involvement on radiography favors a diagnosis of TB, a bilateral involvement and involvement of other epiphysis favors MED (*see* Page 392). Transient synovitis of the hip is another close differential and has been discussed later. One must also not miss

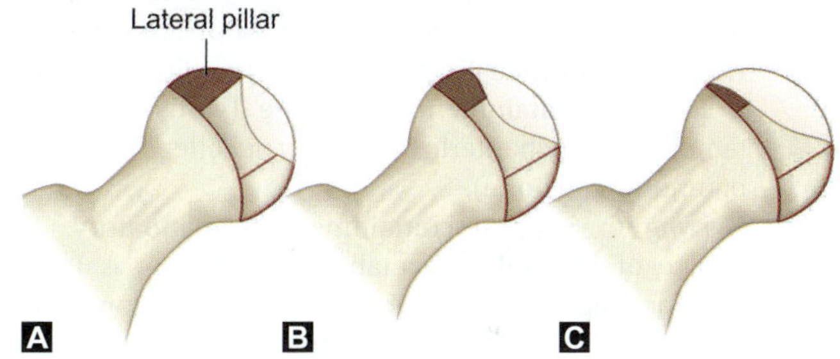

Figs 12.67A to C: Herring's classification

excluding causes that may cause AVN of femoral head in adults (*see* Page 446).

Management

Perthes disease is a self-limiting condition and treatment of the condition revolves around the concept of biological plasticity of the femoral head. During the avascular phase (stage of ischemia) the head is soft and collapses under the weight-bearing forces. By offloading the head (by bed rest) compressive forces can be redistributed to initiate spontaneous repair (owing to growth potential in pediatric age group) and by ensuring containment of head within the acetabulum (abduction braces or surgery) remodeling can be facilitated. However, if weight-bearing is continued, a pathological dislocation will eventually ensue as a flat head cannot be contained in a curved acetabulum. Keeping in mind the above principles, treatment can simply be summarized as per the age of presentation.

Age Less Than 6 Years

Conservative treatment suffices in this age. Bed rest is advocated to the child (skin traction can be applied to ensure this in a child) to ensure no pathological dislocation occurs. Analgesics may be given for a short period to alleviate the pain.

Age 6–9 Years

In this category bone age of the patient is calculated and Herring's lateral pillar classification is used to decide appropriate treatment.

Box 12.5: Catterall head at risk signs (seen on X-ray)

- Gage sign present
- Calcification present lateral to the femoral head epiphysis
- Lateral subluxation of head there
- Horizontally lying growth plate
- Cysts visible in metaphysis of femur

- *Bone age less than 6 years:*
    - *Herring A*: Conservative treatment as mentioned above is followed.
    - *Herring B and C*: An abduction orthosis is additionally prescribed to ensure head remains contained in the acetabulum. A variety of orthoses are available. They can be weight-relieving but non-ambulatory (e.g. Broomstick plaster cast) or those allowing ambulation (e.g. Petrie cast, Scottish rite orthosis, etc.).
- *Bone age more than 6 years:*
    - *Herring A and B*: Abduction brace generally suffices in most patients. However, those who have "head at risk" signs on their X-ray **(Box 12.5)** additionally need a surgical containment procedure (varus derotation femoral subtrochanteric osteotomy or Salter's osteotomy of innominate bone).
    - *Herring C*: Surgical containment is mandatory. The choice of femoral or acetabular osteotomy is largely surgeon-dependent. While a femoral osteotomy **(Fig. 12.63A)** is a simpler procedure yet it offers better containment, it may result in Trendelenburg limp (as trochanter is pushed up) and limb shortening. Acetabular osteotomy **(Fig. 12.63B)** on the other hand offers better hip mobility and less alterations in limb length, however, it is technically more demanding and may result in chondrolysis (necrosis of joint cartilage) owing to increased pressure over the femoral head.

Age More Than 9 Years

The results are highly guarded after this age and surgery often needed is a combination of both femoral and acetabular osteotomies.

Prognostic Factors

Presence of following factors marks a bad prognosis in Perthes disease:

- *Higher age at onset (most important factor):* While children below 6 years have mild disease, those above 9 years have worst outcome)
- Patients with bilateral disease
- Presence of Catterall head at risk signs **(Box 12.5)**
- Extensive subchondral fracture lines seen
- Aspherical incongruent head (Stulberg classification)
- Lateral pillar C (Herring classification).

TRANSIENT SYNOVITIS (TOXIC SYNOVITIS/OBSERVATION HIP/ IRRITABLE HIP)

Introduction

It is a self-limiting acute inflammation of synovium of hip joint (synovitis) occurring commonly in children between the age group of 4–10 years (mean age at onset is 6 years). Most cases are unilateral (95%), occur twice as frequently in boys as in girls. Right and left hips are equally affected.

Etiology

The exact cause is unknown. Most children give a history of viral upper respiratory tract infection. History of trauma may also be there.

Clinical Features

Child presents with an acute onset of hip pain and limp (antalgic gait). Hip is held in flexion, abduction and external rotation due to the effusion (position of ease as joint volume is maximum). The terminal ranges of movements at hip are painful and restricted. Condition is characterized by conspicuous absence of a high-grade fever. Temperature is rarely more than 38.5°C. Laboratory investigations [white blood cell (WBC) counts, erythrocyte sedimentation rate (ESR), C-reactive protein (CRP), etc.] are generally within normal limits. Child is not as toxic looking as in a fulminant condition like septic arthritis. Blood culture is sterile. Joint aspirate is sterile.

Investigations

X-rays: Usually are normal, except for the widening of medial joint space due to effusion in some cases.

Ultrasonography: Shows effusion of hip (non-echogenic). USG-guided aspiration of the hip is the investigation of choice to support the diagnosis and more importantly, to exclude a possible septic arthritis of hip.

Differential Diagnosis

- *Septic arthritis*: The most important differential diagnosis is septic arthritis. It is important to differentiate between the two because the diagnosis of septic arthritis warrants emergent surgery (arthrotomy with joint lavage) to save the hip joint, whereas synovitis can be managed conservatively. The most definitive way of differentiating between the two is aspiration of the hip and analysis of aspirate. Joint aspirate reveals more than 50,000 WBCs/mm^3 with 90% neutrophils. Gram stain and culture of joint aspirate may show bacteria. Although Kocher's criteria **(Box 12.6)** reliably differentiates the two condition, few points that favor septic arthritis over transient synovitis are:
    - Sick looking or toxic child
    - Fever greater than 38.5°C
    - All range of movements are painful (cf terminal range of movements painful)
    - Raised CRP, ESR, WBC counts
    - Positive blood culture
    - Ultrasonography showing echogenic effusion.
- *Osteomyelitis of proximal femur*: Features suggesting diagnosis of it are swelling of proximal thigh, elevated WBC count, elevated ESR and CRP, febrile child, X-rays showing initially soft tissue swelling and later periosteal reaction and bone destruction.
- *Perthes disease*: The course is more protracted (usually more than 6 weeks in Perthes as opposed to a week or so in transient synovitis). Radiographic widening of joint space is more characteristic of Perthes disease than of transient

Box 12.6: Kocher's criteria*

Patient not able to bear weight on affected extremity
- Fever > 38.5°C
- Erythrocyte sedimentation rate (ESR) > 40
- White blood cell (WBC) count > 12,000/mm^3

* Score ≥ 3 signifies > 90% probability of septic arthritis.

synovitis. All laboratory work-up is within normal limits in Perthes disease also, so differentiation is best made on X-rays (smaller femoral head and subsequently increased density of head). It is said that 1–3% of children with an episode of transient synovitis may progress to Perthes disease.
- *Juvenile rheumatoid arthritis (JRA)*: See chapter 16 for details about this condition.

Treatment

Patient is advised bed rest with traction and nonsteroidal anti-inflammatory drugs (NSAIDs) (for relieving muscle spasm and reducing pain). The patient must be kept under observation (observation hip). The condition is self-limiting. Most patients are symptom-free by 2 weeks and condition resolves by itself.

HIGH-YIELD POINTS

- Transient synovitis > Septic arthritis > Perthes disease is the most common cause of painful limp in a child less than 10 years of age.
- Order of investigations when an inflammatory hip joint swelling is suspected:
  X-ray → USG-guided aspiration of joint fluid → MRI.
- *Caffey's sign*: This refers to loss of sphericity of femoral head along with presence of a subchondral fracture line typically in weight-bearing anterolateral part of the femoral head on radiograph of patients with Perthes disease.
- Arthrodiastasis (distraction of a joint) is a relatively new treatment for Perthes disease. Here a distraction force is maintained across hip joint by an external fixator. It is postulated that by creating a space between the articulating surfaces, mechanical stress is minimized and the synovial circulation improves. This encourages fibrous repair of defects of articular cartilage and preservation of a congruent femoral head.

SLIPPED CAPITAL FEMORAL EPIPHYSIS

Introduction

Slipped capital femoral epiphysis (SCFE) refers to displacement or slipping of the femoral capital epiphysis (femoral head epiphysis) from its normal position relative to the neck. In true sense, the capital epiphysis (femoral head) remains seated in the acetabulum, the physis disrupts and the neck rotates anteriorly **(Figs 12.68A and B)**. The slip characteristically occurs during the period of rapid growth spurt (puberty) when the physis is relatively weak and excessive body weight results in excessive shear forces on the physis, causing it to disrupt.

Incidence

- Boys of age 12–15 years and girls of age 11–13 years are commonly affected
- Male: female = 2:1
- Bilateral in 20–40% cases.

Etiology

Majority of patients have no underlying cause. But some have associated conditions like hypothyroidism (most common), panhypopituitarism, hypogonadism, growth hormone excess, craniopharyngioma. Single most important risk factor for SCFE is obesity.

Typical body habitus is short, fat and sexually immature child nearing puberty. There is disparity between the growth hormone (pituitary) and gonadal hormone levels. While the former try to cause physeal hypertrophy the latter try to achieve physeal maturation. Imbalance makes the physis unable to resist shearing stresses generated by body weight thereby causing slipping of capital epiphysis **(Flow chart 12.3)**.

Clinical Features

Slips are classified as (Loder classification): Stable (child can bear weight on extremity) or unstable slip (child not able to bear weight). They can also be classified as "acute (<3 weeks)", "chronic (>3 weeks)", or "acute on chronic". Chronic slips are the most common. In acute slips classical presentation is an adolescent

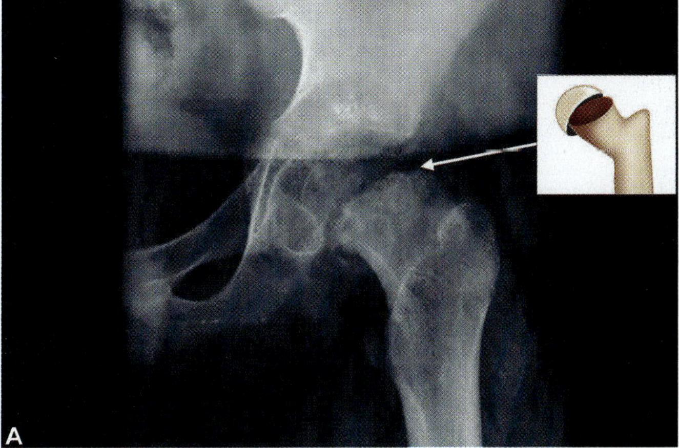
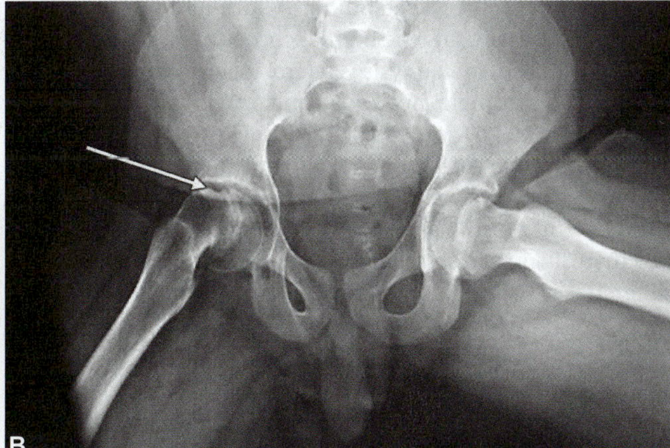

Figs 12.68A and B: (A) X-ray left hip; and (B) X-ray pelvis with both hips anteroposterior (AP) view showing slipped femoral epiphysis (arrow)

Courtesy: Dr Nitin Agarwal (JN Medical College, AMU).

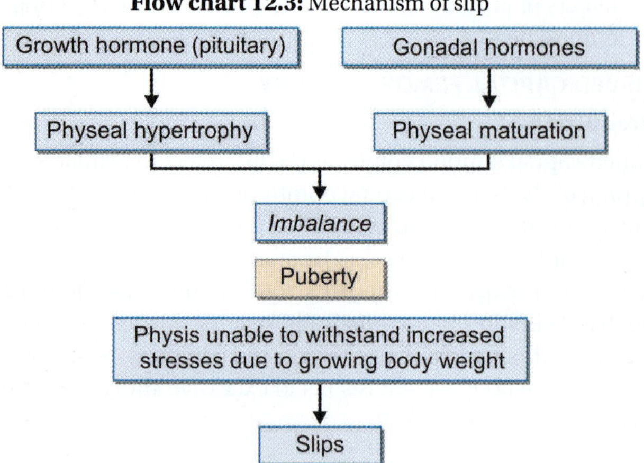

Flow chart 12.3: Mechanism of slip

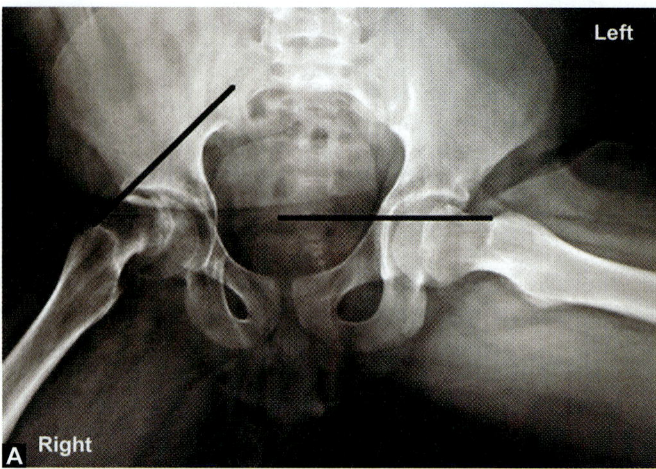

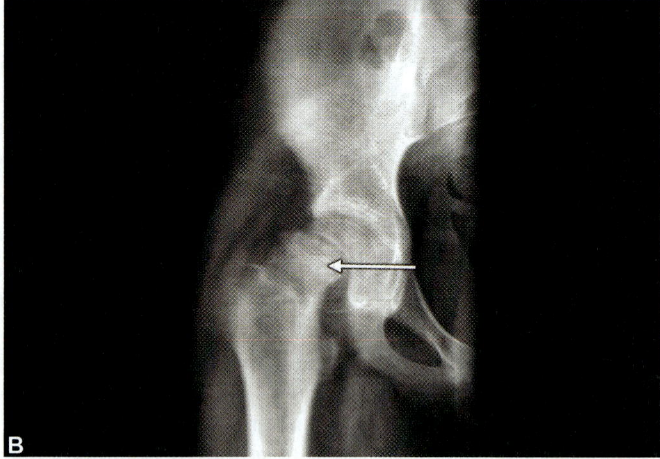

Figs 12.69A and B: (A) Trethowan sign (on right side); (B) Metaphyseal blanch sign (arrow)

child, typically short and fat, complaining of groin pain and antalgic limp. Excessive external rotation of involved side during walking (out-toeing gait) is characteristic. Restricted abduction and internal rotation are noted on examination. When the hip is flexed it goes into obligatory external rotation, this is called as "axis deviation". Some degree of shortening of affected extremity is there.

Radiographic Features

X-rays: Earliest sign is wide and irregular physis with rarefaction in its juxtaepiphyseal region (preslip). Slip is best seen in a frog leg lateral X-ray view of the affected hip. Grading can also be done based on distance of slip. Up to one-third slip is mild, one-third to two-thirds is moderate and more than two-thirds is severe.

Some other important X-ray signs in SCFE include:
- Trethowan sign: Normally, a line drawn along the superior border of neck (Klein's line), should intersect some part of epiphysis (head). But is SCFE, this line intersects a very small part of epiphysis or not at all **(Fig. 12.69A)**.
- Metaphyseal blanch sign of steel **(Fig. 12.69B)** is a crescent-shaped area of increased density overlying the metaphysis (neck) adjacent to physis. It is due to posterior slippage of epiphysis in relation to metaphysis.
- Scham sign is the loss of dense triangular appearance of inferomedial neck (normally appears dense as it overlaps the posterior wall of acetabulum). Normally the posterior acetabular margin cuts the medial corner of metaphysis, but in SCFE whole of metaphysis is lateral to acetabular margin.
- Southwick's slip angle (head shaft angle in both AP and lateral views) **(Fig. 12.70)** is a measure of severity of slip. It is an angle between axis of femoral shaft and a line perpendicular to the base of epiphysis. The difference between affected and contralateral normal side depicts the severity. Difference of less than 30° is mild slip, 3060° is moderate and more than 60° difference is severe slip.

Computed tomography: It is usually not necessary for diagnosis. However, it can provide a more accurate measurement of slip angle than plain radiographs.

Magnetic resonance imaging: It detects physeal widening and irregularity when X-rays and CT are negative. It can detect disease in preslip stage and hence provides the earliest diagnosis.

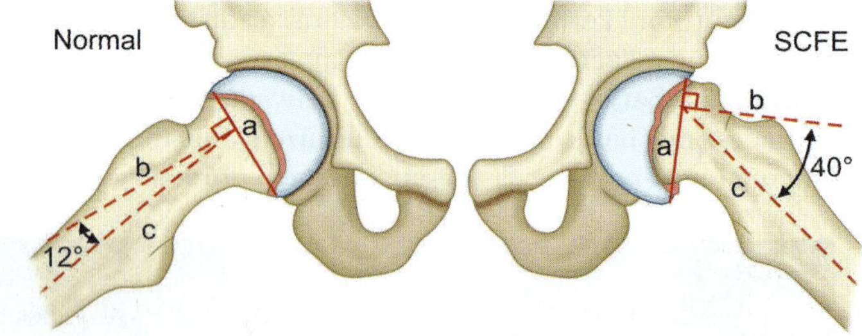

Fig. 12.70: Southwick's angle

Ultrasonography: It is relatively least useful but may show joint effusion and a step between head and neck of femur.

Treatment

Primary aim is to prevent further slip and promote closure of physis. Reduction of existing slip is not always possible and may even be harmful (causes AVN). So, *in situ* pinning (fixing slip with smooth pins or screws) is the preferred treatment in chronic slips that are mild or moderate grade **(Fig. 12.71)**. Severe chronic slips may need corrective osteotomy. In acute slips, gentle reduction may be tried, followed by in situ pinning.

HIGH-YIELD POINTS

- The physeal disruption in SCFE occurs through the hypertrophic zone of the cartilage.
- Important complications of unstable slips: avascular necrosis of head and chondrolysis (lysis of the articular cartilage of hip joint diagnosed radiologically by less than 3 mm wide joint space).
- *Idiopathic chondrolysis of hip (ICH)*: In some cases, more commonly in females, loss of articular cartilage (joint space on X-ray < 3 mm) occurs without obvious reasons and they constitute the entity ICH. Condition is postulated to be autoimmune but exact etiology is unknown.

CONGENITAL COXA VARA

Introduction

Normal neck shaft angle of proximal femur in an adult is 125–135°. An angle less than 125° is called "coxa vara". Congenital coxa vara **(Table 12.7)** is caused by a primary cartilaginous defect in the inferomedial part of femoral neck (the cartilage remnant being called as "Fairbank's triangle"), which causes a defect in ossification of femoral neck **(Fig. 12.72)**. There is relative overgrowth of greater trochanter and a short femoral neck causing coxa vara with progressive shortening of the affected extremity. The varus deformity develops only once the child starts walking.

Incidence

- Males = Females
- Bilateral in 30–50% cases.

Clinical Features

Painless limp is the characteristic feature. Trendelenburg gait occurs due to upriding of greater trochanter with short limb component in unilateral cases, waddling gait is seen in bilateral cases. LLD in unilateral cases is mild (shortening is not more than 3 cm). The patient has restricted abduction and internal rotation. Absence of telescopy differentiates the condition from DDH, a close differential diagnosis.

Radiographic Features

- Neck shaft angle is decreased (<125°). The proximal femur gives appearance of a shepherd crook deformity (*see* Page 314).
- Triangular piece of bone in the medial femoral neck (Fairbanks triangle) bounded by two radiolucent lines forming an inverted V or inverted Y is a characteristic sign **(Fig. 12.72)**.
- *Hilgenreiner epiphyseal angle **(Fig. 12.73)***: This is an angle between Hilgenreiner line (horizontal line through triradiate cartilage) and a line parallel to physis. Normal is between 0° and 25°. It has prognostic value, more the Hilgenreiner epiphyseal angle poorer the prognosis.

Treatment

Treatment is based on Hilgenreiner epiphyseal angle:
- *Hilgenreiner epiphyseal angle less than 45°*: Observation (shortening is usually mild and can be dealt with shoe lift)
- *Hilgenreiner epiphyseal angle 45–59°*: Surgery or observation depending on symptoms (symptomatic limp or progressive deformity)
- *Hilgenreiner epiphyseal angle greater than 60°*: Surgery.

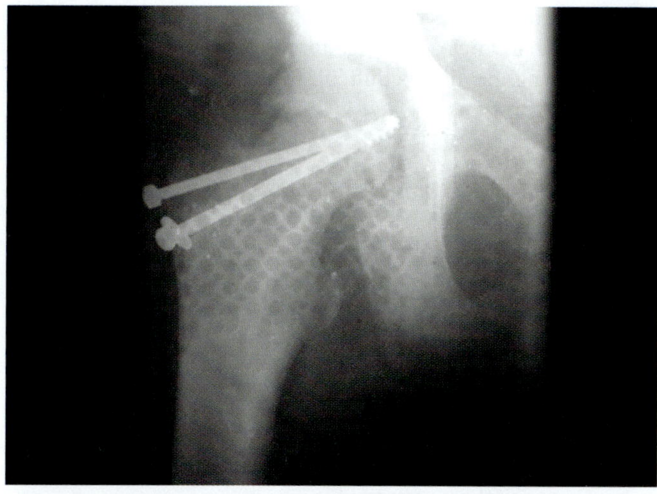

Fig. 12.71: *In situ* fixation of slipped capital femoral epiphysis (SCFE)

Table 12.7: Values of neck shaft angle in different age groups	
Age	*Neck shaft angle*
Birth	150°
3 years	145°
9 years	138°
Adult	125–135°

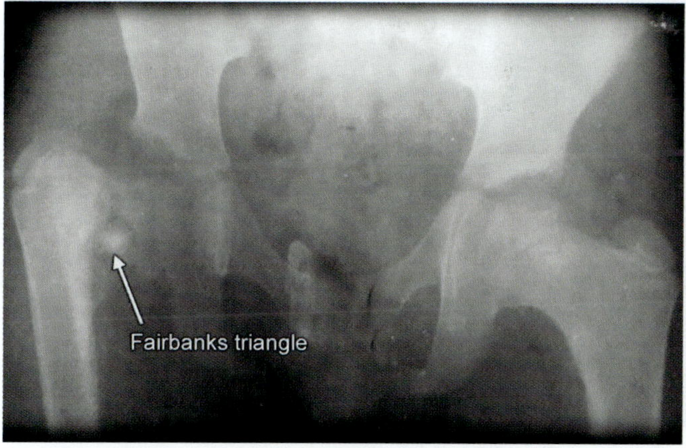

Fig. 12.72: Congenital coxa vara showing Fairbanks triangle

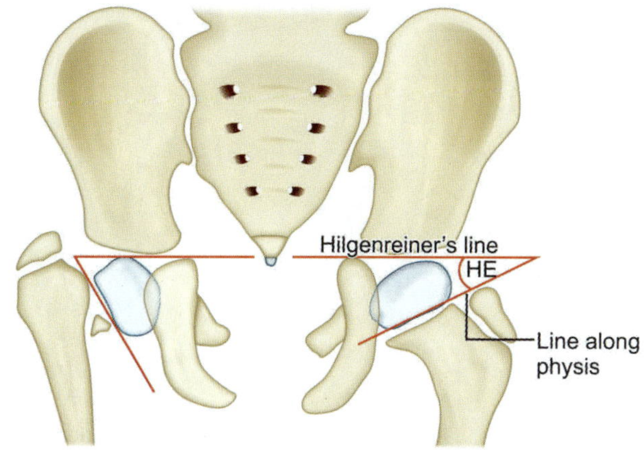

Fig. 12.73: Hilgenreiner epiphyseal (HE) angle

Surgery: Subtrochanteric valgus osteotomy is done **(Fig. 12.74)** to restore neck shaft angle. Ideal age for surgery is 4–5 years. Before this age, internal fixation is difficult in the cartilaginous femoral head.

HIGH-YIELD POINTS

- *Acquired coxa vara may be seen in:*
  - Perthes disease
  - Slipped capital femoral epiphysis
  - Developmental dysplasia of hip
  - Post-traumatic (neck femur fracture)
  - Postinfective (septic arthritis)
  - Fibrous dysplasia
  - Renal osteodystrophy
  - Osteogenesis imperfecta.
- *Cases where Fairbanks triangle is present:*
  - Congenital coxa vara
  - Nonunion fracture neck of femur
  - Perthes disease.

PROXIMAL FEMORAL FOCAL DEFICIENCY

Proximal femoral focal deficiency (PFFD) is a rare congenital deficiency that is characterized by varying degree of femoral and acetabular hypoplasia causing limb shortening. It is often associated with other abnormalities like fibular aplasia or hypoplasia (fibular hemimelia is the most common association), foot abnormalities, cruciate ligament deficiencies, patellar abnormalities, shortened tibia and fibula, etc. Child presents with short, flexed, abducted and externally rotated limb. Feet are usually normal.

On X-rays, hypoplasia ranges from short femur with coxa vara and bowing to complete absence of acetabulum and proximal femur **(Fig. 12.75)**. Aitken classification **(Figs 12.76A to D)** is used to classify the disease.

Treatment: Treatment should be individualized according to deformity. Children with bilateral deformities may be observed. In other children, treatment is usually difficult and may include amputation or arthrodesis and knee prosthesis, extension prosthesis, femoropelvic fusion, limb lengthening and contralateral epiphysiodesis and Van Ness rotation plasty (tibia is attached to the hip joint with the foot facing backward. A prosthesis is attached to foot such that now it acts as the knee, **Fig. 12.77**).

LIMB LENGTH DISCREPANCY

Inequality of limb length is a frequent concern with which many patients come to an orthopedic surgeon. While the scenario

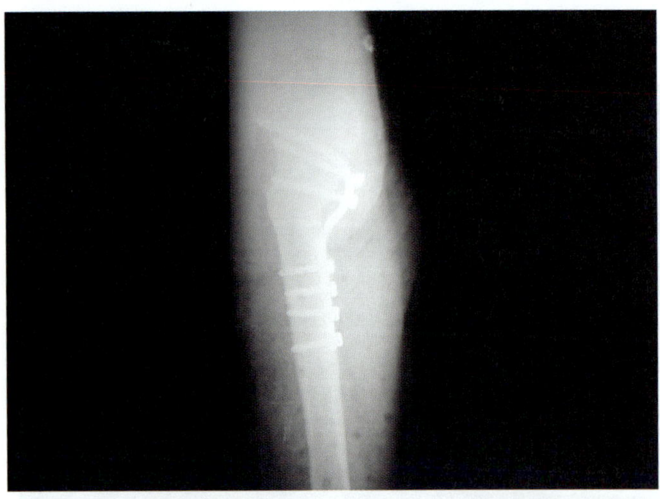

Fig. 12.74: Valgus osteotomy for coxa vara

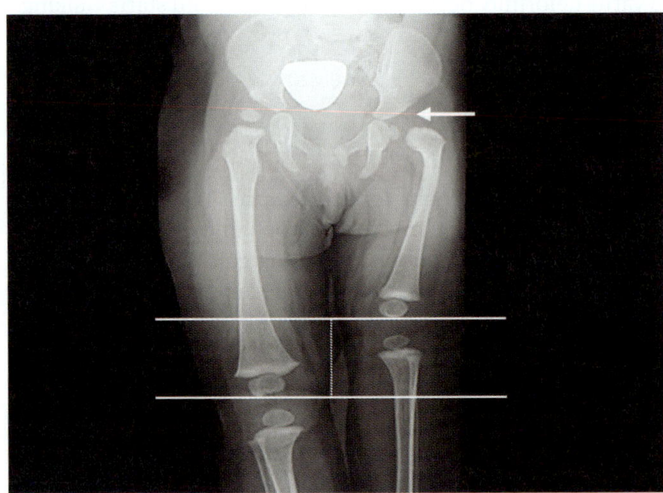

Fig. 12.75: Proximal focal femoral deficiency

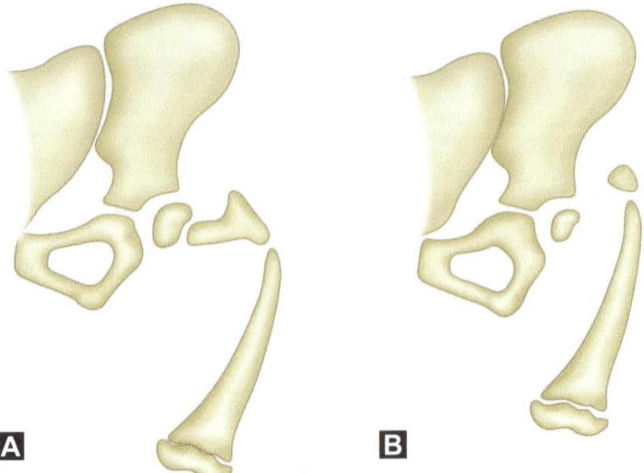

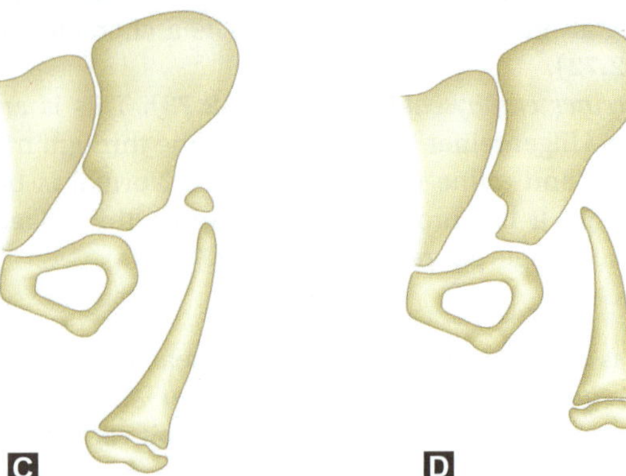

Figs 12.76A to D: Aitken's classification. In types A and B, femoral head and acetabulum are present but with varying amounts of dysplasia. In types C and D, there is no effective hip joint

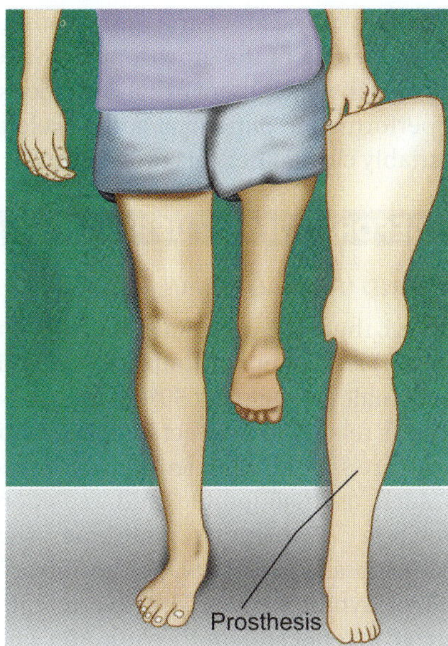

Fig. 12.77: Rotationplasty

commonly results as the pathological process causes shortening in the involved extremity, in rare cases, the cause may be lengthening on involved side. The common causes implicated in causing the discrepancy have been tabulated in **Box 12.7**.

Although the discrepancy in the upper limb is rarely a concern, limb length inequality in the lower limb may cause serious gait problems. The short leg compensates with toe walking (ankle equinus) or to balance patient may flex the knee on the normal side which over time may lead to fixed contractures. There may be increased chances of developing a chronic low back pain or a postural scoliosis. Hence, a surgeon needs to be familiar with methods of assessment of inequality and with methods that can predict the final discrepancy in skeletally immature people so that he can advise appropriate management.

Assessment of Limb Length Discrepancy

Assessment can be made on clinical as well as radiological grounds.

Clinical assessment: The best way to make clinical estimation of limb length inequality is by the graduated block method **(Figs 12.78A and B)**, where blocks of set height are placed under the affected side until the pelvis is leveled. An Allis/Galeazzi test **(Fig. 12.55B)** can then be performed to decipher whether the shortening is in femur or tibia.

Radiological assessment: Special full length AP radiographs of bilateral lower limbs (scanogram/orthoroentgenograms, **Fig. 12.79**) can be obtained while the patient stands on the graduated blocks to document the discrepancy. CT scan is even more accurate and is less sensitive to patient malpositioning. The latter is specifically indicated in case the patient has a knee flexion contracture (developed due to compensation).

Predicting the Discrepancy in Skeletally Immature

Growth at distal femur on an average is 9 mm/year. A number of methods have been described to predict the amount of growth remaining in the femur and the tibia in skeletally immature children.

Box 12.7: Causes of limb length inequality

Causes of shortening in affected limb
- Congenital causes
  - Congenital limb deficiencies (PFFD, hemimelia, etc.)
  - Congenital deformities (DDH, Perthes disease, coxa vara, congenital pseudoarthrosis, Blount's disease, etc.)
- Acquired causes
  - Trauma (amputations, fracture malunions, compound fractures with bone loss, physeal injuries, etc.)
  - Infections (osteomyelitis)
  - Tumors that may disrupt growth across physis (osteochondroma, bone cyst, enchondroma, etc.)
  - Paralytic disorders (e.g. poliomyelitis)
  - Irradiation

Causes of lengthening in affected extremity
- Postfemoral or tibial shaft fracture (especially in children)
- Soft tissue overgrowth syndromes (e.g. hemihypertrophy*, *Proteus* syndrome, Klippel-Trenaunay syndrome†, Beckwith-Wiedemann syndrome, etc.)

Abbreviations: PFFD, proximal femoral focal deficiency; DDH, developmental dysplasia of hip.

*The condition has strong association with neurofibromatosis and renal abnormalities (Wilms tumor).

†Klippel-Trenaunay syndrome involves overgrowth of extremities due to arteriovenous malformations occurring in association with cutaneous hemangiomas and varicosities.

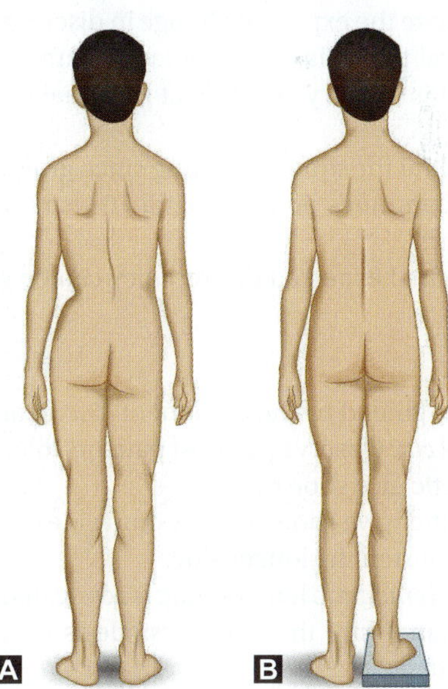

Figs 12.78A and B: Graduated block method to assess limb length discrepancy (LLD). Leg length inequality results in asymmetric iliac crest or posterior superior iliac spine heights when the patient is made to stand erect with knees straight and the feet flat on the floor. Graduated blocks of set height are put under the shorter limb till the pelvis is leveled. The height of block gives the estimation

- *Green-Anderson growth remaining method*: This calculation is based on data tabulated in complex tables that provide growth remaining in the extremity at different ages which can be matched to the patient to make a prediction.
- *Moseley' straight line graph*: Considered to be more accurate than Green-Anderson method. Data interpretation is simpler owing to graphic presentation.

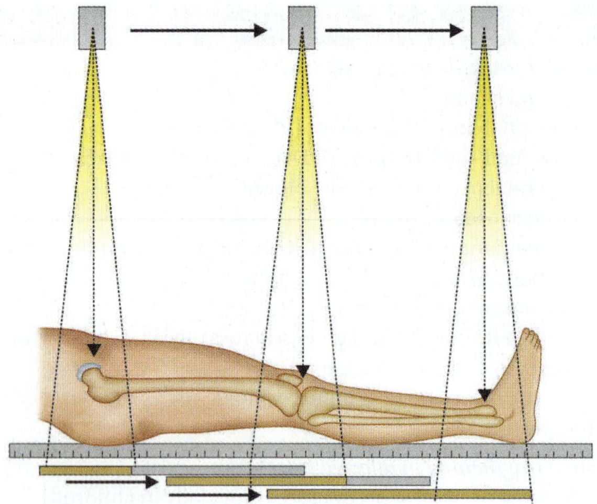

Fig. 12.79: A scanogram being performed. The tube is moved to take exposures at hip, knee and ankle while the cassette slides along to capture the image. In contrast, in orthoroentgenogram, the tube moves in similar fashion but a single long film is placed under the patient to capture radiograph of entire lower limb

- *Menelaus' method*: This is the most accurate method that is based on a mathematical formula:
  - Calculate the existing discrepancy, E
  - Calculate the expected change in discrepancy, C (growth at distal femur is on an average 9 mm/year, at proximal tibia it is 6 mm/year while at proximal femur it is 3 mm/year)
  - Calculate the time remaining since growth, T (growth in boys continues on average till 16 years while in girls till 14 years)
  - Now, final expected discrepancy can be given by: E + (T × C).

Management

Management is guided by the amount of discrepancy present:
- *Less than 2 cm:* Observe (as most patients tolerate this well). If symptomatic give shoe raise.*
- *2–5 cm:* Either give shoe raise on short side or go for epiphysiodesis to shorten the longer side.†
- *More than 5 cm:* Limb lengthening is advocated. If discrepancy is more than 7 cm, then epiphysiodesis on the longer side may be added.
- *More than 15–20 cm:* Lengthening of this amount is difficult to achieve. Consideration for a primary amputation followed by prosthetic fitting may be considered.

Methods of Limb Lengthening

- Distraction osteogenesis (*see* Chapter 2 for details)
- *Chondrodiastasis*: It is a recently introduced method to achieve limb lengthening and deformity correction based on Hueter Volkmann's law that states "tensile forces across physes stimulate growth and vice versa". This method employs gradual physeal distraction (without producing fracture) and opening of the growth plate (Salter and Harris type I epiphyseal detachment) that lengthens the limb. It should be performed in patients nearing skeletal maturity as physis invariably closes after this procedure.

DEFORMITIES OF UPPER LIMB

RADIAL CLUB HAND (RADIAL HEMIMELIA)

In radial club hand, there is congenital deficiency (hemimelia) of the radial (preaxial) side of upper limb. The condition is slightly more common in males and almost 50% of the cases are bilateral.

Pathogenesis is related to a defect in apical ectodermal ridge (AER). Most cases are sporadic, but few may be linked to exposure to teratogens such as thalidomide and radiation. Associated syndromes include Holt-Oram syndrome [heart defects, commonly atrial septal defect (ASD)], thrombocytopenia with absent radius (TAR) syndrome, VACTERL (vertebral, anal, cardiac, tracheal, esophageal, renal and limb) syndrome, coloboma of the eye, heart defects, atresia of the nasal choanae, retardation of growth or development, genital or urinary abnormalities, and ear abnormalities and deafness (CHARGE) syndrome and Fanconi anemia.

Clinical Features

Children (slightly more common in males) with this anomaly present with absence of radius that may be partial or complete (more common). Forearm is short and radially deviated (manus valgus, **Figs 12.80A and B**). In complete absence of radius, hand is almost perpendicular to the forearm. It is commonly associated with hypoplastic or absent thumb. Carpals (scaphoid and trapezium commonly) may be absent as well. Flexor muscles of forearm are underdeveloped.

Treatment

Surgical reconstruction involves centralization of the wrist (carpus) on the ulna. An absent thumb can be reconstructed by a procedure called as "pollicization". Passive stretching should be done before surgery to ensure good surgical outcome. It is also wise to always rule out cardiac defects (which may need to be treated earlier).

MADELUNG DEFORMITY

In this deformity the lower end of radius curves forward carrying with it the carpus and the hand but leaving the ulna sticking out on the back of the wrist **(Figs 12.81A and B)**. The left out ulna can be balloted like a piano key (piano key sign). The deformity may be congenital or post-traumatic. In congenital type also even though the pathology is present since birth, the deformity becomes obvious by 10 years as growth occurs. Function is excellent and only severe cases need corrective osteotomy.

RADIOULNAR SYNOSTOSIS

Radioulnar synostosis refers to osseous fusion between these two bones. It may be congenital (rare) or traumatic.

---

*Up to 1 cm lift may be incorporated inside the shoes but more than 1 cm lift should better be fixed to the sole.
†If one has to choose between shortening and lengthening, it is better to leave a shortening in limb than lengthening. A short limb can be managed by a shoe raise on the same side; however, if lengthening is to be managed, then procedures would involve manipulating the normal limb that is not easily accepted by patients.

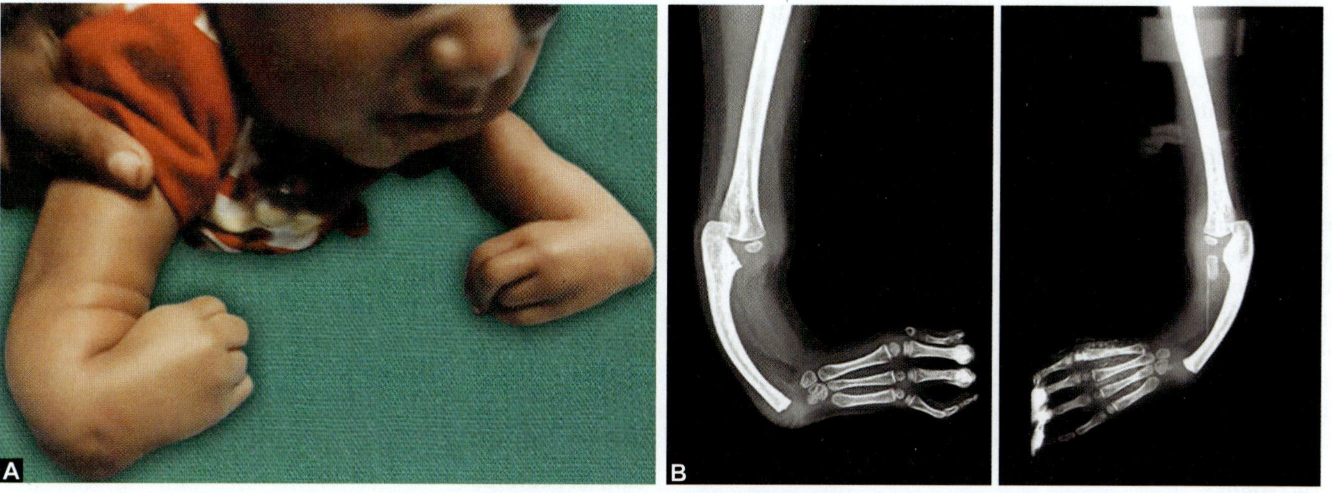

Figs 12.80A and B: Radial club hand

Courtesy: Dr Matad Lokeshwaraiah Chetan (SS Institute of Medical Sciences, Davangere, Karnataka).

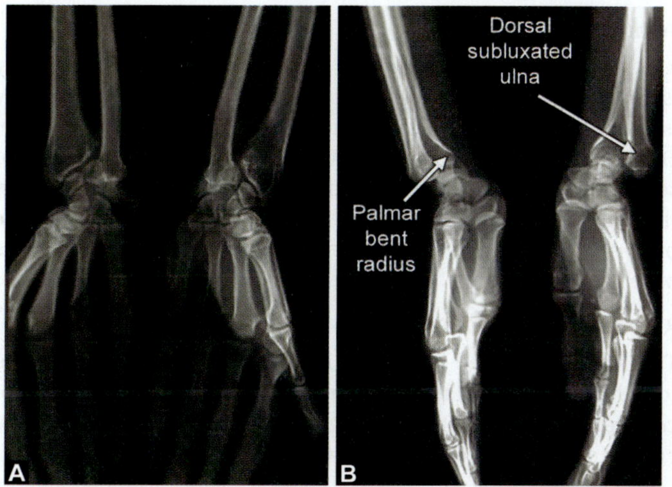

Figs 12.81A and B: X-ray of both wrists anteroposterior and lateral views showing Madelung deformity (radius has grown volarwards and ulna is sticking out dorsally)

Fig. 12.82: Radioulnar synostosis

Courtesy: Dr Deepak Raghav (JN Medical College, AMU).

Congenital Radioulnar Synostosis

It occurs due to a defect in the longitudinal segmentation of radius and ulna. Both sexes are affected with equal frequency, with 60% cases being bilateral. Fusion commonly is found in proximal one-third of forearm **(Fig. 12.82)** and the forearm is fixed in pronation. Muscles and fascial tissues in the forearm are also anomalous to varying degrees, so simple resection of the bony bridge does not restore motion (supination and pronation). Rather surgery is not indicated in most patients as most patients are able to carry on daily activities well with some adjustments. Only rarely when deformity is bilateral and severe, surgery may be done. Aim of surgery is to reposition forearm in a useful position rather than to provide movement. Osteotomy is done to place one forearm in neutral and other in slight pronation (10–20°).

Traumatic Radioulnar Synostosis

Traumatic radioulnar synostosis is mostly iatrogenic and results from operatively maltreated forearm fracture. Highly comminuted and open fractures, especially with both bones fractured at same level pose a greater risk. Patients with a concomitant head injury are more likely to land up with this complication (owing to greater growth factors released after injury). Treatment is indicated when the restriction of forearm rotation is disabling. Resection of synostosis along with interposition of fat/muscle/fascia/silicone is done. Unlike in congenital variety, the results of resection are good.

DEFORMITIES OF THE TRUNK AND VERTEBRAE

TORTICOLLIS (WRY NECK)

Derived from Latin words tortus (twisted) and collum (neck), torticollis refers to abnormal and asymmetric neck position. Most often it is due to painful lesions of the neck causing reflex muscle spasm. Strictly speaking it can be of following types:

- Congenital muscular torticollis
- Acquired [cervical lymphadenitis, tonsillitis, adenoiditis, retropharyngeal abscess, tuberculosis (TB) of cervical spine,

cervical spine tumors, cervical prolapsed disk and cerebellar tumors]

- Idiopathic cervical dystonia
- Compensatory (squint).

Congenital (Infantile) Muscular Torticollis (Sternomastoid Tumor)

It is a painless condition caused by fibromatosis of the sternocleidomastoid (SCM) muscle, resulting in the formation of a palpable mass (palpable at birth or within 4 weeks of birth) in the muscle. Association with DDH and metatarsus adductus points toward the condition likely occurring as a result of packaging problem. Increased pressure in-utero leads to a perinatal compartment syndrome localized to the neck that causes ischemia of the SCM muscle ending in fibrosis. An increased incidence also has been reported in breech delivery and first born cases.

Clinical Features

The deformity is usually apparent at birth or shortly thereafter. More commonly right side is involved. Head is tilted toward the involved muscle and chin is rotated toward opposite side (Cock Robin appearance) **(Fig. 12.83A)**. As the head is tilted towards opposite side of contracture such that ear touches the shoulder, contracted SCM feels tight and hard and stands out **(Fig. 12.83B)**. A palpable mass may be felt in middle to lower third of the sternal portion of the SCM muscle within the first 4 weeks of life. Mass spontaneously regresses in a few months leaving behind a fibrosed muscle (that may remain palpable as a cord), but the deformity persists. As the fibrous tissue fails to elongate with growth, the deformity rather becomes progressive. Infant may also have a "bat ear" due to folding in-utero. Asymmetrical development of face (plagiocephaly) may occur later in life, because child always sleeps on one side causing flattening of that side. Radiography of the cervical spine should be done to rule out segmentation defects of cervical spine.

Treatment

Most cases especially those in first year can be treated with a conservative regime of regular stretching. Severe deformity may be treated with surgery. Unipolar release (at clavicular attachment only) or bipolar release of SCM (Z plasty at clavicular side and release at mastoid attachment, preferred method) followed by physiotherapy is done. Surgery is ideally done at 4–6 years of age. Surgery in infants is rather avoided as scar tethers to deeper structures.

SPRENGEL SHOULDER

Congenital elevation of the scapula is known as "Sprengel shoulder". Scapula actually forms at higher level and descends. Interruption in normal caudal descent of scapula results in this deformity. One-third of patients have an extra bone (omovertebral bar) connecting scapula to cervical spine that obstructs the normal descent that is thought to be pathogenic. Associated congenital anomalies include cervical rib, Klippel-Feil syndrome, congenital scoliosis and renal anomalies.

Clinical Features

Scapula is hypoplastic and lies more superior in relation to chest cage **(Fig. 12.84)**. Head is often deviated to the affected side and shoulder abduction is limited.

Treatment

Mild-to-moderate cases require no treatment. Only if deformity is causing severe cosmetic and functional impairment, surgery is indicated. Surgery is done once child reaches 3 years of age. Operative techniques include Green's procedure (excision of supraspinatus portion of scapula) and Woodward's procedure (bringing down of scapula after shifting the origin of trapezius; preferred procedure). Most important complication of surgery is brachial plexus injury.

KLIPPEL-FEIL SYNDROME

This is characterized by congenital fusion of cervical spine due to failure of segmentation. There is failure of normal division of cervical somites at 3–8 weeks of gestation. It may even involve the craniocervical junction (occiput C1-C2).

Clinical Features

Classical triad consists of short-webbed neck, low posterior hairline and restriction of neck movements. Segment of spine near the

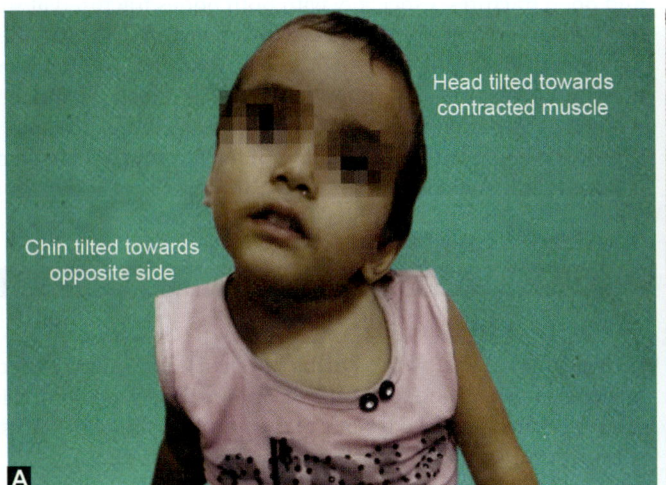

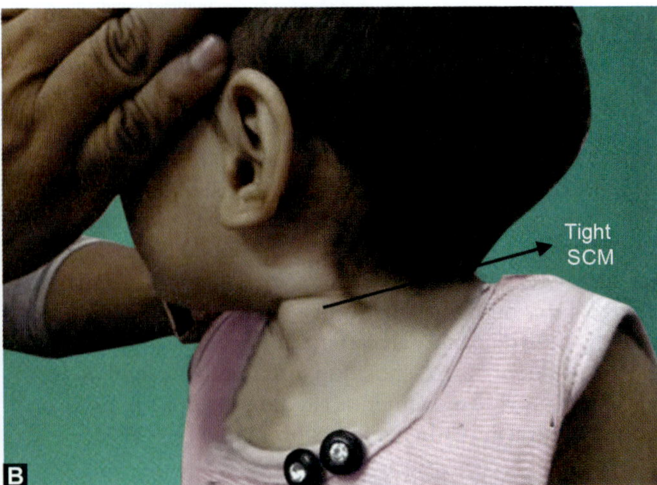

Figs 12.83A and B: (A) Congenital muscular torticollis; (B) SCM becomes tight as head in tilted towards opposite side in an attempt to make ear touch the shoulder

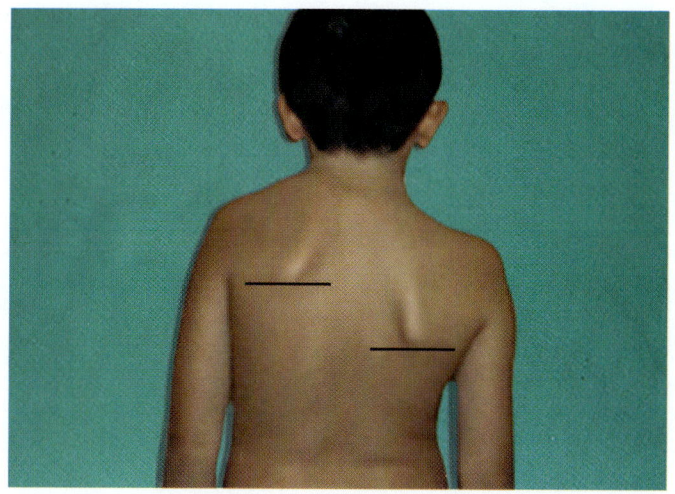

Fig. 12.84: Sprengel shoulder (left side)

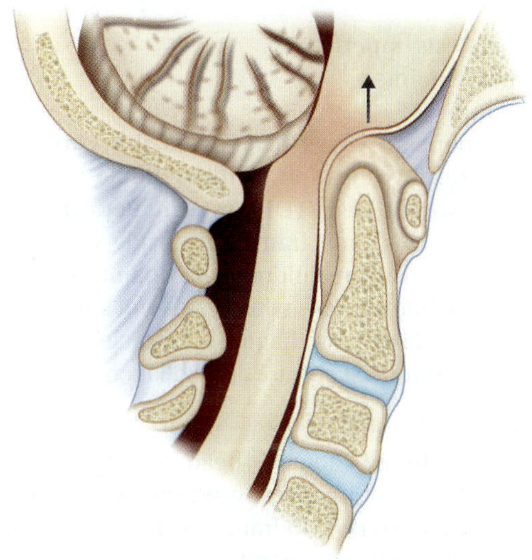

Fig. 12.85: Diagrammatic representation of basilar impression

fused part becomes hypermobile, causing degenerative changes, which may lead to radiculopathy or myelopathy in young adult life. Torticollis is present. Scoliosis (congenital or idiopathic) occurs in 60% of patients. Sprengel deformity of shoulder accompanies the syndrome in 50% cases. Other associated conditions include genitourinary abnormalities (structural abnormalities such as double collecting system, horseshoe-shaped kidney, renal aplasia, etc.), congenital heart defects, hearing loss, synkinesis, ocular anomalies and cervical canal stenosis.

Treatment

Symptomatic children with cervical instability require fixation with halo vest or surgical fusions. Patients should be advised to avoid collision sports.

BASILAR IMPRESSION

In this condition, there occurs upward migration of the upper cervical spine (i.e. tip of the odontoid process) into the floor of the skull, i.e. into the foramen magnum **(Fig. 12.85)**. Cause can be a primary bony abnormality in the vertebra (e.g. Odontoid anomalies, Morquio syndrome, Klippel-Feil syndrome, etc.) or

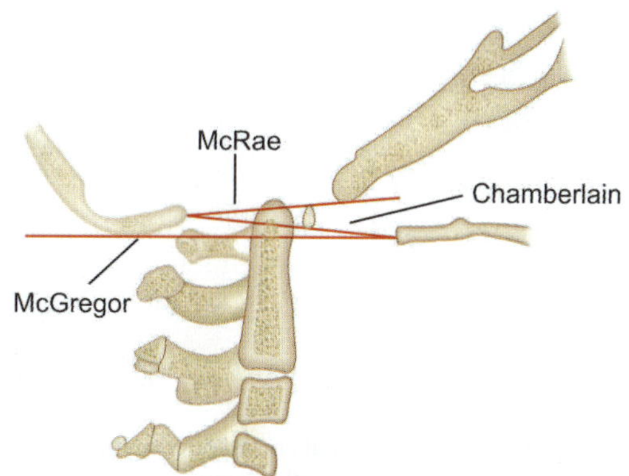

Fig. 12.86: Some criteria to identify basilar impression

softening of the base of the skull (due to osteomalacia, rickets, rheumatoid arthritis, etc.). In the latter case, the term used is Basilar invagination.

Most patients are in their second or third decade of life and present with quadriparesis or paraesthesias of limbs due to cord compression. There may be symptoms of increased intracranial pressure (due to blockade of aqueduct of Sylvius). The diagnosis can be confirmed on AP and lateral radiographs. Many criteria (Chamberlain, McGregor, McRae, Fischgold, Metzger lines and Clark, Redlund-Johnell and Ranawat indices) have been described **(Fig. 12.86)** that can be used as a reference to determine upward migration. Treatment involves surgical decompression and stabilization.

MISCELLANEOUS CONDITIONS OF INTEREST IN CHILDREN

BATTERED BABY SYNDROME

Child abuse (battered baby) and neglected or nonaccidental injury in children was first described by Kempe et al. in 1962. They had reported that as many as 10–15% of fractures in children younger than 3 years may be a result of child abuse. Owing to such a high incidence, soon "battered baby syndrome (BBS)" became a recognized clinical entity. It is characterized by physical injuries (skin injuries, multiple fractures, subdural hematomas, sexual abuse, etc.) caused by nonaccidental trauma in children. Most cases of BBS are seen before the age of 3 years (more than 50% are younger than 1 year). Accidental fractures are rare before age of 1 year.

Pattern of Injuries

The most common physical injuries are skin injuries (bruises, scrapes and burns).

Fractures, generally multiple, are the second most common presentation. Although no particular fracture pattern, morphology or location is pathognomonic, most common bone fractured is humerus followed by tibia and femur (King et al.). A single transverse fracture in the diaphysis is generally classical in these long bones. Metaphyseal corner fractures and metaphyseal bucket-handle fractures **(Fig. 12.87)** are almost pathognomonic of child abuse, but less commonly seen than diaphyseal fractures. Skull fractures (eggshell fractures, occipital impression fractures,

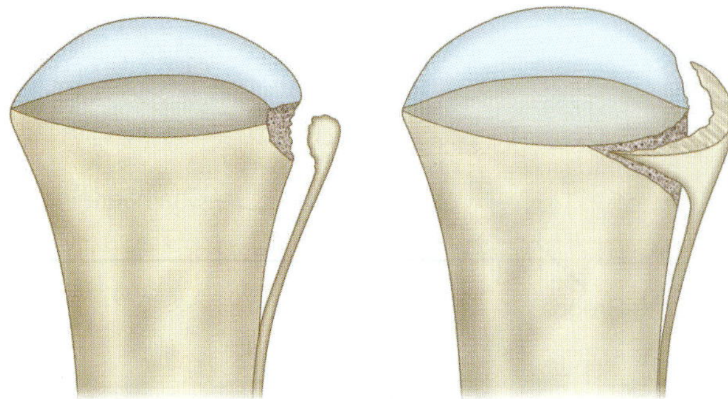

Fig. 12.87: Metaphyseal corner and metaphyseal bucket-handle fractures

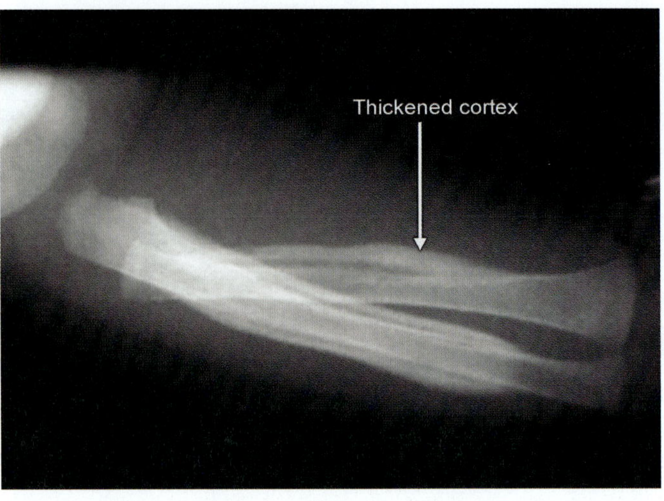

Fig. 12.88: X-ray forearm lateral view showing thickened cortices due to Caffey's disease

fractures crossing suture lines) and subdural hemorrhages are common in severe cases.

Sexual abuse is estimated to occur in approximately 10% of these children.

Diagnosis

The diagnosis is challenging as the infant or child often cannot provide adequate information. Suspect the condition if history obtained from parents does not correlate with the clinical examination and radiological dating of fractures (e.g. parents claim injury is 1 day old but callus is visible on X-rays; fracture callus appears roughly between 5 days and 14 days after fracture in children and fracture definition may be lost as early as 2–3 weeks). Children in high-risk family (divorced or separated parents; maternal history of depression, alcohol abuse, drug abuse, uneducated parents, etc.) are often a victim of abuse.

A skeletal survey (AP and lateral views of skull and chest, lateral view of spine, AP view of spine and long bones of all four extremities and PA oblique views of the hand and feet) is recommended in any child younger than 1 year with a fracture suspected of child abuse, a child with previous history of one or more fractures, a child with multiple fractures and a child with family history of fragile bones (OI). Rib fractures are often difficult to detect and if suspected the skeletal survey should be repeated at 2 weeks (callus may be appreciated).

Differential Diagnosis

Differentials are metabolic and inherited conditions related to fragile bones. These include OI, rickets and renal diseases, disuse osteopenia (e.g. cerebral palsy in a child) or medications (e.g. corticosteroids) leading to fragile bones.

The closest differential undoubtedly is OI. Although it may be very difficult at times to differentiate between the two, some features might be useful to arrive at a particular diagnosis. A transverse femur fracture in a child less than 1 year old and a transverse humerus fracture in a child less than 3 years old should highly be suspected of child abuse. Characteristic pattern of bruising (multiple bruises in clusters; bruising at places away from bony prominences; uniformly shaped bruises; imprint bruising; ligature marks, cigarette burns to the palms of hands and soles of feet) may help in identification. Else the following factors may point toward OI being the greater possibility:

- Positive family history
- Blue sclera
- Dentinogenesis imperfecta
- Hypermobile joints
- Short stature
- Abnormal bone on X-rays (osteopenia, thin cortices, etc.).

A very useful investigation to differentiate the two is dual energy X-ray absorptiometry (DEXA) scan. Perform a DEXA 4–6 months apart. In this time frame this study classically shows increase in bone density in children who do not have a metabolic bone syndrome while patients with OI will not show this increase in bone density. Still in case diagnosis is unclear, best course of action is to get a fibroblast culture and collagen analysis.

HIGH-YIELD POINT

Shaken baby syndrome (abusive head syndrome) is a clinical entity where the triad involves subdural hematomas, retinal hemorrhages and posterior rib fractures. The clinical outcome is poor in this condition if it is missed.

CAFFEY'S DISEASE (INFANTILE CORTICAL HYPEROSTOSIS)

This is a self-limiting inflammatory disease of unknown etiology, seen mainly in infants less than 6 months old. It is characterized by intense diaphyseal periostitis **(Fig. 12.88)** and hyperostosis (thickening of cortex of bone often leading to doubling of width of bone), occurrence of soft tissue nodules and growth abnormalities. The characteristic triad includes cortical bone thickening, painful soft tissue swellings and systemic symptoms (irritability and fever). Clinically the disease is often confused with osteomyelitis. Most common site of involvement is mandible and its presentation in mandible often mimics jaw tumors. Other common sites include the clavicle, ribs, scapula and the long bones.

Two forms of the condition are known: (1) familial (AD inheritance) and (2) sporadic (more common).

Treatment

The condition is self-limiting and usually resolves in 6 months to 1 year time. NSAIDs (indomethacin and naproxen) may be used. Corticosteroids are reserved for extensive disease. Antibiotics have no role, but some patients might be given antibiotics early as fever and leukocytosis suggest a systemic infection.

Neuromuscular Disorders

CEREBRAL PALSY

INTRODUCTION

Cerebral palsy (CP) is defined as "a nonprogressive neurological disorder primarily affecting movement and muscle coordination, due to insult to the developing brain before, during or just after birth". An insult to the developing brain during the course of birth process results in neurological deficit. This neurological deficit is nonprogressive, as the damage that has once occurred is static but the clinical picture worsens with growth. As the muscles are fibrotic and contracted, they cannot lengthen and adapt to growing bones, resulting in progressively worsening joint contractures as the child grows. By definition, the onset of the condition must be before the age of 2 years.

A number of classifications have been proposed for the condition:

- *Geographic classification*: Based on the extent of neurological deficit:
  - *Monoplegia (rare)*: Only one extremity is involved (commonly lower)
  - *Hemiplegia*: Ipsilateral upper and lower extremities (upper > lower), 50% patients are mentally retarded
  - *Paraplegia*: Both lower extremities involved equally
  - *Quadriplegia*: All four extremities involved equally
  - *Diplegia (most common)*: All four extremities involved (lower > upper)
  - *Double hemiplegia*: All four extremities involved (upper > lower)
  - *Total body*: Severe involvement all four extremities, along with absent head and neck control (resulting in drooling, dysphagia, dysarthria).
- *Physiological classification*: Based on the part of brain involved:
  - *Spastic type (most common form 80%)*: This is characterized by corticospinal tract involvement. Lack of coordination and balance, joint contractures and joint subluxations and dislocations are common. Clonus and Babinski sign are present. There is hyperreflexia and jack-knife spasticity.
  - *Extrapyramidal type*: Here extrapyramidal system is involved and the category is further subdivided into various subtypes depending on different areas of involvement (basal ganglia, thalamus, cerebellum, and substantia nigra):

- *Athetoid type*: Dyskinetic, purposeless worm-like movements. Reflexes are normal and joint contractures are uncommon
- *Choreiform type*: Continuous purposeless movements of wrist, fingers, ankles, and toes
- *Rigid type*: Cogwheel or lead-pipe rigidity* without hyperreflexia or clonus. It is the most hypertonic type of CP
- *Ataxic type*: Very rare type due to damage to cerebellum. Patient has tremors and drunken gait
- *Hypotonic type*: Weakness accompanied by hypotonia and normal deep reflexes. It may later evolve into spastic or ataxic types
- Mixed type.

- *Etiological classification*: Based upon the cause of the insult:
  - *Prenatal (most common 70%)*: Infection [TORCH (Toxoplasmosis, Other agents, i.e. HIV, measles, varicella, etc. Rubella, Cytomegalovirus, and Herpes simplex) agents], toxins (e.g. methyl mercury), Rh incompatibility (kernicterus), congenital malformations of brain, vascular insult
  - *Perinatal*: Traumatic delivery, prematurity, birth asphyxia, and chorioamnionitis
  - *Postnatal*: Infection (meningitis, encephalitis), hypoxic-ischemic encephalopathy, child abuse, and traumatic brain injury.

CLINICAL FEATURES

Children with this condition present with varied forms of neurological involvement as discussed above. Abnormalities of tone, posture, and movement are there. Developmental milestones are delayed or never appear **(Table 13.1)**. Primitive reflexes persist longer than usual **(Table 13.2)**. Affected children may display some characteristic of gait patterns and joint deformities.

Common gait patterns seen in children with CP: Toe walking (equinus), crouched knee gait (hip flexion, knee flexion and ankle dorsiflexion), jump knee gait (hip flexion, knee flexion and ankle plantar flexion) **(Figs 13.1A and B)**, scissoring gait (due to spasm of hip adductors) **(Fig. 13.2)** and Stiff knee gait.

Common deformities seen in children with CP:
- *Upper extremity deformities*: Internal rotation contracture of shoulder, flexion deformity of elbow, flexion and ulnar deviation of wrist, thumb in palm deformity **(Fig. 13.3)** and flexion of fingers.

Difference between spasticity and rigidity: Spasticity is velocity dependent increase in muscle tone with passive stretch, caused by exaggeration of muscle stretch reflexes while in rigidity the tone is equally increased throughout the range of motion independent of velocity of stretch.

Table 13.1: Appearance of some important milestones

Parameters	Usual time of appearance
Head control	3–6 months
Sit without support	6–9 months
Crawling	8–9 months
Walking without support	2–18 months

Table 13.2: Some important primitive reflexes and their usual time of disappearance

Primitive reflexes	Usual time of disappearance
Palmar grasp	Appears at 34 weeks gestation and disappears by 2–4 months
Plantar grasp	Disappears by 9–12 months
Asymmetric tonic neck reflex	Disappears by 4–6 months
Moro reflex	Appears at birth and disappears by 4–6 months
Placing reflex	Appears at birth and disappears by 5–9 months
Stepping reflex	Appears at birth and disappears by 1–2 months
Parachute reflex	Appears at 6–9 months and thereafter persists

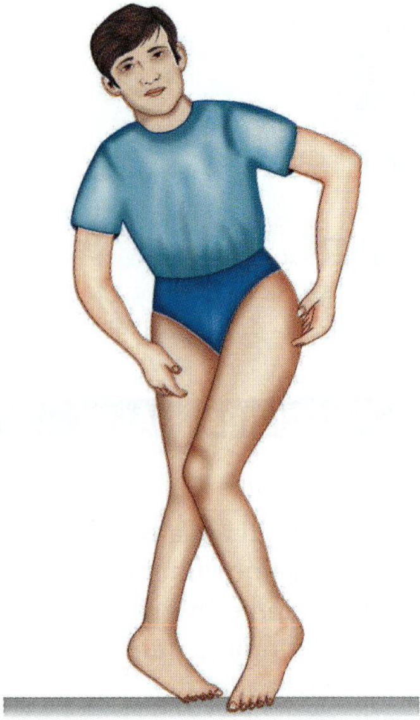

Fig. 13.2: Scissoring gait

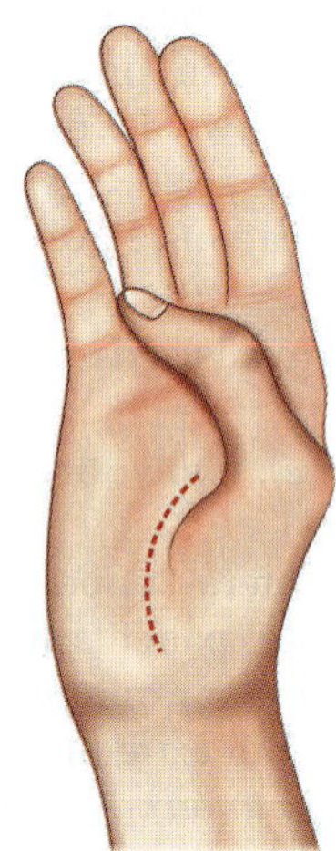

Fig. 13.3: Thumb in palm deformity. The thumb is acutely flexed into the palm due to contracture of flexor pollicis longus, thenar muscles and adductor pollicis

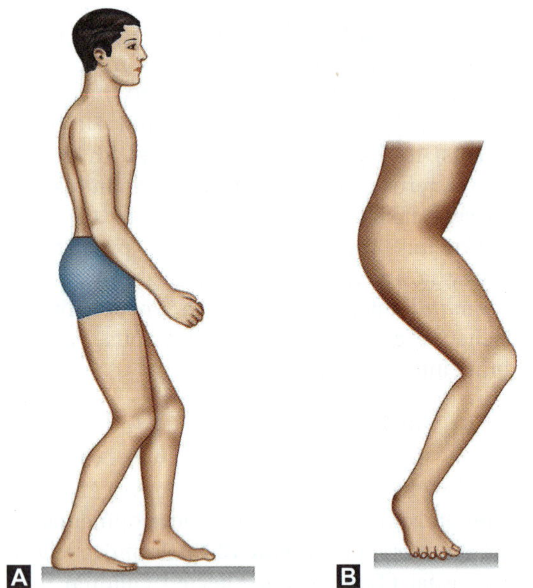

Figs 13.1A and B: (A) Crouched knee; and (B) Jump knee gaits

- *Lower extremity deformities*: Subluxation and dislocation of hip (mostly posterior), flexion contracture of knee (due to hamstring spasm), variable deformities of foot and ankle (equinus, equinovarus, equinovalgus, cavus).
  Associates conditions in children with CP:
- Mental retardation [low intelligent quotient (IQ)]: 40–60%
- Seizures: 40%.
- Visual impairment
- Constipation
- Dysphagia
- Hearing impairment
- Osteoporosis
- Hydrocephalus.

DIAGNOSIS

The diagnosis is largely clinical and is reached by eliciting proper history which may reveal a low IQ, disappointing school performance and delayed developmental milestones. A thorough clinical examination greatly aids if one examines for muscle tone and documents power charting. Finding of primitive reflex patterns persisting longer than usual also helps in clinching the diagnosis.

MANAGEMENT

Management can be described under the following headings:

- *Mechanical measures and medical management*: Spasticity can be managed by physical therapy, gait training, bracing and splinting, and by drugs. Effective drugs include:

– *Dantrolene*: It acts at the level of skeletal muscle (peripherally acting) by inhibiting release of calcium ions. It is used less frequently because of the potential to result in profound weakness and liver toxicity.

– *Baclofen*: It is a gamma aminobutyric acid (GABA) agonist, which acts at level of spinal cord (centrally acting) and inhibits the release of excitatory transmitters. It can be administered orally or via intrathecal route. Intrathecal infusion dose is 1/30th of oral dose and can be delivered via an implantable subcutaneous pump to ensure continuous delivery. Important complications include pump and catheter infection, spinal fluid leak and respiratory depression.

– *Botulinum A toxin*: It acts at the neuromuscular junction (peripherally acting) to inhibit the release of acetylcholine. It is directly injected into spastic muscles where the effect may last up to 6 months. The goal is to use the effect obtained to facilitate physiotherapy and mobilization, and delay surgical intervention. However, the efficacy of repeated injections may reduce due to development of antibodies. Inadvertent systemic injection has the potential of causing severe respiratory depression. Contraindications to its use include known resistance or antibodies, failure of previous response, myasthenia gravis, fixed contracture and concomitant use of aminoglycosides.

- *Surgical management*:
  – *Selective dorsal rhizotomy*: One of the pathogenetic mechanisms behind CP is that end organs generate abnormal sensory impulses that lead to excessive stimulation of excitatory fibers. In this procedure, the rootlets carrying excessive stimulatory information to dorsal sensory fibers are cut. Goal is to reduce the stimulatory input that goes from dorsal sensory fibers to efferent motor fibers. Ideal patient is 3–8-year-old child with spastic diplegia, voluntary trunk and motor control, pure spasticity and no fixed contractures. It is not recommended in spastic quadriplegia and hemiplegia.
  – Muscle-tendon lengthening/release procedures or tendon transfers or rarely osteotomies may be done as per the clinical scenario.

Some notable procedures include:
- Equinus in CP patients is generally due to selective contracture of soleus muscle and is treated by vulpius release.
- Equinovarus deformity at foot can also occur and tendon transfer of Kaufer (tibialis posterior to peroneus brevis) and Hoffer (tibialis anterior to medial cuneiform) are useful for correction. On the contrary, equinovalgus if occurs is corrected by tendon transfers of Perry (peroneus brevis to tibialis posterior).
- Hip dislocation in CP occurs due to flexion adduction-contracture at hip and can be managed by San Diego procedure.
- Scissoring **(Fig. 13.2)** occurs due to adductor spasm at hip and is managed by adductor tenotomy if abduction is less than 30°.

POLIOMYELITIS

INTRODUCTION

Polio is an acute infectious disease caused by poliovirus. The target population is the pediatric age-group and the target organs include the spinal cord (anterior horn motor cells) and the brainstem (bulbar nuclei).

EPIDEMIOLOGY

In the past, polio was an epidemic occurring mainly in the summer months. Most of the countries are now free from the disease due to effective preventive measures (effective immunization and surveillance). Only three countries are endemic as of 2014: Pakistan, Nigeria and Afghanistan, although sporadic cases have been reported in few other countries also.

India's last case (due to type 1 virus) was reported on January 13, 2011 from Howrah, West Bengal. As of now India is free from new cases. This does not mean that the disease is no longer of significance to healthcare providers. Patients with sequelae of disease are still abundant and although these cases are not infectious, many of them are crippled and are considered outcast in the modern society. The role of orthopedic surgeon is not during acute phase, but to effectively treat its sequelae to help these people lead a more normal life.

ETIOPATHOGENESIS

Infection is caused by poliomyelitis virus, which belongs to group *Enterovirus* and family *Picornavirus*. Lipid envelope encloses a single-stranded ribonucleic acid (RNA) core. Three different strains of virus are known (type I, II and III) with no cross-immunity. It enters body via feco-oral route, multiplies in intestine where it may manifest as episode of diarrhea and then reaches the nervous system through bloodstream. The virus has special affinity for some brainstem nuclei (bulbar polio) and anterior horn cells of the spinal cord (especially the lumbar and cervical enlargements of the cord). Damage to these neurons produces flaccid type of paralysis. The proportion of motor units destroyed is variable and the resultant weakness depends on the percentage of motor units that have been destroyed.

COURSE OF DISEASE

The disease process is divided into three phases:

1. *Acute phase*: The child presents with fever, mild headache, malaise, sore throat and diarrhea. This is preparalytic stage that lasts for 5–10 days. Diagnosis in this stage is very difficult unless the area is endemic.

   Soon muscle weakness appears, generally after 2–3 days of onset of fever and peaks over another 2–4 days and in rare cases may progress to cause dyspnea and dysphagia (bulbar polio affecting motor neurons of the respiratory and cardiovascular centers of the medulla). This is the paralytic stage. If patient does not succumb to respiratory paralysis, fever subsides after 7–10 days and patient enters convalescent stage.

2. *Convalescent phase*: Also known as phase of recovery, this lasts up to 16–24 months. Maximum recovery occurs in 3–6 months and no recovery beyond 24 months. This phase is divided into sensitive and insensitive phases. In sensitive phase, muscles are tender and in spasm while in insensitive phase muscles are nontender but still in period of recovery.

3. *Chronic residual phase*: This phase is also known as the stage of post-polio residual paralysis (PPRP). It is seen after 24 months when maximum recovery has occurred and residual paralysis persists. The paralysis is lower motor neuron (flaccid) type which is asymmetrical and patchy in distribution with no sensory loss and no bladder bowel involvement. In PPRP, the major causes of deformity are: muscle imbalance, faulty posture and continuous growth of bones against fibrotic contracted muscles.

DIAGNOSIS

The diagnosis of polio must be considered in endemic areas whenever a child presents with acute flaccid paralysis after ruling out the other conditions that may present in similar manner **(Table 13.3)**.

POLIO AND ORTHOPEDICS

The orthopedic surgeon is primarily expected to deal with the extensive muscle paralysis that may ensue and protect the patient from developing resultant deformities. Almost any pattern of paralysis in the involved muscles of limb is possible; however, some important points of consideration are as follows:

Polio most commonly involves the muscles of the lower limb; acute fatality is because of the involvement of the respiratory muscles generally. The most common muscle to be affected is quadriceps femoris, which is partially paralyzed in majority of cases. The most common completely paralyzed muscle in polio is tibialis anterior. In the upper limb most commonly involved muscle is deltoid. Although hand muscles are rarely involved, the most common affected muscle of hand is opponens pollicis.

Important Deformities in Polio

The major deformities in polio occur in lower limb due to the iliotibial band (ITB) contracture.

Relevant anatomy (Fig. 13.4): The ITB is a longitudinal fibrous reinforcement of the fascia lata. Three muscles give origin to ITB: (1) tensor fascia lata (TFL), (2) gluteus medius and (3) gluteus maximus, and it inserts at lateral condyle of the tibia at Gerdy's tubercle. The action of the ITB and its associated muscles is to extend, abduct and externally rotate the hip. In addition, the ITB contributes to lateral knee stabilization.

Tensor fascia lata is an abductor and medial rotator of hip while it extends the knee. This muscle originates from iliac crest and inserts into the iliotibial tract.

Deformities: The ITB contracture can lead to:
- Flexion, abduction and external rotation deformity at hip (most common)
- Flexion and valgus at knee or sometimes triple deformity at knee (flexion, posterior subluxation and external rotation of tibia on femur)
- Equinovarus at ankle and foot
- Lumbar scoliosis and pelvic obliquity at spine and pelvis, respectively.

To test for ITB contracture, Ober's test is done **(Fig. 13.5)**. To perform this test, make the patient lie in the lateral position, support the knee and flex it to 90°. Then extend and abduct the

Table 13.3: Differentials of poliomyelitis	
Guillain-Barré syndrome	It is an ascending symmetrical myelopathy that occurs a bit later in life. Facial nerve involvement can be seen. Most cases have complete recovery
Acute transverse myelitis	There is acute sensory and motor paralysis below a particular level at which the vascular supply to cord has been interrupted
Traumatic paraplegia	There is history of trauma and radiograph may show the fracture
Neuropathy	Usually presented with both motor and sensory loss that is generally bilateral. Treating the cause may lead to improvement
Myopathy	Since the paralysis is lower motor neuron type with no sensory loss, the condition is an important differential. Mostly this condition is genetic. The pattern is predictable and generally symmetrical. The paralysis tends to worsen over time. Creatine phosphokinase (CPK) levels may be raised and a muscle biopsy may provide the diagnosis
Spinal dysraphism	Patients tend to have tuft of hair or swelling at the back. There may be both motor and sensory loss and the paralysis may deteriorate with growth

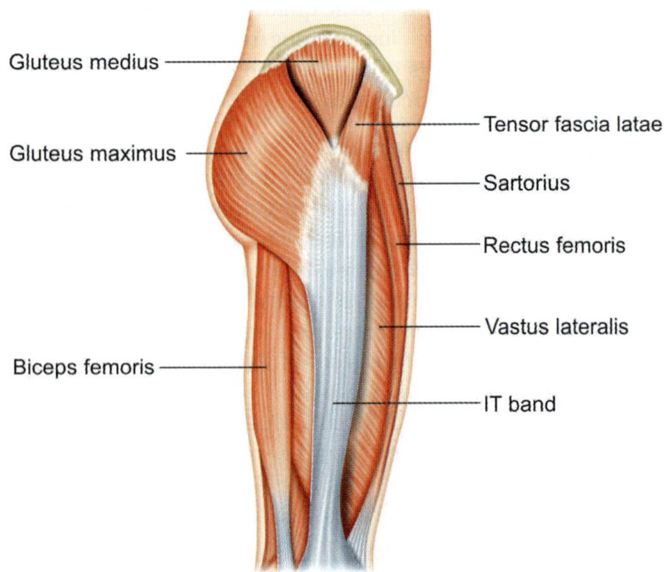

Fig. 13.4: Iliotibial band (ITB)

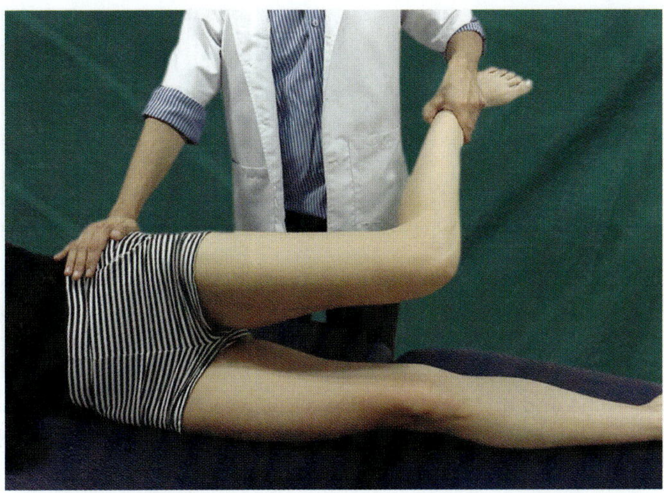

Fig. 13.5: Ober's test for iliotibial band (ITB) contracture

hip. Then release the knee support. Failure of the knee to adduct is a positive test.

MANAGEMENT

The management of polio is subdivided into prevention and treatment of the disease.

Prevention

Polio is best prevented by immunization. Two types of vaccines are available: oral polio vaccine (OPV) and inactivated polio vaccine (IPV). OPV is more effective and is included in National Immunization Program. Even if a patient has had an attack of polio, he should be immunized as there are three strains of the virus and he can get another attack due to infection by another strain. Intramuscular injections should be avoided in children in the polio endemic zones.

Treatment

Treatment depends on the phase of the disease:
- *Acute phase*: The aim of treatment in the acute phase is to provide symptomatic treatment and to avoid the deformities. Patient is given rest and paralyzed limbs are supported in splints to reduce the pain and muscle spasm. Active movements are avoided. Respiratory muscle paralysis warrants ventilatory support. Hot fomentation and analgesics are given for pain relief.
- *Convalescent phase*: Joints are splinted to reduce pain and adequate joint mobilization exercises are begun to gain the range of motion and prevent occurrence of deformities.

Once infection occurs there is no way to limit the severity of paralysis or prevent it. The aim is to limit the resultant deformities and comorbidities.

Treatment of Post-polio Residual Paralysis

Once the paralysis is established and recovery has halted, the aim of treatment in this stage is to correct the deformities if they have developed and to provide maximum attainable function.
- *Nonoperative methods*: Use of splints and traction to prevent and correct the existing deformities.

- *Operative procedures*:
  - *Soft-tissue release operations*: The ITB contracture is corrected by release of contracted soft tissue (Ober-Yount's fasciotomy of the ITB).
  - *Tendon transfers*: Muscle imbalance is corrected by transferring the tendon of normal muscle to the site which provides the function of paralyzed muscle.

Some important tendon transfers include:
- *Saha transfer (for deltoid paralysis)*: Trapezius to deltoid transfer.
- *Steindler's flexorplasty (for loss of elbow flexion)*: Shifting flexor origin proximally for about 5 cm to strengthen elbow flexion.
- *Sharrard/mustard transfers (for paralysis of hip abductors and extensors, i.e. gluteus medius and maximus)*: Transfer of iliopsoas to greater trochanter.

Tendon transfers are not to be done before 4 years of age as the rehabilitation exercises cannot be taught to a child of less than 4 years of age. However, an undue delay should be avoided as a delay in tendon transfers in case there is a muscle imbalance would lead to a progressive deformity.

Bony Procedures

Joint stabilization procedures (arthrodesis): Fixed deformities cannot be corrected by soft-tissue procedures alone, it is important to correct the deformity and then stabilize the joint by arthrodesis, e.g. in deformities of ankle and foot, triple arthrodesis may be needed in which talocalcaneal, talonavicular and calcaneocuboid joints are fused or a flail subtalar joint may need to undergo the Grice-Green subtalar arthrodesis.

HIGH-YIELD POINTS

- The first description of polio was given by Underwood in 1789.
- Although polio has been a disease of the past, recent attention is focused on new cases caused by oral vaccine, so-called vaccine-associated poliomyelitis. The risk of contracting polio from vaccine is however extremely low.
- Another manifestation that has received attention over recent years has been the post-polio syndrome. This is characterized by generalized weakness, fatigue and multiple body aches in people who contracted polio a couple of decades earlier.
- In polio, the most common bone fracture is supracondylar femur fracture. Femur is also the most common bone fractured in muscular dystrophies and arthrogryposis.
- Fractures in polio heal rapidly.

SPINA BIFIDA AND OTHER RELATED CONDITIONS (MYELODYSPLASIAS)

SPINA BIFIDA

It is a neural tube defect (NTD) characterized by failure of fusion of the neural tube posteriorly. The spinal cord may lie exposed from the back due to incomplete closure of the vertebral arches and patient may land up with a progressive neurological impairment. The condition is often associated with maldevelopment of spinal cord and the membranes.

The severity of the defect varies and based on the same, the condition is divided into following types:

- *Spina bifida occulta*: This is the most common but fortunately mildest form. The laminae fail to fuse to form spinous processes resulting in bifid spinous processes. The meninges do not herniate through the bony defect and the defect is covered with skin. It is the most common type but not usually diagnosed, as it is asymptomatic. Overlying skin may have stigmata, such as a hairy patch, hemangioma, dermal sinus, nevus, or a lipoma, which is an indicator of underlying spina bifida. It is the most common in lumbosacral region ($S_1 > L_5$) and usually diagnosed incidentally on radiographs in adults. In rare cases there may be neurological impairment due to tethering of the cord to the undersurface of the skin by a fibrous membrane (membrana reunions), tethering of the cord to filum terminale (*see* tethered cord syndrome), a presence of septum dividing the spinal canal (*see* diastematomyelia) or defective neural development.

- *Spina bifida cystica*: This is the more severe form where the defect not only involves the vertebral arches, but also extends to the overlying meninges, soft tissues and skin. It includes meningocele, myelomeningocele and syringomyelocele.

  - *Meningocele*: It refers to herniation of meninges through the bony defect to form a posterior midline sac containing cerebrospinal fluid (CSF). Nerve roots and cord do not herniate into the sac, hence the child is neurologically normal. The meninges are covered by skin (closed defect). It is the most common in lumbosacral region.

  - *Meningomyelocele/myelomeningocele*: The spinal cord or nerve roots (cauda equina) along with the meninges herniate through the bony defect. The sac is not covered by skin (open defect). The cord is usually splayed open within the sac and is referred to as neural placode. It is commonly accompanied by other anomalies such as Chiari malformation and hydrocephalus.

  - *Syringomyelocele*: It refers to a cord with dilated central canal and very thin cord substance herniating through the bony defect. The sac is covered by skin.

Etiology

Risk factors during gestation implicated in causation of NTDs include positive family history, folic acid deficiency, gestational diabetes and anticonvulsants (valproate, carbamazepine).

Diagnosis

An increase in the level of maternal serum AFP (alpha fetoprotein) during 2nd trimester is a sensitive indicator of open NTDs. In fact, the condition can be confirmed by measuring levels of AFP and acetylcholinesterase in amniotic fluid.

Ultrasonography (USG) is also highly specific for detection of NTDs, and can confirm diagnosis as early as 18 weeks of gestation.

Otherwise the classical clinical presentation **(Figs 13.6A and B)**, hair tufts or swelling at the back point towards the diagnosis that is aided by radiography **(Figs 13.7A and B)**.

Treatment

Spina bifida occulta needs no treatment. In other more severe cases, closure of sac and ventriculoperitoneal shunting is done

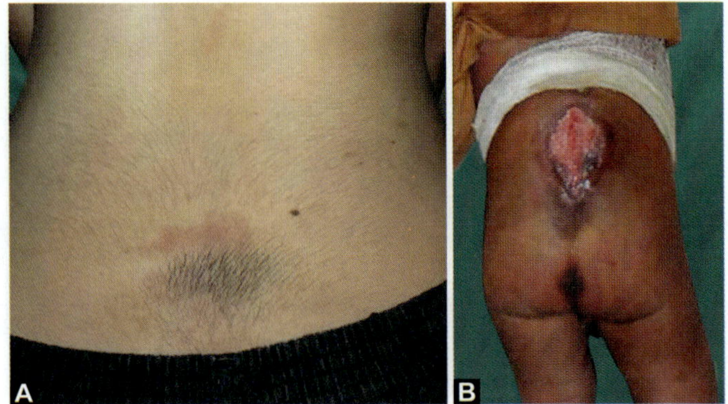

Figs 13.6A and B: (A) Patient with spina bifida occulta having tuft of hair at the back; and (B) A child with spina bifida cystica having a swelling at the back

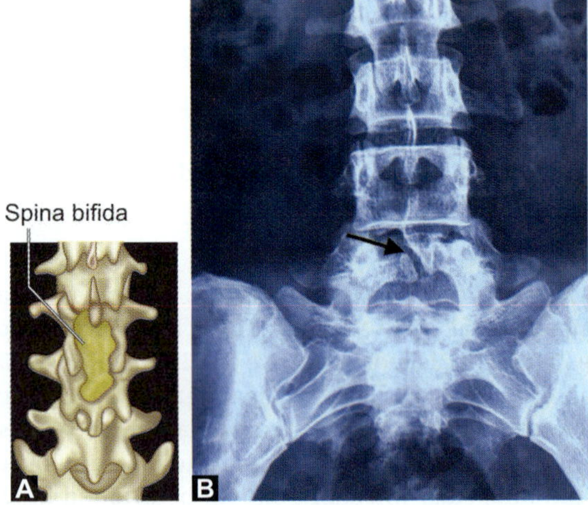

Figs 13.7A and B: X-ray of LS spine showing spina bifida L_5. Note absence of spinous process of L_5 vertebra (arrow) owing to unfused laminae

in perinatal period (preferably within 2–3 days of birth). In-utero closure is also attempted now-a-days, as damage to neural structures can be minimized by early closure.

However, one must remember that most of the defects in children can be prevented by adequate intake of folate by pregnant women. Since neural tube forms during the initial 3–6 weeks of pregnancy, folic acid intake should be started 3 months prior to planned pregnancy and should continue for the 1st trimester (i.e. 3 months after conception). Recommended dose is 400 µg/day, however, in high-risk women (having affected pregnancy with spina bifida or having spina bifida themselves) dose of 4,000 µg/day is recommended.

Spina Bifida and Orthopedics

Role of the orthopedic surgeon comes later when deformities develop due the muscle paralysis caused due to damage to cord and nerve roots.

Common orthopedic problem in such children include hip dislocation, knee flexion or extension contractures, external tibial torsion, and rigid talipes equinovarus. Management of such

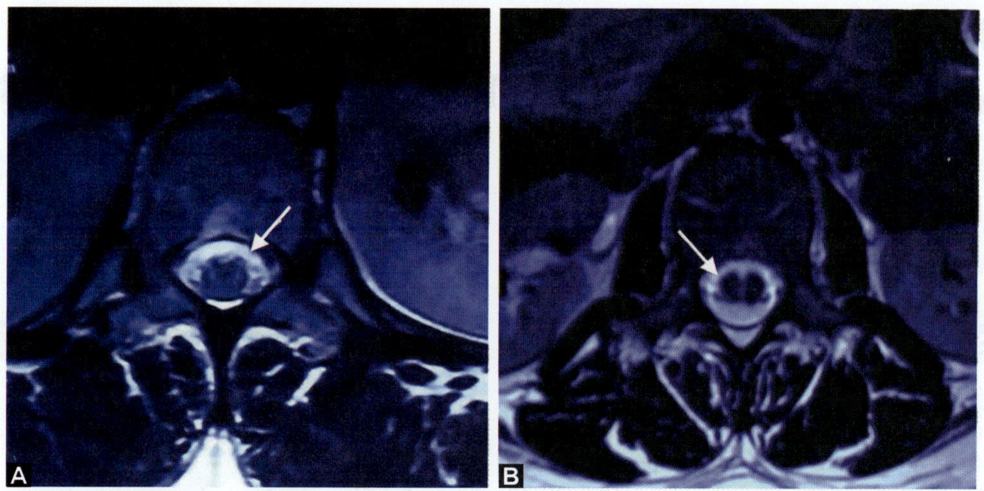

Figs 13.8A and B: (A) Spinal cord (arrow) in axial section of a normal person; and (B) Spinal cord divided into two halves by a septum (arrow) in a child with diastematomyelia

problems is challenging and often not satisfactory, e.g. a rigid clubfoot in meningomyelocele may need decancellation of talus and cuboid (subchondral excision of talus and cuboid, known as Verebelyi-Ogston procedure).

DIASTEMATOMYELIA

It is a congenital malformation in which the spinal cord is split vertically into two halves by a bony, fibrous, or fibrocartilaginous spur **(Figs 13.8A and B)**. It is different from dimyelia which means complete duplication of the spinal cord. Diastematomyelia is most common in lumbar region. Midline cutaneous stigmata like tuft of hair, dimple, lipoma, and hemangioma are common. On X-rays, there is widening of the interpedicular distance on anteroposterior (AP) view, along with any associated vertebral body defects that are commonly seen. Child is usually neurologically normal at birth and neurological defect develops later on. Excision of the septum is recommended only when there is a progressive neurological defect, and not routinely in all patients.

TETHERED CORD SYNDROME

This condition is characterized by tethering/pulling of the spinal cord at the base of the spinal canal. As the child grows, this tethering causes the spinal cord to stretch. Fluid pressures in the cord fluctuate leading to cyst formation and hence syringomyelia. Tight filum terminale may be a causative factor.

Clinical symptoms may be in the form of hairy patches, dimples or fatty tumors on the lower back, back pain, weakness in legs, bladder bowel involvement and scoliosis. The symptoms are progressive and worsen with growth. Magnetic resonance imaging (MRI) is the investigation of choice and provides the diagnosis.

Treatment is largely supportive. One may attempt at cutting the affected nerve roots in order to provide pain relief in patients in severe pain. The prognosis is very poor.

HIGH-YIELD POINT

- *Writer's cramps (Mogigraphia/Scrivener's palsy):* This is a task specific focal dystonia of the hand seen in those using the hand in repetitive activities like writing, typing, playing musical instruments, etc. The patients complain of spasm in hand muscles during specific activities like writing that involve fine motor movements. The cause is poorly understood and treatment is tailored to symptoms. NSAIDs, muscle relaxants, baclofen and botulinum toxin have a role apart from avoidance of repetitive activity and physiotherapy to correct muscle tone and hand posture.

Genetic and Developmental Disorders

SKELETAL DYSPLASIAS

INTRODUCTION

Skeletal dysplasias are a heterogeneous group of developmental disorder of bone with a wide spectrum of manifestations ranging from early onset of osteoarthritis with normal survival to death in utero or in early infancy. These are characterized by disordered growth of bone, resulting in abnormalities of the long bones, skull, chest, pelvis and spine. More than 300 skeletal dysplasias have been described, all are rare, but some are extremely rare. Osteogenesis imperfecta is the most common skeletal dysplasia while thanatophoric dysplasia is the most common lethal skeletal dysplasia. Common skeletal dysplasias are listed in **Box 14.1**.

CLASSIFICATION

Skeletal dysplasias are classified based on the part of the bone that is predominantly involved, i.e. epiphysis, metaphysis or diaphysis **(Table 14.1)**. The word "spondylo" is used as prefix to indicate the involvement of spine.

Most skeletal dysplasias are associated with short stature (defined as the height less than the 3rd percentile, for the chronological age of the patient). Hence, skeletal dysplasias can also be classified based on which portion of the bone is shortened:

- Rhizomelia indicates shortening of the proximal portion of a limb due to shortening of femur or humerus.
- Mesomelia indicates shortening of the middle portion of a limb due to shortening of leg or forearm bones.
- Acromelia is due to the shortening of foot and hand bones.

Achondroplasia is the most common variety associated with abnormally short stature (dwarfism).

DIAGNOSIS

Diagnosis of many skeletal dysplasias can be made by using prenatal ultrasound and postnatal X-ray of the baby. Diagnosis can be confirmed by molecular testing of mother and child.

HIGH-YIELD POINTS

- *Dysostosis*: It is isolated dysplasia of a bone or a group of bones, i.e. craniofacial dysostosis, polydactyly, syndactyly, etc.
- Phocomelia (meaning seal like limbs) is a birth defect wherein the proximal bones of the limbs are shortened, such that the hands and the feet are located very close to the trunk **(Fig. 14.1)**. It was the prime concern in children whose mothers had been on antiemetic drug Thalidomide, which led to the stoppage of the drug.

Box 14.1: Common skeletal dysplasias

- Osteogenesis imperfecta—most common
- Multiple epiphyseal dysplasia (MED)
- Spondyloepiphyseal dysplasia (SED)
- Achondroplasia
- Pseudoachondroplasia
- Metaphyseal chondrodysplasia

Table 14.1: Classification of dysplasias based on which part of the bone is predominantly involved

Epiphyseal dysplasias	• Spondyloepiphyseal dysplasia (SED) • Multiple epiphyseal dysplasia (MED) • Dysplasia epiphyseal hemimelica (Trevor's disease) • Chondrodysplasia punctata
Physeal and metaphyseal dysplasia	• Achondroplasia • Hypochondroplasia • Hereditary multiple exostosis • Enchondromatosis
Metaphyseal and diaphyseal dysplasia	• Metaphyseal dysplasia (Pyle's disease) • Diaphyseal dysplasia (Engelmann's disease) • Osteopetrosis (marble bone disease) • Pycnodysostosis • Craniometaphyseal dysplasia
Mixed dysplasia	• Cleidocranial dysplasia • Nail-patella syndrome • Diastrophic dysplasia • Pseudoachondroplasia
Connective tissue disorders	• Ehlers-Danlos syndrome • Osteogenesis imperfecta • Larsen's syndrome

Storage disorders and metabolic defects	• Gaucher's disease
	• Homocystinuria
	• Alkaptonuria
	• Mucopolysaccharidoses:
	  – Hunter's disease
	  – Hurler's syndrome
	  – Morquio syndrome

Chromosomal disorder	• Down syndrome

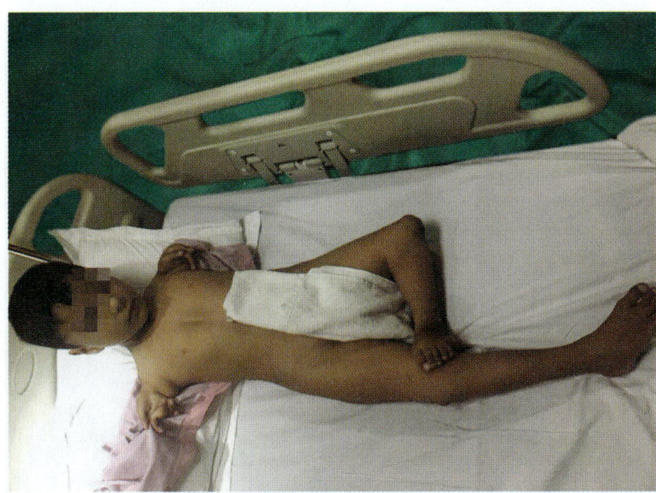

Fig. 14.1: Clinical picture of a child with phocomelia

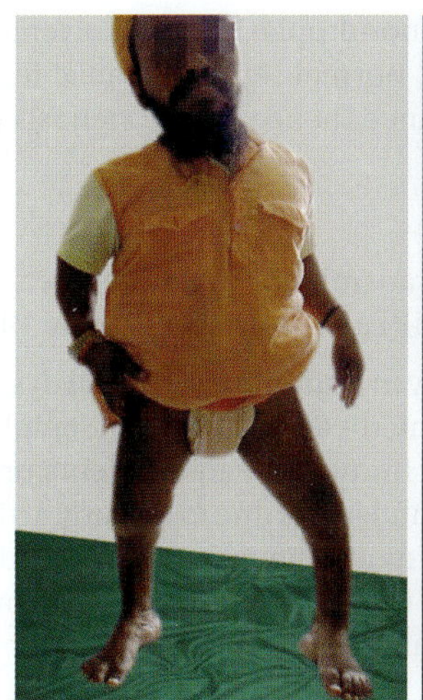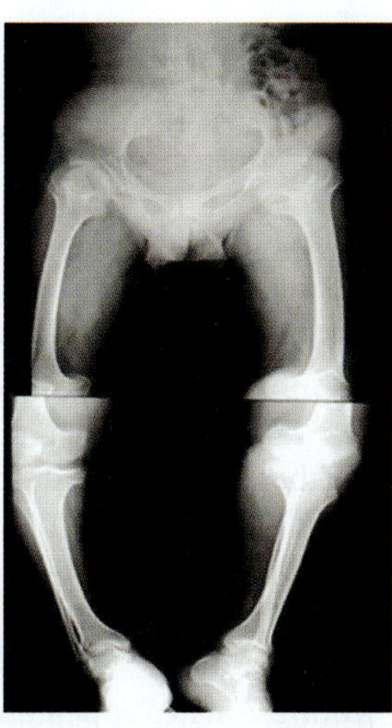

Fig. 14.2A: Typical clinical appearance and X-ray of achondroplasic patient showing classical deformities in thigh and legs

SOME COMMON SKELETAL DYSPLASIAS AND RELATED ORTHOPEDIC DISORDERS

Achondroplasia

Genetics: Autosomal dominant transmission; mutation in fibroblast growth factor receptor gene-3 (FGFR-3).

Clinical features: Normal intramembranous ossification leads to normal skull and clavicles, whereas abnormal endochondral ossification results in shortening of the long bones. Patients classically have rhizomelic micromelia, i.e. arms and thighs are most severely shortened **(Fig. 14.2A)**. Short stature is apparent at birth. Hands are short and broad. All fingers are approximately of the same length (starfish hand) with wide separation between the middle and ring finger (trident hand, **Fig. 14.2B**). Elbow contracture, broadening of the ends of long bones, angular deformities of the lower limbs and waddling gait are often present. There may be protuberant belly and obesity. Facial features are also characteristic. Achondroplasics have large head with prominent mandibles, small maxillae and depressed nasal bridge. However, these children have normal intelligence (circus dwarf).

X-ray features: Bones are short and thick. In the spine, there are posteriorly scalloped vertebrae, short pedicles and short interpedicular distance. Bullet-shaped vertebrae are seen in infants. Pelvis is broad and flat (champagne glass pelvis, i.e. width is greater than depth) with squared iliac wings, horizontal acetabular roofs and narrow sciatic notches. Epiphyses of bones are, however, normal.

Treatment: Orthopedic consultation is usually required for cervical and lumbar canal stenosis, angular deformities of knee and for limb lengthening.

Hypochondroplasia

It is similar to achondroplasia, but less severe. It cannot be detected at birth and may remain undiagnosed until puberty when a child fails to achieve his growth spurt. Final height is shorter but relatively these children are taller than those with achondroplasia. X-ray features are however, similar to achondroplasia.

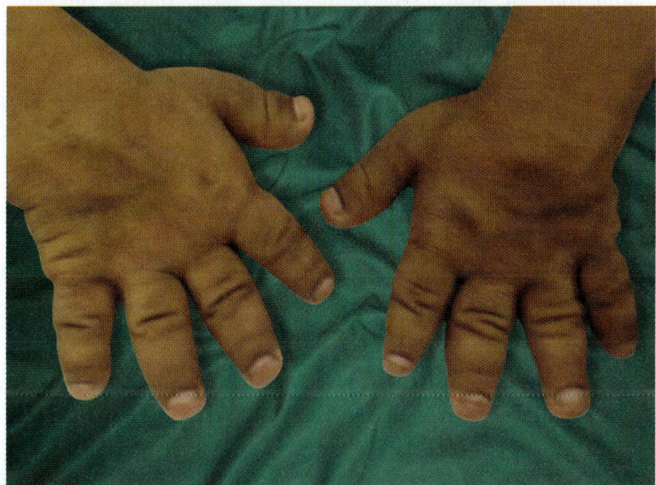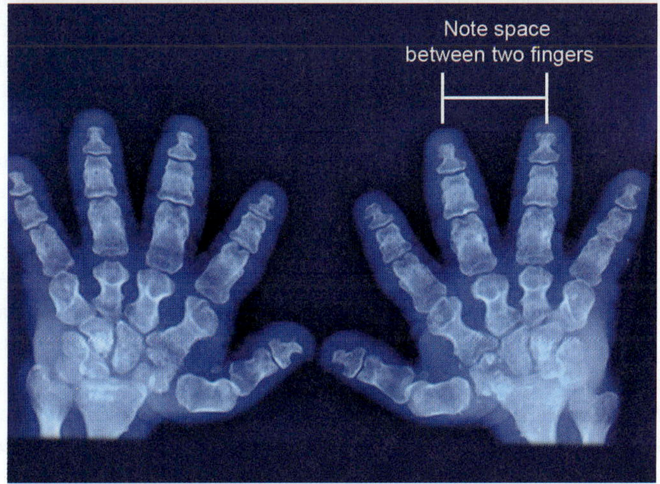

Fig. 14.2B: Clinical picture and X-ray (AP view) showing trident hand in achondroplasic

Pseudoachondroplasia

It is also a type of rhizomelic dwarfism. The child is normal at birth and shortening may not become apparent until after infancy.

Distinguishing features from achondroplasia are involvement of both epiphysis and metaphysis, normal skull and facial features and normal interpedicular distance (hence, spinal stenosis is not a feature).

Multiple Epiphyseal Dysplasia

Genetics: Autosomal dominant transmission, mutation in cartilage oligomeric matrix protein (COMP) gene on chromosome 19.

Clinical features: Basic pathology in multiple epiphyseal dysplasia (MED) is abnormal fragmented and flattened epiphyses, especially those of femoral and humeral heads. Patients present in early childhood with stiff, painful joints due to an early arthritis. Bilateral hip involvement may make them walk with waddling gait. Height is mildly short and true dwarfism (height below the 3rd percentile for height) is usually not present.

X-ray features: Late appearance of ossification centers and fragmented and flattened epiphyses and premature osteoarthritic changes are characteristic features. Coxa vara and double-layered patella may be seen. Flat bones like skull, pelvis, mandible, clavicles, ribs, scapulae and sternum are normal. There is no vertebral involvement.

Treatment: Orthopedic consultation is usually required for painful hip joints due to early arthritic changes. Due to fragmentation of the femoral head epiphysis and coxa vara picture may look like a case of bilateral Perthes disease.

Spondyloepiphyseal Dysplasia

Spondyloepiphyseal dysplasia (SED) is of two types: (1) SED congenita and (2) SED tarda.

Spondyloepiphyseal Dysplasia Congenita

Genetics: Autosomal dominant transmission, mutation in COL2A1 locus on chromosome 12.

Clinical features: It is characterized by abnormal epiphyses that result in a short trunk dwarfism (i.e. rhizomelic and mesomelic dwarfism of limbs). Affected children have a short neck and wide set eyes. Limb deformities, viz. genu valgum and coxa vara are common. Clubfoot deformities may also be seen. These children generally have excessive lumbar lordosis with a protuberant abdomen.

X-ray features: Epiphyses are irregular and flattened. There is late appearance of ossification centers of carpal and tarsal bones. Secondary ossification centers of long bones also have a delayed appearance. Small iliac wings, flat acetabulam and coxa vara are commonly seen in pelvis X-ray. Spinal involvement is seen in form of odontoid dysplasia that puts the patient at risk of atlantoaxial dislocation. Platyspondyly, i.e. flattened vertebral bodies are present on a spine X-ray.

Treatment: Patients seek orthopedic consultation usually for spine abnormalities, viz. cervical instability, excessive lumbar lordosis, scoliosis, etc. or at other times for lower limb deformities, like coxa vara and genu valgum.

Spondyloepiphyseal Dysplasia Tarda

Genetics: Inheritance is autosomal recessive or X-linked recessive.

Clinical features: It is a less severe form which manifest later in childhood or adolescence. Height is minimally affected. The child presents with complaints of bilateral hip pain (hip osteoarthritis) and short height.

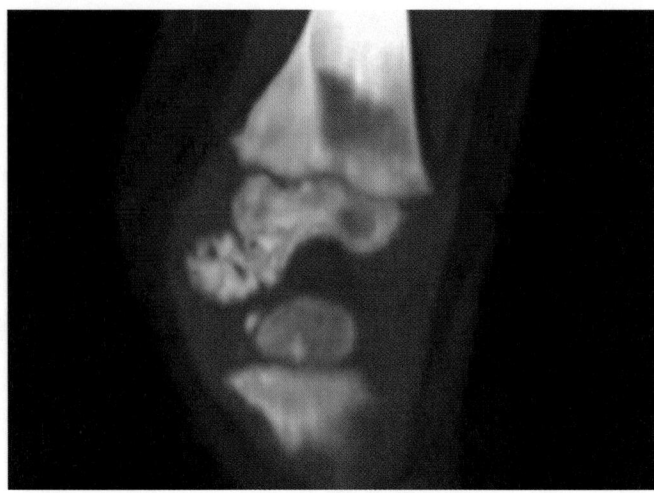

Fig. 14.3: CT scan of knee joint showing half-epiphyseal involvement characteristic of Trevor's disease
Source: Dr Yuranga Weerakkody, Radiopaedia.org.

X-ray features: X-rays show abnormal hip joints and other epiphyses. Platyspondyly may also be seen.

Dysplasia Epiphysealis Hemimelica (Trevor's Disease/Fairbank's Disease)

Trevor's disease is characterized by involvement of only one-half of the epiphysis on only one side of the body. This leads to an asymmetrical limb deformity due to asymmetrical enlargement of the epiphysis **(Fig. 14.3)**. The lesion is very similar to osteochondroma but always affects a single limb. Knee and talus are the most common sites. Excision of enlarged epiphyseal cartilage is required if it interferes with the joint function.

Osteopetrosis (Marble Bone Disease, Albers-Schönberg Disease)

Osteopetrosis is characterized by defective osteoclastic bone resorption due to defects in their carbonic anhydrase type II proton pump. Defective bone resorption interferes with normal bone remodeling leading to thickened, radiologically dense (white) bones and hence the term, marble bone disease.

Clinical features: Patients present with features of pancytopenia (abnormal bleeding, anemia, infections and failure to thrive) due to encroachment of the marrow cavity by bone overgrowth. Osteomyelitis is common due to decreased immunity. Although bones are thickened but they are defective as there is no remodeling due to lack of osteoclastic activity which makes them susceptible to fracture. Bone pain and pathological fractures are thus common. Healing of fractures is generally normal, but abnormal bones are difficult to fix surgically making internal fixation difficult in these patients. Two types have been described, malignant osteopetrosis (autosomal recessive) and benign osteopetrosis (autosomal dominant). Benign form is usually symptom-free and diagnosed incidentally on X-rays prescribed for other reasons.

X-ray features: Thickened, sclerotic (white) bones are characteristic features. Endobones **(Fig. 14.4A)** or bone-within-a-bone appearance (radiodense tissues inside the cortices of long bones) is pathognomonic for osteopetrosis. Defective bone remodeling around the knee joint causes typical Erlenmeyer flask deformity **(Fig. 14.4B)**. Rugger jersey spine (*see* Page 412) may be a feature as well.

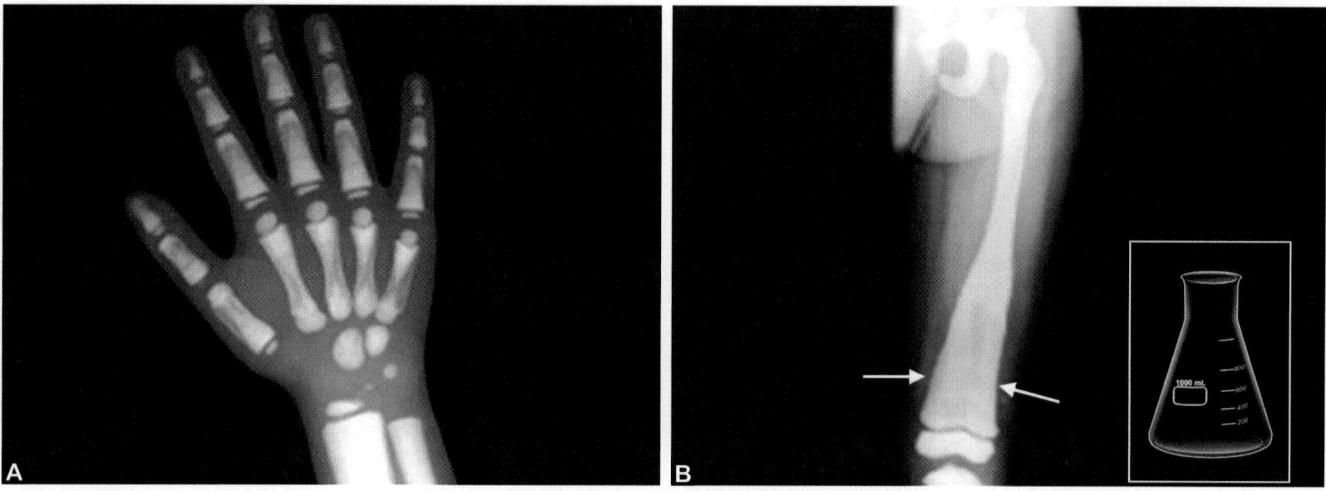

Figs 14.4A and B: X-ray of hand AP view showing bone within bone appearance in a patient of osteopetrosis (*Source:* Apy Liu, YK Ng, APW Hui, et al. Clinical quiz: answer. HK J Paediatr [New Series]. 2011;16:293-4.); (B) Thickened sclerotic bone with typical Erlenmeyer flask deformity (arrows) in osteopetrosis (*Source:* Orphanet Journal of rare diseases published by BioMed Central).

Treatment: It can be treated by early bone marrow transplantation.

Chondrodysplasia Punctata (Stippled Epiphyses)

Chondrodysplasia punctata is a group of disorders characterized by calcific stippling of the epiphyses and surrounding periarticular soft tissues. Most common is Conradi-Hünermann syndrome, which is an X-linked dominant disorder.

Clinical features: Important clinical findings in this condition include ichthyosis, coarse hair, frontal bossing, epicanthic folds, down slanting palpebral fissure, depressed nasal bridge, rhizomelic shortening of limbs, developmental dysplasia of the hip (DDH), congenital talipes equinovarus (CTEV), scoliosis, congenital cataract and sensorineural deafness.

X-ray features: Punctate calcification of epiphyses **(Fig. 14.5)** is typical but may disappear after 1st year of life.

Cleidocranial Dysostosis

Genetics: Autosomal dominant, mutation in *CBFA* gene on chromosome 6 leading to defective intramembranous ossification, so that clavicle, skull and pelvis are abnormal.

Clinical features: Patients are short-statured and have the typical appearance with small faces (Elfin facies), wide skull and drooping shoulders. One or both clavicle may be underdeveloped or even missing. Sometimes bilaterally affected child is able to bring both the shoulders in front of chest and touch them together. Other defects include high and narrow palate, small scapulae, pectus excavatum and delayed permanent dentition.

X-ray features: Clavicles are hypoplastic or absent (most commonly lateral end of clavicle is absent). Skull X-ray shows wide suture lines, small maxilla, hypoplastic or absent facial bones and multiple wormian bones **(Fig. 14.6)**. X-ray pelvis shows a wide symphysis pubis, wide sacroiliac joint, small iliac wings and thin rami. Other features include coxa vara, spina bifida and hypoplastic terminal phalanges. X-ray hand shows pseudoepiphyses of the metacarpal and metatarsal bones (epiphyses present at both ends of the second through fifth metacarpal and metatarsals) resulting in characteristic lengthening of the second metacarpal.

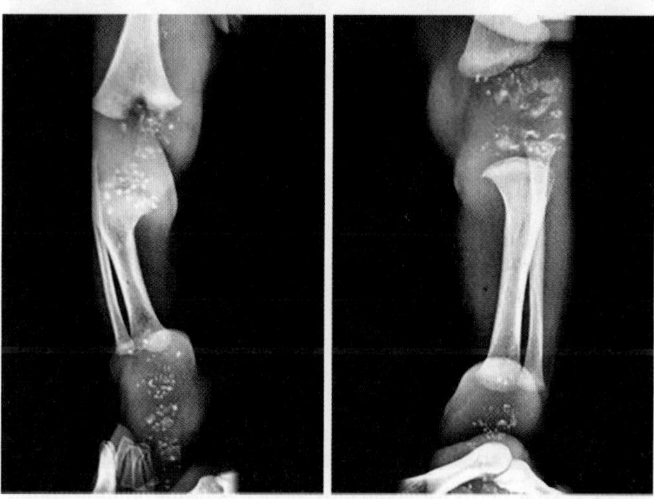

Fig. 14.5: X-ray of lower limb showing calcific stippling of the epiphyses of the knee and ankle joints characteristic of chondrodysplasia punctata

Source: Dr Tim Luijkx, Radiopaedia.org.

Osteopoikilosis (Spotted Bones)

It is an autosomal dominant benign disorder (mutations in gene LFMD3) characterized by presence of multiple bone islands or multiple enostosis (cartilage remnants) across the skeleton. X-rays demonstrate multiple round or oval radioopacities **(Fig. 14.7)** in metaphyseal and epiphyseal region of long bones, carpals, tarsals and acetabulum. Axial skeleton (except pelvis) is generally spared and hence there's rare ribs, skull or spine involvement. On histopathology bone is cortical like, with well developed haversian system. Condition is asymptomatic and often just an incidental finding in young adults, requiring no treatment. An important caution is to rule out presence of a blastic metastasis. While Osteopoikilosis lesions are mostly regular sized, blastic metastasis are generally irregular in size.

Melorheostosis/Leri's Disease (Candle Bone Disease)

It is a rare sclerosing bone disorder characterized by cortical hyperostosis (thickening of cortex of bone). The gene mutated in

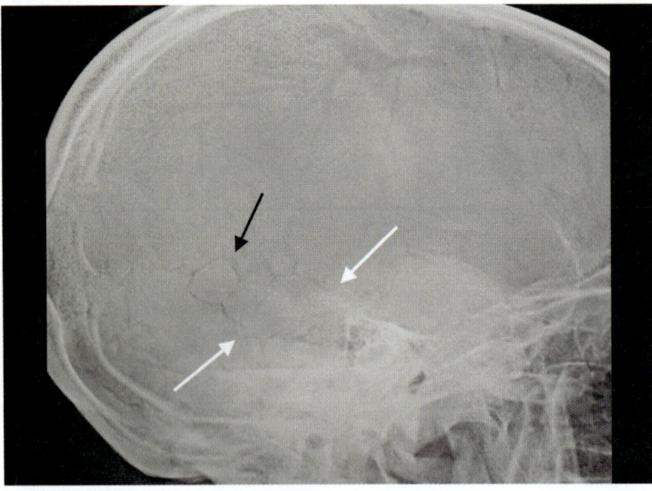

Fig. 14.6: X-ray skull lateral view showing Wormian bones
Source: LearningRadiology.com.

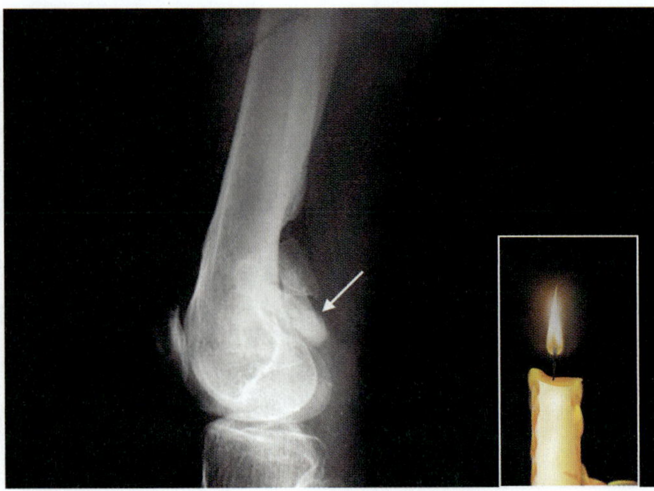

Fig. 14.8: Irregular cortical sclerosis in melorheostosis. Note the dripping candle wax appearance (arrow)

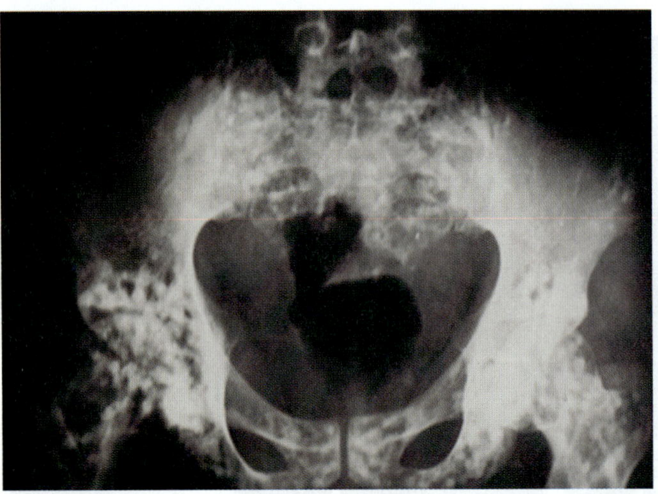

Fig. 14.7: X-ray pelvis with both hips AP view showing multiple round opacities characteristic of osteopoikilosis

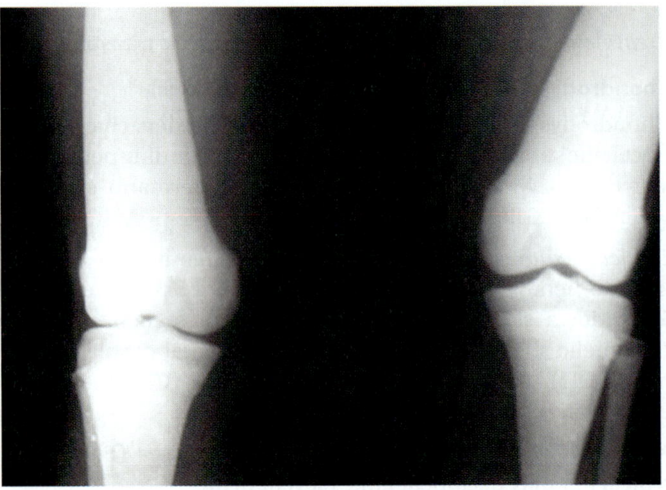

Fig. 14.9: Generalized osteosclerosis in pycnodysostosis

this condition is LFMD3, same as in Osteopoikilosis. The disease may be monostotic or polyostotic. Patients often present with bone pain and soft-tissue contractures that lead to deformities of the joints.

X-ray picture is characteristic **(Fig. 14.8)** showing asymmetrical, irregular cortical sclerosis giving the appearance of wax dripping down the side of a candle appearance.

Pycnodysostosis

This is a mixed skeletal dysplasia that is best known for being the closest differential of osteogenesis imperfecta. It is also characterized by blue sclera and proneness to fracture. These patients have short-limbed short stature, triangular facies, hypoplastic facial bones and mandibles and abnormal dentition. Lateral end of clavicle is hypoplastic or absent, terminal phalanges of fingers are also hypoplastic. This autosomal recessive disorder is supposedly caused by a mutation in the gene present on chromosome 1 that codes the lysosomal enzyme cathepsin K, present in osteoclasts.

X-ray features: Generalized osteosclerosis **(Fig. 14.9)** is a characteristic feature. X-ray of the skull shows widened sutures and open fontanels. Spine X-ray may show failure of segmentation of vertebrae in cervical and lumbar region.

Metaphyseal Chondrodysplasia (Pyle's Disease)

It is a heterogeneous group of disorders with both autosomal dominant and recessive inheritance, characterized by abnormal bulbous metaphyses (with normal epiphyses) due to defective osteoclastic remodeling in metaphyseal areas of long bones. The Schmidt type is the most common type amongst this metaphyseal dysplasia. It is characterized by short stature, genu varum and coxa vara and waddling gait. Thickening of the basilar skull bones may result in cranial nerve entrapments.

X-rays classically show cupping and splaying (widening) of metaphyses, resembling the Erlenmeyer flask deformity **(Fig. 14.4B)** seen in osteopetrosis. However, in comparison the cortices are thinner and the bone is more osteopenic.

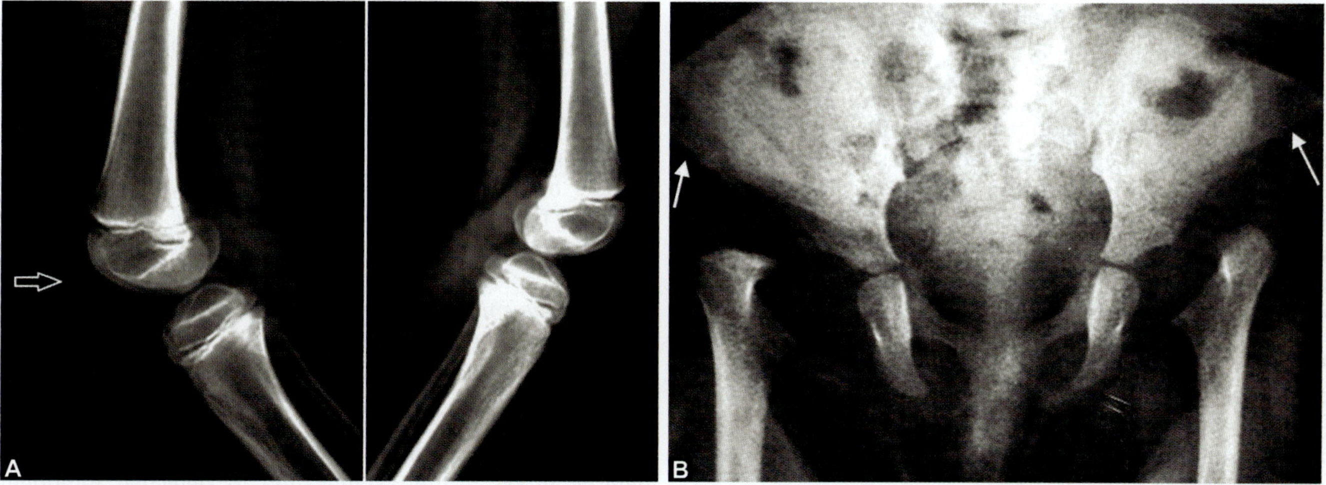

Figs 14.10A and B: (A) X-ray both knees lateral views showing hypoplastic patella on right side (arrow) and absent patella on left side in a patient of nail-patella syndrome; (B) Bilateral iliac wings (arrows) in nail-patella syndrome

Diaphyseal Dysplasia (Camurati-Engelmann Disease)

This rare disease is characterized by bilateral symmetrical increased density (sclerosis) of shaft of long bones. The child usually presents with muscle weakness and bilateral leg pain. Skull bone thickening may cause cranial nerve palsies.

Nail-patella Syndrome (Onycho-osteo-dysplasia)

It is a rare autosomal dominant disorder, characterized by dystrophy of the nails (greatest in thumbnail and least in a little finger nail which is rarely affected) and hypoplastic or absent patellae. Genu valgum and hypoplastic lateral femoral condyle usually lead to recurrent dislocation of patella. Lateral half of the elbow joint is hypoplastic which causes cubitus valgus deformity. Open angle glaucoma, nephropathy, clubfoot, DDH, scoliosis and Plummer-Vinson syndrome are other associated features.

X-ray features: Hypoplastic or absent patella **(Fig. 14.10A)**, bilateral posterior iliac horns (Fong's prongs, **Fig. 14.10B**) and prominent anterior iliac spine are characteristic features.

HIGH-YIELD POINTS

- Spondyloepiphyseal dysplasia and MED have a remarkable resemblance with Perthes disease. Symmetrical involvement of bilateral hips favors a diagnosis of MED and SED.
- Erlenmeyer flask deformity refers to a radiographic appearance of relative constriction of the diaphysis and flaring of the metaphysis. It is typically seen on femoral X-ray (*see* **Fig. 14.4B**). It is seen in many conditions, like osteopetrosis, achondroplasia, metaphyseal dysplasia (Pyle's disease), fibrous dysplasia, rickets, rheumatoid arthritis, Ollier's disease, thalassemia, Gaucher's disease, Niemann-Pick disease, etc.
- Bone within bone appearance (Endobones, **Fig. 14.4A**) can be seen in osteopetrosis, sickle cell anemia, thalassemia, Paget's disease, acromegaly, lead poisoning, growth arrest lines (infancy), Gaucher's disease and congenital syphilis.
- Wormian bones (*see* **Fig. 14.6**) are intrasutural skull bones resembling puzzle pieces that form because of detachment of portions of primary ossification centers of adjacent membranous bones. They are most commonly located within the lambdoid suture. The most common cause is idiopathic > Osteogenesis imperfecta > Cleido-cranial dysplasia. The list of causes can be remembered by the Mnemonic "SODA PORCH".

  S–Syndrome-Kinky hair syndrome
  O–Osteogenesis imperfecta
  D–Down syndrome
  A–Acro-osteolysis
  P–Pycnodysostosis
  O–Otopalatodigital syndrome
  R–Rickets
  C–Cleidocranial dysostosis
  H–Hypothyroidism/hypophosphatasia

- *Sclerosing bone (white bone) disorders*: These are characterized by varying sclerosis (whitening) of bones. These include osteopetrosis, osteopoikilosis, osteomyelitis, osteopathia striata, melorheostosis, Caffey's disease and pycnodysostosis.
- Osteopoikilosis is often found concurrently with melorheostosis (both have same gene mutation, i.e. LFMD3) and some people feel that they represent a spectrum of the same disorder.

OSTEOGENESIS IMPERFECTA (LOBSTEIN-VROLIK'S DISEASE/BRITTLE BONE DISEASE/FRAGILITAS OSSIUM)

INTRODUCTION

Osteogenesis imperfecta (OI) is a rare connective tissue disorder cum a skeletal dysplasia characterized by brittle bones which fracture easily. Basic defect is hindered crosslinking of immature collagen, leading to impaired formation of mature polymerized collagen.

INHERITANCE

It is transmitted both in autosomal dominant (predominant) and autosomal recessive patterns. Around 90% of these patients have genetic mutation in the *COL1A1* and *COL1A2* genes resulting in glycine substitution in procollagen molecule, which causes abnormal collagen crosslinking.

PATHOLOGY

Not only is the collagen abnormal but also there is decreased production of collagen. Both these factors result in insufficient osteoid production by osteoblasts. Consequently, bone remodeling is abnormal leading to changes like increased diameter of Haversian canals and osteocyte lacunae, replicated cement lines, increased number of osteoblasts and osteoclasts and paucity of trabeculae. The cortex of the bone is also thinner than normal.

CLINICAL FEATURES

Type I collagen is present in skin, ligaments, bone, teeth and sclera and consequently these are the tissues that are defective. Hence, patients present with a constellation of symptoms involving multiple systems.

Bone and Joint Involvement

There is marked osteopenia that leads to frequent fractures after trivial trauma. Fractures can even occur in utero or at the time of birth with severe forms presenting as stillbirths. With time course, the fractures become recurrent due to brittle bones, disuse osteopenia, progressive long bone deformity and joint stiffness occurring due to immobilization. Frequency of fractures usually declines after puberty but in women rises again after menopause. Bone remodeling is defective and results not only in progressive bowing of long bones (**Figs 14.11A and B**) but also the saber shin appearance of the tibia, short stature, scoliosis, cod fish vertebra (*see* Page 401, **Fig. 15.1**), basilar invagination and olecranon apophyseal avulsion fractures. Fracture healing, however is normal, but fractures tend to heal with abundant callus, although the callus is of poor quality. Hyperplastic callus may sometimes be difficult to differentiate from osteosarcoma. New bone is pliable for long time due to defective osteoid formation resulting in malunion and deformities. Hyperlaxity of ligaments with hypermobility of the joints is also present. Wormian skull bones (*see* **Fig. 14.6**) are characteristically found. Other features include scoliosis and protrusio acetabuli. Basilar invagination, i.e. softening of base of skull may be present and

patients may present with apnea, altered consciousness, ataxia or myelopathy. It is usually seen in the third or fourth decade of life, but can manifest as early as in teenage years.

Ocular Involvement

As a consequence of the thin collagen layer in the sclera, sclera appears blue owing to the hue of underlying uveal vessels. Following features may be present in addition:

- *Saturn's ring:* White sclera immediately surrounding the cornea
- *Arcus juvenilis:* White opacity concentric to limbus in the periphery of cornea
- Hypermetropia and retinal detachment.

Auditory Involvement

Conductive hearing loss is due to otosclerosis (abnormal bone material grows around stapes due to defective remodeling) and leads to deafness. Onset is in adolescence or adulthood. Sensorineural hearing loss can also coexist due to pressure on the auditory nerve as it emerges through the skull.

Dental Involvement

Dentinogenesis imperfecta (dentin dysplasia) is characteristic. Yellowish brown/bluish gray discoloration of teeth is seen. Enamel, which is ectodermal in origin, is normal. Deciduous and permanent teeth both are involved, they break easily and are prone to carries. Lower incisors are particularly more severely affected.

Skin and Muscle Involvement

The skin is thin and translucent and is prone to subcutaneous hemorrhages. Muscles are hypotonic due to multiple fractures and deformities. Hernias are common.

Metabolic Features

A hypermetabolic state exists, resulting in excessive sweating and heat intolerance. The patient is susceptible to hyperthermia during general anesthesia.

CLASSIFICATION

Sillence described seven types of osteogenesis imperfecta. Salient features of each type are given in **Table 14.2**. Type V, VI and VII

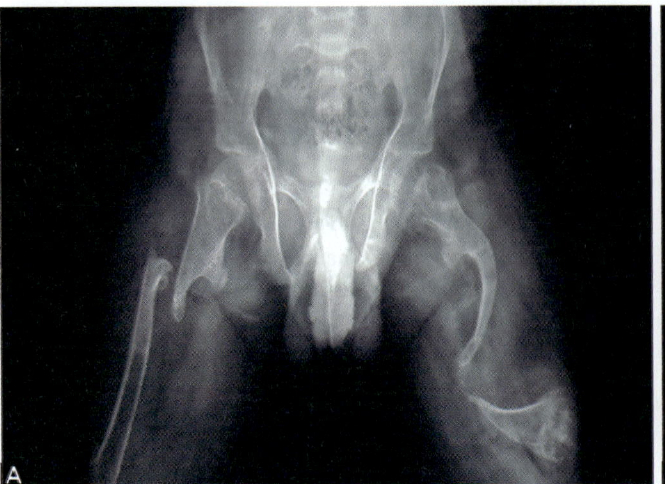
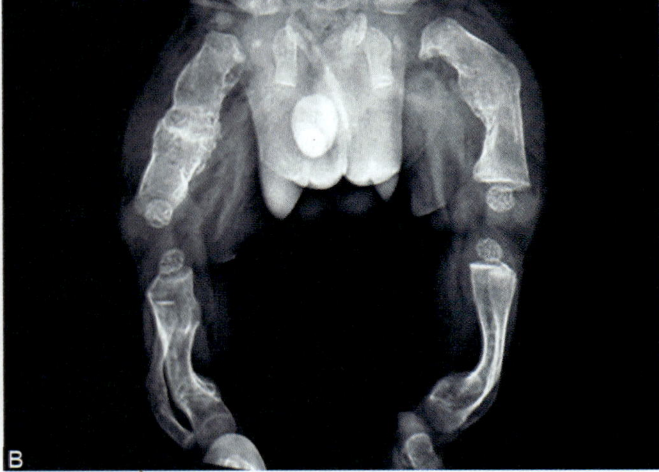

Figs 14.11A and B: Osteogenesis imperfecta—see multiple fractures in various stages of healing, callus formation and bony deformities

Table 14.2: Sillence classification of osteogenesis imperfect (OI)

Type	Inheritance	Sclera	Features
I	Autosomal dominant (AD)	Blue	Mildest form. The most common form Presents at preschool age Hearing deficit in 50%
II	Autosomal recessive (AR)	Blue	Lethal in the perinatal period (hence living cases not seen)
III	AR	Normal	Fractures at birth Progressively short stature Most severe survivable form
IV	AD	Normal	Moderately severe form Bowing bones and vertebral fractures, common No hearing loss
V			Hypertrophic callus after a fracture Ossification of interosseous membrane between radius and ulna and tibia and fibula
VI			Moderate severity Similar to type IV
VII			Associated with rhizomelia and coxa vara

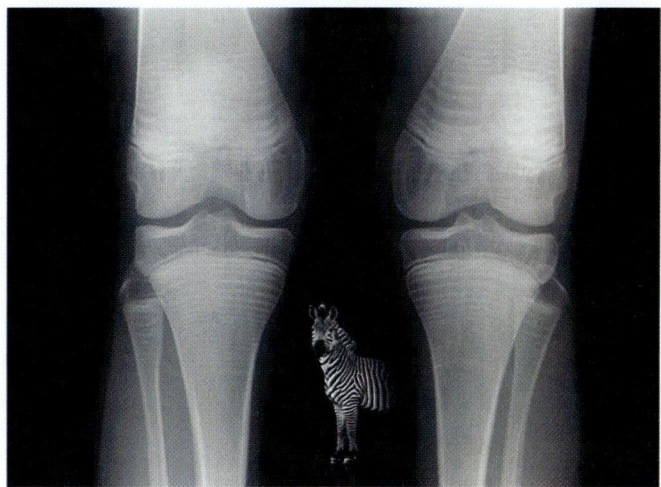

Fig. 14.12: Zebra strip sign following bisphosphonate therapy in osteogenesis imperfecta

Source: Radiology Signs @RadiologySigns (Education Website).

have no Type I collagen mutation, but have abnormal bone on microscopy and a similar phenotype. Cases can also be classified into congenital form (fractures present at birth) and tarda form (less severe, fractures occur later on).

DIAGNOSIS

Prenatal Diagnosis

Although prenatal USG may show multiple fractures in severe forms, polymerase chain reaction (PCR) can be conducted on chorionic villi biopsy at 8–12 weeks, demonstrating the synthesis of abnormal proalpha collagen chains.

Postnatal Diagnosis

Skeletal survey (radiographs) shows multiple fractures in various stages of healing, abundant callus formation and bony deformities **(Figs 14.11A and B)**. Bone cortices are thin with generalized osteopenia. The skull has a mushroom appearance with a very thin calvarium. Wormian bones (*see* **Fig. 14.6**) may be seen in the skull X-ray. They are said to be significant if more than 10 in number, measure at least 6 mm × 4 mm and are arranged in a general mosaic pattern. Iliac crest biopsy may be done which shows a decrease in cortical widths and cancellous bone volume, with increased bone remodeling. Although a positive family history, characteristic clinical features and typical radiographic findings are usually sufficient for a diagnosis, the most definitive proof comes by detection of defective collagen or identification of the mutation. A molecular defect in type I procollagen is detected by incubating the skin fibroblasts with radioactive amino acids and analyzing the proalpha chains by polyacrylamide gel

electrophoresis. It shows a decreased rate of synthesis of proalpha 1 chains and abnormal proalpha chains.

Screening of Family Members

Polymerase chain reaction is a useful method for screening other family members at risk of having the disease.

MANAGEMENT

Fracture Prevention

Early bracing is done to reduce deformities and lessen the chance of fractures. Growth hormone may be used due to its anabolic effects. Bisphosphonates are the preferred drugs, given to reduce fracture rate and pain and to increase cortical thickness by inhibiting osteoclast function. They do not prevent development of scoliosis. Chronic use causes horizontal metaphyseal bands on radiographs. In fact, patients who receive cyclical bisphosphonate therapy may show Zebra strip sign **(Fig. 14.12)** on X-rays. It is seen prior to closure of the physis as transverse sclerotic bands due to reduced bone resorption and turnover caused by bisphosphonate therapy alternating with bands of normal lucency in the metaphysis of distal femur, proximal tibia, proximal fibula, pelvis, acetabulum, vertebral bodies, forearm bones, metacarpals and phalanges. Zebra lines appear after 8–10 weeks of therapy and progressively migrate toward diaphysis and disappear after physeal closure.

Fracture Treatment

Treatment is mostly nonoperative if the child is less than 2 years of age. For children above the age of 2 years, fixation with special implants like Bailey-Dubow rods (telescoping rods that can telescope and increase in size with growth) is preferred. This splints the whole bone to reduce further fracture risk and also allows long bone growth to continue uninterrupted. Bowing deformities of long bones are treated with multiple realignment osteotomies with rod fixation (Sofield-Miller procedure/Seek-kebab treatment, **Fig. 14.13**).

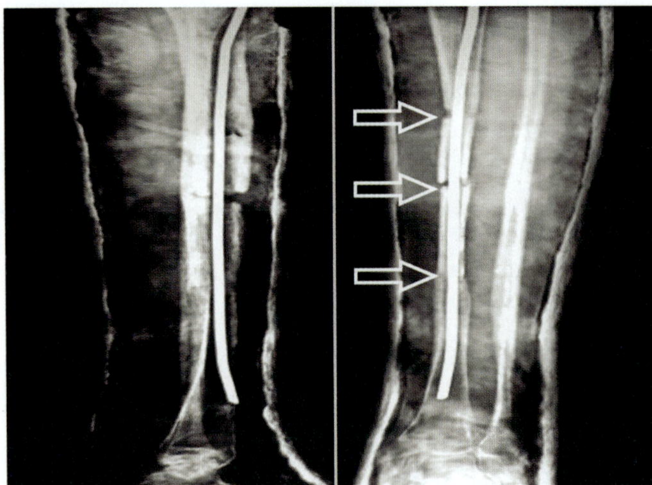

Fig. 14.13: Seek kebab treatment: See osteotomies at multiple levels (arrows)

Table 14.3: Diagnostic criteria for neurofibromatosis (NF)-1 and 2 (Two or more than two criteria of NF-1 should be met for diagnosis of NF-1 and any one of NF-2 criteria should be present to make a diagnosis of NF-2)	
NF-1 (Peripheral)	*NF-2 (Central)*
• More than or equal to six café-au-lait spots each over 5 mm in diameter before puberty or over 15 mm in diameter in older individuals • More than or equal to two neurofibromas or a single plexiform neurofibroma • Freckles in inguinal/axillary region • Optic glioma • More than or equal to two lisch nodules (hamartomas of the iris) • Sphenoid bone dysplasia • Osteoporosis • First degree relative with NF	• Bilateral eight nerve masses (acoustic neuromas) • A first-degree relative with NF type II and either a unilateral 8th nerve mass or any two of the following: Meningioma, glioma, neurofibroma, schwannoma and posterior subcapsular lenticular opacity

NEUROFIBROMATOSIS

Neurofibromatosis (NF) is a hereditary genetic disorder characterized by multisystem manifestations due to hamartomatous growths affecting the central and peripheral nervous system, skeletal system and the skin and subcutaneous tissues.

It can be classified into following varieties:
- Single neurofibroma
- Generalized NF (Von Recklinghausen's disease)
- Plexiform NF (affects the fifth cranial nerve). A further variety of plexiform NF is the pachydermatocele where a large mass is formed that hangs from the face onto the neck.
- Elephantiasis neurofibromatosa (involves leg, causing thickening of the subcutaneous tissue of the limb).

VON RECKLINGHAUSEN'S DISEASE

This is a generalized NF that is further subdivided into peripheral (Type I) and central (Type II) types.

Type I (Peripheral, Neurofibromatosis-1)

It is an autosomal dominant condition with 100% penetrance characterized by mutations in tumor suppressor gene "Neurofibromin" present on chromosome 17 whose function is to inhibit p21 ras oncoprotein. Most commonly, these patients present with multiple café-au-lait spots (with smooth edges—coast of California) or at other times with axillary or inguinal freckling (Crowe's sign). In later stages, skeletal abnormalities may be seen which include scoliosis (most common), congenital pseudarthrosis of the tibia, hypertrophy of a limb, verrucous hyperplasia, i.e. thickened overgrown skin, etc. The patients tend to have cognitive deficits and it is not uncommon to get a history of seizures. Hydrocephalus may be seen at birth, hormonal dysfunctions may be evident as they grow and they may also develop optic gliomas.

Type II (Central, Neurofibromatosis-2)

The central variety is the less common subtype being an autosomal dominant condition involving mutations in the gene *Merlin* present on chromosome 22. The musculoskeletal abnormalities encountered in NF-1 are generally not present in type II. These patients classically develop bilateral acoustic neuromas and have visual symptoms due to posterior subcapsular lenticular opacities. Facial nerve involvement may also be seen and not uncommon are brain and spinal cord tumors (meningioma is seen in almost every second patient).

The diagnostic criteria for the two varieties are given in **Table 14.3**.

HIGH-YIELD POINTS

- *Giraffe spots/Café-au-lait spots (meaning coffee with milk)*: These are light brown colored macules present anywhere on body mostly on the face and scalp. These are seen in NF-1, von Hippel-Lindau syndrome, tuberous sclerosis, McCune Albright syndrome, ataxia telangiectasia, Bloom's syndrome, Chediak-Higashi syndrome, Peutz-Jeghers syndrome.
- Pseudarthrosis (false joint formation) can be congenital or acquired. The most common cause of acquired pseudarthrosis is a nonunion of a fracture. However, the most common cause of congenital pseudarthrosis is idiopathic followed by NF. The latter is mainly an association and not exactly a cause. Other causes include osteogenesis imperfecta, ankylosing spondylitis, cleidocranial dysplasia, fibrous dysplasia, postsurgery (e.g. after triple arthrodesis).

STORAGE DISORDERS AND ORTHOPEDICS

Storage disorders are a group of rare metabolically inherited diseases characterized by the accumulation of abnormal substances in body tissues owing to enzyme defects eventually leading to multiple organ dysfunction. Important ones from an orthopedic perspective are the lysosomal storage disorders that are discussed below:

GAUCHER'S DISEASE

This belongs to a category called sphingolipidoses or lipid storage disorders (others in this list are Niemann-Pick disease, Fabry disease, etc.) where sphingolipids accumulation occurs

Table 14.4: Mucopolysaccharidosis

Features	Hurler's syndrome (MPS–I)	Hunter's syndrome (MPS–II)	Sanfilippo syndrome (III)	Morquio's syndrome (IV)	Scheie's syndrome (I–S)	Maroteaux-Lamy syndrome (VI)
Defective enzyme	α-1-iduronidase deficient	Sulfoiduronate sulfatase low	N-heparan sulfatase or α-acetyl glucosaminidase low	N-acetylglucosamine-6-sulfate sulfatase	α-L iduronidase	N-acetylgalacto-samine-4-sulfatase
Increased in urine	Dermatan sulfate > heparan sulfate	Heparan sulfate> dermatan sulfate	Heparan sulfate	Keratin sulfate	Dermatan sulfate > heparan sulfate	Dermatan sulfate
Inheritance	AR (Autosomal recessive)	Sex linked recessive, all male patients	AR	AR	AR	AR
Age of presentation	First few months of age	6–12 months	Early childhood	2–4 years	Late childhood	Early-to-late childhood
Orthopedic manifestations	Dorsolumbar kyphosis, anterior inferior beaking of body of vertebral bodies (L1, L2), moderately short stature, odontoid hypoplasia, acetabular dysplasia and joint contractures in hand (PIP contractures)	Manifestations are similar to mucopolysaccharidosis (MPS) I, but are milder. There is an absence of thoracolumbar kyphosis. Carpal tunnel syndrome may be seen in these patients	Only noticed because of short stature. There is no kyphosis. There may be minimal widening of clavicles at medial ends	Markedly short stature (severe skeletal dysplasia), thoracolumbar kyphosis, flat vertebral bodies (platyspondyly), central anterior beaking of vertebral bodies, marked manubriosternal angle, Wine glass pelvis odontoid hypoplasia, atlantoaxial instability, acetabular dysplasia, coxa valga, genu valgum, pes planus, pectus carinatum are seen. Joint contracture and stiffness are absent (instead joint hyper- mobility is seen)	Just a less severe version of hurler syndrome. There are small epiphysis in the hands of these children	Same as Hurler's syndrome
Mental retardation	Severe	Late in onset and less severe	Severe	Absent	Absent	Absent

in lysosomes. It is an autosomal recessive disorder. There is a deficiency of a lysosomal enzyme glucocerebrosidase causing accumulation of glucocerebroside in the reticuloendothelial system, mainly in liver, spleen and bone marrow.

Orthopedic manifestations include abnormal bone remodeling leading to classical Erlenmeyer flask deformity of distal femur **(Figs 14.4A and B)** and proximal tibia, delayed healing and pathological fractures. Patients of Gaucher's disease are at increased risk of osteomyelitis and avascular necrosis.

MUCOPOLYSACCHARIDOSIS

Mucopolysaccharidoses (MPS) are a heterogeneous group of inherited disorders characterized by progressive lysosomal storage of glycosaminoglycans. Orthopedic manifestations have common features across all forms of MPS **(Table 14.4)**.

HIGH-YIELD POINTS

- Dysostosis multiplex is the name given to a broad constellation of skeletal abnormalities (X-ray features) commonly seen in all mucopolysaccharidosis. These include abnormal bone thickening and irregular epiphyseal ossification, dysplastic femoral heads, acetabular dysplasia, iliac hypoplasia with iliac wings, coxa valga and genu valgum deformities, flattened vertebral bodies (platyspondyly) with anterior beaking, odontoid hypoplasia, kyphosis, scoliosis, short thickened clavicles, bullet-shaped phalanges, a large skull with a thickened calvarium and J-shaped sella turcica.
- Carpal tunnel syndrome is the most common entrapment neuropathy in mucopolysaccharidoses.

HOMOCYSTINURIA AND ORTHOPEDICS

It is an autosomal recessive disorder of amino acid metabolism characterized by deficiency of enzyme cystathionine synthase.

Orthopedic manifestations include dolichostenomelia (excessively long and thin limbs), flexion contractures of digits and elbow, arachnodactyly, planovalgus feet, broadening of the metaphyses and epiphyses of long bones, high-arched palate, pectus carinatum, pectus excavatum and generalized osteopenia.

Metabolic Bone Diseases

OSTEOPOROSIS

INTRODUCTION

Normal bone is composed of approximately two-third parts mineral (calcium hydroxyapatite) and one-third part organic matrix/osteoid (mainly collagen type I). Osteoporosis refers to a condition when there is a decrease in both the bone matrix as well as the bone mineral content. It is different from osteomalacia where the prime problem is a deficient mineralization while the bone matrix is adequate. By and far it is the most common metabolic bone disease.

EPIDEMIOLOGY

A number of risk factors exist for the disease. **Table 15.1** gives the list of some important risk factors implicated in causation of osteoporosis.

CLASSIFICATION

Osteoporosis can be classified as primary and secondary.
- Primary osteoporosis is further subclassified into type I and type II.
  Type I (postmenopausal osteoporosis) is characterized by accelerated bone loss after menopause (due to decrease in endogenous estrogen production). The loss is largely from trabecular bone (approximately 2–3% of the total bone/year) rather than cortical bone. This predisposes the patient to vertebral fractures and distal radius fractures.
  In Type II (senile) osteoporosis, the bone loss is more gradual (0.5–1%/year), and involves both cortical and trabecular bone. This increases the risk of hip and vertebral fractures in both men and women over the age of 70 years.
- Secondary osteoporosis is caused by external factors as depicted in **Box 15.1**.
  A detailed history of drug intake must be elucidated from every patient with osteoporosis. Corticosteroids are very frequent cause when prednisolone is given in a dose greater than 7.5 mg/day for a long duration. The loss is largely from trabecular bone, more so in the first 6 months of therapy. Heparin can cause a reversible osteoporosis at doses more than 15,000 units/day for more than 4 months. It causes a hypocalcemia-induced increase in parathyroid hormone (PTH) activity that leads to the condition. Diuretics need a special mention. While furosemide causes calciuria and leads to osteoporosis, thiazides decrease urinary calcium excretion and are considered to be protective. In fact, they have been recommended as add-on therapy in recalcitrant cases of steroid-induced osteoporosis.

CLINICAL FEATURES

Most patients with the disorder are asymptomatic. Back pain is considered the earliest symptom. Decrease in bone mass causes reduction in strength of bones, thereby leading to pathological fractures. Distal radius is the most common site in patients less than 70 years old while in those more than 70 years age, it is the dorsolumbar spine that is the most common site. However, overall vertebral fractures are more common. Multiple compression fractures develop with resulting loss of height and a progressive kyphosis obvious at the back (called as the Dowager's hump). Neurological deficit is however uncommon. Other common osteoporotic fractures include distal radius (Colles' fracture) and hip fractures (fracture neck of femur and trochanteric fractures).

INVESTIGATIONS

Serum calcium, phosphorus, alkaline (ALK) phosphatase and vitamin D levels are usually normal.

X-rays: At least 30% of the bone mass must be lost for osteoporosis to be apparent on the radiographs. The findings on a spine radiograph that point toward the diagnosis **(Fig. 15.1)** include loss of vertebral body height, multiple compression fractures, cod fish appearance or fish mouth appearance of vertebral body (biconcave upper and lower vertebral margins, **Fig. 15.1**).

Table 15.1: Factors affecting osteoporosis	
Risk factors	*Protective factors*
• Old age	• Estrogen replacement therapy
• Thin built	
• Female sex	• Oral contraceptive use
• Early menopause or late menarche	• Thiazide diuretic use
• Prolonged amenorrhea >1 year	
• Oophorectomy during reproductive years	
• Treatment with osteoporosis causing drugs	
• Smoking	
• Alcohol consumption	
• High caffeine intake	
• Inactivity	
• History of recurrent falls and fractures	

Box 15.1: Causes of secondary osteoporosis

- Drugs:
    - Corticosteroids
    - Heparin
    - Anticonvulsants
    - Furosemide
    - Gonadotropin-releasing hormone agonist
    - Cyclosporine
    - Lithium
    - Excessive thyroxine intake
- Prolonged immobilization
- Excessive alcohol intake/cigarette smoking
- Systemic diseases:
    - Endocrine abnormalities:
        - Hyperthyroidism
        - Hyperparathyroidism
        - Cushing's syndrome
        - Hypogonadism
    - Rheumatoid arthritis
    - Osteogenesis imperfecta
    - Multiple myeloma
    - Anorexia nervosa

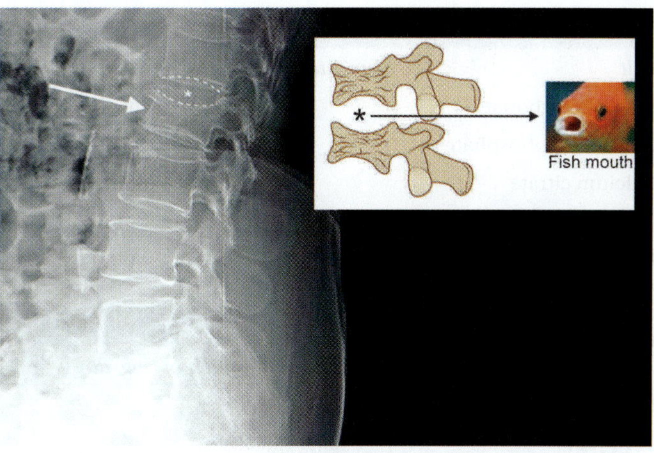

Fig. 15.1: X-ray LS spine of a patient with osteoporosis showing cod fish/ fish mouth appearance of vertebral body (arrow). Note the biconcave vertebral margins generating a fish mouth like shadow (marked with asterisks). Some people refer it to as cod fish vertebrae in reference to salmon spine vertebrae that are biconcave

Table 15.2: Osteoporosis—diagnostic criteria

	BMD T-score
Normal	<1 SD below normal
Osteopenia	1–2.5 SD below normal
Osteoporosis	≥2.5 SD below normal with no h/o fractures
Severe osteoporosis	≥2.5 SD below normal with h/o nonviolent fractures

Osteoporosis can be graded on the basis of hip X-ray by a special index called as Singh's index. The index is based upon the visible number of trabeculae in the femoral neck and grades osteoporosis into six types, type I being most severe and type VI being normal.

Quantitative CT: This is a better indicator, but is the most expensive method and exposes patients to maximum radiation.

Single photon absorptiometry (SPA): It is an inexpensive method that measures cortical bone mineral density (BMD) at one site (usually distal radius) by calculating the ratio of photons absorbed and transmitted. Unfortunately, this method is not applicable to entire skeleton.

Dual energy X-ray absorptiometry (DEXA) scan: Based on a similar principle as SPA, this test measures the quantity of mineral salts in the bone. Generally, lumbar spine and hip (neck of femur) measurements are taken, but the wrist and ankle can also be evaluated.

The test grades the disease based upon a T-score and a Z-score.
- *T-score*: It compares the highest value of BMD obtained from a particular site (i.e. spine, hip, forearm, etc.) to a reference value of 30 years old of same sex and ethnicity.
- *Z-score*: It compares the BMD value obtained with a subject of the same age and sex.

The World Health Organization (WHO) has given the diagnostic criteria for osteoporosis based upon the BMD T-score, measured on a DEXA scan whereby osteoporosis is defined as a T-score of greater than or equal to 2.5 standard deviations (SD) below normal (*see* **Table 15.2** for details).

This test has emerged as the gold standard method for screening of bone mineral mass and diagnosis of the disease in the presenting population. Cost-wise, it is moderately expensive but delivers a very low radiation dose to the patient and the scan time is generally less than 5 minutes. The values tend to correlate well with the fracture risk. An openly available fracture risk calculator called FRAX Tool can be used to estimate the probability of an individual sustaining an osteoporotic fracture over next 10 years. It is based on assessment of some important clinical risk factors and BMD (T-score) at femoral neck.

The Food and Drug Administration of USA (FDA, US) approved indications for DEXA include: Primary hyperparathyroidism, estrogen deficient women at risk of osteoporosis, patients on glucocorticoid treatment, history of osteoporotic vertebral fractures, monitoring response to treatment wherein repeat evaluations are suggested at every 2 years thereafter.

MANAGEMENT AND PREVENTION

Treatment focuses on preventing further bone loss and decreasing the risk of fractures.

Medical Treatment

Calcium Supplements

The daily necessary calcium intake, below which the body has to attain calcium from bone, is 400 mg. A number of calcium preparations are available **(Table 15.3)** and can be prescribed to match the patient requirements depending upon age and sex **(Table 15.4)**. In the absence of excess of vitamin D, calcium supplementation is rarely associated with renal stones. However, one must remember that dietary fibers and iron therapy impair

Table 15.3: Calcium preparations

Salt	Elemental calcium (%)	Solubility
Calcium carbonate	40	Insoluble
Tricalcium phosphate	39	Insoluble
Calcium citrate	21	Soluble
Calcium lactate	18	Soluble
Calcium gluconate	9	Soluble

Table 15.4: Recommended calcium intake

Age	Elemental calcium (mg/day)
Infants	400–600
1–10 years	800–1,200
Adolescents	1,200–1,500
Adults: men	1,200–1,500
Women 19–24 years	1,200–1,500
25–50 years	1,000
>50 years	1,500
Pregnant and lactating	1,500

calcium absorption as do tetracyclines. It is recommended that simultaneous tetracyclines should be administered with at least a gap of 2 hours between the two drugs.

Bisphosphonates

These are the drugs of choice for both senile and postmenopausal osteoporosis. They exert their action by selectively inhibiting osteoclastic activity and reduce the risk of both vertebral and nonvertebral fractures. Three generations of these drugs are currently available:

1. *First generation*: Etidronate: was the first bisphosphonate to be introduced but not for osteoporosis. It primarily has a role in Paget's disease.
2. *Second generation*: Alendronate and risedronate: both of them are FDA-approved for treating osteoporosis in men and women (postmenopausal and steroid-induced osteoporosis). Alendronate is generally given orally in a dose of 70 mg/week. The patient is advised to take the medicine empty stomach with one glass of water and not to lie down for at least half an hour as these can cause esophageal complications.
3. *Third generation*: Ibandronate and zoledronic acid: newer long-acting additions that are given as slow IV infusions on monthly and yearly basis, respectively. Ibandronate can also be given 150 mg tablet once a month.

Long-term use of these drugs (generally over 5 years) has recently caught attention due to special atypical fractures that have been reported in the subtrochanteric area of the femur. These are generally transverse insufficiency fractures with thickening of the lateral femoral cortex and are associated with slow healing (**Fig. 15.2**). Another peculiar side effect of the bisphosphonate therapy is *osteonecrosis of the jaw (ONJ)*. It is caused by both oral and IV bisphosphonates and may be related to the inhibition of osteoclast-mediated resorption of bone. ONJ manifests as exposed, nonvital

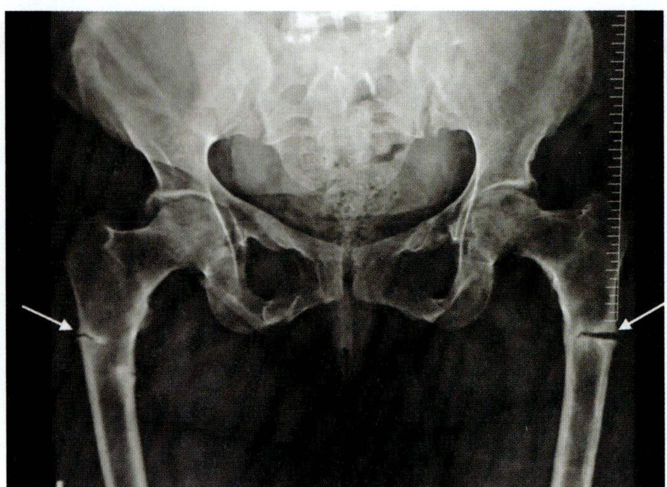

Fig. 15.2: Bisphosphonate-induced bilateral subtrochanteric insufficiency fractures (arrows)

bone involving the maxillofacial structures. Other drugs that can also cause ONJ (medication-related osteonecrosis of the jaw) include antiresorptive (denosumab) and antiangiogenic medications.

Hormone Replacement Therapy

Hormone replacement therapy (HRT) can be particularly indicated in postmenopausal osteoporosis. The daily dose of unconjugated estrogens that has been shown to improve BMD is 0.625 mg (for esterified estrogens, the dose is 0.3 mg) and can be given in combination with progestin (5–10 mg medroxyprogesterone acetate).

Other beneficial effects apart from osteoporosis prevention include relief from vasomotor symptoms of menopause, favorable lipid profile, decreased risk of cardiovascular events and a decreased risk of colorectal cancer.

Most common side effects of HRT include breast tenderness and headaches. The potential risks of prolonged exposure include endometrial cancer, thromboembolic phenomena and risk of getting cholecystitis. There have been concerns over increased risk of breast cancer, but not proven. Adding progestin seemingly decreases this risk. Women receiving combination therapy can get withdrawal bleeding. Due to these side effects HRT is not used primarily to prevent osteoporosis.

Selective Estrogen Receptor Modulators

Selective estrogen receptor modulators (SERMs) are synthetic compounds (**Box 15.2**) that exhibit estrogenic properties in some tissues and antiestrogenic properties in others. Tamoxifen is used in breast cancer and raloxifene has been approved for treatment of osteoporosis. Raloxifene is commonly used in a dose of 60 mg daily. Side effects include hot flashes and leg cramps. Risk of thromboembolism increases, especially in the first 4 months of therapy. Raloxifene is usually chosen for osteoporosis prevention when there is an independent need for breast cancer prophylaxis. Raloxifene reduces the risk of vertebral fractures only. Newer SERM like lasofoxifene has been shown to reduce the risk of nonvertebral fractures as well.

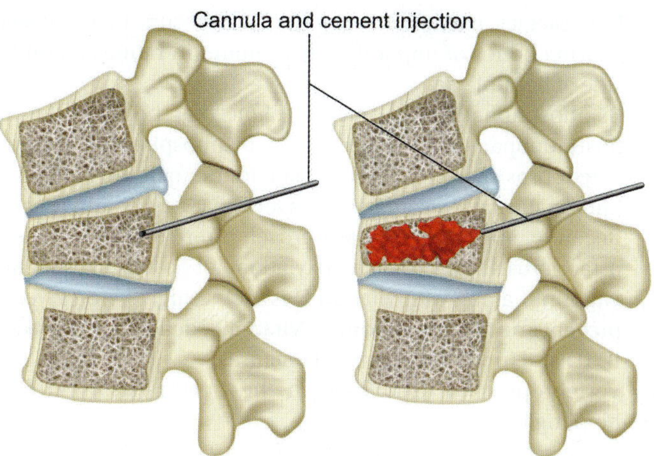

Fig. 15.3: Vertebroplasty diagrammatic representation

Box 15.2: Commonly used selective estrogen receptor modulators

- Tamoxifen
  - *Agonist:* Bone, lipoprotein system, uterus (increased thromboembolic events and endometrial cancer are side effects)
  - *Antagonist:* Breast (used in breast cancer)
- Raloxifene
  - *Agonist:* Bone, lipids
  - *Antagonist:* Breast, endometrium

Anabolic Steroids

These are synthetic derivatives of testosterone. They inhibit osteoclastic bone resorption and increase bone formation through the androgen receptors in bone tissues.

Calcitonin

It prevents bone resorption by inhibiting osteoclastic activity and also has an analgesic effect. Calcitonin reduces the risk of vertebral fractures only, with no effect on peripheral fractures. Routes of administration can be subcutaneous, intramuscular and intranasal. Dose for nasal route is 200 IU/day. Rhinitis is the most common reported side effect.

Vitamin D

Vitamin D3 at doses of 400–800 IU/day or calcitriol 0.5 μg/day is recommended as add-on therapy to calcium supplementation for established disease. It primarily increases the absorption of calcium from the gut.

Sodium Fluoride

Not approved by the FDA yet, but used in Europe. It replaces the hydroxyl ion in crystal lattice forming fluoroapatite that forms dense bone. Most of the effect is on trabecular bone as it has a higher turnover rate. Therapeutic amounts of calcium have to be administered to ensure beneficial effect. The dose is 30 mg/day (decrease in renal failure patients). Gastrointestinal side effects are the main problem. Twenty percent patients may experience a painful lower extremity syndrome due to cortical bone stress fractures.

Strontium

Replaces calcium in hydroxyapatite and is thus anabolic apart from having antiresorptive properties. In a dose of 2 gm/day it reduces risk of both vertebral and nonverterbral fractures.

Recombinant Parathormone (Teriparatide)

Parathyroid hormone directly acts on osteoblasts. Although a continuous infusion of PTH stimulates bone resorption, small pulses in the form of once daily subcutaneous injections (20 μg/day) have been shown to improve bone formation and reduce the risk of both vertebral and nonvertebral fractures. Long-term therapy (20 μg s/c daily) for 1.5–2 years is advised for both men and postmenopausal women who have T score <3.0 with presence of two or more modifiable risk factors or those who have T score <2.5 with a history of fragility fracture. The cost is high and its anabolic effects are masked in patients on bisphosphonates, so best is to give as monotherapy. Also, it is the drug of choice in patients with bisphosphonate-resistant osteoporosis. Side effects include gastric intolerance, dermatitis and arthralgias.

Denosumab (Prolia, Xgeva)

Developed by the biotechnology company Amgen for treatment of giant cell tumor and metastasis to bone, Denosumab is a fully human monoclonal antibody that acts against receptor activator of nuclear factor k-beta (RANK) ligands (RANKL) receptors and inhibits osteoclast function (*see* **Fig. 15.8**). It has been recently advocated for osteoporosis treatment but long-term results are awaited. Common side effects are muscle and joint pains, allergic reactions, infections, atypical hip fractures and osteonecrosis of jaw (but unlike bisphosphonates the incidence drops to zero, 6 months after injection). It is contraindicated in people with hypocalcemia.

Surgical Treatment

Vertebroplasty and kyphoplasty are minimally invasive percutaneous procedures used for symptomatic compression vertebral fractures (without neurological impairment), refractory to medical treatment.

Vertebroplasty **(Fig. 15.3)**: It refers to injecting bone cement, i.e. polymethyl methacrylate (PMMA), in vertebral body via a transpedicular route to strengthen the collapsing vertebrae, and to avoid further compression.

Kyphoplasty: In kyphoplasty a balloon is inflated inside the vertebral body. After restoration of vertebral height balloon is retracted and cement PMMA is injected under continuous fluoroscopic control. Both vertebroplasty and kyphoplasty provide immediate and significant pain relief. In addition kyphoplasty also reduces the vertebral deformity (kyphosis).

Absolute contraindications to vertebroplasty and kyphoplasty are local or generalized infection, untreated bleeding disorder, healed osteoporotic fractures, allergy to bone cement and spine tumors with cord compression.

HIGH-YIELD POINTS

- *Disuse osteoporosis*: Prolonged immobilization due to any cause reduces muscle mass and BMD. In elderly stroke causing hemiplegia is an important cause of disuse osteoporosis. In hemiplegics maximum drop in BMD occurs in nonweight bearing bones of upper limb (maximum in humerus) on the side of hemiplegia.

- Bisphosphonates are drugs of choice for both senile and postmenopausal osteoporosis. In bisphosphonate-resistant osteoporosis teriparatide has been found to be very effective.
- Etidronate may prevent bone loss secondary to heparin therapy.
- Recently, many studies have proven the role of vitamin K in osteoporosis (gamma-carboxylation of osteocalcin), and vitamin K along with vitamin D is increasingly being given to prevent and treat osteoporosis. Vitamin K deficiency decreases BMD and increases the risk of fractures.
- Vertebroplasty is also used in the treatment of vertebral hemangiomas.
- *Some newer drugs for osteoporosis:*
  - *Cathepsin-K inhibitors:* Odanacatib is a once weekly oral treatment for osteoporosis. It inhibits cathepsin-K, a cysteine protease expressed in osteoclasts which degrades type 1 collagen (not yet approved by FDA, phase 3 trial completed)
  - *Monoclonal antibody to sclerostin (Romosozumab):* Sclerostin, an osteocyte-secreted protein, negatively regulates osteoblasts and inhibits bone formation through the LRP5/Wnt signaling pathway. Romosozumab has shown promising results in phase 2 trials.

RICKETS

INTRODUCTION

Rickets is a disorder of defective mineralization of the growing skeleton (before epiphyseal closure), the pediatric counterpart of osteomalacia. There is a deficiency of vitamin D that disturbs the calcium and phosphorus homeostasis and produces the characteristic manifestations. To understand the disorder, it is necessary to understand the metabolism of calcium and vitamin D in the body.

VITAMIN D METABOLISM (FLOW CHART 15.1)

Vitamin D is synthesized primarily in the body (90%) from 7-dehydrocholesterol present in the epidermis upon exposure to sunlight while small amounts (10%) are added by the dietary sources (vitamin D_3 or cholecalciferol from animal sources and vitamin D_2 or ergocalciferol from plant sources). The raw compound enters in the liver, where hydroxylation occurs, leading to the formation of 25-hydroxy vitamin D (calcidiol) which enters the renal tubules. In kidney, 1-alpha hydroxylase (an enzyme stimulated by PTH) acts on it and converts it into the active form, i.e. 1,25-dihydroxycholecalciferol (active vitamin D3 or calcitriol). This 1-alpha hydroxylation is the rate limiting step in vitamin D metabolism. The active vitamin D3 so generated increases absorption of calcium and phosphorus from the intestines,

Flow chart 15.1: Vitamin D metabolism in body

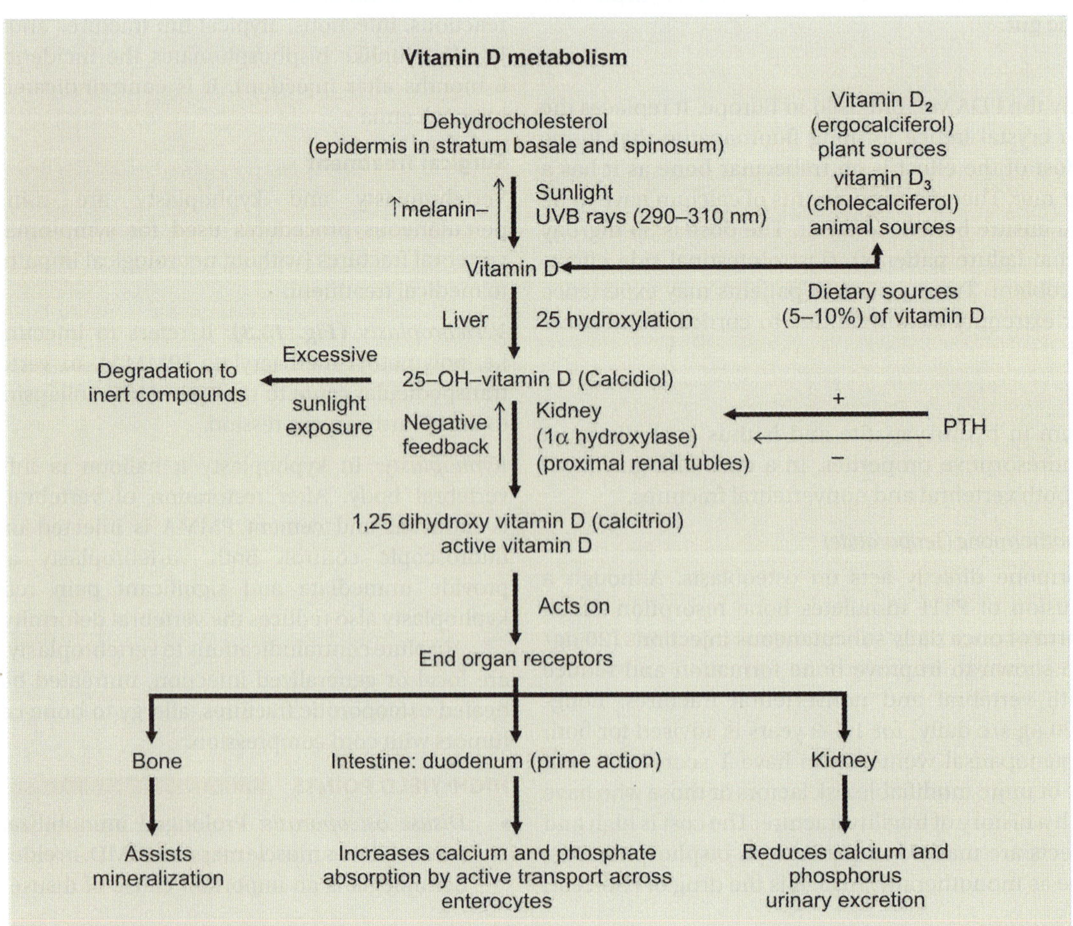

Flow chart 15.2: Causes of vitamin D deficiency

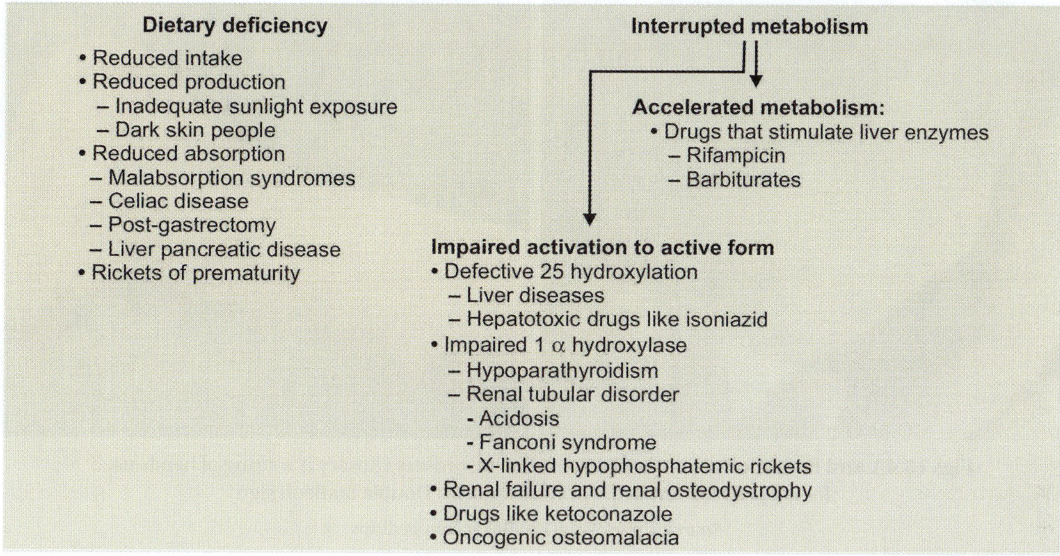

increases absorption of these compounds from the renal tubules and also acts on bone to assist in mineralization.

CAUSES OF DEFICIENCY

The deficiency of vitamin D in rickets results secondary to a number of causes as shown in **Flow chart 15.2**.

PATHOPHYSIOLOGY

The prime pathology in rickets is inadequate mineralization or calcification of physis (growth plates) in growing bones due to deficiency of vitamin D. Hence, the zone of provisional calcification is inadequately mineralized and bony trabeculae become weak. Under increasing stresses of body weight, the physis gets deformed, leading to defective growth and bony deformities.

SIGNS AND SYMPTOMS

Nutritional rickets generally manifests in infants and preschool children. Generalized features are failure to thrive, muscle weakness, listlessness and lethargy. The child may present with tetany (positive Trousseau or Chvostek sign) or convulsions because of hypocalcemia. Pathological fractures may result due to weak bones. Once the patient starts walking, bony deformities may develop like bow legs (genu varum, most common), knock knees (genu valgum, occurs in older children), windswept deformity of the legs (varum at one knee and valgum at the other).

Some other classical clinical features are:
- Frontal bossing (thickening of frontal bone), usually evident after the age of 6 months
- Delayed closure of fontanel
- *Craniotabes (usually first manifestation)*: Refers to soft skull bones that can be pressed like a ping-pong ball
- Delayed dentition
- *Broadening of ankle, wrist and knee joints*: Due to deformed physis
- *Enlarged costochondral junctions (rickets rosary **Fig. 15.4A**)*: Due to subluxation of the physis
- Indentation over the lower chest at attachment of diaphragm (Harrison's sulcus)
- *Pot belly*: Due to abdominal muscle hypotonia
- *Pigeon chest (pectus carinatum)*: Refers to a protruding sternum
- *Double malleoli sign (**Fig. 15.4B**)*: It is seen due to metaphyseal widening.

RADIOGRAPHIC FEATURES (FIGS 15.5A AND B)

There may be delayed appearance of the epiphysis. The physis is widened (normal thickness is 2–4 mm) due to nonmineralized osteoid that accumulates in the area. There is no zone of calcification due to defective mineralization and the area is filled by irregularly arranged cartilage cells, so the metaphyseal margins touching the growth plate look irregular and frayed. Due to weight-bearing stresses, the metaphysis becomes cup-shaped and splayed (flat and wide). Generalized osteopenia may be visible and the cortex may thin out. Deformities of bones may be visible in the later stages.

LAB INVESTIGATIONS

To order appropriate lab investigations, one needs to know the various types of rickets.

Types of Rickets (Table 15.5)

Nutritional Rickets

This is the most common variety in developing countries. The recommended daily intake of vitamin D is 400 IU for infants, 600 IU from 1 year to 70 years of age, and 800 IU for those over

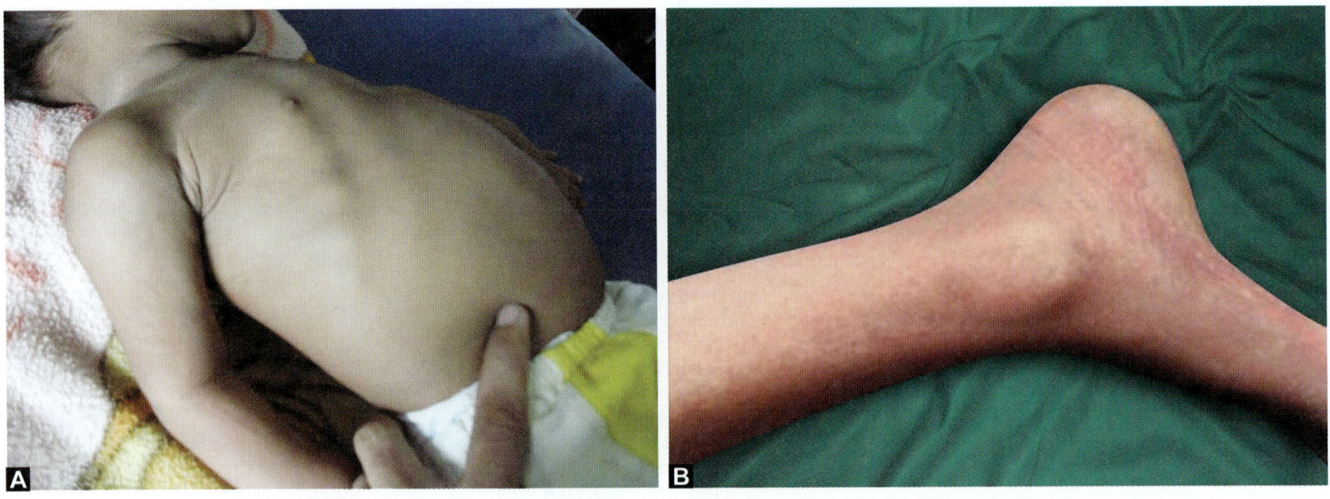

Figs 15.4A and B: Clinical signs of rickets. (A) Rachitic rosary (Rosary is a string of beads used for keeping a count while prayers) and (B) Double malleoli sign

Source: Courtesy by Kondekar.com peditips.

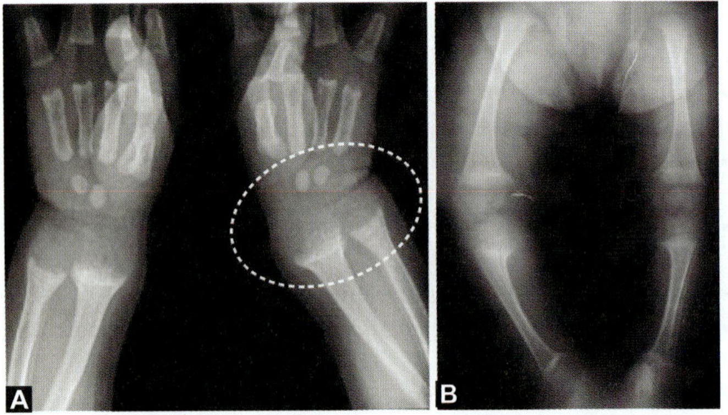

Figs 15.5A and B: (A) X-ray of both wrist joint AP views showing the widening of wrist joint with cupping and fraying of metaphysis (dotted circle); (B) X-ray of both lower limbs AP view showing cupping and fraying of metaphyses around the knee joint

Abbreviation: AP view, anteroposterior view.

70. Inability to take these recommended levels leads to dietary deficiency of vitamin D, so active vitamin D [1,25(OH)$_2$D] levels are low. This leads to inability to absorb calcium and phosphorus. PTH is elevated in response to hypocalcemia, corrects the serum calcium, so calcium levels are normal to low while phosphate levels may be low to normal. Alkaline phosphatase (ALP) is elevated.

Cut-off value for vitamin D deficiency: Most investigators have used different cut-off levels to define vitamin D deficiency **(Table 15.6)**. Most commonly used cut-off value to define vitamin D deficiency is 25(OH)-vitamin D less than 20 ng/mL, insufficiency as 20–29 ng/mL and sufficiency as more than or equal to 30 ng/mL. Severe deficiency is defined as a level less than 5 ng/mL.

Vitamin D-dependent Rickets

In this variety, the dietary intake of vitamin D is normal, but there is a problem in its metabolism or action.

Vitamin D-dependent rickets (VDDR) type I: It is an autosomal recessive disorder due to deficiency of 1-alpha-hydroxylase renal enzyme. It is necessary for the formation of the active metabolite of vitamin D which is not formed in adequate amount [1,25(OH)$_2$-vitamin D levels low]. This leads to inability to absorb calcium and phosphorus and levels of both minerals are low in serum. PTH is elevated in response to hypocalcemia. ALP is also elevated. To differentiate it from nutritional rickets, levels of 25(OH)-vitamin D and 1,25(OH)$_2$-vitamin are measured. In nutritional variety, both will be low while in vitamin D-dependent rickets (VDDR) type I, the levels of 25(OH)-vitamin D will be increased while the active form [1,25(OH)$_2$-vitamin D] will be markedly decreased. The rachitic features appear early with renal tubular dysfunction.

Vitamin D-dependent rickets (VDDR) type II: It is vitamin D receptor insensitivity disease due to mutation of VDR gene. End organs are insensitive to 1,25(OH)$_2$-vitamin D, so calcium and phosphorus cannot be absorbed leading to low levels. PTH will be elevated in response to hypocalcemia. To differentiate it from above two situations, vitamin D metabolite levels are used. Here, both 25(OH)-vitamin D and 1,25(OH)$_2$-vitamin D would be elevated to increase calcium absorption as there is no problem in the metabolic pathway (mnemonic: in type II, the two metabolites are elevated). Alopecia is present in association with the rachitic features.

Vitamin D-Resistant Rickets (Renal Tubular Rickets)

This is also known as familial hypophosphatemic rickets. Here, the basic abnormality is renal tubules' inability to retain phosphate. Large amounts of phosphorus are excreted in the urine, leading to hypophosphatemia; the calcium levels are however normal. Defective mineralization results as both calcium and phosphorus are needed for mineralization. Since calcium levels are normal, PTH is not stimulated and its blood levels remain unchanged, so would be the case with vitamin D metabolites as the metabolic pathway is not affected. ALK phosphatase is elevated as in all above forms. The diagnosis is established by documenting a low urinary pH and decreased urinary calcium and increased levels of urinary phosphates. Rachitic features in this type appear early,

Table 15.5: Biochemical abnormalities in various types of rickets

	Nutritional rickets	*Vitamin D-dependent rickets I (hydroxylations problem)*	*Vitamin D-dependent rickets II (end organ insensitivity)*	*Vitamin D-resistant rickets (renal tubular rickets)*	*Renal osteodystrophy*
S. Calcium	N–↓	↓	↓	N	N–↓
S. Phosphorus	↓–N	↓	↓	↓↓	↑
Alkaline Phosphatase	↑	↑	↑	↑	↑
PTH	↑	↑	↑	N	↑↑↑
25 (OH) vitamin D	↓↓	↑↑	↑↑	N	N
1,25 (OH)$_2$ vitamin D	↓	↓↓	↑↑↑	N	↓↓
Urine Ca	↓	X	X	↓	↓
Urine phosphorus	↓			↑↑	↓

Table 15.6: Definition and classification of vitamin D deficiency*

US Institute of medicine classification/American Academy of Pediatrics definition:	*US Endocrine Society classification*
Severe deficiency < 5 ng/mL	–
Deficiency < 15 ng/mL	Deficiency < 20 ng/mL Insufficiency 21–29 ng/mL
Sufficiency > 20 ng/mL	Sufficiency > 30 ng/mL
Risk of toxicity > 50 ng/mL	Toxicity > 150 ng/mL

*It is suggested to determine the 25(OH)-vitamin D level in the patients. Vitamin D taken orally and which is produced in the skin is rapidly converted to 25(OH)-vitamin D, but in serum only a fraction of 25(OH)-vitamin D is converted to its active metabolite 1,25(OH)$_2$-vitamin D.

just after infancy. Children lag behind in growth have severely deformed bones, but no myopathy and no hypocalcemia.

This situation can occur in renal tubular defects like Fanconi anemia and renal tubular acidosis where there is a problem with the kidney to reabsorb phosphorus. In acidosis, the body has to excrete fixed base, i.e. bicarbonate and calcium phosphate are excreted along.

X-linked hypophosphatemic rickets is another condition in this category which is a genetic disorder with dominant inheritance characterized by mutations in the phosphate-regulating gene (PHEX gene-having homology to endopeptidases) present on chromosome X. This leads to excessive urinary excretion of phosphate by restricting the ability of proximal renal tubular brush border to reabsorb phosphorus and calcium.

Renal Osteodystrophy

Renal osteodystrophy is seen in children who have a chronic renal disease that leads to renal failure. The problem begins with a damaged renal glamorous inability to excrete phosphorus leading to hyperphosphatemia. Because of kidney failure, less of 1,25(OH)$_2$-vitamin D is produced which eventually leads to hypocalcemia. This stimulates PTH and causes secondary hyperparathyroidism. Increased PTH resorbes calcium from bone in heavy amount, leading to osteitis fibrosa cystica (multiple cysts in the bone). Spine radiograph may show alternate bands of sclerosis and lysis referred to as the rugger jersey spine. Ectopic

calcification can occur due to high phosphate levels. Prolonged stimulation of PTH secretion leads to hyperplasia of the parathyroid glands. Parathyroid gland becomes autonomous and insensitive to changes in calcium, phosphate and vitamin D. This causes hypercalcemia and known as tertiary hyperparathyroidism. Diagnosis is never a problem. High serum phosphate level, markedly raised PTH levels and decreased active vitamin D levels with low urinary calcium and phosphorus, in the presence of other features of renal failure are enough to establish the diagnosis.

MANAGEMENT OF RICKETS

Treatment depends upon the type of rickets.

Nutritional rickets may be treated gradually over several months with daily dose regimen or with a radical approach using high-dose regimens. Single-day dose (Stoss therapy) of 15,000 mcg (or 600,000 IU) of vitamin D is the commonly used high-dose regimen. The single-day therapy is easy to administer and has better compliance. The single day high-dose can be given orally or intramuscularly. With single day high-dose therapy, radiographic healing becomes visible in 6–10 days. Single day high-dose therapy is followed by a daily based maintenance dose of vitamin D. Another high-dose regimen is 50,000 IU of vitamin D weekly for 8 weeks orally followed by a daily maintenance dose. The maintenance dose is 400 IU/day for infants and 600–1000 IU/day for children more than 1 year old. High-dose vitamin D may be repeated (after 3 months) if poor compliance persists. Commonly recommended daily dose regimen of vitamin D is 1,000 IU daily for newborns, 1,000–5,000 IU daily for infants 1–12 months old, and 5,000–10,000 IU daily for children of 1 year and older. Calcium intake should be maintained at approximately 1,000 mg/day (30–75 mg/kg of elemental calcium per day in three divided doses). The patient is also advised to take diet rich in calcium-containing foods like fish oil, egg yolk and margarine.

Estimation of serum calcium, phosphorus and serum alkaline phosphatase levels is recommended 1 month after initiation of therapy. To monitor the effect of treatment, ALP levels and 24-hours urinary calcium can be used, but the best sign to comment on healing in rickets is healing of the growth plate on X-rays. 24 hours urinary excretion of calcium should be in the range of 100–250 mg/24 hours. Lower value indicates persistent vitamin D deficiency. Treatment is continued until 24 hours urinary calcium and ALP return to normal. Radiological healing is usually evident after 1 month. Usually it takes 1–2 months for serum 25(OH)-vitamin D levels to normalize and 3–6 months for ALP to return to normal. In later stages of healing as mineralization proceeds in the provisional zone of calcification, a white line appears on X-rays, next to the metaphysic, called the white line of Frankel.

In VDDR type I, active form of vitamin (calcitriol) has to be given since 1-hydroxylation is defective. VDDR type II has end organ insensitivity and requires very large doses of vitamin D. Vitamin D-resistant rickets is treated by treating the underlying problem along with phosphate administration to correct hypophosphatemia in association with calcium supplementation.

Treatment of renal osteodystrophy involves serum phosphate reduction (dietary restriction, use of phosphate binders, calcium salts and dialysis), use of vitamin D analog and renal replacement therapy. Sodium bicarbonate is used to correct acidosis. Cinacalcet, a calcium receptor sensitiser (calcimimetic) that inhibits PTH release is usually used in patients on dialysis with advanced disease. Parathyroidectomy may be required for tertiary hyperparathyroidism.

Approach to a patient with rickets has been nicely summarized in **Flow chart 15.3**.

Flow chart 15.3: Approach to a patient with rickets

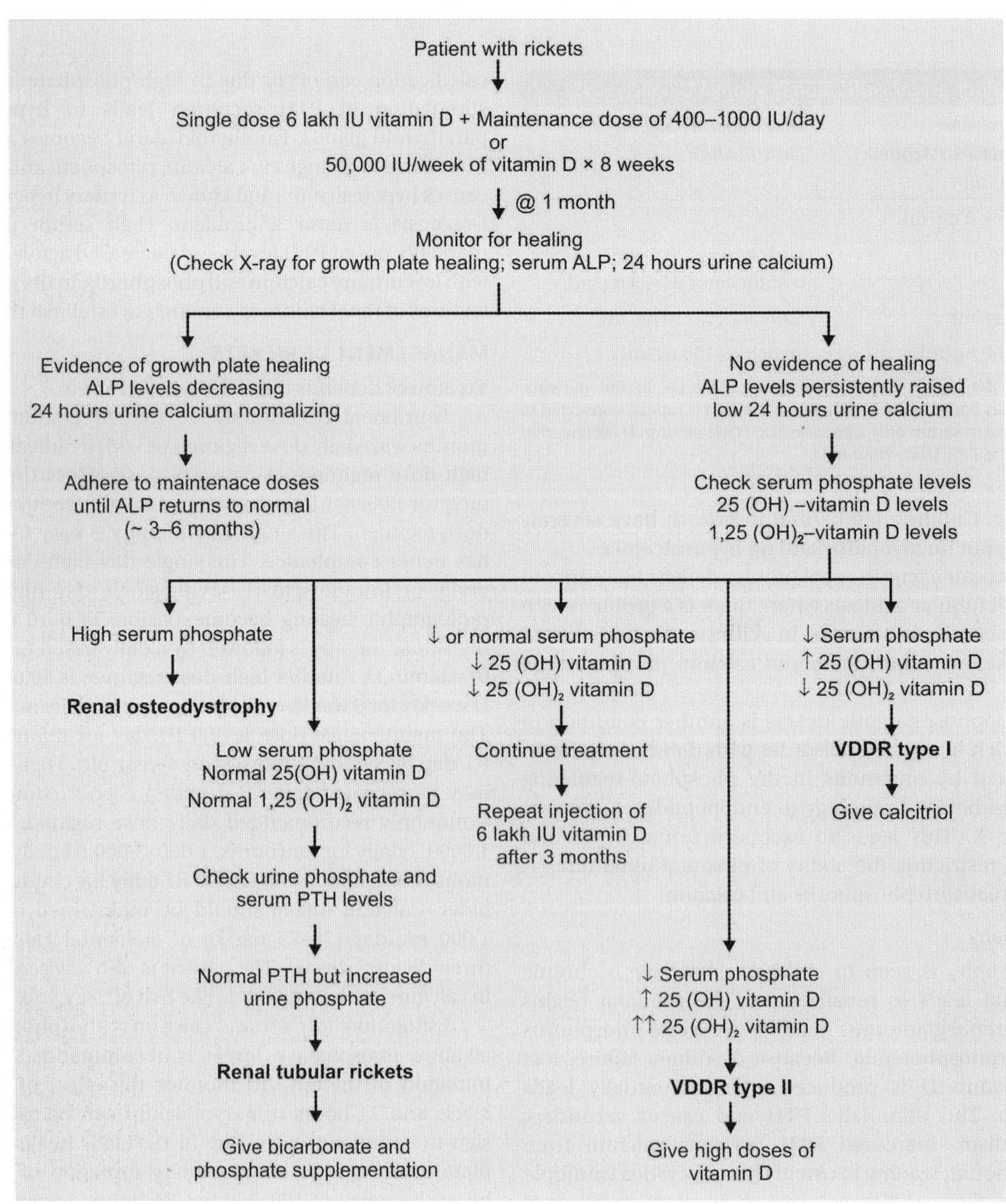

Abbreviations: ALP, alkaline phosphatase; VDDR, vitamin D-dependent rickets.

Treating Rickets with a Deformity (e.g. Genu Valgum/Club Foot)

Resolution of skeletal deformities occurs completely with treatment with vitamin D and calcium. If the deformity persists even after radiological healing (the best way to predict healing) in rickets, surgery (i.e. corrective osteotomy) to correct that deformity can be done. However, surgery should be done only after the levels of ALP are brought to normal as when ALP is raised, bone is soft and not in a state to hold the fixation implant.

HIGH-YIELD POINTS

- Vitamin D content of human milk is low approximately 30–40 IU/L, so breastfed infants if not exposed to adequate sunlight tend to develop rickets.
- Mother's supplementation of vitamin D and mother's sunlight exposure if increased also increases the vitamin D content of breast milk.
- The clinical evidence of florid rickets may not be evident in children with severe protein-energy malnutrition, since rickets is a disease of growing bones and growth is retarded in severe malnutrition.
- Magnesium deficiency also causes rickets (magnesium-dependent vitamin D-resistant rickets) which does not respond to high-dose vitamin D therapy. In these patients excellent response is seen with oral magnesium-chloride supplementation. Therefore, serum magnesium levels should be assessed in all cases of vitamin D resistant rickets.
- In renal osteodystrophy (tertiary hyperparathyroidism) metaphyseal changes resembling rickets are seen in children. Together with cortical erosions this gives a "rotting fence-post" appearance especially at the femoral neck.
- Serum ALP is elevated in rickets (all forms), osteomalacia, Paget's disease, primary hyperparathyroidism and chronic renal failure (CRF) with secondary hyperparathyroidism, renal osteodystrophy and lytic bone neoplasms. The levels are normal in osteoporosis, osteopetrosis, fibrous dysplasia, multiple myeloma and hypoparathyroidism. Decreased levels may be seen in achondroplasia, hypophosphatasias and cretinism.

INTRODUCTION

Osteomalacia is basically a disorder of inadequate mineralization of bone that occurs "in adults" due to deficiency of vitamin D in the body. The osteoid production however is unaffected, but inadequately mineralized osteoid leads to soft and weak bones and hence the term osteomalacia. It is different from osteoporosis where there is decreased osteoid as well as mineral content, or in other words where the whole bone mass is reduced.

ETIOLOGY

The primary cause is vitamin D deficiency in the body. Since most of the required vitamin D is synthesized in the body by the action of sunlight, the deficiency is common in Muslim women who follow the custom of "purdah". Other causes may include decreased intake as in malnourished individuals, conditions where absorption is inadequate like malabsorption syndromes, celiac disease or when the requirement may be increased like multiple pregnancies, and lactating mothers. Drugs that interfere with the metabolism like anticonvulsants (phenytoin, phenobarbitone, carbamazepine), phosphate-binding antacids, cholestyramine, fluoride and heavy metals may also lead to this clinical condition.

SIGNS AND SYMPTOMS

Diffuse bone pains, backache and a generalized muscular weakness are common features. The most common symptom is dull aching pain in lower back, pelvis and hips. Pathological fractures can occur, especially in the spine leading to progressive kyphosis.

RADIOGRAPHIC FEATURES

The characteristic X-ray findings of osteomalacia are Looser's zones (named after Emil Looser, Swiss surgeon) also known as cortical infarctions, Milkman's fractures, increment fractures, umbauzones or pseudofractures **(Figs 15.6A and B)** that occur due to incomplete healing of stress fractures by a calcium-deficient callus. They appear as thin transverse lucencies, running at right angles to the involved cortex since the indentations are caused by

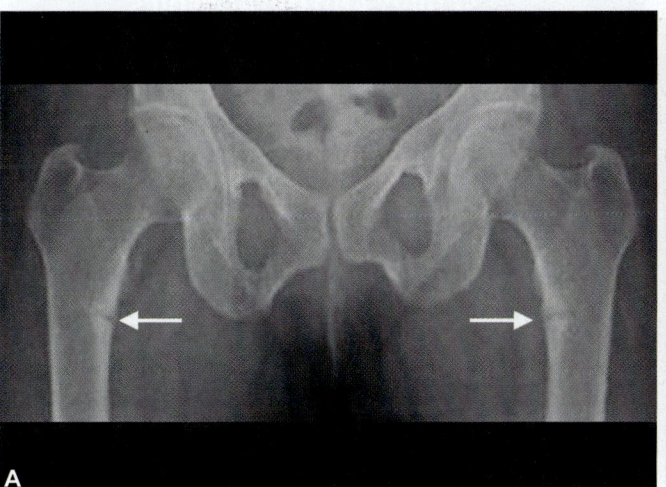
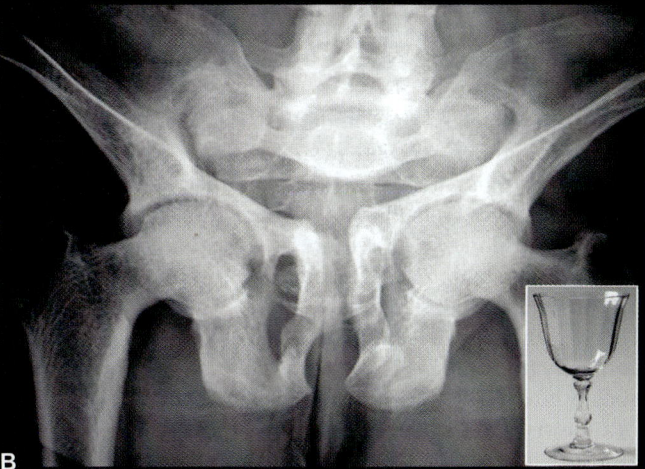

Figs 15.6A and B: X-ray features of osteomalacia. (A) Figure showing Looser's zone in the subtrochanteric region (arrows) in both femur and (B) Bilateral coxa vara and champagne glass pelvis

vascular crossings pressing on a soft bone. The margins may be irregular and sclerotic. Often, they are multiple and symmetrical.

Common sites include: Pubic and ischial rami (most common site), medial proximal femur, axillary edge of scapula immediately below the glenoid, lumbar vertebrae, ribs and clavicle.

Other X-ray findings that point the diagnosis include:
- *Biconcave codfish vertebrae*: Due to indentation on vertebral bodies by the intervertebral disk
- Trefoil or champagne-glass pelvis
- Protrusio acetabuli and coxa vara (atraumatic).

LAB INVESTIGATIONS

The values of serum and urinary calcium are low and phosphate levels are also on the lower side. There is an increase in alkaline phosphatase and PTH levels. To confirm the diagnosis, one can document reduced levels of vitamin D in the body (*see* **Table 15.6**). Demonstration of excessive uncalcified osteoid on histopathology (biopsy) is the gold standard method to confirm the diagnosis, but is seldom needed.

DIFFERENTIAL DIAGNOSIS

Following conditions that can present with multiple site bone pains should be excluded while finalizing the diagnosis:
- Osteoporosis
- Fibromyalgia
- Polymyositis and polymyalgia rheumatica
- Rheumatoid arthritis
- Multiple myeloma
- Metastatic bone disease.

MANAGEMENT

Vitamin D deficiency is highly prevalent in patients who present with musculoskeletal symptoms, such as vague bone pain, generalized myalgia and weakness. High-risk individuals with serum 25(OH)-vitamin D concentrations less than 20 ng/mL should be treated with 50,000 IU of vitamin D_2 or D_3 orally once per week for 6–8 weeks or 6,000 IU daily for 8 weeks, followed by 800 units of vitamin D daily thereafter. For individuals with serum 25(OH)- vitamin D levels of 20–30 ng/mL, initial supplementation with 800 units of vitamin D3 daily may be sufficient to maintain levels in the target range. All patients should consume total calcium of at least 1,000–1,200 mg/day.

HIGH-YIELD POINTS

- Most common cause of osteomalacia (vitamin D deficiency) is lack of adequate exposure to sunlight.
- Sunscreen lotions with a sun protection factor of 30, reduce vitamin D synthesis in the skin by more than 95%.
- People with darker skin require at least three to five times longer exposure to make the same amount of vitamin D as a person with a white skin tone.
- There is an inverse association of serum 25(OH)-vitamin D and body mass index (BMI) greater than 30 kg/m², and thus, obesity is associated with vitamin D deficiency.
- Otto pelvis or arthrokatadysis refers to primary (idiopathic) protrusio acetabuli (head crosses medial to ilio-ischial line). It is commonly seen in young women and is usually a bilateral finding. Secondary protrusio acetabuli can result

from trauma (e.g. central fracture dislocation of hip) or can be non-traumatic. Most common cause of non-traumatic protrusio acetabuli in India is osteomalacia and in the world is rheumatoid arthritis. Other important causes include: Paget's disease, osteoarthritis, ankylosing spondylitis, osteogenesis imperfecta, trauma, tubercular arthritis, Marfan's syndrome and psoriatic arthritis.

- *Hypovitaminosis-associated proximal myopathy (osteomalacic proximal myopathy)*: Several studies report an association between vitamin D deficiency and proximal myopathy. Patients may present with predominant proximal muscle weakness (difficulty in getting up from squatting position or climbing stairs), generalized muscle wasting with preservation of sensation and deep tendon reflexes, generalized bone pain and waddling gait. Infants may manifest features of muscle weakness and hypotonia. Exact pathogenesis is not clear but patients have low serum calcium, very low serum vitamin D and raised PTH. Treatment is same as for osteomalacia.
- Conditions with Looser's zones:
  - Osteomalacia (characteristic)
  - Renal osteodystrophy
  - Fibrous dysplasia
  - Hyperthyroidism
  - Paget's disease of bone
  - X-linked hypophosphatemia
  - Osteogenesis imperfect.

ONCOGENIC OSTEOMALACIA/RICKETS

Oncogenic osteomalacia is an unusual paraneoplastic syndrome characterized by mesenchymal tumors that secrete the fibroblast growth factor that apparently produces osteomalacia/hypophosphatemic rickets with biochemical abnormalities consisting of hypophosphatemia, normocalcemia, and increased levels of ALP. These tumors include fibrous dysplasia, hemangiopericytoma (most common), osteosarcoma, chondroblastoma, chondromyxoid fibroma, malignant fibrous histiocytoma, giant cell tumor, metaphyseal fibrous defect and hemangioma. Most tumors producing this condition are benign and slow growing in nature.

SCURVY AND ORTHOPEDICS

INTRODUCTION

Normal recommended intake of vitamin C for an infant is 30–40 mg and for a child is 40–70 mg. An inadequate intake leads to deficiency of vitamin C, causing the disease called scurvy.

PATHOPHYSIOLOGY

Ascorbic acid (vitamin C) is necessary for the synthesis of collagen (collagen type I is a major constituent of bone) as it acts as a cofactor in the hydroxylation of the lysine and proline. These two amino acids are important for cross-linking of triple helix of collagen. Defective collagen synthesis leads to impaired wound healing, fragile capillaries causing abnormal bleeding and defective bone formation.

SIGNS AND SYMPTOMS

The deficiency develops after 6–12 months of deprivation, so neonates generally get spared. Affected children usually are

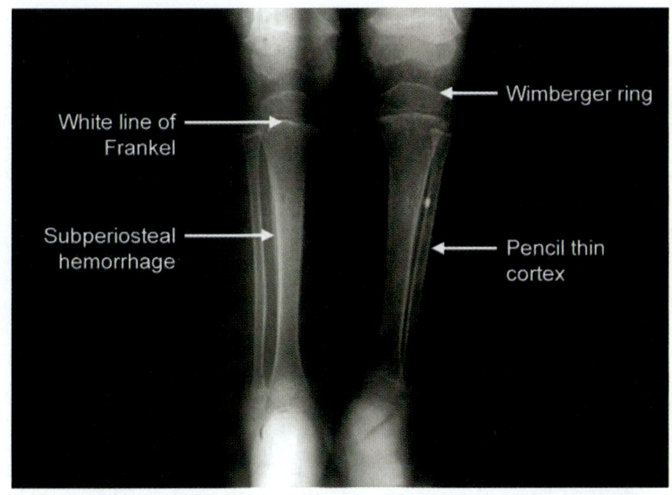

Fig. 15.7: X-ray showing characteristic signs of scurvy

lethargic, anemic, having malaise and may come with bleeding spongy gums or with a history of bleeding from the alimentary tract. Wound healing is impaired in these children.

Orthopedic manifestations are characterized by exquisite bone pains due to subperiosteal hemorrhages mostly occurring beneath the periosteum of the metaphyseal growing ends of long bones of the lower extremity. The child may minimally move the limb owing to extreme pain and the condition simulates a pseudoparalysis. Pathological fractures may be reported but more commonly there occur epiphyseal separations.

RADIOGRAPHIC FEATURES (FIG. 15.7)

- Pencil thin cortex
- *Subperiosteal hemorrhages*: Lower end of the femur and tibia are most commonly involved. It is visualized in the healing phase of scurvy.
- *White line of Frankel*: Dense zone of provisional calcification in metaphysis.
- *Wimberger ring*: Circular, opaque, dense band around the epiphysis of a long bone.
- *Pelkan spur*: Metaphyseal spurs leading to cupping of the metaphysis.
- *Trummerfeld zone*: Lucent metaphyseal band underlying the Frankel's line.

MANAGEMENT

Scurvy is treated with vitamin C administered by mouth or injection. 100–250 milligrams of vitamin C are given by mouth four times daily for 1 week. Joint pain disappears in 48 hours and symptoms of scurvy are completely cured in 7–10 days.

HIGH-YIELD POINTS

- *Barton's disease*: It includes features of both rickets and scurvy.
- Infantile scurvy is also known as Barlow's disease. The infants with scurvy remain alert, but motionless from fear of pain and scream upon handling. They present with painful, swollen limbs or swelling of joints, particularly about the knees, spongy gums.

- Causes of white line of Frankel:
  – Scurvy
  – Healing rickets
  – Lead poisoning
  – Acute leukemia
  – Growth arrest lines due to chronic diseases like bronchial asthma, cystic fibrosis
  – Methotrexate therapy
  – Healing in renal osteodystrophy.
- Conditions where "Ring shaped epiphyses" can be seen on radiographs are Rickets, Scurvy, Osteogenesis Imperfecta, Hypothyroidism and Osteopetrosis.

HYPERPARATHYROIDISM

INTRODUCTION

Hyperparathyroidism is a condition of excessive secretion of PTH or parathormone, either by the parathyroid glands or by an ectopic focus (generally a malignant tumor like breast, lung or pancreatic carcinoma) leading to multisystem manifestations. Bone disease occurs in approximately half of the patients with the disorder.

Parathormone: Action and Effects

The main effect of PTH is to increase the serum calcium concentration by increasing intestinal absorption of calcium, decreasing its renal tubular excretion and mobilizing calcium from bone to make it enter the circulation. While it elevates the calcium concentration in blood, it decreases serum phosphate levels and increases phosphate excretion.

The mechanism by which the hormone mobilizes calcium from bone needs special mention. Osteoclasts, the bone resorbing cells, have RANK receptors on their surface while osteoblasts have the complimentary RANK Ligand (RANKL) on their surface, that remains covered by special proteins called osteoprotegerins. PTH attaches to osteoblasts via its own receptors (PTHr) and makes the osteoprotegerins dissociate exposing the RANKL, thereby enabling the osteoclasts to attach to them via their RANK receptors thereby activating them. These activated osteoclasts cause bone resorption bringing about the manifestations of hyperparathyroidism. Although bone resorption is caused by PTH, it acts via its receptors on osteoblasts that eventually stimulate the bone resorbing cells, i.e. the osteoclasts **(Fig. 15.8)**.

CLASSIFICATION

Hyperparathyroidism can be classified into three types:

1. Primary hyperparathyroidism is due to adenoma (most common cause) or hyperplasia of parathyroid gland that leads to increased parathormone production. Most commonly it is seen in females (female:male 3:1) in the middle age group (40–65 years). For long, patients may remain asymptomatic and hypercalcemia may be the only finding in blood tests. Due to hypercalcemia, patient presents with anorexia, nausea, depression, abdominal pain, muscle weakness and fatigue (not tetany). Increased glomerular filtration and tubular absorption of calcium causes kidney stone (nephrocalcinosis), polyurea, recurrent urinary infection and impaired renal function. Osteitis fibrosa cystica (replacement of bone marrow by fibrous tissue) and hemorrhages in this fibrous tissue,

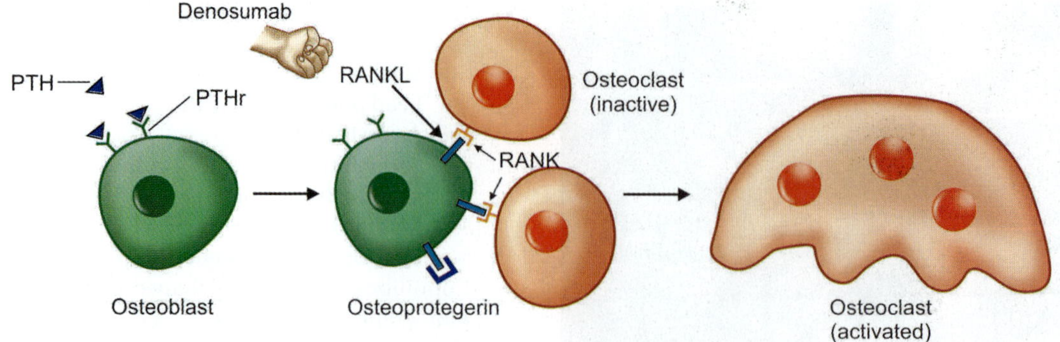

Fig. 15.8: Mechanism of action of PTH. Denosumab knocks down RANKL preventing osteoclast activation and is hence a drug useful in treating osteoporosis (*see* Page 403)

producing brownish, fluid-filled cystic, tumor-like masses in bones, called Brown's tumors, are characteristic.

2. In secondary hyperparathyroidism, the elevated PTH levels result secondary to some disease that produces a persistent state of hypocalcemia in the body like vitamin D deficiency. Since the raised PTH levels are in reflex to the hypocalcemia, serum calcium is usually low (tetany can occur) and phosphate usually high, but the levels can be variable depending upon the cause.

3. In tertiary hyperparathyroidism, the parathyroid gland becomes autonomous, free from any inhibitory feedback control and produces excessive amounts of the hormone into the circulation. In CRF, hyperphosphatemia and decreased renal production of $1,25(OH)_2$-vitamin D initially produces a decrease in ionized calcium. The parathyroid glands are stimulated (secondary hyperparathyroidism) and may enlarge, becoming autonomous (tertiary hyperparathyroidism). The bone disease seen in this setting is known as renal osteodystrophy (*see* above).

ORTHOPEDIC MANIFESTATIONS

- Generalized osteopenia secondary to diffuse bone resorption.
- *Generalized bone pains*: The bones may even be tender to palpation.
- *Pathological fractures*: Generally involve the dorsolumbar spine, neck and shaft of femur and pubic rami.
- *Brown tumors*: In regions where bone loss is particularly rapid, hemorrhage, reparative granulation tissue, and vascular, fibrous tissue replace the normal marrow, resulting in a brown tumor. Since hemosiderin is present in the area, it gives the characteristic brown color on histology. The lesion has a collection of osteoclasts and giant cells.

RADIOGRAPHIC FEATURES (FIGS 15.9A TO D)

- Generalized osteopenia leading to diffuse rarefaction of bones.
- *Brown tumors*: Appear as expansile cystic lytic lesions seen mostly in mandible, maxilla, ribs, clavicle and pelvis. Multiple brown tumors may be present in advanced stage leading to multiple cysts scattered throughout the skeleton, a condition referred to as osteitis fibrosa cystica/Von Recklinghausen disease of bone.
- Subperiosteal resorption of the phalanges is diagnostic (commonly seen on radial sides of middle phalanges). There may be resorption of the lateral ends of the clavicle.

- *Loss of lamina dura of the teeth*: Lamina dura is a thin cortical shell of bone that surrounds the tooth socket. This may be resorbed in hyperparathyroidism.
- Diffuse stippling may be seen in the skull called the salt and pepper appearance. This is due to intermingling of areas of decreased radio-opacity and sclerotic radio dense areas.
- *Rugger jersey spine*: It refers to appearance of horizontal striped vertebrae seen as a result of alternate bands of bone loss and osteosclerosis in patients with renal osteodystrophy. The changes are also commonly seen at the base of skull apart from vertebrae.

LAB INVESTIGATIONS

Blood tests show increased serum PTH concentration, hypercalcemia, hypophosphatemia and increased serum ALK phosphatase level in primary variety. In secondary variety, the PTH and ALK levels are high, but calcium and phosphorus levels are variable.

Renal investigations may be done to detect calculi. Investigations are tailored to detect the cause of hypersecretion, to look for a parathyroid tumor or to locate any ectopic focus if suspected.

MANAGEMENT

Management is largely supportive. Adequate hydration is maintained and the patient is advised to decrease calcium intake. Surgical excision of the ectopic focus or a parathyroidectomy may be required in severe case of unresolved long-standing hypercalcemia, recurrent kidney stones and severe osteoporosis.

An important postoperative complication of parathyroidectomy can be the hungry bone syndrome. Hungry bone syndrome refers to the rapid, profound and prolonged hypocalcemia associated with hypophosphatemia, and hypomagnesemia that result because of suppressed PTH levels, which follows parathyroidectomy. It is a relatively uncommon but serious adverse effect of parathyroidectomy. The severe hypocalcemia is believed to be due to the increased influx of calcium into bone, due to the sudden removal of the effect of high circulating levels of PTH. Various risk factors have been suggested for the development of a hungry bone syndrome, including older age, weight/volume of the resected parathyroid glands, radiological evidence of bone disease and vitamin D deficiency. Treatment is aimed at replenishing the severe calcium deficit by using high doses of calcium supplemented by high doses of active metabolites of vitamin D.

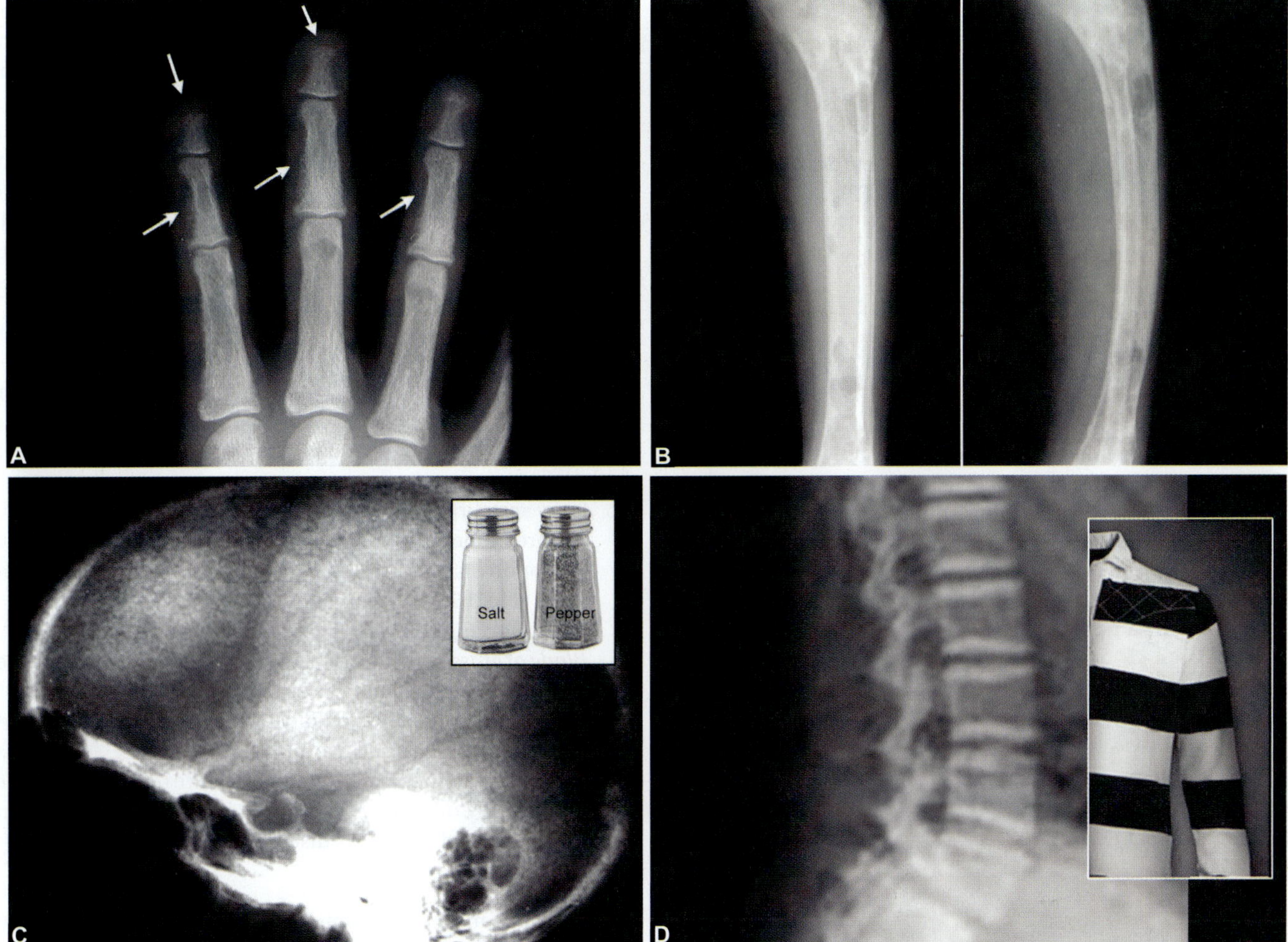

Figs 15.9A to D: X-ray features of hyperparathyroidism. (A) X-ray of hand AP view showing subperiosteal resorption; (B) X-ray of leg AP and lateral views showing multiple Brown's tumor; (C) X-ray of skull showing diffuse stippling, i.e. the salt and pepper appearance; (D) X-ray of LS spine (lateral view) showing the classical Rugger Jersey spine

Source: Courtesy by Learning radiology.com.
Abbreviations: AP view, anteroposterior view; LS, lumbosacral.

Adequate correction of magnesium deficiency is also essential. Preoperative treatment with bisphosphonates has been suggested to reduce postoperative hypocalcemia.

- Metacarpal sign describes a relatively short length of 4th and 5th metacarpals in relation to other metacarpals **(Fig. 15.10)**. It is seen associated with Turner syndrome, Albright's hereditary osteodystrophy, pseudohypoparathyroidism, pseudopseudohypoparathyroidism, sickle cell disease, hereditary multiple exostosis and homocystinuria.
- Hyperparathyroidism can be part of multiple endocrine neoplasia 1, 2A and 2B.
- In hyperparathyroidism due to malignancy, the serum levels of PTH are low. Instead, one can detect high levels of PTH-related peptide.
- Rugger jersey spine is seen in renal osteodystrophy and osteopetrosis (marble bone disease).
- Acroosteolysis refers to bony erosions of terminal tufts of phalanges. Important causes include:

  - Primary acroosteolysis (Hajdu Cheney syndrome)
  - Psoriatic arthritis
  - Hyperparathyroidism
  - Polyvinyl chloride exposure
  - Ergot poisoning
  - Thermal injury
  - Extreme cold; frost bite
  - Leprosy
  - Juvenile chronic arthritis
  - Raynaud disease
  - Scleroderma.

PAGET'S DISEASE (OSTEITIS DEFORMANS)

INTRODUCTION

Paget's disease is a disorder of abnormal bone turnover. There is increased osteoblastic activity followed by increased osteoclastic activity leading to deformed and brittle bones (osteitis deformans) that easily fracture. The most common age group is more than 40 years, and males and females are equally affected.

ETIOPATHOGENESIS

Etiology of the disease is still unknown, although paramyxovirus and respiratory syncytial virus have been implicated. The course of the disease, however, is divided into three phases:

1. *First phase (osteolytic phase)*: Characterized by increased bone resorption and hypervascularization seen on radiograph as an advancing blade of grass appearance **(Fig. 15.11D)**.
2. *Second phase (phase of bone formation)*: The resorbed bone is replaced by structurally weak bone that is brittle and breaks easily.
3. *Third phase (sclerotic/burnout phase)*: Bone resorption declines progressively resulting in hard, dense, avascular pagetic/mosaic bone.

SIGNS AND SYMPTOMS

Pelvis followed by tibia is the most commonly affected bone, but other bones like the femur, clavicle, spine and skull are also affected. The disease can be monostotic (affecting single bone) or polyostotic (multiple bones involved). Patients are usually asymptomatic and diagnosed incidentally with increased serum ALK phosphatase level. Pain is usually dull ache but still the most common presenting symptom. The patient presents with short neck because of flattened base of skull, kyphotic deformity and bowing of tibia and femur or at times with pathological fractures. Rarely, features of cranial nerve compression or spinal stenosis may also be seen. Deafness results due to VIII nerve compression and otosclerosis. It has been postulated that the senorineural hearing loss in Paget's disease is due to loss of BMD in the cochlear capsule. In patients with Paget's disease an increase in blood flow to extremities involved by Paget's disease can lead to vascular steal phenomenon, wherein blood is diverted from internal organs to skeleton leading to cerebral ischemia and spinal claudication.

RADIOGRAPHIC FEATURES

Radiographs initially show flame-shaped osteolysis and later on bone becomes deformed and expanded with thickened and sclerotic cortex. Some characteristic X-ray signs of this disease include:

- Ivory vertebrae (diffusely sclerotic vertebrae)
- Picture frame vertebrae **(Fig. 15.11A)**
- Osteoporosis circumscripta/osteoporotic patch/cotton wool spots **(Fig. 15.11C)** seen in the skull
- *Brim sign (Fig. 15.11B)*: Sclerotic iliopectineal line
- *Blade of grass appearance*: It is "V"-shaped radiolucency seen in the diaphysis of long bones **(Fig. 15.11D)**.
- Biopsy of bone characteristically shows the mosaic pattern, but is rarely indicated.
- A banana fracture or incremental fracture refers to a complete, horizontally oriented pathological fracture seen in deformed bones affected by Paget's disease.

LAB INVESTIGATIONS

Serum calcium and phosphorus levels are usually normal. Markers of bone formation and bone resorption (*see* **Box 2.6**, Page 17) show elevated levels. Urinary N-telopeptide (bone resorption marker) is a sensitive marker and can be used to monitor response to treatment.

DIFFERENTIAL DIAGNOSIS

All diseases with white sclerotic bones come under the differentials, viz. osteopetrosis, fluorosis, diffuse idiopathic skeletal hyperostosis (DISH).

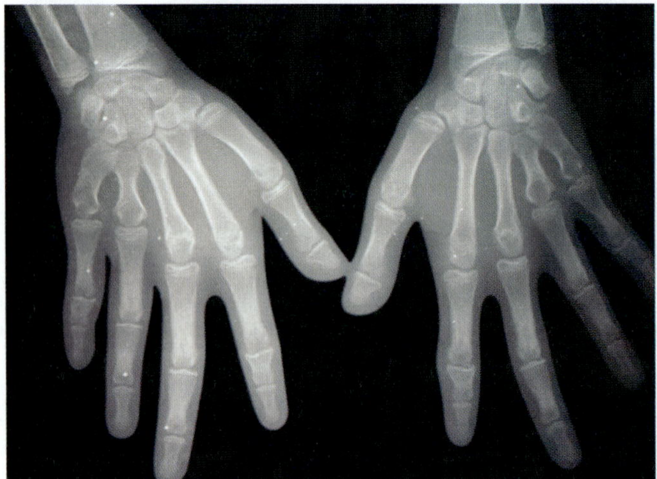

Fig. 15.10: Metacarpal sign (see small 4th and 5th metacarpals)

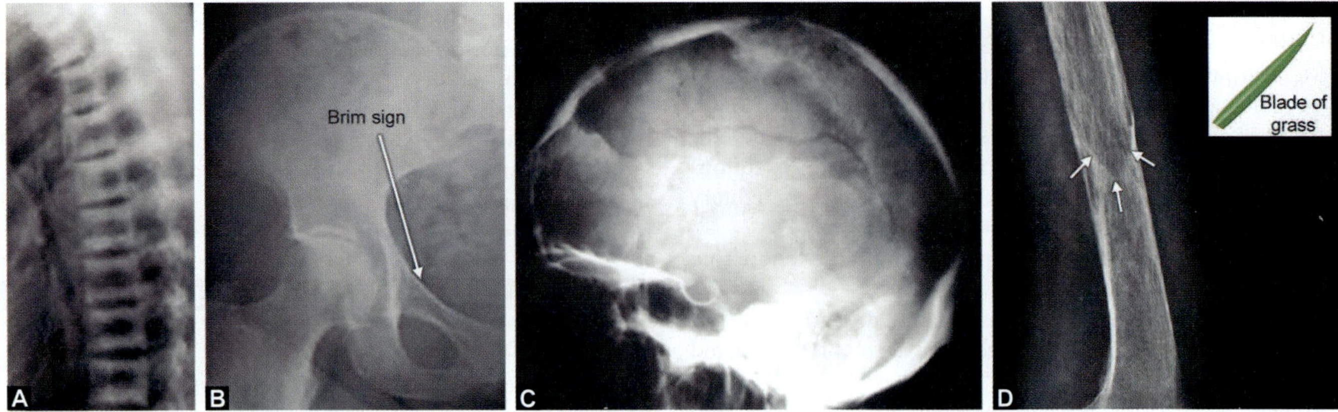

Figs 15.11A to D: Showing X-ray signs of Paget's. (A) Picture frame vertebra; (B) Brim sign (arrow); (C) Osteoporosis circumscripta; (D) X-ray femur lateral view showing blade of grass appearance of Paget's disease (arrows)

Source: Courtesy by Dr Keith H. Wittenberg, RSNA Radiology.

MANAGEMENT

Plicamycin (Mithramycin), an anti-neoplastic agent (is toxic to osteoclasts) was the first effective drug introduced for the treatment of Paget's disease. However, it is seldom used now due to high rate of adverse reactions. Drug of choice in Paget's disease are the bisphosphonates, which reduce bone turnover and increase lamellar bone formation. Etidronate was first implied for the treatment, but risedronate is more preferred now. Calcitonin has been recently found to be very effective in relieving the pain in Paget's disease and decreasing bone resorption but the effect is only temporary. Calcium and vitamin D should also be supplemented. Pathological fractures usually require surgery and internal fixation.

COMPLICATIONS

- Deafness occurs due to VIII cranial nerve compression and otosclerosis.
- Impaired vision, facial palsy and trigeminal neuralgia all can occur due to cranial nerve compression due to skull enlargement.
- High output cardiac failure can occur due to increased and prolonged blood flow to the bone.
- Osteosarcoma is seen in less than 1% of cases.

FLUOROSIS

INTRODUCTION

Although fluoride is the most abundant element in nature, being highly reactive it is seldom found in abundance in a free state. In very small amounts less than 1 parts per million (ppm), the mineral is essential for the formation of dental enamel and for mineralization in the bones. While inadequate ingestion leads to dental caries, over ingestion is also characterized by serious problems.

Fluorosis is a state of chronic fluoride intoxication (more than 10 ppm in body tissues) seen in some parts of India (Punjab, Andhra, Tamil Nadu) and Africa, where the fluoride content of drinking water is high (2–4 ppm), as opposed to most other places where drinking water fluoride content is less than 1 ppm.

PATHOPHYSIOLOGY

High fluorine concentration in water is responsible for increased osteoblastic activity and deposition of fluoroapatite crystals in the bones. They are not adequately removed by osteoclasts and this leads to osteosclerosis (white bones) evident in spine, ribs, pelvis and long bones (forearm and leg). Bony attachment of tendons, ligaments and fascia are also thickened due to new bone formation (hyperostosis).

SIGNS AND SYMPTOMS

In the human body, almost 95% of fluoride is contained in the bones and teeth. Thus, the symptoms of this disorder primarily span over these two systems.

Dental fluorosis: Teeth lose their shiny appearance and become chalk white. Over time, the white patches become yellow resulting in mottling of teeth. It is characteristically seen first up in the incisors of the upper jaw, and occurs only in permanent teeth when they are erupting. It is not seen after they are completely formed.

Skeletal fluorosis: Backache, joint pain and stiffness are common clinical features. The bone becomes weak and pathological fracture may occur and later on bones may deform and bowed. Calcification of the posterior longitudinal ligament occurs in the spine and leads to narrowing the spinal canal. In advanced stages, this may lead to compression of the cord leading to spastic paralysis. Genu valgum is particularly common in the fluoride endemic areas **(Fig. 15.12)**.

RADIOGRAPHIC FEATURES

Thickening and sclerosis of bone (due to increased density), the subperiosteal new bone formation and heterotrophic ossification of ligament and tendons (especially posterior longitudinal ligament in the spine and the pelvic ligaments) may be visible **(Figs 15.12A and B)**. Calcification of the interosseous membrane of the forearm and leg is characteristic **(Fig. 15.12C)**.

LAB INVESTIGATIONS

Elevated fluoride levels in blood, urine samples and in drinking water point toward the diagnosis. Otherwise, patient from an

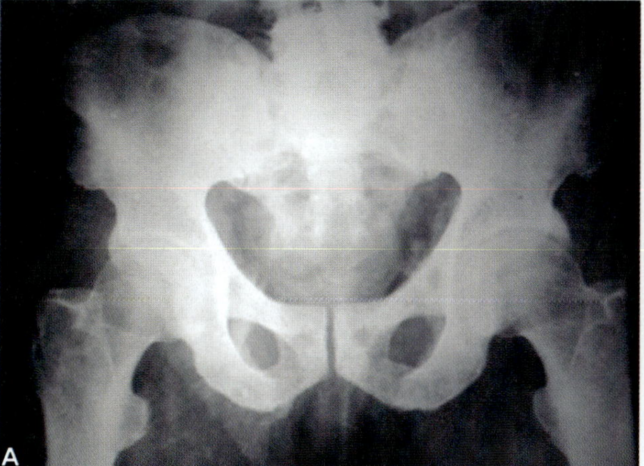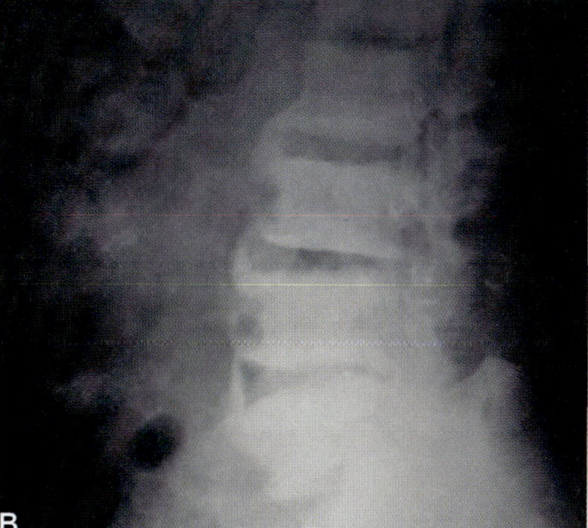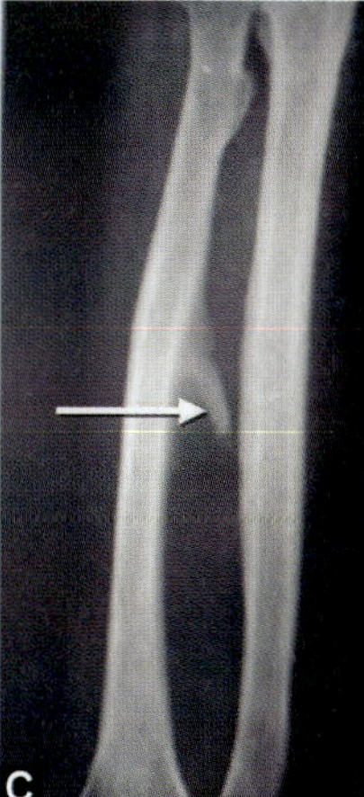

Figs 15.12A to C: X-ray features of fluorosis. (A) X-ray of pelvis AP view showing calcification and sclerosis; (B) X-ray of lumbar spine lateral view showing calcification of spinal ligaments; (C) X-ray forearm AP view showing calcified interosseous membrane (arrow). Note intensely white bones

Abbreviation: AP view, anteroposterior view.

endemic area with characteristic X-ray changes is enough to tell the tale.

DIFFERENTIAL DIAGNOSIS

All conditions leading to osteosclerosis (white bones) come under the differential. These include Paget's disease, DISH, osteopetrosis, renal osteodystrophy, secondaries from prostate and Engelmann disease.

MANAGEMENT

No specific treatment is available and management has to be tailored to the symptoms. In fact, prevention is the best treatment. Deflorination of the water is advocated. Patients improve markedly on using deflorinated water. Children less than 6 years should avoid fluoride tooth pastes (advised for prevention of dental caries). Affected patients should be advised to avoid fluoride-rich foods like fish, cheese and tea.

HIGH-YIELD POINTS

- *Nalgonda technique*: This is the deflorination method developed by National Environmental and Engineering Research Institute.
- Bone disease in fluorosis is more severe in those with concurrent calcium deficiency.

DIFFUSE IDIOPATHIC SKELETAL HYPEROSTOSIS

It is an idiopathic condition characterized by calcification and ossification of soft tissues, mainly ligaments and enthesis. It generally affects people in their 5th or 6th decades and has a predilection for thoracic spine, although any joint of the body may be involved.

The calcification in this disorder tends to involve the anterior ligaments of the spine (usually more than four contiguous vertebrae) characteristically giving the radiological appearance of

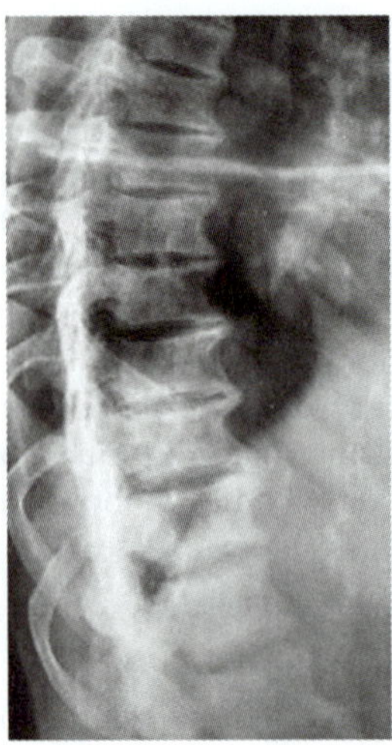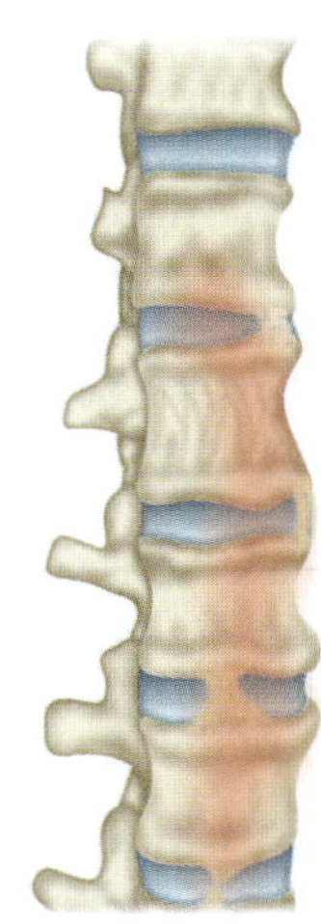

Fig. 15.13: Flowing calcification in diffuse idiopathic skeletal hyperostosis

melted candle wax dripping down the vertebral bodies (flowing calcification) **(Fig. 15.13)**. The picture sometimes simulates ankylosing spondylitis and the two often need to be differentiated (*see* **Table 16.6**, Page 430).

In DISH, lumbar spine and sacroiliac joint involvement is very infrequent. The condition is absolutely noninflammatory and hence features like morning stiffness and reduced range of motion are not very severe and neither is the erythrocyte sedimentation rate raised. There is no human leukocyte antigen B27 positivity, and on X-rays of DISH, osteophytes seen are nonbridging.

Mostly, the disease is discovered as an incidental finding and treatment is largely supportive. It includes nonsteroidal anti-inflammatory drugs for reducing pain and inflammation and physiotherapy for reducing stiffness.

Arthritis and Related Disorders

RELEVANT ANATOMY

The basic structure common in all synovial joints in the body is depicted in **Figure 16.1**. There are two articulating surfaces, with the ends of each bone being covered by hyaline cartilage referred to as articular cartilage. A fibrous capsule encircles all around the joint. The inner side of the capsule is lined by special membrane called as the synovium. The synovial membrane (made of Types I and III collagen) contains specialized cells called as synovial cells that secrete a viscous yellowish fluid called synovial fluid that lubricates the joint cavity. The synovial cells are of two types: Type A (macrophage-like cells) is primarily involved in phagocytosis while Type B (fibroblast-like cells) possesses a rich network of endoplasmic reticulum and secretes hyaluronic acid, proteins and prostaglandins present in synovial fluid.

SYNOVIAL FLUID

This specialized fluid is basically an ultradialysate of blood plasma to which hyaluronic acid has been added by the synovial cells. An absence of basement membrane in the synovium allows an easy passage of fluid from capillaries into the joint cavity. The normal average amount is 0–4 mL varying from joint to joint. The composition of the fluid is relatively similar in all places with a water content of 96% and a pH of 7.3–7.6. Hyaluronic acid is the most important component that gives it its thixotrophic properties (its viscosity decreases with increased rate of shear) and thereby allows it to follow non-Newtonian kinetics (viscosity is shear rate-dependent). Synovial fluid does not clot on standing as there is no fibrinogen.

An aspiration of the synovial fluid sample and its analysis forms the cornerstone in a number of conditions as shown in **Table 16.1**.

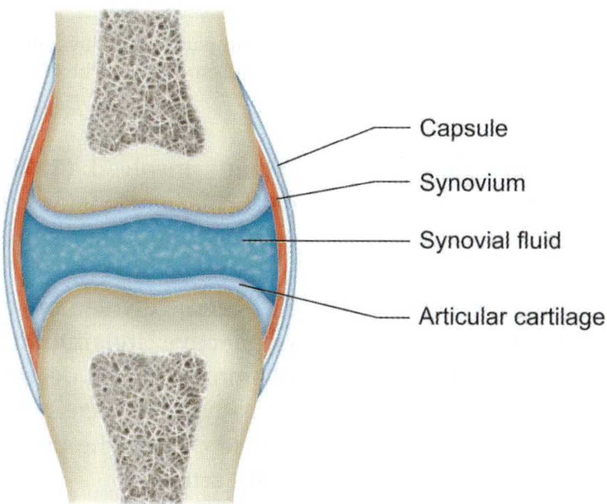

Fig. 16.1: Normal joint anatomy

ARTICULAR CARTILAGE

Composition

The average thickness of articular cartilage is 1.5–3 mm. The exact composition is well depicted in **Figure 16.2A**. Chondrocytes constitute less than 10% of the total volume of cartilage; consequently, the functional properties of cartilage, including stiffness, durability and distribution of load rely primarily on the extracellular matrix. However, the synthesis and maintenance of the extracellular matrix depend on the chondrocytes.

Zones

For the purpose of description, articular cartilage is typically depicted in four zones **(Fig. 16.2B)**.

- Zone 1 (*superficial zone*) is the thinnest and forms the gliding surface of the joint. The upper part of this layer in fact has no cells. It only has sheets of fine fibrils that make it look like a clear film, and hence the name Lamina splendens. The deeper layer consists of flattened ellipsoid chondrocytes that are almost inactive. The collagen fibrils and chondrocytes here are organized with their axis parallel to the articular surface.
- Zone 2 (*transitional zone*), as the name suggests it indicates a transition whereby the collagen and proteoglycan content increases (least in superficial zone), while the water content goes down. The diameter of collagen fibrils of this zone is larger than that in the superficial zone. The chondrocytes are relatively more active and start assuming spheroidal shape. In this layer, collagen fiber orientation and chondrocyte arrangement transitions from parallel to columnar (arranged in columns).
- Zone 3 (*Middle/deep/radial zone*) is the largest of all zones. It contains chondrocytes that are more spheroidal and are organized in a columnar pattern perpendicular to the joint surface. The cells here are synthetically most active having abundant cell organelles viz Golgi apparatus, mitochondria and hold large amounts of intermediate filaments and glycogen granules. Furthermore, the largest collagen fibrils of articular cartilage and the highest content of proteoglycans are also contained here. As the number of proteoglycans increases, the amount of water decreases from the superficial to the deep zone.
- *Tidemark* is a basophilic line which forms the boundary between calcified and uncalcified cartilage. It is considered to be a part of Zone 4, i.e. calcified zone only, although the exact reason for its existence is still unknown.
- Zone 4 (*Calcified zone*) is the deepest zone of calcified cartilage that divides the softer cartilage from underlying subchondral bone. The cells from the deep zone bore directly

Table 16.1: Synovial fluid analysis

Parameters	Normal	Degenerative Osteoarthritis	Inflammatory Gout	Inflammatory Rheumatoid arthritis	Infectious Pyogenic arthritis	Infectious Tuberculous arthritis
Appearance	Straw or clear yellow	Clear yellow	Yellow to turbid milky	Yellow, cloudy	Purulent	Yellow, turbid
Viscosity	Normal	Normal	Decreased	Decreased	Decreased	Decreased
Total white blood cell (WBC) count	≤200	≤2,000	2,000–50,000	2,000–50,000	>50,000	10,000–20,000
Polymorphonuclear leukocytes	<20%	<20%	60–70%	50–60%	90%	60%
Crystals	Negative	Negative	Urate crystals	Negative	Negative	Negative
Glucose level	A bit lower than plasma level	↓	↓	↓	↓↓	↓↓

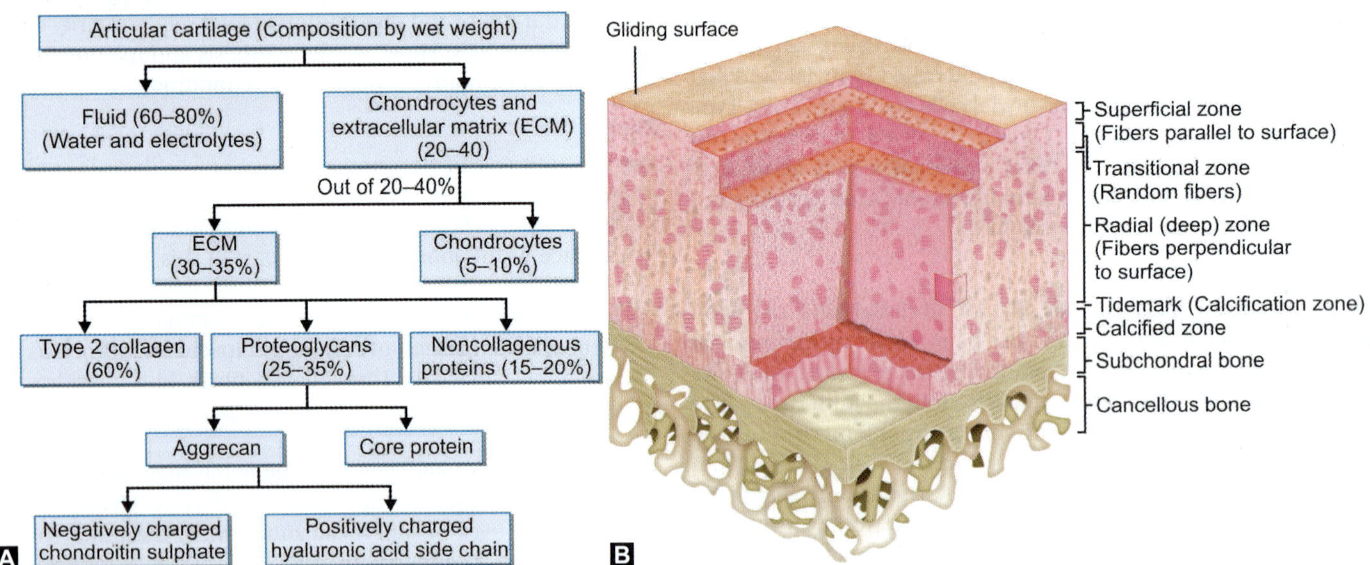

Figs 16.2A and B: (A) Composition of articular cartilage; (B) Zones of articular cartilage

into the calcified cartilage. These chondrocytes contain very little cytoplasm and almost no endoplasmic reticulum (metabolically least active) but connect the articular cartilage to the underlying bone.

Age-related changes in the articular cartilage include: Decreased number of chondrocytes, decreased water content, decreased proteoglycan content due to increased enzymatic degradation and accumulation of pentosidine, an advanced glycation end product (AGEs).

ARTHRITIS

Arthritis (inflammation of the joint) practically refers to a condition where there is destruction of the articular cartilage of the joint (cf. arthralgia that refers simply to a painful joint from any cause). The articular cartilage is not visible on X-ray and manifests as clear space between the articulating surfaces on the radiograph. When this joint space is reduced, a radiological diagnosis of arthritis can be made.

Table 16.2: Classifying arthritis on the number of joints involved

Monoarthritis	Gout, infective and trauma
Oligoarthritis	Gout, SSAs, JIA and reactive arthritis
Polyarthritis	RA, JCA, SLE and PsA

Abbreviations: SSAs, seronegative spondyloarthropathies; JIA, juvenile idiopathic arthritis; RA, rheumatoid arthritis; JCA, juvenile chronic arthritis; SLE, systemic lupus erythematosus; PsA, psoriatic arthritis.

Based upon the number of joints involved **(Table 16.2)** arthritis can be classified as monoarthritis (single joint involved), oligoarthritis (two to four joints involved) and polyarthritis (five or more than five joints involved).

Based upon the etiology arthritis can be divided broadly into infective (septic/tubercular), noninfective inflammatory (i.e. rheumatoid arthritis) and non-inflammatory (i.e. degenerative) categories. Infectious arthritis has already been discussed in detail in Chapter 9. In this chapter, we would discuss the degenerative and the inflammatory varieties of joint arthritis.

INFLAMMATORY ARTHRITIS

Inflammatory arthritis is comprised of two main categories of arthritis.

1. Rheumatoid arthritis (*seropositive**)
2. *Spondyloarthropathies (seronegative):* These diseases include ankylosing spondylitis (AS), psoriatic arthritis, the arthritis associated with inflammatory bowel disease (IBD), and reactive arthritis. These diseases have common features such as the involvement of the sacroiliac (SI) joints (sacroiliitis) and axial spine (spondylitis); oligoarthritis, inflammation at the attachment of tendon, fascia, and ligament insertion sites (enthesitis); association with human leukocyte antigen (HLA) B27 and extraskeletal features such as eye involvement (uveitis), cardiac and other system involvement.

RHEUMATOID ARTHRITIS

Rheumatoid arthritis (RA) is an autoimmune multisystem disorder of young and middle-aged adults characterized by an erosive chronic symmetric arthritis that mostly involves peripheral joints and at times the axial skeleton and may show extra-articular and systemic manifestations.

Incidence

The overall prevalence in the general population is 0.8%. Mostly affected are young and middle-aged adults (20–50 years) with male : female ratio 1 : 3.

Etiopathogenesis

The exact cause is unknown. The current hypothesis says that an initiating antigen (mainly viruses such as rubella, Epstein Barr and mycoplasma) triggers a self-perpetuating chronic inflammation in genetically predisposed individuals (associated with HLA DRB1*04) that leads to the formation of immune complexes made up of immunoglobulins and complements. Cellular events are initiated when antigen-presenting cells present complexes of class II major histocompatibility complex (MHC) molecules and peptide antigens which bind to their receptors on the T-cells. A cascade of cellular events leads to the secretion of various proinflammatory cytokines, including key cytokines interleukin 1 (IL-1) and tumor necrosis factor alpha (TNF-α). These cytokines cause synovial cells and chondrocytes to secrete enzymes that degrade articular cartilage and periarticular tissues.

These immune complexes are deposited in the synovium, where they initiate inflammation and primary synovitis sets which eventually cause synovial hypertrophy. The hypertrophied synovium surrounds the periphery of the articular cartilage and gives rise to an inflammatory mass called pannus. Pannus is rich in osteoclasts and buries into the junction between the articular cartilage and subchondral bone and detaches the cartilage to expose the raw bone that gradually gets eroded by the enzymatic products released in the inflammatory cascade. Adhesions develop between opposing areas leading first to a fibrous ankylosis that later transforms into bony ankylosis. In advanced disease, the joint gets distended by hypertrophic synovium and increased amount of synovial fluid and the supporting ligaments get stretched and may spontaneously rupture causing a subluxation or dislocation.

Diffuse vasculitis, commonly affecting the arterioles is very often associated. Lymph nodes show hyperplasia. Muscles show nodular polymyositis. Subcutaneous nodules (rheumatoid nodules) form over the extensor surfaces of limbs and show central area of fibrinoid necrosis surrounded by fibroblasts arranged radially and a surrounding fibrous capsule. Nerves show perineural fibrosis.

Clinical Presentation

This multisystem disorder is characterized by symmetrical polyarthritis with an acute onset in 10%, subacute in 20% and insidious in around 70% patients. Problem generally starts with the involvement of the small joints of hand (less commonly feet) which include the metacarpophalangeal (MCP) joints and proximal interphalangeal (PIP) joints with classical sparing of the distal interphalangeal (DIP) joints in a female who is in her thirties. Soon thereafter, the metatarsophalangeal (MTP) joints of the foot may be involved. Involvement of the large joints (knee, elbow, hip, shoulder, etc.) is not uncommon but occurs relatively later. Although most of the axial skeleton is generally spared, the cervical spine (especially C1-C2 articulation) may be at times involved, leading to atlantoaxial instability or even subluxation. Less commonly, there may be superior migration of the odontoid (basilar invagination, *see* Page 381). The involved joints are painful, swollen and stiff. In fact, morning stiffness, especially of at least 1-hour duration is a characteristic feature of the disease.

The 14 specified joints (both sides) that are commonly involved in RA are:

1. Proximal interphalangeal joint
2. Metacarpophalangeal joint
3. Wrist joint
4. Elbow
5. Knee
6. Ankle
7. Metatarsophalangeal joints.

Less commonly involved joints: Hip, temporomandibular, subtalar and atlantoaxial joints.

Joints not involved include: DIP, lumbar spine and SI joints.

In RA, the inflammatory destruction is just not limited to the bone. The synovial linings of the tendon sheaths may be thickened and inflamed aggravating chances of tendon rupture, especially in the hands and feet. Vaughan Jackson lesion refers to the serial disruption of the digital extensor tendons. It begins from the ulnar aspect, first involving the extensor digiti minimi (EDM) and progresses radially to involve ring, middle and index fingers subsequently. Mannerfelt syndrome refers to the rupture of the flexor pollicis longus tendon from attrition caused by a bony spur in the carpal tunnel (scaphoid).

The disease course is characterized by remissions and exacerbations. Over years, the disease process may become less active, but it generally, leaves a number of joints damaged and permanently deformed. The characteristic deformities of various joints seen in RA are discussed further.

---

*Seropositivity refers to the condition where patients tend to have rheumatoid factor (RF), an autoantibody against the Fc portion of immunoglobulin G (IgG), detectable in their serum.

Hand

*Boutonniere deformity (**Fig. 16.3A**)*: Flexion contracture of PIP joints and extension of DIP joint. It is due to rupture of the central extensor expansion of the fingers.

*Swan neck deformity (**Fig. 16.3B**)*: Hyperextension of PIP joints with flexion of the DIP joint. It is due to rupture of the volar plate of the PIP joint.

*Z-deformity (**Figs 16.4A and B**)*: Radial deviation of the wrist with ulnar deviation of the digits.

Caput ulnae syndrome: It refers to the destructive process initiated by the synovitis of the distal radioulnar joint (DRUJ), which includes stretching of the tendon sheath of wrist extensors and volar subluxation of the carpal bones. Trigger finger and trigger thumb may result due to nodules over the tendons.

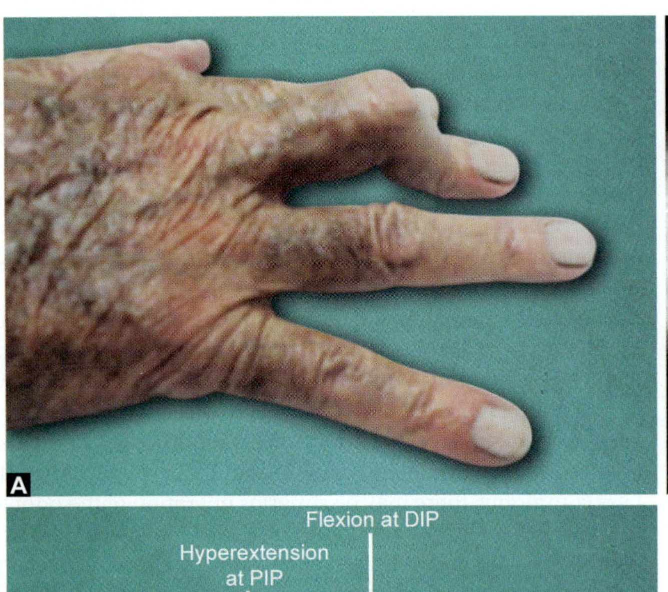

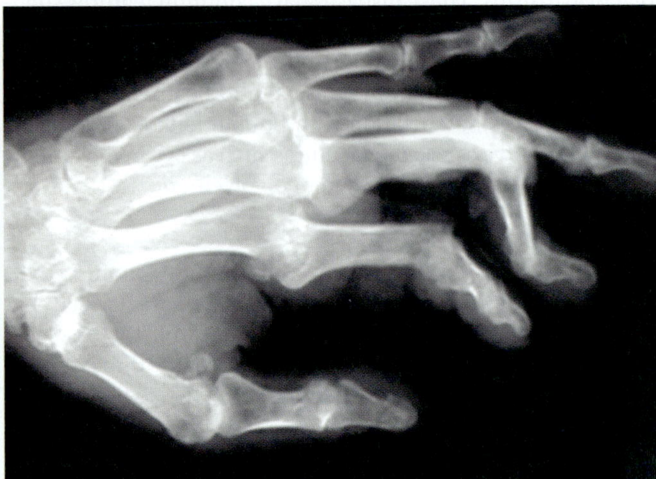

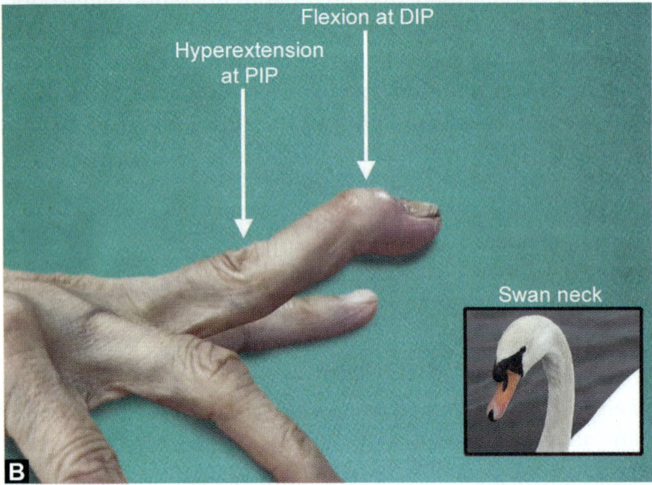

Figs 16.3A and B: (A) Boutonniere deformity of middle finger and X-ray of same patient showing advanced arthritic changes of proximal interphalangeal joint of middle finger; (B) Swan neck deformity of middle finger

Courtesy (Fig. 16.3A): Dr Charlie Goldberg, UCSD, California.

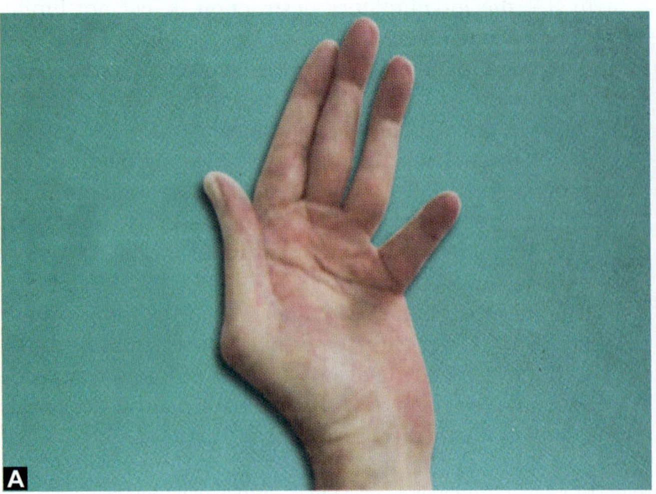

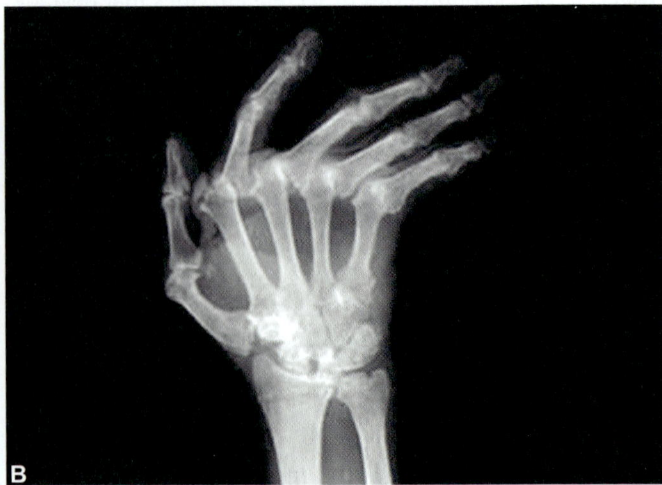

Figs 16.4A and B: Z-deformity—Radial deviation of the wrist with ulnar deviation of the digits

Vaughan-Jackson syndrome: In RA, sequential disruptions of the digital extensor tendons may occur beginning on the ulnar side of the hand and wrist. Extensor tendons of EDM and extensor digitorum communis (EDC) are involved first, and if the underlying pathology is not treated, sequential rupture of the EDC tendons of the ring, long and index fingers occurs. Rupture of the extensor indicis proprius (EIP) occurs in the last.

Mannerfelt syndrome: It refers to the rupture of the flexor pollicis longus tendon from attrition caused by a bony spur on the volar side of scaphoid in the carpal tunnel.

Hitchhiker thumb deformity: It refers to flexion of the MCP and extension of DIP joint of the thumb.

Foot

Hallux valgus (most common; **Fig. 16.5**), claw toes, hammer toes, bunion, callosities under PIP joints and over dorsum, flattening of longitudinal arch, Achilles tendinitis.

Knee

Genu valgum is more commonly seen in rheumatoid knees.

Windswept deformity **(Fig. 16.6):** Genu varum at one knee and valgum at the other.

Extra-articular Manifestations

Besides the articular manifestations discussed earlier, the disorder also has some characteristic extra-articular manifestations that rarely may be the presenting mode. These extra-articular features may be seen in up to one-third of the patients and are as follows:

- *Systemic manifestations*: Generalized fatigue, low-grade fever, weight loss, etc.
- Diffuse osteoporosis is almost always associated
- *Rheumatoid nodules*: These are the most pathognomonic extra-articular feature and appear as nontender subcutaneous nodules seen in around 25% of the cases. They present mainly over pressure areas or periarticular extensor surfaces with olecranon being the most common site **(Fig. 16.7)**. Rarely, nodules may form in pleura and meninges

- Rheumatoid vasculitis is widespread and can involve any organ. Vasculitis of vasa nervorum (the vessels supplying nerves) leads to mononeuritis multiplex, an asymmetric asynchronous painful motor-sensory peripheral neuropathy involving at least two separate nerves
- Nerve entrapment syndromes may be there (like carpal tunnel syndrome, cubital tunnel syndrome, tarsal tunnel syndrome, etc.)
- *Eye changes*: Keratoconjunctivitis sicca (most common eye manifestation), episcleritis, scleritis (most severe eye manifestation) and secondary glaucoma
- *Cardiac manifestations*: Pericarditis (most common cardiac manifestation), cardiomyopathy, arrhythmias, heart block, etc.
- *Pulmonary manifestations*: Pleurisy, effusion, fibrosing alveolitis, pneumonitis and Caplan's syndrome
- Pleural and pericardial effusions (with a very low glucose content)
- Anemia of chronic disorder, leukocytopenia, thrombocytosis, marrow hypoplasia, splenomegaly, generalized lymphadenopathy, pitting edema of foot and Felty's syndrome.

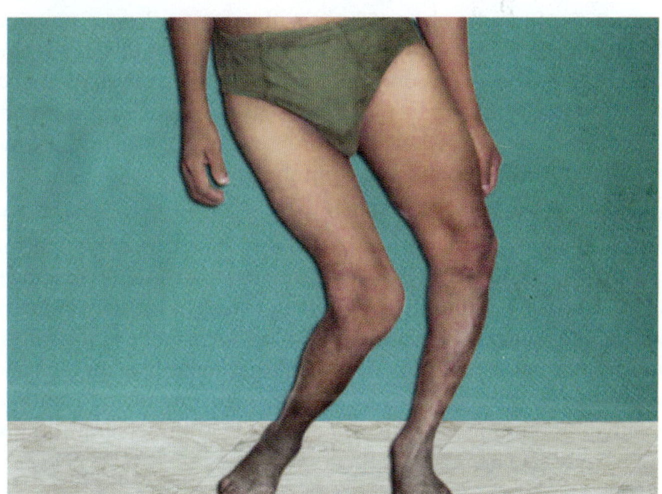

Fig. 16.6: Windswept deformity

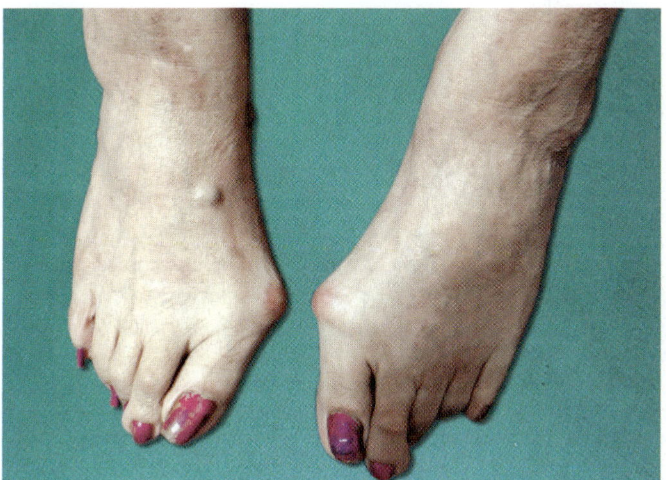

Fig. 16.5: Hallux valgus

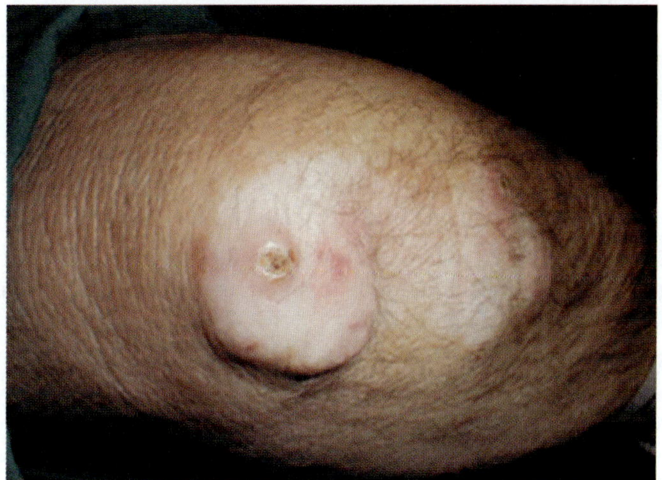

Fig. 16.7: Rheumatoid nodules at the extensor surface of elbow

Investigations

Based on the characteristic clinical presentation, the diagnosis is suspected and further strengthened by making use of the following investigations:

Routine blood investigations: Hemoglobin (Hb) may be low; white cell counts are raised along with a raised erythrocyte sedimentation rate (ESR) and C-reactive protein (CRP) levels.

Rheumatoid factor: The RF is an IgM autoantibody against an Fc region of IgG, seen in almost two-third patients with RA. RF is detected by latex fixation assays (sera with titers of >1:40 are considered positive) and nephelometry (≥20 international units are considered positive). Its detection can suggest the diagnosis. However, early in the disease the levels are lower, therefore the sensitivity is lower and hence it is not useful for screening purposes. RF is positive in about 50% of cases at presentation and in up to 70–80% cases after 6 months of diagnosis. The presence of RF is also not specific for RA as it can be seen in 5% of healthy population and in diseases such as systemic lupus erythematosus (SLE), tuberculosis (TB), Sjögren's syndrome, syphilis, chronic liver disease, sarcoidosis, leprosy, infectious mononucleosis and malaria. The prevalence of positive RF also increases with age and up to 25% of people above 65 years of age may show a positive RF. So above 65 years only high titer (>1:640) should suggest the diagnosis. However, a good prognostic significance is attached to RF, as the levels often parallel disease activity with patients displaying high titers having more severe disease and extra-articular manifestations more commonly.

Anti-cyclic citrullinated polypeptide (Anti-CCP): Anti-CCP antibodies are positive in up to 98% of cases. It has superior specificity and similar sensitivity compared to RF for the diagnosis of RA. Anti-CCP antibodies are often present in the serum years before RA is diagnosed, whereas RF may be negative at the initial presentation of the disease. This test is particularly useful in case of chronic hepatitis infection, which is also associated with a positive RF but not with positive anti-CCP. Antinuclear antibody (ANA) may also be raised in RA.

Radiological evaluation: The survey should include the X-rays of both hands and the affected joints. The classical features are **(Fig. 16.8)**:
- Soft tissue swelling (earliest radiological feature)
- Juxta-articular osteopenia (an early feature)
- Symmetrical reduction of joint space (cf. asymmetrical; mostly medial joint collapse in degenerative arthritis)
- Subchondral erosions and cysts (cf. subchondral sclerosis in degenerative arthritis)
- Deformities of hands and foot joints.

Synovial fluid analysis: In RA, synovial fluid aspirate is yellowish green, cloudy, turbid due to high amounts of leukocytes **(Table 16.1)** and its sugar content is low.

Synovial biopsy: Although diagnostic criteria for RA **(Table 16.3)** well establishes the diagnosis on most occasions, synovial biopsy remains the gold standard and can be taken arthroscopically or by open methods to confirm the diagnosis in cases of a dilemma.

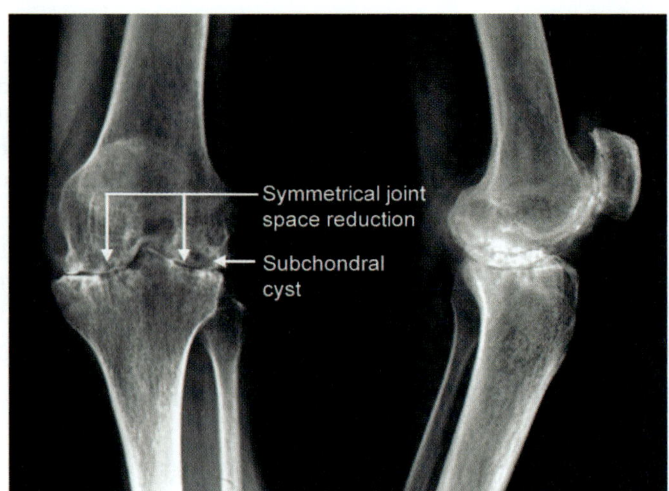

Fig. 16.8: Knee X-rays of a patient with rheumatoid arthritis

Table 16.3: Diagnostic criteria of rheumatoid arthritis (RA)

Revised American Rheumatism Association Criteria for Diagnosis of RA 2010

- *Joint involvement*:*

– 1 large joint	0
– 2–10 large joint	1
– 1–3 small joints (with or without large joint involvement)	2
– 4–10 small joints	3
– >10 joints (at least 1 small joint)	5

- *Serology:*

– Negative RF and negative anti-CCP	0
– Low positive RF or low positive anti-CCP	2
– High positive RF or high positive anti-CCP	3

- *Acute phase reactants:*

– Normal CRP and normal ESR	0
– Abnormal CRP and abnormal ESR	1

- *Duration of symptoms†*

– <6 weeks	0
– ≥6 weeks	1

Result:
- Score ≥6 positive
- Patients with score <6/10 are not classified as having RA; their status can be reassessed and the criteria may be fulfilled cumulatively over time

Target population:
- Patients who have at least one joint with definite clinical synovitis (swelling)

**Large joints:* Shoulder, elbow, hips, knee, ankle, etc. *Small joints*: MCP, PIP, 2nd to 5th MTP, thumb, IP joints, wrists.

†With synovitis not better explained by another disease.

Abbreviations: anti-CCP, anti-cyclic citrullinated polypeptide; RF, rheumatoid factor; CRP, C-reactive protein; ESR, erythrocyte sedimentation rate; MCP, metacarpophalangeal; PIP, proximal interphalangeal; MTP, metatarsophalangeal; IP, interphalangeal.

Differential Diagnosis

Important conditions to exclude are: osteoarthritis (OA), SLE, psoriatic arthritis, Reiter's syndrome and viral arthropathy.

Prognostic Factors

Poor prognostic factors in RA include:

- Young females have a poorer prognosis than males
- Family history of RA
- High titers of RA
- Positive serum anti-CCP
- Presence of HLA-DR4
- Presence of erosion on X-ray early in the course of disease
- Persistent synovitis
- Presence of extra-articular manifestations
- Elevated ESR, CRP.

Assessment of disease activity in patients with RA: There are many scores based on patient, clinician and laboratory data, which are used for assessment of disease activity in RA patients, e.g. patient activity scale (PAS); routine assessment of patient index data with three measures (RAPID-3); clinical disease activity index (CDAI), disease activity score with 28-joint counts (DAS-28) and simplified disease activity index (SDAI). DAS-28 is a commonly used score, which ranges between 0 and 9.4. Scores below 2.6 indicates remission, between 2.6 and 3.2—low disease activity, between 3.2 and 5.1—moderate disease activity and scores above 5.1 indicate high disease activity.

Treatment

Most of the patients with RA require lifelong treatment. Treatment should be started early in the course of the disease for a better outcome. Medical treatment is guided by the presence or absence of poor prognostic factors, response to treatment and disease activity. Treatment should be aggressive in patient with poor prognostic factors such as positive RF and anti-CCP, erosive disease and high disease activity.

Medical Treatment

Nonsteroidal anti-inflammatory drugs (NSAIDs) and steroids: NSAIDs and steroids are used mainly for induction of remission as both these agents have a rapid onset of action. NSAIDs provide symptomatic relief (but not halt disease progression) from pain, especially in the prediagnosis stage when one is awaiting the results of investigations. Intra-articular steroids may be added in this situation in case the pain relief is partial. Once the diagnosis is established, the disease-modifying antirheumatic drugs (DMARDs) are introduced to decrease the progression of the disease. However, DMARDs are very slow acting and take 3–6 months to reach their peak effect, so during this stage, oral steroids may be given to halt the inflammatory process. Low dose glucocorticoid therapy* (prednisone 5–10 mg daily) provides rapid symptomatic relief and also retards the radiographic progression of RA. But since long-term steroid therapy may be hazardous in terms of the likely side effects. The paradigm is to shift toward DMARDs for long-term control and taper the steroids over a 2–3 month period.* High-dose glucocorticoids are the mainstay in cases where extra-articular manifestations such as vasculitis (especially mononeuritis multiplex), scleritis, pericarditis or endocarditis are there.

Disease-modifying antirheumatic drugs: DMARDs are slow-acting drugs and are meant for maintenance of remission[†] and preventing acute exacerbations in both early and established RA.[‡] Synthetic DMARDs [methotrexate (MTX), sulfasalazine (SSZ), hydroxychloroquine (HCQ), leflunomide (LEF) and minocycline and biologic DMARDs **(Table 16.4)** are mainstay of antirheumatoid therapy. Synthetic DMARDs are generally the first line to be started and most doctors prefer to start with a combination therapy in form of MTX (most preferred DMARDs) with SSZ and HCQ.

Methotrexate is started as a single dose once a week (7.5–30 mg/week). The dose is escalated from 7.5–15 mg/week to 20–30

Table 16.4: Biological disease-modifying antirheumatic drugs (DMARDs) in rheumatoid arthritis (RA)	
Agents	*Comments*
Infliximab	It is a chimeric mouse-human IgG1 monoclonal antibody which targets TNF-α
Etanercept	It is a dimeric fusion protein of human p75 TNF receptor and human IgG1-Fc targeted against TNF-α and lymphotoxin-α
Adalimumab (Exemptia)	It is a recombinant human IgG1 monoclonal antibody directed to human TNF-α
Abatacept	It is a fusion protein of human CTLA4 and Fc domain of human IgG1
Golimumab	It is a recombinant human IgG1 monoclonal antibody directed to human TNF-α
Rituximab	Rituximab is a chimeric mouse-human IgG1 monoclonal antibody that targets CD20
Certolizumab pegol	Humanized antigen-binding fragment (Fab) of a monoclonal antibody conjugated to polyethylene glycol. It targets TNF-α
Tocilizumab	Chimeric mouse-human IgG1 monoclonal antibody against IL-6
Anakinra	Anakinra is a recombinant protein and IL-1 inhibitor

Abbreviations: IgG, immunoglobulin G; TNF, tumor necrosis factor; IL, interleukin.

---

*Low-dose glucocorticoids <10 mg/day prednisolone; high-dose glucocorticoids 10–60 mg/day prednisolone; short-term glucocorticoids <3 months duration.
[†]*Remission*: Tender/swollen joint count, CRP and patient global assessment score each ≤1 or simply DAS-28 ≤ 2.6.
[‡]*Early RA*: Symptom duration <6 months; *established RA*: Symptom duration >6 months.

mg/week, if improvement is not seen in 3 months. If response to oral MTX is not optimal, it can be given as a subcutaneous injection. Oral folic acid tablets are given at doses of 5–10 mg/week, 24–48 hours after MTX, to avoid toxicities secondary to inhibition of rapid cell turnover. MTX is contraindicated in pre-existing liver disease, hepatitis B or C infection, ongoing alcohol use, renal failure, bone marrow suppression and in women of childbearing potential who are not using contraception.

Hydroxychloroquine is the least toxic but also the least effective DMARD so not used as monotherapy. It is given in combination with MTX at a dose of 200–400 mg daily. Retinal toxicity is a serious side effect with prolonged treatment and patients should undergo a baseline ophthalmological examination within 1 year of the start of the treatment and yearly screening is required after 5 years of the treatment.

Sulfasalazine is usually prescribed along at a dose of 1–2 g/day in combination with the above two drugs. Gastrointestinal intolerance is the most common side effect of SSZ.

Minocycline is also an effective DMARD to be used early in RA in doses of 100 mg twice daily. Cutaneous hyperpigmentation may occur with prolonged therapy.

Leflunomide has an efficacy comparable to MTX and is a viable alternative in patients who are intolerant to MTX. It is given daily in a dose of 10–20 mg orally. Diarrhea is a common side effect which may require reduction of the dose. Baseline liver function tests are done before starting the drug as it is also hepatotoxic (though less than MTX). Contraindications are same as with MTX including hepatic disease, pregnancy and ongoing alcohol use. However, it can be used in patients with mild-moderate renal insufficiency. Women who wish to conceive must have their blood levels drawn as it is teratogenic and has exceptionally long half-life of up to 4 weeks (even if the therapy was administered years ago).

Since serious side effects may be associated with DMARD use, laboratory monitoring is integral component of DMARD therapy. American College of Rheumatology (ACR) criteria for laboratory monitoring while on DMARDs is given in **Box 16.1**.

Patients with established RA should receive at least 3 months of synthetic DMARD therapy before switching in-between DMARDs or while switching from synthetic DMARDs to biological DMARD agents. Biological DMARDs **(Table 16.4)** have revolutionized the treatment of RA. They all are very effective drugs and reduce the sign and symptoms of synovitis and halt the radiographic progression of the disease. They are effective in patients who do not respond optimally to MTX. Onset is also rapid compared to synthetic DMARDs and is seen within 4 weeks. Although they are effective as monotherapy, but greater efficacy is seen when used in combination with MTX. The major disadvantages are cost and concerns about long-term toxicities (demyelinating diseases, reactivation of latent TB, etc.). Because of the cost and side effects (*see* **Box 16.2** for contraindications), currently they are recommended in patients who do not respond to monotherapy or combination therapy of synthetic DMARDs given for a minimum of 3 months. A TNF blocking agent, which includes adalimumab (Exemptia), infliximab, etanercept and the newer golimumab and certolizumab is the first choice among biological DMARDs. Non-TNF biological DMARDs, e.g. rituximab, abatacept, tocilizumab and anakinra are recommended in patients who

---

Box 16.1: American College of Rheumatology recommendations (2008) for laboratory monitoring intervals for rheumatoid arthritis (RA) patients receiving non-biologic disease-modifying antirheumatic drugs (DMARDs)

1. Baseline monitoring is required for all DMARDs before initiation of therapy and includes complete blood count, serum creatinine and liver transaminase levels
2. No laboratory monitoring is required after baseline for hydroxychloroquine and minocycline
3. For methotrexate, leflunomide and sulfasalazine, all baseline tests should be repeated every 2–4 weeks for first 3 months and then every 3 months till the drugs are continued

---

Box 16.2: Contraindications and concerns to the use of biological disease-modifying antirheumatic drugs (DMARDs)

1. Contraindicated in New York Heart Association (NYHA) class III or IV heart failure or in those with an ejection fraction of 50% or less
2. Increased risk of opportunistic bacterial and fungal infections, e.g. fatal *Legionella and Listeria infections*
3. *Increased risk of viral and bacterial infection*: It is recommended that before the start of the biological therapy, the inactivated influenza vaccine, recombinant human papillomavirus vaccine, live attenuated herpes zoster vaccine and recombinant pneumococcal vaccine should be administered to patients. Live vaccines are contraindicated during biological therapy
4. Patients should be screened for latent tuberculosis (TB) infection with either the tuberculin skin test or interferon-gamma-release assay (IGRA) and chest X-ray. History of TB infection and active TB are contraindications to use of biological DMARDs
5. Lymphoproliferative disease, hepatitis B or C infection, pregnancy and lactation are contraindications to use of biologic DMARDs

---

do not adequately respond to conventional DMARDs and anti-TNF medications (*see* **Flow chart 16.1** for summary of medical management of RA). Before administration of rituximab intravenous (IV) methylprednisolone (100 mg or equivalent) is given to prevent infusion reactions.

Future drugs for RA: Janus kinases (JAKs) inhibitor "Tofacitinib" has demonstrated efficacy in patients who were not responsive to DMARDs or TNF inhibitors. Fostamatinib, an oral inhibitor of spleen tyrosine kinase has produced a response in combination with MTX in patients who were not optimally responsive to MTX alone.

Orthopedic Treatment

Physiotherapy should be advised to all to maintain joint mobility and muscle strength and splints may be used to prevent and correct deformities. Hot fomentation or wax bath for pain relief and lifestyle modification like use of western toilet, high chair, proper posture and avoiding squatting are other supportive measures. Following surgical options may need to be resorted to in indicated patients:

Synovectomy: It has a preventive role in joints where destruction is minimal and synovitis is the main cause of pain. It can be done arthroscopically assisted or by open methods. The synovectomy should be virtually complete so as to avoid recurrence of symptoms.

Osteotomy: It is indicated when a joint is partially destroyed. The goal is to shift the body's weight off the damaged articular surface, e.g. a high tibial varus osteotomy in genu valgum/varum arthritic knees.

Arthrodesis: Surgical fusion of damaged joints gives good pain relief at the cost of the joint function. So, it is commonly performed in the peripheral joints such as the wrist, ankle, interphalangeal (IP) joints of hands and feet where functional loss is less disabling and arthroplasty is less reliable.

Joint replacement surgeries: In advanced stages, arthroplasty remains the only way to alleviate pain and correct deformity.

HIGH-YIELD POINTS

- Rheumatoid arthritis has a strong association with HLA DR4. Other HLAs associated with RA include HLA DR1, DR9 and DR10, DR14. The HLAs that are thought to be protective against RA include HLA DR5, DR2, DR3 and DR7.
- Most common joints involved in RA are MCP > wrist > PIP > knee.
- Rheumatoid nodules are most common extra-articular feature. However, following diseases must be considered in patients with subcutaneous nodules and arthritis: gout, sarcoidosis, rheumatic fever, SLE and amyloidosis.
- *Seronegative RA:* These are patients who have clinical picture of RA but have negative RF. They generally have better prognosis and fewer extra-articular manifestations. However, when followed over time a number of such patients actually are found to have some other related arthritis such as psoriatic arthritis, SLE, gout or another crystal deposition disease, etc. Hence, the clinician must be vigilant in them.
- *Rheumatoid arthritis and pregnancy:* The disease improves during pregnancy, although postpartum it flares up. MTX, LEF and biological DMARDs are contraindicated while HCQ and SSZ are allowed. Steroids may be given to control flares, if required.
- *Ball Catcher's view (hands in ball catching position):* Special X-ray view to detect early erosive changes in RA of hand.
- *Caplan's syndrome:* RA associated with coal workers pneumoconiosis involving the upper lobes of the lung. The multiple pulmonary nodules in these patients show cavitation and specks of calcification.
- *Felty's syndrome:* It comprises a triad of RA, splenomegaly and neutropenia. It is seen in patients with severe seropositive disease. Treatment is focused on treating RA. If neutropenia is severe, splenectomy may be needed.
- Rheumatoid arthritis tends to spare the central nervous system (CNS). Neuropathies are generally due to vasculitis.
- Although mononeuritis multiplex is a common extra-articular manifestation of RA, the most common cause of the same in India is leprosy.

JUVENILE IDIOPATHIC ARTHRITIS

It is an autoimmune, noninfective, inflammatory arthritis involving one or more joints, usually of more than 6 weeks duration in children less than 16 years of age. Juvenile idiopathic arthritis (JIA) is the most common chronic rheumatic illness of childhood.

Flow chart 16.1: Summary of medical management of Rheumatoid Arthritis (simplified from American College of Rheumatology, 2015 Guidelines)

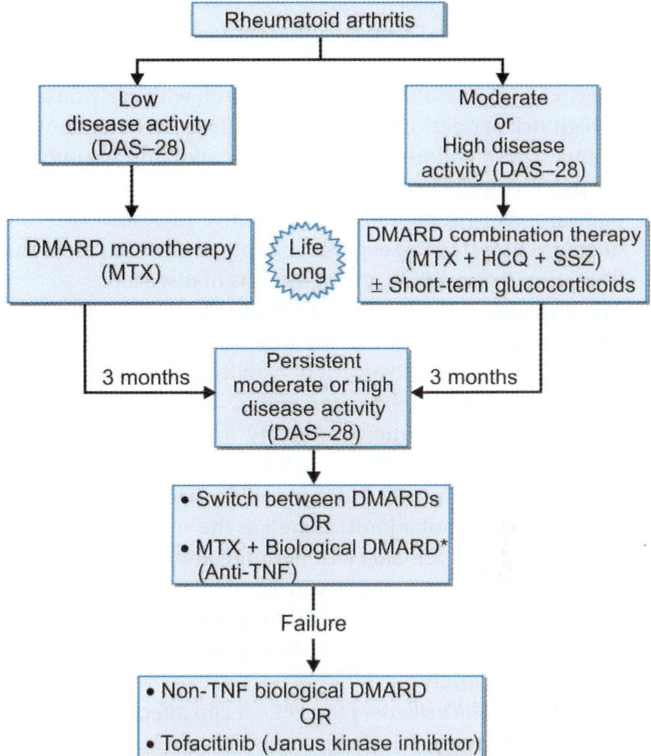

*Inj Exemptia (Adalimumab) 40 mg subcutaneous twice a month.
Abbreviations: MTX, methotrexate; HCQ, hydroxychloroquine; SSZ, sulfasalazine; DMARD, disease-modifying antirheumatic drug; TNF, tumor necrosis factor.

Juvenile chronic arthritis (JCA) and juvenile rheumatoid arthritis are commonly used to describe juvenile arthritis in Europe and North America, respectively. In the updated system of the International League of Associations for Rheumatology (ILAR), term JIA was recommended to replace all other terms.

Pathogenesis

Exact etiopathogenesis is not clear and multifactorial, but like RA, antigen-driven autoimmune process plays a key role in the inflammatory pathology of oligoarthritis and polyarthritis in genetically susceptible individuals. Association between multiple polymorphisms in HLA genes and different forms of JIA has been confirmed by many studies. Oligoarthritis is associated with HLA A2 and HLA DRB1, RF positive polyarthritis with HLA DR4 and enthesitis-related arthritis with HLA B27. It has been proposed that pathogenesis is different in different types of JIA but overproduction of proinflammatory cytokines play a key role in clinical manifestations in all types of JRA.

Clinical Presentation

Based upon age at onset, number of joints involved and presence of extra-articular symptoms, ILAR classifies JIA into six types:

1. *Oligoarticular JIA (40%):* Affects four or fewer joints (in half of these cases, only one joint is involved) in the first 6 months of illness. Oligoarticular JIA commonly occurs in younger children,

ages 1–7 years. It is the most common clinical subtype (40%) and is more common in girls. The knee joint is most commonly involved joint, followed by subtalar and then elbow joint. Small joints of hand and feet are rarely involved. The cervical spine is also mostly spared. The involvement is generally not symmetric but a history of morning stiffness is usually present and the affected joints are often swollen. Children with early onset are at high risk of developing a chronic iridocyclitis or an anterior uveitis. These children require regular slit-lamp examination for painless iridocyclitis. Approximately 70% of children with pauciarticular JIA demonstrate a positive ANA test. Extended oligoarticular JIA is an aggressive subtype in which more than four joints get involved after 6 months of disease.

2. *Polyarticular JIA (30–35%)*: It affects five or more joints in the first 6-month course of the disease. It can affect children of any age. Seropositive variety usually affects teenage girls. Seropositive JIA is characterized by a positive RA factor, symmetrical involvement of joints, morning stiffness and association with HLA DR4, thus the clinical picture resembles RA. Iritis is uncommon and the neck (cervical spine) and jaw (temporomandibular joint) as well as the small joints of hand and feet usually are affected. Seronegative polyarticular JIA (negative RA factor) affects younger children aged between 8 years and 12 years. There are no associated extra-articular features and iritis is rare. It has a better prognosis than seropositive variety.

3. *Systemic JIA/Still's disease (10–20%)*: It can affect both children and adult at any age. It is characterized by systemic features such as daily spiking fever in a quotidian pattern, lymphadenopathy, hepatosplenomegaly and a salmon pink rash located over the trunk, face, palm and soles. Diagnostic criteria include fever of at least 2 weeks duration plus arthritis in one or more joints plus at least one of the following systemic features: rash, lymphadenopathy, hepatosplenomegaly or serositis. Arthritis is just one manifestation of the generalized disorder and may not manifest until months after the onset of fever. Pericarditis and pleural effusions are present in almost 10% of the children. Laboratory investigations reveal high leukocyte count, raised ESR and elevated ferritin levels. Most children are less than 3 years of age and this variety has an equal incidence in both boys and girls. The long-term prognosis is worst even though cardiac manifestations are transient and presence of pericarditis is not related to severity of disease.

4. *Psoriatic JIA*: It is characterized by psoriatic rash or positive family history of psoriasis along with arthritis of one or more joints, sacroiliitis with prominent involvement of DIP joint, sacroiliitis, dactylitis, sausage digits and nail pitting. It can occur at any age and ANA is positive in up to 60% of cases. Anterior uveitis is common and require regular slit-lamp examination.

5. *Enthesitis-related JIA*: It is commonly seen in children between 10 years and 12 years of age and characterized by inflammation at the sites of attachment of ligaments and tendons to bone. Inflammation at the attachment of tendons and ligaments often leads to stiffness. Raised ESR, CRP and positive HLA B27 are found in a majority of cases. Heel pain, sacroiliitis, tight iliotibial band leading to positive Ober's test

are common features along with arthritis. Reactive arthritis, arthritis associated with IBD and juvenile-onset spondylitis are also included in this group.

6. *Undifferentiated arthritis*: This group includes patients which do not fit into any category or have features of more than one group.

Diagnosis

There is no single or definitive test. Rather, the diagnosis is made from clinical findings, coupled with laboratory findings and analysis of aspirated joint fluid. ANA is most commonly found positive immunological marker in JIA and its presence increases the risk for the development of uveitis. HLA B27 may be positive in children with symptoms of enthesitis-related arthritis. Rarely anti-CCP and RF can also be positive. X-ray may show erosions and loss of joint space. Magnetic resonance imaging (MRI) shows synovial hypertrophy, joint effusion and cartilage damage.

Treatment

The arthritis has a waxing and waning course with remissions and relapses. Up to 50% of children may have continued disease into adulthood. Symptomatic treatment is generally enough to tide over the exacerbations. Fortunately, most children with JRA recover from the arthritis and are left with only mild deformities. Those who are RF positive and have multiple joint involvement tend to land up with an adult rheumatoid-like disease and a poorer prognosis. Management principles are almost same as for RA with NSAIDs, glucocorticoids and DMARDs.

SERONEGATIVE SPONDYLOARTHROPATHIES

It is a group of autoimmune disorders with onset usually below the age of 40 years characterized by inflammatory arthritis of predominantly axial skeleton with or without large peripheral joints, absence of RF in serum (hence seronegative) but having a strong association with HLA B27 with the presence of uveitis in the patients.

The group includes (mnemonic: PEARS):
- Ankylosing spondylitis
- Reiter's syndrome
- Psoriatic arthritis
- Enteropathic arthritis (associated with ulcerative colitis/Crohn's disease)
- Synovitis, acne, pustulosis, hyperostosis and osteitis (SAPHO) syndrome.

ANKYLOSING SPONDYLITIS (MARIE-STRUMPELL DISEASE/BECHTEREW'S DISEASE)

Ankylosing spondylitis is a chronic progressive inflammatory seronegative spondyloarthropathy, involving mainly the axial skeleton (spine and the sacroiliac joints) with variable involvement of root joints (hip and shoulder).

Incidence

Age of onset is mostly 15–25 years. Males are affected 2–10 times more commonly than females.

Etiopathogenesis

The primary site of pathology in AS is the enthesis (site of attachment of tendons and ligaments to bone). Autoimmune attack leads to enthesitis with edema in the adjacent bone that may result in erosive lesions in the affected joints. The joints involved undergo first fibrous and eventually bony ankylosis. Ossification also occurs in the ligaments that are ending up as enthesis, especially the ligaments of the spine that gradually get ossified, progressively leading to stiffness.

The disease has been noted to have a striking association with the presence of a genetic marker HLA B27. This marker is present in 1–6% of the general population, but positive in almost 90% of the patients with AS. Antineutrophil cytoplasmic antibodies (ANCAs) are also associated with AS.

Clinical Features

The patient is usually a young male, presenting with gradual onset of pain and stiffness of the lower back and often walks to the clinician with a straight stiff back. The symptoms are more prominent in the morning after getting from bed or after a period of inactivity and the pain is classically relieved by activity.

Sacroiliac joint is the first joint to be involved followed by the lumbar spine. Eventually, the whole spine may be involved in severe cases (cervical spine is involved late). In late stages, the patient's spine adopts a "question mark" posture due to hyperkyphosis of thoracic spine and straightening of the lumbar spine (sniffing dog posture). Some patients may complain of pain over manubrium sterni, pubic symphysis and sternocostal joints. Rarely, the patient may present with involvement of shoulders or hip or peripheral joints first. Arthritis in the root joints (hips and shoulders) occurs in approximately 25% of patients while peripheral joint involvement may be seen in up to one-third of cases. In decreasing frequency peripheral joints involved are hip, shoulder, knee, wrist, MCP, MTP and PIP joints. Enthesitis is a prominent feature and chronic inflammatory enthesitis leads to chest wall pain (costosternal joints), heel pain (TA insertion) and sole pain (plantar aponeurosis insertion).

Not uncommon is to find a patient with a pathological fracture secondary to a minor trauma. Most acute spinal fractures in the AS population occur in the cervical spine, particularly at C5-C6 and C6-C7 levels. Vertebral fractures are four times more common while the risk of cord damage is 11 times greater in patients with AS. The most common injury mechanism in such cases is hyperextension.

A patient with AS may also have some extra-articular manifestations. Most common extra-articular manifestation is acute anterior uveitis (iridocyclitis) occurring in almost one-third of cases. However, the list is large and includes: pericarditis, aortic incompetence, pulmonary complications, bilateral apical lobe fibrosis, ulcerative colitis and Crohn's disease and generalized osteoporosis.

Examination

A thorough examination of these patients means evaluating for the involvement of SI joints, lumbar spine, thoracic spine and lastly cervical spine.

Tests for Sacroiliac Joint Involvement

- Tenderness localized to the posterior superior iliac spine (PSIS), as PSIS overlies SI joints.

- *Sacroiliac side-to-side compression test (**Fig. 16.9**)*: The patient is in the side lying position and the examiner's hands are placed over the upper part of the iliac crest, pressing toward the floor. The movement causes strain in the SI joint. A positive test is indicated by pain in the SI joint.
- *Gaenslen's test (**Fig. 16.10**)*: The patient lies on his or her back, the examiner maximally flexes the hip on the normal side (by pushing the knee toward patient chest) and extends the affected hip (by allowing it to fall over the side of the table). The test is considered positive, if the patient complains of pain over the SI joint.
- *Pump handle test (**Fig. 16.11**)*: The patient lies supine, the examiner grasps the affected side knee of the patients with one hand and flexes the knee and hip, and forces it toward the opposite shoulder across the chest. Pain over involved SI joints indicates a positive test.
- *Patrick test/FABER test (**Fig. 16.12**)*: The test is performed by keeping the limb flexed, abducted and externally rotated (FABER). If pain is elicited on the ipsilateral side anteriorly, it is suggestive of hip joint pathology of same side. If pain is

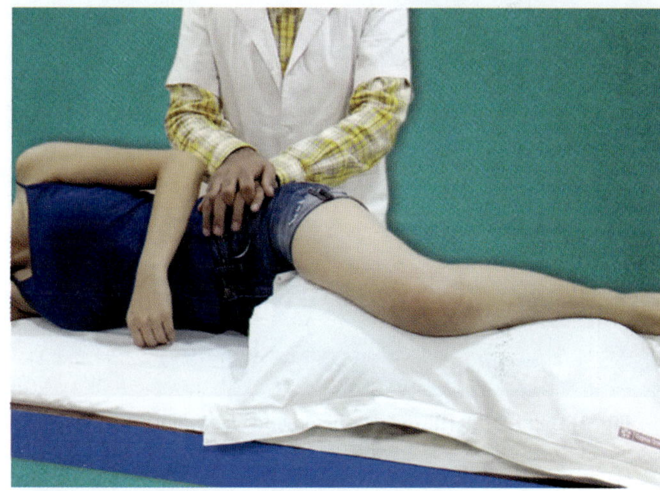

Fig. 16.9: Sacroiliac joint side-to-side compression test

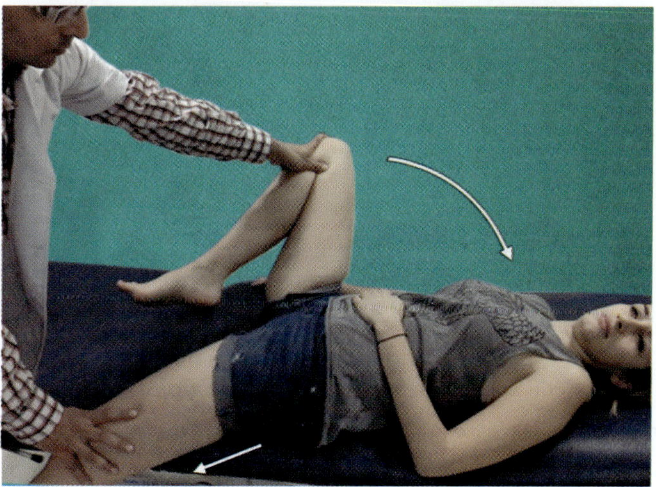

Fig. 16.10: Gaenslen's test

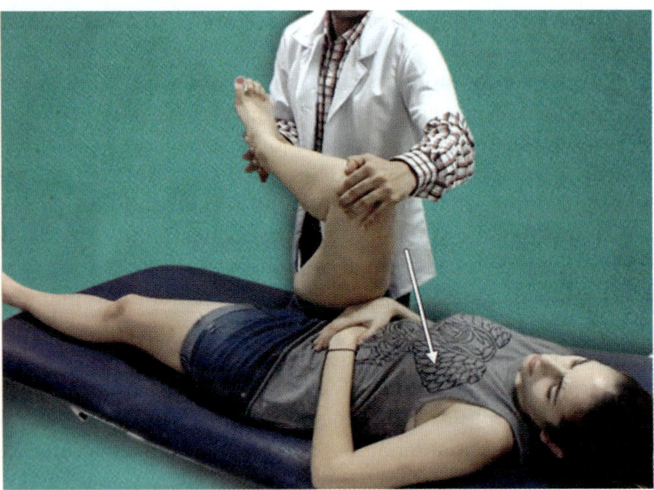

Fig. 16.11: Pump handle test

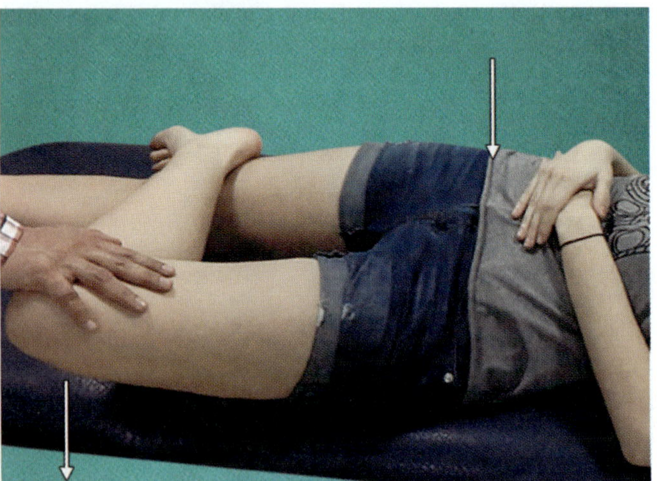

Fig. 16.12: FABER (flexed, abducted and externally rotated) test

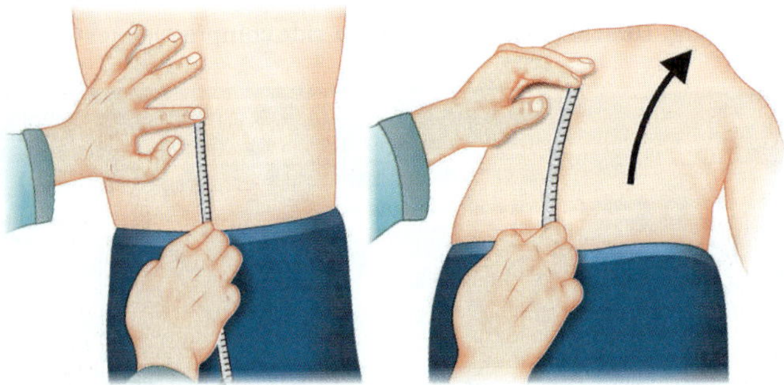

Fig. 16.13: Modified Schober's test

elicited on the contralateral side posteriorly around the SI joint, it is suggestive of pain arising from the SI joint.

Test for Lumbar Spine Involvement

- Look for loss of lumbar lordosis.
- *Check for restricted lumbar spine motion (modified Schober's test; Fig. 16.13)*: With the patient in standing posture, two bony points are marked on the lumbar spine, one at the

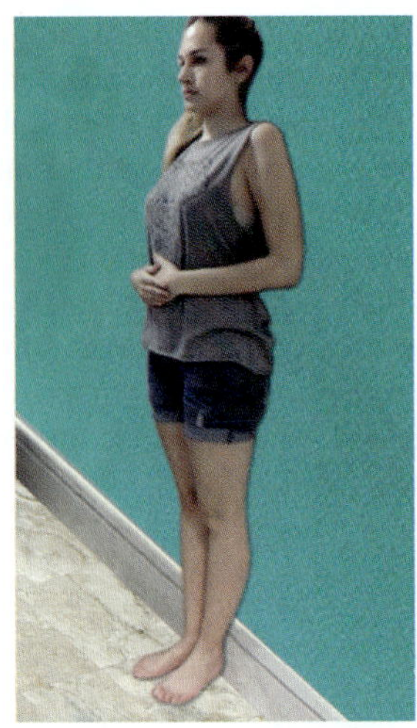

Fig. 16.14: Fleche test

level of the sacral dimples and second 10 cm apart from it; the patient is asked to touch his toes with knees extended. Normally, the two points should be separated by more than 5 cm; if the lumbar excursion is less than 5 cm, it implies a loss of lumbar flexion suggestive of AS.

Test for Thoracic Spine Involvement

Measure chest expansion: An expansion of less than 5 cm during full inspiration, at the level of nipples suggests involvement of the costovertebral joints.

Test for Cervical Spine Involvement

In severe cases, the cervical spine involvement may also be present. It can be detected by the Fleche test **(Fig. 16.14)**. The patient is asked to stand against a wall and to simultaneously touch the heels, the back and the back of head against the wall. If the patient is unable to touch the back of head against the wall, it indicates cervical spine involvement.

Investigations

Blood investigations show an elevated ESR, positive serum HLA B27 and mild anemia.

Radiographic Examination

Bilateral symmetrical sacroiliitis is the hallmark of AS. An anteroposterior view of the pelvis is often adequate to show sacroiliitis. Changes typically start in the lower third of the SI joint. Haziness and widening of the joint due to subchondral erosions is the earliest change. Destruction is first evident on the iliac side. This is usually accompanied by variable osteoporosis around the SI joint. As the disease progresses sclerosis, new bone formation and calcification of SI and sacrotuberous ligaments around the SI joint occur, leading to ankylosis (fibrous then bony) of the SI joint as the end result **(Fig. 16.15)**.

Radiographs of the lumbosacral spine show loss of lumbar lordosis, diffuse osteoporosis, calcification of the anterior and posterior longitudinal ligaments, squaring of the vertebral bodies and bridging osteophytes (k/a syndesmophytes). Eventually, the spine in advanced stages gives the classical bamboo spine appearance **(Fig. 16.16)**. *Dagger sign* refers to a single central radiodense line in the anteroposterior (AP) radiographs of spine

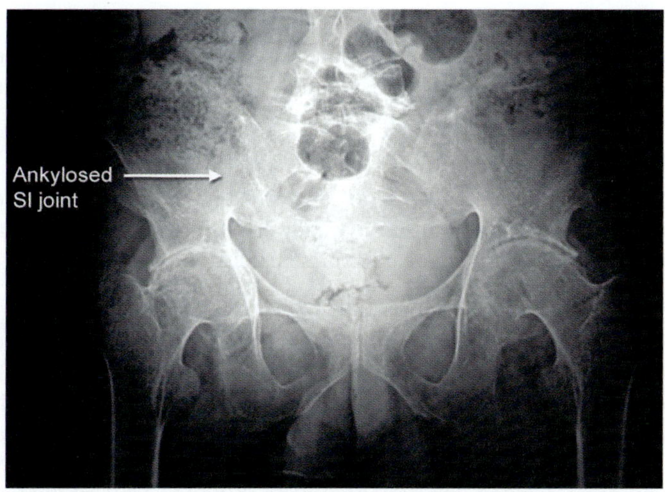

Fig. 16.15: X-ray pelvis anteroposterior view showing sacroiliac (SI) joint ankylosis in ankylosing spondylitis

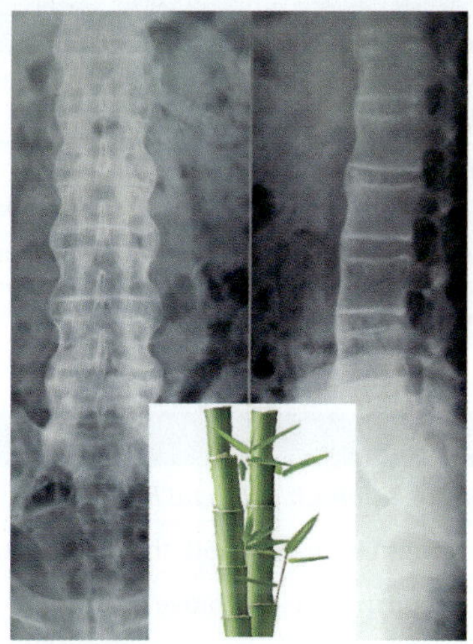

Fig. 16.16: X-ray lumbosacral spine anteroposterior and lateral views showing bamboo spine appearance in ankylosing spondylitis

related to ossification of supraspinous and interspinous ligaments **(Fig. 16.17)**.

Earliest diagnosis, however, is made by MRI [short TI inversion recovery (STIR) sequence or with gadolinium-enhanced MRI]. For active sacroiliitis, a dynamic MRI with fat suppression, is considered to be best. Some important MRI signs in AS **(Figs 16.18A and B)** are:

- *Romanus lesion (shiny corner sign)*: This in an early MRI finding and represents small erosions at the anterosuperior and the anteroinferior margin (corners on lateral radiograph) of the vertebral bodies, with surrounding reactive sclerosis.
- *Anderson lesion (spinal pseudoarthrosis)*: Refers to the inflammatory involvement of the intervertebral disks (spondylodiscitis) in the AS.

Diagnosis

Modified New York criteria **(Box 16.3)** have conventionally been used to establish the diagnosis of AS. The Assessment of Spondyloarthritis International Society (ASIS) has proposed a separate criteria to facilitate an earlier diagnosis for axial spondyloarthritis **(Table 16.5)**.

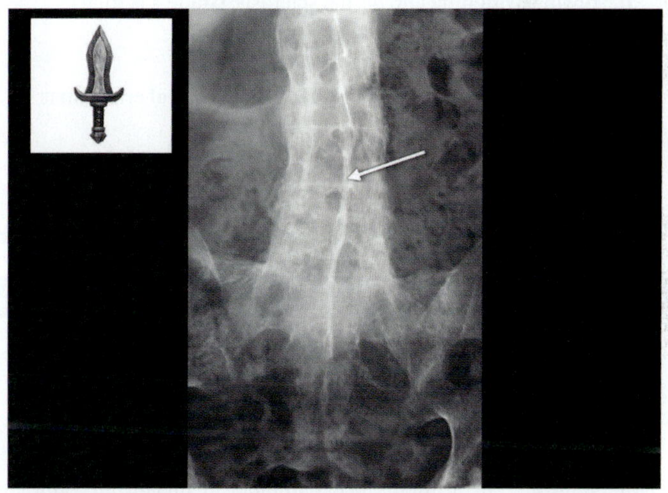

Fig. 16.17: Dagger sign

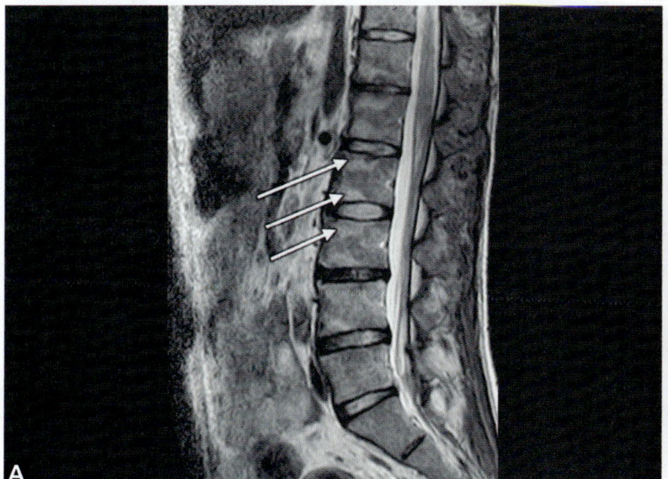

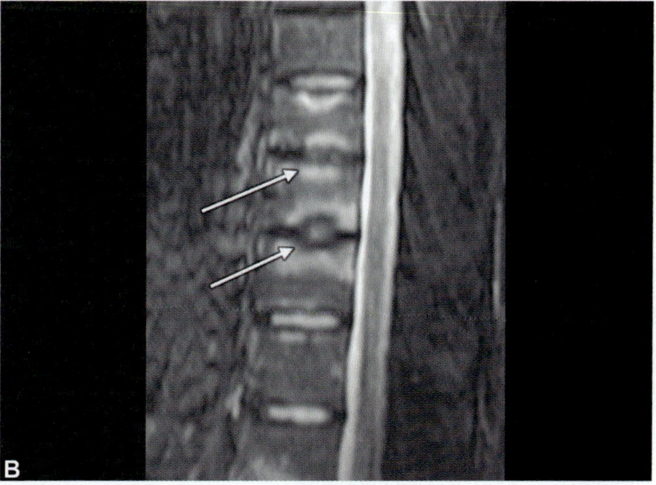

Figs 16.18A and B: Early magnetic resonance imaging (MRI) signs of ankylosing spondylitis (AS). (A) Sagittal section of MRI of lumbosacral spine showing shiny corner sign (arrows); (B) MRI of lumbar spine showing spondylodiscitis (arrows)

Differential Diagnosis

Although all common causes of low backache (see Chapter 7) need to be excluded, diffuse idiopathic skeletal hyperostosis (DISH) presents a challenging differential **(Table 16.6)**.

Treatment

Although no treatment modality exists to eradicate the disease process, but a number of disabilities that the disease produces can be tackled by timely intervention.

General Measures and Physical Therapy (Box 16.4)

Patients are encouraged to do regular exercises and stay active so as to maintain joint mobility. They are educated to maintain a proper posture and advocated spinal extension exercises.

Medical Management

Nonsteroidal anti-inflammatory drugs form the first line of treatment. Indomethacin (most commonly used), phenylbutazone (most effective, but discontinued owing to high incidence of neutropenia) and diclofenac provide relief from pain and stiffness. If NSAIDs need to be given for longer or if toxicity symptoms develop, the patient may be shifted to TNF inhibitors. The anti-TNF agents currently approved are adalimumab

---

Box 16.3: Modified New York criteria (1984) for the diagnosis of ankylosing spondylitis (AS)

Clinical criteria
- Low back pain and stiffness for more than 3 months that improves with exercise but not with the rest
- Limitation of lumbar spine mobility in both the sagittal and frontal planes
- Limitation of chest expansion to 2.5 cm (1 inch) or less, measured at the level of the fourth intercostal space

Radiological criteria
- Unilateral sacroiliitis of grade 3–4 or
- Bilateral sacroiliitis of grade ≥2 (grade 1 is suspicious changes, grade 2 is minimal erosion or sclerosis, grade 3 is moderate-to-severe sacroiliitis with one or more of these erosions, sclerosis, narrowing, widening and partial sclerosis. Grade 4 is total ankylosis)

Grading
- Definite ankylosing spondylitis if: The radiological criterion is associated with at least one clinical criterion
- Probable ankylosing spondylitis if: Three clinical criteria are present or the radiologic criterion is present without any signs or symptoms satisfying the clinical criteria

---

Table 16.5: The Assessment of Spondyloarthritis International Society (ASIS) criteria for axial spondyloarthritis (SpA)

In patients with back pain ≥3 months and age at onset <45 years AS is the diagnosis when either of these is present

Sacroiliitis on imaging plus ≥ 1 SpA feature*	HLA B27 Plus ≥ 2 other SpA features*

**Spondyloarthropathy (SpA) features:* back pain, peripheral arthritis, uveitis, dactylitis, psoriasis, inflammatory bowel disease, good response to nonsteroidal anti-inflammatory drugs, family history of SpA, HLA B27, or elevated C-reactive protein.

Table 16.6: Comparison of ankylosing spondylitis and diffuse idiopathic skeletal hyperostosis

	Ankylosing spondylitis	*Diffuse idiopathic skeletal hyperostosis*
Sex/age	Common in males of 15–40 years of age	Common in males in 5th to 6th decade
Etiology	It is chronic progressive inflammatory seronegative spondyloarthropathy	It is a form of degenerative arthritis
Pathogenesis	The primary site of pathology in ankylosing spondylitis is the enthesis (site of attachment of tendons and ligaments to bone). Ossification also occurs in the ligaments that are ending up as enthesis, especially the ligaments of the spine that gradually get ossified, progressively leading to stiffness	Characterized by ossification at sites of tendon, ligaments and joint capsule insertion (enthesitis) anterior longitudinal ligament of the spine is most commonly involved
Distribution	SI joint, lumbar spine (eventually whole spine), the hip joint is commonly involved	Marked predilection to the axial skeleton; mainly involve thoracic spine
Course	All patients invariably present early with pain and stiffness of back	It is usually asymptomatic and discovered incidentally
SI joint	Bilateral, symmetrical involvement (sacroiliitis) In late cases, erosion may cause pseudo widening of the SI joints	Not involved
ESR	Elevated	Normal
HLA B27	Positive in 90% cases	Negative
Disability	Marked disability of the spine and hip joints in advanced cases	Usually no disability
X-ray features	Bamboo spine, squaring of vertebrae, syndesmophytes	Candle wax appearance due to calcification along the anterior and lateral portion of the vertebral bodies (separated from vertebral bodies)
Treatment	NSAIDs, TNF inhibitors	Usually not required

Abbreviations: SI, sacroiliac; ESR, erythrocyte sedimentation rate; HLA, human leukocyte antigen; NSAIDs, nonsteroidal anti-inflammatory drugs; TNF, tumor necrosis factor.

(Exemptia), etanercept, infliximab and golimumab. The response is generally attained by 6–12 weeks, but cost and long-term safety are limiting factors. It is crucial to go to a tubercular screening of the patient as these drugs may activate latent TB. SSZ, a DMARD used in RA, is effective in patients of AS with peripheral joint involvement. The evidence does not currently support the use of other DMARDs, corticosteroids or radiotherapy in AS.

Surgical Management

Surgery is tailored to correct the debilitating deformities that form part of the spectrum of this disease. Spinal osteotomies are done to correct deformities of spine (e.g. Smith-Peterson osteotomy—an extension osteotomy to correct kyphosis of spine, pedicle subtraction osteotomy). Ankylosed joints are salvaged by joint arthroplasty **(Figs 16.19A and B)**. There is increased risk of heterotopic ossification after joint arthroplasty in AS and radiotherapy has been proposed to have a prophylactic role in this situation.

REACTIVE ARTHRITIS (REITER SYNDROME)

Reactive arthritis is an inflammatory polyarthritis that occurs after infection (nonpurulent) elsewhere in the body away from the affected joints. Two forms are recognized: a dysenteric form and a sexually transmitted form. The former occurs with infection after the Shigella, *Salmonella* and *Campylobacter* species, while the latter is seen in cases of urogenital tract infections with *Chlamydia trachomatis*, *Mycoplasma genalium* or *Lymphogranuloma venereum*. Most common triggering organisms are *Chlamydia followed by Shigella*. Pathophysiology

involves initial immune system activation by the infecting organism triggering an autoimmune reaction that involves the joints, eye, skin and the urinary system. A strong association exists with HLA B27 with almost 25% patients testing positive with the genetic marker (as opposed to 1% of the general population who develop dysentery or urogenital infection).

Reiter syndrome is a clinical triad (described by Hans Reiter in 1916) of nonerosive reactive arthritis, urethritis and conjunctivitis occurring generally after 1–3 weeks of the gastrointestinal or genitourinary infection. The usual age of onset is 20–40 years with men being affected more commonly than women (10:1).

Clinical Features

Acute asymmetric oligoarthritis (knee, ankle, etc.) develops after 1–4 weeks after acquisition of gastrointestinal or urogenital infection. Although up to 25% patients do not have a history of any preceding infection. Low back pain is a common feature due to axial skeletal involvement. SI joint involvement is often unilateral (cf AS). Disease span is often interrupted by remissions after several weeks or months of symptoms while other times some patients may have chronic disease. Like other spondyloarthropathies patients with reactive arthritis also have features of enthesitis. Extraskeletal features include ocular involvement (i.e. conjunctivitis, iritis, scleritis, episcleritis and keratitis) and mucocutaneous lesions in the form of circinate balanitis (inflammatory lesion of the glans or shaft of the penis) and keratoderma blennorrhagicum (papular rash on the palm and soles).

Radiographic Findings

Proliferative changes along the shaft of bones present as fluffy periostitis. Radiographic changes of sacroiliitis are often unilateral. Bony erosions are often present at the site of enthesitis. Less often osteolytic destruction and bony ankylosis may be seen.

Treatment

Most patients can be managed with symptomatic treatment with NSAIDs. Intra-articular glucocorticoids may be considered for peripheral arthritis involving a few joints. Rarely antibiotics are required to treat infections. DMARDs (SSZ) may be considered in

---

Box 16.4: Activity advice to a patient of ankylosing spondylitis

1. Sleep on a firm bed and use a thin pillow to prevent neck flexion deformity
2. Erect posture should be encouraged while sitting or standing
3. Sleeping in prone position should be adopted to prevent spinal flexion deformity
4. Do not sleep on the side in a curled-up position
5. Active exercise program: Swimming, jogging, spinal and peripheral joint ROM, spinal extension exercises, etc.

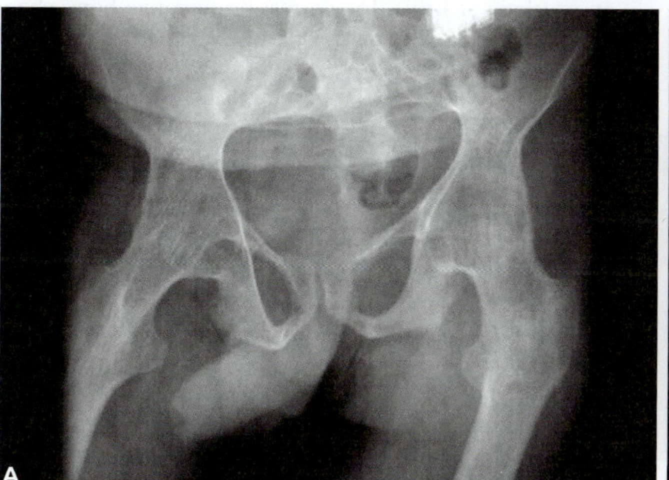
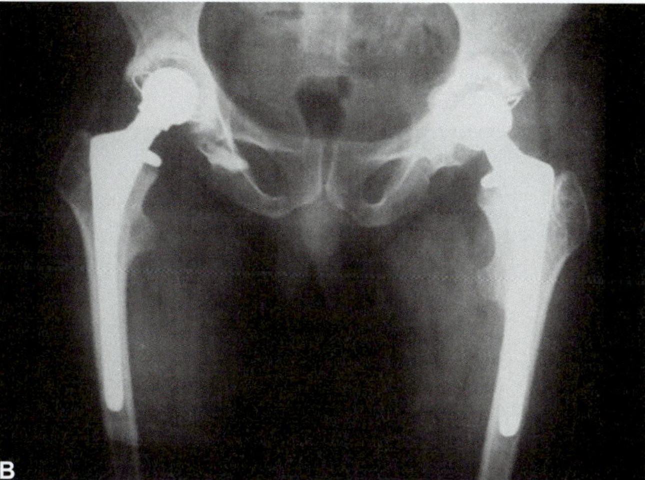

Figs 16.19A and B: Total hip replacement (THR) for bilateral ankylosed hip joints

chronic patients with reactive arthritis refractory to NSAIDs and glucocorticoids.

PSORIATIC ARTHRITIS

Psoriasis is an inflammatory skin disorder characterized by recurrent episodes of erythema and itching; thick, dry and silvery scales on the skin along with nail abnormalities. Joint symptoms are seen in approximately 20–30% of adults with psoriasis. Cases of psoriasis and characterized by a seronegative polysynovitis that follows into an erosive arthritis, sacroiliitis and spondylitis. The usual age of onset is 30–50 years with an equal male-to-female ratio.

Pathophysiology

Pathophysiology is much similar to RA with initial lesion being a chronic synovitis with cell infiltration that leads to an erosive destructive arthritis. Group A streptococcal infection has been implicated as an initial trigger in inciting an immune response in guttate psoriasis. Destruction may sometimes be unusually severe (hence k/a arthritis mutilans). There is a strong genetic predisposition; family history of psoriasis is often present and almost 60% patients who have a concomitant sacroiliitis or spondylitis lesion are positive for HLA B27. Other associated major histocompatibility alleles are HLA B7, HLA B13, HLA B17, HLA B57 and HLA Cw*0602.

Clinical Features

The skin lesions mostly precede arthritis, but about 20% patients may present with an initial arthritis in one of the five patterns as described by Wright and Moll (Wright and Moll classification):

1. *Symmetrical polyarthritis*: It is the most common form of psoriatic arthritis. Resembles RA, but is milder than RA.
2. *Asymmetrical oligoarthritis*: Less than five tender and swollen joints are involved. It involves small or medium-sized joints in an asymmetric distribution. It is second most common form after symmetrical polyarthritis.
3. *Distal arthritis*: Classic presentation involves DIP and the PIP joints. Erosion of the terminal tufts (acro-osteolysis) in association with nail changes. Dactylitis, or "sausage digit", is a characteristic feature of the spondyloarthropathies and it is seen in up to 50% patients with psoriatic arthritis. It refers to the complete swelling of a single finger or more commonly a toe.
4. *Arthritis mutilans*: In this rare subtype extreme destruction of the phalanges and MCP joints is seen, giving rise to shortened and subluxated digits that can be telescoped producing the "doigt en lorgnette" or opera glass deformity and classical "pencil in cup deformity" on X-rays **(Figs 16.20A and B)**.
5. *Spondyloarthropathy*: Almost in one-third of the cases, SI joint (usually unilateral) and spine involvement is seen. The predominance of cervical spine involvement over thoracolumbar spine distinguishes it from AS.

Almost any peripheral joint can be involved in psoriatic arthropathy. The disease has greater tendency to produce ankylosis of the small joints of hand and feet as compared to RA. Shortening of the digits producing telescoping due to underlying osteolysis is characteristic of the disease. Enthesitis (inflammation at the insertion of the tendons to bone) is a distinctive feature of all spondyloarthropathies and occurs in up to 40% of psoriatic arthritis patients. Enthesitis commonly involve tendon inserting on the foot (TA and plantar fascia) and pelvis leading to heel, foot and hip region pain.

Associated nail changes **(Fig. 16.20C)** that may be seen in 90% patients with psoriatic arthropathy include: pitting, horizontal ridging, yellowish discoloration of the margin, subungual hyperkeratosis and onycholysis (separation of the nail from the nail bed). Eye symptoms may be present in up to one-third cases and may include uveitis, blepharitis, blepharoconjunctivitis and dry eye (keratoconjunctivitis sicca).

Diagnosis

Wright and Moll provided the diagnostic criteria **(Box 16.5)** for psoriatic arthropathy. Some characteristic features of this erosive arthropathy that help to clinch the diagnosis in clinic include:

- Joint-space narrowing and erosions involving the distal and PIP joints
- Distal interphalangeal involvement with the classical "pencil in cup" deformity
- Small joint ankylosis
- Severe osteolysis of the phalanges and metacarpal bones (arthritis mutilans)
- Periostitis and proliferative new bone at sites of enthesis
- Periarticular osteopenia, which is seen in RA is usually absent in psoriatic arthritis. In contrast proliferative bony changes are seen along the shaft of the metacarpal and metatarsal

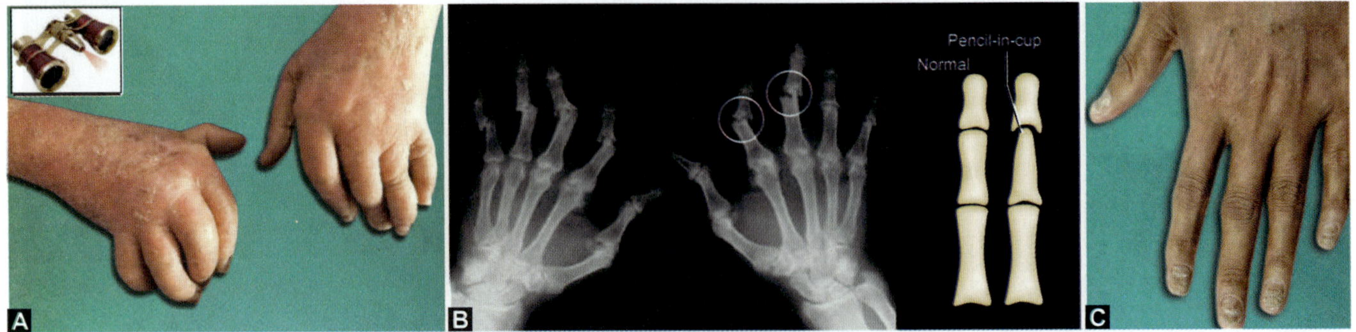

Figs 16.20A to C: (A) Opera glass deformity of hand (opera glasses are theater binoculars and hand deformity simulates as if a person is holding them); (B) Pencil in cup deformity (in circle); (C) Nail changes in psoriatic arthritis patient

bones adjacent to erosive changes leading to fluffy periostitis. This is also known as "whiskering".

Treatment

Antipsoriatic medicines form the mainstay of treatment. MTX is the drug of choice. Retinoids, psoralens and psoralens and ultraviolet A (PUVA) therapy all have a role in management. For orthopedic lesions, NSAIDs provide the pain relief. DMARDs (MTX, SSZ and LEF) are second line therapy after NSAIDs. Anti-TNF drugs are indicated for advanced arthritis with unstable or painful joints. TNF inhibitors that have been approved for psoriatic arthritis include adalimumab (Exemptia) etanercept, infliximab, golimumab and certolizumab pegol. Arthrodesis of DIP joint helps in relieving pain and improving function in terminal stages.

HIGH-YIELD POINT

- Arthritis mutilans is seen in Psoriatic arthritis, RA, JIA, diabetes, leprosy, neuropathic arthropathy and Reiter's syndrome.

ENTEROPATHIC ARTHRITIS

It occurs in association with both ulcerative colitis and Crohn's disease and presents either as peripheral arthritis or sacroiliitis and spondylitis. In about 15% patients with IBD, this peripheral arthritis is seen. The peripheral arthritis is often migratory and nonerosive. Extra-articular features like iritis, skin lesions such as erythema nodosum and pyoderma gangrenosum may be present. About 10% of patients with IBD present with sacroiliitis/spondylitis (AS-like symptoms). Often treatment of the underlying bowel disease leads to remission of the peripheral arthritis. DMARDs are useful in this condition, particularly SSZ because of its additional effect on IBD. NSAIDs should be avoided as they can exacerbate IBD. TNF inhibitors are useful in resistant cases. Differentiating features of spondyloarthropathies are given in **Table 16.7**.

CRYSTAL DEPOSITION ARTHROPATHIES

GOUT

It is a disorder of purine metabolism characterized by hyperuricemia (>6.8 mg/dL) that leads to deposition of monosodium urate crystals in joints and periarticular tissues and thereby precipitates recurrent attacks of acute synovitis and eventually leads to arthritis. The disorder is predominantly seen in middle-aged alcoholic men or at rare times in postmenopausal women.

The hyperuricemia in gout may be due to:

- *Underexcretion of uric acid (90%)*: Patients on drugs like thiazide diuretics, cyclosporine, salicylates, pyrazinamide, ethambutol; hypertensive or diabetic patients
- *Overproduction of uric acid (10%)*: Patients having a condition like lymphomas, leukemias, Paget's disease, hemolytic anemia, hypoxanthine-guanine phosphoribosyltransferase (HGPRT) deficiency (Lesch-Nyhan syndrome)
- *Both overproduction and underexcretion*: Alcohol abuse cases.

Factors predisposing to gout:

- Obese, alcoholic middle-aged (usually over 30 years) male patient
- Dietary excess of purine-rich foods: Meat, beans, peas, cauliflower, lentils, spinach, mushrooms, alcohol and fructose containing diet
- Trauma, post-surgery
- Chronic inflammatory diseases
- Hemolytic disorders, myeloproliferative disorders
- Long-term use of aspirin, diuretics.

Pathogenesis

Central to the pathogenesis of gout is the high blood urate levels that cause deposition of monosodium urate crystals (called as tophi) into the synovium of joints. When there are fluctuations in uric acid levels, the microtophi break apart and liberate the crystals into the synovial fluid. This incites a foreign body kind of reaction inviting the macrophages. The macrophages ingest the crystals and initiate an inflammatory synovitis that produces the acute exacerbation. Recurrent attacks lead eventually to the destruction of joint cartilage that culminates in chronic tophaceous gouty arthropathy.

Table 16.7: Differentiating features of various seronegative spondyloarthropathies

Spondyloarthropathy	AS	Psoriatic arthritis	Enteropathic arthritis	Reactive arthritis
Male-to-female ratio	More common in men	1:1	1:1	More common in men
Arthritis	Oligo, mono	Oligo, poly	Oligo, mono	Oligo, mono
Joint involvement	Hip, shoulder, knee	DIP, PIP and knee	Knee, ankle	Knee, ankle
SI joint involvement	Bilateral	Unilateral	Bilateral	Unilateral
Dactylitis	Uncommon	Common	Uncommon	Common
Cutaneous changes	None	Nail pitting Onycholysis Rashes	Erythema nodosum, Pyoderma gangrenosum	Circinate balanitis, Keratoderma blennorrhagica

Abbreviations: AS, ankylosing spondylitis; DIP, distal interphalangeal; PIP, proximal interphalangeal; SI, sacroiliac.

Although hyperuricemia is a sine qua non for the development of gout, all patients with the disease may not have raised uric acid levels. Hyperuricemia is present even in 5% of the normal population, but they do not ever develop gout. What has been seen the gouty attacks seem more to be associated with fluctuations in the uric acid levels (either increase or more often decrease) rather than on absolute levels. So, it is quite possible that the measured levels of uric acid at the time of the attack may well be within normal limits. Nevertheless, the occurrence of gout is directly related to the magnitude and duration of hyperuricemia. The higher the serum urate levels, the more likely an individual is to develop gout. And moreover, measuring uric acid levels is a good way to monitor the effect of treatment therapy.

Clinical Presentation

The disease course is characterized by recurrent acute attacks that end up into the stage of chronic gouty arthropathy. On an average, it takes about a decade between initial acute attack and the development of chronic arthropathy.

Acute gout: It is characterized by sudden onset, severe joint pain with red, hot, swollen, shiny overlying skin that mimics septic arthritis. Pain increases to most intense level in 8–12 hours. The attack may be precipitated by local trauma, intermittent illness, unaccustomed exercise or alcoholic binge. The most common site of involvement (50% cases) is the MTP joint of the great toe (podagra; **Fig. 16.21**). Other joints like the ankle, small joints of the hand, knee and elbow may be involved.

Chronic gout: Recurrent acute attacks in due course lead to chronic gout. It is asymmetric and polyarticular. Joints become eroded, painful and eventually stiff and deformed. Uric acid crystals deposited in and around the joints (over synovium, articular cartilage, tendons, ligaments and bursae) to form clumps of chalky material called "tophi" **(Figs 16.22A to C)**. They vary in size from 1 mm to several centimeters in diameter and are commonly seen around the MTP joint of the big toe, Achilles tendon, olecranon bursae and pinnae of ears. Although muscles and skin are spared from the deposition, large tophi, can ulcerate through the skin and discharge the chalky material. Prolonged hyperuricemia by this time often leads to uric acid nephropathy secondary to formation of stones, due to precipitation of uric acid in urine.

Investigations

- *Serum uric acid*: It may or may not be raised. Nevertheless, it should be documented to monitor the treatment effect.
- Twenty-four-hour urinary uric acid excretion of greater than 800 mg/day indicates overproduction of uric acid. It is not required in all patients with gout, but is useful before starting uricosuric therapy, since this form of therapy is effective only in underexcreters.
- X-ray changes include:
    - Soft tissue swelling (may be the only sign during acute attack)
    - Periarticular deep erosions
    - Joint space narrowing
    - *G sign/Martel sign* **(Fig. 16.22B)**: Punched out lesion of bone with overhanging bony edges.
    - Conspicuous absence of osteoporosis.

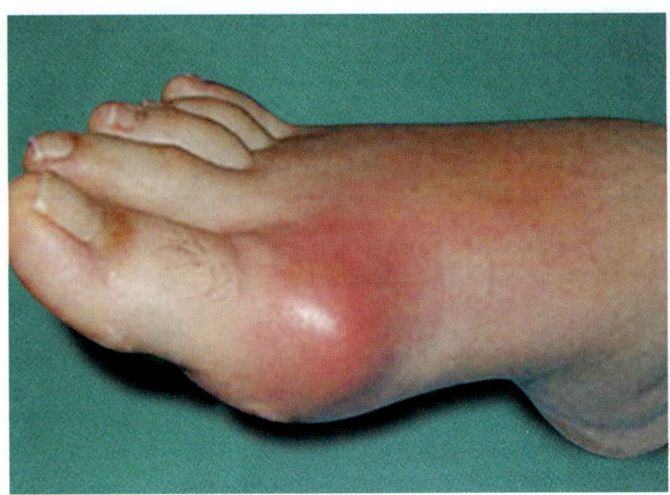

Fig. 16.21: Acute attack of gout at great toe (also called as podagra)

- Ultrasonography can also be used to make the diagnosis. It shows a superficial, hyperechoic band on the surface of the articular cartilage, known as "double contour sign". Joint aspiration and synovial fluid analysis **(Table 16.1)** is the gold standard to confirm the diagnosis by demonstrating characteristic strongly negative birefringent, needle-shaped urate crystals on polarizing microscopy.

The American College of Rheumatology criteria for the diagnosis of gout are given in **Box 16.6**.

Treatment

Asymptomatic hyperuricemia: No treatment is needed.

Acute attack: It is treated with rest to the joint, ice fomentation and NSAIDs (naproxen, indomethacin, etc. are very effective) for acute pain relief. NSAIDs should be started as early as possible after the attack to terminate it. After termination NSAIDs should be continued for next 2–3 days. The fastest acting drug to halt the acute attack is colchicine but nausea, vomiting, abdominal cramps and bloody diarrhea remain dose limiting side effects and hence it is not preferred now. Rather in such patients, corticosteroids (prednisone 20–40 mg/day tapered over 1–2 weeks) are preferred. Urate-lowering drugs are contraindicated in an acute attack of gout as sudden changes in uric acid levels in serum may itself precipitate gout.

Chronic gout (with or without renal complications): Any drug causing hyperuricemia should be withdrawn. General measures like reduction of weight, good hydration, avoiding alcohol and a low purine diet should be advocated. After the first attack, the likelihood of further attacks is reduced by prophylactic therapy, which include NSAIDs and a urate-lowering drug. The drug of choice is allopurinol or febuxostat—xanthine oxidase inhibitors. Allopurinol is started at 100 mg/day for a week and then the dose is gradually increased to 300–400 mg/day. Febuxostat is started at a dose of 40 mg/day. If serum uric acid levels are still elevated after 2 weeks, then the dose can be increased to 80 mg/day. A pegylated mammalian (porcine-like) recombinant uricase pegloticase is given to those patients who have severe gout with tophaceous deposits despite prophylactic therapy. Prophylactic therapy with urate-lowering drugs is continued

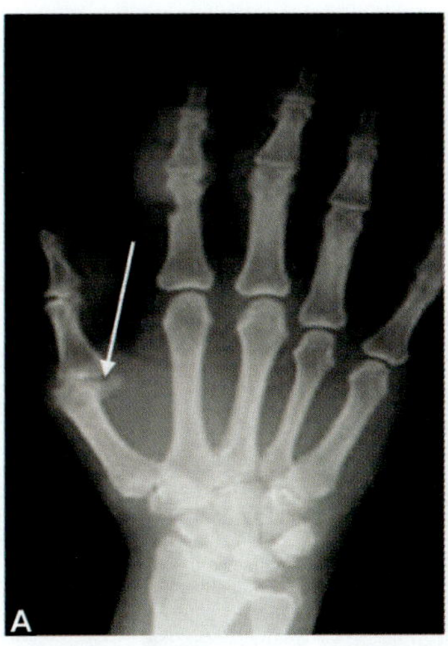
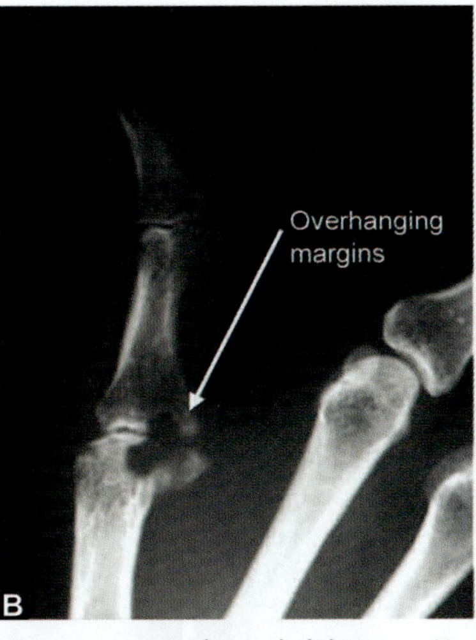

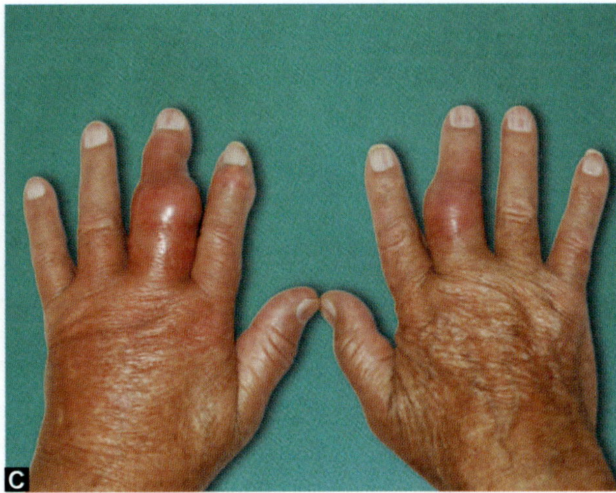

Figs 16.22A to C: (A) X-ray of hand showing gouty tophi (arrow); (B) X-ray of hand anteroposterior view showing Martel sign in gout; (C) Gouty tophi
Courtesy (Fig. 16.22C): Dr Charlie Goldberg, UCSD, California.

Box 16.6: The American College of Rheumatology criteria for the diagnosis of gout

- Presence of characteristic urate crystals in joint fluid, or
- Presence of urate crystals in a tophus, or
- The presence of any 6 or more of the following 12 clinical, laboratory and radiographic features:
    - Monoarticular arthritis, >1 attack of arthritis, joint redness, maximum redness developing within 1 day, painful and swollen first MTP joint, U/L involvement of first MTP joint, U/L involvement of tarsal joint, tophus, hyperuricemia, sterile joint fluid culture during acute episode, subcortical cyst without erosion on X-ray and symptomatic swelling within a joint on X-ray

Abbreviation: MTP, metatarsophalangeal.

---

indefinitely to prevent fluctuation in serum uric acid. Uricosuric drugs (probenecid, sulfinpyrazone, etc.) are effective only in underexcretors with good renal function. The target should be to keep the serum urate level at 6.0 mg/dL or less. Surgical treatment (curettage) may be needed for ulcerating tophi not responding to conservative treatment.

HIGH-YIELD POINTS

- Renal manifestations are seen in 10–25% of gout patients at some time of their life.
- Although the incidence of nephrolithiasis correlates with serum uric acid levels, the level of uric acid in urine is a stronger predictor.
- Even though the majority of calculi in gout is predominantly composed of uric acid, even calcium-containing stones are more common in gout patients than in the general population.

CALCIUM PYROPHOSPHATE DIHYDRATE ARTHROPATHY

This disorder is characterized by deposition of calcium pyrophosphate crystals in the articular tissue. Pyrophosphate that shows elevated intra-articular concentrations is most likely generated by abnormal cartilage, which combines with calcium

ions in the matrix and leads to crystal nucleation on collagen fibers.

Aging is the most common risk factor for calcium pyrophosphate dihydrate (CPPD) deposition disease and its spectrum includes three overlapping conditions:

1. *Chondrocalcinosis*: It is the asymptomatic appearance of calcific material in articular cartilage, intervertebral disks and knee menisci. The condition is generally seen in elderly people and is mostly incidental finding on X-rays. A number of disorders are there where chondrocalcinosis is an associated finding: hemochromatosis, hyperparathyroidism, hypothyroidism, hypophosphatasia, hypomagnesemia, hepatolenticular degeneration (Wilson's disease) and alkaptonuria (ochronosis).

2. *Pseudogout*: This is acute synovitis due to CPPD crystals, typically affecting middle-aged women. Larger joints like knee (most common site), wrist, shoulder, ankle and elbow are commonly involved. The involved joint is tense and tender and the diagnosis is often confused with acute gout. Confirmation comes with the demonstration of positively birefringent, rhomboid-shaped crystals in the synovial fluid on joint aspiration.

3. *Chronic pyrophosphate arthropathy*: Usually, a patient is an elderly female, presenting with chronic arthritis of joints like hip, knee, ankle, shoulders, elbows and wrist. It resembles OA, but the X-ray features are distinctive.

Blood Investigations

Evaluation of serum calcium, urate, phosphorous, alkaline phosphatase, magnesium, iron/transferrin, thyroid-stimulating hormone (TSH) and parathormone (PTH) levels is done to know the etiology.

Radiological Features

The characteristic X-ray feature is chondrocalcinosis—calcification of articular cartilage in joints, the menisci in the knee, pubic symphysis, intervertebral disks **(Figs 16.23A and B)** and at times tendons and bursae around joints.

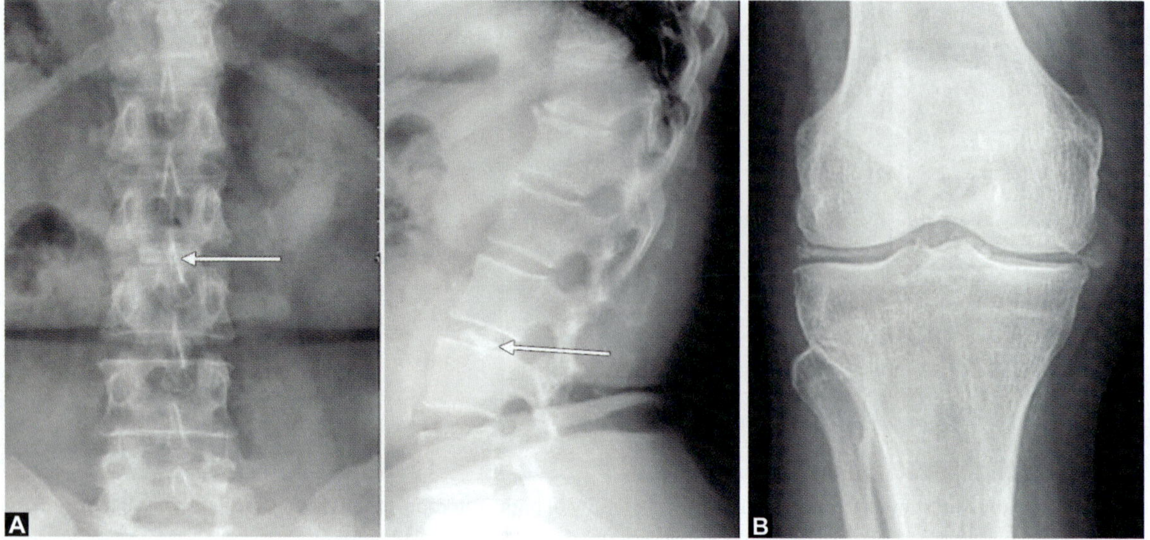

Figs 16.23A and B: (A) Intervertebral disk calcification (arrow); (B) Meniscal calcification in chondrocalcinosis of the knee

Courtesy (Fig. 16.23B): Radiopedia.org.

In chronic stages, degenerative changes (joint space narrowing, subchondral sclerosis, osteophytes, etc.) are seen, but notably involving the unusual site like the patellofemoral compartment of the knee, talonavicular joint. In advanced stages, marked joint destruction with the loose body formation may be seen.

Treatment

Rest to the joint, ice fomentation in acute attacks, aspiration in cases of tense joint swelling, NSAIDs/coxibs for pain relief, oral/intra-articular steroids are the treatment modalities used.

Surgical treatment (arthrodesis/arthroplasty) may be needed for advanced arthritis.

CALCIUM OXALATE DEPOSITION ARTHROPATHY

It is a rare crystal deposition disorder seen mainly in patients either with a metabolic enzyme defect (primary hyperoxaluria) causing increased oxalate production or with end-stage renal failure leading to decreased oxalate excretion. Other rare causes include short bowel syndrome, thiamine or pyridoxine deficiency, diet rich in spinach and ascorbic acid, etc. Patients present with monoarthritis or oligoarthritis affecting mainly joints of hand and feet. Other features include miliary skin calcium oxalate deposits, synovial calcification and vascular calcifications of hand and foot vessels. Diagnosis can be confirmed by identifying the crystals of oxalate (bipyramidal, positively birefringent) in synovial fluid. Rest to the joint and NSAIDs are the mainstay of treatment.

TUMORAL CALCINOSIS

It is a familial condition of dysfunction of phosphate metabolism (not a tumor) that results in periarticular extra-capsular soft tissue deposition of inorganic calcium phosphate. Commonly seen in young black males, it commonly affects the shoulders, hips and elbows **(Fig. 16.24)** and rarely even knees. On knee X-rays, one finds ossification around the knee, but not in joint menisci. The condition is frequently seen in patients undergoing renal dialysis.

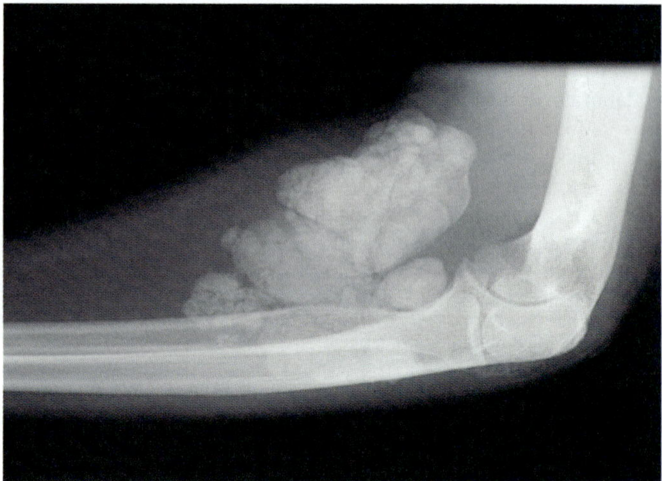

Fig. 16.24: X-ray showing extra-capsular calcification around elbow in a case of tumoral calcinosis

Courtesy: Learningradiology.com.

The depositions are clinically painless, but result in swelling around joints. These masses have a tendency to enlarge and may even ulcerate through the overlying skin and extrude. Treatment involves normalizing the serum phosphate levels.

HIGH-YIELD POINTS

- The most reliable means of distinguishing inflammatory from noninflammatory arthritis is by analyzing the cell count of the synovial fluid.
- Pain and stiffness in inflammatory arthritis generally improve with activity while in degenerative arthritis it settles to rest.
- Commonly involved joints in different forms of arthritis are depicted in **Figure 16.25** and summarized in **Table 16.8** while differences between rheumatoid and seronegative spondyloarthropathies are given in **Table 16.9**.

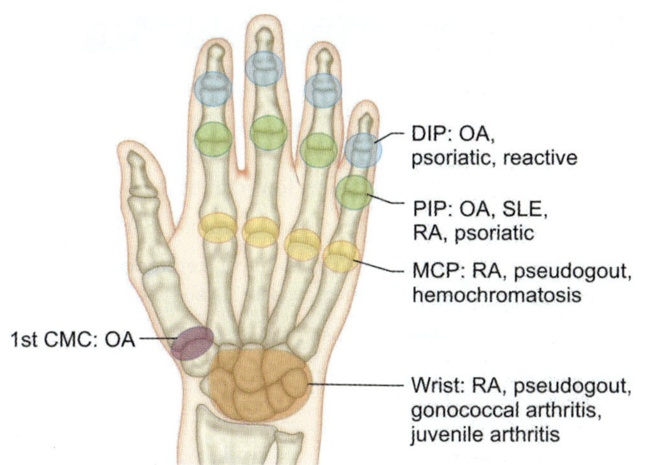

Fig. 16.25: Involvement of various joints in different arthritis types

Abbreviations: CMC, carpometacarpal; DIP, distal interphalangeal; OA, osteoarthritis; SLE, systemic lupus erythematosus; PIP, proximal interphalangeal; RA, rheumatoid arthritis; MCP, metacarpophalangeal.

Table 16.8: Different joints involved in various forms of arthritis

Disease	*Commonly affected joints*
Gout	MTP joint of great toe
Pseudogout	Knee
Rheumatoid arthritis	MCP, PIP, wrist Not involved: DIP
Osteoarthritis	Knee, hip, PIP, DIP, 1st CMC Not involved: MCP, wrist
Ankylosing spondylitis	Sacroiliac joints > lumbar spine
Hemophilic arthritis	Knee: most common
Septic arthritis	Knee: most common
Charcot arthropathy	Foot (mid tarsal joints): most common
Reactive arthritis	Knee
Psoriatic arthritis	DIP and PIP joints

Abbreviations: MTP, metatarsophalangeal; MCP, metacarpophalangeal; PIP, proximal interphalangeal; DIP, distal interphalangeal; CMC, carpometacarpal.

- Pseudo-AS and pseudorheumatoid arthritis are presentations of chondrocalcinosis that mimic the native disorders, respectively.

DEGENERATIVE ARTHRITIS

OSTEOARTHRITIS

Osteoarthritis is a chronic, age-related degenerative disorder of joints in which there is progressive softening and destruction of articular cartilage accompanied by new growth of bone at the joint margins (osteophytes), cyst formation in subchondral area, sclerosis in the subchondral bone, mild synovitis and capsular fibrosis. Although there are some signs of inflammation it is not primarily an inflammatory arthritis.

Etiopathogenesis

There is imbalance between normal cartilage repair mechanisms and its degradation which leads to net loss of cartilage. The cartilage loss is "asymmetric", greater where the stress on the joint is the greatest (e.g. in the knee, medial compartment being more commonly affected than the lateral compartment). Once the cartilage is lost, the denuded bone surfaces rub against each other, the process is called "eburnation". Subchondral cysts form in areas beneath the eburnated surfaces. The subchondral bone shows marked osteoblastic activity and manifests as subchondral sclerosis in the most stressed part of the joint.

Risk factors for OA: Advanced age, trauma to the joint (old malreduced intra-articular fracture), occupation (footballers are more prone to have OA knee, baseball pitchers are more prone for OA shoulder), obesity, smoking and a positive family history.

Joints commonly involved: Knee (most common), hip, DIP, PIP, first CMC, first MTP, facet joints of the cervical spine and lumbosacral spine.

Clinical Features

Patients usually present after middle age, the weight-bearing joints are commonly involved (knee > hip). Characteristically, symptoms of OA show a waxing and waning course. Pain is the usual presenting complaint. The pain is typically aggravated on exertion and relieved on taking rest unlike rheumatoid and other inflammatory arthritis. Possible causes of pain are synovial inflammation, muscle spasm, medullary hypertension and microfractures in the subchondral bone, stretching of periosteal nerve endings by osteophytes and distension of fibrosed capsule by joint effusion. Stiffness is also a common presenting complaint, which occurs with periods of inactivity.

On examination, crepitus may be felt around the involved joint. Deformities are seen in late stages due to capsular fibrosis or joint instability, e.g. genu varum in OA knees. Sometimes, the joints appear deformed/swollen because of excessive osteophyte formation around joint margins, e.g. Bouchard's nodes (PIP joint) and Heberden's nodes (DIP joint) **(Fig. 16.26A)**. Irregular joint space narrowing and marginal osteophytes of IP joints resemble a flying seagull and is called as Seagull wing deformity **(Fig. 16.26B)**. Bony ankylosis is uncommon except in IP joints of fingers where it may be the end result.

Investigations

X-ray of the knee joint orthogonal views (AP and lateral) are sufficient to make the diagnosis. Hallmark radiological features **(Fig. 16.27)** are:
- Decreased joint space (asymmetric, medial > lateral)
- Subchondral sclerosis
- Subchondral cysts
- Marginal osteophytes
- Loose bodies
- *In late stages*: Deformities of the joint and joint subluxations.

ESR, CRP and serum uric acid are usually normal. Elevated homocysteine levels have recently been documented and may have a role in pathogenesis.

Treatment

Principles of management are to provide pain relief, to maintain joint mobility and muscle strength and to protect joints from eccentric loads (unloading joint) by modification of lifestyle and advising specific precautions. Treatment is best guided by grading the disease **(Box 16.7)**.

Table 16.9: Differences between rheumatoid arthritis (RA) and seronegative spondyloarthropathies (SSA)

Features	RA	SSA
No. of joints involved	Polyarthritis	Oligoarthritis
Enthesitis	No	Yes
Limbs	Both upper and lower limbs	Predominantly lower limbs
Spine	Cervical spine	Lumbar spine and sacroiliac (SI) joints
Lesions in skin and mucus membrane	Palmar erythema, subcutaneous nodules	Oral ulcer, genital ulcer, keratoderma blennorrhagica, psoriasis
Lung lesions	Interstitial lung disease, pleural effusion, nodules	Apical fibrosis
Eye lesions	Scleritis, episcleritis, scleromalacia performance	Conjunctivitis, uveitis
Rheumatoid factor	Positive	Negative

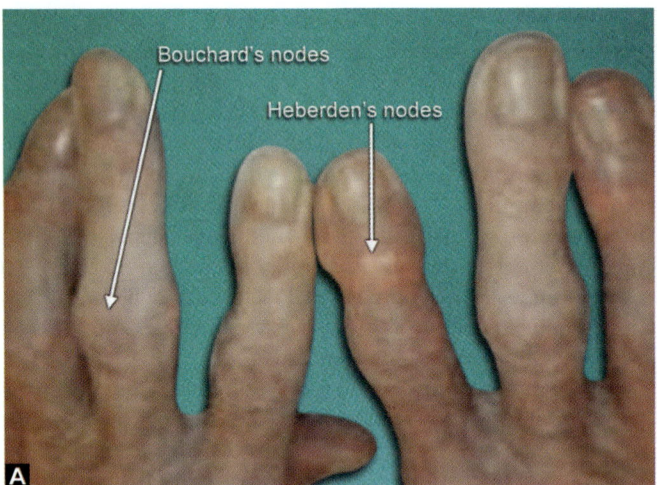

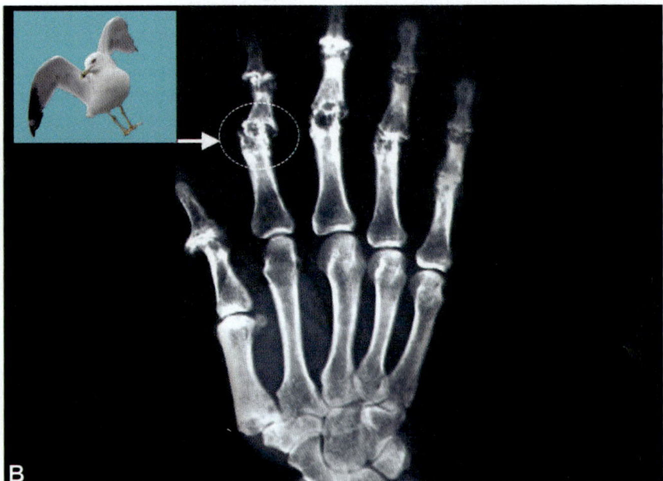

Figs 16.26A and B: (A) Clinical picture showing Bouchard's and Herbenden's nodes; (B) X-ray hand of a patient with osteoarthritis changes showing Seagull wing deformity
Courtesy: Radiologykey.com.

Early Stages of Osteoarthritis

Treatment is primarily conservative for the early grades of OA (stage 1) and includes lifestyle modifications and pharmacotherapy.

Lifestyle modifications: These include avoiding climbing stairs, sitting cross-legged and squatting to off load the joint from excessive forces. Weight reduction and use of braces (e.g. knee caps) and walking aids also assist in the process. Quadriceps strengthening and aerobic exercises are advised to improve muscle strength around the joints. Hot fomentation and transcutaneous electrical nerve stimulation (TENS) may provide pain relief.

Pharmacotherapy: Role of pain killers, steroids and chondroprotective agents has been a subject of much debate.

- *Nonsteroidal anti-inflammatory drugs*: Advised for pain relief on a short-term basis. Acetaminophen is recommended by most guidelines as the first-line therapy, although NSAIDs (diclofenac) have been shown to provide better improvement in pain and function. Selective Cox-2 inhibitors (etoricoxib) are generally preferred by clinicians because of their better side effect profile and almost a matchable efficacy. Opioids (tramadol) can be given where NSAIDs are not suitable.

- *Chondroprotective agents*: Diacerein, chondroitin sulfate, glucosamine, all are controversial drugs used for OA knee. Many trials have failed to show their efficacy in OA knee. Currently they are not recommended by American Academy of Orthopaedic Surgeons (AAOS) as per their latest guidelines for OA knee treatment. Intra-articular hyaluronic acid (a component of articular cartilage, *see* **Fig. 16.2A**), although is widely used in the early grades of OA; AAOS recently downgraded the recommendations on hyaluronic acid in the 2013 edition of its guidelines. Intra-articular injections of platelet-rich plasma (PRP), which contains many growth factors have rather emerged as a promising potential treatment. PRP stimulates proliferation and synthesis of collagen (*see* Page 474 for details).

- *Selective serotonin reuptake inhibitors (SSRIs)*: Duloxetine (SSRI) has been approved by Food and Drug Administration (FDA) for management of chronic musculoskeletal pain including OA. It has proven its efficacy in OA pain in patients who have failed or have intolerance to other commonly used drugs.

- *Intra-articular steroids*: OARSI (Osteoarthritis Research Society International) and American College of Rheumatology recommend use of intra-articular steroids in moderate-to-severe OA knee and OA hip patients who do not respond to oral analgesics.

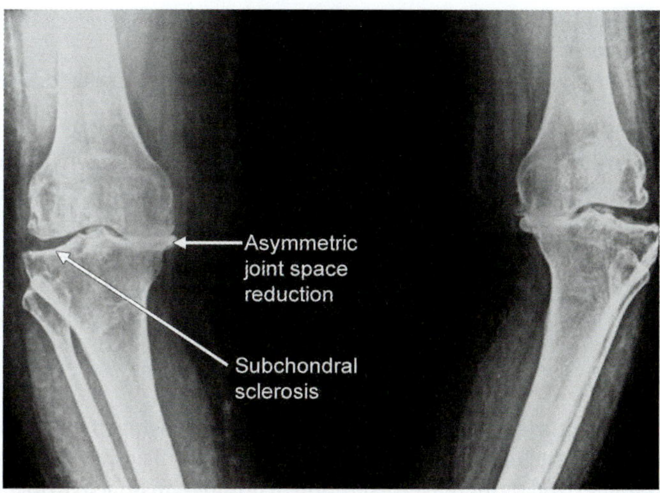

Fig. 16.27: X-ray knee showing signs of osteoarthritis

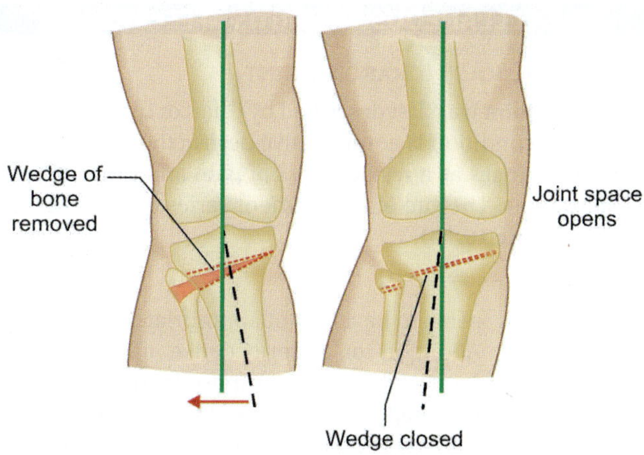

Fig. 16.28: Lateral closing wedge high tibial osteotomy for varus deformity of osteoarthritis knee

> **Box 16.7:** Ahlback grading for osteoarthritis knee
>
> I.   Joint space narrowing
> II. Joint space absent
> III. Bone attrition or loss

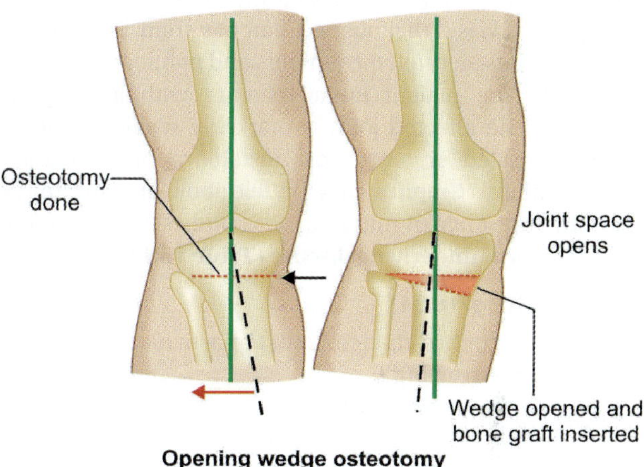

Fig. 16.29: Medial opening wedge high tibial osteotomy for varus deformity of osteoarthritis knee

Advanced Stages of Osteoarthritis

At advanced stage correction is mostly amenable to surgery. High tibial osteotomy (read below) is an excellent option in cases where only medial joint space is lost and lateral and patellofemoral compartments are preserved. Total knee replacement (Chapter 19) is generally the best option for advanced arthritis when the cartilage loss is complete. Arthroscopic debridement and balancing of a meniscal tear can provide temporary relief in OA knee where symptoms can be localized to a degenerative meniscus (e.g. locking, medial joint line tenderness, etc.). Arthrodesis can be opted in small joints of hand and feet.

High tibial osteotomy: High tibial osteotomy (HTO) is commonly done for medial OA with varus knee deformity (less commonly done for valgus deformity). The aim of HTO is to unload the involved joint compartment by correcting the mechanical axis of the lower limb. The osteotomy changes the bony alignment and redistributes weight from the medial to the lateral compartment in degenerative OA of knee which mostly affects medial compartment.

To correct the malalignment, a laterally based wedge of bone can be removed from the proximal tibia and distal tibia shifted laterally to close this wedge, when the technique would be called a lateral closing wedge osteotomy **(Fig. 16.28)**. Else an osteotomy can be made in proximal tibia, distal bone shifted laterally to open a wedge-shaped gap medially, that can be filled with bone graft, when the technique would be called medial opening wedge osteotomy **(Fig. 16.29)**. While the open wedge technique avoids a need for concurrent fibula to be cut, requirement of a bone graft and higher chances of non-union are demerits. On the contrary, close wedge technique needs fibula to be cut for allowing the shift of axis and may shorten the limb. The choice is hence largely surgeon-dependent although most surgeons prefer the opening wedge technique.

The ideal candidate for HTO is one who is young (<60 years), active, with isolated involvement of medial compartment with a varus deformity, good range of motion and without ligamentous instability. It is relatively contraindicated in patients with inflammatory arthritis (RA) that generally involves both compartments, body mass index (BMI) more than 35, flexion contracture more than 15°, knee flexion less than 90° and varus deformity more than 20°.

The indications for HTO also overlap to a great extent with unicondylar knee replacement (*see* Page 479). Authors prefer to go with HTO when the alignment on a scanogram is varus while they prefer to opt for unicondylar knee replacement when alignment is near to normal.

HIGH-YIELD POINTS

- The most common bone involved in OA knee is the patella
- The most common muscle weakness seen in OA knee is of the quadriceps
- The first diagnostic sign of OA on X-ray is reduction of joint space.

MISCELLANEOUS ARTHRITIS AFFECTIONS

NEUROPATHIC JOINT (CHARCOT JOINT)

Neuropathic joint was first described by Charcot in tabes dorsalis in 1868. The condition is a progressive destructive (but painless) arthritis that arises as a result of loss of pain and proprioceptive joint sensations. The site of involvement varies depending upon the cause **(Table 16.10)**.

Pathogenesis

The basic factor seems to be a lack of appropriate sensory input from the joint. Abolition of proprioceptive and/or sensory impulses from the joint leads to it being exposed to unusual trauma for a prolonged time. Repetitive trauma leads to fragmentation and destruction of the joint cartilage, loose body formation and pronounced bone destruction along with attempted evidence of new bone formation (osteophytosis) in abnormal sites.

Clinical Presentation

Although a number of popular terms are in use in context of this condition, the classic diagnostic Charcot's triad includes gross joint swelling, exaggerated movements and painless presentation **(Fig. 16.30)**. The patient initially comes with a single joint involvement. The affected joint is markedly swollen, deformed, may be subluxated or have gross instability, but is classically minimally painful. Crepitus may be felt about moving the joint owing to the presence of multiple loose bodies. The patient may exhibit features of underlying disease **(Table 16.11)**.

X-ray Features (Fig. 16.31)

- Marked destructive changes with periarticular erosions
- Joint space narrowing
- Osteophyte formation
- Subchondral sclerosis
- Loose bodies.

The changes simulate OA, but the absence of pain is diagnostic.

Management

The principle in the management of neuropathic joint consists of minimizing the trauma to which the unstable and insensitive joint is exposed, by efficient bracing, weight-relieving calipers or leather corset. Large effusions may be aspirated and in troublesome cases, joint debridement (arthrocentesis) and arthrodesis may be necessary, although the results are often disappointing. Joint arthroplasty is relatively contraindicated in Charcot's disease.

ALKAPTONURIC ARTHRITIS (OCHRONOSIS)

Alkaptonuria (AKU) is an inherited disorder of tyrosine metabolism occurring due to deficiency of enzyme homogentisic acid oxidase characterized by increased excretion of homogentisic acid in urine (urine turns black on standing, due to oxidation of homogentisic acid) and deposition of homogentisic pigment in the soft tissues (ochronosis).

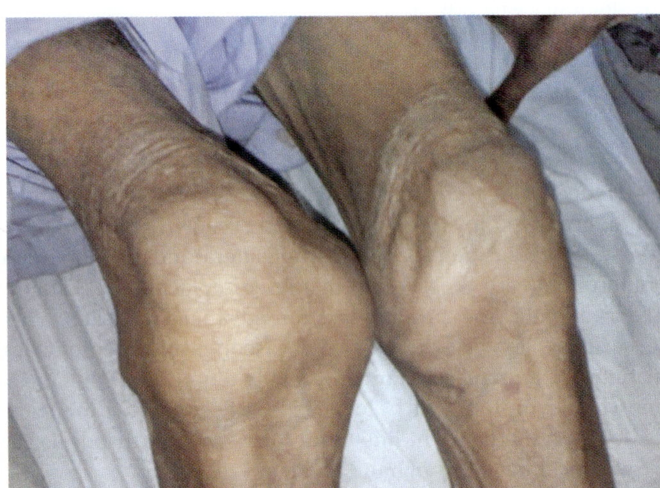

Fig. 16.30: Clinical photograph of patient with Charcot joints (knee). Note marked joint swelling in right knee

Table 16.10: Neuropathic joints—site predilection varies with the disease

Causative disorder*	Joints involved
Diabetes (most common cause)	Tarsus and tarsometatarsal (most common) Metatarsophalangeal Ankle joint > knee and spine
Tabes dorsalis (2nd most common cause)	Knee (most common) Hip Ankle Lumbar spine
Leprosy	Interphalangeal (hand) Metatarsophalangeal (feet) Lower limbs
Syringomyelia	Shoulder (most common) Elbow Wrist Cervical spine
Myelomeningocele	Ankle Intertarsal joint

Miscellaneous causes: Amyloidosis, multiple sclerosis, peripheral nerve disorders, intra-articular steroid injections in weight-bearing joints and Charcot Marie tooth disease.

Table 16.11: Some terms in relation to neuropathic joint disease

Term	Definition
Bag of bones	Clinical term to describe the palpable signs of an advanced neuropathic joint
Charcot's Joints	Physical appearance of a neuropathic joint of any cause owing to disorganization, debris and distension
Clutton's joints	Physical appearance of bilateral nonpainful swelling, usually in the knees owing to congenital syphilis
Licked candy stick	Generalized pencil-like tapering of a long bone towards a joint owing to atrophic resorption
Tumbling building block spine	Multisegmental subluxated vertebral bodies simulating falling building blocks
Jigsaw vertebra	Fragmented appearance of a vertebral body owing to multiple fractures

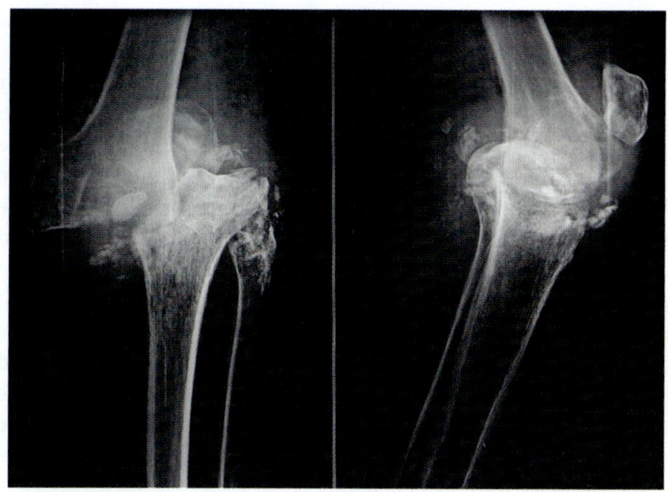

Fig. 16.31: Knee X-ray showing marked destructive changes in Charcot's disease of knee

Orthopedic Manifestations

Joint symptoms occur, usually after the age of 40 years. The pigment deposits (**Figs 16.32A and B**) in articular cartilage, synovium, menisci and intervertebral disks cause periarticular, meniscal and intervertebral disk calcifications. Spine and shoulder joints are common sites of affection. Symptoms simulate OA.

Management

Arthropathy is treated on a symptomatic basis. Later stages may need joint replacement. Vitamin C supplementation may have a role in the treatment. Nitisinone is a newer disease modifying drug for AKU. It inhibits 4-hydroxy-phenyl-pyruvate-dioxygenase and could prevent or slow the progression of disease in AKU.

HEMOPHILIC ARTHRITIS

Hemophilia is an X-linked recessive disorder that manifests generally in males (females are carriers) and is characterized by the deficiency of clotting factors VIII (hemophilia A, 80% cases) and IX (hemophilia B, Christmas factor). The deficiency results in spontaneous hemorrhages into the joints that initiate a chronic synovitis that eventually culminates in progressive destructive arthritis.

Orthopedic Manifestations

Patients with plasma clotting factor levels more than 40% tend to lead a normal life while those with levels less than 5% have prolonged bleeding after an injury or surgery. Those with severe hemophilia (level <1%) form the main clinical spectrum as they are the ones who are prone to spontaneous joint and muscle hemorrhages. Problems discussed below may be encountered in these patients.

Intramuscular Bleeding

Although bleeding into muscles is relatively less common than joint bleeding, it can lead to muscle necrosis, fibrosis and development of contractures. In the lower limb, most common site is quadriceps followed by triceps surae while in the upper limb, bleeding generally occurs into the deltoid. In abdomen hemorrhages into iliopsoas may occur mimicking appendicitis while retroperitoneal hemorrhages may simulate renal colic.

Intra-articular Bleeding (Hemarthrosis)

These are the more common manifestations that bring these patients to the doctor. Weight-bearing joints are commonly involved. In decreasing frequency the joints involved are the knee, ankle, elbow, shoulder and hip joints. Involved joints are intensely swollen and warm and may simulate an infective etiology. Recurrent hemorrhage precipitates the hyperplasia and fibrosis of synovium causing chronic synovitis. The articular cartilage is damaged by pannus formation and by the action of proteolytic enzymes.

Hemophilic Pseudotumors

Uncontrolled bleeding in a confined place of musculoskeletal system produces cystic swellings which can cause pressure changes of surrounding structures. Pseudotumor can develop within the muscle fascia without producing bony changes or may cause cortical thinning, but more commonly they are caused by subperiosteal hemorrhages. Thigh is the most common site of pseudotumor formation followed by abdomen and pelvis. The quadriceps is the most common muscle to develop pseudotumor.

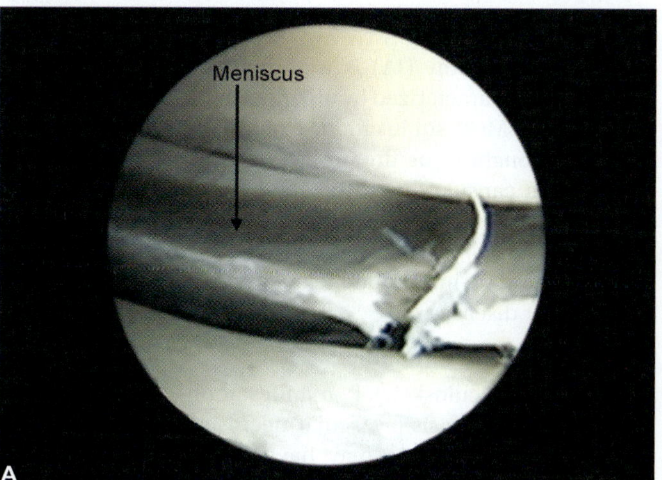

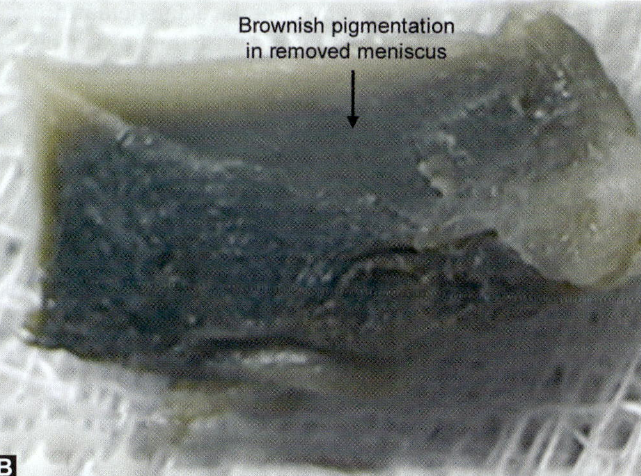

Figs 16.32A and B: (A) Degenerative meniscal tear due to ochronotic arthritis (arthroscopic view); (B) Black pigment deposition in removed meniscus

Courtesy: Dr JVS Vidyasagar, Global Hospital, Hyderabad.

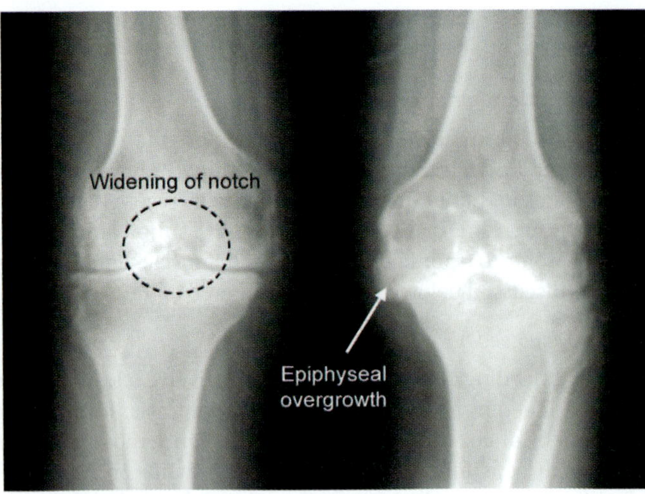

Fig. 16.33: Anteroposterior X-ray view of both knees showing signs of hemophilic arthropathy

Nerve Palsies

Hematomas may cause compression neuropathies (generally transient). Femoral nerve followed by median nerve is the most common nerve involved. Not uncommon is bleeding into the peripheral nerve sheath that causes peripheral neuropathy.

X-ray Features (Fig. 16.33)

X-ray features are diagnostic and include:

- Soft tissue swelling
- Juxta-articular erosions (no sclerosis) and subchondral cysts
- Narrowing of the joint space
- Epiphyseal overgrowth
- Widening of the intercondylar notch and squaring of the patella in knee
- Enlargement of the proximal radius.

Management

Medical management of hemophilia aims at factor VIII or IX replacement. Factor level should be raised to 30–40% of normal to control intramuscular and soft tissue bleeding. NSAIDs should be used cautiously in these patients. Pseudotumor should not be aspirated or biopsied. Management of the acute hemarthrosis involves factor replacement primarily and RICE therapy (involves the rest of the limb, ice fomentation, compression by applying a crepe bandage and elevation of the affected part to reduce swelling). Aspiration is performed only in severe distension; it is usually avoided. Traction is effective in relieving muscle spasm and maintaining range of motion. The joint is temporarily immobilized in the correct position and active ROM is encouraged. For disabling hemophilic arthropathy synovectomy, arthrodesis or arthroplasty may be required. During surgery factor level should be maintained at 100% of normal value. Synovectomy may be arthroscopic, open or by radiation. Yttrium is most commonly used for radiosynovectomy (radiation synoviorthesis).

SOME OTHER IMPORTANT ARTHRITIC AFFECTIONS

Post-chikungunya Rheumatic Disorder

Chikungunya (CHIK) (*ref.* stooped posture patient adopts due to severe polyarthritis) is a rapidly spreading viral illness caused by CHIK virus, a single stranded ribonucleic acid (RNA) virus of the genus Alphaviridae. Outbreaks have been particularly common in tropical Africa and Indian ocean islands.

The infection is transmitted to humans by mosquito vector Aedes (*Aedes aegypti* and *A. albopictus*). After an incubation period of 2–4 days, the infection manifests in two successive phases. An initial presentation is with high grade fever, pruritic skin rash (50% cases), gastrointestinal symptoms and severe symmetrical polyarthritis involving small joints of hands and wrists and ankles. The subsequent phase is unique with a spectrum of rheumatic and musculoskeletal manifestations that may last up to an year (up to 8 years have been reported). These include persistence of polyarthralgia and morning stiffness and development of plantar fasciitis, tunnel syndromes, multiple tendinitis and tenosynovitis. Lesions of psoriatic arthritis may be exacerbated while 5% of the patients eventually go on to fulfill the ACR criteria for diagnosis of RA.

Diagnosis of the condition is primarily by blood investigations. Leukocyte count may be reduced and there may be mild thrombocytopenia. Elevated ESR or CRP levels are not frequently seen. The primary diagnostic tool in initial phase is IgM-anti CHIK virus antibody test (enzyme-linked immunosorbent assay, ELISA). RT-PCR is more specific during initial viremic phase (1 week). Detection later in the course (>2 weeks) involves identification of IgG antibodies that may persist up to years. X-rays initially may be non-specific but articular erosions on MRI have been reported by few studies in persistent arthritis stage.

Treatment is largely symptomatic and involves use of NSAIDs in acute stage. Persistent arthralgias are difficult to handle and in absence of specific evidence-based guidelines, NSAIDs remain the first-line choice. Steroids may be tried but rebound symptoms after therapy stops have been a concern. Role of DMARDs is also unclear. Hydroxychloroquine has no effect but MTX may be beneficial in chronic stage and especially in patients who develop RA.

Parvovirus Arthropathy

Human parvovirus arthropathy in young adults is characterized by transient sudden onset of polyarthropathy involving multiple small joints but absence of rashes. In few patients it can also lead to chronic arthritis. Symptomatic management mostly suffices.

Jaccoud Arthropathy

Jaccoud arthropathy (JA) is a chronic, deforming non-erosive arthropathy characterized by ulnar deviation of the second to fifth fingers with MCP subluxation. Exact pathogenesis is not clear, but it is thought to be due to ligamentous laxity or contracture of the joint capsule due to repeated episodes of inflammation. It is commonly associated with rheumatic fever, SLE, psoriatic arthritis, AS, Sjögren's syndrome, mixed connective tissue disease, human immunodeficiency virus (HIV) infection and many other diseases.

HIV-associated Arthropathy

Although musculoskeletal manifestations in HIV infection include osteonecrosis [avascular necrosis (AVN)], vasculitis and myositis; HIV infection may have articular manifestations in 40–50% cases but most of the times they skip being diagnosed. Articular syndromes that have been described in association with the infection include HIV-associated arthropathy, seronegative spondyloarthropathies (reactive arthritis, psoriatic arthritis, undifferentiated spondyloarthropathy, etc.), rheumatoid arthritis and painful articular syndrome.

The HIV-associated arthropathy may appear at any stage of the disease and may have a varied pattern of involvement. Among various patterns of joint involvement in HIV arthropathy, asymmetric oligoarthritis is most common form. It most commonly involves knee and ankle joints. Symmetrical non-erosive polyarthritis mimicking RA is next common pattern. It causes same hand and foot deformities as in RA. Mostly HIV-associated arthropathy is non-erosive and short-lived but many patients develop chronic erosive arthritis. X-ray features may include joint space narrowing, periarticular osteopenia and erosion. RA factor, HLA B27 and ANA are usually negative.

Painful articular syndrome is characterized by a self-limited disorder of bone and joint pain lasting for less than 24 hours in patients with HIV infections. Pain of severe intensity occurs in asymmetric pattern and knees, shoulders and elbows are most commonly involved joints.

Systemic Lupus Erythematosus-associated Arthritis

Joint involvement is one of the early features and arthritis and arthralgias are noted in up to 95% of SLE patients. Like RA, a symmetrical polyarthritis is most common pattern of joint involvement and small joints of hands, wrist and knee joint are frequently involved. However, in contrast to rheumatoid arthritis, SLE arthritis or arthralgia is migratory and non-erosive. SLE produces similar deformities of hand as in RA but these are believed to be due to ligaments laxity and muscle contracture and not due to articular destruction.

Kashin-Beck Disease

Kashin-Beck disease (KBD) is a chronic, degenerative disease of joints and muscle causing skeletal deformities and short stature. It is endemic in North-central China, North Korea, Tibet and South Eastern Siberia. Exact etiology is not known but many factors have been postulated to be contributory to the disease including selenium deficiency, mycotoxin contamination of grains and water pollution with organic material. Mostly it affects children and adolescents. It is characterized by symmetrical epiphyseal destruction leading to dwarfism and metaphyseal enlargement. Patients present with multiple joint pain and swelling, decreased range of motion of joints, morning stiffness, shortened fingers, decreased muscle strength, general fatigue and growth retardation. Ankle, knee, wrist and elbow joints are commonly affected. There is no cure for the disease and treatment is mostly palliative.

Mseleni Joint Disease

Mseleni joint disease (MJD) is a type of crippling chondrodysplasia endemic in the Mseleni population in northern Kwazulu Natal, South Africa. It symmetrically involves multiple joints leading to pain, stiffness and decreased range of motion. Hip joints are most noticeably involved and hip dysplasia and protrusion acetabuli are two distinct features of hip involvement by Mseleni disease.

CHONDROMALACIA PATELLAE

The term chondromalacia coined by Alleman basically refers to "softening of cartilage". Chondromalacia patellae is an idiopathic disorder affecting mostly young females. It is characterized by degeneration of the articular cartilage on the back of the patella producing patellofemoral pain. The disease results due to decrease in sulfated mucopolysaccharides (ground substance) in deep layers of patellar articular cartilage (as opposed to OA where the superficial layers of cartilage are affected). Central ridge area at the back of the patella is the classically involved area. Although the exact etiology is unknown, the most important predisposing factor seems to be malalignment of the extensor apparatus (patella alta, etc.). Overuse and trauma may have a role.

Diagnosis: These patients classically present with anterior knee pain. The pain occurs on squatting, climbing stairs and after getting up from periods of prolonged sitting (theater/movie sign). X-rays initially are normal, although a skyline view (**Figs 5.76A and B**, *see* Page 147) is more informative. MRI may be normal in early stages (as softening is not visible) but findings become evident in moderate-to-severe cartilage loss. Arthroscopic examination is considered the gold standard for establishing the diagnosis but one should be careful to palpate the lesion as initial stages involve softening of deeper layers of cartilage that is not visible to naked eye.

Management: Treatment is largely conservative as the lesions seldom progress to frank OA. Patients are advised vastus medialis obliquus and quadriceps strengthening exercises to strengthen the knee muscles. In cases where cartilage loss is severe, arthroscopic debridement or cartilage transplant surgeries may be required.

OSTEOCHONDROSIS

INTRODUCTION

Osteochondrosis (synonym osteochondritis) includes a group of disorders which involve degeneration or necrosis of the osteochondral (bone-cartilage) part of a joint, i.e. the articular cartilage and it's underlying subchondral bone. Since mostly involved are young people, they are disorders of growing epiphysis and hence also called as epiphysitis.

As per the probable etiology, the lesion in different locations is named differently:

- *Crushing type*
  - *Freiberg's disease*: Metatarsal heads **(Fig. 16.34A)**
  - *Kohler's disease*: Navicula **(Fig. 16.34B)**
  - *Kienbock's disease*: Lunate
  - *Panner's disease*: Capitulum
  - *Scheuermann's disease*: Ring epiphysis of vertebrae (see Chapter 7)
  - *Calve's disease*: Central bony nucleus of vertebrae
  - *Thiemann's disease*: Phalangeal epiphysis
- *Traction/pulling type*
  - *Tibial tuberosity*: Osgood-Schlatter's disease **(Fig. 16.35)**
  - *Calcaneal epiphysis*: Sever's disease
  - *Patellar ligament (at its lower pole patellar attachment)*: Johansson-Larson syndrome
  - *Base of fifth metatarsal*: Iselin's disease
  - *Medial epicondyle of humerus*: Adam's disease
- *Splitting type*
  - Osteochondritis dissecans (see below).

OSGOOD SCHLATTER'S DISEASE

It is a traction apophysitis of the proximal tibial apophysis. It is a common cause of knee pain in growing children and commonly

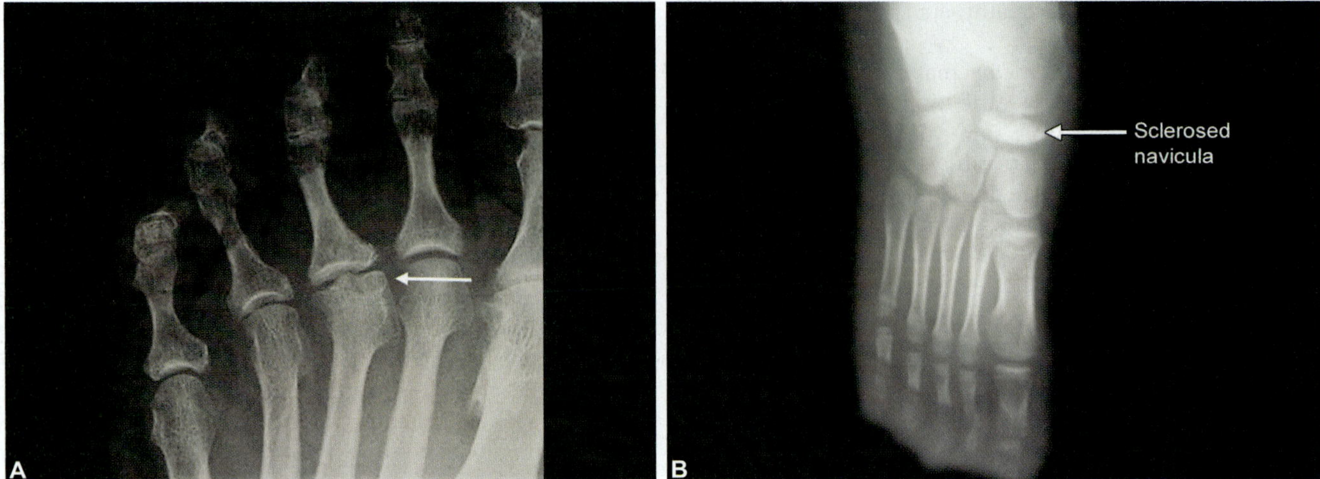

Figs 16.34A and B: (A) X-ray of foot showing Freiberg disease; (B) X-ray of foot showing sclerosed navicula in a patient with Kohler's disease

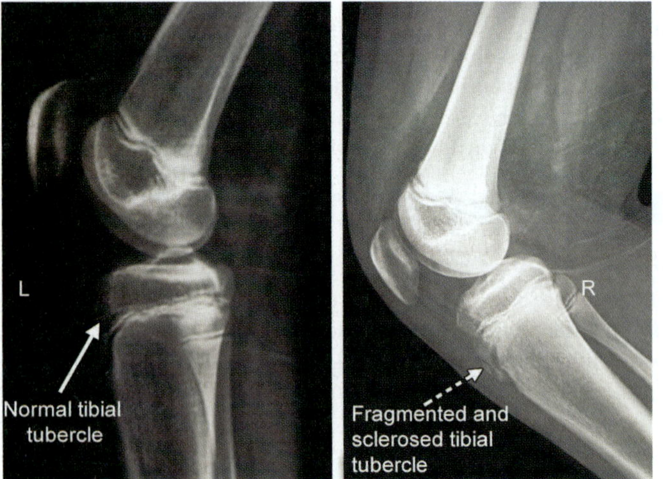

Fig. 16.35: Lateral X-rays of knee joint showing comparison of a normal tibial tubercle (arrow) with a fragmented and sclerosed tubercle (dotted arrow) in Osgood-Schlatter syndrome

affects boys between 12 years and 15 years of age. Exact etiology is not known, but repeated forceful contractions of the quadriceps may cause small avulsion fractures of the secondary ossification center of the tibial tuberosity. It is particularly common in adolescents playing sports like football, basketball, jumpers, runners, gymnastics, etc. which involve repeated forceful knee extension. Approximately 30% cases are bilateral. Patients present with complaints of anterior knee pain and tenderness can be elicited at the tibial tuberosity. X-ray **(Fig. 16.36A)** may show enlarged, fragmented or sclerosed tibial tubercle or calcification at the insertion of the patellar tendon.

Treatment: It is a self-limiting disease and mostly pain subsides with bony fusion of the tibial tubercle. Management requires limitation of the pain provoking activity, quadriceps stretching and strengthening exercises and analgesics.

KIENBOCK'S DISEASE

It is osteochondritis of lunate that occurs possibly due to a chronic stress injury. Approximately 70% of these patients have a negative ulnar variance (ulna ending far short of radius) that tends to stretch the ulnolunate ligament causing a chronic stress injury to lunate **(Fig. 16.37)** that eventually starts degenerating, collapsing and fragments, the condition, culminating in secondary OA of the wrist.

Affected patients are in the age group 15–40 years, mostly being manual laborers who present with pain usually in the dominant wrist. On examination, one may find tenderness over lunate. X-rays are done that initially may be normal, but later on show increased density of the lunate **(Fig. 16.36A)** followed by evident collapse and fragmentation. MRI **(Fig. 16.36B)** provides the earliest diagnosis and is the investigation of choice.

Management in early stages (before the collapse) involves radial shortening/ulnar lengthening procedures to correct ulnar variance along with a vascularized pronator quadratus-based muscle pedicle graft to increase vascularity. In advanced stages with collapse, arthrodesis of the wrist is performed.

OSTEOCHONDRITIS DISSECANS

This is a special type of osteochondritis in which an osteochondral fragment separates from the rest of the bone and forms a loose body in the joint. Knee (lateral surface of medial femoral condyle) is the most common site affected, but a few other areas can also be involved like talus (anteromedial corner), femoral head (superomedial part), elbow (capitellum) and first metatarsal head.

The disease is two times more common in males and occurs generally during adolescence (10–20 years). Approximately 30% cases are bilateral. Patients generally tend to come with a vague aching discomfort in the knee present for months. When these patients are made to sit on a couch with legs hanging, there is pain on internal rotation of the leg, which disappears as the leg is externally rotated (Wilson's test).

X-rays classically reveal a loose body or may show a loosely attached osteochondral fragment **(Fig. 16.38)** in the joint that clinches the diagnosis. An intercondylar or tunnel view is more informative. Bone scan can provide early diagnosis, but MRI is the investigation of choice, provides earliest diagnosis and also aids in management.

Management depends upon the size of the defect created by separation of the fragment. In smaller lesion, multiple drilling of

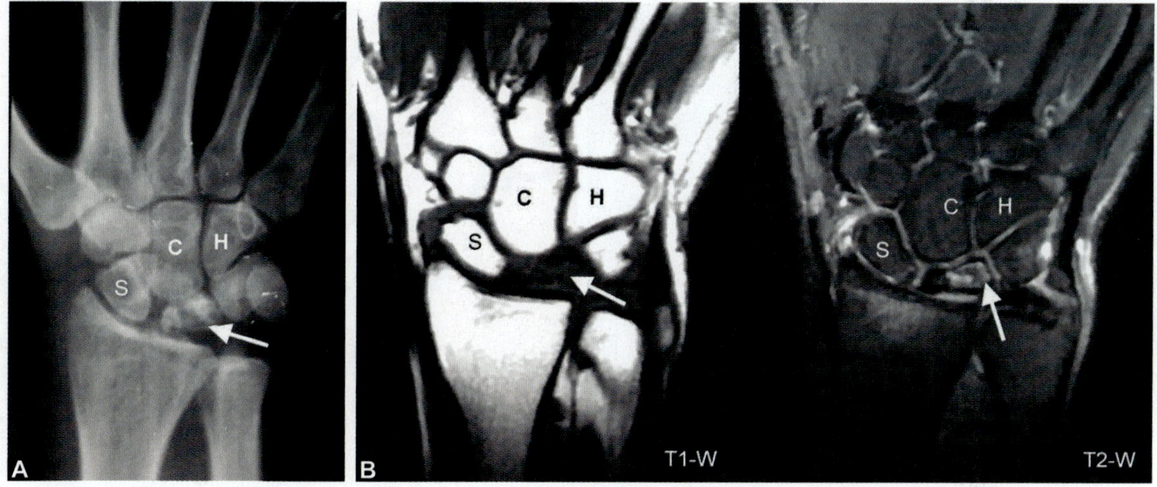

Figs 16.36A and B: Kienbock's disease. (A) X-ray of hand AP view showing increased sclerosis and cystic changes in lunate; (B) MRI (T1 and T2-W) images showing degeneration of lunate

Abbreviations: S, scaphoid; C, capitate; H, hamate.

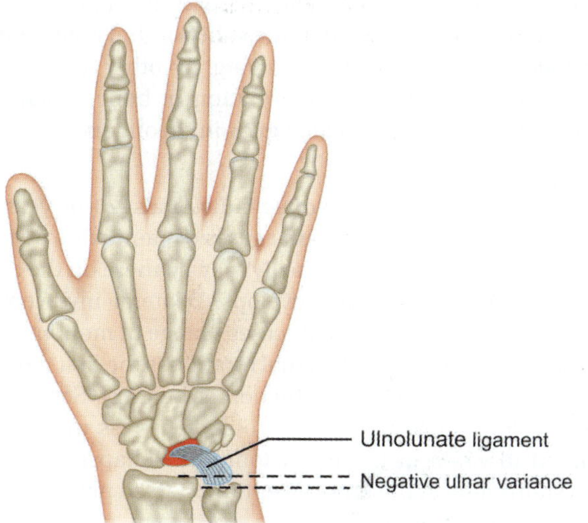

Fig. 16.37: Negative ulnar variance in pathogenesis of Kienbock's disease

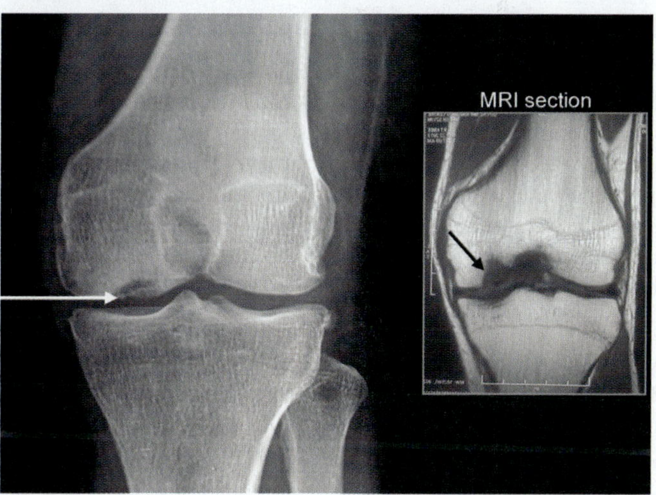

Fig. 16.38: X-ray of knee joint anteroposterior view showing osteochondral fragment loosely attached to the medial femoral condyle (white arrow). Magnetic resonance imaging (coronal section of the knee joint) further confirms the diagnosis (black arrow)

the crater is performed. Drilling leads to fresh pool of bleeding from marrow and the inflow of growth factors that cause the lesion to heal. In larger defects, a mosaicplasty or osteochondral autologous transplantation surgery is performed wherein an osteochondral graft is harvested from non-weight-bearing area of the knee and is transplanted into the crater (**Fig. 6.55**, *see* Page 194).

SYNOVIAL CHONDROMATOSIS

In this condition, there occurs cartilaginous metaplasia in the synovium of the joint, leading to formation of multiple (may be even more than 50) loose bodies **(Figs 16.39A and B)**. Knee followed by hip is the most common site of affection and this disease is the most common cause of multiple loose bodies in the knee. The term "Snow storm appearance" is used to describe the appearance of this condition on arthroscopic evaluation of the knee. Symptomatic cases may need removal of loose bodies and synovectomy.

HIGH-YIELD POINTS

- *Finsterer's sign*: Diagnostic for Kienbock's disease. The patient is asked to make a fist. There is tenderness at the base of the third metacarpal on tapping and its normal prominence is absent in patients with the disease.
- Negative ulnar variance is associated with Kienbock's disease, whereas positive ulnar variance is associated with ulnar impaction syndrome and injury to TFCC (triangular fibrocartilage complex).
- The most common cause of loose bodies in the knee joint is OA of knee. However, the most common cause of loose body in knee joint in young patient is osteochondritis dissecans of knee. And the most common cause of multiple loose bodies in the knee joint is synovial chondromatosis.

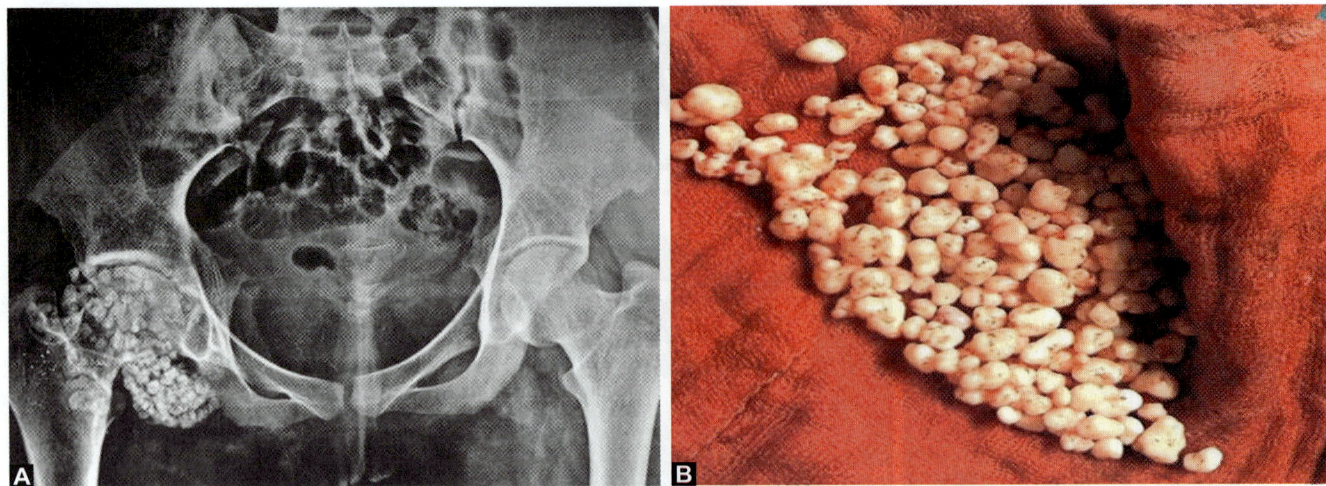

Figs 16.39A and B: (A) Synovial chondromatosis of the hip joint; (B) Multiple loose bodies after removal
Courtesy: Dr Umesh Meena (SMS Medical College, Jaipur)

AVASCULAR NECROSIS OF HEAD OF FEMUR (CHANDLER'S DISEASE)

The femoral head is prone to AVN that might occur after a dislocation or after a fracture of neck of femur, due to its precarious blood supply, as already discussed in Chapter 5. However, apart from traumatic causes, a number of cases present with spontaneous osteonecrosis (AVN) of the femoral head without any antecedent traumatic event or fracture and without any evident infection or sepsis. The femoral head is the most common site for this atraumatic AVN, a condition called as Chandler's disease.

ETIOLOGY

Although a number of factors have been implicated as shown in **Box 16.8**, the most common cause remains idiopathic. Steroids and alcohol intake are next most common causes for AVN.

PATHOPHYSIOLOGY

The factors mentioned above either lead to intravascular thrombosis of sinusoidal vessels or produce an extravascular marrow swelling (like steroids, alcohol that increase fat content), that eventually causes ischemia. The subarticular areas lie at the most distant part of the bone's vascular territory and are largely enclosed by cartilage, restricting their access to local blood supply.

Box 16.8: Causes of avascular necrosis (AVN) femoral head

- Idiopathic (most common cause)
- *Coagulation disorders:* Familial thrombophilias, hypolipoproteinemia, thrombocytopenic purpura, nephrotic syndrome
- *Thrombosis:* Hemoglobinopathies (Sickle cell disease), storage disorders (Gaucher's disease), pancreatitis, pregnancy, polycythemia, anticancer drugs, postrenal transplant
- *Embolic occlusion of vessels:* Caisson's disease
- *Vasculitis:* Irradiation, SLE (antiphospholipid antibodies)
- *Miscellaneous:* High-dose steroid therapy, i.e. more than 2 g of prednisone or its equivalent for 2–3 months (occlusion of vessels by fat emboli and increased marrow pressure due to fat accumulation), alcohol intake, HIV, etc.

Abbreviations: SLE, systemic lupus erythematosus; HIV, human immuno-deficiency virus.

Thereby even on minimal insult, the subchondral trabeculae get affected (generally anterolateral part of superior weight-bearing zone of femoral head in the subchondral region involves first), followed by changes occurring in other compromised areas eventually leading to deformation of bone, collapse and fragmentation which if untreated ends in secondary OA.

CLINICAL PRESENTATION

Mostly, the disease is seen in young individuals (20–40 years age), and it is one of the most common causes of painful hip in a young adult. Pain in the groin area initially may be there on the activity, but later on even rest pain develops. Bilateral involvement is common and seen in about 75% cases. Range of motion also gets affected during the course. Internal rotation is the first movement to be restricted followed by abduction. When the "Sectoral sign" is positive, the range of internal rotation is less in hip flexion compared to when in hip extension. The collapse of the head causes shortening of the limb. Over time, a fixed pelvic deformity may eventually develop.

INVESTIGATIONS

X-ray is usually the first investigation ordered that may be normal in the initial stages. As disease progresses, one may find patchy areas of increased density or sclerosis in the superolateral part of the femoral head (as decalcification does not occur in avascular bone that appears white). As the disease progresses irregularity of the head, fragmentation and collapse may be noted **(Fig. 16.40)**. In the end stages, the joint space is lost and the hip ends up in secondary OA.

Bone scan can provide an early diagnosis. In the early phase there is decreased uptake of radiotracer, producing a "cold area" on the scan. Once the reparative process begins, there is increased uptake of the radio tracer in the area surrounding the cold spot, creating the classical "Donut sign" **(Fig. 16.41)**. The earliest diagnosis is provided by MRI which is also the investigation of choice. MRI signs of AVN are serpiginous areas of low signal intensity around an avascular area on T1 image and double line sign made up of two concentric high and low signal intensity areas on T2 images **(Fig. 16.42A)**. In the initial stages, there may be edema in the marrow but as the disease progresses, subchondral fracture lines (crescent sign, **Fig. 16.42B**) and

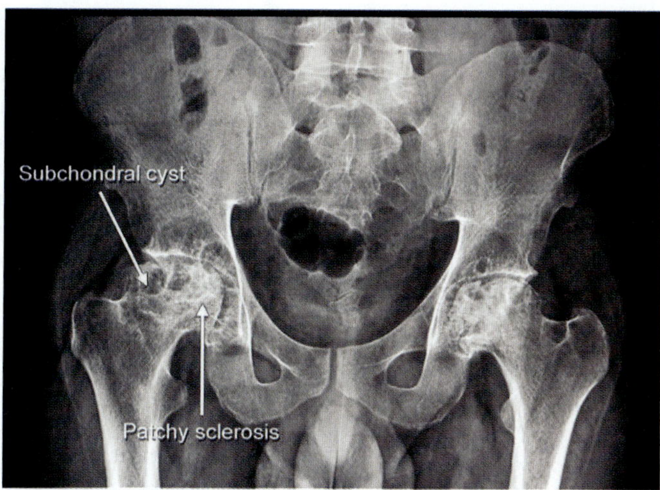

Fig. 16.40: X-ray pelvis anteroposterior view showing fragmentation and collapsing of head of both femurs due to avascular necrosis

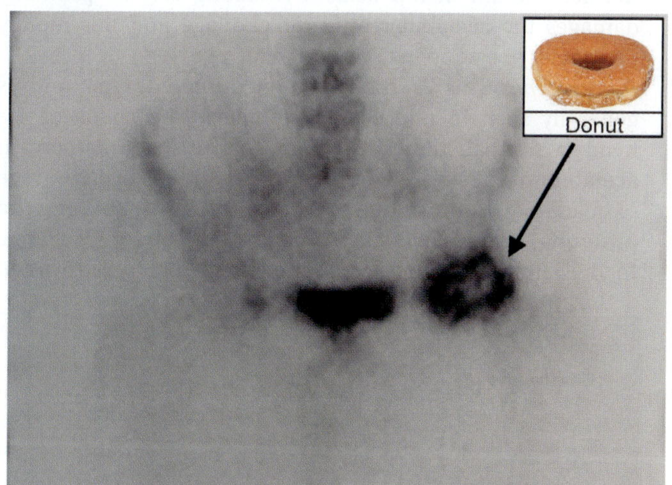

Fig. 16.41: Donut sign visible in bone scan in left femur in a patient with avascular necrosis (AVN) of left femoral head

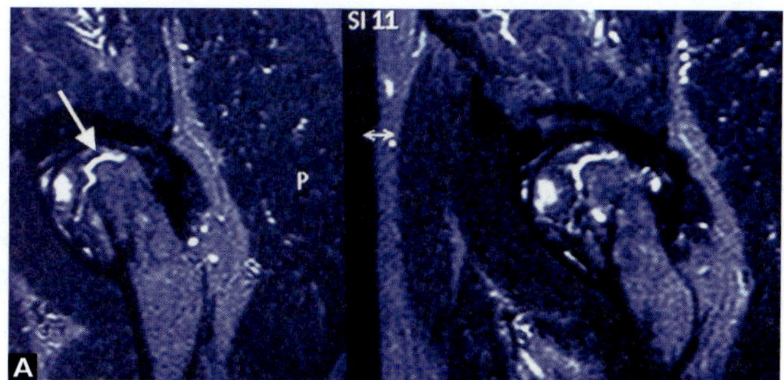

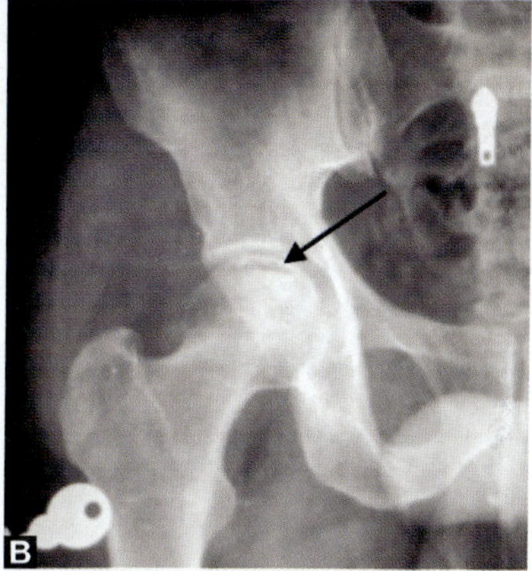

Figs 16.42A and B: (A) Double line sign (arrow) of avascular necrosis femoral head on magnetic resonance imaging; (B) Crescent sign. Note the subchondral lucency (arrow)

Table 16.12: Staging of osteonecrosis by modified Ficat-Arlet staging system

Stage	Radiograph findings
0	None (bone scan may show decreased uptake)
1	Normal (bone scans show cold spot)
2A	Diffuse or localized osteoporosis, cyst or sclerosis
2B	Crescent sign (subchondral collapse with maintained sphericity, Fig. 16.42B), flattening
3	Loss of sphericity
4	Joint space narrowing, arthritic changes

eventually fragmentation and collapse may be noted. Another investigation tailored to cause may be needed.

STAGING

Many systems are currently in use to grade the severity of the disease, modified Ficat-Arlet is most commonly used classification for grading of AVN of the femoral head. It is based on the radiograph findings (**Table 16.12**) of the osteonecrosis.

DIFFERENTIAL DIAGNOSIS

The disease has to be differentiated from all possible causes of chronic arthritis of hip like TB, primary and secondary OA.

MANAGEMENT

Management is dictated by the presence of the collapse of the bone.

In the precollapse stage, the preferred treatment is a surgery called core decompression (**Fig. 16.43**). The sclerotic focus is reamed to decompress the marrow and relieve pressure in an attempt to improve vascularity and a fibular bone graft is inserted into the reamed area.

If the collapse has started, but is an only patchy area, then one can go for a vascularized fibular or muscle pedicle grafting or a realigning osteotomy (abduction/adduction hip osteotomy or Sugioka's transtrochanteric rotational osteotomy) to make the affected area become non-weight-bearing. In case there is advanced collapse or superimposed arthritic changes, then replacement arthroplasty remains the preferred choice.

HIGH-YIELD POINTS

- *Transient osteoporosis in pregnancy*: Transient osteoporosis of pregnancy is a rare condition of unknown etiology that affects otherwise healthy pregnancy in the third trimester. The patient presents with sudden onset of pain with mild restriction of hip range of motion. Radiological investigations show bone marrow edema and transient osteoporosis of the hip. Radiological findings and symptoms usually resolve within weeks of labor.

- *Ahlback's disease*: It is spontaneous AVN of the femoral condyles (knee) in an adult.
- Avascular necrosis changes classically start in the sub-chondral area of the femoral head.
- In HIV patients incidence of AVN of the femoral head is higher than the general population. Anti-retroviral therapy (mainly protease inhibitors), steroid intake, IV drug abuse, alcohol intake, smoking and hyperlipidemia all have been implicated in causation of AVN of femoral head in HIV patients.

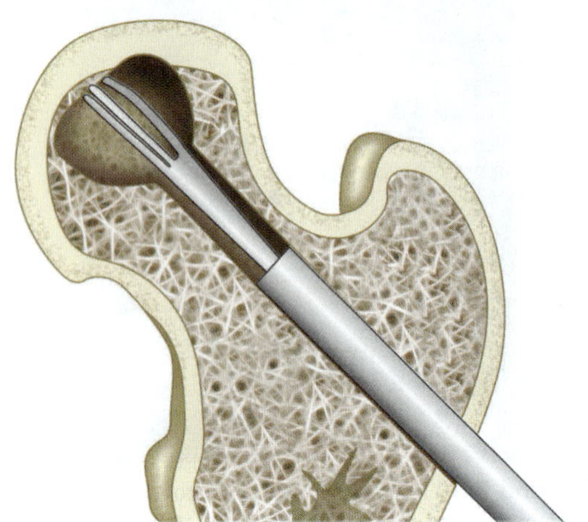

Fig. 16.43: Schematic representation of core decompression for non-traumatic avascular necrosis of femoral head

Femoroacetabular impingement (FAI) or hip impingement syndrome refers to a condition where there are morphological abnormalities in femoral head or neck region or surrounding acetabulum causing an abnormal contact between the two, thereby resulting in pain and limited range of motion at the hip. Considerable interest has recently aroused in this topic owing to the condition being recognized as an important modifiable precursor of OA of the hip in young and middle-aged adults.

TYPES

Femoroacetabular impingement can be of following types **(Fig. 16.44)**:

i. *Cam type*: This is the more common type (than Pincer) seen commonly in young males. The problem here is abnormal aspherical head shape with a bony prominence usually present anterosuperiorly at the head neck junction (giving pistol grip appearance on X-ray, **Fig. 16.44**) that impinges against the acetabulum in hip flexion. Resulting contact primarily damages the acetabular articular cartilage and this rapidly progresses to end up in OA of hip joint.

ii. *Pincer type*: This is the least encountered type and is generally seen in middle-aged females. The shape of the head is normal, rather, problems of version are there in acetabulum causing overcoverage of head. The overcoverage of head may be global due to a deep acetabular socket (coxa profunda) or overcoverage of head may involve a focal area. In the latter situation, acetabulum is generally retroverted

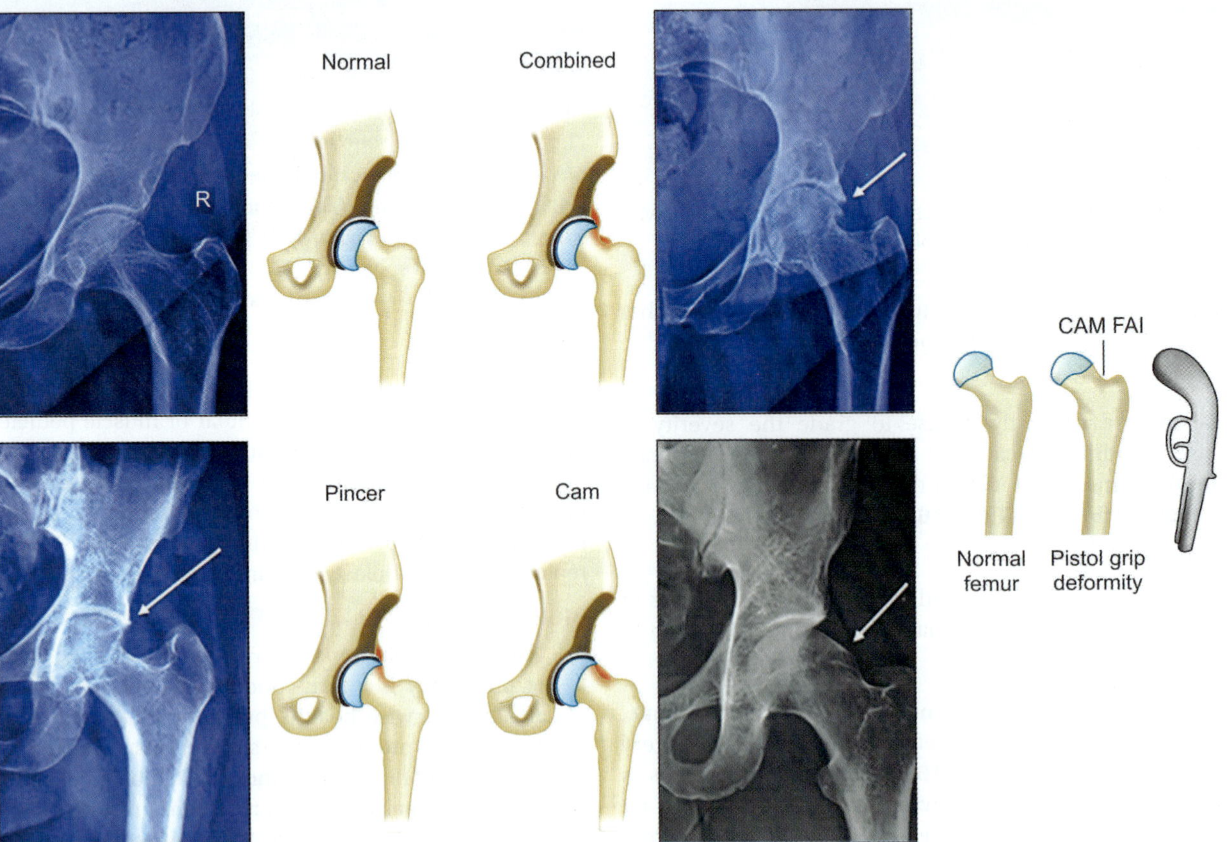

Fig. 16.44: Types of femoroacetabular impingement (FAI). Note the classical pistol grip deformity in Cam-type FAI

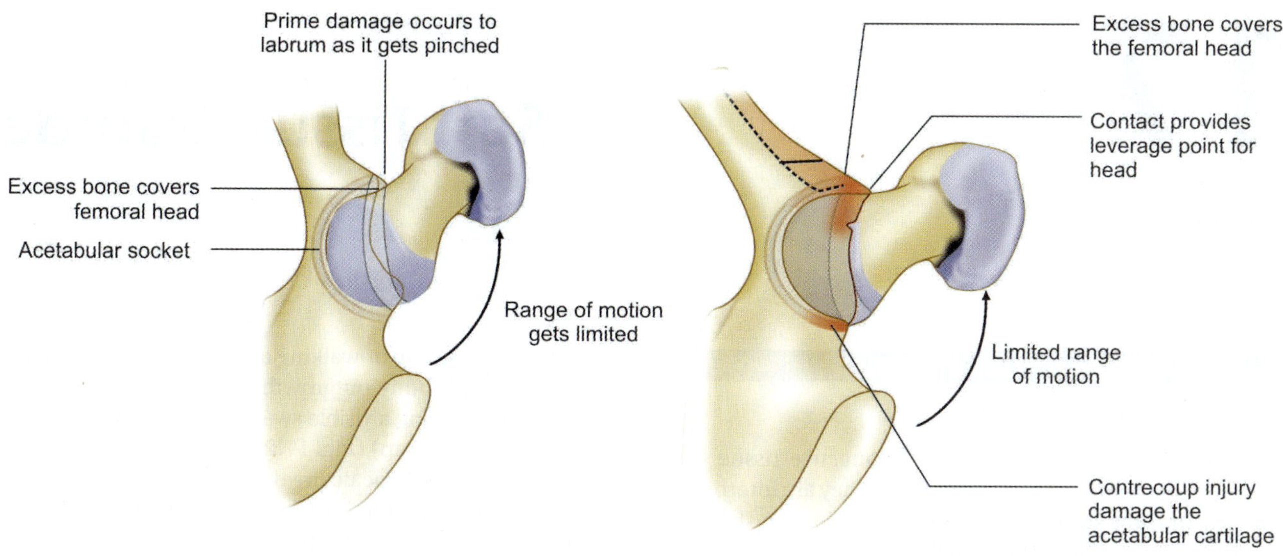

Fig. 16.45: Mechanism behind contrecoup injury in pincer-type of femoroacetabular impingement

and as the antero-supero-lateral acetabular rim contacts the head, the labrum (prime site of damage) gets crushed. The progression is slow but as the condition worsens head gets levered from acetabular socket causing chondral damage in posteroinferior acetabulum (contrecoup injury, **Fig. 16.45**), the end result again eventually being OA of hip.

iii. *Mixed type*: This has mixed features of both types and is the most common variety.

DIAGNOSIS

Groin pain of insidious onset is the complaint that brings these patients to the doctor. The affected hip generally has limited internal rotation. Impingement test at hip is performed by making the patient lie supine and moving the hip into 90° flexion and then adducting and internal rotating it. Reproduction of patient's pain signifies a positive test. On taking the hip into FABER (flexion, abduction and external rotation) position, one may find increased knee to table distance.

Radiographic Features

i. Pistol grip deformity **(Fig. 16.44)** is classical in cam-type and provides a spot diagnosis.
ii. Coxa profunda and protrusio may be evident in pincer FAI. Coxa profunda refers to a deep acetabular socket that is recognized by medial acetabular rim lying medial to ilioischial line. Protrusio refers to a condition where the femoral head migrates medially to lie medial to the ilioischial line.
iii. Crossover sign may be appreciable. This occurs in pincer impingement where the anterior wall shadow (that is normally medial) crosses lateral to the posterior wall shadow on AP hip X-ray.
iv. Central edge angle of Wiberg (*see* Page 365) is less than 25°.
v. Alpha angle **(Fig. 16.46)** may be increased.

MANAGEMENT

Initial management is conservative tailored to symptoms. Persistent symptoms may require removal of impingement source to re-establish head neck offsets. Hip arthroscopy offers an

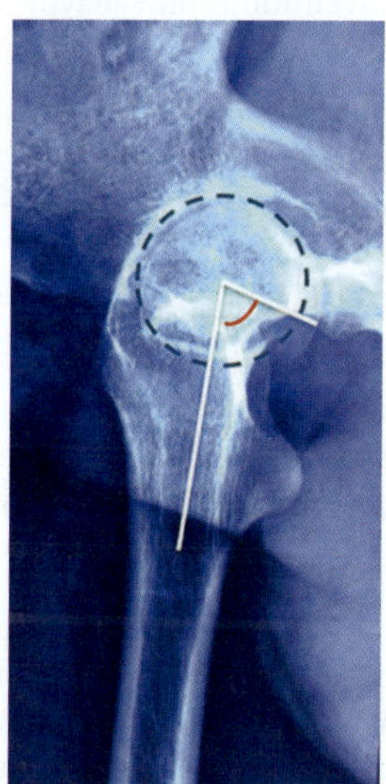

Fig. 16.46: Pincer-type femoroacetabular impingement showing increased alpha angle (almost 80°). The angle is formed by a line through the center of femoral head and neck and a second line from the femoral head center to the point where the head exits a concentric circle drawn around it

attractive approach as one can also address the labral pathology (labral repair) and concomitant chondral damage in same sitting.

HIGH-YIELD POINTS

- First radiological sign in cam-type FAI is anterolateral migration of femoral head while in pincer-type FAI it is posteroinferior joint space narrowing.
- Acetabular labral tears (traumatic or with FAI) are now increasingly being recognized as a precursor of OA hip. Although the tears are well evident on MRI, clinically patients with labral tears demonstrate "C" sign of Byrd. When asked to mark their pain, they often cup their hands forming a "C" over the greater trochanter.

Soft Tissue Disorders

ADVENTITIOUS BURSITIS

INTRODUCTION

True or anatomical/synovial bursae are connective tissue sacs lined by synovium, containing a viscous fluid. They are interposed between two moving structures to reduce friction or shear or they may be present at sites of unusual pressure like many bony prominences.

Adventitious bursa refers to a bursa that is not normally present at that site. Adventitious bursae typically develop in areas of chronic frictional irritation.

Following are the important sites of adventitious bursitis:
- *Student's elbow*: Olecranon bursitis **(Fig. 17.1A)**
- *Tailor's ankle (bunionette)*: Lateral aspect of fifth metatarsal head **(Fig. 17.1B)**
- *Weaver's bottom*: Ischial bursitis
- *Clergyman's knee*: Infrapatellar bursitis
- *Housemaid's/coal miner's knee*: Prepatellar bursitis
- *Baker's/popliteal cyst*: Semimembranosus bursitis
- *Retrocalcaneal bursitis*: Achilles tendon bursitis.

RETROCALCANEAL BURSITIS

It refers to inflammation of the retrocalcaneal bursa that lies between the posterior aspect of the calcaneum and anterior aspect of Tendo Achilles **(Fig. 17.2A)**. The most likely etiology is the back of the heel repeatedly rubbing against the shoes. It commonly occurs in females in their twenties and thirties. The pain is aggravated by running or walking and relieved by rest. When this is associated with bony outgrowth of the posterosuperior part of the calcaneum causing a visible swelling, it is known as Haglund's deformity (pump bump) **(Fig. 17.2B)**.

Treatment of retrocalcaneal bursitis consists of nonsteroidal anti-inflammatory drugs (NSAIDs), modification of activity, changing to soft footwear or backless shoes and local ice application or a contrast bath (hot and cold fomentation alternatively in a ratio of 3:1 or 4:1 starting from hot fomentation for a period of 15–30 minutes). Haglund's deformity can also be treated with such conservative measures, but when refractory, it may require surgery in the form of resection of the superior aspect of the tuberosity.

MORRANT BAKER'S CYST (POPLITEAL CYST)

Popliteal cyst presents as a swelling in the popliteal fossa **(Figs 17.3A and B)** formed due to egress of fluid through the normal communication between the knee joint and the semimembranosus bursa or the bursa beneath the medial head of gastrocnemius. It can be seen both in children as well as in adults (especially those having osteoarthritis changes in the knee). Swelling, pain or discomfort in the region usually brings these patients to doctors.

Diagnosis

Transillumination test is positive, but can be negative at times due to thick muscle cover on the back. In these cases, ultrasonography (USG) can establish the diagnosis and distinguish effectively between popliteal cyst and other lesions in the location such as

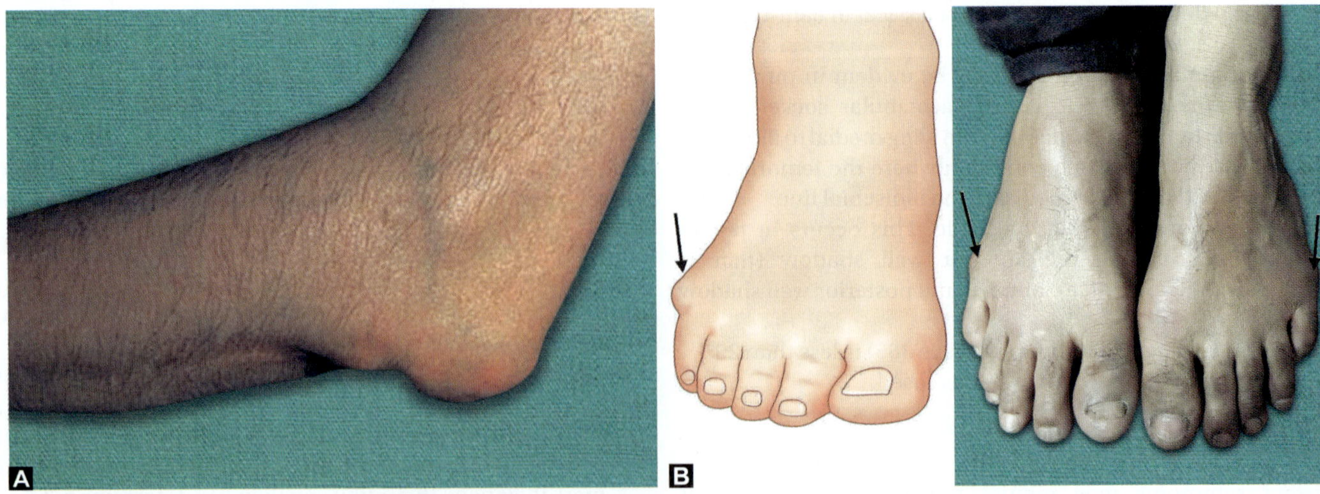

Figs 17.1A and B: (A) Student's elbow; (B) Bunionette (arrows)

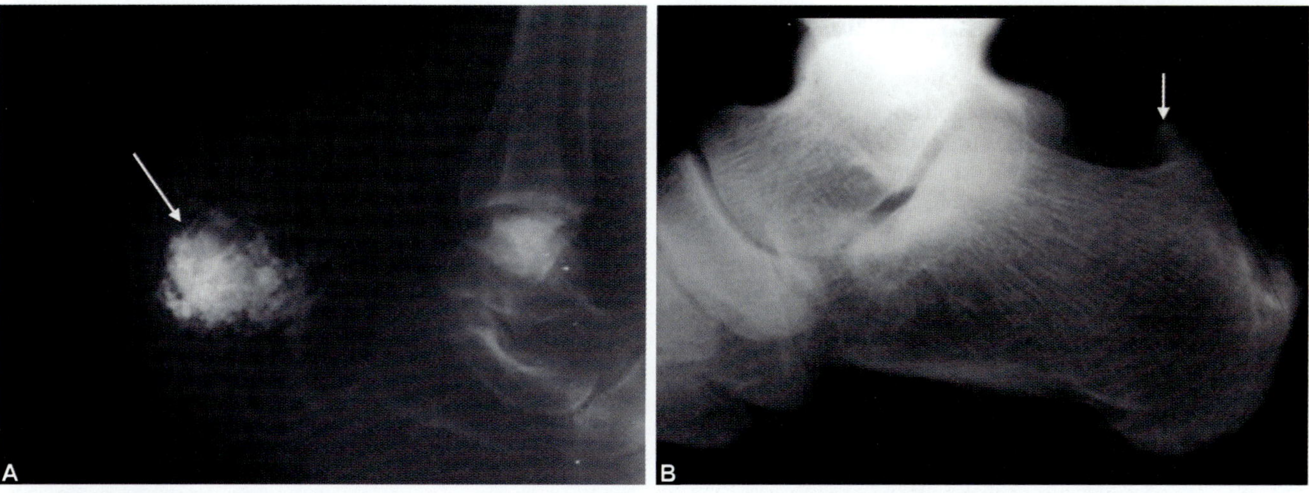

Figs 17.2A and B: (A) X-ray ankle lateral view showing heavily calcified retrocalcaneal bursa (arrow); (B) Haglund's deformity (arrow)

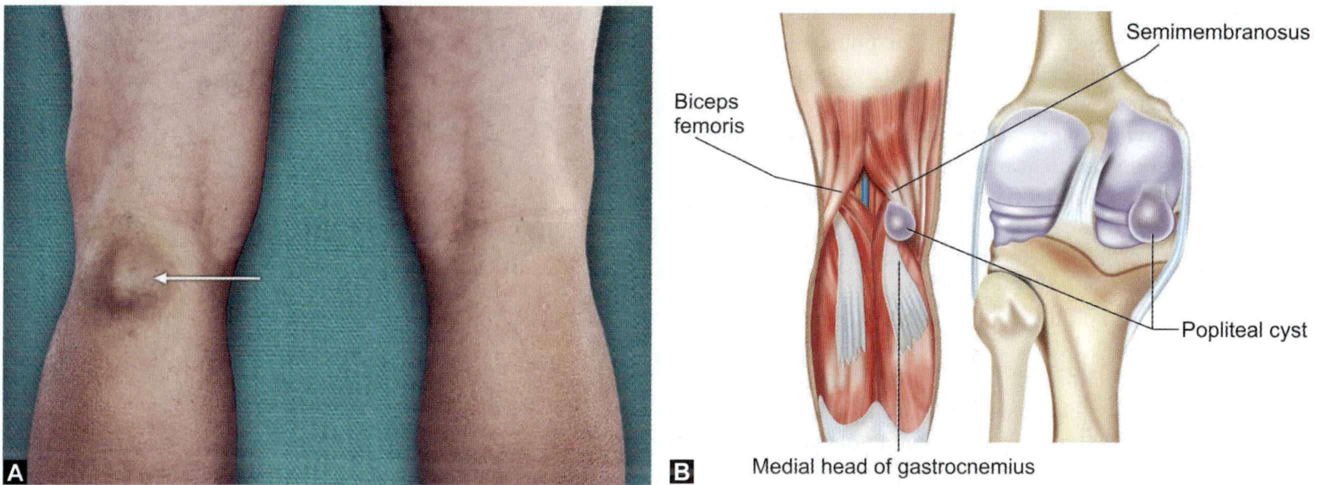

Figs 17.3A and B: (A) Clinical picture showing Baker's cyst (arrow) in the popliteal fossa; (B) Diagrammatic depiction of a Baker's cyst

lipoma, fibrosarcoma, vascular tumors, xanthomas, etc. X-rays are not of much use. Computed tomography (CT) can effectively delineate the extent of the cyst, but magnetic resonance imaging (MRI) is best and can also elucidate associated intra-articular pathology, that is common in adults.

Treatment

Treatment of the cyst differs in children and adults.

In adults, the cyst is often associated with an intra-articular pathology (e.g. tear in the posterior one-third of medial meniscus). Hence, an arthroscopic decompression of the cyst is mostly performed in symptomatic cases along with the required treatment of the associated intra-articular pathology. Not dealing effectively with the intra-articular pathology often leads to recurrence of the cyst. However, if no significant intra-articular pathology is present, an open excision can also be performed.

In children, intra-articular pathology is rare and cyst infrequently communicates with the knee joint. In them prolonged neglect is wise as many cysts spontaneously regress. In nonresolving cysts, aspiration and injection of steroid is effective.

Surgery is rarely required, and if performed, even incomplete excision affects a cure.

- Largest bursa in the body: Iliopsoas bursa.
- The most common site of bursitis is the shoulder, i.e. subacromial bursitis (*read below*).
- The most common patellar bursitis is the prepatellar bursitis.
- Swellings around the knee:
  - In front of knee—prepatellar and infrapatellar bursitis
  - Medial side of knee—pes anserine bursitis
  - On back of knee—Baker's cyst.
- *Bursae around the knee that communicate with the knee joint*: Suprapatellar bursa, popliteal bursa, gastrocnemius bursa and pes anserine bursa.
- The infrapatellar bursa is divided into superficial and deep bursa. The clergyman's knee is inflammation of the superficial infrapatellar bursa.
- *Hoffa's syndrome*: Inflammation in infrapatella fat pad leading to anterior knee pain.

WRIST AND HAND AFFECTIONS

GANGLION

It is a cystic degeneration of the tendon sheath or joint capsule. It presents mostly as a unilocular cystic structure filled with thick gelatinous fluid. Dorsum of the wrist is the most common site **(Fig. 17.4)** and it usually develops from the dorsal aspect of the scapholunate ligament. The swelling becomes more prominent on flexion of the wrist. Mostly it is a painless mass, but rarely may it become painful. Treatment initially involves aspirating the cyst and injecting steroid (hyaluronidase). Recurrent cases may need surgical excision.

DE QUERVAIN'S DISEASE

Tendons in the body are enclosed in double-walled sheaths with an inner visceral layer and an outer vaginal layer. Inflammation of the complete tendon sheath is called tenosynovitis while isolated involvement of the outer layer is called tenovaginitis.

De Quervain's disease is tenovaginitis affecting the common tendon sheaths of the extensor tendons of the first extensor compartment of the forearm, viz. abductor pollicis longus and extensor pollicis brevis **(Fig. 17.5)**. Common age group is 30–50 years with women affected six times more frequently than men.

It is an overuse syndrome related to the frequent maneuvering of the wrist in ulnar deviation as in lifting heavy pan off the stove, pushing a luggage trolley and inflating a blood pressure (BP) cuff.

On examination, these patients classically have tenderness at the radial styloid process. The pathognomoic (not diagnostic) clinical test is Finkelstein's test **(Fig. 17.6)**. In this test, on grasping the patient's thumb and pulling it ulnarward, excruciating pain is felt over the styloid tip.

X-rays are usually normal and clinical examination and history point the main diagnosis. Arthritis at the base of the thumb, superficial radial nerve entrapment or neuroma and intersection syndrome (tenosynovitis at the crossing of the extensor pollicis brevis and abductor pollicis longus over the extensor carpi radialis longus and brevis) are main differentials. Tenderness and crepitus in intersection syndrome is felt 4–6 cm proximal to the extensor retinaculum.

Management

Initially conservative. Activity may be restricted by giving a thumb spica splint. Nonresponders may be given local heat therapies and steroid injections into the tendon sheaths. Since local steroid injection accidentally into the tendon may lead to it's rupture, corticosteroids are better applied topically and then driven into the subcutaneous tissues using ultrasound (phonophoresis) or electrically charged ions (iontophoresis). Recalcitrant cases may need surgery to release the first dorsal compartment to relieve pressure (splitting open the thickened tendon sheaths).

TRIGGER FINGER/THUMB

It is a stenosing tenosynovitis of the flexor tendon sheaths of the fingers/thumb that mostly affects people older than 45 years of age. The flexor tendon sheath is thickened and constricted so that free gliding of the tendon in the sheath does not occur freely. Often the constriction is present at the mouth of the tendon sheath, i.e. at the level of metacarpophalangeal (MCP) joint or at the level of A1 pulley (*see* Page 107 for details on pulley system), so that the tendon becomes trapped right at the point of entry into the sheath **(Fig. 17.7)**. This produces the characteristic snapping of

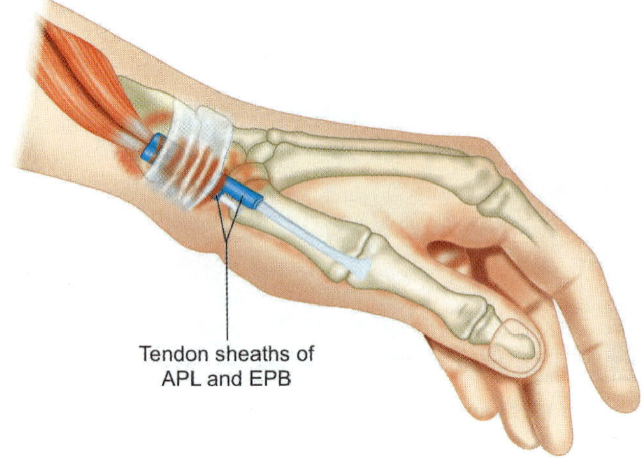

Fig. 17.5: De Quervain's disease

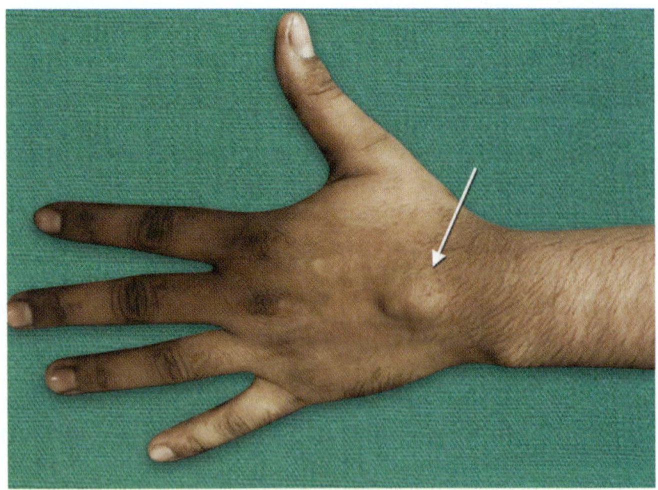

Fig. 17.4: Ganglion cyst (arrow)

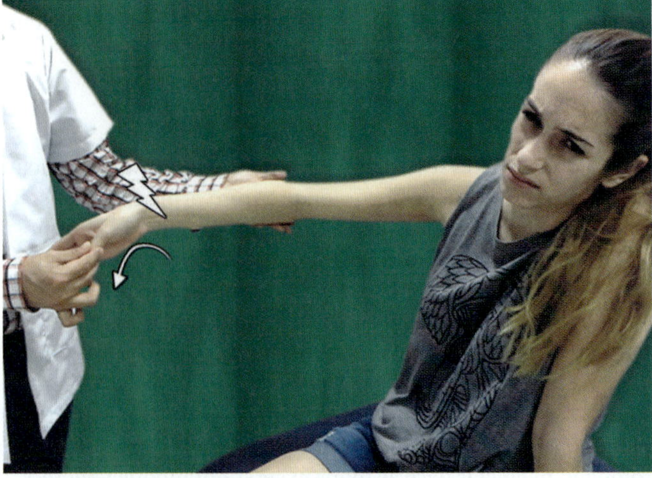

Fig. 17.6: Finkelstein's test

the finger on trying to flex and extend it, referred to as triggering. Triggering is more pronounced in the morning time.

Although the condition is idiopathic, important predisposing factors include: local trauma, rheumatoid arthritis, gout and diabetes.

The middle and ring fingers are the most commonly involved areas and constriction is most commonly found in front of the MCP joints in trigger finger and interphalangeal (IP) joints in trigger thumb. On examination, one may palpate a tender nodule in front of the MCP joints.

Initial treatment usually is nonoperative and includes stretching, night splinting, and ultrasonic heat therapy. Corticosteroid injections are also effective. Patients with diabetes mellitus may be more refractory to nonoperative management, in all such cases, surgical release reliably relieves the problem.

DUPUYTREN'S CONTRACTURE

Dupuytren's disease is a proliferative fibrometaplasia of the subcutaneous tissue of the palm. Palmar fascia is replaced by fibrous tissue (palmar fibromatosis) in the form of nodules and cords that may result in secondary progressive and irreversible finger joint flexion contractures. Ring finger is usually first to be involved followed by little and other fingers **(Figs 17.8A and B)**. Flexion contractures most commonly occur at the MCP joints, followed by proximal interphalangeal (PIP) joints and then distal interphalangeal (DIP) joints.

In a few patients of Dupuytren's disease, similar lesions may be found in the plantar fascia (Ledderhose's disease) and in the penile fascia (Peyronie's disease).

Predisposed Individuals

The condition is commonly seen in men of Scandinavian and Celtic origin (Male:Female = 10:1) in their fourth to sixth decade of life. People those who are diabetics, alcoholics, smokers and who are on antiepileptic drugs are at greater risk of affection. Although the exact cause remains unknown, hand trauma and heavy manual labor performed by an individual may be contributing factor. Hereditary predisposition is present in some families.

Clinical Presentation

The involvement is commonly bilateral (45%), but it is rarely symmetrical. In the early stages, thickening of palmar aponeurosis or nodules may be felt at the base of the ring or little fingers while in later stage flexion deformity of the fingers develops. Nodules are typically painless, although larger ones may be painful due to associated tenosynovitis. Garrod's nodules or "knuckle pads" are common on the dorsum of the PIP joints in these patients.

Treatment

An elderly patient with minimal deformity needs no treatment. But when flexion contractures of the fingers at PIP joints exceed 15° and at the MCP joints exceed 30°, then contracted fascia has to be resected (total/partial fasciectomy). An amputation also rarely is indicated in case incorrectable recurrent flexion contractures have made the finger nonuseful.

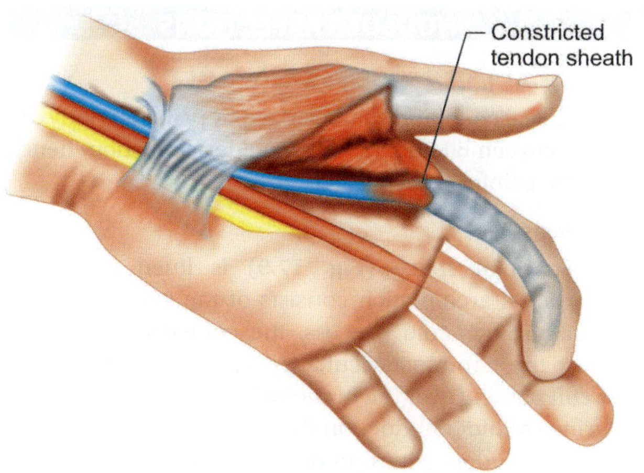

Fig. 17.7: Trigger finger

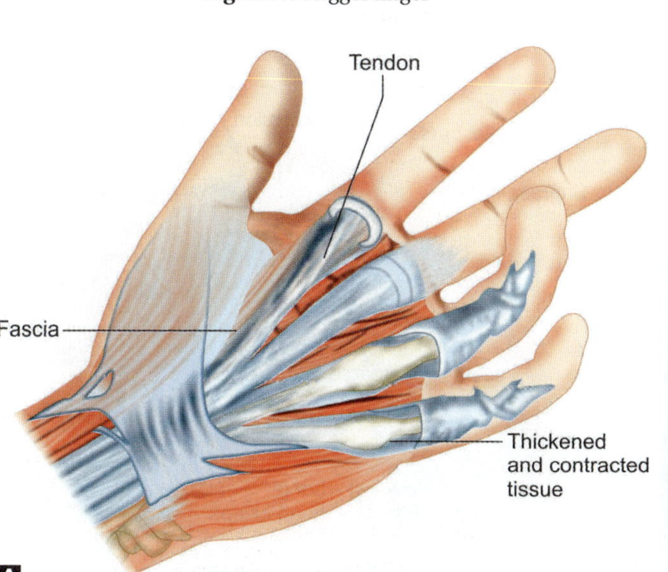

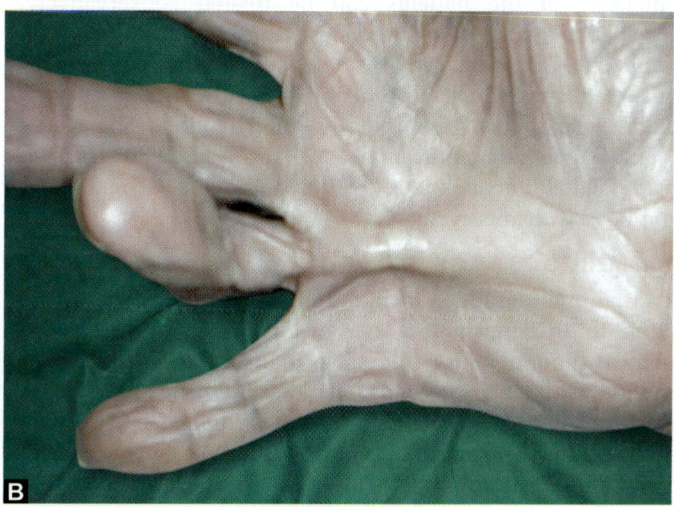

Figs 17.8A and B: (A) Dupuytren's contracture; (B) Dupuytren's contracture developing in the ring finger
Courtesy: Figure 17.8B: Dr Charlie Goldberg, UCSD, California.

HYPOTHENAR-HAMMER SYNDROME

The hypothenar-hammer syndrome is an uncommon cause of digital ischemia caused as a result of occupational or sports activities which involve repetitively striking objects with the heel of the hand.

Pathogenesis

The superficial branch of the ulnar artery passes over the hypothenar muscles before penetrating the palmar aponeurosis. This superficial position makes it susceptible to injury. Repeated blunt trauma to the hypothenar aspect of the hand occurs in professions (automechanics, metal workers, carpenters, and brick layers) and sports (baseball, golf, volleyball) where occupation demands for repeated use of the hypothenar portion of the palm to hammer, push or twist objects. Blunt trauma to the hypothenar aspect of the palm in these occupations causes this superficial branch to be injured and compressed against the adjacent boney hook of the hamate resulting in ischemia of the second, third, fourth or fifth digits. The thumb is usually spared.

Diagnosis

Patients present with pain, paresthesia, discoloration and cold sensitivity. Repeated injury may cause callus formation at the hypothenar aspect of the palm. Diagnosis can be established by positive Allen's test (*see* Page 280) and Doppler ultrasound. Doppler ultrasound measures digital brachial index, which, if less than 0.7 suggest vascular reconstruction. The Allens's test checks the patency of the ulnar artery and it is performed by compressing the radial artery with one thumb and the ulnar artery with the other thumb. Now the hand is exsanguinated by rapidly clenching and opening the fist several times. Now the ulnar artery is released, if it is patent, the hand becomes pink again within 5 seconds. If it is occluded hand becomes pink only after releasing the radial artery. Angiography is the gold standard in making the diagnosis and may reveal thrombus occlusion, tortuous "corkscrew" ulnar artery, aneurysm or embolus in the superficial palmar arch or distal ulnar artery.

Management

A majority of the patients can be treated conservatively. Conservative treatment includes lifestyle modification, cessation of smoking, avoidance of further trauma and padding of hand. Medicines which have been tried with variable success include calcium channel blockers and antiplatelet agents or anticoagulation. Indications for vascular reconstruction include digital brachial index less than 0.7, digital ischemia and thrombosis with aneurysm.

DRUMMER BOY'S PALSY

It is a chronic tendinitis of the extensor pollicis longus (EPL) tendon. In drummer boy, it is an overuse injury to EPL due to repetitive motion injury (repetitive palmar flexion and ulnar deviation). Tendon rubs against the dorsal tubercle of the radius and with accumulative trauma, it may get attenuated or in extreme cases rupture may occur. Treatment is usually conservative with activity modification. Transfer of extensor indicis to substitute EPL may be required in cases of rupture.

HIGH-YIELD POINTS

- Ganglion is the most common swelling/soft tissue mass of the hand.
- Compound palmar ganglion (*see* Page 296) is due to chronic inflammation of the common sheath of flexor tendons both above and below the flexor retinaculum causing an hourglass like swelling in front of the wrist. Both rheumatoid arthritis and tuberculosis are common causes.
- Congenital trigger thumb is also a known entity. In this triggering in the thumb resolves mostly by the age of 1 year. However, an important differential to exclude in congenital clasped thumb (absence of the extensor tendons of thumb).
- In Dupuytren's contracture structures contracted in the fingers can be remembered by mnemonics: "**No GPS Location**" (**N**atatory ligament, **G**rayson ligament, **P**retendinous band, **S**piral band and **L**ateral digital sheath).
- Most common causes of rupture of the extensor pollicis longus tendon are fractures around the wrist joint and rheumatoid arthritis.

SHOULDER AFFECTIONS

SUBACROMIAL IMPINGEMENT SYNDROME

This is a clinical condition characterized by pain anteriorly over the shoulder between 60 and 120° of shoulder abduction, hence also called as the painful arc syndrome.

Pathogenesis

The subacromial space **(Fig. 17.9)** is lined above by the coracoacromial arch, which consists of the anterior part of the acromion, the coracoid process, the coracoacromial ligament (CAL), and the acromioclavicular (AC) joint and below by the the rotator cuff passing over the humeral head.

During shoulder abduction the greater tuberosity along with rotator cuff tendon slides under the acromion (subacromial space), the movements being smoothened by the presence of the subacromial bursa in the subacromial space between the

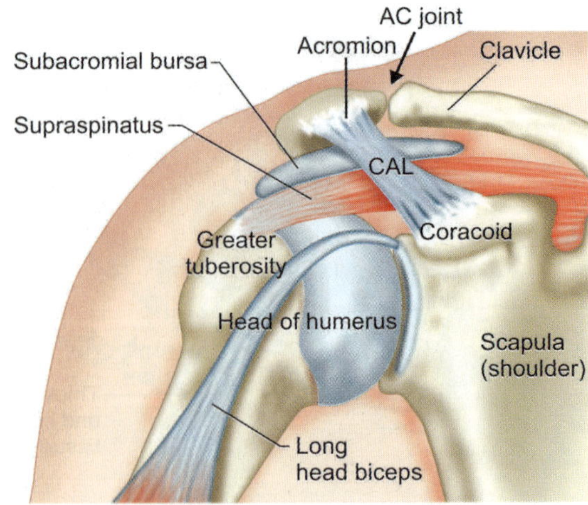

Fig. 17.9: Subacromial space
Abbreviations: AC, acromioclavicular; CAL, coracoacromial ligament.

opposing bony surfaces. Any condition that compromises this space may result in subacromial impingement which is the most common cause of shoulder pain.

Neer described three progressive stages of impingement **(Box 17.1)** signifying that untreated the impingement eventually ends with rotator cuff tears, leading the shoulder disabled.

Etiology and Classification

Subacromial impingement can be divided into primary (intrinsic and extrinsic), secondary, depending on the causes.

(A) *Primary impingement*: This is the classic version where the cause is located within the subacromial space. It can be intrinsic or extrinsic depending on the causes.

1. *Intrinsic causes:* In this category, the structures passing beneath the coracoacromial arch become enlarged. For example, rotator cuff tendon calcification occurring due to age-related degeneration (calcific tendinitis, **Figs 17.10A and B**), thickening of a subacromial bursa (subacromial bursitis), etc.

2. *Extrinsic causes:* In this category due to various causes, the space in the subacromial region available for smooth gliding of the rotator cuff is reduced. These causes are related to alterations in the anatomy of the coracoacromial arch (also known as outlet impingement) and have been tabulated in **Box 17.2**.

(B) *Secondary impingement*: Secondary impingement is related to weakness of shoulder muscles, postural abnormalities, shoulder instability and scapular dyskinesia (see Chapter 6). These all factors alter the normal scapula-humeral rhythm leading to impingement.

Clinical Testing

Following clinical tests may help in reaching the diagnosis:

Neer's impingement sign: Examiner passively raises the arm in forward flexion while stabilizing the scapula (to prevent scapulothoracic movement) **(Fig. 17.11)**. This causes pain in the shoulder anteriorly.

Neer's impingement test: 5 mL of 1% lidocaine is injected into the subacromial space. After several minutes, Neer maneuver is again performed and this time pain is absent or significantly reduced, indicating that subacromial impingement was the cause of pain.

Hawkins-Kennedy test: Forward flexion of shoulder to 90° with forcible internal rotation reproduces the impingement pain. This test is sensitive, but not very specific **(Fig. 17.12)**.

Scapular assistance test **(Fig. 17.13):** Examiner pushes the inferior medial scapular angle during shoulder elevation to assist scapular upward rotation and posterior tilt. A positive result is indicated by relief of painful symptoms related to the subacromial impingement and increased arc of motion.

Imaging

X-rays may show calcific deposits **(Figs 17.10A and B)** or fracture. MRI is the investigation of choice and reveals bursitis or tendinitis in the region.

Treatment

Initial treatment is conservative with anti-inflammatory medicines and restriction of overhead activities. Local heat

---

Box 17.1: Stages of impingement syndrome (Neer)

- *Stage I:* Subacromial bursitis with subacromial edema and hemorrhage
- *Stage II:* Rotator cuff tendinopathy with a partial-thickness tear
- *Stage III:* Progression to a full-thickness rotator cuff tear

---

Box 17.2: Extrinsic causes for subacromial impingement (outlet impingement)

- Hooked acromion
- Horizontal acromion with decreased tilt
- Osteoarthritis of AC joint
- Fracture of acromion or clavicle
- *Os acromiale:* Unfused acromial ossification center **(Fig. 17.10B)**

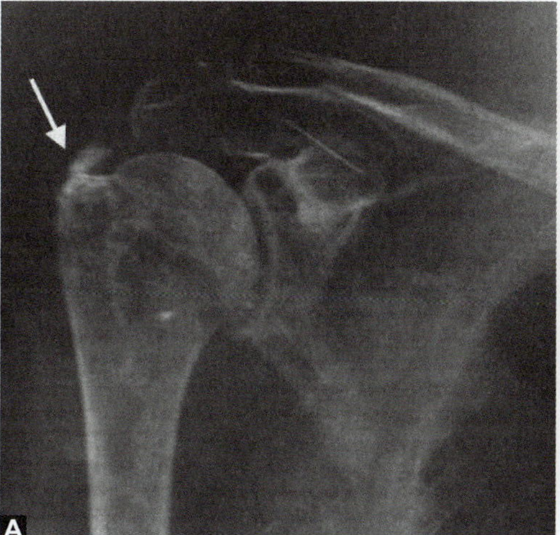

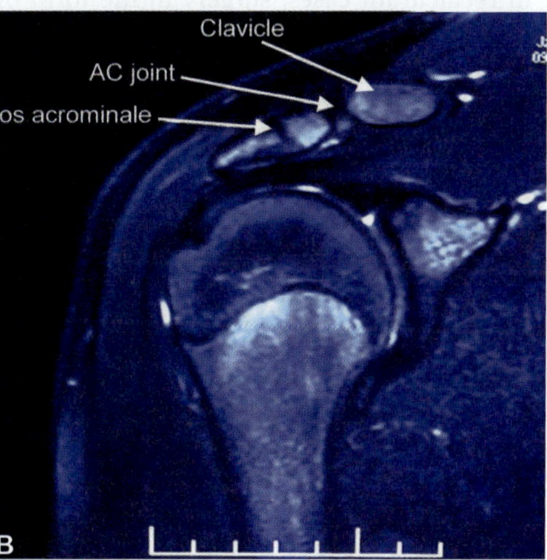

Figs 17.10A and B: (A) Calcific tendinitis, see calcification in the insertion of rotator cuff tendon at the greater tuberosity (arrow); (B) MRI of shoulder depicting unfused acromion ossification center (os acrominale)

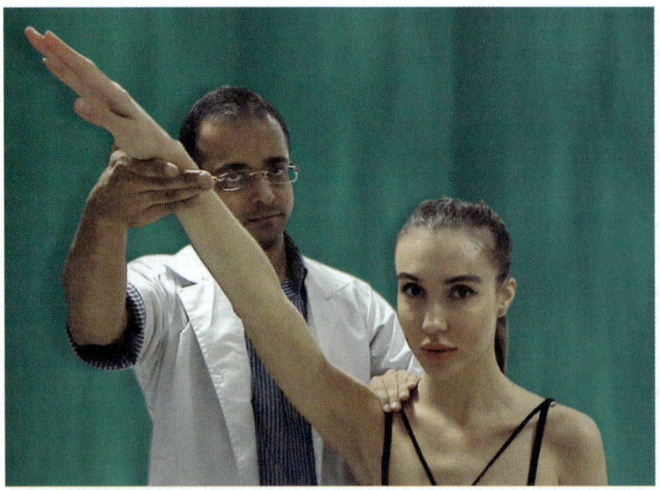

Fig. 17.11: Neer's impingement test

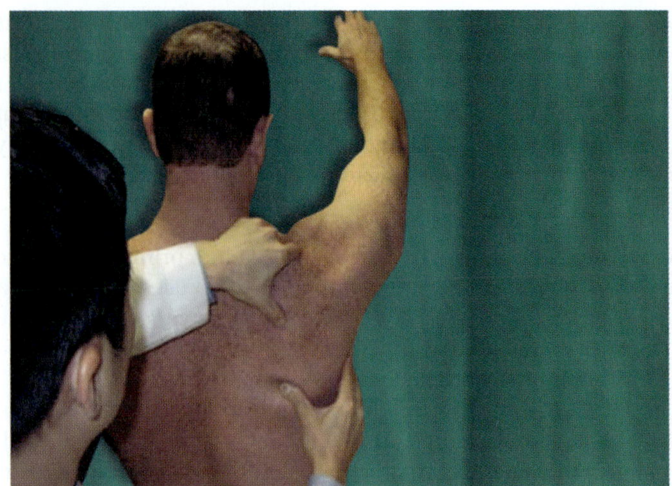

Fig. 17.13: Scapular assistance test

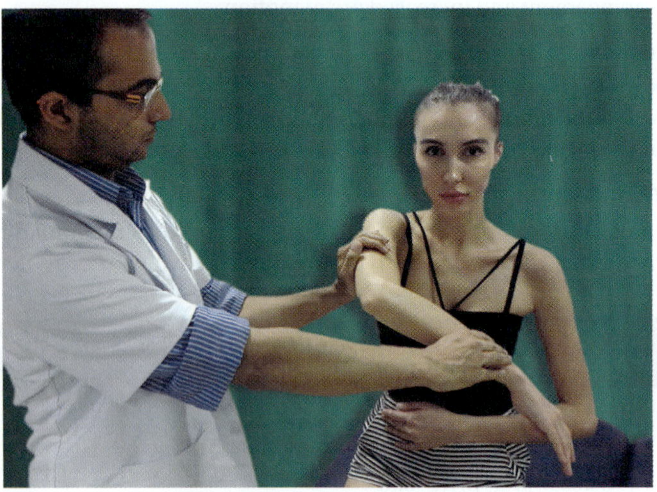

Fig. 17.12: Hawkins-Kennedy test

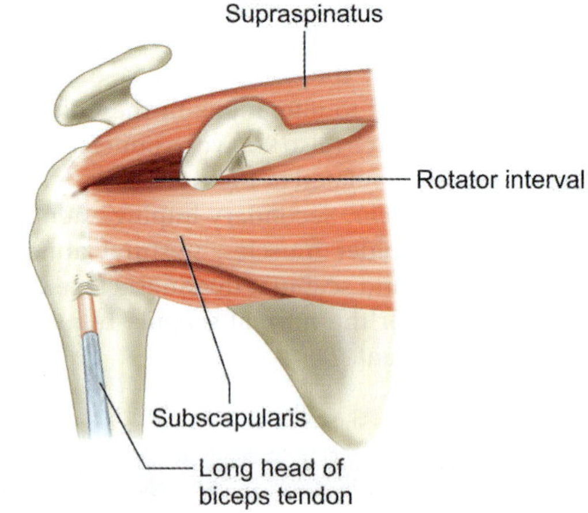

Fig. 17.14: Rotator interval (a triangular space bounded above by the supraspinatus tendon, below by the subscapularis and, medially the apex is formed by the coracoid process of scapula). It contains the coracohumeral ligament that is most prominently involved

therapies may be added to provide relief. Steroids may be given as local injections. In recalcitrant cases, surgery in the form of arthroscopic subacromial decompression and debridement and removal of impinging osteophyte/bony fragments (acromioplasty) is usually indicated. Stage III impingement additionally requires arthroscopic or open rotator cuff repair.

PERIARTHRITIS SHOULDER (FROZEN SHOULDER)

Periarthritis shoulder, also known as frozen shoulder, refers to a situation where the patient has painful restriction of shoulder motion in all planes but on X-ray everything seems to be normal. The pathology in such cases is often attributable to a condition more appropriately called as 'Adhesive capsulitis'. In this condition, there is chronic inflammation followed by fibroblastic proliferation in the shoulder joint capsule (precisely the subsynovial layer), decreased synovial fluid in the joint and consequently stiffness and pain on attempted movement. The changes more severely involve an area in the anterior part of capsule called the rotator interval **(Fig. 17.14)** and coracohumeral ligament.

Associations

The condition generally affects people of 40–60 years of age and is more common in females. It is almost five times more common in diabetics. It is bilateral in 20–30% cases. Other important associations include hyperthyroidism, hypothyroidism, prolonged immobilization, cervical disk disease, Parkinson's disease, myocardial infarction and stroke.

Clinical Presentation

Patients present with severe pain and stiffness in the affected shoulder. There is a global restriction of movements in all directions affecting both passive and active range of motion (unlike rotator cuff tear where only active movements are lost). The first movement to be lost is external rotation then abduction.

Course of the Disease

The disease is self-limiting with a chronic course that spans over a period of 6–12 months passing through three characteristic phases:

1. *Painful phase (few weeks to months)*: Dull pain occurs at rest. Shoulder motion are painful with pain radiating to deltoid insertion. Pain is usually worse at night. Range of motion is still well maintained or only slightly reduced. These symptoms are usually present for less than 10–16 weeks.
2. *Phase of progressive stiffness/freezing phase (10 weeks–12 months)*: There is progressive loss of range of motion. With the progression of disease, gross reduction of movement occurs, with almost no external rotation possible.
3. *Resolution/thawing phase*: This is usually seen 12 months after the onset of the disease. Improvement in pain and range of motion occurs, but some loss of range of motion usually persists.

Diagnosis

Diagnosis is mainly clinical. Insidious onset of painful restriction of both passive and active external rotation and other movement without any crepitus is the hallmark of frozen shoulder. Radiographs are mostly normal. MRI may show thickening in the area of rotator interval.

Differential Diagnosis

Important conditions to exclude are caries sicca (tuberculosis of shoulder, *see* Page 310) and rotator cuff tears (*read above*).

Treatment

The disease is self-limiting and initial treatment is thus conservative. NSAIDs can relieve pain. Intra-articular steroid injection is beneficial in painful stage, but the effect might persist only for short-term and not well maintained. It is, however, more effective when used in combination with physiotherapy. Physical therapy and stretching are most effective in patients presenting with stages I and II of frozen shoulder.

Cases where conservative treatment fails manipulation under anesthesia can pain and range of motion. The shoulder is sequentially manipulated (forward elevation in the sagittal plane while fixing the scapula, external rotation in 0° of abduction, external rotation in 90° of abduction, internal rotation in 90° of abduction, and lastly cross-body adduction). Over enthusiastic manipulation may result in fracture of the humerus and should be avoided.

Arthroscopic release of the rotator interval and the anterior-inferior capsule has become the standard procedure where conservative treatment or manipulation under anesthesia has failed. Diabetic status should be controlled.

HIGH-YIELD POINTS

- Codman's paradox method is used for manipulation under anesthesia in frozen shoulder that is effective in preventing a damaging rotational torque to the humerus and hence avoiding a proximal humerus fracture.
- Frozen pelvis refers to marked inflammation of the pelvic tissue. The most common cause is endometriosis and the condition is dealt by gynecologists.
- *Internal impingement*: This is a special condition that is found in sportsmen involved in throwing sports. Due to repeated throwing actions damaging the posterior capsule leading to its contracture, such people loose some amount of internal rotation movement in their shoulders. On attempting a throw, owing to a contracted capsule, humeral head slides back and contacts the posterosuperior labrum and rotator cuff causing pain during throwing action. This is called internal impingement. The details have been discussed in Chapter 6.

FOOT AFFECTIONS

BUNION

A bunion is a bony bump that forms over the dorsal surface of the first metatarsal head **(Figs 17.15A and B)**. It mainly results due to imbalance between two tendons: (1) peroneus longus (that depresses the first metatarsal) and (2) tibialis anterior (that elevates the first metatarsal). It can also result from paralysis of the gastroc-soleus. In this situation, the long toe plantar flexors exert more force to give added strength to plantar flexion as gastroc-soleus is weak.

MORTON'S NEUROMA

It is basically a neuritis and perineural fibrosis of common digital nerves of foot. The term is a misnomer as histopathologically it is not a neuroma. Third interspace is most commonly affected, followed by a second.

Typical symptoms are pain and paresthesia in web space and adjoining toes. Compression of interspaces by compressing the foot results in a palpable click (Mulder's click).

A trial of conservative treatment which includes wide toe box shoes, metatarsal bars or pads, local steroid injections should be

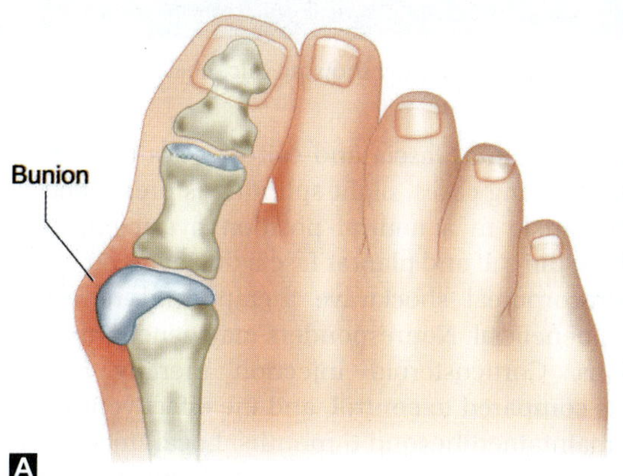

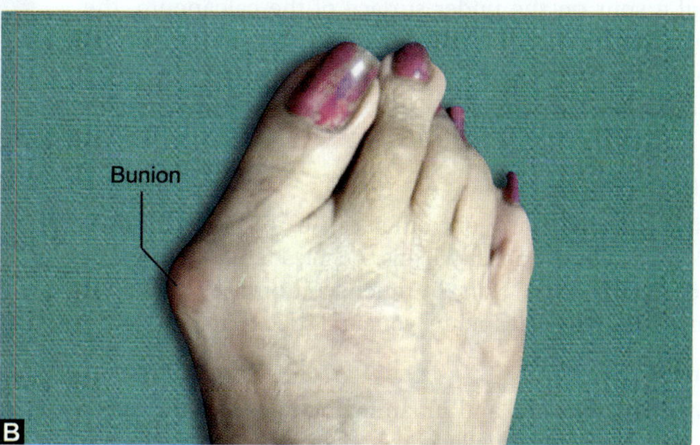

Figs 17.15A and B: Bunion

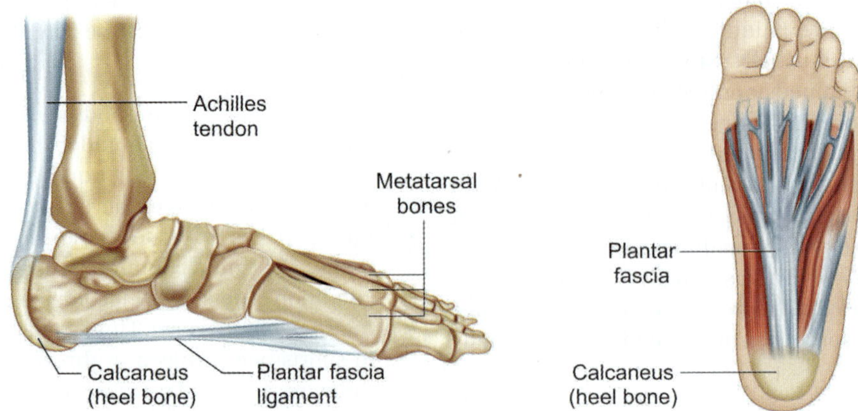

Fig. 17.16: Diagrammatic representation of plantar fascia

tried at first, but they are commonly not very effective. Surgery includes decompression or resection of nerve, which gives complete relief.

PLANTAR FASCIITIS

Plantar fascia is a thick aponeurosis present on the bottom side of the foot that originates at the medial calcaneal tubercle and runs to the heads of the metatarsal bones **(Fig. 17.16)**. Plantar fasciitis results due to repetitive tensile overload on the plantar fascia from prolonged standing or running or other sports activity. Histological changes suggest degenerative changes rather than inflammation as a cause of pain. So plantar fasciosis (degenerative process) is a more appropriate term to describe it rather than plantar fasciitis (inflammatory process). Risk factors for plantar fasciitis are given in **Box 17.3**.

Clinical Presentation

The condition is one of the most common causes of heel pain. Patients classically present with heel pain that is worst in the morning when the patient takes the first few steps. The pain, reduces as the day goes by but worsens late in the day with continued activity. On examination, there may be tenderness usually localized to the medial aspect of the calcaneal tuberosity. Passive dorsiflexion of the first toe is painful.

Diagnosis

Diagnosis is usually clinical. X-rays are usually normal, but may reveal a spur on the under surface of the calcaneum, the significance of which is doubtful **(Fig. 17.17)** as many normal persons also have heel spur without any pain. On USG, thickness of plantar fascia greater than 4.0 mm is diagnostic of plantar fasciitis.

Differential Diagnosis

Differentials include ruling out other causes of heel pain like calcaneal spur, retrocalcaneal bursitis, Achilles tendinitis, Sever's disease (osteochondritis), tarsal tunnel syndrome, bone tumor or osteomyelitis of the calcaneum, gout and rheumatoid arthritis.

Management

Management involves oral anti-inflammatory medications, use of heel pads to relieve pressure, local ice application and stretching

Box 17.3: Risk factors for plantar fasciitis

- Obesity
- Pes planus and pronated feet
- Pes cavus
- Tight Achilles tendon and limited dorsiflexion
- Weak plantar flexors
- Prolonged weight bearing/running on hard surface
- Poor biomechanics or limb malalignment

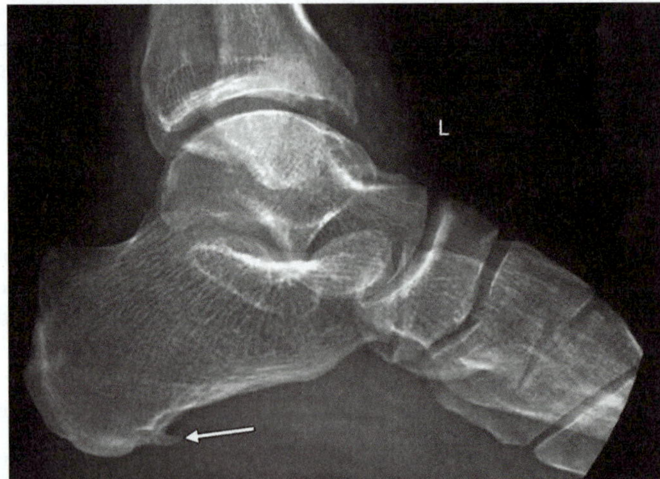

Fig. 17.17: X-ray showing calcaneal spur (arrow)

exercises of plantar fascia and calf muscles **(Figs 17.18A to C)**. In long-standing cases, night splinting is prescribed to keep the patient's ankle in a neutral position overnight, and passively stretching the calf and plantar fascia during sleep.

Extracorporeal shockwave therapy and ultrasonic therapy are also beneficial. Nonresponders may benefit from local steroid injections. Corticosteroid injection therapy has short-term benefits compared to control, and the effectiveness of treatment is not maintained beyond 6 months. Local injection of platelet-rich plasma provides significant relief of pain and improvement of

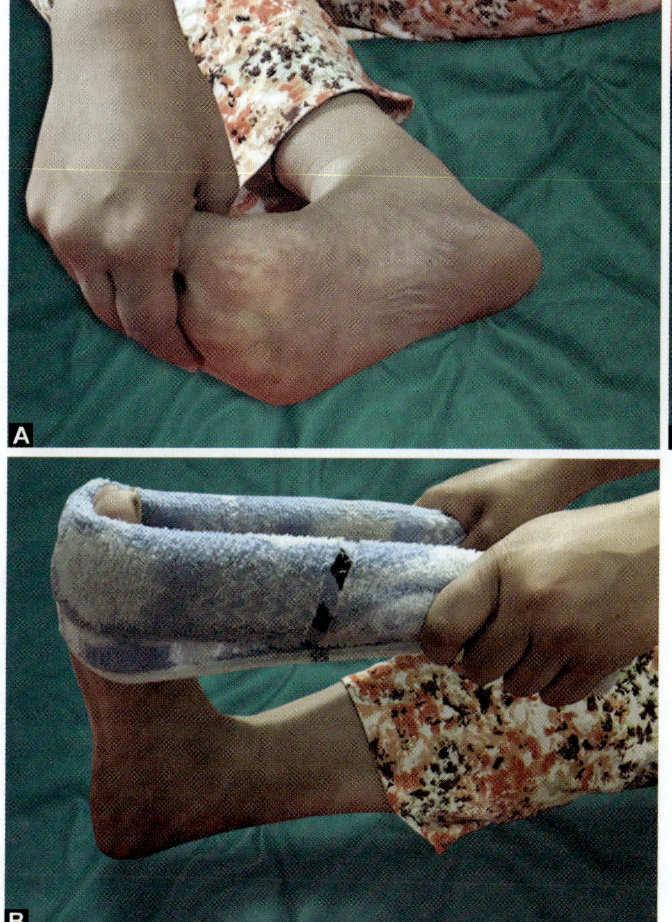

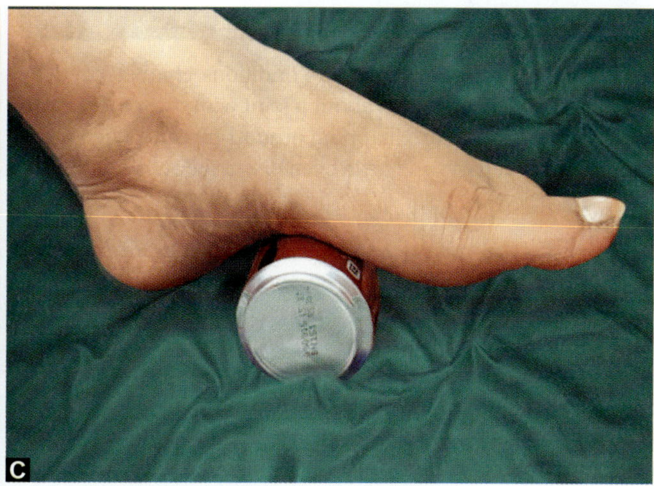

Figs 17.18A to C: (A) Stretching of the plantar fascia, dorsiflex the toes to stretch the plantar fascia; (B) Towel stretching of the calf muscles. Keep the plantar fascia and calf muscles stretched for 30 seconds three times with 30 seconds of rest in between; (C) Roll stretching: roll plantar fascia for 1 minute three times with 30 seconds of rest in between. These stretching exercises are done before going to sleep and before taking first steps in the morning

function, and the results seem to be comparable, and sometimes superior to local steroid injection. In recalcitrant cases, excision of the calcaneal spur or release of fascia may be opted.

METATARSALGIA

It refers to pain in the forefoot region due to increased stress over metatarsals, mainly the head region. It is a symptom which has multiple etiologies. Common causes include Morton's neuroma, stress fracture, foot deformities (hammer toes, hallux valgus), poor footwear, intense training, arthritis, etc. Investigations include X-rays to rule out stress fracture and arthritic changes, inflammatory markers (erythrocyte sedimentation rate, C-reactive protein, rheumatoid factor) to rule out rheumatoid arthritis or an inflammatory pathology. MRI is more specific and sensitive for stress fractures. Treatment is based on the underlying cause. If no cause can be found general measures include changing footwear, using supportive metatarsal bars in foot **(Fig. 17.19)**, weight loss and reducing activity.

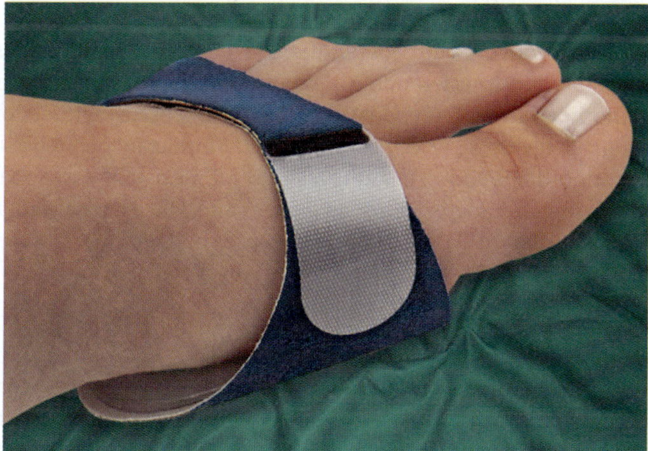

Fig. 17.19: A supportive metatarsal bar prescribed for complaint of metatarsalgia

HIGH-YIELD POINTS

- *Ainhum (dactylolysis spontanea)*: This is a condition classically seen in people of African descent where a constriction spontaneously forms at the base of a toe (most commonly 5th toe) and over a few months or years it progresses to lead to an autoamputation of the digit. The condition is likely to be genetic and in around 75% cases it is bilateral.
- Plantar calcaneal spurs are also sometimes seen in rheumatoid arthritis and in seronegative spondyloarthropathy cases (like ankylosing spondylitis, psoriatic arthropathy, etc.).

SNAPPING SYNDROMES

Snapping syndromes are a group of conditions characterized by audible or palpable snap (click) about a joint with movement, with or without associated pain. Snapping around hip and knee are a common clinical scenario and have been discussed subsequently.

SNAPPING HIP SYNDROME

Snapping hip syndrome (coxa saltans/dancer's hip) occurs in persons who demand heavily on their hip joint (e.g. ballet dancers and athletes requiring repetitive and extreme hip flexion and abduction). Snapping of the hip is divided into extra-articular and intra-articular snapping based on the etiology. Intra-articular snapping occurs due to lesions inside the joint, viz. labral tears, loose bodies, and osteochondral fragments. Patients often complain of catching and locking sensation into the hip joint with movement. Extra-articular snapping (more common) occurs due to causes outside the joint. It is further divided into internal and external forms. In internal form, snapping usually occurs anterior to the hip joint and is commonly attributed to impingement of iliopsoas muscle or its tendon against iliopectineal eminence. In external form, snapping occurs lateral to the hip joint and is attributed to movement of iliotibial band (ITB) over the greater trochanter.

Patient with the condition usually comes with complaint of an audible click. Snapping may be associated with pain if underlying tendon gets inflamed. Examiner can reproduce snapping by some provocative movements like internally and externally rotating the extended and adducted hip, flexing the extended hip and extending the flexed hip or a combination of these movements. Diagnosis is mainly clinical in extra-articular snapping, but dynamic ultrasound and MRI are helpful in making diagnosis of intra-articular snapping and to reveal the tendon and ITB pathology in extra-articular snapping.

Conservative treatment in the form of ice, rest, NSAIDs, ultrasonic and interferential therapies along with stretching of the iliopsoas and ITB is effective in the majority of cases. Injection of a local anesthetic with a corticosteroid into the involved bursa or around the tendon sheath is also useful. Resistant cases may require lengthening of iliopsoas tendon and ITB. Intra-articular snapping due to labral tear and loose body often requires arthroscopic repair of the labrum or removal of loose body.

SNAPPING KNEE SYNDROME

Snapping knee syndrome refers to the feeling of clicking, snapping or abrupt movement during knee flexion or extension. Snapping may be produced by abnormal movement of the loose intra-articular structure like a torn meniscus (intra-articular snapping) or by friction of a tendon, muscle or fascial band over a bony prominence (extra-articular snapping).

Structures which can cause snapping around the knee are:
- *Intra-articular snapping*: Meniscal pathology, synovial plicae, and loose bodies
- *Extra-articular snapping*:
  - *Lateral snapping:* Snapping of biceps femoris over fibular head, patellar dysplasia, ITB friction over lateral tibial condyle

  - *Posteromedial snapping:* Flicking of gracilis and semitendinosus tendons over the muscle belly of semimembranosus when the knee is moved from full flexion to extension (snapping pes syndrome).

Clinical examination may reveal tenderness at bony prominences (fibular head or lateral epicondyle) or joint line. Snap may be visible at times on joint movement. Clinical examination can be supported by real-time ultrasound, which remains the most sensitive tool for extra-articular knee snapping. For intra-articular snapping, MRI is the investigation of the choice.

Treatment initially is conservative with NSAIDs and stretching exercises. If medical treatment is unsuccessful surgical excision of either snapping structure or bony prominence is required.

HIGH-YIELD POINTS

- Hallux saltans is palpable triggering of flexor hallucis longus tendon in foot along the medial wall of calcaneum.
- Dancer's tendinitis is tendinitis of flexor hallucis longus in dancers.

MUSCULAR CYSTICERCOSIS

Cysticercosis is infestation by larva of pork tapeworm (*Taenia solium*) that humans develop by eating undercooked pork. It is an important public health issue, especially in the developing world.

The most common manifestation that the larva produces in humans is neurocysticercosis. Isolated muscular cysticercosis, however, is rare and usually associated with nervous system involvement. Only a few cases of isolated involvement of biceps, brachialis, trapezius and gastrocnemius have been reported. Symptomatic muscular cysticercosis presents with pain, swelling and spasm of the involved muscle.

Diagnosis of isolated muscular cysticercosis poses a challenge to clinicians because of the rarity of the disease. Most of the time patients correlate the pain with the trauma or intense exercise which further delays the diagnosis. Apart from immunochemical studies (including detection of anticysticercal antibodies), CT, MRI and USG are important diagnostic modalities. MRI may show fluid equivalent signal and peripheral rim enhancement, suggesting parasitic cyst involvement or abscess.

Successful treatment has been reported with albendazole 15 mg/kg/day for 7–30 days along with prednisolone 2 mg/kg/day for 2 weeks tapering in the next 1 week. Recalcitrant cases can be taken up for excision.

FUNCTIONAL PAIN SYNDROMES

Functional pain syndromes (FPS) or functional somatic syndromes include those conditions where patients present with localized or diffuse muscle-joint pains, without any identifiable organic cause. These include fibromyalgia syndrome (FMS), chronic fatigue syndrome (CFS) and chronic low back or pelvic pain, apart from pain associated with conditions like irritable bowel syndrome, migraine and tension-type headaches and temporomandibular joint disorders.

FIBROMYALGIA (FIBROSITIS)

Fibromyalgia syndrome is a chronic musculoskeletal pain syndrome of unknown etiology (noninflammatory, nonautoimmune) that

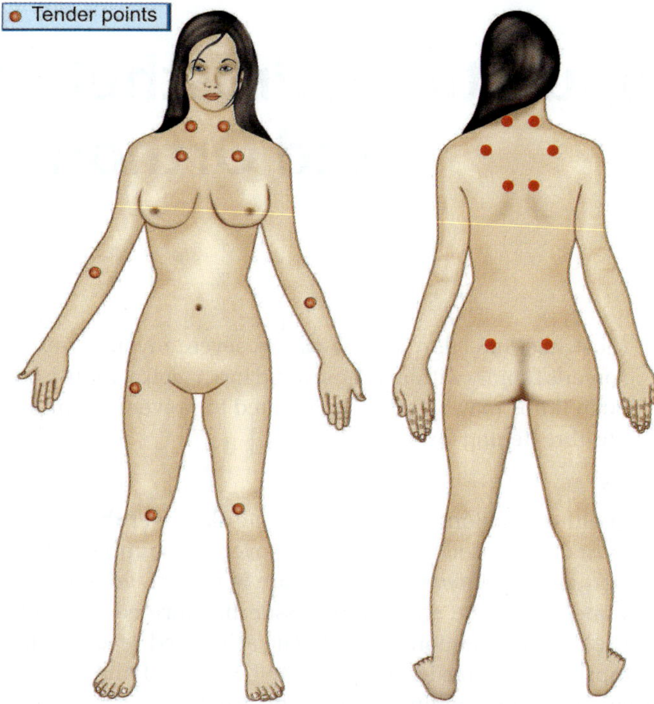

Fig. 17.20: Tender points in fibromyalgia

Table 17.1: Diagnostic criteria for fibromyalgia syndrome (FMS)

Always present	*Often present*
• Chronic and diffuse pain	Morning stiffness
• Characteristic tender	Fatigue
points on examination	Paresthesias
• Normal laboratory	Raynaud's phenomena
investigations	Headache
	Sleep disturbances
	Anxiety
	Depression

is classified under nonarticular rheumatism. The proposed mechanism is amplification of pain perception in central nervous system (CNS) and muscle deconditioning. It affects all age groups and is more prevalent in females of middle age. Patients present with gradual onset widespread pain (pain in all four limbs and trunk for at least 3 months), multiple tender points (11 out of 18 tender points, **Fig. 17.20)** and other frequently-associated symptoms (generalized fatigue, sleep disturbances, depression, anxiety, bowel upset, etc.). Tenderness on digital palpation over tender points (with pressure applied being just enough to blanch your finger nail, i.e. 4 kg/cm²) is a characteristic feature. Diagnostic criteria for FMS is given in **Table 17.1**.

Patients usually fail to respond to one form of therapy so multimodality treatment is required for fibromyalgia. Patient

Box 17.4: Diagnostic criteria for chronic fatigue syndrome (CFS)

- *Presence for more than 6 months of* "clinically evaluated, unexplained, persistent or relapsing fatigue that is new or definite onset; is not from ongoing exertion; is not alleviated by rest and results in reduction of occupational/social/personal activities"
- *PLUS Four of the following eight symptoms:*
  1. Postexertion malaise of at least 24 hours
  2. Impairment of short-term memory
  3. Sore throat
  4. Tender cervical/axillary nodes
  5. Muscle pains
  6. Multi-joint pains
  7. Headaches
  8. Unrefreshing sleep

Source: Brukner and Khan, Sports Medicine.

education, psychological support, low-dose NSAIDs, physical therapy for pain (interferential therapy, transcutaneous electric nerve stimulation) and exercise program are the mainstay of treatment. Aerobic exercises improve the muscle deconditioning while low-dose antidepressants (combination of 20 mg fluoxetine in morning and 25 mg amitriptyline at bedtime) take care of disturbed sleep pattern and amplified CNS pain pathways. Manipulative (Manual) therapy is another excellent mode of treatment where a physical or massage therapist uses his hands to pressurize muscles in order to break tissue adhesions and reduce muscle tension. Nonresponders may need corticosteroid injection at tender areas. A psychiatric referral may be needed to rule out a psychiatric disorder.

CHRONIC FATIGUE SYNDROME

Chronic fatigue syndrome (also called as neurasthenia or myalgic encephalomyelitis) is a heterogeneous group of disorders rather than a single disease entity. It is defined as widespread fatigue that interferes with activities of daily living (ADL) for at least 6 months. It is very common in affluent societies amongst women and young adults. Acute infective illnesses, anxiety traits, family history of the condition, history of a depressive episode are some important precipitating factors.

Patients classically present with overwhelming fatigue after physical activity or exercise with headaches, sore throat, diffuse muscle pains and sleep disturbances. Diagnosis is largely clinical and the diagnostic criteria has been given in **Box 17.4**.

Important differentials to consider are FMS, hypothyroidism and depression. FMS is differentiated by presence of characteristic tender points as outlined above causing widespread pain but relatively much less fatigue.

Exercise is the cornerstone of management in these patients. Aerobic activity should be encouraged and intensity in a slow graduated manner. Psychological support, low-dose NSAIDs and antidepressants may also have a role.

18

CHAPTER

Amputations, Prosthetics and Orthotics

INTRODUCTION

Amputation is an iatrogenic or a traumatic removal of all or part of a limb when its blood supply is irreversibly compromised by a disease or severe injury. When the removal occurs through a joint, the term used is disarticulation.

Overall, most common cause of amputation in India is road traffic accidents while chronic peripheral vascular disease (PVD) and diabetes mellitus (DM) remain the most common causes in the world. In children, the most common cause of amputation is a congenital limb deficiency followed by trauma.

EMERGENCY CARE OF A TRAUMATIC AMPUTATION

All traumatic amputations are managed in emergency, according to the advanced trauma life support (ATLS) guidelines. But here first priority is an immediate control of major bleeding. A combat-related casualty or a victim of traumatic amputation is much more likely to die of hemorrhage than an airway problem. So in this situation guidelines change from "ABC" (Airway, breathing and circulation) to "CABC" where "C" stands for catastrophic bleeding (life-threatening hemorrhage). Any major bleeding should be immediately controlled by tourniquet application which should be fixed as distal on the stump as possible. After control of bleeding, next comes the care of airway, breathing and circulation. This is essentially same as emergency care for any trauma victim (*see* Chapter 3). The amputated stump should also be transferred to the hospital as at times it can be reimplanted (*see* Page 108 for details). The part should be cleaned with saline and wrapped in sterile saline soaked gauze and placed in an iced saline container. The amputated part should not come in direct contact with ice.

INDICATIONS

The absolute indication for an amputation is irreversible ischemia in a diseased or traumatized limb due to any cause. At times amputation is needed in malignant neoplasms and fulminant infections (like clostridial gas gangrene) in view of saving the patient's life over the limb. A rare but important situation is a congenital anomaly in a child that has a severely malformed limb that needs amputation for improving cosmesis and function.

However, one must exercise caution in some special situations:

- In cases of crush limb injury, Mangled Extremity Severity (MES) Score (*see* Page 58) is a valuable predictor of limb salvage.
- Frostbite is an indication for amputation, but one should delay amputation until viable tissue is clearly demarcated.

- Clostridial infection of limb causes severe myonecrosis that spreads rapidly within 24 hours and has a typical mousy odor. Such limbs may better be amputated to prevent a fulminant life-threatening toxemia.

TYPES

It can either "guillotine/open" when the skin over the stump is not closed or "closed" when the skin over the stump is sutured. In open amputations, the skin closure is performed after a few days once adequate granulation tissue has formed (secondary closure). In amputation, bone is cut at desired level (with an attempt to save maximum possible bone) and the stump is covered with surrounding muscles and skin flaps.

For stabilization of stump muscles either of the two methods is used:

- *Myodesis*: Here the muscles are attached to bone end by drill holes. This is the preferred method, but contraindicated in patients with severe limb ischemia (e.g. PVD).
- *Myoplasty*: Here muscle is sutured to periosteum, fascia or muscle of an antagonist group. Muscles should preferably be divided around 5 cm distal to the bony resection level.

Once muscles have been stabilized, the skin flaps can be fashioned in either of the following ways:

- *Skewed*: When there is a long posterior flap; commonly preferred method for below knee amputation.
- *Scandinavian*: Where there are equal medial and lateral flaps; mainly used in cases of PVD.

One must also know how to handle the neurovascular bundle. The blood vessels must be doubly ligated with nonabsorbable sutures to prevent any accidental bleeding postoperatively. Nerves are gently pulled and transacted with a sharp knife to ensure that end retracts proximal to the bone ends, thereby preventing the formation of a painful neuroma at the stump. Large nerves like sciatic nerve carry their vasa vasora along and hence should be ligated before transacting.

USE OF TOURNIQUET

The use is desirable as it lessens the blood loss and provides a clear surgical field. But, the limb must be properly exsanguinated before inflating the tourniquet. However, exsanguination is contraindicated in cases where indication is an infection or malignancy for the fear of spreading the pathology proximally.

RECOMMENDED LEVELS IN VARIOUS AMPUTATIONS

Above knee amputation: 18 cm below the tip of greater trochanter or 12 cm from the medial joint line.

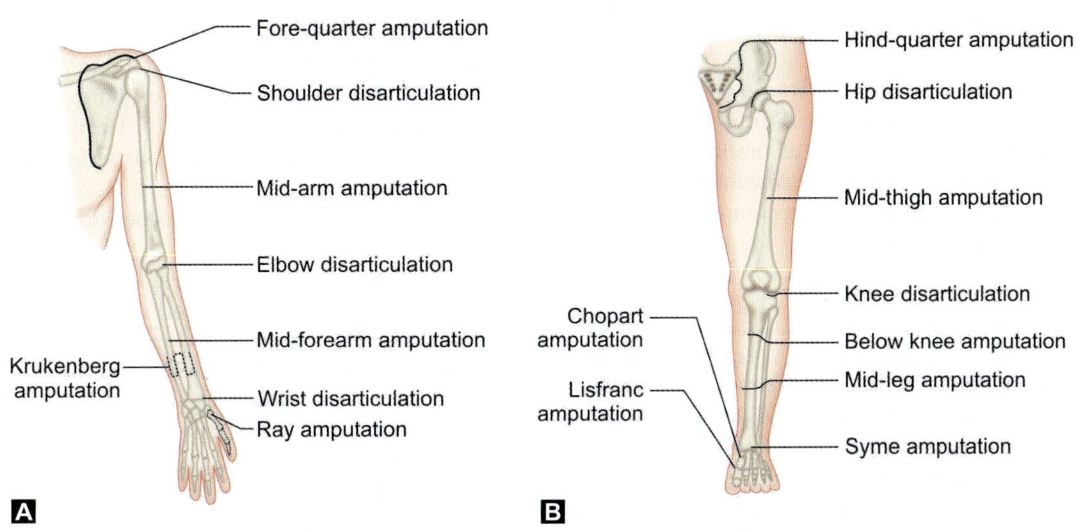

Figs 18.1A and B: Levels of various amputations. (A) Upper limb; (B) Lower limb

Below knee amputation: 15 cm from the medial joint line (ideally at the musculotendinous junction of gastrocnemius).

Above elbow amputation: 20 cm from the acromion.

Below elbow amputation: 18 cm from the tip of olecranon.

NOMENCLATURE FOR SOME SPECIFIC AMPUTATIONS (FIGS 18.1A AND B)

Lower Limb Amputations

Hindquarter amputation: Whole of the lower limb with half of the ilium is removed.

Lisfranc amputation (Lisfranc, France; 1815): Amputation at tarsometatarsal junction.

Chopart amputation: Midtarsal joint amputation.

Syme's amputation: Talus and calcaneus are removed with rotation of heel pad to close the stump through the dome of the ankle. Distal tibia and fibula 0.6 mm proximal to the periphery of the ankle joint are also removed.*

Modifications of Syme's amputation:
- *Sarmiento's amputation:* Distal tibia and fibula are cut 1.3 mm proximal to the ankle joint with excision of medial and lateral malleoli.
- *Boyd's amputation:* In Boyd's amputation, after telectomy calcaneus is shifted forward and calcaneotibial arthrodesis is done.
- *Pirogoff's amputation:* Vertical section of the calcaneus is performed through the middle and calcaneus is rotated forward to fuse to the tibia. Talectomy is performed as well.
  Basically, both Boyd and Pirogoff's amputation involve calcaneotibial arthrodesis.

Upper Limb Amputations

Forequarter amputation: Removal of scapula along with a portion of clavicle and whole of the upper limb.

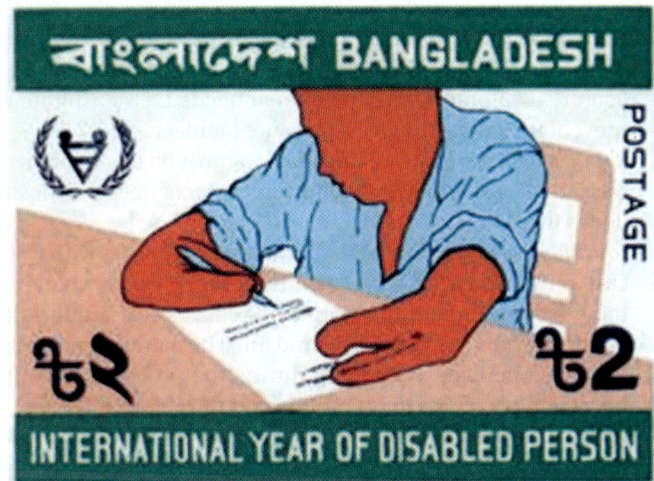

Fig. 18.2: Stamp published by Bangladesh government showing Krukenberg amputation

Krukenberg amputation: It is done in below elbow amputation to provide a pincer grasp. It is primarily indicated in blind bilateral hand amputee. This amputation separates the radius and ulna in a shape of forceps (motored by pronator teres muscle) to be used as a makeshift pincer **(Fig. 18.2)**.

Ray amputation: Removal of a finger/toe with respective metacarpal/metatarsal.

AFTER TREATMENT

Once the amputation has been completed, the stump is dressed. Two types of dressings are in use. A soft dressing is the traditional dressing with gauze, cotton and bandage. A rigid dressing involves application of a molded Plaster of Paris slab over the conventional dressing to cover the stump. This helps in restricting blood loss and also enhances wound healing. Another major advantage is that a temporary prosthesis called a Pylon (endoskeletal

---

*Knee disarticulation and Syme's amputation have end bearing stumps. End bearing stumps are those stumps where bone ends are metaphyseal and weight can be taken through the end of the stump.

prosthesis) can be fitted to the stump and the patient can be mobilized immediately.

Wrapping a crepe bandage over the stump is also advisable to promote shrinkage and maturation. Stump exercises are immediately started to maintain range of motion of adjacent joints and build up the strength of muscles controlling the stump. Prosthetic fitting and gait training can be accomplished in about 2–3 months time after the amputation.

SPECIAL CONSIDERATIONS IN CHILDREN

For performing an amputation in children, Krajbich principles are often looked at. In children, aim should be to preserve the growth plates and all length possible. In lower limb amputations, where ever possible knee joint should be preserved. Disarticulation is preferred over transosseous amputation. The most common issue that bothers in most cases is the terminal bone growth that sometimes needs revision. One way of dealing with this problem is to use epiphyseal caps to cover medullary canals.

COMPLICATIONS

The complications include:
- *Bleeding*: Bleeding from stump can occur due to inadequate hemostasis achieved during surgery or from slipping of a ligature. Exploration may be done if needed, else aspirate to prevent infection and give a pressure bandage.
- *Skin flap necrosis*: Suture line tension must be low to prevent this. Small areas may heal while large area of necrosis mostly needs revision flaps.
- *Infection*: Mostly seen in diabetic patients or in cases with PVD. One must always prefer a secondary skin closure whenever there is doubt about the viability of soft tissues around the stump. Any discharge from wound must be handled seriously. Excessive periosteal stripping during the procedure should be avoided as if this gets complicated further by infection, a ring sequestrum may form at the stump.
- *Postamputation neuroma*: To prevent postamputation painful neuroma the nerves are generally pulled before cutting them during amputation and in case it forms, the best treatment is excision. While ultrasonic therapy is not much effective, pulsed radiofrequency ablation, interferential therapy (IFT) and transcutaneous electrical nerve stimulation (TENS) may have a role. TENS is most preferred and works by inhibiting pain gate pathway.
- *Phantom sensations*: It refers to a situation where the patient feels that the amputated part is still present and he is getting discomforting sensations from that part. Phantom sensations are extremely distressing and are present in 30–80% patients. More proximal is the amputation, more are the sensations felt. The problem tends to diminish with time. By the end of the first year phantom limb gradually shortens to stump end (known as Telescoping). Treatment is difficult and antidepressants, opioids, ketamine, TENS and increased prosthetic use all have been reported to provide some benefits.
- *Joint contractures*: These result from improper positioning of stump and inadequate physiotherapy. Contractures preclude the appropriate use of prosthesis and hence must be prevented.

HIGH-YIELD POINTS

- Interesting historical facts about amputations:
  - Amboise Pare, a French military surgeon, introduced the use of ligatures in 1529. He is called the Father of amputation surgery. He also performed the first elbow disarticulation.
  - First hip disarticulation was performed by William Kerr of England in 1774.
  - Antiseptic techniques were introduced by Joseph Lister (Father of antiseptic surgery, 1867).
- Most common amputation overall—transtibial.
- Risk of wound complications is increased when the patient has a low total lymphocyte count (TLC) level and a low serum albumin level.
- In diabetics, a below knee amputation is relatively contraindicated due to vascular issues.
- Lisfranc and Chopart amputations have a severe tendency to go into equinus.
- Amputees are advised to walk slow and take longer steps rather than taking several short steps to lower their energy consumption.
- *Jactitation*: Refers to a distressing phantom limb pain with involuntary jerking of stump.
- There is no phantom limb sensation in congenital limb deficiencies and patients with brain damage.
- Syme's amputation (*Edinberg, James Syme, 1843*):
  - It is more energy efficient than mid-foot amputation even though it is more proximal
  - Stable heel pad is the most important factor in Syme's amputation as migration of the heel pad is the most important complication. It has been used successfully to treat forefoot gangrene in diabetics, but the patent tibialis posterior artery is a prerequisite.
- Energy expenditure with amputation at various levels is inversely proportional to length of remaining limb:
  - Long below knee amputation—10%
  - Medium below knee amputation—25%
  - Short below knee amputation—40%
  - Average above knee amputation—65%
  - Hip disarticulation—100%.

PROSTHETICS AND REHABILITATION OF AN AMPUTEE

INTRODUCTION

For an amputee the duty of a surgeon extends way beyond performing the procedure. In fact, a much bigger challenge is rehabilitation of these patients. It is imperative to integrate emotionally with the patient, provide him psychological counseling and make his disability socially acceptable by providing an appropriate replacement for the lost part.

Prosthesis (plural: prostheses, a Greek word meaning an addition, application or attachment) is an artificial device (metallic or non-metallic) that replaces a body part. It is a functional replacement for an amputated or congenitally malformed or missing limb. A prosthesis can replace an internal body part (e.g. hemiarthroplasty prosthesis) or replaces the part externally (e.g.

artificial limb). It is easier to design a prosthesis for a lower limb, but in upper limb, considering the dexterity, functional demand and cosmesis, still a lot of advancement is needed to achieve satisfactory designs.

TYPES

A prosthesis may be provided at times only for a cosmetic problem while at most other times the aim is to improve functional performance. Since the prosthesis lacks proprioception and muscle power, the power forces are provided to the prosthesis by movement of either the residual limb or the normal limb on the other side. Such prostheses are called as body powered prosthesis. In other cases, one can opt for an externally powered prosthesis (battery-operated prosthesis or myoelectric prosthesis).

Some commonly used prostheses are:
- *Above knee prosthesis*: Quadrilateral socket prosthesis
- *Below knee amputation*: Patellar tendon bearing prosthesis
- *Syme's amputation*: Canadian Syme's prosthesis
- *Partial foot amputations*: Shoe fillers.

PARTS OF PROSTHESIS

A prosthetic device is broadly divided into the following parts **(Fig. 18.3)**:
- *Socket*: It is the part of the prosthesis that contacts the stump. These could be end bearing sockets where whole weight is borne by the end of the stump or total contact sockets where weight is distributed throughout the surface of the socket. They are custom made to fit the stump.
- *Suspension*: It holds the socket in contact with the stump.
- *Prosthetic extension with substitutive joints (Shank/Pylon*)*: Some prosthesis may have additional joints depending upon the length of the prosthesis and parts of the limb to be replaced.
- *Terminal device*: This is the distal most part of the prosthesis. The traditional terminal device for lower limb prosthesis (i.e. the foot) has been the solid ankle cushion heel (SACH) foot (introduced by University of California in 1995). It has a compressible heel cushion wedge that provides "pseudo-plantar

flexion" after heel strike and a rigid keel **(Fig. 18.4)**. Ankle action is provided by the soft rubber heel which gets compressed under load during the early part of the stance phase of walking **(Figs 18.5A and B)**. This SACH foot has been modified by an Indian doctor, Dr PK Sethi, to make it suitable for barefoot walking. The same has been named as Jaipur foot **(Fig. 18.6,** for differences *see* **Table 18.1)**. Another modern day innovation has been the SAFE (solid ankle-flexible-endoskeletal) foot. It has the same principle as the SACH foot with the ability for the sole to conform to slightly irregular surfaces and thus makes it better suited for the amputee to walk over uneven terrain. Feet of this type make walking easier because of the flexibility, and are sometimes called "flexible keel" feet **(Fig. 18.7)**. Most recent developments include the dynamic response feet, which are indicated where the gait patterns generate enough energy to be worth storing. For this reason, they are called "energy storing feet". They incorporate elastic keel structures that absorb energy during midstance and terminal stance, and then "release" it during preswing and initial swing.

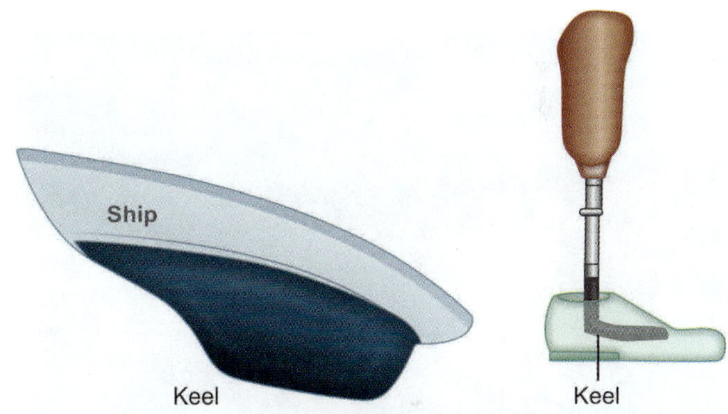

Fig. 18.4: Keel of a ship compared with keel of foot

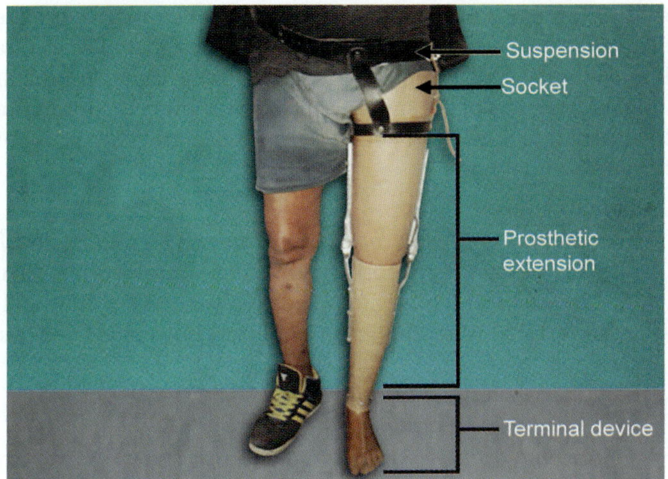

Fig. 18.3: Parts of a prosthesis

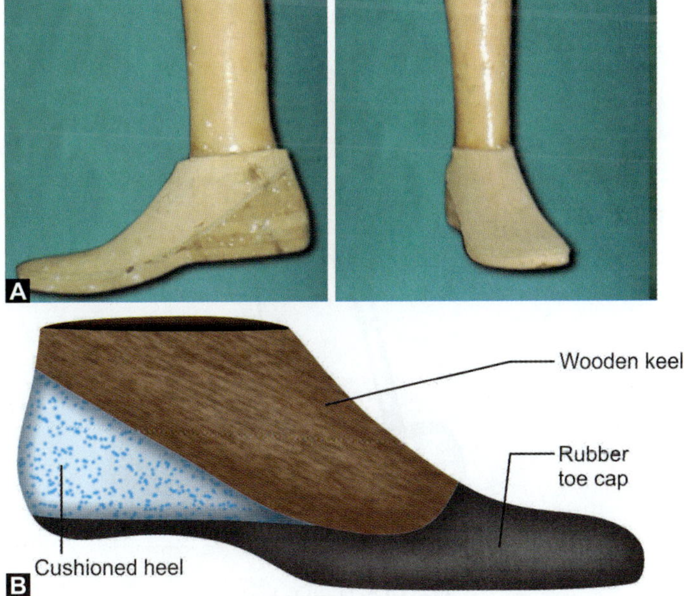

Figs 18.5A and B: Solid ankle cushion heel foot

---

*'Pylon' word here should not be confused with a temporary endoskeletal prosthesis used immediately after an amputation that is also called Pylon.

Table 18.1: Differences between Jaipur and solid ankle cushion heel (SACH) foot

Jaipur foot	SACH foot
It looks like a normal foot so the patient does not need to wear shoe over it. However, amputee can use shoe satisfactorily over it. For the same reason barefoot walking is possible	It requires a shoe over it for walking and also to hide it. Barefoot walking is not possible
It has metallic keel which is confined to the ankle only and allows for dorsiflexion and plantar flexion to take place and thus allowing for squatting	It has a rigid wooden keel which does not allow for dorsiflexion and plantar flexion and thus, squatting is not possible
Jaipur foot allows for adequate inversion and eversion of terminal piece so walking on uneven and muddy surface is comfortable	Walking only on level ground is comfortable as it does not allow for inversion and eversion at "sub tarsal" level
Cross-legged sitting is possible due to adequate forefoot adduction and transverse rotation of the foot	Cross-legged sitting is not possible
It is very cheaper than a SACH foot. It can be made from locally available material by rural artisan	It is very costlier than Jaipur foot. Modern technology with skilled personnel is required to manufacture it
Shock absorbing capacity is less than a SACH foot	The shock absorbing capacity is more than a SACH foot
It meets the sociocultural needs (bare foot walking, cross legged sitting) of Indian and many Asian populations	It does not meet such needs

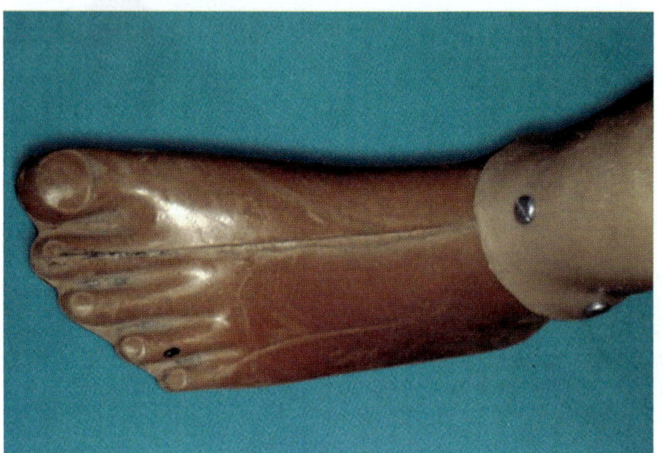

Fig. 18.6: Jaipur foot

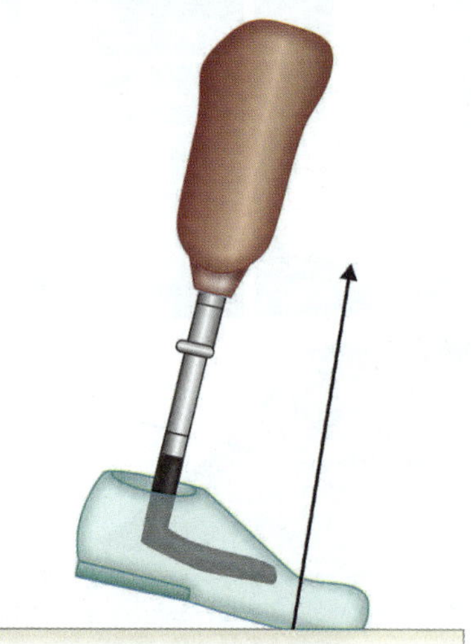

Fig. 18.7: Flexible keel

ORTHOTICS AND OTHER RELATED DEVICES

INTRODUCTION

Orthosis (plural: orthoses) is a device that aids or supports a body part and enhances the structural and functional characteristics of the skeletal system.

They can be classified as "static" or "dynamic" types. Static orthosis is rigid and gives support without allowing any movements. It basically supports a fractured limb, a painful joint or is used to prevent joint contractures by keeping limbs in functional position. A Dynamic orthosis device allows movements in some directions.

NOMENCLATURE OF ORTHOTICS

Earlier, various orthoses were called by different names, viz. braces, calipers, splints, corsets, etc. To avoid confusions a systematic nomenclature was developed in 1972 to name the orthoses. This terminology uses the first letter of each joint crossed by the orthosis in sequence, with letter "O" fixed at last (signifying orthosis). For example, an orthosis for foot drop crosses the ankle and is called ankle-foot orthosis and designated as AFO, a thoracolumbosacral orthosis (TLSO), affects the thoracic, lumbar and sacral regions of the spine. Orthoses are now classified as per the different regions at which they are applied and named as per the above guidelines.

- Spinal orthosis*:
  - *Cervical and cervicothoracic orthoses (Figs 18.8A to E)*: Cervical and cervicothoracic orthoses, previously known as cervical collar, four post-collars, SOMI (Sternal-Occipital-Mandibular Immobilizer) brace, halo devices, etc.
  - Thoracolumbar orthoses **(Figs 18.9A to C)**
  - Lumbosacral orthoses.
- *Upper limb orthoses:* Wrist Hand Orthosis (WHO, previously known as cock-up splint).

*Spinal orthosis used in scoliosis have been discussed in Chapter 7.

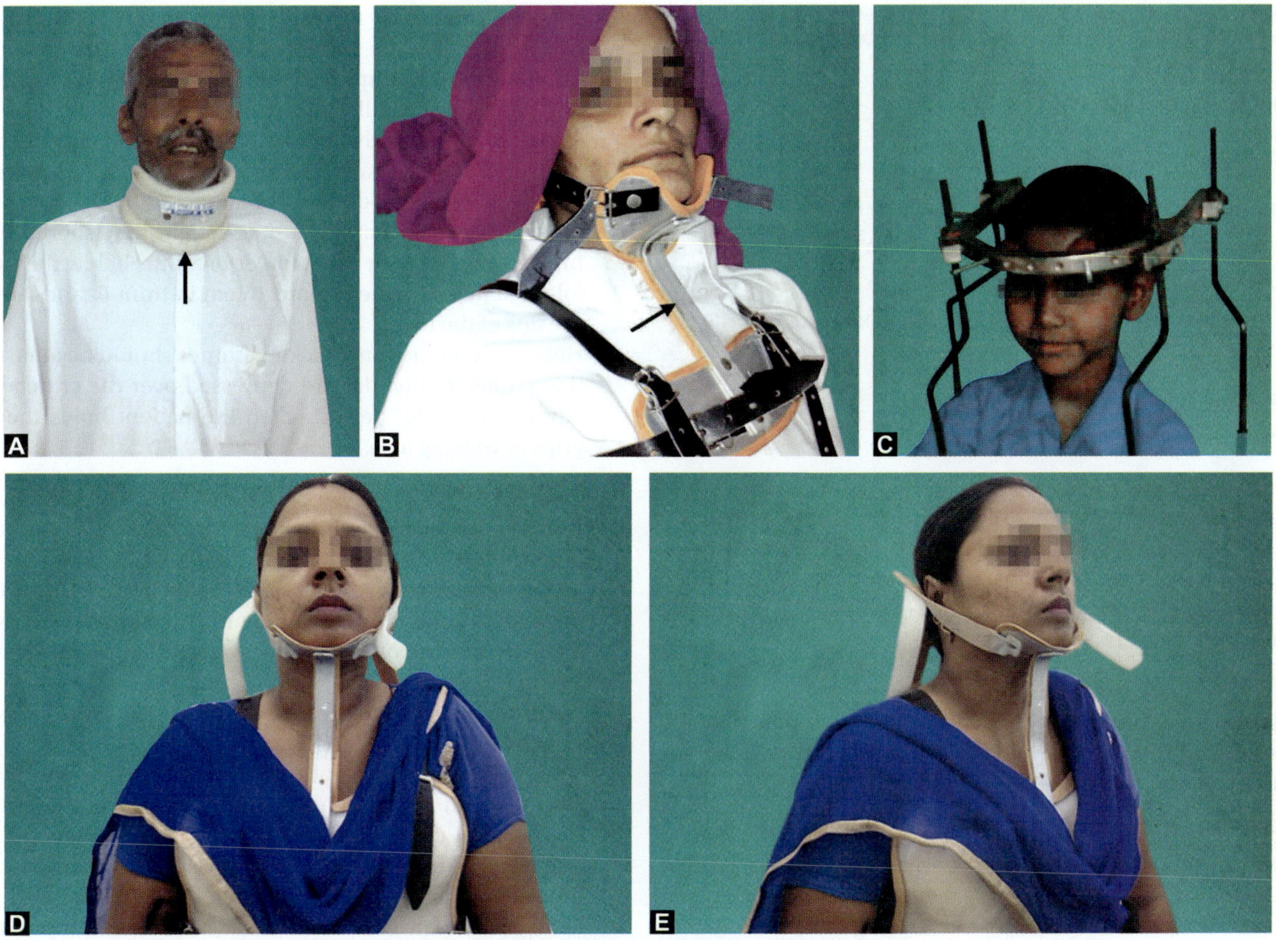

Figs 13.8A to E: Cervical and cervicothoracic orthoses. (A) Hard cervical collar; (B) Four post collar; (C) Halo device; (D and E) SOMI (Sternal-Occipital-Mandibular Immobilizer) brace

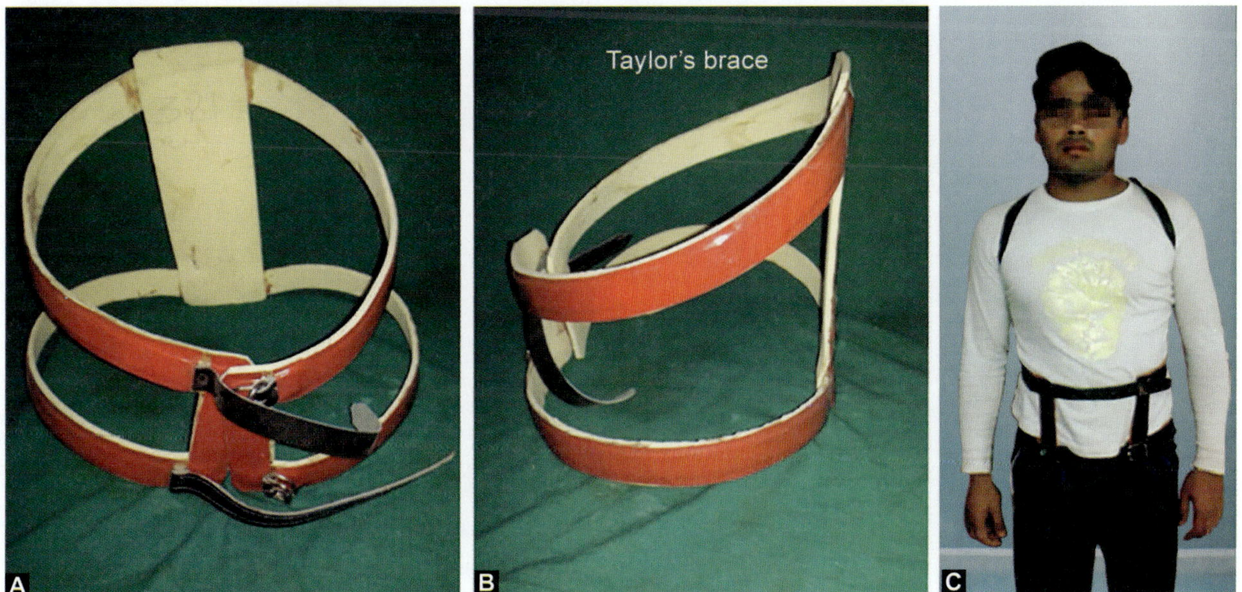

Figs 18.9A to C: Thoracolumbar orthosis

Table 18.2: Footwear modifications for various indications

Footwear	Indications
Thomas heel (Crooked and Elongated heel)	Flat foot
CTEV shoes	Clubfoot
Silicone heel pad	Plantar fascütis
Metatarsal bar	Metatarsalgia
Inner/medial border raise	Genu valgum
Outer/lateral border raise	Genu varum and osteoarthritis
Metatarsal pad	Corn
Arch support	Flat foot

Abbreviation: CTEV, congenital talipes equinovarus.

- *Lower limb orthoses:* Ankle Foot Orthosis (AFO, previously called as below knee caliper), Knee Ankle Foot orthosis (KAFO, previously known as above knee caliper), Hip Knee Ankle Foot Orthosis (HKAFO), Knee orthosis (KO, previously known as knee brace), etc.

FOOTWEAR MODIFICATIONS

Footwear can also be modified to relieve or improve pain in many foot problems. The footwear modifications that are available for various indications are given in **Table 18.2**.

AMBULATORY AIDS

An ambulatory (walking) aid is a device that helps a patient to maintain functional independence by increasing the area of support and maintaining the center of gravity within that area. Walking aids are used for ambulation of injured or disabled patients who are not able to bear body weight on their lower limbs. Walking aids enable the patients to bear some- body weight on their upper limbs. Examples of walking aids are sticks, crutches, walking frames and parallel bars.

A cane or crutch is always carried in the hand opposite to the side of pathology (*see* Page 119 for explanation). Adjustment of height of walking aids is done as follows:

- If axillary crutches are of proper height they should extend from a point 5 cm or three finger breadths below the axillary fold to a point on the ground 15 cm in front of and lateral to the tips of the toes.
- Height of crutches and walking frames should be adjusted so that patient's shoulder are depressed over the crutches and elbows are at 30° flexion when the patient holds the hand grips of walking aids.

HIGH-YIELD POINTS

- In India first artificial limb center was started in the Armed Force Medical College, Pune.
- Jewett brace is a hyperextension thoracolumbar orthosis that prevents a patient from bending forwards. It may be used to facilitate healing of an anterior wedge fracture involving the T10 to L3 vertebrae.
- Weight transmission in single cane is 20–25%, but in axillary crutch it is up to 80%.
- Floor reaction orthosis (also called Ground Reaction AFO): A floor reaction AFO is generally used with patients affected by neurological conditions such as spina bifida, cerebral palsy, and post-polio paralysis. In these cases, the floor reaction AFO functions to maintain the affected joints in proper alignment, to accentuate knee extension at midstance and compensate for weak or absent gastroc-soleus (calf) muscles.

promotes callus formation, speeding-up union. Dynamization around 10–12 weeks of fracture fixation generally gives good results.

- *Reduced working length (WL):* WL is the length of the unsupported part of the nail between the proximal and the distal firm grip of the nail and the bone. Stability of fixation against the bending forces is inversely proportional to WL. In comminuted fractures supported length of the nail is small and working length increases. Static locking in modern interlock nails reduces working length **(Fig. 19.3B)** and thus increases stability.

BONE PLATING

INTRODUCTION

The journey of plating of long bone fractures has been more than 100 years long. The earliest references in literature for application of a metal plate credited to Carl Hansmann (Germany, 1886) and William Lane (England, 1895). However, innovations in design and technique by Lambotte and Sherman in the early years of the 19th century were behind the great expansion of this unique method of internal fixation. Surprisingly, most of these plates were soon abandoned, owing to problems with corrosion, strength and high rates of failure.

Success shortly ensued as greater understanding of the aims and technique developed. In the earlier part of the plating era, designs aimed to achieve rigid fixation of fracture to ensure absolute stability (zero movement at fracture site). This was achieved at the expense of surgical exposure and hence open reduction of fractures was the standard method for plate application which involved significant soft tissue stripping from bone. Fractures in such cases healed with primary healing (no callus formation) owing to rigid fixation. As entire plate rested against bone surface, there was excessive plate-bone contact. Researchers hypothesized that this excessive plate-bone contact interfered with cortical perfusion. Hence, absence of callus formation, cortical bone loss under the plate (due to disruption of periosteal blood supply by excessive plate-bone contact) and risk of refracture after plate removal were among limitations associated with these designs. This lead to a revolutionary era of changing concepts and biological fixation (preservation of soft tissue and blood supply of bone) became the aim. Target was to minimally disturb the fracture site (attempt closed reduction), limit the plate-bone contact area and aim for relative stability (micromotion remains at fracture site). Healing in such cases was secondary with callus formation. Results improved and this method of fracture fixation became an integral component of the orthopedic treatment.

EVOLUTION OF THE PLATING TECHNIQUE

Better understanding of the plating concepts generated a string of plating designs, each with its own unique legacy.

Dynamic Compression Plating

In mid-19th century, concept of dynamic compression plating with interfragmentary compression came in vogue. In 1958, Bagby and Janes presented a plate they called dynamic compression plate **(DCP, Fig. 19.4A)**, with especially designed oval holes (as opposed to circular holes) to provide dynamic interfragmentary compression. These oval-shaped holes (cut-out of double cylinder) had inclined edges. Due to this feature, when the screw is threaded into the hole eccentrically, it causes movement of the plate, thereby bringing compression at the fracture site (*see* Page 31 in Chapter 2 for details). The limitations with this method were cortical bone loss under the plate due to high plate-bone contact area and lack of a biological approach (periosteum and soft tissue preservation), hence with time advancements ensued.

Biological Plate Osteosynthesis

In 1958, Arbeitsgemeinschaft für Osteosynthesefragen (AO) group (read later) was formed, that developed a new plate which was claimed to reduce interference with cortical perfusion. They called it as the limited contact-dynamic compression plate **(LC-DCP, Fig. 19.4B)**. LC-DCP combined both principles of dynamic compression and biological fixation. In addition to compression holes as in a DCP, it has multiple furrows (cut-outs) on the undersurface, thereby limiting the contact surface with the bone **(Fig. 19.4A)**. By limiting the contact surface, less of periosteum is damaged and hence large surface is allowed for the ingrowth of bone and periosteal blood vessels. Limited compression of the periosteal blood supply (biological fixation) not just improves healing at the fracture site but also avoids the stress risers at implant removal.

Locked Compression Plating

The initial encouraging results and optimism with LC-DCP were contradicted by many cadaveric and clinical studies which failed to show any difference in cortical blood flow between DCP and LC-DCP group. This led to the development of the point-contact fixator (PC-Fix, not available in market now) and the LISS (Less Invasive Stabilization System, 2001) that eventually surfaced as the modern day locking compression plate (LCP) system in 2003. LCP not just further reduced the plate bone contact area, it also brought a new concept of self-tapping monocortical screw fixation due to provision for locking holes in the plate into which screw head gets locked **(Fig. 19.4A)**. The screw holes of this plate have threads with high pitch and screws for this plate (locking screws) also have threads in their heads that can be locked to the holes in the plates. This feature enables some salient advantages as outlined here:

- Since screws hold on to the plate by locking in the plate holes, it affords a rigid fixation even if the quality of bone is poor. In fact, locking plate is especially designed for rigid fixation in cases of periarticular fractures and fractures of osteoporotic bones, where screws hold to the plate (as hold in bone might not be good) and provide rigid fixation. Most modern LCPs allow insertion of multiple locking screws in converging and diverging directions to provide an excellent angular stability.
- LCP act as an internal fixator **(Fig. 19.4B)**, where the screws (c.f. pins of external fixator), which are the principal load-transferring elements, are locked in the plate (c.f. tubular rods of external fixator). As plate is not compressed against the bone (low plate-bone contact area) and the forces are transferred to the plate across the screws, periosteal blood supply is preserved. Hence, less cortical bone loss under the plate and no risk of stress fractures on implant removal.

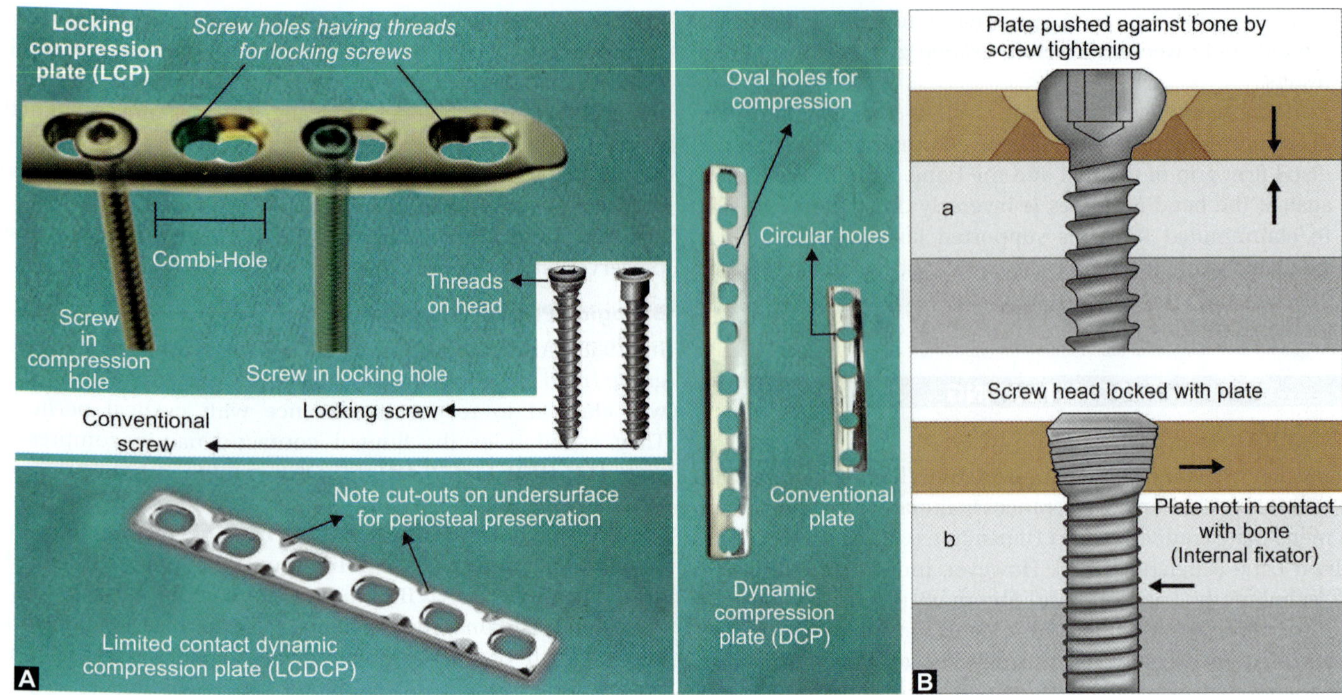

Figs 19.4A and B: (A) Different types of plates; (B) Diagram depicting locking plate acting as an internal fixator. Note how conventional plate is pushed by a screw to contact the entire bone surface (a) causing periosteal damage while a locking plate stays at few millimeters distance from bone (b) due to locking of screw head in locking hole

- Modern LCPs classically have "combi-holes" where one part of the hole has locking threads to incorporate locking screws while the other part of the hole is similar to DCP (oval hole cut-out of double cylinder). This allows it to be used in locking mode where needed offering the above advantages but also at the same time it can also be used to provide compression at fracture site by inserting eccentric screws in oval holes **(Fig. 19.4B)**.

Minimally Invasive Plate Osteosynthesis

While plating concepts were evolving, simultaneously implantation methods were also changing, focusing on minimizing operative dissection, preserving the periosteal blood supply and fracture hematoma and causing less damage to the soft tissue envelope around the fracture. All these efforts led to the development of less traumatizing percutaneous approach (with minimal skin incisions). Both LISS and LCP can be put, using minimally invasive plate osteosynthesis (MIPO) technique. These plates are anatomical or precontoured according to shape of bone and particularly used to fix comminuted metaphyseal fractures.

MIPO Technique

Locking compression plates, anatomically contoured to periarticular bone, are introduced through small incisions **(Figs 19.5A and B)** in epiperiosteal plane.

Fracture site is not opened, and fracture reduction is done by indirect techniques using traction and reduction forceps. Plate bridges the comminuted metaphyseal fracture and screws are put proximal and distal to this comminution (Bridge plating mode, *see* Page 31).

Advantages of MIPO Technique

Locked compression plate does not compress the periosteal blood supply. Thus, the fracture's biological environment is largely maintained and it improves the healing rates and reduces complications. Faster healing, less nonunion rates, reduced complication rates, shorter operative time and smaller skin incisions are advantages of MIPO technique.

HIGH-YIELD POINTS

- Less invasive stabilization system and LCP, both are types of locked compression plates. While LISS plates have only locking holes, LCPs have holes for both conventional screws and locking screws (Hybrid holes or combi-holes). Thus, LCP can be used as a compression as well as hybrid locking plate and is an advanced version from LISS.
- LCP can be fixed or variable angle plates. In fixed angle LCPs, screws have to be put only at a preguided angle so that they can lock with the plate. Variable angle locked compression plates are provided with some mechanism (e.g. expansion ring or a locknut) which allows the screw to be angled 10–15° within the hole and yet lock with the plate.
- Screws in a DCP or LC-DCP can be angled maximum up to 40°.

AO/ASIF'S LATEST CONCEPTS IN FRACTURE FIXATION

In 1958, a group of Swiss orthopedic surgeons formed an organization that they named the Arbeitsgemeinschaft für Osteosynthesefragen (AO), German term for the Association for

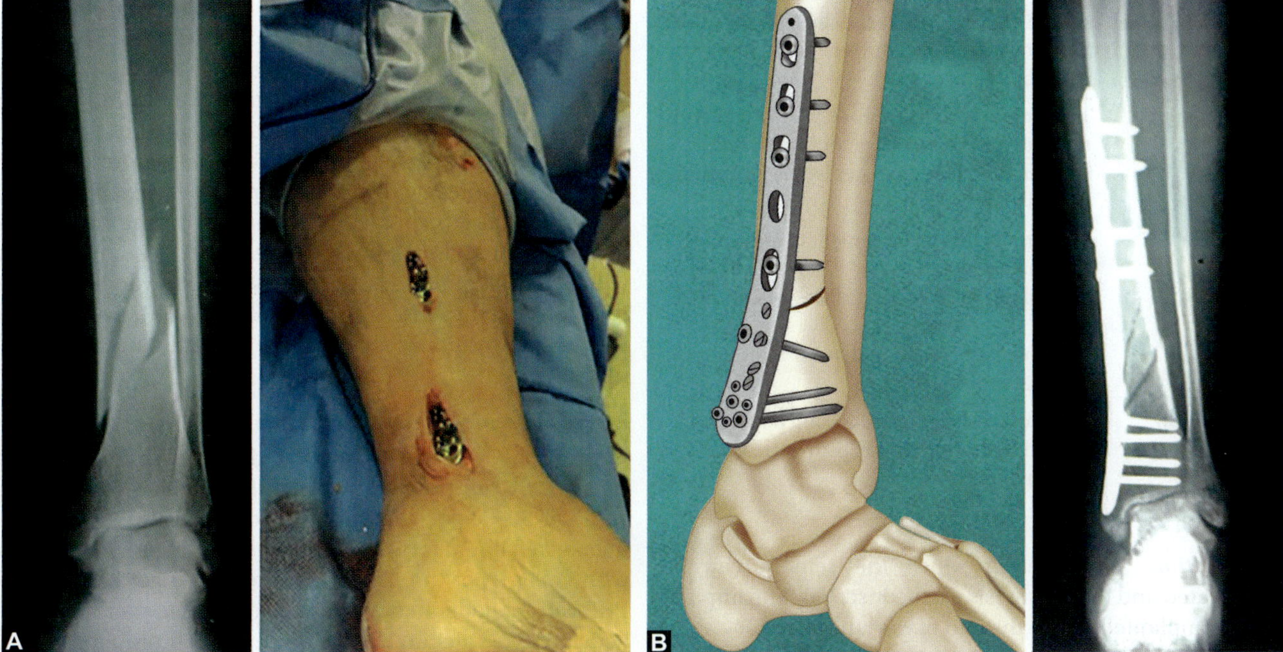

Figs 19.5A and B: Minimally invasive plate osteosynthesis (MIPO) technique. Anatomical precontoured locking plate inserted in epiperiosteal plane without opening the fracture site. Bridge plating performed using MIPO technique. See that no screw has been put in fractured/comminuted part of the bone. Only small skin incisions have been given at two ends to enable screw insertion for plate fixation

the Study of Internal Fixation (ASIF). Eminent members in the founding group were Maurice Muller [main proponent of the internal fixation concept, Orthopedic Surgeon of the century, a title conferred to him by the International Orthopedic Society (SICOT)], Robert Danis and Ruedi Allgower.

This foundation is involved in conducting research, developing new techniques for fracture fixation and in designing high quality orthopedic implants. It also runs training courses on internal fixation of fractures for orthopedic surgeons across the world. The organization has propagated standard principles for fracture fixation **(Box 19.2)** that all orthopedic surgeons are advised to follow.

BONE CEMENT

INTRODUCTION

Bone cement is one of the biggest inventions that have revolutionized orthopedic surgeries.

CONSTITUENTS

Commercially available bone cement has one liquid (methyl methacrylate monomer) and one powder component [polymer, polymethylmethacrylate (PMMA)]. Mixing of polymer to monomer produces a dough that can be modulated. Bone cement actually acts as a grout (space filler, no adhesive properties) by producing interlocking fit between surfaces.

HOW TO USE

It is prepared during surgery by mixing the monomer liquid and polymer powder. After mixing in a bowl, it is stirred well. It takes

Box 19.2: Current AO principles of fracture care

1. Reduction of fracture to restore anatomy*
2. Fracture fixation to provide absolute or relative stability depending on the fracture and the patient**
3. Preservation of blood supply to soft tissues and the bone
4. Early and safe mobilization of the injured part and the patient as a whole

*In articular fractures and in metaphyseal and diaphyseal fractures of forearm bones (which act as an articular unit), anatomical reduction is required. However, in metaphyseal and diaphyseal fractures of any other bone perfect anatomical reduction is not required and the relationship between main proximal and distal fragments should restored along with maintenance of length, alignment and rotation. This is called functional/acceptable reduction.

**Absolute stability means that fracture site is so fixed that there is no movement at the fracture site. It is required in articular fractures and forearm fracture. Means to achieve it includes lag screw and compression plating. In absolute stability, callus formation is not seen and bone unites by primary healing. Relative stability is characterized by a little movement at the fracture site. It is required in metaphyseal and diaphyseal fractures of the long bones. It is achieved by bridging plate, intramedullary nail and external fixator. Micromotion at the fracture site promotes callus formation and fracture heals by secondary healing.

few minutes to become dough when it is ready to apply to the bone surfaces or to insert into the femoral canal. After application of bone cement on the bone surfaces (or putting bone cement into femoral canal) implantation is done.

The whole process is divided into four phases:

1. *Mixing time*: Time taken by the powder and liquid to fully integrate.
2. *Dough time*: From the beginning of mixing to the point when the cement no longer sticks to surgical gloves.

Table 19.1: Mixing techniques

First generation	Hand mixing of cement, it is put in the canal by a finger
Second generation	The femoral canal is prepared by brush and made dry. Cement restrictor is inserted into the canal and then cement is put using cement gun
Third generation	Vacuum-mixing of the cement to reduce cement porosity Pulsatile lavage of bone surfaces and femoral canal Cement pressurization for better bone penetration
Fourth generation	The prosthesis is inserted using distal and proximal centralizers to ensure an even cement mantle

3. *Working time*: Time during which the cement can be manipulated and the prosthesis can be inserted. The implant must be implanted before the end of working time.
4. *Setting time*: Time from the beginning of mixing until the time at which the exothermic reaction heats the cement (usually 10–12 minutes).

Mixing Techniques

Mixing techniques have been discussed in **Table 19.1**.

HIGH-YIELD POINTS

- Barium sulfate is added to bone cement to make it radiopaque.
- *Antibiotic impregnated bone cement*: Many antibiotics (which are heat stable) can be added to bone cement to be delivered at surgical sites. Gentamicin, tobramycin, cefuroxime, vancomycin are commonly added antibiotics.
- Factors increasing bone cement dough and setting time:
  - Decreased temperature of OT
  - Decreased humidity
  - Slow mixing.
- *Bone cement implantation syndrome:* It occurs at the time of cementation, reaming, prosthesis insertion or at the time of tourniquet deflation in replacement surgeries (mostly during hip replacement) and is characterized by hypoxia, hypotension and/or loss of consciousness. Although exact cause is unknown, recent theories that have been proposed for its occurrence relate it to the release of cement particles/emboli into the circulation during cementation and resultant right ventricular failure.

ORTHOBIOLOGICS

INTRODUCTION

"Orthobiologics", refers to the relatively new treatment modality for healing of musculoskeletal injuries by the use of biological substances, viz. bone grafts, autologous blood, platelet-rich plasma (PRP), and stem cells. They are mainly used for treatment of injured tendons, ligaments and bone nonunion. Bone grafts have already been discussed in Chapter 2 and this chapter will focus on role of other orthobiologics.

AUTOLOGOUS BLOOD AND PLATELET-RICH PLASMA

Autologous blood injection (ABI) involves injecting one's own blood at the site of pathology. PRP on the other hand is a fraction of autologous blood having a platelet concentration 4–5 times above baseline. Platelets contain alpha granules which release clotting and growth factors (transforming growth factor beta, vascular endothelial growth factor, platelet-derived growth factor, and epithelial growth factor) and speed up the healing process in the diseased area. Since ABI delivers RBCs and WBCs along with platelets, the platelets are delivered in a very low concentration compared to PRP. So the results of ABI have been variable with mixed results. Hence, PRP is currently the more preferred modality.

Preparation of Platelet-rich Plasma

Approximately 3 cc or 6 cc of PRP is made after about 10–12 minutes of centrifugation (first a hard spin followed by a soft spin) of 30–60 mL of venous blood. The PRP so produced is inactivated liquid form that gets activated after coming in contact with collagen of the tissues. To produce a gel like consistency, PRP can be generated as an activated form after addition of an activator like calcium chloride or topical thrombin that activates the clotting cascade.

Orthopedic Applications of Platelet-rich Plasma

Platelet-rich plasma is increasingly used in the treatment of chronic nonhealing tendon injuries including medial and lateral epicondylitis, patellar tendinitis, Achilles tendinitis and rotator cuff tendinopathy and tear. It has also been used with favorable results in early osteoarthritis of the knee.

STEM CELLS IN ORTHOPEDICS

For a cell to be called as a stem cell it must have the capacity to differentiate into the desired daughter cell with the self-renewal capacity of the daughter cell. Off late there has been considerable interest in stem cell treatment as the potential it holds may be revolutionary.

Types of Stem Cells

Totipotent stem cells are most powerful stem cells, which can differentiate to form all of the embryonic and extraembryonic cells. Totipotent stem cells are obtained within a few hours of cell divisions after fertilization (at, or before, the morula stage). At the blastocyst stage the embryo contains pluripotent stem cells, which can divide either into embryonic cells or extraembryonic cells. Adult stem cells are multipotent, i.e. they can produce cells of a specific cell lineage only. Mesenchymal stem cells (MSCs) have attracted maximum attention of orthopedic surgeons because of their ability to differentiate into bone and cartilage. MSCs have been obtained from bone marrow, adipose tissue, synovium and periosteum.

Orthopedic Applications of MSCs

Mesenchymal stem cells are either injected directly at the site of repair or a carrier of suitable biomaterial can be used to deliver the stem cells. Collagen, fibrin, gelatin, and hyaluronic acid are most frequently used as a scaffold to deliver stem cells at the site of repair. Current research on use of stem cells in orthopedics is focusing on areas such as tendon and ligament repair, cartilage regeneration, atrophic nonunion of a fracture and bone defects.

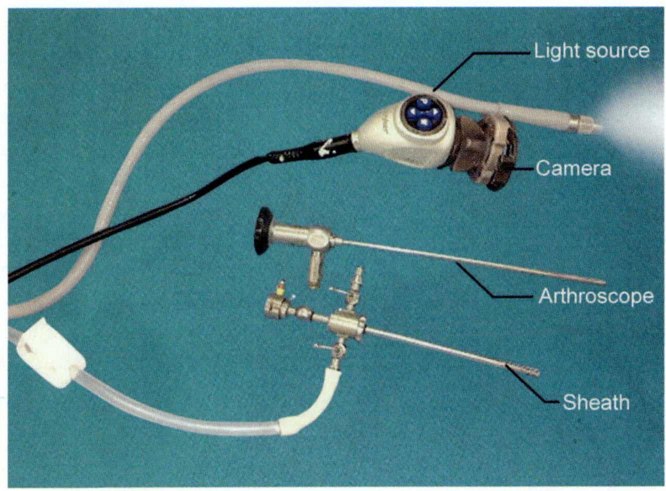

Fig. 19.6: Arthroscope—camera and light source

ARTHROSCOPIC SURGERY

INTRODUCTION

Arthroscopic surgery is a minimally invasive surgical procedure, which allows examination and management of many joint disorders using an arthroscope and arthroscopic instruments. An arthroscope is an endoscope that is inserted into the joint through a very small incision (called the viewing portal) to visualize the interior of the joint. The arthroscope is attached to a camera and a light source to see inside the joint **(Fig. 19.6)**. Arthroscopic instruments are especially designed instruments that are inserted into the joint through another small incision (the working portal) to perform the procedure. The working and the viewing portals, though, are fixed for every joint, they can be switched as per the surgeon's convenience.

Arthroscopic surgery has various advantages over conventional surgery:

- *Small incisions and scars*: Usually stab incisions are given for making portals which heal with minimal scarring.
- Less postoperative pain.
- *Faster rehabilitation and faster return to work*: Selected arthroscopic procedures can be performed under local anesthesia.

- Reduced hospital stay.
- *Making the diagnosis*: Arthroscopy is the gold standard in making diagnosis of knee ligament and cartilage injuries.
- Reduced complication rate.
- *Dynamic assessment of joint*: Though functional magnetic resonance imaging has now been launched in many centers, to assess the status of the joint during various movements, arthroscopic evaluation of the joint in motion, has been done for long to assess the same.
- Perform procedures which cannot be performed through open surgery, e.g. partial meniscectomy, meniscus repair.

Indications

With the development of newer instruments and better understanding of the mechanism of injuries, the indications of arthroscopic surgery are on an increase. The knee is the most common joint to undergo arthroscopic procedures, followed by shoulders, though virtually every major joint in the body (viz. elbow, wrist, hip and ankle) are being "scoped" for diagnostic and therapeutic purposes. The common indications for arthroscopic surgery of the knee and shoulder are listed in **Table 19.2**.

Complications of Arthroscopic Surgeries

Hemarthrosis and an iatrogenic damage to the articular cartilage are the common complications of the arthroscopic surgeries. Extravasation of fluid through a rent in capsule or a prolonged tourniquet time is often associated with development of compartment syndrome in these surgeries. Improper portal placement may lead to damage to neurovascular structures.

ARTHROSCOPY OF KNEE

Knee arthroscopy **(Fig. 19.7A)** is performed with the patient supine, and under tourniquet applied over proximal thigh. Firstly diagnostic arthroscopy is performed. With the use of a 4-mm diameter, 30-degree oblique viewing arthroscope introduced through the anterolateral portal (viewing portal), almost all of the structures within the knee joint can be seen. Anteromedial portal (working portal) is next established to insert the desired instruments and start the planned procedure. **Box 19.3** gives the list of various portals used in knee arthroscopy **(Fig. 19.7B)**.

Table 19.2: Common indications for arthroscopic surgeries	
Joints	*Common indications*
Knee joint	To confirm the diagnosis (diagnostic arthroscopy), partial or complete meniscectomy, meniscal repair, cruciate ligament reconstruction (most common indication), microfracture/OATS/ACI for osteochondral lesions, synovectomy, synovial biopsy, arthrolysis (lysis of adhesions) for stiff knee, loose body removal
Shoulder joint	Rotator cuff repair, Bankart's repair, SLAP repair, arthroscopic capsular release in frozen shoulder, Acromio-Clavicular joint reconstruction, loose body removal, subacromial decompression, debridement of joint, etc.
Ankle joint	Loose body removal, correction of anterior impingement, microfracture/OATS/ACI for osteochondral lesions (most common indication), debridement and synovial biopsy
Elbow joint	Arthrolysis for stiff elbow, loose body removal (most common indication), synovial biopsy
Wrist joint	The triangular fibrocartilage complex repair (TFCC), excision of wrist ganglion, synovial biopsy, radiocarpal fractures, etc.
Hip joint	Labral tears (most common indication), femoroacetabular impingement (FAI), snapping hips, loose body removal, synovial biopsy

Abbreviations: OATS, osteochondral autograft transfer system; ACI, autologous chondrocyte implantation; SLAP, superior labral tear from anterior to posterior.

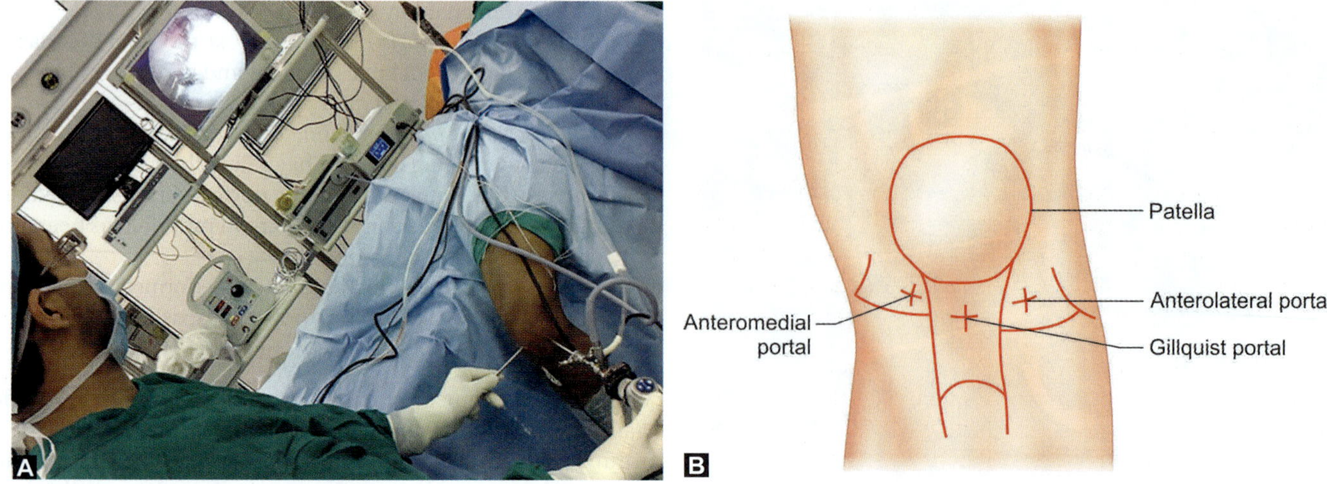

Figs 19.7A and B: (A) Knee arthroscopy; (B) Knee arthroscopy portals

Box 19.3: Important knee arthroscopy portals

- *Anterolateral*: This is the main viewing portal (main diagnostic portal) and first portal to be made. It is made 1 cm above the lateral joint line and 1 cm lateral to the patellar tendon. It can view all structures except anterior horn of the lateral meniscus, periphery of posterior horn of the medial meniscus and posterior cruciate ligament (PCL)
- *Anteromedial*: This is a main working portal. It is made 1 cm above the medial joint line and 1 cm medial to the patellar tendon. It is used for viewing lateral compartment and also for inserting arthroscopic instruments inside the knee
- *Posteromedial*: It is used for repair of posterior horn meniscal tears, PCL tears and loose body removal from posterior compartment
- *Superolateral portal*: It is used for viewing the patellofemoral articulation
- *Central transpatellar portal of Gillquist*: It is located in midline 1 cm inferior to lower pole of patella. It is used in anterior cruciate ligament (ACL) reconstruction after the graft has been harvested

Box 19.4: Important portals for shoulder arthroscopy

- *Posterior portal*: The posterior portal is the primary entry portal for shoulder arthroscopy. It allows examination of most of the joint and assists in the placement of subsequent portals. This portal is located approximately 2 cm inferior and 1 cm medial to the posterolateral tip of the acromion
- *Anterior portal*: It is established after the posterior portal. It passes through the anterior soft spot, which is a triangle bounded by the biceps tendon superiorly, the subscapularis tendon inferiorly, and the anterior edge of the glenoid at the base

ARTHROSCOPY OF SHOULDER

The shoulder is the second most common joint to undergo arthroscopic procedures. Shoulder arthroscopy is performed in either beach chair position or lateral decubitus position. Posterior portal is established first as the viewing portal and then subsequent portals **(Box 19.4)** are established as the need of the intended procedure demands.

HIGH-YIELD POINTS

- *Triangulation*: This is a fundamental arthroscopic skill that a surgeon needs to develop to properly maneuver instruments inside the joint. It is developed, once the surgeon can imagine the tip of the instrument inside the knee and the arthroscope in other hand is forming a "triangle".
- Professor Kenji Takagi (Japanese surgeon) performed the first arthroscopic examination of the knee joint (Tubercular knee), and is credited with the discovery of the arthroscope.
- Masaki Watanabe (Japanese surgeon), developed the first commercial arthroscope, was the first to develop the concept of triangulation and perform a successful arthroscopic surgery.

ARTHROPLASTY

INTRODUCTION

Arthroplasty refers to a surgery whereby the natural articulating surfaces of the joint are replaced with artificial surfaces. It can be of three types:

1. *Excision arthroplasty:* Classical example is the hip joint where the femoral head is excised, creating a pseudo joint (Girdlestone's arthroplasty). It relieves pain, but limp persists. Other sites, where excision arthroplasty is performed, include elbow and great toe (Keller's operation).
2. *Interposition arthroplasty:* This outdated method involved interposition of natural/synthetic material between articular surfaces, e.g. muscle, fascia, fat or synthetic membranes.
3. *Replacement arthroplasty:* In replacement arthroplasty or joint replacement surgery, one or both of the articulating surfaces of a joint are replaced with metal prosthesis. If only one articulating surface is replaced, it is called *hemiarthroplasty* (partial joint replacement) and if both the articulating surfaces are replaced, it is called *total joint arthroplasty* (total joint replacement). The most commonly done total joint replacement is knee followed by the hip. The most common partial joint replacement is hip, followed by the shoulder.

REPLACEMENT ARTHROPLASTY OF THE HIP JOINT

Hip joint is a common joint to undergo both total joint replacement and hemiarthroplasty.

Hemiarthroplasty

In this procedure only the femoral head (and neck) is replaced by artificial prosthesis and the natural acetabular surface is retained **(Fig 19.8)**. The indication for hemiarthroplasty of hip is a fracture neck of femur in an elderly patient, though it can also be done for intertrochanteric fracture where fixation is either not possible or anticipated to be weak.

Types of Hemiarthroplasty Prosthesis

The prosthesis used for replacement of the femoral head can be unipolar or bipolar. Unipolar prosthesis **(Fig. 19.9A)** is one where the head is fixed to stem (i.e. no movement occurs between head and stem) as a single piece, whereas a bipolar prosthesis **(Fig. 19.9B)** is one in which there is an outer acetabular metallic shell that contains inside it a component called liner (made of polyethylene), inside which the head revolves. In unipolar

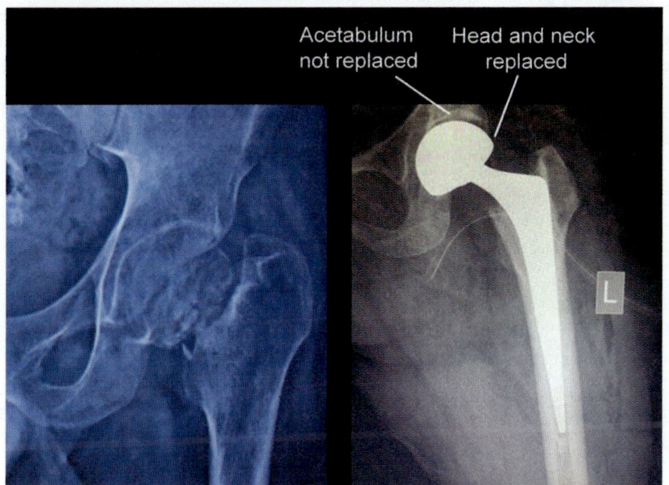

Fig. 19.8: X-ray hip AP view showing fracture neck femur treated with a hemiarthroplasty

prosthesis the motion occurs only at one interface, i.e. between the femoral head and acetabular surface while in bipolar prosthesis (head within a cup design) motion occurs at two surfaces, viz. the femoral head and the liner and the acetabular shell and the acetabulum. The disadvantage of unipolar design is that since there is only one motion interface, acetabular erosions result due to continuous rubbing of the prosthetic femoral head with the acetabulum, leading to anterior thigh pain and acetabular protrusio. Bipolar prosthesis on the other hand experiences less wear and tear, thereby increasing the longevity.

A hip prosthesis can be fixed to bone by either of two methods:

1. *Cemented fixation:* Here bone cement (i.e. PMMA) is used to fix the prosthesis. Use of bone cement provides immediate stability to implanted prosthesis whereas a noncemented prosthesis will not provide such good immediate stability. However, stability may be short lived and loosing may set up early as cement mantle may develop cracks with time.

2. *Uncemented fixation:* Here initial stability is achieved by a "press fit" mechanism, i.e. a slightly oversized component (i.e. prosthesis) is driven into a relatively smaller sized hole (i.e. femoral canal). It becomes fully stable once there is ingrowth of bones into the groves of the implant. The stability so attained may be longer lasting than cemented fixation.

Details regarding the designs of commonly used hemiarthroplasty prostheses are given in **Box 19.5**.

Total Hip Replacement

In this procedure, both the femoral head and the acetabular surface are replaced **(Figs 19.10A and B)**. Dr John Charnley is credited for performing the first total hip replacement (THR) in 1960. The great success achieved by the procedure with technological advancements led to an enormous expansion of its indications with time **(Box 19.6)**.

Total Hip Replacement Prosthesis: Components and Bearing Surfaces

Total hip replacement prosthesis **(Fig. 19.11)** has a femoral component (femoral head and a femoral stem with an offset neck) and an acetabular component (an acetabular cupshell and an insert/liner). Bearing surface simply means surfaces of

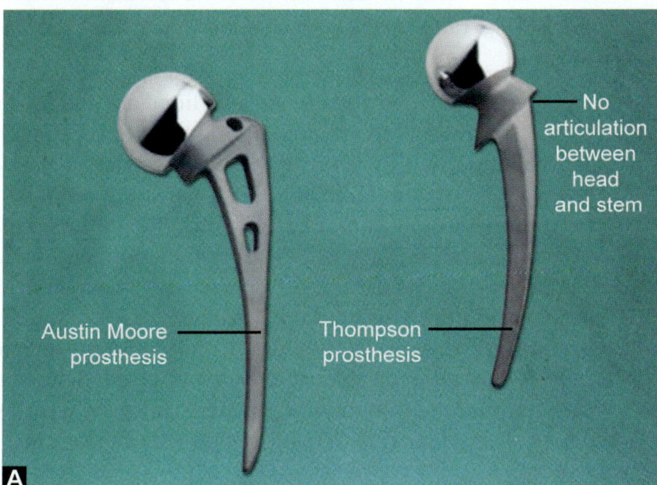

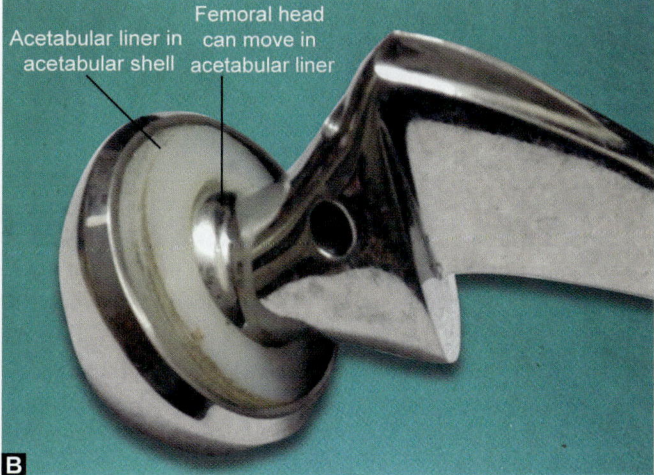

Figs 19.9A and B: (A) Unipolar hip prostheses; (B) Bipolar hip prosthesis

Box 19.5: Commonly used hemiarthroplasty prostheses

- *Austin Moore prosthesis (Fig. 19.9A)*: It is a unipolar, noncemented hip prosthesis. It is used in fracture neck of femur in an elderly patient with a large intramedullary canal. It has a head, a short neck, a shoulder and a stem. The stem has two holes in which, ingrowth of bone occurs, fixing the prosthesis
- *Thompson's prosthesis (Fig. 19.9A)*: It is also a unipolar prosthesis without holes in the stem and without a shoulder. It can be used with or without cement in cases of fracture neck of femur in an elderly patient. It is particularly useful in cases where the neck has been resorbed completely
- *Bipolar prosthesis (Fig. 19.9B)*: Bipolar prostheses are two component prostheses with a "head in a cup design", as explained earlier. It is also used for replacement arthroplasty (hemiarthroplasty) in neck femur fractures

Box 19.6: Indications and contraindications of total hip replacement (THR)

Indications
- Degenerative arthritis (primary osteoarthritis; secondary osteoarthritis as in SCFE, DDH, Perthes disease, Paget's disease, post-traumatic)
- Osteonecrosis
- Inflammatory arthritis (rheumatoid arthritis, ankylosing spondylitis, juvenile rheumatoid arthritis)
- Failed reconstruction [osteotomy, previous total hip replacement (THR), resurfacing arthroplasty]
- Bone tumor of proximal femur
- Tuberculosis (healed)

Contraindications
Absolute contraindications
- Active infection
- Medical ailment with poor tolerability for surgery
Relative contraindications
- Charcot arthropathy
- Abductor insufficiency
- Rapidly progressive neurological diseases

Abbreviations: DDH, developmental dysplasia of the hip; SCFE, slipped capital femoral epiphysis.

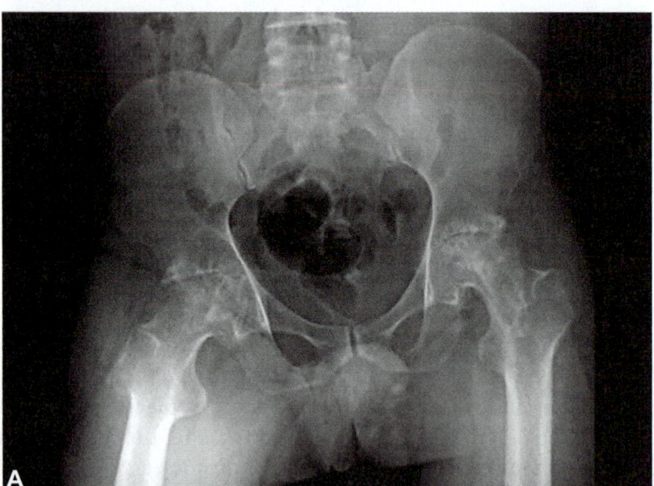

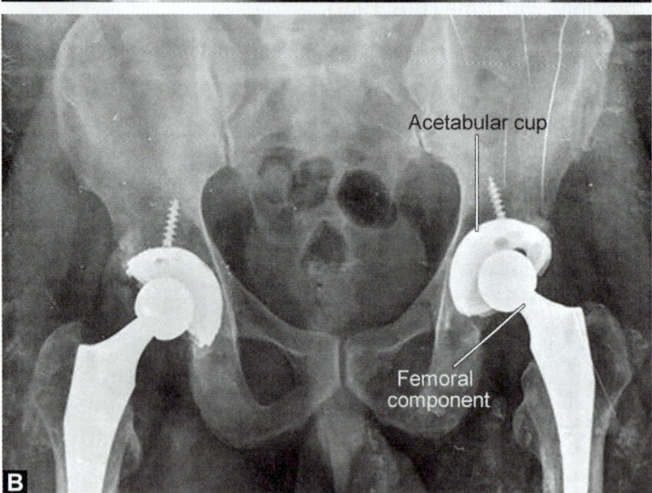

Figs 19.10A and B: (A) X-ray pelvis with AP views showing bilateral avascular necrosis (AVN) of head of femur; (B) Bilateral total hip arthroplasty

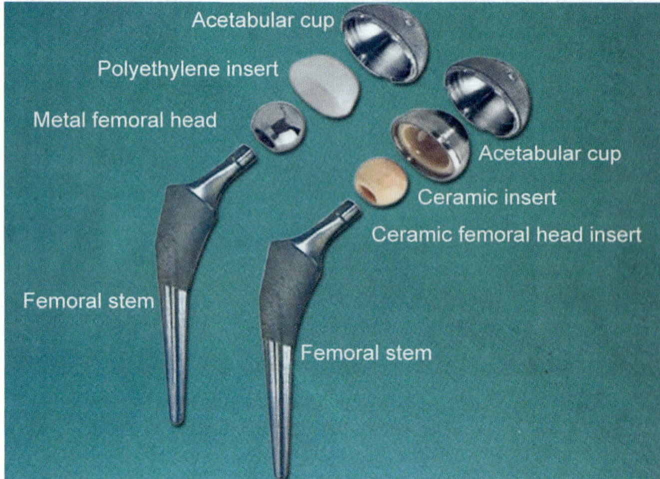

Fig. 19.11: Total hip prosthesis components

acetabular insert/liner and femoral head. Depending upon the material used, bearing surfaces may be one of the following:

- *Metal on polyethylene* (i.e. femoral head if of metal and acetabular liner is made of polyethylene): Polyethylene is a relatively softer material and hence its early wear is the major concern with this bearing surface.
- *Metal on metal* (i.e. both head and liner are made up of metal): This design allows the femoral head to be of a larger size, limiting the dislocation rate. The wear rate is also low. However, increased levels of metal ions (i.e. cobalt and chromium) in blood are a concern and hence this surface is contraindicated in patients with renal failure and women of childbearing age group. A hypersensitivity reaction may cause pseudotumor around the prosthesis.
- *Ceramic on polyethylene* (i.e. ceramic head and polyethylene liner): A hard ceramic against a resilient polyethylene makes this a popular combination in practice. However, wearing of softer polyethylene due to contact with a harder ceramic is a concern.
- *Ceramic on ceramic* (i.e. both head and liner are made up of ceramic): This combination offers the least wear rates as

ceramic is the hardest substance of all bearing materials. However, ceramic is brittle (i.e. not ductile) and chip fractures occur if neck and acetabular liner make contact in extreme range of joint motions. A complication unique to ceramic on ceramic bearing is squeaking (clicking sounds coming from the joint).

Fixation Methods for the THR Prosthesis

Fixation in THR can be cemented where both acetabular and femoral components are fixed with cement, uncemented where both the components are uncemented (fixation initially is press fit and over time by bone ingrowth over a porous surface) or hybrid, where one of the components is cemented and the other is uncemented. Uncemented THR has longer life and is done for younger and active individuals and cemented THR are done for elderly low demand patients. Since cemented acetabular components have exceedingly high rates of failure, they have gone out of use and rather a hybrid fixation where acetabular component is uncemented and femoral component is cemented generally serves the best bargain.

Complications of THR

- *Thromboembolism*: Venous thromboembolism is one of the most common serious complications arising from total hip arthroplasty. Preventive measures for thromboembolic complications include administration of low molecular weight heparin, DVT pumps, early mobilization and ankle pump exercises.
- *Nerve injuries*: The sciatic nerve is the most common nerve injured during posterior approach to the hip, but femoral, obturator and superior gluteal nerves can also be injured, depending upon the approach used. Important causes include direct surgical trauma, excessive retraction, and injury during implant positioning.
- *Heterotopic ossification*: It occurs in the soft tissues around a hip. Risk factors include anterior or anterolateral approach, post-traumatic arthritis and male patients with hypertrophic osteoarthritis. Current areas of attention in the prevention of heterotopic bone are low-dose radiation and nonsteroidal anti-inflammatory drugs (NSAIDs).
- *Limb length discrepancy*: Shortening or lengthening of the limb is possible due to inaccurate resection of femoral neck, choosing inappropriate offset and improper implant position.
- *Subluxation or dislocation*: The incidence of dislocation, post-THR is 3%. Contributing factors include posterior approach to hip, history of previous hip surgery, improper implant positioning, inadequate soft-tissue tension and malpositioning of the limb in early postoperative period.
- *Periprosthetic fractures*: Fractures of the femur or acetabulum can occur during and after the surgery. Femoral fractures are more common and require treatment, unlike their acetabular fractures which are usually not clinically apparent. A fracture may occur during dislocating the hip, during femoral canal reaming or during implant insertion. Late onset fractures may occur due to stress concentration.
- *Infection*: Infected joint replacement is a disaster. Meticulous sterility and proper infection control measures should be undertaken before the joint replacement surgery. If infection occurs, erythrocyte sedimentation rate (ESR) and C-reactive

protein (CRP) value are raised. ESR and CRP values may be used in monitoring also, however, one must know that ESR may not return to normal until 6 months (at times a year) after surgery while CRP values may also take up to 3 weeks to normalize. Recently, raised serum interleukin-6 level has been documented as the most valuable marker for the diagnosis of periprosthetic infection in patients who have had a total hip or total knee arthroplasty.

- *Aseptic femoral and acetabular loosening:* This is the most serious long-term complication of THR and the most common indication for which a revision is required. The prosthesis components loosen due to a hypersensitivity reaction to wear debris (mostly of polyethylene liner) that are generated over years of use.

REPLACEMENT ARTHROPLASTY OF THE KNEE

Knee is the most common joint to undergo a replacement procedure. Indications and contraindications for the procedure are given in **Box 19.7**.

Unicondylar Knee Replacement

When only one compartment of the three compartments (medial tibiofemoral, lateral tibiofemoral and patellofemoral) of the knee is affected, unicondylar knee replacement (UKR) is indicated. In this procedure, articulating bones of only one compartment (either medial or lateral tibiofemoral compartment) are resurfaced and polyethylene insert is placed. Both the cruciates are retained. Varus/valgus deformities greater than 10°, torn cruciate ligaments, inflammatory arthropathy (i.e. rheumatoid arthritis) and morbid obesity are contraindications to UKR.

Total Knee Replacement

It is basically a resurfacing arthroplasty, where the articular surfaces of the femur and tibia are replaced with artificial components **(Figs 19.12A and B)**. The patella may/may not be resurfaced. The surgery involves accurate bony cuts and soft tissue releases, so at the end of the surgery appropriate limb alignment is attained. The recent introduction of computer navigation total knee replacement (TKR) system allows the bone cuts to be made even more precisely.

TKR Prosthesis: Components

Insall is credited with developing the modern knee replacement prosthesis designs. In a standard TKR **(Fig. 19.12C)** three components are used: (1) metal tibial baseplate, (2) metal femoral component, and (3) polyethylene liner/insert (kept between the femoral and tibial components).

Box 19.7: Indications and contraindications for total knee replacement (TKR)

Indications
- Painful disabling arthritis of knee
- Osteonecrosis with subchondral collapse of femoral condyle
- Disabling deformity
- Chondrocalcinosis and pseudogout causing disabling pain

Contraindications
- Septic knee
- Remote or ongoing sepsis
- Knee extensor mechanism insufficiency
- Severe recurvatum secondary to muscular weakness

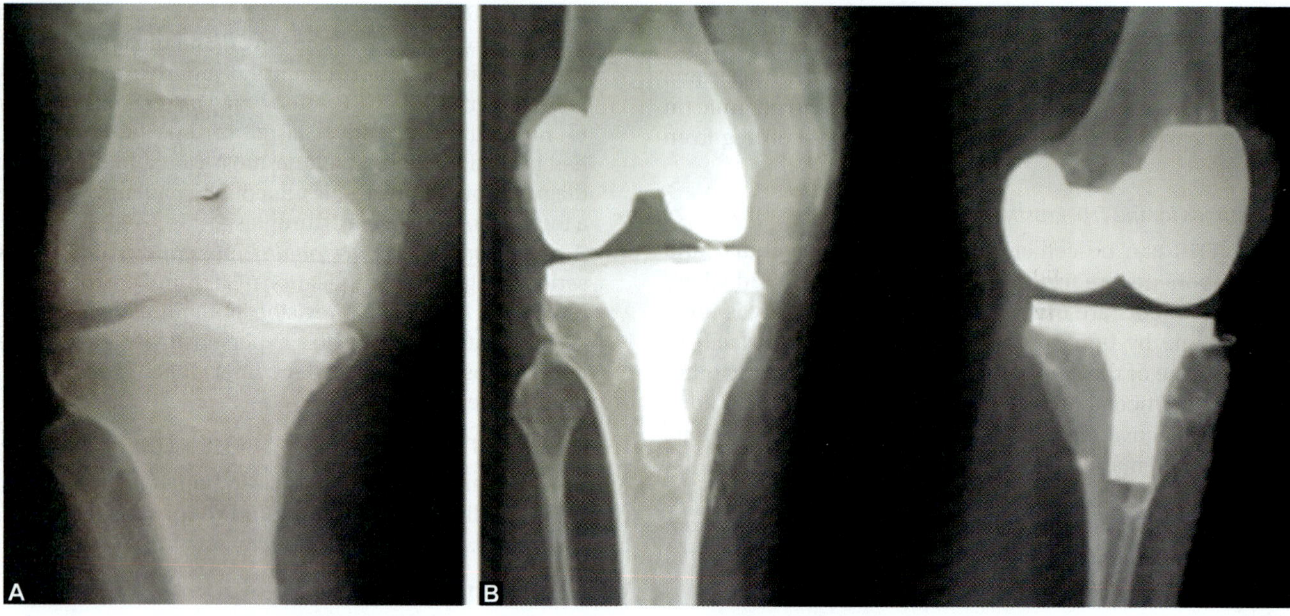

Figs 19.12A and B: (A) X-ray knee AP view showing advanced osteoarthritic changes; (B) X-ray knee AP and lateral views showing total knee arthroplasty

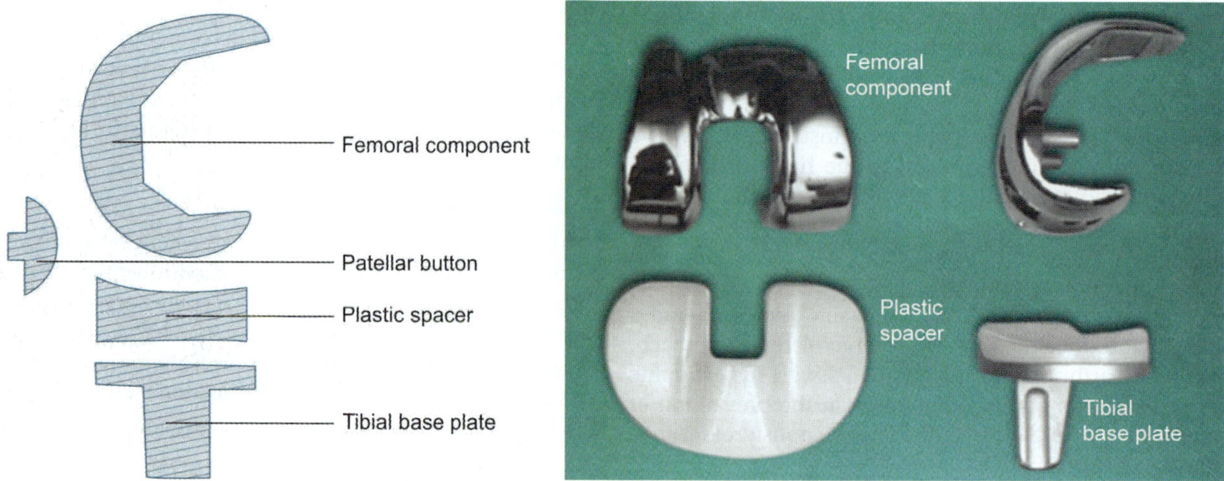

Fig. 19.12C: Different components of total knee arthroplasty

Types of TKR

- On the basis of cementing:
    - *Cemented*: Conventional procedure as of today
    - *Uncemented*: Not been a success yet
- On the basis of bearing surface:
    - *Fixed bearing*: The polyethylene insert is fixed on the tibial base plate.
    - *Mobile bearing*: The polyethylene insert rotates within the tibial base plate (rotating platform). This allows for errors in rotational malpositioning and reduces wear rates.
- On the basis of cruciate retention:
    - *Cruciate retaining:* Spares more bone (i.e. less of bone removed) and allows greater postoperative knee flexion. Problem is retaining the cruciates makes the technique more difficult.
        - Bicruciate retaining (both PCL and ACL retained)
        - Single cruciate (PCL) retaining
    - *Cruciate sacrificing* (both PCL and ACL sacrificed): Here a special mechanism (cam-post) is built in the prosthesis to ensure good postoperative knee flexion. Main drawback is that more bone resection is needed to fit in cam-post mechanism. Technique is easier. Its further two categories are:
        - Posterior stabilized design
        - Ultracongruent (deep dish design).

Complications of TKR

Complications for the procedure are much the same as in THR, with loosening of the prosthesis due to polyethylene wear being the major matter of concern. It is the tibial component that generally becomes loose and merits revision.

REPLACEMENT ARTHROPLASTY OF THE SHOULDER

Three types of arthroplasties are done in shoulder joint commonly:

Hemiarthroplasty: Only the humeral head is replaced. It is done in severely comminuted fractures of the proximal humerus, especially in elderly patients.

Total shoulder arthroplasty (TSA): It is done is painful arthritic shoulder. A plastic "cup" is fitted into the shoulder socket (glenoid), and a metal "ball" is attached to proximal humerus. It relies on rotator cuff muscles to function properly.

Reverse shoulder arthroplasty (RSA): It is done in patients with chronic irreparable rotator cuff tears, failed TSA, and relies on deltoid to function properly. In it, the glenoid cup is placed on the humeral head and the humeral ball on the glenoid surface. This unnatural articulation established in irreparable rotator cuffs (*see* Page 172) allows the joint's center of rotation to be shifted down and medially, stretching the deltoid **(Fig. 19.13)**, making it more powerful thereby enabling it to over take the function of supraspinatous (i.e. to carry out the first 15° of abduction).

HIGH-YIELD POINTS

- The most common cause of death following THR is myocardial infarction > pulmonary embolism.
- In THR it is mostly the acetabular component that fails first while in TKR it is the tibial component that fails more commonly.
- There is an apprehension regarding arthroplasty procedure that when a joint is replaced the proprioceptive receptors are damaged and hence the final gait of the patient gets affected. However, most scientific studies have rather found that the leftover receptors get up regulated and eventually there is no effect on the gait pattern after both hip or knee arthroplasty.
- Dr John Charnley who performed the first THR in 1960 is regarded as the Father of Arthroplasty surgery. He gave the principles of low friction arthroplasty.

Treatment of musculoskeletal malignant tumors has come a long way from amputation as the sole treatment to limb salvage surgery. Limb salvage surgery is a surgical procedure whereby a diseased bone is reconstructed to yield a functional limb by using combination of bone grafts (autografts or allografts) and special metal prosthesis called megaprostheses. Megaprosthesis is a larger prosthesis that is designed to replace a large segment of bone and adjacent joint. A customized megaprosthesis is made according to patient's dimensions. With modern endoprosthetics, it is possible to replace the whole of the bone with adjacent joints **(Figs 19.14A to C)**.

Work-up of Patient

All patients should undergo an array of imaging modalities to know the extent of disease. MRI is the most important tool to see the local extension of the disease. A bone scan is used to screen for skipping lesions and involvement of other bones. Computed tomography (CT) scan of the chest is done to rule out pulmonary metastases as the lung is the most common site for metastasis from musculoskeletal tumor. PET-CT has revolutionized the way of doing tumor staging. Histopathological diagnosis should be made by biopsy. It is important to plan the biopsy site so as the entire biopsy track could be excised en bloc along with the tumor.

Indications and Contraindications for Limb Salvage

Osteosarcoma is the most common tumor for which the limb salvage surgery is needed. However, any tumor that can be adequately removed with a safe margin and leaving behind a functional limb should be the candidate for limb salvage. Involvement of major nerves and/or vessels, pathological fracture and inadequate motors (muscles) after resection are relative contraindications for limb salvage surgery.

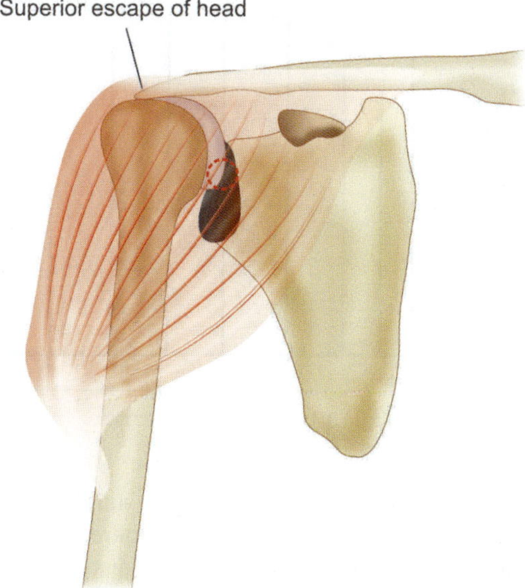

Fig. 19.13: Schematic representation of the mechanics behind Reverse Shoulder Arthroplasty. Note the center of rotation (red dotted circle) shifted downwards by the new articulation

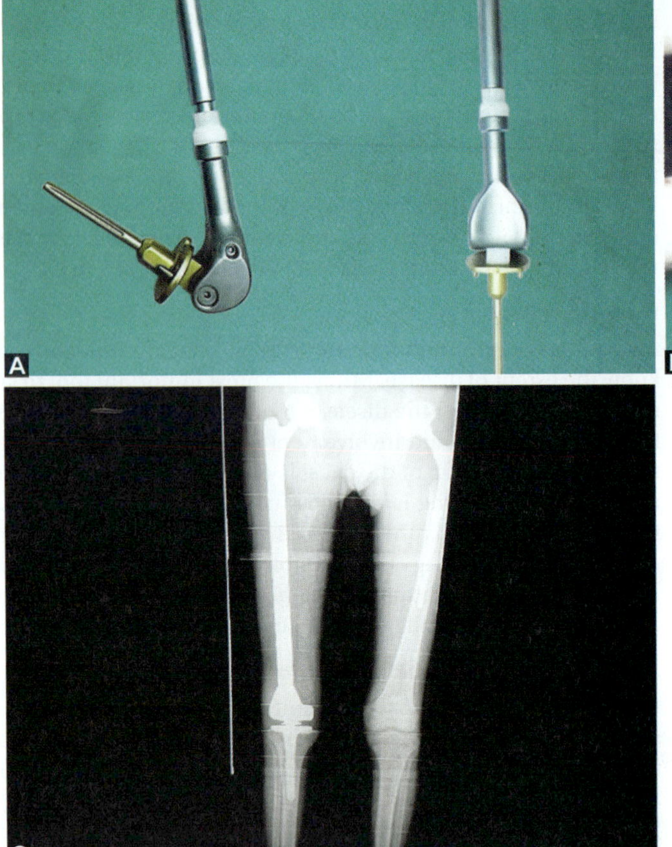

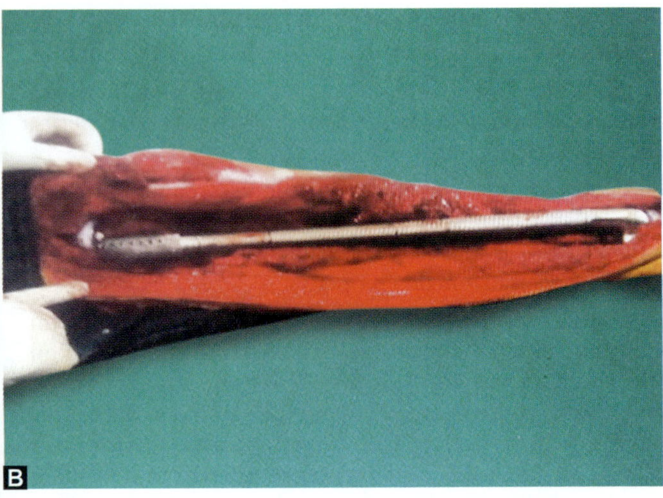

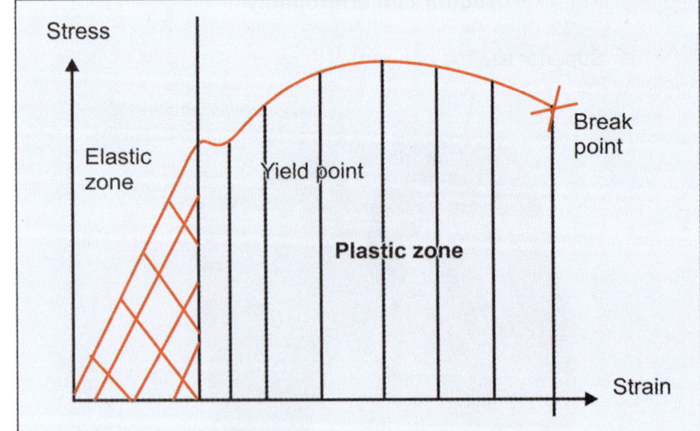

Figs 19.14A to C: (A) Megaprosthesis; (B) Replacement of whole femur with knee and hip joints with megaprosthesis; (C) AP view of the thigh with hip joint and knee joint showing megaprosthesis (on right side) left side is showing total hip replacement

Courtesy: Dr RK Sharma (Indraprastha Apollo Hospital, New Delhi).

ORTHOPEDIC BIOMATERIALS

A biomaterial is a substance (biological or synthetic) that can be introduced into the body tissues. Three types of biomaterials are mainly used for orthopedic implants, viz. metals (stainless steel, titanium alloys and cobalt-chromium alloys), ceramics (aluminum oxide, calcium phosphate, etc.) and polymers [ultra-high molecular weight polyethylene (UHMWPE)]. To understand their applications, one needs to be familiar with following properties of a biomaterial:

- *Biocompatibility:* It is the property of being compatible (i.e. causing no immunological or toxic reaction) with body tissues.
- *Stress-strain relationship (Fig. 19.15):* When a load (stress) is applied to an implant, changes may occur in its shape (strain). Initially, these changes are reversible and implant returns to its original shape when the load is removed. This is called elastic deformation. The ability of an implant to resist this deformation is a measure of its stiffness. It is mathematically given by a ratio of stress over strain called Young's modulus of Elasticity (Y). Higher the value of "Y", stiffer is the implant. A substance like a rubber band has very low value of "Y" and hence is very flexible. Important biomaterials arranged in their increasing order of stiffness (Y) are: polymers <bone

Fig. 19.15: Stress-strain curve

cement < bone (cortical) < titanium < stainless steel <cobalt-chromium < ceramics. Although, apparently one may feel that a stiffer substance would be strongest and should be the material of choice to manufacture an implant, the decision is not that simple. If fixation material is much stiffer than bone (e.g. cobalt-chromium), then, most of the body weight gets transmitted through the implant (as stiffer structures bear more weight). This offloads the bone, leading to a reduction in bone density (osteopenia), a phenomena called *stress shielding*. Stress shielding causes bone atrophy leading to the loosening of the implant and refracturing of the bone. So, Young's modulus nearer to that of bone (low value of "Y") is a desirable feature of the implant device.

Now, when the load applied to an implant is continually increased, such that it rises above the yield point **(Fig. 19.15)**, irreversible changes may occur in the shape of implant, which is known as plastic deformation. Breaking point occurs when the continued load causes implant to break. A substance that cannot handle the plastic deformation is termed brittle and breaks easily while a substance that is ductile can absorb considerable energy and handle lot of plastic deformation prior to mechanical failure. Ductility is an important property that aids plate "contouring" for fracture fixation without putting the plate strength at risk.

- *Fatigue:* It refers to failure of an implant due to repeated stress at magnitudes lower than ultimate stress. High fatigue resistance is a desired property of orthopedic implant material. Increasing order of fatigue limit and tensile strength of common biomaterials is as follows: stainless steel < cobalt-chromium < titanium.

CHARACTERISTICS OF COMMON ORTHOPEDIC BIOMATERIALS

Stainless Steel (Cr, Ni, Mo)

Internal fixation implants used for fractures are commonly made up of stainless steel. The form of stainless steel which is used in orthopedic implants is 316L (suffix L indicates low concentration of carbon, i.e. 0.03%). Carbon is added for the strength and chromium is added to provide resistance to corrosion (it forms an oxide layer which prevents corrosion; this is known as passivation. It is a cheap, biocompatible, strong and relative ductile material, but susceptible to crevice corrosion.

Titanium and Cobalt-Chromium Alloys

Titanium alloys are more biocompatible (causes less tissue reaction) than stainless steel and cobalt-chromium alloys. They are more resistant to corrosion, ductile, have high fatigue resistance and low Young's modulus, but also more sensitive to cracks and scratches (notch sensitivity) and have poor wear characteristics. Titanium alloys are used for internal fixation implants and joint replacement prostheses.

Cobalt-chromium alloys have very high Young's modulus, so make the bone susceptible to stress shielding. They are mainly used for joint replacement prostheses. When a cemented fixation is used, to offload the cement, a stiff implant (cobalt-chromium) is chosen so that cement mantle does not develop cracks. However, in cementless fixation, stiff implants may offload bone causing stress shielding **(Fig. 19.16)**, so in such cases titanium alloys with a lower Young's modulus are preferred to avoid stress shielding.

Ceramics

These are inorganic, nonmetallic, crystalline oxides/carbides/nitrides of metallic elements, formed by the application of heat. Common ceramics used as orthopedic biomaterials are alumina (aluminum oxide), zirconia (zirconium oxide), hydroxyapatite and silica. They are chemically inert and have best biocompatibility.

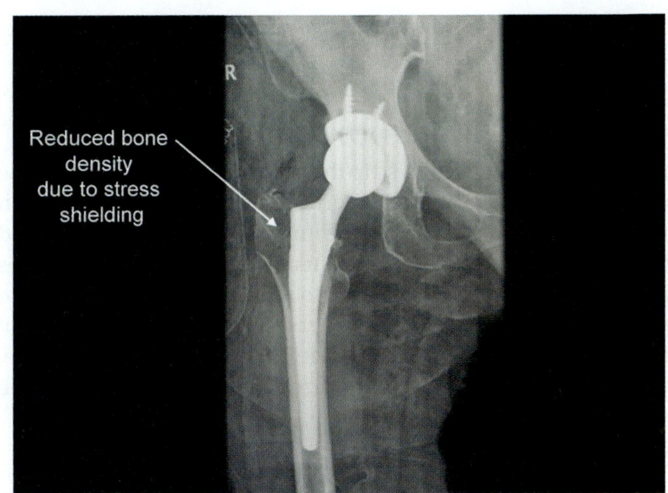

Fig. 19.16: Stress shielding by implant in uncemented total hip replacement. Note the osteopenia in the region of greater trochanter. Titanium alloys should be preferred in such cases as their Young's modulus (Y) is nearer to bone than cobalt-chromium alloys

They are very strong but brittle (i.e. break easily), so not useful for implants used for fracture fixation. They are used for coating of metal implants to increase their biocompatibility. Off late they have become popular bearing surfaces for total hip arthroplasty prostheses.

Polymers

Bone cement, i.e. PMMA and UHMWPE are most commonly used polymers in orthopedic implants. UHMWPE has high abrasion resistance, low friction and high impact strength. These properties make it a popular biomaterial to be used as liners of acetabular cups in total hip arthroplasties, in the tibial insert and patellar component in total knee arthroplasties and as a spacer in intervertebral artificial disk replacement.

HIGH-YIELD POINTS

- Bone is anisotropic structure in terms of Young's modulus of elasticity, i.e. its modulus of elasticity depends on the direction of the loading. It is weaker in shear, then tension and then compression.
- Tribology is the branch of science and technology that deals with the study of friction, wear and lubrication characteristics of materials. It has its implications in long-term survival and function of the orthopedic implants and prostheses.
- "Creep" is the phenomenon of progressive deformation of a material over time, when constant stress is applied at high temperature, below the elastic limit of that material.
- *Biodegradable implants*: These implants provide sufficient strength to the bone until fracture heals and then degrade spontaneously, thus eliminating need for second surgery for their removal. These are mainly made up of polyglycolic acid, polydioxanone acid and polylevolactic acid.

COMMON INSTRUMENTS AND IMPLANTS USED IN ORTHOPEDICS

INTRODUCTION

Concepts of nailing and plating and prostheses for hip and knee arthroplasty have already been discussed earlier in this chapter.

Other instruments and implants commonly used in orthopedic surgeries will be discussed here.

GENERAL INSTRUMENTS

Periosteum Elevator (Fig. 19.17)

It is an instrument used to strip the periosteum off the bone to be worked with. By elevating the periosteum, we get a safe plane in the operative field, because all the important structures like blood vessels, nerves and tendons are outside the periosteum. Muscles attached to the bone are attached to the periosteum which has to be elevated to get a smooth surface of the bone for the purpose of internal fixation. Periosteal elevator has one blunt beveled edge. It can be of different shapes and sizes depending upon the bone where they are used.

Osteotome (Figs 19.18A and B)

It is the instrument used in osteotomy (the process of cutting the bone). It has a sharp end, which is beveled on both sides and a broad end for hammering. It is also of various sizes and shapes.

Bone Chisel (Fig. 19.19)

It looks very much similar to an osteotome except that its sharp end is beveled on only one side. It is used to level an irregular bony surface as in removing excessive callus or in removing osteophytes in knee replacement surgery.

Bone Levers (Fig. 19.20)

They are used to lift or lever out the bone from the depth of the surgical wound or to keep the soft tissues away from the working field. Bone levers are of different sizes depending on the bone where they are used.

Bone Nibblers (Fig. 19.21)

Bone nibblers are used to nibble bone or fibrous tissues. They are used in spinal surgeries and surgeries for nonunion.

They are of various shapes:
- *Straight nibbler*: For general use
- *Curved nibblers*: For spinal surgeries
- *Double action nibbler*: Straight and curved.

Bone Cutter (Fig. 19.22)

It is used to cut the bones into smaller pieces as in preparing a bone graft or removing osteophytes in joint replacement surgeries. It is also available in various shapes and sizes.

Mallet/Hammer (Fig. 19.23)

It is used for hammering a chisel or an osteotome.

Bone Curette (Fig. 19.24)

It is a spoon-shaped instrument used to curette out a bony cavity as in a giant cell tumor or in preparing a fracture end for fixation.

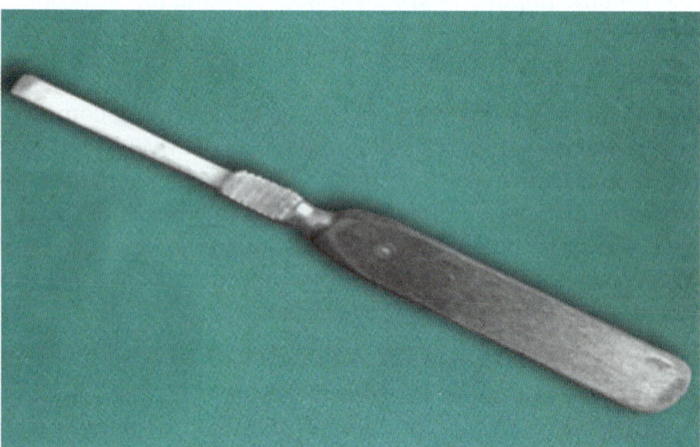

Fig. 19.17: Periosteal elevator

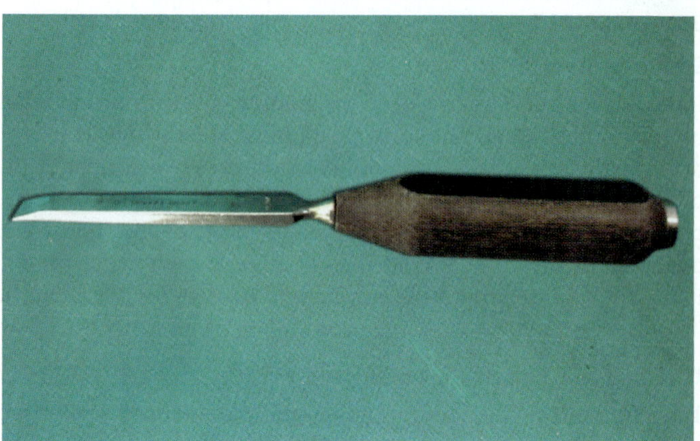

Fig. 19.19: Bone chisel

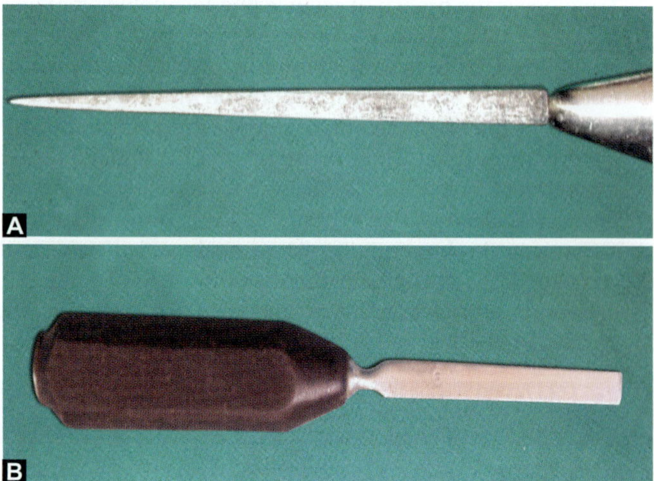

Figs 19.18A and B: Osteotomes

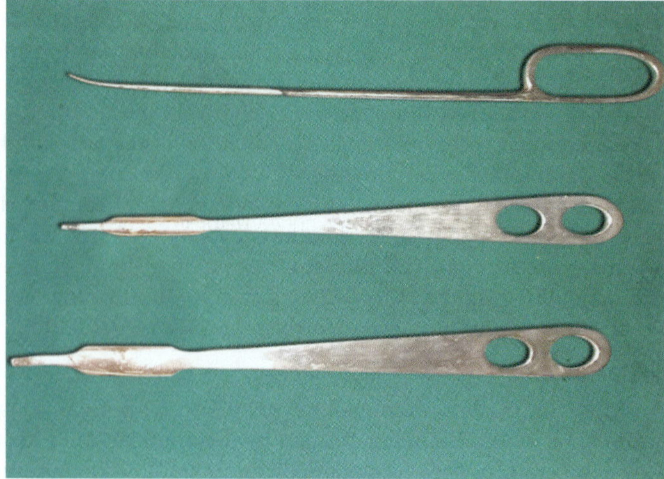

Fig. 19.20: Bone levers

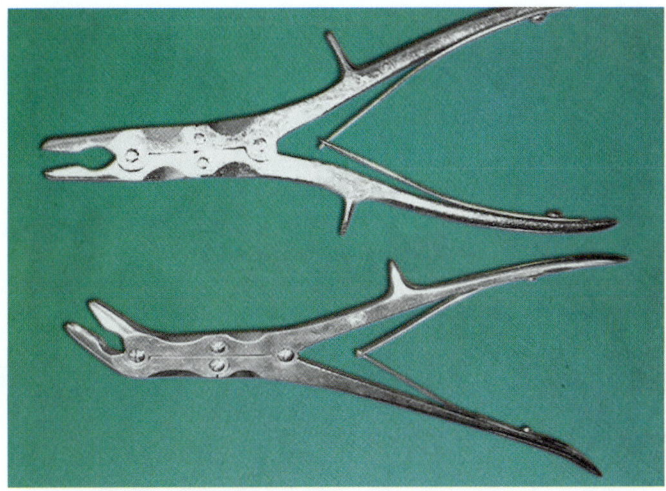

Fig. 19.21: Straight and curved bone nibblers

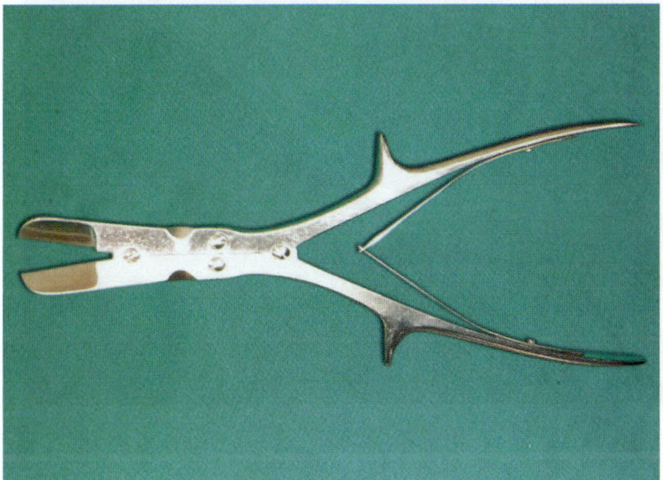

Fig. 19.22: Bone cutter

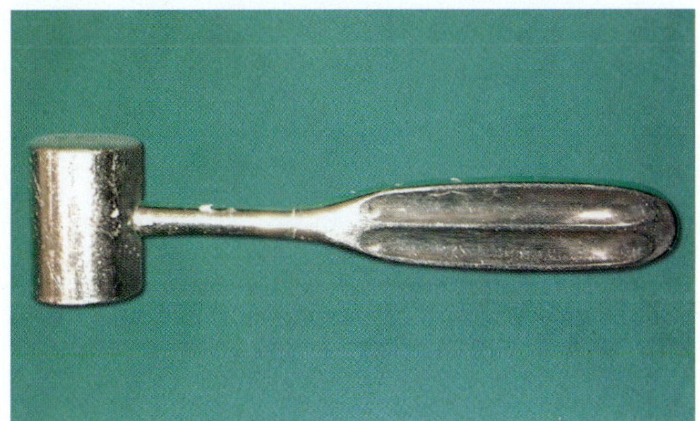

Fig. 19.23: Hammer/mallet

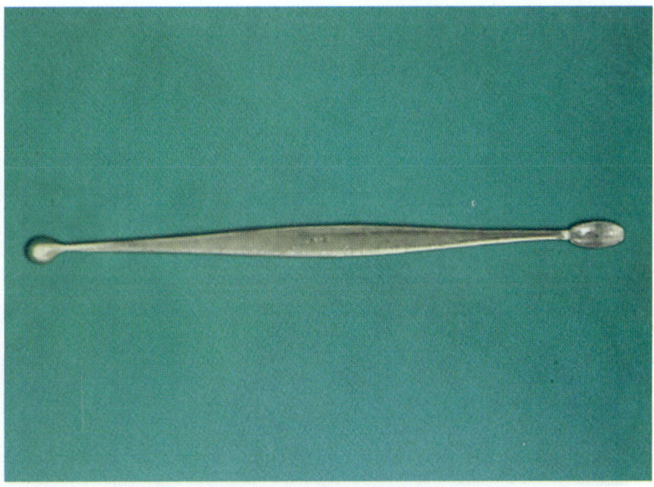

Fig. 19.24: Bone curette

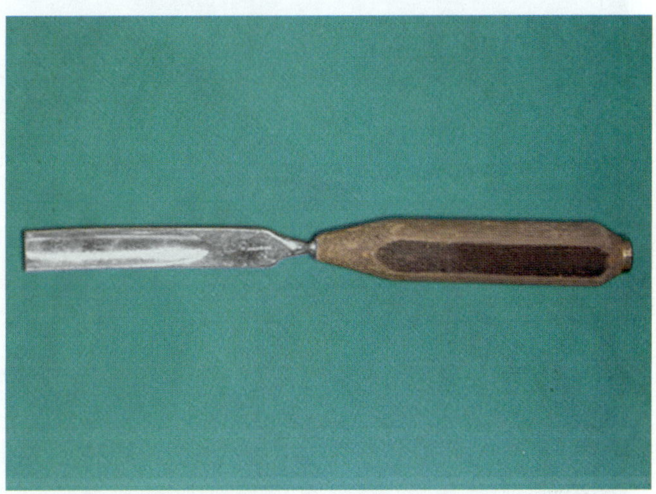

Fig. 19.25: Bone gouge

Bone Gouge (Fig. 19.25)

It is a concave-bladed chisel used mainly in the process of harvesting bone grafts (for cutting cortical bone or for scooping cancellous bone).

Bone Holding Forceps (Figs 19.26A to F)

It is an instrument used to hold the bone for manipulation. It is of various types:

- Lane's forceps (**Fig. 19.26A**) for holding femur and tibia
- Ferguson forceps or lion jaw forceps (**Fig. 19.26B**) for holding fibula and forearm bones
- Self-retaining reduction forceps of AO type (**Fig. 19.26E**), which have an arrangement for locking and self-retaining
- Reduction forceps like patella reduction forceps (**Fig. 19.26C**), malleolar reduction forceps (**Fig. 19.26D**), and pelvic reduction forceps (**Fig. 19.26F**). These are used to hold the reduction of the fractured fragments during surgery.

Plate Holding Forceps (Figs 19.27A and B)

Once the bone is reduced, the plate is placed over it and held with a plate holding forceps before it is fixed with screws. It can be a self-retaining forceps (**Fig. 19.27A**) or a Lowman's clamp (**Fig. 19.27B**).

Right Angle Retractors (Fig. 19.28)

These are used to retract different tissue layers during surgery.

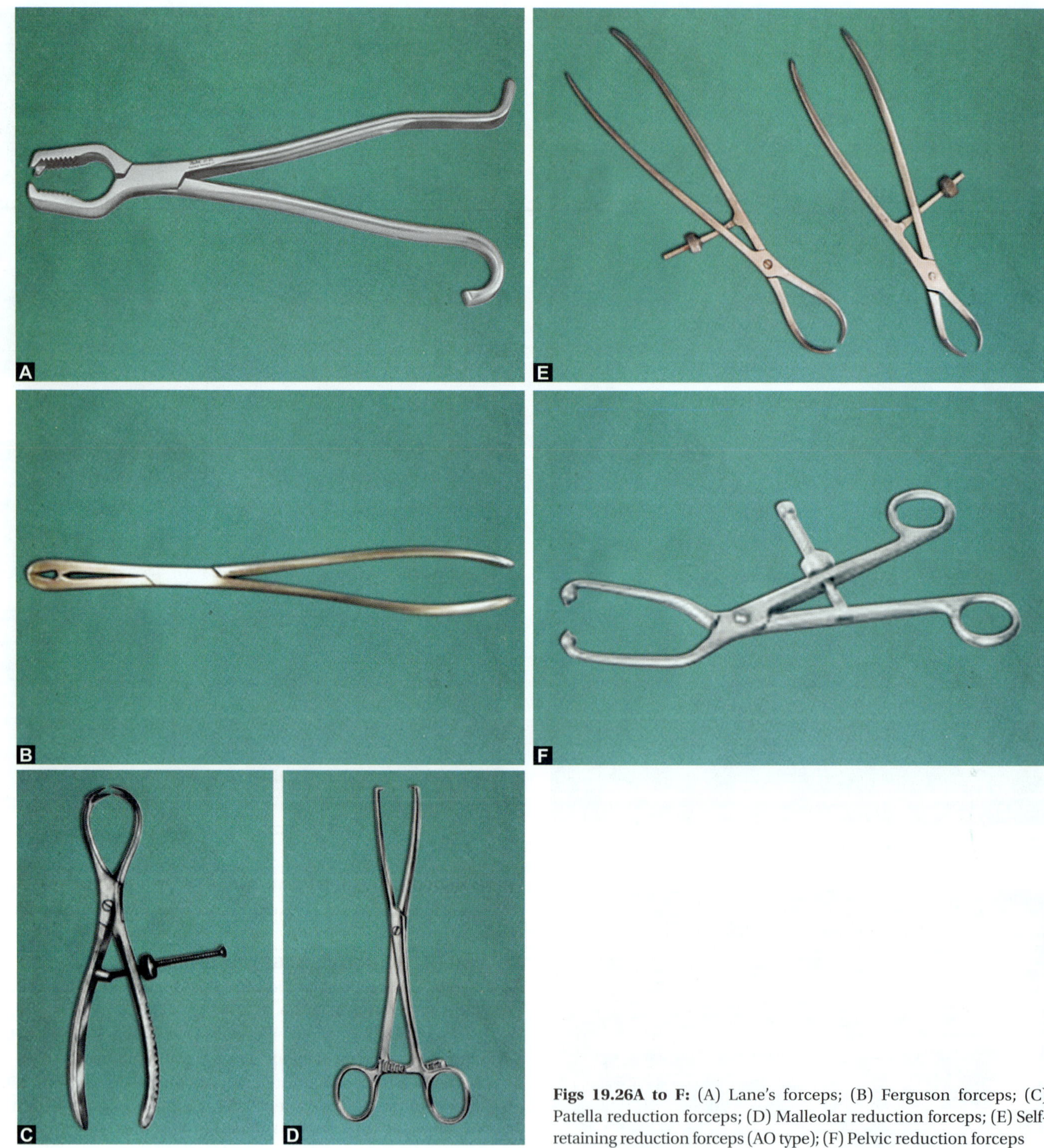

Figs 19.26A to F: (A) Lane's forceps; (B) Ferguson forceps; (C) Patella reduction forceps; (D) Malleolar reduction forceps; (E) Self-retaining reduction forceps (AO type); (F) Pelvic reduction forceps

Drill Bit (Fig. 19.29A)

It is an instrument used to drill a hole in the bone so that screws can be inserted. Depending upon the sizes of the screws, drill bits of varying sizes are used.

Depth Gauge (Fig. 19.29B)

Once a hole is drilled, next its depth is measured with an instrument called depth gauge, so that only a proper size screw is inserted.

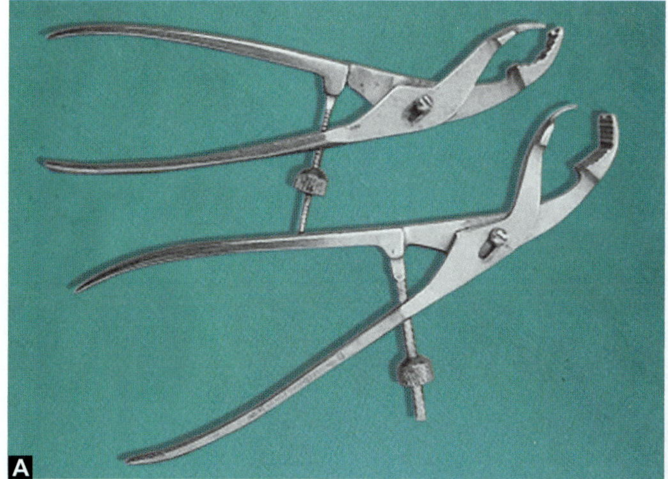

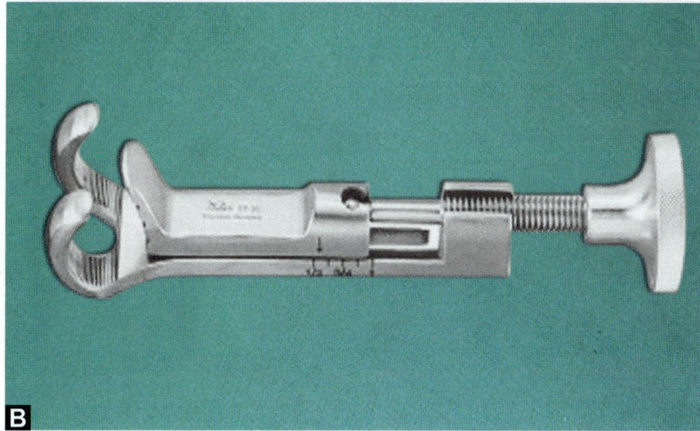

Figs 19.27A and B: (A) Plate holding forceps; (B) Lowman's clamp

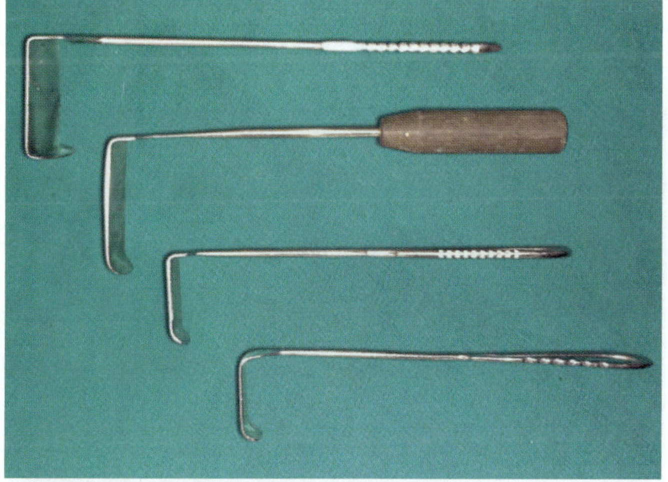

Fig. 19.28: Right angle retractors

Screw Tap (Fig. 19.29C)

Screw tap is used to create threads in the screw hole so that the screw can be inserted easily. Tapping should be done only after estimation of screw size, else, insertion of depth gauge after tapping will destroy the taps (threads) cut by the screw tap.

Screw Driver (Fig. 19.29D)

It is an instrument used to drive a screw into the screw hole. It usually has a hexagonal tip for driving the screws with hexagonal head.

Tooth and Non-toothed Forceps (Fig. 19.30)

It is used for grasping and holding tissues during surgery and to pick-up the tissue layers while suturing. Non-toothed forceps are used to hold delicate tissues and to dissect out nerves and vessels.

Sponge Holding Forceps (Fig. 19.31)

It is used to hold sponge or swab during surgery. In orthopedic surgery, it is mainly used to hold the sponge for cleaning and painting of the part to be operated before the surgery.

Kocher's Forceps and Allis Forceps (Figs 19.32A to C)

Kocher's forceps has serrated blades with interlocking teeth at the tips. It is used to hold tissues and for compression of bleeding tissues. Allis tissue forceps has inward curved and toothed blades, but no serrations. It is mainly used for grasping tough tissues like fascia, tendons, etc.

TRACTION INSTRUMENTS

Steinman's Pin (Fig. 19.33A)

It is a straight, stout pin of varying diameter from 3 mm to 6 mm. One end is flat and the other end is sharp. It is used to apply skeletal traction, i.e. distal femur and proximal tibial skeleton traction.

Kirschner's Wires (Fig. 19.33B)

Kirschner's wires (K-wires) are straight stainless steel wires which are sharp at both ends. These are available in different diameters ranging from 1 mm to 3 mm. Both the ends are sharp. They are used in: (1) internal fixation of small bones of hands and feet; (2) internal fixation of bones in children; (3) for the purpose of traction in children; (4) for temporary fixation of fracture fragments (to hold the reduction) in adults during surgery; (5) in Ilizarov's fixation system.

Denham's Pin (Fig. 19.33C)

It looks exactly similar to Steinman's pin except that it has threads in the middle. The purpose of these threads is to get a firm grip on the bone in which it is inserted. It is used to apply traction in osteoporotic bones and cancellous bones like calcaneum.

Bohler's Stirrup (Fig. 19.34)

It is an instrument used to hold the Steinman's pin for applying traction. It has two screws at both the ends which will hold the pin tight. The direction of the traction can be altered without rotating the pin inside the bone by varying the direction of the Bohler's stirrup.

Crutchfield Tong (Figs 19.35A and B)

It is a type of skull tong, which is used to apply skeletal traction through the skull in cases of cervical spine instability. It has two sharp prongs used for insertion into the outer table of the skull and a slot in the middle for applying traction.

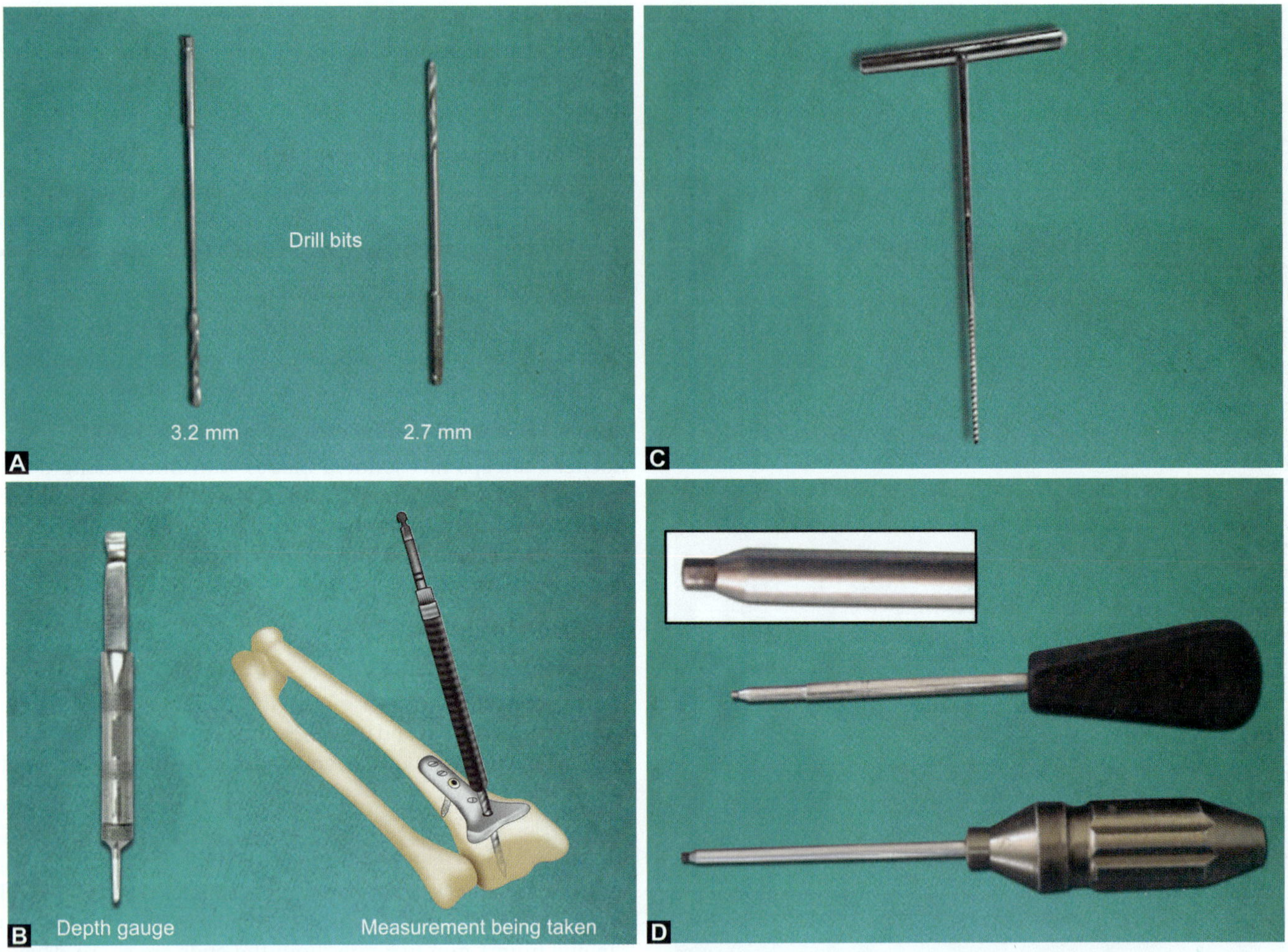

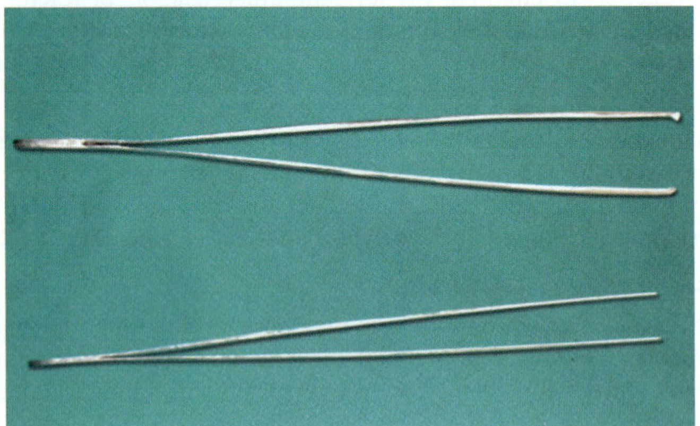

Figs 19.29A to D: Drill bits, depth gauge, bone tap and screw driver (See hexagonal tip of orthopedic screw driver)

Fig. 19.30: Tooth and non-toothed forceps

Fig. 19.31: Sponge holding forceps

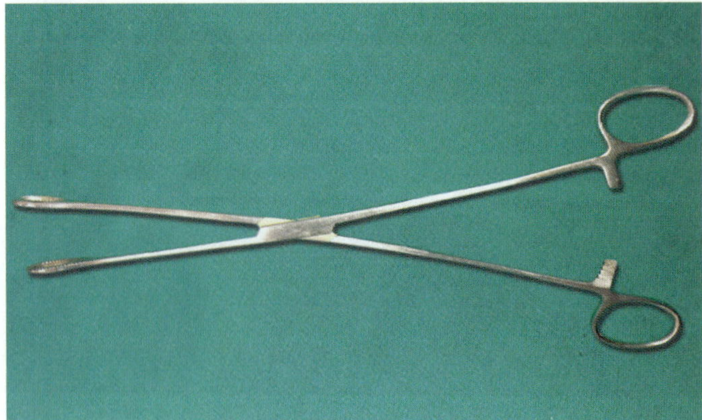

EXTERNAL FIXATOR ASSEMBLY

It is a set of implants used for external fixation of bones. External fixation is used in case of open fractures (Gustilo Anderson Grade II and above), infected nonunion, deformity correction, etc. where we do not want to fix the bone internally.

The external fixator assembly consists of **(Figs 19.36A and B)**:

Schanz pins: Straight pins of varying sizes with threads at the tip. They are inserted into the bone percutaneously.

Tubular rods: These are used to span the Schanz pins and connected to them and to each other by clamps.

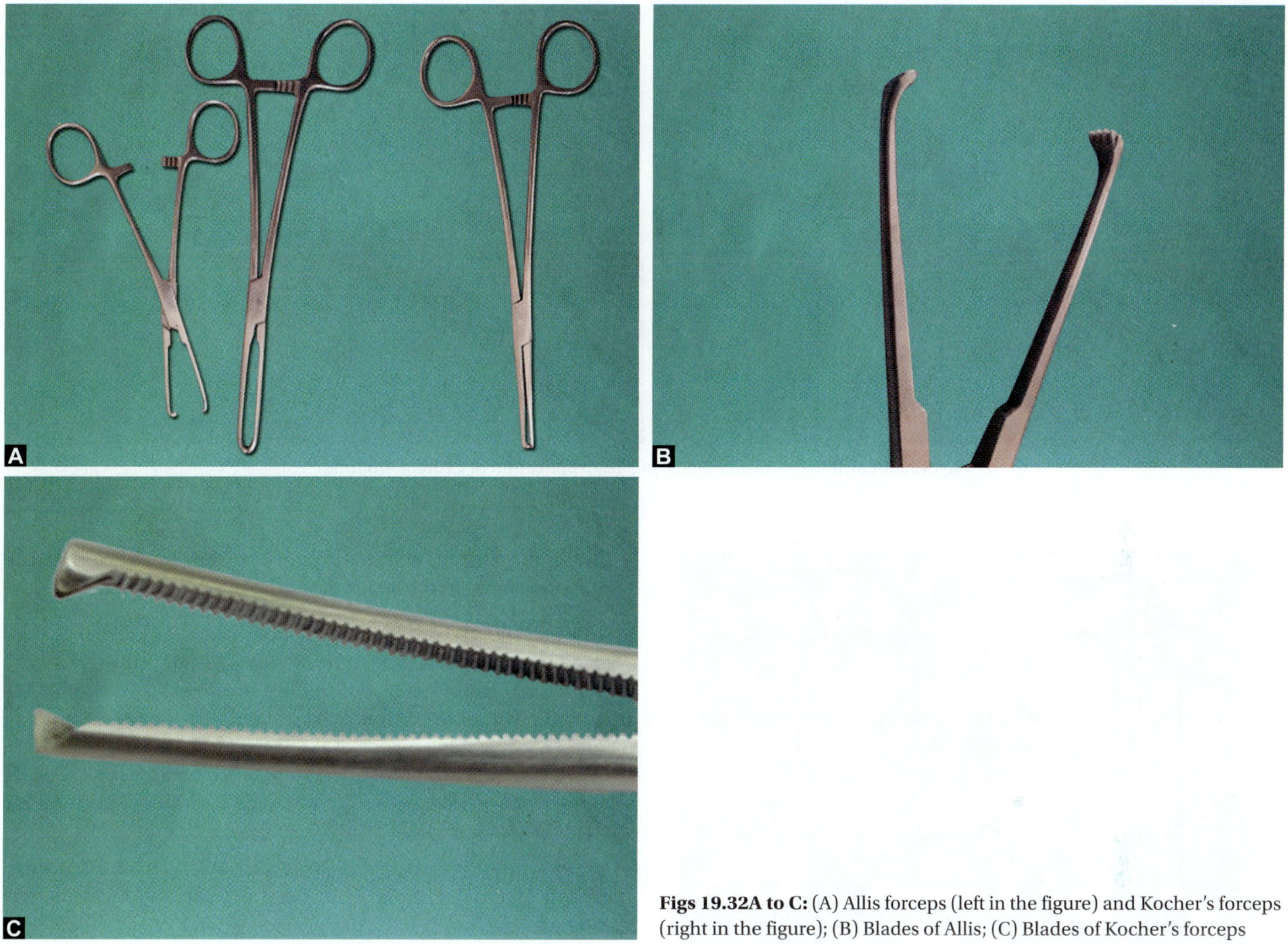

Figs 19.32A to C: (A) Allis forceps (left in the figure) and Kocher's forceps (right in the figure); (B) Blades of Allis; (C) Blades of Kocher's forceps

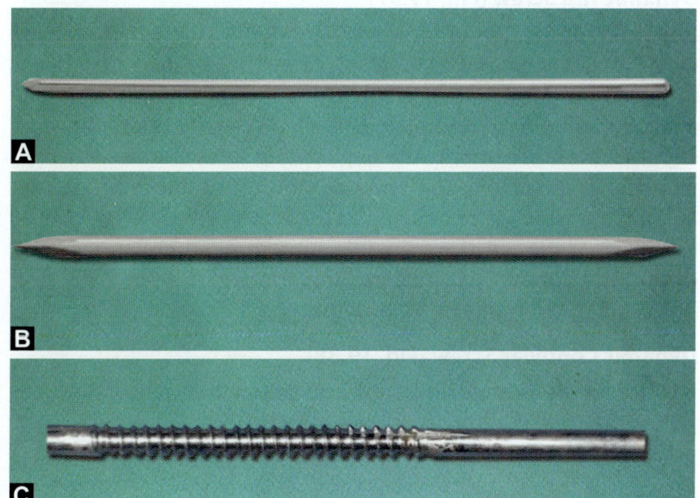

Figs 19.33A to C: (A) Steinman's pin; (B) Kirschner' wire; (C) Denham's pin with threads in the middle

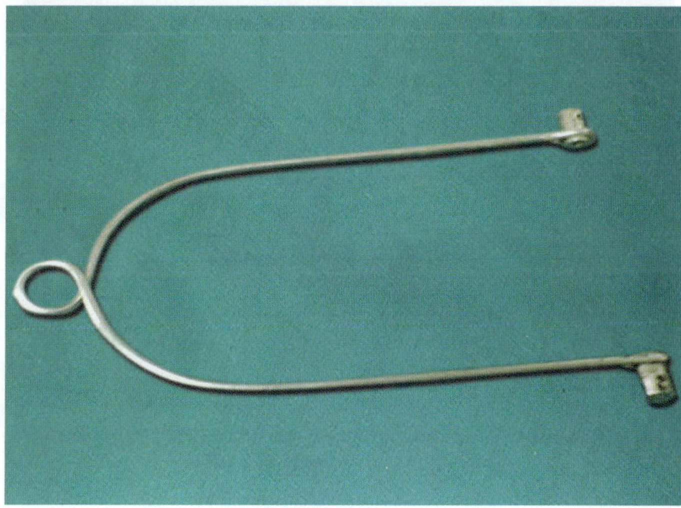

Fig. 19.34: Bohler's stirrup

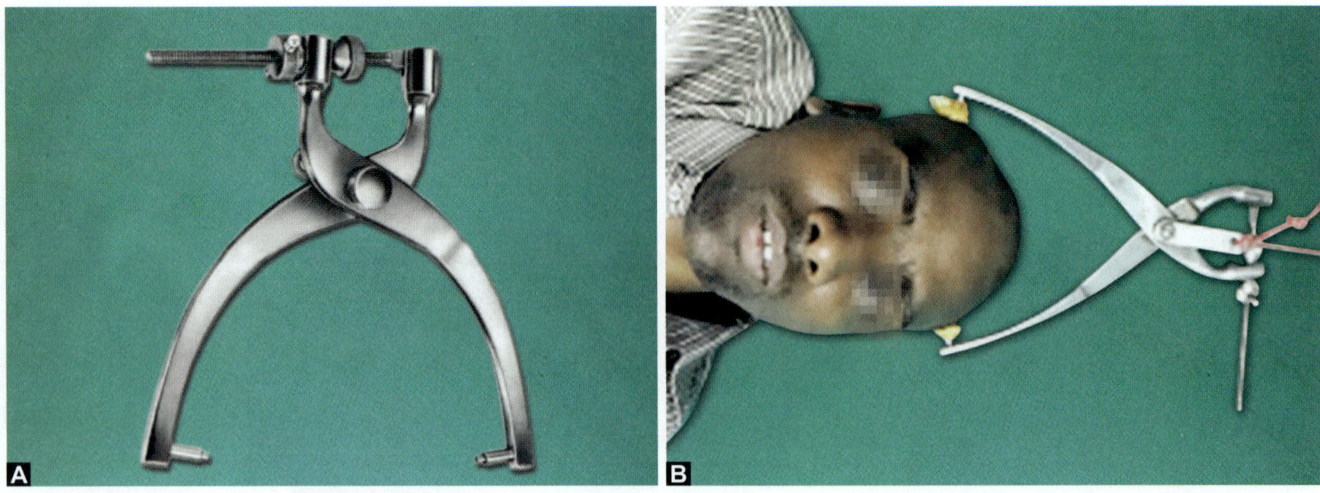

Figs 19.35A and B: (A) Crutchfield tong; (B) Application of Crutchfield tong

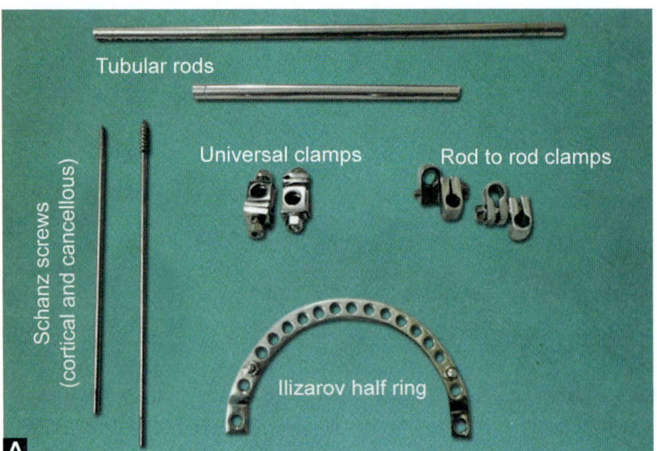

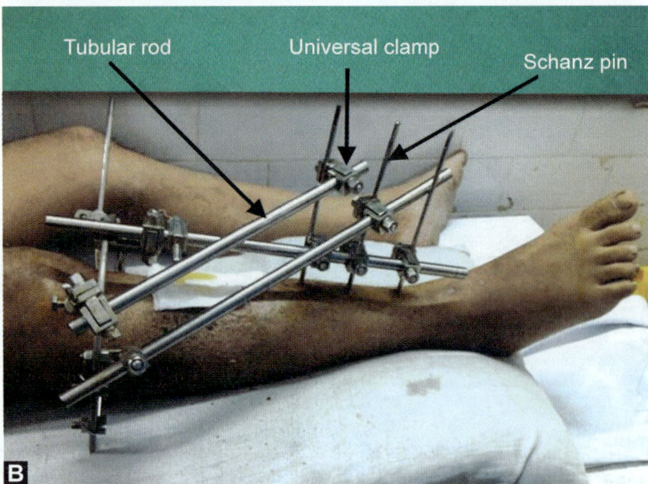

Figs 19.36A and B: (A) External fixator assembly; (B) External fixator applied for an open fracture of tibia

Clamps: These are used for connecting rods to Schanz pins or to interconnect rods to each other. Two tubular rods are connected to each other with a tube to tube clamp while a universal clamp connects a rod to a Schanz pin.

With these parts, external fixators can be constructed to any length and shape as per requirement.

Expandable Fixators

JESS (Joshi's external stabilization system) fixator: This is a modified external fixator that works on the concept of ligamentotaxis. It is commonly used in comminuted distal radius fractures (*see* Page 34 and 96 for details). A special JESS has also been designed to be used in cases of clubfoot [congenital talipes equinovarus (CTEV) where it works by distracting contracted soft tissues of posteromedial side of foot (*see* Page 346).

Ilizarov and LRS (limb reconstruction system) fixators: These modified external fixators work on the principle of distraction osteogenesis. The details have been discussed in Chapter 2 (*see* Page 30).

IMPLANTS FOR FRACTURE FIXATION AROUND HIP

Dynamic Hip Screw (Fig. 19.37)

It is used for fixation of intertrochanteric fractures. It comprises of a sliding screw and an angled plate. The sliding screw has a threaded portion which gets engaged into the femoral head and a nonthreaded part. The plate is angled (usually in the range of 125–145, most commonly the angle being 135°) and has a barrel, which slides over the nonthreaded portion of the sliding screw and a plate which is to be fixed to the femoral shaft with cortical screws. It works on the principle of controlled collapse of the cancellous bone in the intertrochanteric region, thereby aiding union and preventing any malunion.

Dynamic Condylar Screw (Fig. 19.38)

It is similar to dynamic hip screw except that the angle of the plate is 95° and is used in the treatment of subtrochanteric fractures in proximal femur or supracondylar fractures in the distal femur.

Blade Plate (Fig. 19.39)

It is also an implant used for fixation of trochanteric fractures. It consists of a blade attached to a plate at an angle. It comes in variable angles. The blade is inserted into the femoral head and the plate is fixed to the femoral shaft. It also comes as a

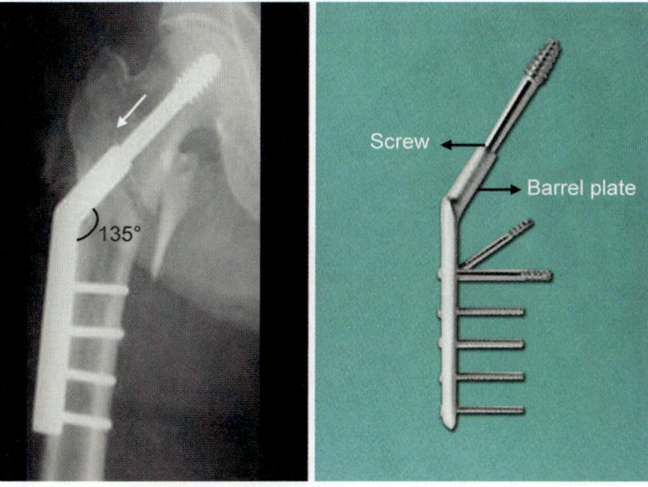

Fig. 19.37: Dynamic compression screw

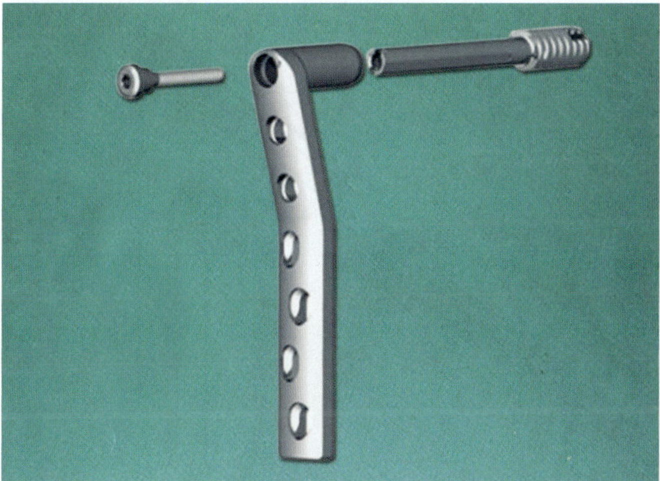

Fig. 19.38: Dynamic condylar screw

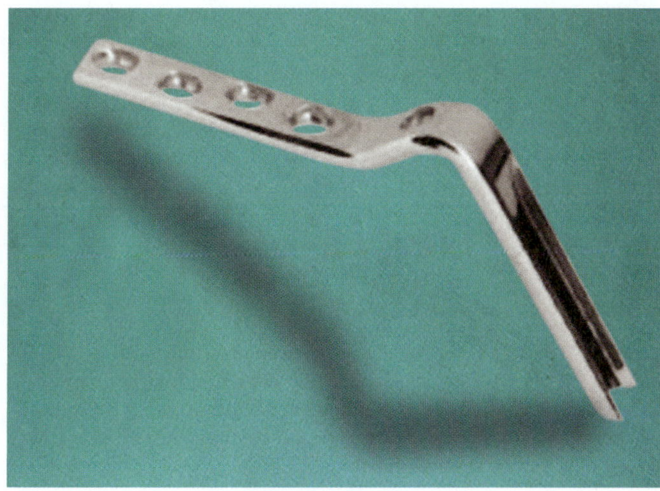

Fig. 19.39: Blade plate

double-angled plate, which is used in cases of valgus osteotomies (e.g. Pauwels' osteotomy).

BONE SCREWS

A screw is a mechanical device that converts rotation into linear motion. Screws are used to fix the plates to the bones or fixing the bone directly.

Parts of a Bone Screw

A bone screw conventionally has four parts **(Fig. 19.40A)**: (1) head (with a hexagonal slot for engagement with a screw driver), (2) shaft (core), (3) threads, and (4) a tip. The shaft diameter pertains to the minimum diameter of a screw recorded at the base of its threads. The diameter of drill bit to be used to drill screw hole should pertain to this shaft diameter. Threads are engraved on this shaft to increase purchase of screw in bone. The thread diameter is thus, the widest diameter of a screw. Screws with wide threads are used in soft cancellous bones to obtain firm purchase. The distance a screw will advance on a single turn of screw driver is also dependent on the threads. The distance between any two adjacent threads is called *pitch of screw*. A screw advances by a pitch distance (called "lead" of a screw) on single turn of a screw driver. The tip of a screw, on the other hand, is an important part deciding the ease of its insertion. Depending on the tip, there can be three types of screws:

1. *Nontapping screw:* They have smooth and conical tips. A bone tap is used after drilling for easing the insertion of these screws.
2. *Self-tapping:* Tip of these screws has cutting flutes for creating a channel, so no taping of the bone tunnel is required after drilling **(Fig. 19.40B)**.
3. *Self-tapping and self-drilling:* These screws sharp polygonal tip and flutes. Drilling and taping are not required before insertion of the screw.

Types of Bone Screws

A number of screw types are available for various applications in orthopedics:

- *Cortical screws (**Fig. 19.41A**):* These are used for fixing a plate to the cortical bone. They have a shaft with smaller threads over it.
- *Cancellous screws:* These are used for fixation in cancellous bones. Their threads are deeper so as to get a firm hold. Cancellous screws can be fully threaded or partially threaded **(Fig. 19.41A)**. The use of partially threaded cancellous screws (also called lag screws) is to bring about interfragmentary compression as explained in **Figure 19.41B**. The threaded portion of the screw engages to the distal fragment (thread hole) while the non-threaded portion of screw just slides through a gliding hole (drilled with slightly oversized bit) as the screw head pushes the proximal fragment towards the distal part, thereby compressing the fracture.

The introduction of cannulated (i.e. hollow from inside) cancellous screws has been another modern day development. These are especially popular for fixation of neck femur fractures in young patients **(Fig. 19.41C)**. First fracture is temporarily stabilized with thin wires (guidewires)

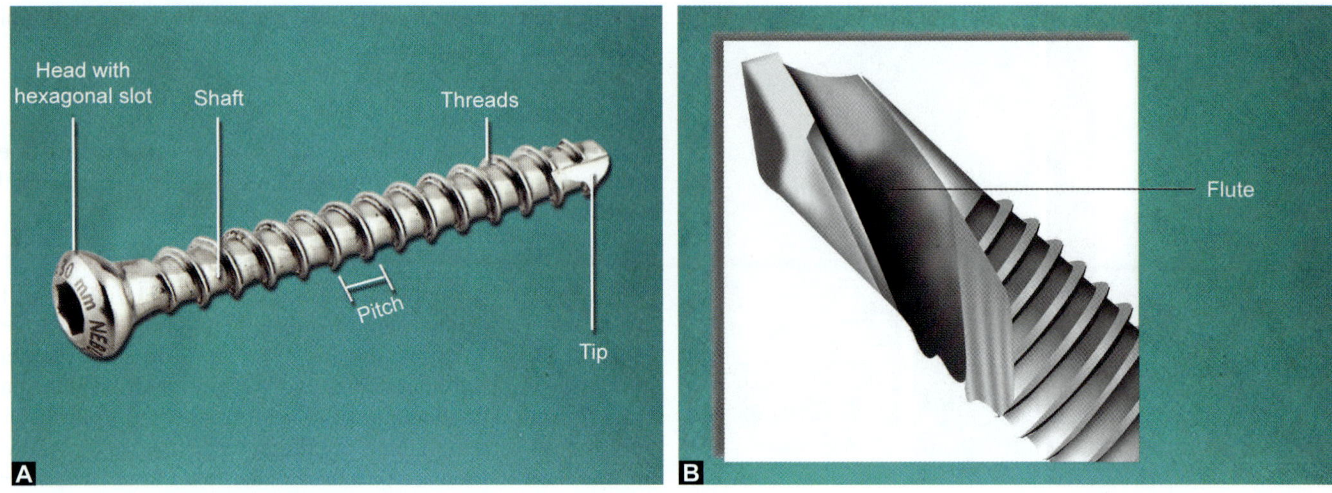

Figs 19.40A and B: (A) Parts of a bone screw; (B) Tip of a self-tapping screw depicting the characteristic flute

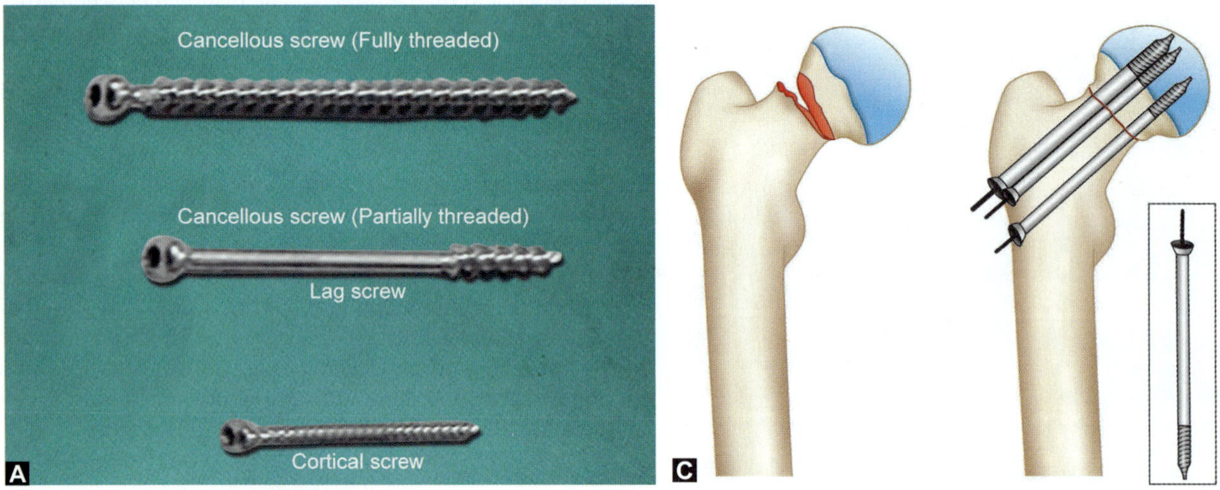

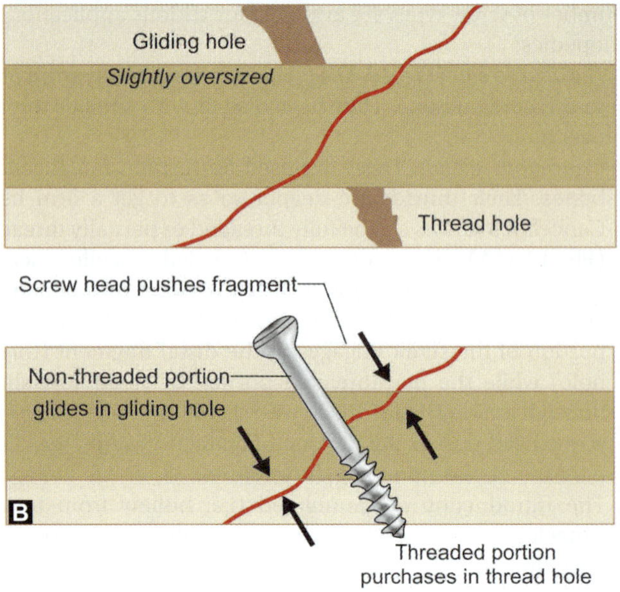

Figs 19.41A to C: (A) Cortical and cancellous (fully and partially threaded) screws; (B) Lag screw principle depicting interfragmentary compression using a partially threaded cancellous screw; (C) Fixation of neck femur fracture using cannulated cancellous screws (i.e. hollow from inside) threaded over guidewires

Table 19.3: Commonly used cortical and cancellous screw sizes (diameters)

Types of screw	Thread diameter (mm)	Shaft/core diameter (mm)	Drill bit diameter* (mm)
Cortical screw	4.5 mm	3.2 mm	3.2 mm
	3.5 mm	2.7 mm	2.7 mm
Cancellous screw	6.5 mm	3.2 mm	3.2 mm
	4.0 mm	2.7 mm	2.7 mm
Locking screw	4.5 mm	4.0 mm	4.0 mm

*As mentioned earlier the size of drill bit corresponds with the shaft diameter of screw. Path for threads that are wider than core is created by "screw tap" to ensure firm purchase.

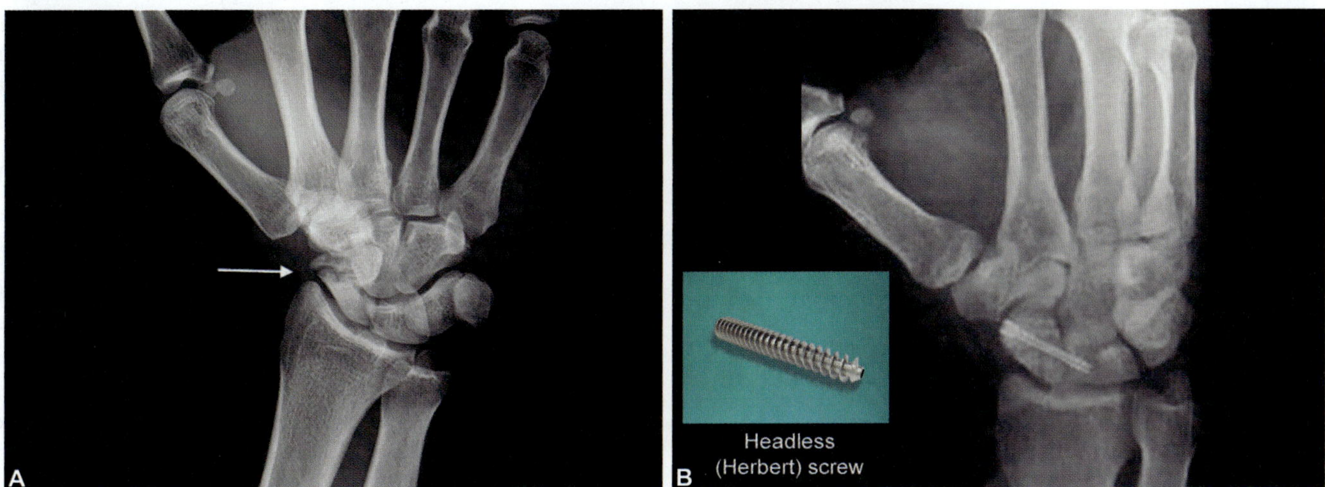

Figs 19.42A and B: X-ray wrist showing fracture of scaphoid (arrow); (B) Fracture fixation with a headless screw
(note the screw head buried inside bone)

positioned in acceptable location and thereafter cannulation allows these screws to be simply channeled over the already inserted guidewires, making the procedure simpler and easier.

- *Locking screws:* These screws have threads extending on to the screw heads. They are especially designed for insertion in a locking plates where their heads lock on to the plate holes for a firmer grip in osteoporotic bones (*see* **Figs 19.4A and B)**.

Common cortical and cancellous screw diameters used in orthopedics are given in **Table 19.3**.

- *Headless screws:* These were introduced by Herbert (Herbert screw, **Fig. 19.42A**) and characterized by variable pitch and the absence of the head. Greater pitch of the distal threads compared to proximal threads results in variable lead of screw at either end. With each turn, distal threads advance more than the proximal threads, leading to interfragmental compression. These are used for fixation of small bones like capitellum, scaphoid **(Fig. 19.42B)** and other carpal bones, tarsal bones, etc.

- *Interference screws* **(Figs 19.43A and B)**: They are most commonly used to secure tendons into bone tunnels in ligament reconstruction surgeries (ACL, PCL reconstruction). These are cannulated, fully threaded variable pitch headless screws. These are different from headless Herbert screws as they do not cause interfragmentary compression. They rather fix the tendon/ligament by pressing it against the tunnel wall, thereby generating resistance against axial movement of the tendon inside a bone tunnel.

IMPORTANT SURGICAL APPROACHES

SHOULDER AND UPPER ARM

These areas are generally opened from anterior aspect by Henry's approach. The plane is between the deltoid (lateral) and pectoralis major (medial).

LOWER ARM

Lower arm is generally opened from posterior approach. The plane is between lateral (lateral) and long (medial) head of triceps muscle.

FOREARM

- To open from anterior aspect, follow Henry's approach for the forearm. The plane is between the brachioradialis (lateral) and flexor carpi radialis (medial). This approach is particularly preferred in distal forearm.
- To open from posterior aspect, follow Thompson's approach. It is generally used for operations on proximal forearm.

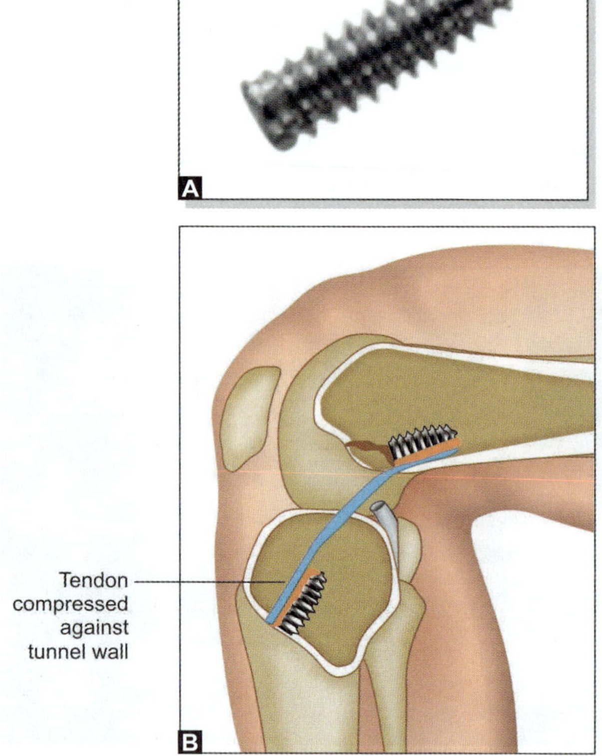

Figs 19.43A and B: (A) Interference screw; (B) Diagrammatic representation of a tendon fixed in tunnel using interference screw for fixation

PELVIS AND ACETABULUM

- *Kocher-Langenbeck approach*: It is a nonextensile posterior approach to the acetabulum, which provides visualization of posterior wall and lateral aspect of the posterior column of the acetabulum. Posterior approach to the hip joint (Moore's approach) uses the same incision and tissue planes.
- *Ilioinguinal approach and iliofemoral approach*: These are anterior approaches.

HIP

Hip can be approached from all sides depending upon indication for surgery.
- *Anterior approach (Smith Peterson approach)*: Surgical plane is present between the sartorius medially (femoral nerve) and tensor fascia lata laterally.
- *Posterior approach (Moore's or Southern approach)*: Incision is identical to Kocher-Langenbeck, except localized posterior to the greater trochanter. After incising TFL and gluteal fascia, gluteus maximus is bluntly divided and then external rotators are cut to expose the joint.
- *Anterolateral approach (Watson-Jones approach)*: This approach utilizes the surgical plane between the tensor fascia latae in front and the gluteus medius behind.

- *Direct lateral or transgluteal approach (Hardinge's approach)*: In this approach periosteum is elevated covering the greater trochanter and the anterior one-third of the gluteus medius and vastus lateralis insertions on the greater trochanter are split longitudinally and sharply separated from the greater trochanter.
- *Medial approach (Hoppenfeld and deBoer approaches)*.

Total hip replacement can be performed from either of anterior, posterior or lateral approaches. The posterior approach provides the best exposure and is approach of choice in revision surgeries. However, it carries a higher dislocation rate. The dislocation rate is least with anterior approach but the exposure is limited and there are higher chances of heterotopic ossification. The lateral approach is a balance between the two. There is still no approach of choice and the approach to choose is surgeon dependent.

In case of developmental dysplasia of the hip (DDH), the hip joint is opened from the anterior side by special approach called as Somerville approach.

KNEE

Generally, knee is opened from anterior aspect by medial parapatellar approach. Lateral (Henderson) approaches are used in rare circumstances.

Common approaches for total knee replacement:
- *Medial parapatellar approach*: Most commonly used. Medial patellar retinaculum is excised and patella is retracted laterally to expose the joint.
- *Subvastus approach*: Here vastus medialis is lifted from its insertion on medial intermuscular septum and retracted laterally along with patella. It is a modification that is especially less damaging to the vascularity of the patella and the quadriceps muscle, but has the disadvantages that exposure is not as good so cannot be used in obese patients and in revision knee arthroplasties.
- *Midvastus approach*: This approach involves splitting the vastus medialis in line with its fibers.

ANKLE

- *Colona and Ralston (posteromedial approach)*: Incision is given behind the medial malleolus. It is used particularly for fixing Pott's fractures (bimalleolar fractures).
- *Gatellier and Chastang (posterolateral approach to ankle)*: For fixing Cotton's fractures (trimalleolar fractures where the posterior malleolus also has to be fixed).
- *Ollier's approach*: It is a special approach where the incision is on the anterolateral aspect of the ankle and foot in an area called sinus tarsi (a depression seen on anterolateral aspect of proximal foot). It can be used to expose three joints: (1) subtalar, (2) calcaneocuboid, and (3) talonavicular in single incision and hence would be the approach to perform triple arthrodesis in patients with CTEV who are older than 10 years.

Synopsis of Orthopedics

FRACTURE EPONYMS

UPPER LIMB

Mallet finger: Avulsion or rupture of extensor tendon from the base of the distal phalanx.

Jersey finger: Avulsion of flexor tendon (FDP) from base of distal phalanx.

Gamekeeper's/Skier's thumb: Avulsion of the ulnar collateral ligament at metacarpophalangeal (MCP) joint of thumb from base of proximal phalanx.

Bennett's fracture dislocation: Oblique, displaced intra-articular fracture of the base of the first metacarpal with subluxation of the trapeziometacarpal joint such that the shaft of the first metacarpal is displaced laterally by abductor pollicis longus.

Rolando fracture: Intra-articular Y-shaped fracture of the base of the first metacarpal with same but relatively less of diaphyseal displacements as a Bennett's fracture.

Boxer's fracture: Fracture through the neck of the 5th metacarpal, usually occurs in boxers.

Kaplan's dislocation: Dislocation of the MCP joint (classically of index finger).

Colles fracture: A fracture at the corticocancellous junction of the distal end of the radius with dorsal tilt of distal fragment, commonly seen in postmenopausal osteoporotic females.

Smith's fracture: A fracture at the corticocancellous junction of the distal end of the radius with ventral tilt of distal fragment (also called as Reverse colles fracture).

Barton's fracture: Intra-articular fractures through the distal articular surface of the radius, taking a margin of radius with the carpals, displaced anteriorly or posteriorly.

Chauffeur fracture: A fracture of the styloid process of the radius.

Die punch fracture: A comminuted impacted fracture of distal radius.

Torus fracture: Special fracture pattern seen in children where a single cortex of bone is buckled inside. It is mostly seen in distal radius.

Green stick fracture: A special fracture pattern seen classically in children (due to elastic bones and a thick periosteum) where there is break in a single cortex of bone and on X-ray one finds only bending of bones.

Night stick fracture: A fracture of the shaft of ulna sustained while trying to protect from a stick blow.

Monteggia fracture: Fracture of the proximal third of the ulna with dislocation of the radial head.

Galeazzi fracture (Piedmont fracture): Fracture of the distal third of radius with subluxation of the distal radioulnar joint.

Side-swipe injury (Baby car fracture): It is an elbow injury sustained when one's elbow is projecting out of a car and is side swept by another vehicle. The patient sustains fractures of the distal end of humerus with fractures of proximal ends of radius and ulna.

Nurse maid's elbow/Malgaigne's subluxation: Refers to Pulled elbow which is subluxation of radial head out of the annular ligament.

Hotchkiss terrible triad of elbow injury: Comminuted fracture of the radial head, fracture of the coronoid process of ulna and posterolateral dislocation of elbow.

Luxatio erecta: Refers to inferior dislocation of shoulder.

Hume's fracture: Monteggia variant occurring in children where there is fracture of olecranon (i.e. proximal ulna) along with anterior dislocation of radial head.

PELVIS AND LOWER LIMB

Dashboard fracture: A fracture of posterior lip of the acetabulum, often associated with posterior dislocation of the hip (other concomitant injuries can involve femoral condyles, patella and posterior cruciate ligament).

Straddle fracture: Bilateral superior and inferior pubic rami fractures.

Open book fracture: A pelvic fracture due to anteroposterior compression of pelvis where the pubic symphysis is disrupted and pelvis opens up like a book.

Malgaigne's fracture: A type of pelvis fracture due to side-to-side compression of pelvis where there is fracture of pubic rami anteriorly and sacroiliac (SI) joint or ilium posteriorly but on the same side.

Bucket handle fracture: A type of pelvis fracture due to side-to-side compression of pelvis where there is fracture of pubic rami anteriorly and sacroiliac joint or ilium posteriorly but on the opposite side.

Crescent fracture: Iliac wing fracture in pelvis that enters into SI joint.

Jumper's fracture: Transverse fracture of sacrum seen in patients who have a fall from height during a suicidal attempt. It is characterized by 'H 'or 'U' shaped fracture line involving upper sacrum (S1 and S2).

Wind swept pelvis: It is a lateral compression injury of ipsilateral hemipelvis and open book or external rotation type injury of contralateral hemipelvis.

Duverney fracture: Isolated iliac wing fracture.

Unresolved fracture: Neck femur fracture.

Underwear fracture: Intertrochanteric fracture.

Hoffa fracture: Fracture of the condyles of femur in coronal plane.

Bumper fracture: A fracture of the tibial plateau.

Toddler's fracture: A spiral fracture of the tibial shaft seen in toddlers due to twisting injury.

Pott's fracture: Bimalleolar ankle fracture.

Cotton's fracture: Trimalleolar ankle fracture.

Bosworth fracture: A fracture dislocation at ankle where fibula is trapped behind tibia.

Massonaie's fracture: In this an ankle fracture is associated with fracture of the neck of fibula.

Runner's fracture: Stress fracture of the distal fibula.

Pilon fracture: It is a comminuted intra-articular fracture of the distal end of tibia.

Tillaux fracture: This is avulsion of anterior tibial margin by the anterior tibiofibular ligament (Salter-Harris type III injury).

LeForte-Wagstaffe fracture: This is fibular avulsion fracture of the anterior tibiofibular ligament (counterpart of Tillaux fracture).

Aviator's fracture: Fracture of neck of talus.

Lover's fracture/Don Juan fracture: Calcaneum fracture when there is fall from height.

Chopart fracture–dislocation: A fracture–dislocation through intertarsal joints.

Lisfranc fracture–dislocation: A fracture–dislocation through tarsometatarsal joints.

Jones fracture: Avulsion fracture of the base of the 5th metatarsal due to pull of peroneus brevis at the metaphyseo-diaphyseal junction.

Pseudo-Jones/Dancer's fracture: Avulsion fracture of the tip of 5th metatarsal.

March fracture: Stress fracture of the shafts of 2nd or 3rd metatarsal.

Chalk stick fractures: In these fractures, the fracture line is transverse to the long-axis of the bone, like a broken stick of chalk. They are seen mostly in long bones (also in vertebrae) in Paget's disease and osteopetrosis and ankylosing spondylitis.

Banana fracture or incremental fracture: It refers to a complete, horizontally-oriented pathological fracture seen in deformed bones affected by Paget's disease.

Triplane fractures: Salter-Harris type IV injuries of distal tibia seen classically in adolescents. The fracture line characteristically runs in all three planes—vertically across epiphysis, horizontally in physis and obliquely across metaphysis.

SPINE

Jefferson's fracture: Burst fracture of the first cervical vertebra.

Whiplash injury: Cervical spine injury where sudden flexion followed by hyperextension (main damaging force) takes place.

Chance fracture: Also called seat belt fracture, the fracture line runs horizontally through the body of the vertebra, through and through, to the posterior elements.

Burst fracture: It is a comminuted fracture of the vertebral body where fragments "burst out" in different directions often entering the canal and injuring cord.

Clay-Shoveller's fracture: It is an avulsion fracture of spinous process of one or more of the lower cervical or upper thoracic vertebra (usually C7 or T1).

Hangman's fracture: It is a fracture through the pedicle and lamina of C2 vertebra, with spondylolisthesis of C2 over C3, sustained in hanging (less commonly) or in road traffic accidents (more commonly).

Growing fractures: These are skull fractures seen mainly in infancy and early childhood characterized by progressive diastatic enlargement of the fracture line. A complication can be a cystic mass filled with CSF, called as a "leptomeningeal cyst".

Motorcyclist's fracture: It is a fracture of the floor of the skull. The base of the skull is divided into two halves, anterior and posterior, each moving independent of each other as if connected via hinge, hence also called as "Hinge fracture".

Undertaker's fracture: It is basically a postmortem fracture which occurs due to careless handling of the dead body by undertakers, most commonly at C6–C7 level.

IMPORTANT DEFORMITIES WITH PNEUMONICS

(Note—In fractures, describing deformity means defining the position of distal fragment in respect to proximal fragment)

Fracture supracondylar humerus: Cubitus varus (Gun stock deformity).

Fracture lateral condyle humerus: Cubitus valgus.

Colles' fracture: Dinner fork deformity.

Smith's fracture: Garden spade deformity.

Nonunion scaphoid: Hump back deformity.

Anterior dislocation shoulder (FABER): Flexion, Abduction and External rotation.

Posterior dislocation shoulder (FADIR): Flexion, Adduction and Internal rotation.

Inferior dislocation shoulder: Hyperabduction (Salute position).

Anterior dislocation hip (FABER): Flexion, Abduction, External rotation.

Posterior dislocation hip (FADIR): Flexion, Adduction, Internal rotation.

Central fracture dislocation hip: Abduction/Adduction and IR/ER both are possible depending upon injury mechanism plus there is significant shortening.

Fracture NOF (intracapsular) (PDE): Proximal migration, Adduction, External rotation.

Fracture NOF (extracapsular) (PDE): But more exaggerated deformities as compared to intracapsular and also there is coxa vara, i.e. reduced femoral neck shaft angle.

Fracture shaft of femur (PBF-E): Proximal fragment is abducted, flexed and externally rotated.

Pulled elbow: Arm by the side, forearm pronated.

OA of hip (DEF): Adduction, Flexion, External rotation.

OA of knee: Genu varum.

TB knee: Triple deformity, i.e. flexion, external rotation and posterior subluxation of tibia on femur.

TB hip
   Synovitis: (FABER) with apparent lengthening
   Early arthritis: (FADIR) with apparent shortening
   Late arthritis: (FADIR) with true shortening.

RA knee: Genu valgum, wind swept deformity.

RA hand: Swan neck deformity, Boutonniere's deformity, Z deformity of wrist.

RA foot: Hallux valgus, claw toes, hammer toes.

Rickets: Genu varum, valgum and wind swept deformity.

Blount's disease: Bilateral genu varum with genu recurvatum and internal tibial torsion.

IMPORTANT CLINICAL SIGNS AND TESTS

UPPER LIMB

- *Impingement at shoulder*:
  - Neer's test
  - Hawkins-Kennedy test.
- *Supraspinatus testing (most common tendon rupture)*: Jobe's empty can sign, Drop arm test.
- *Subscapularis testing*:
  - Belly press test
  - Left off test
  - Bear hug test.

- *Infraspinatus and Teres Minor testing*: Drop sign, Hornblower sign, External rotation lag sign.
- *Axillary nerve testing (in shoulder dislocation or fracture neck humerus)*: Regiment batch sign.
- *Shoulder instability*:
  - *Anterior instability*: Apprehension sign
  - *Posterior instability*: Posterior drawer/Jerk test
  - *Inferior instability*: Sulcus sign.
- *Anterior shoulder dislocation clinical tests*:
  - Dugas test
  - Callaway's test
  - Hamilton ruler
  - Bryant test.
- *SLAP (superior labral tear from anterior to posterior) tear at shoulder*: O'brien's test, Dynamic labral shear, Biceps load tests (I and II).
- *Elbow dislocation*: Bowstring of triceps and disturbed three point relationship.
- *Tennis elbow*:
  - Cozen's test
  - Maudsley's test
  - Mill's maneuver.
- *Biceps tendinitis*:
  - Speed test
  - Yergason test.
- *VIC*: Volkmann's sign.
- *Piano key sign*: Distal radioulnar joint instability (e.g. Madelung deformity, Malunited colles fracture, etc.).
- *De Quervain's synovitis*: Finkelstein test.
- *Scaphoid fracture*: Watson's test.
- *Flexor tenosynovitis*: Kanavel's signs.
- *Finsterer sign*: Kienbock's disease.
- *Opera glass deformity of hand*: Psoriasis.

NEUROLOGY

- *Tinel's sign & motor march*: Signs of nerve regeneration.
- *Serratus anterior/Rhomboides/trapezius palsy*: Winging of scapula.
- *Erb's palsy*: Porter tip hand.
- *Claw hand*:
  - Klumpke's paralysis
  - Ulnar nerve palsy
  - Combined median & ulnar nerve palsy.
- *Radial nerve palsy*: Finger drop (better) > wrist drop.
- *Ulnar nerve palsy*:
  - Book test (Froment sign) for adductor pollicis
  - Card test for palmar interossei
  - Egawa's test for dorsal interossei.
- *Median nerve palsy*:
  - Pointing sign/Clasping sign/Pope's sign
  - Pen test for abductor pollicis brevis
  - Ape thumb deformity due to paralysis of abductor pollicis brevis
  - Schaeffer's test for Palmaris Longus.
- *Carpal tunnel syndrome*:
  - Phalen's test (conventional test)
  - Durkan's direct nerve compression test (most sensitive)
  - Hand diagram (most specific)
  - Semmes-Weinstein monofilament test.
- *Sciatic/Common peroneal nerve palsy > Deep peroneal nerve palsy*: Foot drop.
- *Mulder's click*: Morton's neuroma.
- Tests for thoracic outlet syndrome
  - Adson's test
  - Wright's test/hyperabduction test
  - Military maneuver
  - Roos test.
- *Patency of radial & ulnar artery*: Allen's test.
- *Signs of nerve root compression*:
  - SLR (passive)
  - Well leg/cross leg SLR (large disk)
  - Lasegue's test
  - Bragard sign
  - Bowstring sign of Mcnab.
- *Modified Schober's test*: For testing lumbar spine flexion (as in Ankylosing spondylitis).
- *Scoliosis*: Adam's test for determining fixity of a curve.

LOWER LIMB

- *Signs of supratrochanteric shortening (Neck femur fracture, hip dislocation acute or chronic)*:
  - Nelaton's line (can detect shortening in bilateral conditions)
  - Chinese line
  - Shoemaker's line
  - Bryant's triangle.
- *Fixed flexion deformity at the hip*: Thomas test.
- *Iliotibial band contracture*: Ober's test.
- *Posterior dislocation of hip*: Vascular sign of Narath.
- *SCFE*: Axis deviation.
- *AVN hip*: Sectoral sign.
- *Siffert-Katz sign*: Blount's disease.
- *CDH (leg length discrepancy)*: Allis'/Galeazzi test.
- *Unstable hip (CDH, Non-union NOF fracture, Neglected dislocation of hip)*: Telescopy + gluteus medius weakness: Trendelenburg test.
- *Iliopsoas tendonitis*: Ludloff sign.
- *SI joint involvement (Ankylosing Spondylitis)*:
  - Gaenslen's test
  - Patrick/FABER test
  - Pump handle test.
- *Ankylosing Spondylitis with cervical spine involvement*: Fletche test.
- *CDH screening*:
  - Ortolani's test
  - Barlow's test (better).
- *Osteochondritis Dissecans knee*: Wilson's test.
- *Chondromalacia patellae*: Movie/theatre/cinema sign.
- *Pes cavus*: Coleman block test.
- *Tendo Achilles rupture (second most common tendon rupture)*: Simmonds Thompson test.

MISCELLANEOUS

- *Chvostek's sign*: Tetany.
- *Beighton's criteria*: Generalized ligamentous laxity.
- *Sausage digits and arthritis mutilans*: Psoriatic arthritis.
- *Scurvy*: Pseudo-paralysis of parrot.
- *Trident hand*: Achondroplasia.
- *Blue sclera/Dentinogenesis imperfecta*: Osteogenesis imperfecta.

RADIOLOGY EPONYMS

IMPORTANT X-RAY SIGNS

General Orthopedics

X-ray signs in scurvy: Wimberger ring, White line of Frankel (also seen in healing rickets and lead poisoning, methotrexate therapy and renal osteodystrophy), Trummerfeld zone, Pelkan spur, Pencil thin cortex, Corner sign.

X-ray signs in rickets: Widening/splaying of the physis and cupping of the metaphysis.

X-ray signs in osteomalacia: Pseudofractures/looser's zones, triradiate and champagne glass pelvis, cod fish vertebrae.

Conditions with Looser's zones: Osteomalacia (characteristic), Renal osteodystrophy, Fibrous dysplasia, Hyperthyroidism, Paget's disease of bone, X-linked hypophosphatemia, Osteogenesis imperfecta.

X-ray signs in Perthes disease: Sagging rope sign, Gage sign and Crescent sign (also seen in avascular necrosis of head of femur).

X-ray signs in SCFE: Trethowan sign, metaphyseal blanch sign of steel.

X-ray features in Achondroplasia: Short interpedicular distance, bullet-shaped vertebra, champagne glass pelvis.

X-ray features in nail patella syndrome: Hypoplastic or absent patella, bilateral posterior iliac horns (Fong's prongs) and prominent anterior iliac spine.

Dripping candle wax appearance/Flowing calcification: Melorheostosis (Leri's disease).

X-ray signs in Trochlear dysplasia: Crossing sign, Double contour sign.

Rugger jersey spine: Hyperparathyroidism, osteopetrosis.

X-ray signs in hyperparathyroidism: Pepper pot skull, Salt and pepper appearance (skull), sclerosis at the base of skull, Brown's tumors, Rotting fence postappearance of femur, subperiosteal resorption of radial side of terminal and middle phalanges (For other causes of acroosteolysis *see* page 336).

X-ray signs in ankylosing spondylitis: Romanus lesions of the spine (Shiny corner sign), Anderson's lesion (Spinal pseudarthrosis), Squaring of vertebrae, Bamboo spine appearance, Dagger spine appearance.

Pencil in cup appearance: Psoriatic arthropathy.

Ivory phalanx: Psoriatic arthropathy.

Martel/ G sign: Gouty arthritis.

Kissing spines: Baastrup's disease (A degenerative change, bony proliferation between the spinous processes of closely approximated adjacent vertebrae).

X-ray signs of Paget's disease: Osteoporosis circumscripta (cotton wool spots in skull), Tam O' Shanter sign (skull), Picture frame vertebra, Ivory vertebrae, Blade of grass or flame appearance (long bones), Brim sign.

Bone within bone appearance (Endobones): Osteopetrosis, sickle cell anemia, thalassemia, Paget's disease, acromegaly, lead poisoning, Growth arrest lines (infancy), Gaucher's disease and congenital syphilis.

Erlenmeyer Flask deformity: Osteopetrosis, achondroplasia, metaphyseal dysplasia (Pyle's disease), fibrous dysplasia, rickets, rheumatoid arthritis, Ollier's disease, thalassemia, Gaucher's disease, Niemann-Pick disease.

White bone (sclerotic bone) disorders: Osteopetrosis, osteopoikilosis, osteomyelitis, osteopathia striata, melorheostosis, Caffey's disease, pyknodysostosis.

Fairbank's triangle: Congenital coxa vara (classical), nonunion neck femur in children.

TB hip: Wandering acetabulum, Pestel and mortar appearance.

TB spine: Aneurysmal sign (Anterior TB), Concertina collapse (Central TB).

Wormian bones: Idiopathic > Osteogenesis imperfecta > Cleido-cranial dysplasia.

Vertebrae plana: See bone tumor capsule.

Risser's sign: Scoliosis.

Trauma

Thurston Holland Fracture fragment: Type II and type IV physeal injuries.

Light bulb sign: Posterior dislocation of shoulder.

Hill Sachs lesion: Recurrent shoulder dislocation.

Bankart's lesion: Recurrent shoulder dislocation.

Sourcil sign: Massive retracted rotator cuff tear.

Celery stalk appearance of distal femur: Chronic ACL tears (mucoid degenerations) and Congenital Rubella.

Fat pad sign: Undisplaced supracondylar fracture humerus.

Terry Thomas/David Letterman sign: Scapholunate dissociation due to ligamentous injury.

Spilled tea pot sign: Lunate dislocation.

Hawkins sign: Fracture talar neck for predicting avascular necrosis.

Battered baby syndrome: Metaphyseal Corner fractures, Metaphyseal Bucket handle fractures, Eggshell fractures, Subdural hemorrhages.

Spur sign: Both column fracture acetabulum.

Beheaded scottish dog sign (Oblique view) and Inverted Napoleon Hat sign (AP view): Spondylolisthesis.

SOME IMPORTANT ANGLES, TRIANGLES, LINES AND INDICES

Southwick's angle: SCFE.

Acetabular index: CDH.

Alpha and Beta angles: CDH (on ultrasonography).

Kite's angle: CTEV.

Singh's index: For grading osteoporosis by quantifying trabeculae in neck femur.

Ward's triangle: Femoral neck (significant for osteoporosis grading).

Babcock's triangle: Neck of femur (could be starting point of TB hip).

Reimer's index: CDH.

Center edge angle of Wiberg: CDH.

Fairbank's triangle: Congenital coxa vara (classical), Perthes disease, Nonunion neck femur.

Neck shaft angle: Normal is 127 degrees.

Pauwel's angle: Neck of femur fracture.

Hilgenreiner's epiphyseal angle: Congenital coxa vara.

Shenton's line: Normally a continuous line. Broken in any pathology that affects supratrochanteric area.

Bohler and Gissane'a angles: Calcaneum fractures.

Neutral triangle: Calcaneum.

Meary's angle and calcaneal pitch: Pes planus and cavus.

Bauman's angle and anterior humeral line: Supracondylar humerus fracture.

Distal radius indices: Radial length, Volar tilt, Ulnar variance.

Gilula lines: Congruent arcs in normal wrist X-ray.

Cobb's angle and Mehta's angle: Scoliosis.

Matta's roof arc angle: Acetabular fractures.

Alpha angle: Femoroacetabular impingement.

Metaphyseal-Diaphyseal angle of Drennan: Blount's disease.

SOME X-RAY VIEWS TO REMEMBER

Axillary view: Lateral view of shoulder joint.

West point axillary view: For Bankart's lesion.

Internal rotation view and Stryker notch view: For Hill-Sachs lesion.

Zanca view: Acromioclavicular joint.

Serendipity view: Sternoclavicular joint imaging to detect dislocation.

Green span view: Fractures of radial head and capitellum.

Jones (AP) view elbow: Evaluation of reduction in supracondylar humerus fractures.

Oblique view wrist and PA view wrist in ulnar deviation: Scaphoid fractures.

Brewerton view: Used to see metacarpal head fractures.

Robert's view: Used for thumb CMC joint.

Carpal tunnel view: For hook of hamate fractures.

Ball catcher's view: For visualizing erosions in RA hand.

Judet views (Obturator oblique and Iliac oblique views): Acetabular fractures.

Frog leg view: A modified method of taking lateral view of hip joint intraoperatively.

Von Rosen view: CDH.

Axial view, Skyline view and Merchant's view: Patellar subluxation.

Mortise view (ankle AP view in 15° internal rotation): Ankle injuries evaluation.

Canale view: Talar neck fractures.

Harris view of hind foot: Calcaneum fractures.

Broden views: Intraoperative assessment in calcaneal fractures.

Swimmer's view: Cervical spine lateral view (shoulder pull down) to assess lower cervical spine (C6, C7 and T1 can be visualized).

Ferguson view: This is 20° caudocephalic AP view of lumbar spine used to detect compression of L5 by a large transverse process of L5 vertebra against sacrum (called as Far out syndrome).

Extra Marks

Rule of two: In any injury, X-rays should always include one joint above and one joint below the level of trauma.

Ottawa ankle rule: Used to avoid unneeded radiographs after ankle injury (i.e. which patient needs X-ray after ankle injury?). Ankle X-ray is required if there is pain in malleolar region plus bony tenderness along the distal posterior edge (or tip) of medial or lateral malleolus or inability to bear weight for four steps.

Ottawa foot rule: X-ray foot is required if there is any pain in the midfoot zone plus bony tenderness at the base of the fifth metatarsal or at the navicular bone or inability to bear weight for four steps.

BONE TUMOR CAPSULE

Father of Orthopaedic oncology: Enneking.

Classification system of bone tumors: ENNEKING classification.

As per Bone Part Involved

All bone tumors in metaphysis except.

Epiphyseal: GCT (metaphyseal if occurs before physeal closure), Chondroblastoma.

Diaphyseal: Ewing's sarcoma, osteoblastoma/osteoid osteoma, Fibrous dysplasia sometimes.

As per Age Group

All tumors occur in less than 20 years age group except.

40–60 years: Hemangioma, Chondrosarcoma.

20–40 years: GCT.

Bimodal: Osteosarcoma (Primary in 10–20 years and Secondary in 40–60 years).

Also remember, Ewing's age group is 5–15 years with second decade being more common.

Most Common Sites

Fibrous dysplasia: Neck of femur and craniofacial bones (equal frequency).

Simple bone cyst: Proximal humerus.

ABC: Proximal femur.

Enchondroma: Hand bones.

Chondroblastoma: Distal femur.

Chondromyxoid fibroma: Proximal tibial metaphysis.

Osteochondroma: Distal femur > Proximal tibia.

Osteoid osteoma: Femur > Tibia (diaphysis).

Osteoblastoma: Vertebra (posterior elements) > Femur diaphysis.

Hemangioma: Spine (T4-L4 region) > Skull.

Giant cell tumor: Distal femur > proximal tibia > distal radius.

Osteosarcoma: Distal femur.

Chondrosarcoma: Proximal femur.

Ewing's sarcoma: Femur diaphysis > Flat bones.

Chordoma (tumor of notochord remnants): Sacrum.

Ameloblastoma (also referred as Adamantinoma): Mandible Adamantinoma of long bones is separate entity and its most common site is Tibia.

Eosinophilic granuloma: Skull.

Solitary plasmacytoma: Spine.

Multiple myeloma: Spine.

Glomus tumor: Subungual area of fingers.

Synovial cell sarcoma: Knee.

Pigmented villonodular synovitis (PVNS): Knee.

Some Important One Liners

Most common tumor of bone: Metastasis.

Most common primary tumor of bone: Multiple myeloma > Osteosarcoma > Chondrosarcoma.

Most common benign bone tumor: Osteochondroma.

Most common true benign bone tumor: Osteoid osteoma.

Most common lesion of bone: Fibrous cortical defect.

Most common malignant tumor of bone found in first decade of life: Ewing's sarcoma.

Most common radiation-induced tumor: Osteosarcoma > Fibrosarcoma > Malignant fibrous histiocytoma.

Most radiosensitive and chemosensitive bone tumor: Ewing's sarcoma most common tumor of jaw is squamous cell carcinoma of oral mucosa but most common bone tumor of mandible is Ameloblastoma.

Most common bone tumor of hand bones: Enchondroma (benign tumor).

Most common malignant bone tumor of hand bones: Chondrosarcoma (otherwise, most common malignant tumor of hand-squamous cell carcinoma).

Most common malignant bone tumor of chest wall: Chondrosarcoma.

Tumor with history night pains: Osteoid osteoma.

Tumor showing diagnostic response to Aspirin/NSAIDs: Osteoid osteoma Codman's tumor is Chondroblastoma Pulsatile bone tumors include ABC, Osteoclastoma (GCT), Telangiectatic osteosarcoma, Metastasis from follicular carcinoma thyroid and renal cell carcinoma (most pulsatile).

Egg shell calcification is a clinical sign in: GCT.

Cell of origin of Ewing's sarcoma is: Mesenchymal/mesodermal.

Markers for Ewing's sarcoma: MIC-2 gene, CD-99, trl (11;22).

Mode of inheritance in hereditary multiple exostosis is—autosomal dominant.

Virus associated with osteosarcoma is FBJ murine virus.

Most common extraskeletal manifestation of Fibrous Dysplasia is café-au-lait spots.

The least recurrence rate in extended curettage is seen with the use of liquid nitrogen.

Important X-ray Signs

Fibrous dysplasia: Ground glass appearance, Rind sign (sclerotic margin around tumor), Shephard crook deformity (collapse of medial part of femoral neck so that proximal femur becomes hook shaped, seen in Paget's disease and Osteogenesis imperfect also).

Simple bone cyst: Fallen leaf sign (can be seen in ABC but less often), Trap door sign.

Hemangioma: Corduroy appearance (Jail house sign), Polka dot pattern.

Osteoid osteoma: Nidus < 1.5 cm and osteoblastoma > 1.5 cm.

GCT: Soap bubble appearance.

Osteosarcoma: Codman's triangle, Sunray appearance (due to calcification along sharpey's fibers).

Chondrosarcoma: Popcorn like calcification.

Ewing's sarcoma: Onion peel appearance (intense periosteal reaction in layers), Codman's triangle.

Eosinophilic granuloma: Punched out lytic lesions in skull with double contours.

Multiple myeloma: Punched out lesions without a reactive/sclerotic surrounding zone.

Causes of Vertebrae Plana (Flat Vertebrae)

Langerhan cell histiocytosis (LCH): Most common cause is Eosinophilic granuloma, a subtype of LCH.

Ewing's sarcoma.

Lymphoma/Leukemia.

Gaucher's disease.

Aneurysmal bone cyst.

Infection: Spondylitis.

Some Syndromes Associated with Bone Tumors

McCune Albright syndrome: Polyostotic fibrous dysplasia, Precocious puberty, café-au-lait spots.

Mazabraud syndrome: Polyostotic fibrous dysplasia with intramural myxomas.

Diaphyseal achalasia: Multiple osteochondromatosis/Hereditary multiple exostosis.

Masada syndrome: Multiple osteochondromatosis in forearm.

Ollier's disease: Multiple enchondromatosis.

Maffucci syndrome: Ollier's disease plus multiple cavernous hemangiomas.

Important Biopsy Patterns

Fibrous dysplasia: Chinese letter pattern.

Chondroblastoma: Chicken wire appearance.

Malignant fibrous histiocytoma: Storiform pattern.

Fibrosarcoma: Herringbone pattern.

GCT VARIANTS (where giant cells are there on biopsy): Chondroblastoma, ABC (closest), SBC, Osteosarcoma with giant cells, fibrous dysplasia, non-ossifying fibroma.

Ewing's sarcoma: Small round cells (Also seen in lymphomas, neuroblastoma, pineoblastoma, medulloblastoma, retinoblastoma-so called Primitive neuroectodermal tumors).

Biphasic pattern: Synovial cell sarcoma.

Important Tumor Markers

Ewing's sarcoma: trl 11;22 (present in 85% cases), CD-99 and MIC-2 gene positive.

Synovial cell sarcoma: trl X;18.

Eosinophilic granuloma (LCH): S-100, CD1-a, Neuron specific enolase (Birbeck granules may be seen on electron microscopy).

Bone Metastasis

After lung and liver, skeletal system is the third common site to receive secondary metastatic deposits from a primary site. Infact metastasis form the most common tumors of the bone.

Metastasis can be blastic/sclerotic or lytic. Blastic are seen in prostate carcinoma and seminoma while lytic are seen in Kidney, Thyroid and Lung malignancies. However, the most common metastasis to bone come from breast carcinoma and are mixed and most commonly affect the thoracic spine.

Most common primary sites for metastasis to bone
> *In males:* Prostate > Lung
> *In females:* Breast > Lung
> *In children:* Neuroblastoma
> *Overall:* Breast > Prostate > Lung.

Most common area to be involved in metastasis to bone is spine (thoracic spine).

Bone to bone metastasis is seen with Ewing's sarcoma > Osteosarcoma.

Metastasis distal to the knee and elbow are very rare and generally tend to arise from lung (most common) and tibia is the most common affected bone in these cases.

Metastasis from bone to other organs most commonly involve lung.

The IOC for detecting occult osteoblastic metastasis is bone scan and osteolytic ones is PET-CT.

Femoral neck is the most common site for a pathological fracture in bone metastasis.

Markers of Bone Formation and Resorption

Bone Resorption:
> Urine and serum cross-linked N telopeptides
> Urine and serum cross-linked C telopeptides
> Urine hydroxyproline
> Urine deoxypyridinoline
> Urine hydroxylysine glycosides
> Serum TRAP (Tartarate resistant acid phosphatase)
> Serum bone sialoprotein.

Bone Formation:
> Serum bone specific alkaline phosphatase
> Serum osteocalcin
> Serum carboxy terminal extension peptide of procollagen-1
> Serum type I collagen extension peptide.

Soft Tissue Sarcomas

Most common soft tissue sarcoma in adults: Malignant fibrous histiocytoma followed by liposarcoma.

Most common soft tissue sarcoma in young adults: Synovial cell sarcoma.

Most common soft tissue sarcoma in children: Rhabdomyosarcoma.

Most common site of Rhabdomyosarcoma: Genitourinary followed by extremities.

Most common soft tissue sarcoma of the hand/upper extremity: Epithelioid sarcoma.

Most common soft tissue sarcoma in the foot: Synovial cell sarcoma.

Most important prognostic factor in soft tissue sarcomas: Histological grade.

Most common radiation-induced soft tissue sarcoma: Malignant fibrous histiocytoma (otherwise, most common radiation-induced sarcoma-osteosarcoma).

Extra Marks

(#) Prognostic factors for Ewing's sarcoma: The most unfavorable-prognostic factor in Ewing's sarcoma is the presence of distant metastasis at diagnosis. Other unfavorable prognostic factors include an age older than 10 years, a size larger than 8 cm, more central lesions (as in the pelvis or spine) and poor response to chemotherapy. The histological grade is of no prognostic significance, as all Ewing's sarcomas are of high grade. Fever, anemia, and elevated white blood cell (WBC) count, ESR, and lactate dehydrogenase (LDH) values have been reported to indicate more extensive disease and a poorer prognosis. The presence of trl 11; 22 (present in 90% cases of Ewing's sarcoma) however, does not seem to affect the clinical course.

(#) Extraosseous osteosarcoma and Ewing's sarcoma are also known to occur. These generally involve older adults and have relatively bad prognosis as compared to the osseous counter parts. Most common site for extraosseous Ewing's is paravertebral musculature and chest wall while its thigh for extraosseous osteosarcoma.

(#) The most common site for an extramedullary myeloma is skin and soft tissues > liver. Over 80% of these arise in the region of head and neck, especially the upper respiratory tract.

SPINAL CRASH COURSE

SPINAL INJURIES

Vertebrae with most constant number are cervical while the most variable region is coccygeal.

Most common mode of injury: Fall from height in developing and RTA in developed world.

Most common level of vertebral fracture: D12 > L1App 20% of spinal injuries land up with neurological deficit.

Special X-ray view to visualize lower cervical spine: Swimmer's view.

Dislocations without fractures are most common in cervical spine.

Osteoporosis is the most common cause of compression fractures.

Mechanisms of Vertebral Injury

Most common mechanism of injury: Flexion (Flexion distraction).

Most dangerous: Shear/translation > Flexion rotation > Flexion distraction.

Facet dislocations seen in: Flexion rotation > Flexion distraction.

Burst fractures occur due to: Axial compression.

Tear drop fractures and wedge compression fractures occur in: Flexion compression injuries.

Fracture Eponyms

Jefferson fracture: It is the most common type of atlas fracture. It is a Burst fracture of C1 vertebrae. Despite being a burst fracture, the chances of neurological deficit are considerably low.

Chance fracture (Seat belt injury/Jack knife injury): Seen in head on collision of vehicles. It's a flexion followed by flexion distraction injury. Vertebral column is transacted through and through from front to back causing complete cord injury. Generally T12-L2 vertebrae are involved.

Whiplash injury (Rail road spine): It occurs when a vehicle hits your car from back (rear end collision). There is sudden hyper-flexion of spine followed by hyperextension (main damaging force). The X-rays are mostly normal but sometimes there can be injury to the cord.

Clay Shoveller's fracture: Avulsion fracture of spinous process of vertebrae (C7 > T1).

Jumper's fracture: It's a transverse fracture (U or H shaped fracture line in upper sacrum) of sacrum when there's fall from height.

Hangman's fracture: Technically spondylolisthesis of C2 over C3/or a fracture of pars/isthmus of C2. It is classified by Levine and Edwards classification into three types out of which Type II is the most common and in type II, cervical traction is contraindicated for treatment. Just immobilize with collar, union almost always occurs. Mechanism involves hyperextension followed by distraction in hanging and extension with axial loading (RTAs, more common). It is second most common type of axis fracture (Odontoid being most common). Acute post-admission mortality is low.

SCIWORA: It refers to "spinal cord injury without radiological abnormality". It's an injury pattern classically seen in children < 8 years (classically infants) due to their lax ligaments. During injury there is distraction injury to cord but no visible injury to vertebral column.

Treatment Protocol for Spinal Fractures

Stable fractures are treated with cervical traction with crutchfield tongs.

Unstable fractures (with neurological deficit) initially are managed with traction and once patient is stable, operative decompression with instrument stabilization is performed.

If a polytrauma patient present to emergency now, even before airway management the first recommendation is cervical collar application for stabilizing spine.

Spondylolisthesis

Fracture in pars interarticularis part of vertebra which causes upper vertebra to slip forward over the lower.

Isthmic > Degenerative type is the most common.

Most common level is L5-S1.

X-ray signs include: Inverted napoleon hat sign in AP view and Scottish dog sign in lateral view.

Least useful view for spondylolisthesis is AP view.

SPINAL CORD INJURY

Immediately after injury patient lands up with spinal shock, i.e. there is complete loss of power and sensation below the level of lesion. Spinal shock lasts for app. 24–72 hrs and then recovery starts. During recovery, patient demonstrates increased tone and exaggerated reflexes below the level of lesion.

First reflex to come after spinal shock is over: Bulbocavernosus reflex.

Neurogenic shock: It's a complication of spinal cord injury when the injury is above T6 generally. It refers to fall in BP due to loss of sympathetic support from cord. One has to differentiate it from hypovolemic shock. In neurogenic shock despite low BP, pulse rate is low because of absent sympathetic support but in hypovolemic shock there is tachycardia.

Autonomic dysreflexia: It's another possible complication of spine injury (generally above T6 level). It's characterized by paroxysmal hypertension due to autonomic overstimulation that occurs as a result of misinterpretation of the afferent stimuli from areas below the level of the lesion.

To localize level of any spinal cord injury important things to remember:

DERMATOMES	
Upper limb	*Lower limb*
C4—Shoulder	L1—Groin
C5—Lateral arm	L2—Anterior thigh
C6—Thumb and lateral fore arm	L3—Anterior knee
C7—Index to ring finger	L4—Medial leg and foot
C8—Little finger	L5—Lateral leg and foot
T1—Medial forearm	S1—Plantar surface of foot and calf
	S5—Perianal area
MYOTOMES	
Upper limb	*Lower limb*
C5—Deltoid	L2—Hip flexor (Iliopsoas)
C6—Wrist extensors	L3—Knee extensors (Quadriceps)
C7—Wrist flexors/Elbow extensor	L4—Ankle dorsiflexor (Tibialis anterior)
C8—Finger flexors to the middle finger	L5—Long toe extensors (EHL)
T1—Small finger abductors	S1—Ankle plantar flexors (Gastrosoleus)
REFLEXES	
Upper limb	*Lower limb*
Biceps—C5	Knee—L3, L4
Triceps—C7	Ankle—S1, S2
Supinator—C6	Plantar—L5, S1

Beevor's sign: (T7-T12)- Patient is asked to sit up from supine position with hands on back of head and movement of umbilicus is noted.

Complete versus Incomplete Cord Injury

To know if some part of cord is spared look for SACRAL SPARING represented by intact perianal sensations, voluntary rectal motor function and great toe flexor activity. This signifies that at least some part of cord (sacral being innermost) is intact and hence its incomplete cord injury and one can expect some functional return.

Incomplete/Partial Spinal Cord Injury Syndromes

Brown-Séquard syndrome: Hemitransection of cord. I/L loss of muscle power, I/L loss of proprioception, sense of vibration AND C/L loss of pain and temp sensation. Prognosis for recovery is best with 90% patients improving.

Central Cord Syndrome: Most common syndrome. Patients have quadriparesis involving UL (FLACCID PARALYSIS > LL (SPASTIC PARALYSIS). It results from hyperextension injury in older person with preexisting OA of spine. The SC is pinched between the vertebral body ant and buckling ligamentum flavum post affecting the centrally placed UL tracts prognosis is second best with > 50% patients recovering BB function, ambulation.

Anterior Cord syndrome: Typically after hyperflexion. Predominantly patient has motor loss and pain and temperature loss. Dorsal column (sensations) preserved. Recovery rate poorest!

Cauda Equina syndrome (Orthopedic emergency): Refers to multiple hanging lumbar nerve root compression in spinal canal occurring in vertebral injury level below L1 (where spinal cord ends and nerve roots are there in canal. Clinical features include saddle anesthesia, bilateral radicular pain, asymmetrical flaccid paralysis in both lower limbs with areflexia and loss of voluntary bladder and bowel function.

Conus Medullaris syndrome: Seen in T12-L1 injuries. There is loss of bladder bowel control due to injury to sacral part of spinal cord with perianal anesthesia (cf saddle in cauda). Knee reflex is always preserved which can be lost in Cauda equina. The bulbo cavernous reflex may be permanently lost.

Most common incomplete spinal cord injury syndrome: Central cord syndrome.

Incomplete spinal cord injury syndrome with worst prognosis: Anterior cord syndrome.

Incomplete spinal cord injury syndrome with best prognosis: Brown-Séquard syndrome.

Disk Prolapse

The most common level is L4-L5 > L5-S1. In cervical spine the most common level is C6-C7 > C7-C8.

In disk prolapse, for example in L5-S1 prolapse, always lower level nerve root is compressed, so here S1 will be compressed. Same formula applies to disk prolapse in cervical spine.

RED and YELLOW FLAG SIGNS: Red flag include signs that are possible indicators of serious spinal pathology while yellow flags include pyschosocial factors indicative of problem ending up in long-term chronicity and disability.

Treatment: In disk prolapse generally those patients are advised operative decompression (laminectomy) who either present with progressively increasing neurological deficit or those who do not respond to conservative treatment for minimum of 6 weeks.

Spinal Canal Stenosis

Refers to condition where mostly due to facet joint degeneration there is narrowed diameter of spinal canal (< 10 mm), mostly affecting the lumbar spine. These patients present with Ape like posture (forward flexed position) and intermittent claudication pain on walking a fixed distance. The clinical sign positive is Shopping cart sign. The patients not responding to conservative treatment need operative decompression for which conventionally laminectomy was advised while a recent option (especially for cervical stenosis) coming up is Laminoplasty. It is a method of spinal decompression mainly used in canal stenosis in cervical spine (use of laminoplasty for disk removal is not advocated). Here the lamina is not removed. Rather bone is cut and swung open to decompress the cord and then repositioned.

Vertebroplasty and Kyphoplasty

VERTEBROPLASTY refers to injecting bone cement (PMMA) in vertebral body via transpedicular route to strengthen the collapsing vertebrae, a treatment for prevention of osteoporotic compression fractures. KYPHOPLASTY is a better form where an inflatable balloon is introduced prior to cement injection to restore the height of the collapsed vertebra in order to correct the deformity.

Vertebroplasty is also employed in treatment of a vertebral hemangioma. However, the procedure is contraindicated in spinal or generalized infections, uncontrolled bleeding disorders, asymptomatic patients and in spinal tumors with cord involvement.

LIGAMENTOUS INJURIES OF KNEE REVISITED

Introduction

Two cruciate ligaments (ACL, PCL): Intra-articular but extrasynovial.

Two collateral ligaments (MCL, LCL): Extra-articular and extrasynovial.

Two menisci (cartilaginous c shaped washers between condyles with medial meniscus being larger than lateral): Intra-articular and intrasynovial.

Mechanisms of Injury

MCL: Valgus thrust to knee.

LCL: Varus thrust to knee.

ACL: Hyperextension of knee (*With tibia grounded, when knee is hyperextended, femur moves back on tibia. This ruptures ACL which prevents tibia moving forwards on femur or vice versa.*

PCL: Dashboard injury to a hyperflexed knee.

Menisci (Medial injured more than lateral): Twisting injury (rotation of condyles).

(A question comes that injury to menisci is impossible until there is no-Flexion, Extension, Rotation etc? Answer is Flexion as in extension knee is locked and no rotation is possible and hence no meniscal injury (prefer flexion as answer more over rotation).

**But please make note that in clinical practice isolated injuries are seldom seen as combination of forces act on knee, resulting in specific patterns of injuries.

Most common combination pattern: O'DONOGHUE'S UNHAPPY TRIAD (ACL, MCL, Medial meniscus).

Other important pattern is SEGOND FRACTURE: ACL tear plus avulsion of capsule from Lateral tibial plateau (*The question that comes refers to chip of avulsed bone on lateral side of tibia and candidate is asked regarding associated ligament injury, answer is ACL*).

Diagnostic Tests

For Collateral ligament injuries: Stress tests (Varus stress test for LCL and Valgus stress test for MCL tear)—most specific for collaterals when done at 30° of knee flexion, Apley's distraction test.

For ACL: Anterior drawer, Lachman test that is done at 15° of knee flexion (most sensitive). Most specific test is Pivot shift test.

For PCL: Posterior drawer, Godfrey's posterior sag, Quadriceps active test.

For Meniscus: Mcmurray test, Bounce home test, Apley's grinding test, Thessaly's test (currently being proposed as best screening test), Duck waddle test (Childress sign), *Joint line tenderness (Best test for meniscal injury).*

**In chronic cases of ligament injuries there is Instability at knee and *tests for instability include*:

Anterolateral instability (more common) (main component is ACL tear): Pivot shift test.

Posterolateral instability (main component is PCL tear): Dial test, Reverse Pivot shift test. [Dial test is performed at both 90° and 30° knee flexion. At 30° positive test indicates posterolateral corner (PLC) injury while at 90° it indicates PCL plus PLC injury].

Management

For Collateral ligament injury: Conservative treatment as they mostly heal by themselves.

For Cruciate ligament injuries: Reconstruction (i.e replace with hamstring tendon graft).

For Menisci: They are avascular (except in peripheral zone, so remove the torn part (meniscectomy).

Competition Points

Most common ligament injury overall: Medial collateral ligament (but most heal conservatively).

Most common surgically managed knee ligament injury: ACL injury.

Ligament best seen on MRI-PCL (but diagnosis and surgery decision is mainly clinical).

Investigation of choice is MRI but the gold standard is Arthroscopy.

Medial meniscal injury is more common than lateral but degenerative changes post-meniscectomy are more in lateral meniscus.

The most common meniscus tear associated with ACL tear at the time of initial injury is lateral meniscus, though in chronic cases medial meniscus is torn more often than the lateral meniscus due to abnormal loading in ACL deficient knee. Over all posterior horn of medial meniscus is the most common meniscal tear and most tears are of longitudinal type (bucket handle tear is a severe variety of longitudinal type).

Locking (pathological): Refers to inability to extend knee to full extent generally due to a chock of bucket handle tear of meniscus lying inside the joint. (*The term locking has entirely separate and unrelated meaning in anatomy*).

Also remember, if one has to walk downhill, knee will need to go into hyperextension so ACL patients will fear instability while if one has to go uphill, PCL patients will have problems as there is pressure on a flexed knee.

Pellegrini-Stieda Lesion: Calcification at femoral attachment site of MCL.

A Bucket handle tear of meniscus gives a Double PCL sign on MRI of knee (not a PCL tear).

Multiligament knee injuries are defined as disruption of at least 2 of the 4 (ACL, PCL, MCL, LCL) major knee ligaments as a result of trauma.

ACL tear is the most common cause of hemarthrosis in the knee joint.

Swelling after cruciate ligament tear is immediate as blood vessels rupture but not so in meniscus which is avascular. In the latter case the swelling generally appears after a day as it is more commonly due to a synovial reaction.

The most pain sensitive structure in the joint is the capsule and least pain sensitive structure in the joint is the articular cartilage.

Although more common to tear is the medial meniscus, a meniscal cyst and a discoid meniscus (that increase chances of meniscal tear) are more commonly seen in lateral meniscus.

Cyst in a meniscus is more common in lateral meniscus and occurs in the posterior horn. The clinically appear as swellings along the posterior joint line and disappear within joint on knee flexion (Pisani sign).

Celery stalk appearance is seen on MRI in cases of chronic ACL tears (due to mucoid degeneration) while a celery stalk metaphysis is seen on X-ray in cases of Congenital Rubella.

Screw home mechanism: Tibia external rotates in extension while in flexed knee it internal rotates such that the tibial tuberosity comes to lie in line with the patella. This is called Screw home mechanism. It is due to specific bony anatomy of knee (condyles are unequal) and relative difference in lengths of the two cruciate ligaments.

Effusion in the knee joint can be tested by following tests:
    Bulge sign (positive with 10–15 mL of fluid).
    Patellar tap.
    Ballottement of patella.

SURGERIES UNDER ONE ROOF

OPERATIONS WITH SPECIAL NAMES

Upper Limb

Bankart's operation: Anterior shoulder instability due to Bankart's lesion.

Putti plat operation: Anterior shoulder instability due to Hill–Sachs lesion.

Bristow–Latarjet operation: Anterior shoulder instability due to Hill-Sachs lesion.

French osteotomy (modified): Cubitus varus deformity (Malunited supracondylar humerus).

Milch osteotomy: Cubitus valgus deformity (Non-union Lateral condyle humerus).

Maxpage operation: Volkmann's ischemic contracture.

Steindler's release: Plantar fascia release for Pes Cavus.

Fernandez osteotomy: Malunited colles fracture.

Lower Limb

Pelvic osteotomies in CDH
    Salter's osteotomy: Conventional, most commonly done
    Pemberton's osteotomy: Best correction
    Chiari's osteotomy: Salvage procedure.

Varus derotation osteotomy: Perthes disease.

Girdle stone arthroplasty: TB hip.

Core decompression: Nontraumatic AVN femoral head.

Mcmurray's osteotomy: AVN Hip, osteoarthritis hip, non-union fracture neck femur.

Pauwel's osteotomy: Non-union fracture neck femur.

Meyer's/Bakshi's procedure: Non-union neck femur fracture, traumatic AVN femoral head (early stages).

Elmslie Trillat osteotomy: Recurrent dislocation patella.

Yount's release: IT band contracture (Poliomyelitis).

Seek kebab treatment: Osteogenesis imperfecta.

Tension band wiring: Transverse fracture patella, olecranon fracture & malleolar fractures.

Turco's PMSTR: CTEV (1–5 years age).

Dillwyn Evans procedure: CTEV (5–10 years age).

Triple arthrodesis: CTEV (Age > 10 years).

Dwyer's osteotomy: Isolated heel varus (in CTEV).

Lambrinudi arthrodesis: Fixed equinus deformity at foot.

Grice green procedure (subtalar arthrodesis): Congenital Vertical Talus.

Steindler's flexorplasty (shifting flexor origin proximally for about 5 cm to strengthen elbow flexion): For loss of elbow flexion in paralytic disorders.

Vulpius release: Equinus in Cerebral Palsy patients is generally due to selective contracture of soleus muscle and is treated by vulpius release.

Verebelyi-Ogston (V-O) procedure: A rigid clubfoot in meningo-myelocele may need decancellation of talus and cuboid called as VO procedure.

Keller's operation (excision arthroplasty): Hallux valgus.

Mitchell's & Chevron osteotomy: Hallux valgus.

Jone's operation: Claw toes.

Spine

Anterolateral decompression: TB SPINE.

Hong Kong procedure (radical anterior decompression with bone grafting): TB cervical spine.

Smith Peterson osteotomy: Ankylosing spondylitis.

SOME IMPORTANT TENDON TRANSFERS

Omer's transfer: Ulnar nerve palsy.

Jones transfer: Radial nerve palsy.

Saha's transfer (trapezius to deltoid): Deltoid paralysis in polio or brachial plexus palsy.

Camitz transfer (Palmaris longus to Abductor pollicis brevis): Carpal tunnel syndrome.

Zancolli tenodesis: Claw hand.

Sharad/mustard transfer (iliopsoas to greater trochanter): Gluteus medius paralysis (poliomyelitis).

Kaufer (tibialis posterior to peroneus brevis): Equinovarus deformity at foot.

Hoffer (tibialis anterior to medial cuneiform): Equinovarus deformity at foot.

Perry (peroneus brevis to tibialis posterior): Equinovalgus deformity of foot.

IMPLANTS AND THEIR USES

Charnley prosthesis: THR.

Bipolar (Talwalkar) prosthesis: Hemiarthroplasty.

Unipolar prosthesis: Hemiarthroplasty
    Austin Moore prosthesis-young patients
    Thompson prosthesis.

SP (Smith-Peterson) nail: Neck femur fixation.

Knowles and Moore's pins: Neck femur fracture fixation in children.

Dynamic Hip Screw (DHS): Intertrochanteric fractures.

Proximal Femoral Nail: Unstable intertrochanteric fractures.

Reconstruction nail: Concomitant ipsilateral shaft and neck femur fracture.

Condylar blade plate: Distal femoral fractures.

K nail: Femur shaft diaphyseal fracture.

Interlock nails: Femoral and Tibial diaphyseal fractures.

Rush nail: Long bone diaphyseal fractures.

Enders nail: Elastic nails for fixation of long bone diaphyseal fractures.

Talwalkar nails: Diaphyseal fractures of forearm bones.

Insall burstein prosthesis: TKR.

Neer's prosthesis: Shoulder replacement.

Bakshi's prosthesis: Elbow replacement.

Swanson's prosthesis: Small joint arthroplasty in hand.

K wires: Small bone fracture fixation.

Steffi plate: Spine fixation.

Implants for scoliosis correction: Hartshill rectangle, Harrington rods, Luque rods.

Pedicle screws: Fixation of spinal fractures, Scoliosis correction.

THE FIRST-THE LAST; THE SMALLEST-THE LARGEST; THE MOST-THE LEAST; THE BEST-THE WORST!

INFECTIONS

Most common mode of spread of infection to bone—hematogenous.

Most common part of bone involved in osteomyelitis—metaphysis.

Most common etiology in osteomyelitis:
    Overall (in developed and developing countries, all age groups)—*Staph aureus*
    In sickle cell disease patients—*Salmonella*
    In intravenous drug abusers—*Pseudomonas*
    In HIV/immune-compromised—*S. aureus*
    In patients with prosthetic material—*coagulase negative staph > Propionibacterium*
    After animal bite—*Pasteurella multocida*
    After human bite—*Eikenella corrodens*
    Diabetic foot ulcers/Fight bite—*Staph aureus*
    In open fractures and post-traumatic cases—*Staph aureus*
    In postsurgery cases—*Staph aureus.*

First X-ray sign of acute osteomyelitis: Soft tissue shadow > Periosteal reaction.

Investigation for earliest diagnosis of acute osteomyelitis: MRI (Magnetic Resonance Imaging) > Bone scan.

Investigation of choice (IOC) for acute osteomyelitis: MRI.

Gold standard investigation for acute osteomyelitis: Aspiration of pus and culture sensitivity.

Most common complication of acute osteomyelitis: Chronic osteomyelitis.

Most common site for acute hematogenous osteomyelitis (seen predominantly in children) is distal femur.

Most common site of osteomyelitis (acute or chronic) in adults is vertebrae.

Most common complication of chronic osteomyelitis: Acute exacerbation > Pathological fracture.

Most common site of Garre's osteomyelitis is jaw > Diaphysis of tibia.

Most common site for Brodie's abscess is proximal tibia.

Salmonella osteomyelitis most commonly involves: Diaphysis of tibia and forearm bones.

Most common organism causing septic arthritis: S. aureus in all age groups except in young sexually active adults where *Neisseria Gonorrhoea* is the most common cause.

The most common joint affected in septic arthritis: Knee > hip > shoulder.

The most common joint affected in Brucellosis: Hip joint.

Most common organism causing hand infections: S. aureus.

Most common site for felon: Thumb > Index finger.

The most common type of actinomycosis: Oro—cervicofacial.

Overall, most common site of actinomycosis: Mandible.

The most common bone affected in congenital syphilis: Tibia.

In Leprosy, ulnar nerve is the most common nerve involved, followed by common peroneal nerve. Most common cranial nerve involved is facial nerve.

Tuberculosis (TB)

Most common site of skeletal tuberculosis—spine > hip > knee.

Least common site of skeletal tuberculosis—bursal TB.

Amongst bursal TB, most common bursa to be involved—trochanteric bursa.

Most common part of spine to be affected in TB spine—dorsal > lumbar > dorsolumbar (D12-L1).

Most common type of anatomical lesion in TB spine—paradiskal.

In posterior TB, least commonly involved facet joint > spinous process.

Earliest and most common symptom of TB spine—back pain.

Most common cause of paraplegia in TB spine—compression by tuberculous granulation tissue and pus.

Paraplegia in TB most commonly results from disease of upper thoracic spine.

The first clinical sign of TB spine—paraspinal muscle spasm.

The order of neurological involvement in TB spine—ankle clonus (first neurological sign) > plantar extensor > spastic motor weakness > sensory loss > BBI.

Paraplegia is the most common in TB involving dorsal spine.

The first X-ray sign of TB spine—disk space reduction.

The IOC for TB spine—MRI.

The best/gold standard investigation for TB spine—CT-guided biopsy of involved vertebra.

Earliest radiological sign of healing in tuberculosis—sharpening of fuzzy paradiskal margins.

Tuberculosis is the most common cause of kyphosis in India.

Painful limp is the earliest and most common symptom of tuberculosis of hip joint.

The earliest X-ray feature of TB hip is juxta-articular osteopenia > joint space reduction.

TRAUMA AND RELATED AREAS

General

Most mobile joint in the body—shoulder.

Most stable joint in the body—hip.

First clinical stage of union is woven bone while first radiological stage of union is callus (provisional callus that is seen earliest by 3 weeks).

Most common bone to fracture overall and at birth—clavicle > distal end of radius.

Most common fractures in different age groups:
    Birth: Clavicle
    Children: Greenstick fracture of forearm bones > Torus fractures at distal end radius
    Adults: Vertebral fractures > Distal end radius.

Most common fractures when there is history of fall on outstretched hand:
    Child (< 8–10 years old): Supracondylar humerus fracture
    Adolescent: Scaphoid fracture
    Adult: Distal end radius fracture.

Some important facts about dislocations:
    Most common dislocation in adults—shoulder > elbow
    Most common dislocation in children—elbow
    Most common site for Recurrent dislocation—shoulder > Patella
    Most common site for Habitual dislocation—shoulder > Patella
    One of rarest site for recurrent dislocation—ankle
    Most dangerous and one of rarest dislocation—knee
    Most common site of open fractures—tibia.

Most common joint to be involved in open injuries—knee.

Most common site of nonunion—distal Tibia.

Most common cause of nonunion—inadequate immobilization.

The most common joint involved in myositis ossificans is elbow > hip. However, the most common muscle involved in myositis is quadriceps.

In heterotopic ossification the earliest detection can be done by a bone scan. However, the screening investigation for the purpose is alkaline phosphatase levels.

Most common site of physeal injury in a child—phalanx > distal end of radius.

Most common type (Salter-Harris) of physeal injury—Type II.

Weakest zone of growth plate—hypertrophic zone.

Most common site of stress fracture—lower tibia > metatarsals > fibula.

Most common site of stress fracture in foot—metatarsals (2nd > 3rd).

Most common tarsal bone to sustain stress fracture—navicular.

IOC for stress fractures—MRI.

IOC for bilateral stress fractures—bone scan.

IOC for occult fractures—MRI.

Most common cause for destructive bone lesion in adults—metastatic carcinomas.

The most common site of pathological fracture—femoral neck.

In Limb re-implantation the first structure to be re-implanted is bone while the greatest priority is given to vessels.

In Crush injury hand the first to be repaired is bone while greatest priority is given to skin.

Shoulder and Arm

Most common complication of fracture clavicle—malunion.

Most common type of shoulder dislocation—anterior > posterior > inferior (Luxatio Erecta).

Most common subtype of anterior shoulder dislocation—sub-coracoid > subglenoid.

Most common subtype of posterior shoulder dislocation—sub-acromial.

Most common acute complication of shoulder dislocation—axillary nerve injury (circumflex branch).

Most common (overall) complication of shoulder dislocation—recurrent dislocation.

Most common lesion leading to recurrent shoulder dislocation—Bankart's repair.

Most common complication of proximal humeral fractures— stiffness.

The most common complication of fracture shaft humerus—radial nerve palsy.

The most common cause of nonunion in fracture shaft of humerus—distraction at the fracture site.

Elbow and Forearm

The most common type of supracondylar humerus fracture—extension type.

Most common complication of supracondylar humerus fracture—cubitus varus/gun stock deformity (malunion).

The most common fracture associated with vascular injury in child—supracondylar humerus fracture.

Most common nerve involved in supracondylar humerus fractures:
> Overall and in extension type—anterior interosseous nerve > median nerve > radial nerve
> Flexion type—ulnar nerve
> Postsurgery—ulnar nerve
> Posteromedial (more common than posterolateral)—radial
> Posterolateral—median.

The most reliable and earliest sign of compartment syndrome is passive stretch test. The last clinical sign is paralysis and most unreliable is pulselessness.

The most common cause of compartment syndrome is fracture. In children it is supracondylar humerus fracture while in adults it is proximal tibia fracture. Overall compartment syndrome is more common in leg and tibia fractures are the most common cause.

The most common/first muscle involved in supracondylar humerus fracture—FDP > FPL.

The most common nerve involved in Volkmann's ischemic contracture (VIC) is anterior interosseous nerve.

Ipsilateral radius fracture is most commonly associated fracture with supracondylar humerus fracture.

The most common deformity after lateral condyle humerus fracture is cubitus pseudovarus (due to lateral spur formation) > cubitus valgus > cubitus varus.

Lateral condyle fracture is the most common cause of tardy ulnar nerve palsy.

Elbow dislocation is second most common dislocation in adults and the most common dislocation in children.

Most common type of elbow dislocation is posterolateral.

The most common nerve injured in simple elbow dislocation is the median nerve while in complex elbow dislocations (dislocation with fractures) it is the ulnar nerve that is generally injured.

Most common associated fracture with elbow dislocation—medial epicondyle.

The most common complication of distal end radius fractures—stiffness > malunion.

Most common cause of Sudeck's osteodystrophy—distal end radius.

Most common type of Monteggia fracture—Bado Type I.

The most common nerve injured in Monteggia fracture—posterior interosseous nerve.

Wrist and Hand

The most sensitive and specific investigation to detect a fracture of scaphoid—MRI.

Most common type of wrist dislocation—perilunate.

Nerve most commonly involved in perilunate dislocation and lunate fracture—median nerve.

Most common carpal bone to fracture is Scaphoid while least common is Trapezoid.

Neck is the most common site of metacarpal fracture and fifth metacarpal is the most commonly involved metacarpal (Boxer's fracture).

Phalangeal fractures and dislocations are most common hand injuries and fracture of distal phalanx is the most commonly fractured bone in hand.

Thumb followed by fifth finger MCP joints are most commonly dislocated MCP joints. Proximal interphalangeal joint dislocations are more common than distal IP joint dislocation.

Mallet finger is the most common closed tendon injury in sportsmen.

Ring finger is the most commonly involved finger in Jersey finger.

The most common complication of hand injuries is stiffness.

Extensor tendon injuries in hand are more common than flexor tendon injuries. The most common tendon injury in hand is extensor tendon of middle finger. Zone IV (disruption over the metacarpals) is most commonly injured area.

Worst outcome of flexor tendon repair is seen in Zone II (dangerous area or no man's land) because both FDS and FDP run together in common sheath.

Pelvis, Hip and Femur

Most common type of pelvic fractures are rami fractures due to lateral impaction injury.

Posterior wall fractures are the most common type of acetabular fractures.

The most common complication of acetabular fractures is secondary osteoarthritis of the hip joint.

Most common type of hip dislocation—posterior > anterior > central.

Most common acute complication of dislocated hip—sciatic nerve injury (mostly neuropraxia).

Most common complication of dislocated hip—osteoarthritis of hip joint.

Most dangerous complication of dislocated hip is AVN of femoral head.

Although fat embolism is most commonly seen after fracture of femur, it is a rare complication of femur fracture.

Fracture of middle third (transverse fracture pattern) is the most common location of femoral shaft fracture. However, in children the fractures most commonly involve the upper third while pathological fractures especially in elderly involve the relatively weak metaphysio-diaphyseal junction.

Knee ligament injuries are most common associated injury and fracture neck femur is the most commonly missed concomitant fracture with fracture shaft of femur.

Lower limb fractures with maximum shortening are posterior dislocation of hip > femoral shaft fracture > subtrochanteric femur fracture > inter-trochanteric fracture > intracapsular neck femur fracture.

The Leg, Ankle and Foot

In compartment syndrome of tibia the anterior compartment is most commonly involved compartment.

Ankle joint is the commonest site for a ligament injury in the body and ankle sprains are the commonest sports injuries.

The most common ligament injured in ankle sprain is the Anterior Talo Fibular Ligament > Calcaneofibular ligament.

Most common complication of talar fractures—osteoarthritis of subtalar joint.

The most common dislocation of the foot—Lisfranc fracture dislocation.

The most common site of stress fracture in the foot—metatarsals.

The most common bone of the foot to fracture—calcaneum > talus.

Second metatarsal is the longest of all metatarsals and most common site for stress fracture. Fifth metatarsal is most commonly fractured metatarsal.

NEUROLOGY

Largest cord of brachial plexus—posterior cord.

Most common cause of neurological deficit in upper limb—Erb's palsy.

Most common peripheral nerve injury (PNI)—radial nerve.

Most common nerve injuries in athletes—Burners/ Stingers.

Most common cause for nerve injuries—fracture-dislocations.

Most common nerves involved in some common fracture- dislocations
  Clavicular fractures: Lower trunk of brachial plexus
  Shoulder dislocation (all types): Axillary nerve (circumflex branch)
  Surgical neck humerus fracture—axillary nerve
  Shaft humerus fracture (including Holstein Lewis fracture): Radial nerve
  Fracture supracondylar humerus: Median nerve (anterior interosseous branch) > Radial in extension type and ulnar nerve in flexion type
  Medial condyle humerus fractures—ulnar nerve
  Lateral condyle humerus fractures—ulnar nerve (Tardy ulnar nerve palsy)
  Elbow dislocations—median nerve in simple dislocations and ulnar nerve in complex dislocations with associated fractures
  Monteggia fracture dislocation—posterior interosseous nerve
  Lunate dislocation—median nerve
  Hip dislocation—sciatic nerve
  Knee dislocation—common peroneal nerve
  Fibular neck fractures—common peroneal nerve.

Most common infection causing PNI—leprosy.

Most common nerve injured in Total Hip Arthroplasty—sciatic nerve.

Most common nerve injured in intramuscular injections—sciatic nerve followed by Radial nerve.

Most common combined nerve injuries—median plus Ulnar.

Nerve injured during McRobert's procedure for delivery of a child—lateral femoral cutaneous nerve.

Nerve injury with best prognosis—radial nerve.

Nerve injury with worst prognosis—ulnar nerve.

Nerve injury with worst prognosis after repair—sciatic nerve.

Earliest indicator of nerve recovery—electromyography.

Most common sites of nerve compressions—
  Ulnar nerve—Cubital tunnel (behind medial epicondyle)
  Median nerve—Carpal tunnel
  Radial nerve—Fracture shaft humerus
  Posterior Interosseous Nerve—Arcade of Frosche.

Nerve least commonly involved in entrapment neuropathies—femoral nerve.

The most common compression neuropathy overall—Carpal tunnel syndrome > Cubital tunnel syndrome.

Most common cause of Carpal tunnel syndrome—idiopathic > Hypothyroidism.

Most sensitive test for Carpal tunnel syndrome—Durkan's direct nerve compression test.

Most specific test for Carpal tunnel syndrome—hand diagram.

Most common cause of Tarsal Tunnel syndrome—rheumatoid arthritis.

Most common site of nerve grafting—sural nerve while most common site of tendon grafting—palmaris longus.

Most common cause of wrist drop—radial nerve palsy.

RECENT UPDATES

First person to perform arthroscopic procedure—Takaji.

Most common joint to undergo arthroscopic procedures—knee > shoulder.

First person to perform Total Hip Replacement (THR)—John Charnley.

Most common cause of death after THR—myocardial infarction > venous thromboembolism.

MIXED BAG

Most common types of collagen
  In bone—Type I
  In articular cartilage—Type II
  In meniscus—Type I.

The thinnest zone of articular cartilage (with thinnest collagen fibrils) is Zone I (Superficial zone) while the largest is Zone III (Deep zone).

The zone of articular cartilage with synthetically most active chondrocytes—Zone III (Deep zone).

Least active chondrocytes are present in- Zone IV (Calcified zone) of articular cartilage.

The highest content of proteoglycans and the largest collagen fibrils are present in Deep zone (Zone III) of the articular cartilage.

The most abundant cells in bone—osteocytes.

Bone apposition is best seen in Howship's lacunae in normal adult bone while in fractured bone it is best seen in subperiosteal cambium layer.

Most metabolically active mart of bone and part of bone with maximum remodelling—endosteal surface.

In Gait cycle, phase with maximum kinetic energy is heel strike/ loading response while the phase with maximum potential energy is mid-stance.

A bone with no muscle attachment—talus.

The most common congenitally absent muscle—pectoralis major.

Longest muscle in the body—sartorius.

Strongest muscle in the body—gluteus maximus.

Strongest ligament in the body—iliofemoral ligament (Ligament of Bigelow).

Strongest tendon in the body—tendoachilles.

Largest bursa in the body—iliopsoas bursa.

Largest internal organ in the body—skeletal muscles.

Largest avascular structure in the body—intervertebral disk.

The most common site of bursitis is shoulder (subacromial).

Most common site of tendon rupture—supraspinatus > tendoachilles.

Most common cause of tendon ruptures is overuse.

First person to use ligatures—Ambroise Pare (Father of Amputation surgery).

First to use tourniquet—Joseph Lister.

Nerve injury is the most common complication of tourniquet application. Most of these nerve injuries are neuropraxias. And Radial nerve is the most common involved nerve.

The most common amputation performed in orthopedics— transtibial.

The most common indication for amputation—peripheral Vascular Disease.

The best treatment of postamputation neuroma—surgical excision.

METABOLIC DISORDERS

Most common metabolic bone disease—osteoporosis.

The earliest symptom of osteoporosis—back pain.

In osteoporosis, distal radius is the most common site of fracture in patients less than 70-year-old while in those more than 70-year-age, it is the dorsolumbar spine that is the most common site. However, overall vertebral fractures are more common.

Most common complication of osteoporosis—vertebral fractures.

The investigation of choice as well as the gold standard for screening as well as diagnosing and grading osteoporosis is DEXA scan.

The drug of choice for osteoporosis (senile/post-menopausal)—bisphosphonates.

The drug of choice for bisphosphonate resistant osteoporosis—teriperatide.

Most common symptom of osteomalacia—dull aching pain in lower back, pelvis and hips.

Biopsy is the gold standard investigation to make the diagnosis of osteomalacia.

Most common cause of (non-traumatic) protrusio acetabuli in India is osteomalacia and in world is rheumatoid arthritis.

First clinical sign of rickets—craniotabes.

Most common deformity in rickets—genu varum.

The most common subtype of rickets in developing countries—nutritional rickets.

The most common tumor producing oncogenic osteomalacia—hemangiopericytoma.

The most common site for subperiosteal hemorrhages in scurvy—lower end of femur and tibia.

The most common cause of primary hyperparathyroidism—solitary adenoma of the parathyroid glands.

The most common bones affected in Paget's disease of bone—pelvis > tibia.

The drug of choice for Paget's disease—bisphosphonates.

The pain in Paget's disease is best relieved by—calcitonin.

The most common part of spine involved in DISH—thoracic spine.

PEDIATRIC ORTHOPEDICS

The most common congenital anomaly of foot—CTEV.

The prime deformity in CTEV—talonavicular joint subluxation.

Most common type of CTEV—primary idiopathic variety.

Most common deformity to recur in CTEV—equinus > varus.

Most common complication of Triple arthrodesis—talonavicular joint pseudarthrosis.

Most common cause of failure of conservative treatment/relapse in CTEV—noncompliance with bracing.

Most common type of tarsal coalition—talocalcaneal > calcaneo-navicular.

Most common cause of congenital pseudoarthrosis—idiopathic > neurofibromatosis.

Most common cause of acquired pseudoarthrosis—nonunion.

Most common cause of Genu varum—rickets (in India) > Blount's disease (worldwide) in a child and osteoarthritis in an adult.

Most common cause of Genu valgum—idiopathic in a child and rheumatoid arthritis in an adult.

Most common cause of Wind swept deformity—rickets in a child and rheumatoid arthritis in an adult (the term was originally given for rickets).

The prime pathology in CDH—shallow acetabulum.

IOC for CDH in a child less than 6 months is ultrasound (MRI is difficult to get in infants). Thereafter an X-ray can provide the diagnosis in most cases but best anatomical details are given by MRI.

The screening investigation of choice for CDH—ultrasound.

The movements first restricted in CDH abduction and internal rotation.

Acetabular osteotomies for CDH:
    Most commonly performed—Salter
    Best correction—Pemberton
    Salvage procedure—Chiari.

The most common cause of limp in a child less than 10 years of age—Transient synovitis > Septic arthritis > Perthes disease.

In Slipped Capital Femoral Epiphysis (SCFE), slip is best seen in a frog leg lateral X-ray view of the affected hip. The earliest X-ray sign is wide and irregular physis with rarefaction in its juxta-epiphyseal region (preslip stage).

Frequency of affection by hemimelia (congenital deficiencies of long bones)—fibula > radius > femur > tibia.

GENETIC AND NEUROMUSCULAR DISORDERS

Most common permanent disability of childhood is Cerebral Palsy.

Most common type of cerebral palsy—diplegia (geographically), spastic (physiologically), prenatal (etiologically).

Most common muscle involved in Poliomyelitis—quadriceps Femoris (partially paralyzed).

Most common muscle showing complete paralysis in Polio—tibialis Anterior.

Most common muscle of upper limb involved in Polio—deltoid.

Most common hand muscle to be involved in Polio—opponens pollicis.

Most common bone fracture in Poliomyelitis—supracondylar femur fracture.

Most common bone fractured in muscular dystrophies and arthrogryposis—femur.

Most common type of Spina bifida—spina bifida occulta.

Most common site of Spina bifida—S1 > L5.

Most common skeletal dysplasia—osteogenesis imperfect.

Most common lethal skeletal dysplasia—thanatophoric dysplasia.

Most common form of dwarfism—achondroplasia.

ARTHRITIS AND RELATED CONDITIONS

Most pathognomonic feature of RA—rheumatoid nodules.

Most common site for rheumatoid nodules—olecranon.

Most common eye manifestation of rheumatoid arthritis (RA)—keratoconjunctivitis sicca.

The most common cardiac manifestation of RA—pericarditis.

The DMARD of choice and the most commonly used DMARD in RA—methotrexate.

The most common cause of mononeuritis multiplex in India—leprosy.

The first radiological sign of RA—soft tissue swelling > juxta-articular osteopenia.

The most common arthritis to involve wrist—RA.

The most common subtype of Juvenile RA—pauciarticular.

The most common autoantibodies associated with Juvenile RA are anti-nuclear antibodies.

The first joint to be involved in Ankylosing Spondylitis (AS)—SI (Sacroiliac) joint > lumbar spine.

The first X-ray sign of AS—haziness and widening (pseudo-widening) around SI joints (more on the iliac side) due to subchondral erosions that is followed by sclerosis and ossification (first fibrous and then bony ankylosis).

Most acute spinal fractures in the AS population occur in the cervical spine, particularly at C5-C6 and C6-C7 levels.

Most common extra-articular manifestation of AS—acute anterior uveitis (iridocyclitis) occurring in almost one-third of cases.

Most common triggering organism for reactive arthritis—Chlamydia > Shigella.

Most common joint involved in reactive arthritis—knee.

The drug of choice for psoriatic arthritis—methotrexate.

The most common site of Pseudogout—knee.

Psoriatic arthritis most commonly involves—DIP joints of hand.

The joint most commonly involved in primary Osteoarthritis (OA)—knee > hip.

The most common bone involved in OA knee—patella.

The most common muscle weakness seen in OA knee—quadriceps.

Earliest X-ray sign of OA is reduction of joint space.

The first-line drug for osteoarthritis—paracetamol (Acetaminophen).

The most common joint involved in neuropathic/Charcot joint disease—foot (mid tarsal joints).

The most common joint involved in Tabes Dorsalis—knee.

The most common joint affected in ochronosis—spine (inter-vertebral disk) > shoulder.

Most common site for intramuscular bleeding in hemophilia—quadriceps.

In intra-articular bleeding in hemophilia the order of involvement is knee > elbow > shoulder.

Most common region where hemophilic pseudotumors develop—thigh (soft tissue pseudotumors develop in quadriceps while the osseous ones in femur).

Most common nerve compressed by hematoma in hemophilia—femoral nerve.

The most common cause of loose bodies in knee joint—osteochondritis dissecans (OD) in young adults and osteoarthritis in the elderly (overall osteoarthritis).

Most common site of OD—knee (lateral surface of medial femoral condyle is the most common site).

The most common cause of multiple loose bodies in a joint—synovial chondromatosis.

Most common joint affected in synovial chondromatosis—knee.

Most common cause of spontaneous Avascular Necrosis (AVN) of femoral head—idiopathic > steroids.

The earliest diagnosis in AVN is provided by MRI (most sensitive investigation) and it is also the IOC.

The most common cause of monoarthritis in children—TB.

Most common cause of bony ankylosis—septic arthritis.

Practice Session

GENERAL ORTHOPEDICS

1. Adult bone trabeculae are differentiated from fetal bone trabeculae by presence of
   a. Harversian system
   b. Lamellar structure
   c. Certain special staining characteristics
   d. Different types of bone cells in each

2. Most metabolically active part in bone is
   a. Cortical bone   b. Cancellous bone
   c. Periosteal surface   d. Endosteal surface

3. Bone apposition is best seen in
   a. Endochondral ossification
   b. Osteoblastic activity in Howship's lacunae
   c. Subperiosteal cambium layer
   d. Osteoblastic activity at the area of stress

4. Regarding bone remodelling all are true except
   a. Osteoclastic activity at the compression site
   b. Osteoclastic activity at the tension site
   c. Osteoclastic activity and osteoblastic activity are both needed for bone remodeling in cortical and cancellous bones
   d. Osteoblasts transform into osteocytes

5. Callus induction is not hampered in
   a. Hypoxemia   b. Micromovements
   c. Muscle interposition   d. Multiple bone fragments

6. Fracture healing is affected by all except
   a. Osteoporosis   b. Infection
   c. Poor blood supply   d. Soft tissue interposition

7. Provisional callus is seen on X-ray earliest by
   a. 2 weeks   b. 3 weeks
   c. 6 weeks   d. 8 weeks

8. Initial stage of clinical union of bone is equivalent to
   a. Callus formation   b. Woven bone
   c. Hematoma formation   d. Calcification only

9. The most common cause of nonunion is
   a. Infection   b. Inadequate immobilization
   c. Ischemia   d. Soft tissue interposition

10. The most common 1st order site for bone grafting
   a. Iliac crest   b. Tibial metaphysis
   c. Medial malleolus   d. Femoral condyle
   e. Greater trochanter

11. Direct impact on the bone will produce
   a. Oblique fracture   b. Spiral fracture
   c. Transverse fracture   d. Comminuted fracture

12. Most consistent sign of a fresh fracture is
   a. Bony tenderness   b. Crepitus
   c. Deformity   d. Abnormal mobility
   e. Shortening of bone

13. An 8-year-old boy with a history of fall from 10 feet height complains of pain in the right ankle. X-ray taken at that time of injury were normal without any evident fracture line. But after 2 years, he developed a calcaneovalgus deformity in the foot. The missed diagnosis seem to be
   a. Undiagnosed malunited fracture
   b. Avascular necrosis talus
   c. Distal Tibial epiphyseal injury
   d. Ligamentous injury of ankle joint

14. The most common site of Epiphyseal injury in children
   a. Lower end radius   b. Lateral condyle humerus
   c. Upper end femur   d. Lower end femur

15. What is the type of joint seen in the growth plate?
   a. Plane synovial   b. Primary cartilaginous
   c. Secondary cartilaginous   d. Fibrous

16. Traumatic dislocation of the epiphyseal plate of distal femur occurs (PGI type)
   a. Medially   b. Laterally
   c. Posteriorly   d. Anteriorly
   e. Rotationally

17. In children, best remodelling is seen in fractures with
   a. Angulation in diaphysis   b. Angulation in metaphysis
   c. Rotation in diaphysis   d. Rotation in metaphysis

18. The most common fracture in children
   a. Fracture clavicle
   b. Green stick fracture of lower end of radius
   c. Supracondylar fracture
   d. All of the above

19. Salter Harris Type VI (Rang's) injury includes
   a. Thurston Holland's sign
   b. Perichondrial ring injury
   c. Open injury with loss of physis
   d. Transverse fracture of metaphysis with longitudinal extension into the physis

20. A 6-year-old child falls on to his right side and develops a crack in only the dorsal cortex of mid region of radius. The best treatment is
   a. Antibiotics and sedative
   b. Bone plating and external fixation
   c. Slab with wait for bone imperfect
   d. Break the cortex other side and immobilisation by POP

21. Thomas splint was devised by Sir HO Thomas
   a. To splint fracture shaft of femur
   b. To stabilize cervical spine after trauma
   c. For transportation of polytrauma patients
   d. For treating tuberculosis of knee

22. Thomas splint is not used for
   a. Injuries around knee joint   b. Knee dislocation
   c. Infective arthritis of knee   d. Fracture femur

23. Plaster of Paris was discovered by
   a. Percival Potts   b. Abraham Colles
   c. John Charnley   d. Anotonius Mathysen

24. Which side of plaster is manipulated for wedging?
   a. Anterior   b. Posterior
   c. Concave   d. Convex

25. Which of the following is included in the management of intra-articular fracture? (PGI type)
   a. Arthroplasty   b. K wire
   c. Arthrodesis   d. Excision
   e. Plaster of Paris

26. Epiphyseal enlargement occurs in
   a. Scheurmann's disease
   b. Paget's disease
   c. Juvenile rheumatoid arthritis
   d. Epiphyseal dysplasia

27. Epiphyseal dysgenesis is a feature of
   a. Hypothyroidism
   b. Hyperparathyroidism
   c. Hypoparathyroidism
   d. Hyperthyroidism

28. Marker for bone formation is
   a. Serum nucleotidase
   b. Osteocalcin
   c. Urinary calcium
   d. Tartrate resistant acid phosphate

29. Mirel's criteria is developed for the evaluation of
   a. Severity of osteoporosis
   b. Risk of fatigue fracture
   c. Risk of pathological fracture after metastasis
   d. Severity of neurological deficit

30. Treatment of choice in pathological fractures is
   a. Skin traction
   b. Internal fixation
   c. Plaster of Paris casts
   d. External skeletal fixation

31. Most common cause of pathological fracture is
   a. Cyst
   b. Osteoporosis
   c. Carcinoma
   d. All

32. Stress fracture is treated by
   a. Rest
   b. Cast immobilisation
   c. Closed reduction
   d. Internal fixation

33. Fatigue fractures (stress fractures) are most commonly seen in
   a. Metatarsals
   b. Tibia
   c. Fibula
   d. Neck of femur

34. Runner's fracture is a stress fracture of
   a. 2nd metatarsal
   b. 3rd metatarsal
   c. Lower tibia
   d. Lower fibula

35. Bilateral stress fractures are best diagnosed by
   a. X-ray
   b. MRI
   c. CT
   d. Bone scan

36. To detect multiple bone metastasis the preferred investigation is
   a. MRI
   b. CT
   c. Bone scan
   d. PET CT: d > c

37. Most reliable method of detection bony metastasis is
   a. MRI
   b. CT
   c. SPECT
   d. Radiograph

38. Rate of mineralization of newly formed osteoid can be estimated by
   a. Labelled tetracycline
   b. Alzarin red stain
   c. Von Kossa staining for calcium
   d. Immunofluorescence

39. For pronation to occur, which two foot joints must have their axis of rotation in parallel?
   a. Talocrural and subtalar
   b. Lisfranc and talonavicular
   c. Talonavicular and calcaneocuboid
   d. Subtalar and calcaneocuboid

40. Traction system not used in lower limb fractures?
   a. Dunlop traction
   b. Russell traction
   c. Perkin's traction
   d. Bryant's traction

41. Functional cast bracing is not used in fractures of
   a. Humerus
   b. Tibia
   c. Ulna
   d. Thoracolumbar spine

42. A joint is stabilized by all of the following structures except
   a. Synovial fluid tenancy
   b. Bursa
   c. Tendons
   d. Ligament laxity

43. All are true about the metaphysis of developing bone except
   a. Ossifies from primary center of ossification
   b. Is the strongest part of a child's bone
   c. Is a zone of active bone growth
   d. Has hair pin arrangement of blood vessels

POLYTRAUMA

1. A 30 years male suffers from road traffic accident and a car runs over his right leg. On examination, vitals are stable. The right leg is crushed with exposed muscles and bones. The debate about limb survival can be resolved to an extent by MESS score which includes all except
   a. BP
   b. Nerve injury
   c. Velocity of trauma
   d. Distal circulation

2. A person falls from height of 35 feet according to an eye witness. He landed on his feet on the ground which does correlate with his statement, if following fractures are present
   a. Foramen ring fracture with lumbar spine injury
   b. Depressed skull fracture with lumbar spine injury
   c. Gutter fracture with cervical injury
   d. Pelvic fracture with cervical spine injury

3. Permissible ischemia time for a proximal limb amputation is
   a. 4 hours
   b. 6 hours
   c. 8 hours
   d. 12 hours

4. Severely injured patient presents with spinal fracture and unconsciousness. First thing to be done is
   a. GCS scoring
   b. Spinal stabilization by cervical collar
   c. Mannitol drip to decrease ICT
   d. Airway maintenance

5. Which of the following is not a component of the crush syndrome?
   a. Myohemoglobinuria
   b. Massive crushing of muscles
   c. Acute tubular necrosis
   d. Bleeding diathesis

6. Open fracture is treated by
   a. Tourniquet
   b. Internal fixation
   c. Debridement
   d. External fixation

7. A compound fracture is initially treated by antibiotics, wound toilet and
   a. Skin cover
   b. External splintage
   c. Prosthesis
   d. Internal fixation

8. All of the following factors evaluate the chances of amputation in a limb, except
   a. Age
   b. BP
   c. Velocity of trauma
   d. Presence of infection

9. Motorcyclist's fracture is
   a. Ring fracture of base of skull
   b. Comminuted fracture
   c. A hinged fracture where the skull separates into anterior and posterior halves
   d. Fracture base of skull

10. A female child with abuse has fracture pelvis, multiple injuries and is bleeding per vaginum. The immediate step on presenting to the hospital is
   a. Inform the police
   b. Airway assessment
   c. External fixator application for pelvic fracture
   d. Blood transfusion

11. In cardiopulmonary resuscitation, the commonly fractured ribs are
   a. 1st and 2nd
   b. 3rd and 4th
   c. 5th and 6th
   d. 8th and 9th

12. Which of the following structures is fixed first during reimplantation of an amputated digit?
   a. Bone
   b. Artery
   c. Vein
   d. Nerve

13. In crush injuries of hand the greatest priority is given to repair of
   a. Tendons
   b. Skin
   c. Bone
   d. Arteries

14. In an unconscious patient with multiple injuries, best and reliable modality to rule out cervical spine injury is?
  a. MRI
  b. Full AP and lateral view of cervical spine.
  c. While doing CT scan of brain take extra cuts at the cervical spine region.
  d. Clinical examination

UPPER LIMB TRAUMATOLOGY

1. Axis of upper limb passes through
  a. Capitulum
  b. Olecranon
  c. Trochlea
  d. Radial styloid

2. In shoulder X-ray, highest bony landmark is
  a. Head
  b. Greater tuberosity
  c. Lesser tuberosity
  d. Acromion

3. Preferred treatment modality in a 70-year-old male with fracture neck humerus
  a. U slab
  b. Arthroplasty
  c. Analgesic with triangular sling
  d. Open reduction and internal fixation

4. Velpeau bandage and sling and swathe splint are used in
  a. Fracture scapula
  b. Fracture clavicle
  c. Acromioclavicular dislocation
  d. Shoulder dislocation

5. Hanging cast is used in which fracture?
  a. Femur
  b. Tibia
  c. Radius
  d. Humerus

6. Most common cause of nonunion in a fracture shaft of humerus is
  a. Compound fracture
  b. Comminution at fracture site
  c. Distraction at fracture site
  d. Inadequate operative reduction

7. Deformity in posterior elbow dislocation
  a. Extension
  b. Flexion
  c. Both
  d. None

8. Nerve mostly involved in a simple dislocation of elbow is
  a. Median
  b. Ulnar
  c. Radial
  d. Posterior interosseous

9. A 4-year-boy complains of pain around elbow which is held in pronation and extension. X-ray reveals a normal picture. What is the probable diagnosis?
  a. Pulled elbow
  b. Monteggia fracture
  c. Elbow dislocation
  d. Supracondylar humerus fracture

10. Most common elbow injury in adoloscents is
  a. Elbow dislocation
  b. Supracondylar humerus fracture
  c. Physeal injury
  d. Olecranon fracture

11. Fracture supracondylar humerus is usually caused by
  a. Hyperflexion injury
  b. Extension injury
  c. Axial rotation
  d. Hyperextension injury

12. 10-years-old boy presents with cubitus varus deformity and a history of trauma 3 months back. On clinical examination, he has preserved three bony point relationship of elbow, most probable diagnosis would be
  a. Nonunion lateral condylar humerus
  b. Old unreduced dislocation of elbow
  c. Malunited intercondylar fracture of humerus
  d. Malunited supracondylar fracture of humerus

13. In the more common extension type of supracondylar humerus fracture, usual displacement is
  a. Posteromedial
  b. Anteromedial
  c. Anterolateral
  d. Posterolateral

14. All are true regarding compartment syndrome except
  a. Pain on passive stretching is an early sign
  b. Pulse is a reliable indicator
  c. Interstitial pressure > capillary pressure
  d. Paraesthesias are seen late

15. Most common nerve involved in Volkmann's ischemic contracture
  a. Radial nerve
  b. Median nerve
  c. Ulnar nerve
  d. Posterior interosseous nerve

16. Treatment of acute myositis ossificans is
  a. Excision of myositis
  b. Infrared therapy
  c. Passive mobilization
  d. Immobilization

17. The most common site of myositis ossificans is
  a. Knee
  b. Shoulder
  c. Elbow
  d. Wrist

18. False about myositis ossificans progressive is
  a. Life longevity is normal
  b. Pneumonia is common in these cases
  c. Most common site involved is the spine
  d. Onset is usually before 6 years of age

19. Which of the following is true about supracondylar fracture humerus in children?
  a. Anterior displacement of the distal fragment is more common than posterior
  b. Cubitus valgus is more common than cubitus varus during malunion
  c. The neurological complications are transitory
  d. Weakness of elbow flexion is a common complication

20. Traction not used in lower limb
  a. Gallows traction
  b. Bryant's traction
  c. Dunlop traction
  d. Perkin's traction

21. Child presents with a supracondylar humerus fracture with cold and pulseless limb since 3 hours. Next management step is
  a. Immediate exploration
  b. Immediate angiography
  c. ORIF
  d. Closed reduction

22. A 6-years-old child had an accident and developed fracture around elbow. After 4 years, he presented with tingling and numbness in the ulnar side of fingers. Probable fracture, he had was
  a. Olecranon fracture
  b. Dislocation of elbow
  c. Lateral condylar fracture humerus
  d. Supracondylar fracture humerus

23. First sign of compartment syndrome is
  a. Pain on passive stretch
  b. Loss of pulse
  c. Tingling
  d. Loss of movements

24. Indication for surgical compartment release in compartment syndrome in any compartment is absolute compartment pressure greater than
  a. 15 mm Hg
  b. 20 mm Hg
  c. 30 mm Hg
  d. 40 mm Hg

25. Three point symmetry at elbow is not disturbed in
  a. Fracture ulna only
  b. Fracture radius only
  c. Fracture of both bones of forearm
  d. Weak posterior capsule

26. Excision of head of radius in a child should not be done because it
  a. Leads to secondary osteoarthritis of elbow
  b. Causes subluxation of inferior radio ulnar joint
  c. Causes myositis ossificans
  d. Produces instability of elbow joint

27. If head of radius is removed, it will result in
  a. Varus deformity at elbow
  b. No deformity
  c. Valgus deformity at elbow
  d. Lengthening of the limb

28. In fracture of the olecranon, excision of the proximal fragment is indicated in all of the following situations except
  a. Old un-united fractures
  b. Nonarticular fractures

   c. Fracture extending to coronoid process
   d. Elderly patient

29. Essex-Lopresti lesion in upper limb involves
   a. Radial head fracture
   b. Radial shaft fracture
   c. Injury to interosseous membrane
   d. Radial shaft fracture with proximal radioulnar joint dislocation

30. Tension band wiring is done in all except
   a. Fracture patella   b. Fracture olecranon
   c. Fracture medial malleolus d. Colles' fracture

31. Surgical excision is contraindicated in
   a. Patella   b. Head of radius
   c. Lateral condyle humerus d. Olecranon process

32. Terrible triad of elbow injury comprises all except
   a. Elbow dislocation   b. Radial head fracture
   c. Coronoid fracture   d. Olecranon fracture

33. All of the following deformities are seen in a Colles' fracture except
   a. Lateral tilt   b. Volar tilt
   c. Dorsal tilt   d. Supination

34. Not a complication of Colles fracture
   a. Ulna plus deformity   b. Madelung's deformity
   c. Shoulder hand syndrome d. Ulna minus deformity

35. Most important deformity to be corrected in Colles' fracture
   a. Lateral deviation   b. Posterior tilt
   c. Posterior deviation   d. Impaction

36. An elderly female sustained Colles' fracture in her right hand which was properly treated. She now complains of stiffness and severe pain in the wrist with cold sensation and cyanosis in the fingers. X-ray of the hand revealed complete decalcification. She is most likely suffering from
   a. Causalgia
   b. Tubercular arthritis of wrist joint
   c. Traumatic tenosynovitis
   d. Sudeck's atrophy

37. Barton's disease is
   a. Intra-articular fracture of 1st MC
   b. Rickets in presence of scurvy
   c. Fracture neck of 5th MC
   d. Fracture of distal end of radius

38. In children, fracture scaphoid is rare but if it occurs it mostly involves
   a. Waist   b. Neck
   c. Proximal pole   d. Distal pole

39. In treating non-union of scaphoid, vascularized muscle pedicle graft is usually taken from
   a. Pronator teres   b. Pronator quadratus
   c. Brachioradialis   d. Extensor pollicis longus

40. Most common nerve involved in dislocation of lunate is
   a. Median nerve
   b. Posterior interosseous nerve (PIN)
   c. Anterior interosseous nerve (AIN)
   d. Ulnar nerve

41. Boxer's fracture is
   a. Radial styloid fracture   b. Reverse colic's fracture
   c. 5th metacarpal fracture   d. 1st metacarpal fracture

42. A Bennett's fracture is difficult to maintain in a reduced position mainly because of the pull of
   a. Flexor pollicis brevis   b. Extensor pollicis brevis
   c. Abductor pollicis longus d. Adductor pollicis

43. The term Bennett's fracture is used to describe
   a. Fracture dislocation of MCP joint of thumb
   b. IP fracture dislocation of thumb
   c. Anterior marginal fracture of distal end of radius
   d. Fracture dislocation of trapeziometacarpal joint

44. True about mallet finger is
   a. Avulsion of tendon at the base of middle phalanx
   b. Avulsion of extensor tendon at the base of distal phalanx
   c. Fracture of distal phalanx
   d. Facture of proximal phalanx

45. Terry Thomas sign is seen in
   a. Ulnar deviation of wrist   b. Scapholunate dislocation
   c. Scaphoid fracture   d. Colles' fracture

46. In hand surgery, no man's land refers to
   a. Area over the proximal phalanx
   b. Area over the distal phalanx
   c. Area between middle of middle phalanx and distal palmar crease
   d. Area in front of the wrist

47. All are true regarding fracture lateral condyle humerus, except
   a. Salter Harris Type 4 injury
   b. Most common complication of surgically treated cases is cubitus valgus deformity.
   c. Tardy ulnar nerve palsy is a known complication
   d. Cubitus varus occurs more commonly than valgus

48. Treatment of choice for fracture of radius and ulna in an adult
   a. Plaster for 4 weeks
   b. Closed reduction and calipers
   c. Only plates
   d. Fixation with Kuntscher nails

HIP EXAMINATION

1. A patient has been given POP cast for tibial fracture of left leg. He is to be mobilized with a single crutch. It should be advised on which side?
   a. Left   b. Any
   c. Right   d. Both

2. With the hip in 90 degrees flexion a line joining the anterior superior iliac spine (ASIS) and the ischial tuberosity passes through the greater trochanter tip. This line is called
   a. Shoemaker's line   b. Nelaton's line
   c. Cheines line   d. Morel's line

3. A 72-year-old female after hip replacement surgery developed Trendelenburg gait. The nerve likely injured is
   a. Superior gluteal   b. Femoral
   c. Sciatic   d. Inferior gluteal

4. Vascular sign of Narath is seen in
   a. Anterior dislocation of hip b. Central dislocation of hip
   c. Posterior dislocation of hip
   d. Subtrochanteric fracture of hip

5. Telescopic test is useful to diagnose
   a. Perthes' disease
   b. Nonunited intracapsular fracture neck of femur
   c. Ankylosis of hip joint
   d. Malunited trochanteric fracture

PELVIS AND LOWER LIMB TRAUMA

1. Shenton's line is present in X-ray of
   a. Knee   b. Shoulder
   c. Elbow   d. Hip

2. Judet view X-ray are taken for
   a. Pelvis   b. Calcaneum
   c. Scaphoid   d. Spine

3. In pelvic fracture, the approximate amount of blood loss is
   a. 1–2 units   b. 2–4 units
   c. 2–6 units   d. 4–8 units

4. Maximum blood supply to the head of femur is contributed by
   a. Lateral circumflex femoral artery
   b. Medial circumflex femoral artery

   c. Artery of ligamentum teres
   d. Popliteal artery

5. An elderly woman was admitted with a fracture of the neck of right femur which failed to unite. On X-ray evaluation, additionally an avascular necrosis of the head of femur was noted. The condition would have resulted most probably from the damage to
   a. Superior gluteal artery
   b. Inferior gluteal artery
   c. Acetabular branch of obturator artery
   d. Retinacular branches of circumflex femoral arteries

6. Jumper's fracture is seen in
   a. Calcaneum   b. Tibia
   c. Pelvis   d. Neck femur

7. True about crescent fracture is
   a. Anteroposterior compression is the mechanism of injury
   b. Diastasis of pubis with pubic rami fracture
   c. Anteroposterior instability with rotational instability
   d. Fracture of the iliac bone with sacroiliac disruption

8. In fracture neck femur, all the trabeculae of pelvis and femur are in alignment in which stage?
   a. I   b. II
   c. III   d. IV

9. Occult fracture of neck femur is best diagnosed by
   a. X-Ray   b. CT
   c. MRI   d. Bone Scan

10. A 40-year-old female with a history of fall, complaints of pain in right hip and inability to walk. On examination, there is tenderness in Scarpa's triangle. The X-ray is normal, next investigation to be ordered is
   a. Aspiration   b. MRI
   c. CT   d. Bone scan

11. A 60-year-old female lands up in emergency with history of fall, the attitude of limb is extension and external rotation, the probable diagnosis is
   a. Acetabulum fracture
   b. Posterior dislocation of hip
   c. Intertrochanteric fracture
   d. Intracapsular fracture neck femur

12. A 80-year-old man fell in the bathroom and was unable to stand on the right buttock region. He had ecchymosis with external rotation of the leg with the lateral border of the foot touching the couch. The most probable diagnosis is
   a. Anterior dislocation of hip
   b. Extracapsular fracture neck femur
   c. Intracapsular fracture neck femur
   d. Posterior dislocation of hip

13. A patient presents with lower limb in flexion, abduction and internal rotation with shortening. Diagnosis is
   a. Anterior dislocation   b. Central dislocation
   c. Posterior dislocation   d. Lateral dislocation

14. In per rectal examination, femoral head is palpable in
   a. Anterior dislocation of hip   b. Posterior dislocation of hip
   c. Central fracture dislocation of hip
   d. Lateral dislocation of hip

15. A 32-year-old male presented to the casually with pain in the left hip region following RTA. On examination, there is shortening flexion and external rotation deformity. A mass is palpable in the left gluteal region which moves with movement of the femur. Most likely X-ray finding would be
   a. Posterior dislocation of hip with neck in full profile
   b. Dislocation of hip with lesser trochanter in full profile
   c. Fracture roof of acetabulum with central dislocation
   d. Acetabular fracture with posterior dislocation of hip

16. Following RTA a patient presents with flexion and external rotation deformity of the left hip. Shortening of affected limb by 7 cm was also seen. A mass was noted in the left gluteal region which was moving with the movements of the femur. Most likely X-ray finding would be
   a. Thompson-Epstein Type IV dislocation of hip
   b. Dislocated hip with lesser trochanter in full profile
   c. Posterior dislocation of the hip with neck in full profile
   d. Acetabular roof fracture with central dislocation

17. Most common complication of intertrochanteric fracture femur is
   a. Osteoarthritis   b. Malunion
   c. Nonunion   d. Sciatic nerve injury

18. Nonunion is a very common complication of intracapsular fractures of the neck of femur. Which is not an important contributing factor?
   a. Inadequate blood supply
   b. Inadequate immobilization
   c. Inhibitory effect of synovial fluid
   d. Stress at fracture site due to muscle spasm

19. Femoral neck fracture 4 weeks old, in a young adult, should be treated by which one of the following methods?
   a. Pauwel's osteotomy
   b. Reduction of fracture and multiple screw fixation
   c. Excision of hip
   d. Prosthetic replacement of femoral head

20. Treatment of a 50-year-old male with fracture of neck of femur more than 3 weeks old is
   a. Hemiarthroplasty   b. McMurray osteotomy
   c. THR   d. Girdlestone arthroplasty

21. A 65-year-old man presented with fracture neck femur 3 days after injury. Treatment of choice would be
   a. Multiple screw fixation   b. McMurray osteotomy
   c. Hemi-arthroplasty   d. Total hip replacement

22. In a 65-year-old male with history of fracture neck of femur six weeks old, treatment of choice is
   a. SP nailing   b. McMurray's osteotomy
   c. Hemiarthroplasty   d. None

23. Treatment of choice in fracture neck of femur in a 40-year-old male presenting after 2 days of injury is
   a. Hemiarthroplasty
   b. Closed reduction and internal fixation by cancellous screws
   c. Closed reduction and Internal fixation by Austin-Moore pins
   d. Plaster and rest

24. The treatment of choice for a 4 weeks old femoral neck fracture in a 55-year-old man is
   a. Open reduction and internal fixation
   b. McMurray's osteotomy
   c. Hemi-replacement arthroplasty
   d. Total hip replacement

25. Prosthetic replacement of femoral head is indicated in (PGI type)
   a. A fresh intracapsular fracture of neck of femur in old patients
   b. In reduced posterior dislocation of hip
   c. Untreated femoral neck fracture over 65 years
   d. Pathological fracture of NOF due to secondaries

26. In a 10-year-old male, a transcervical fracture neck femur is best treated by
   a. Spica   b. Austin Moore's prosthesis
   c. K- wires   d. Cannulated cancellous screws

27. Avascular necrosis of head of the femur is most common in
   a. Subcapital neck femur fracture
   b. Basal neck femur fracture
   c. Intertrochantric femur fracture
   d. Transcervical neck femur fracture

28. AVN is seen in which types of fracture of femur (PGI type)
   a. Intertrochantric fracture   b. Subcapital fracture
   c. Transcervical fracture   d. Basal fracture

29. Avascular necrosis of head of femur occurs commonly at
   a. Transcervical region
   b. Intertrochanteric region
   c. Subcapital region
   d. Subchondral region

30. Fracture shaft femur is stabilized early in order to
   a. To prevent blood loss
   b. ARDS
   c. Nonunion
   d. Compartment syndrome

31. Blood loss in fracture shaft femur is
   a. 1 units
   b. 2 units
   c. 3 units
   d. 4 units

32. In upper one-third femoral shaft fracture, the displacement of proximal segment is
   a. Flexion, abduction and external rotation
   b. Flexion, adduction and external rotation
   c. Elexion, abduction and internal rotation
   d. Flexion, adduction and internal rotation

33. Fracture shaft of femur in adult unites by
   a. 3 to 4 weeks
   b. 3 to 4 weeks
   c. 3 to 4 months
   d. 4 to 6 months

34. A person with multiple injuries develops fever, restlessness, tachycardia, tachypnea and subconjuctival rash 72 hours after the injury. Probable diagnosis is
   a. Pulmonary embolism
   b. Air embolism
   c. Fat embolism
   d. Bacterial pneumonitis

35. Most common fracture associated with fat embolism is
   a. Humerus
   b. Tibia
   c. Femur
   d. Pelvis

36. In a road-traffic accident four people were injured. Now, person having which trauma should be treated first?
   a. Posterior dislocation of hip
   b. Fracture shaft of femur
   c. Fracture neck of femur
   d. Fracture shaft of humerus

37. Maximum shortening of lower limb is seen in
   a. Fracture neck femur
   b. Fracture shaft femur
   c. Fracture intertrochanteric femur
   d. Posterior dislocation of hip

38. Bulge sign in knee joint is seen after how much of fluid accumulation?
   a. < 30 mL
   b. 100 mL
   c. 200 mL
   d. 400 mL

39. Cylinder cast is applied for
   a. Neck humerus fracture
   b. Neck femur fracture
   c. Patellar fracture
   d. Shaft humerus fracture

40. Transverse fracture of patella with separation of fragments is best treated by
   a. Closed reduction with cylinder cast
   b. Open reduction with screw fixation of the fragments
   c. Blind fixation of the two fragments with K wire
   d. Open reduction with K wire fixation of the fragment with tension band wiring

41. Patellar tendon bearing cast is preferred in which fracture
   a. Patella
   b. Femur
   c. Tibia
   d. Medial malleolus

42. Ankle brachial pressure index value suggestive of critical ischemia is
   a. 1
   b. 0.9
   c. 0.5
   d. 0.4

43. The mechanism of injury in vertical fracture of medial malleolus is
   a. Abduction injury
   b. Adduction injury
   c. Supination external rotation injury
   d. Pronation dorsiflexion injury

44. In posterior compartment syndrome of leg, which passive movement causes pain?
   a. Toe dorsiflexion
   b. Dorsiflexion of foot
   c. Foot inversion
   d. Toe plantar flexion

45. Tillaux fracture is
   a. Stress fracture of the distal fibula 3–8 cm above lateral malleolus
   b. Avulsion fracture of medial femoral condyle at the origin of the medial collateral ligament
   c. Lateral tibial plateau avulsion fracture with anterior cruciate ligament tear
   d. Salter-Harris III fracture of tibia

46. The most common site of March fracture is
   a. Shafts of 2nd and 3rd metatarsals
   b. Avulsion of 5th metatarsal base
   c. Neck of 2nd metatarsal
   d. Neck of 3rd metatarsal

47. Jone's fracture is
   a. Avulsion fracture of base of 5th metatarsal
   b. Avulsion fracture of medial femoral condyle
   c. Bimalleolar fracture of the ankle
   d. Burst fracture of 1st cervical vertebra

48. Bohler's angle is reduced in fracture of
   a. Calcaneum
   b. Navicular
   c. Talus
   d. Cuboid

49. Bosworth's fracture is
   a. Fracture distal end tibia
   b. Fracture distal end femur
   c. Fracture distal fibula with dislocation of distal fragment
   d. Fracture distal fibula with posterior dislocation of proximal fragment

50. Cotton's fracture refers to a
   a. Bimalleolar fracture
   b. Trimalleolar fracture
   c. Wrist subluxation
   d. Knee subluxation

51. Most common complication of fracture neck talus is
   a. Nonunion
   b. AVN
   c. Osteoarthritis of ankle joint
   d. Osteoarthritis of subtalar joint

52. Neutral triangle is seen radiologically in
   a. Neck femur
   b. Calcaneum
   c. Proximal humerus
   d. Talus

53. Most commonly injured tarsal bone is
   a. Talus
   b. Cuneiform
   c. Navicular
   d. Calcaneum

54. Recurrent dislocations are least commonly seen in
   a. Ankle
   b. Shoulder
   c. Hip
   d. Patella

SPORTS MEDICINE (LIGAMENT AND MENISCAL INJURIES OF KNEE, SHOULDER INSTABILITY AND ROTATOR CUFF TEAR)

1. Menisci are connected to tibia by
   a. Arcuate ligament
   b. Coronary ligament
   c. Wrisberg ligament
   d. Oblique ligaments

2. Pellegrini-Stieda lesion is
   a. Calcification at femoral attachment of MCL
   b. Calcification at tibial attachment of MCL
   c. Calcification at femoral attachment of LCL
   d. Calcification at tibial attachment of LCL

3. Torsion of knee most commonly injures
   a. ACL
   b. Medial menisci
   c. Tibial collateral ligament
   d. Fibular collateral ligament

4. A 22-year-old young male, college student, suffered a left knee injury while playing hockey. After 2 months, there was anterior laxity in full extension and it was normal at 90° flexion. What is the most likely injured part?
   a. Anteromedial bundle of anterior cruciate ligament
   b. Posterolateral bundle of anterior cruciate ligament
   c. Posterior cruciate ligament
   d. Anterior part of medial meniscus

5. A dial test that is positive in 30° knee flexion suggests injury to
   a. Posterior cruciate ligament
   b. Posterolateral corner structures
   c. Posterior cruciate ligament as well as PLC
   d. Anteriomedial corner of knee

6. On lateral blow to knee with fracture in intercondylar area, structure damaged is
   a. ACL
   b. MCL
   c. LCL
   d. Menisci

7. In 'bounce home' test of knee 'end feels' are all except
   a. Firm
   b. Empty
   c. Spongy block
   d. Bony

8. Which activity will be difficult to perform in ACL deficient knee joint?
   a. Sit cross leg
   b. Walk uphill
   c. Getting up from sitting
   d. Walk downhill

9. Positive pivot shift test in knee is due to injury to
   a. ACL
   b. PCL
   c. Medial menisci
   d. Lateral menisci

10. Structural integrity of collateral ligaments is best tested by
    a. Varus/Valgus stress test in full flexion
    b. Varus/Valgus stress test in full extension
    c. Varus/Valgus stress test in 30° flexion
    d. Varus/Valgus stress test in 90° flexion

11. Locking of the knee can be due to
    a. Loose body
    b. Menisci
    c. Both
    d. None

12. Which of the following statements about menisci are not true?
    a. Medial menisci is more commonly injured than lateral
    b. Medial menisci is more mobile than lateral
    c. It covers more tibial articular surface than lateral
    d. It is predominantly made of type 1 collagen

13. An 18-year-old boy, while playing football twisted his knee on the ankle and fell down. After 10 min, he got up and again started playing. Next day, he developed swelling and could not move his knee. Probable diagnosis is
    a. Medial meniscal tear
    b. ACL tear
    c. MCL tear
    d. PCL injury

14. Investigation of choice for ligament injuries of the knee is
    a. X-Ray
    b. USG
    c. MRI
    d. Arthroscopy

15. The most common cause of hemarthrosis in knee joint is
    a. Medial collateral ligament tear
    b. Anterior cruciate ligament tear
    c. Fracture patella
    d. Bumper fracture

16. Injury to the medial meniscus is rather impossible when the knee joint dose not
    a. Extend
    b. Flex
    c. Rotate
    d. Abduct adduct

17. It is wise to keep and repair the meniscus rather than removing it when the injury is to
    a. Medial part of meniscus
    b. Mid part of meniscus
    c. Lateral part of meniscus
    d. Associated with collateral ligament injury

18. Injury to cartilage of knee is best diagnosed by
    a. MRI
    b. Arthrography
    c. X-ray
    d. Arthroscopy

19. Most common type of medial meniscal tear is
    a. Radial tear
    b. Longitudinal tear
    c. Oblique tear
    d. Horizontal tear

20. Which of the following acts as the dynamic stabilizer of shoulder joint?
    a. Musculotendinous cuff
    b. Glenoid labrum
    c. Coracohumeral ligament
    d. Glenohumeral ligament

21. Weakest portion of shoulder joint capsule is
    a. Superior
    b. Inferior
    c. Anterior
    d. Posterior

22. Most common sub-type of anterior shoulder dislocation is
    a. Subglenoid
    b. Subcoracoid
    c. Posterior
    d. Subclavicular

23. Which is the true statement regarding shoulder dislocation?
    a. Pain is severe in anterior dislocation
    b. Posterior dislocation is often overlooked
    c. Radiography may be misleading in posterior dislocation
    d. All of the above

24. All are related to recurrent shoulder dislocation except
    a. Lax capsule
    b. Hill-Sachs defect
    c. Bankart lesion
    d. Rotator cuff injury

25. Test for posterior glenohumeral instability is
    a. Fulcrum
    b. Jerk test
    c. Sulcus test
    d. Crank test

26. Nerve injured in inferior dislocation of shoulder
    a. Posterior cord of brachial plexus
    b. Radial nerve
    c. Axillary nerve
    d. Ulnar nerve

27. Bankart's lesion involves the avulsion of labrum from
    a. Anterior lip of glenoid
    b. Superior lip of glenoid
    c. Anterosuperior lip of glenoid
    d. Anteroinferior lip of glenoid

28. Traumatic glenohumeral instability in one direction with Bankart's lesion is treated by
    a. Conservative methods
    b. Surgery
    c. Rehabilitation
    d. Inferior capsular shift surgery

29. Jersey finger is due to rupture of which tendon?
    a. FDS
    b. EDC
    c. Extensor pollicis
    d. FDP

30. A positive Yergason's test indicates
    a. Bicipital tendinitis
    b. Acromioclavicular subluxation
    c. Dislocation of the shoulder
    d. Radial head fracture.

31. What would be the appropriate most treatment for an irreparable tear of rotator cuff in a 30-year-old patient?
    a. Tendon Transfers
    b. Total Shoulder replacement
    c. Acromioplasty
    d. Reverse shoulder arthroplasty

32. Forgotten muscle of rotator cuff is
    a. Supraspinatus
    b. Infraspinatus
    c. Subscapularis
    d. Teres minor

33. Most commonly damaged muscle in rotator cuff is?
    a. Supraspinatus
    b. Infraspinatus
    c. Subscapularis
    d. Teres minor

34. Lift off test is done for?
    a. Supraspinatus
    b. Infraspinatus
    c. Subscapularis
    d. Teres minor

35. Rotator interval is bounded by
    a. Teres major and minor
    b. Supraspinatus and subscapularis
    c. Subscapularis and infraspinatus
    d. Supraspinatus and teres minor

36. Game keepers thumb refers to
    a. Thumb metacarpophalangeal joint ulnar collateral ligament rupture
    b. Thumb metacarpophalangeal joint radial collateral ligament rupture

   c. Thumb interphalangeal joint ulnar collateral ligament rupture
   d. Thumb interphalangeal joint radial collateral ligament rupture

37. The primary pathology in athletic pubalgia is?
   a. Hamstring strain
   b. Abdominal muscle strain
   c. Gluteus medius strain
   d. Rectus femoris strain

38. Most common cause of insertional tendonitis of tendo-Achilles is?
   a. Overuse
   b. Runners and jumpers
   c. Steroid injections
   d. Improper shoe wear

39. Anterior cruciate ligament prevents
   a. Anterior dislocation of tibia
   b. Posterior dislocation of tibia
   c. Anterior dislocation of femur
   d. Posterior dislocation of femur

40. Most common site for ligamentous injuries in the body
   a. Shoulder
   b. Knee
   c. Elbow
   d. Ankle

41. Ligament involved in ankle sprain is
   a. Anterior talofibular ligament
   b. Posterior talofibular ligament
   c. Spring ligament
   d. Calcaneofibular ligament

42. When the foot is suddenly inverted in plantar flexed position, which ligament is most likely injured?
   a. Anterior talofibular
   b. Calcaneocuboid
   c. Posterior tibiofibular
   d. Calcaneofibular

43. In a young male after injury to knee you observed a small piece of avulsed bone from the lateral tibial condyle. What test would you like to do?
   a. Ortolani sign
   b. Telescoping sign
   c. McMurray's test
   d. Lachman test

44. Micro-fracture technique is carried out for
   a. Avascular necrosis
   b. Osteopetrosis
   c. Osteochondral defects
   d. Nonunion

SPINE

1. Vertebra with most constant number
   a. Cervical
   b. Thoracic
   c. Lumbar
   d. Sacral

2. Complete transection of the spinal cord at the C7 level produces all of the following effects except
   a. Hypotension
   b. Limited respiratory effort
   c. Anaesthesia below the level of the lesion
   d. Areflexia below the level of the lesion

3. Wrist flexion and finger extension test the following nerve root
   a. C6
   b. C7
   c. C8
   d. T1

4. A 40-year-old male after RTA attains spinal injury. His lower limb power is greater than that of upper limb and sacral sensations are present. Type of spinal cord lesion is
   a. Central cord syndrome
   b. Anterior cord syndrome
   c. Posterior cord syndrome
   d. Complete spinal cord injury

5. In a patient with head injury, unexplained hypotension warrants evaluation of
   a. Upper cervical spine
   b. Lower cervical spine
   c. Thoracic spine
   d. Lumbar spine

6. Dislocation without fracture is seen in
   a. Sacral spine
   b. Lumbar spine
   c. Cervical spine
   d. Thoracic spine

7. Compression fracture is the most common in
   a. Cervical spine
   b. Upper thoracic
   c. Lower thoracic
   d. Lumbosacral

8. Least helpful investigation for diagnosis of spondylolisthesis
   a. AP view of spine
   b. Lateral X-ray of spine
   c. MRI
   d. CT Scan

9. The number of division in Holdsworth classification for determining stability in thoracolumbar injuries were
   a. 1
   b. 2
   c. 3
   d. 4

10. Spinal injuries without any radiological abnormalities are found in
   a. Young adults
   b. Old people
   c. Teenagers
   d. Infants

11. Regarding Hangman's fracture true statement is
   a. High post admission mortality
   b. Most common axis fracture
   c. Surgical treatment is always necessary
   d. Union almost always occurs

12. Most common mode of injury to spinal cord in head on collision of vehicles
   a. Flexion
   b. Flexion rotation
   c. Extension
   d. Circumduction

13. The first reflex to return once spinal shock is over is
   a. Plantar reflex
   b. Knee reflex
   c. Biceps reflex
   d. Bulbocavernous reflex

14. Which of the following is not included as a yellow flag sign for low back pain?
   a. Radicular impingement
   b. Systemic steroids
   c. Social isolation
   d. High functional limitation at 4 weeks/after 4 weeks

15. Distended bladder, incontinence of urine and priapism are
   a. Signs of injury to the urethra
   b. Signs of injury to cauda equina
   c. Signs of injury to pelvis
   d. Signs of spinal cord injury

16. For removal of vertebral disc all procedures are done except
   a. Laminotomy
   b. Laminectomy
   c. Laminoplasty
   d. Hemi-laminectomy

17. A 52-year-old woman presents to her GP with a long-standing history of lower back pain which has suddenly worsened in severity over the past few days. An urgent MRI scan of the lumbar spine shows a right paracentral disc protrusion at the L4/L5 level. The disc impinges on the lateral recess at this level. The most likely outcome would be
   a. Cauda equine syndrome
   b. Lumbar plexus compression
   c. Loss of ankle dorsiflexion
   d. Loss of function of EHL

18. Turn buckle cast is used for
   a. Scoliosis
   b. Fracture shaft femur
   c. Hangman's fracture
   d. Cervical spine injury

19. Progression of congenital scoliosis is least likely in which of the following vertebral anomaly?
   a. Wedge vertebra
   b. Fully segmented hemivertebra
   c. Unilateral unsegmented bar with hemivertebra
   d. Block vertebra

20. A patient has decreased sensation on the tip of the middle finger and decreased triceps reflex. It is due to disc prolapsed at
   a. C5–C6
   b. C6–C7
   c. C8–T1
   d. T1–T2

21. In spondylolisthesis, there is fracture of vertebra at
   a. Spinous process
   b. Pars interarticularis
   c. Transverse process
   d. Lamina

22. Seat belt injury is
   a. Tear drop fracture
   b. Wedge fracture
   c. Chance fracture
   d. Whiplash injury

23. The most common site of disc prolapse is
   a. L2 – L3
   b. L3 – L4
   c. L4 – L5
   d. L5 – S1

24. A middle-aged lady presents with complaints of neck pain. On examination, there is weakness of extension of right wrist with no sensory impairment. If pathology is a disc prolapse, an MRI of the cervical spine would most probably reveal a prolapsed intervertebral disc at what level?
    a. C3–C4
    b. C5–C6
    c. C4–C5
    d. C1–C2
25. Which is not a deep heat therapy?
    a. Short wave diathermy
    b. Ultrasound therapy
    c. Infrared therapy
    d. Microwave therapy
26. Percutaneous vertebroblasty is indicated in all except
    a. Tuberculosis
    b. Metastasis
    c. Osteoporosis
    d. Hemangioma
27. A 6-year-old child, presents with scoliosis, hairy tuft in the skin of back and neurological deficit. X-ray reveals multiple vertebral anomalies and a vertical bony spur overlying lumbar spine on AP view. The most probable diagnosis is
    a. Dorsal dermal sinus
    b. Diastematomyelia
    c. Tight filum terminale
    d. Caudal regression syndrome
28. Most common type of spondylolisthesis
    a. Congenital
    b. Dysplastic
    c. Degenerative
    d. Isthmic
    e. Traumatic
29. The most common cause of spinal cord injuries in our country is
    a. RTA
    b. Fall into well
    c. Fall from a height
    d. House collapse
30. Most dangerous type of spinal cord injury is
    a. Flexion
    b. Compression
    c. Extension
    d. Flexion–rotation
31. All of the following about the fracture of atlas vertebra are true except
    a. Quadriplegia is seen in 80% of the cases
    b. CT should be done for the diagnosis
    c. Jefferson fractures is the most common fracture of atlas
    d. Atlanto-occipital fusion may sometimes be needed
32. Whiplash injury is caused due to
    a. A fall from a height
    b. Acute hyperextension of the spine
    c. A blow to the top to head
    d. Acute hyperflexion of the spine
33. True regarding Hangman's fracture is
    a. Spondylolisthesis of C2 over C3
    b. Odontoid process fracture of C2
    c. Burst fracture of C1
    d. Fracture of hyoid bone
34. Inverted radial reflex tests which level
    a. C3
    b. C5
    c. L4
    d. L5
35. A patient with a prolapsed disk needs disk removal. Which of the following methods is not used?
    a. Laminectomy
    b. Hemilaminectomy
    c. Laminotomy
    d. Laminoplasty
36. A 50-year-old man presents with acute low back pain radiating down the right lower limb. On examination SLRT < 400, EHL is weak and there is sensory loss on dorsum of first webspace. Likely diagnosis is
    a. PIVD L4-L5
    b. Spondylolysis L5-S1
    c. Lumbar canal stenosis
    d. Spondylolisthesis L4-L5
37. Scheuermann's disease affects which age group?
    a. Adolescents
    b. Adults
    c. Elderly
    d. Infants

PERIPHERAL NERVE INJURIES

1. Finding a slowed conduction time at a specified point along the course of nerve is often valuable in confirming a clinical diagnosis of
    a. Malingering
    b. Neurotmesis
    c. Compression Neuropathy
    d. Myopathy
2. A politician sustained injury at T8 level following a bullet that was fired at him during a rally. All mentioned below are causes of non-recovery except
    a. Absence of endoneural tube
    b. Glial scar formation
    c. Absence of growth factor
    d. Absence of myelin formation inhibitors
3. The H-reflex is important for assessing which of the following?
    a. S1 radiculopathy
    b. L5 radiculopathy
    c. L2 radiculopathy
    d. L4 radiculopathy
4. The most common nerve used for nerve conduction study in H reflex is
    a. Median nerve
    b. Tibial nerve
    c. Ulnar nerve
    d. Peroneal nerve
5. A person was found lying in the right lateral position by the police. He had injuries on his right face, hand and on the right knee. Which of the following nerve injuries can explain the injuries caused in the patient?
    a. Trigeminal nerve
    b. Radial nerve
    c. Femoral nerve
    d. Common peroneal nerve
6. Foot drop due to injury to
    a. Superficial peroneal nerve
    b. Deep peroneal nerve
    c. Common peroneal nerve
    d. Tibial nerve
7. A child sustains supracondylar fracture humerus. On clinical examination, there is extension at MCP joints and flexion at IP joints of hand. Also there is loss of sensations along medial aspect of hand and forearm. The likely cause is injury to
    a. Upper brachial plexus
    b. Lower brachial plexus
    c. Musculocutaneous
    d. Median nerve
8. Following anterior dislocation of the shoulder, a patient develops weakness of flexion at elbow and lack of sensation over the lateral aspect forearm. The nerve that could be injured is
    a. Axillary nerve
    b. Ulnar nerve
    c. Radial nerve
    d. Musculcutaneous nerve
9. Guyon's canal is entrapment neuropathy site for which nerve?
    a. Ulnar nerve
    b. Median nerve
    c. Radial nerve
    c. Axillary nerve
10. Clasping sign is seen in paralysis of
    a. Ulnar nerve
    b. Median nerve
    c. Radial nerve
    d. Axillary nerve
11. The best way to look for PIN palsy is
    a. Loss of sensations over lateral two and a half fingers
    b. Loss of sensations over the thumb web
    c. Wrist drop
    d. Drop at MCP joints of fingers
12. Cheiralgia paraesthetica is compression neuropathy of which nerve
    a. Lateral cutaneous nerve of thigh
    b. Superficial radial nerve
    c. Sural nerve
    d. Lateral cutaneous nerve of forearm
13. Motor march is seen in
    a. Axonotmesis
    b. Neuropraxia
    c. Neurotmesis
    d. All of the above
14. A pole vaulter had a fall during vaulting and had paralysis of the arm muscles. His recovery prognosis can be best assessed by
    a. Strength duration curve
    b. Electromyography
    c. Muscle biopsy
    d. CPK levels

15. All indicate good prognosis in a nerve injury except
- a. Younger age
- b. Neuropraxia
- c. Pure motor nerve injury
- d. Proximal injury

16. Muscles that are paralyzed in Erb's paralysis are all except
- a. Biceps
- b. Brachioradialis
- c. Triceps
- d. Brachialis

17. Klumpke's paralysis involves injury to
- a. C1
- b. C4
- c. C8
- d. T1

18. All are true regarding brachial plexus injury except
- a. Erb's palsy causes paralysis of the abductors and external rotators of the shoulder
- b. In Klumpke's palsy, Horner's syndrome may be present on the ipsilateral side
- c. Preganglionic lesions have a better prognosis than the postganglionic lesion
- d. Histamine test is useful to differentiate between the pre- and postganglionic lesions

19. The most common cause of neurological deficit in the upper limb is
- a. Erb's palsy
- b. Polio
- c. C1-C2 dislocation
- d. Fracture dislocation of the cervical spine

20. Compression of a nerve in the carpal tunnel produces inability to
- a. Adduct the thumb
- b. Abduct the thumb
- c. Oppose the thumb
- d. Flex the distal phalanx of the thumb

21. Ulnar paradox is due to
- a. FDP
- b. FPL
- c. ECRB
- d. A simultaneous radial nerve disease

22. Froment's sign tests
- a. Abductor pollicis brevis
- b. Abductor pollicis longus
- c. Adductor pollicis
- d. Extensor pollicis longus

23. The most common cause of wrist drop is
- a. Dislocation of elbow
- b. Intramuscular injection
- c. Fracture humerus
- d. Dislocation of shoulder

24. Thoracic outlet syndrome is best diagnosed by
- a. MRI
- b. CT
- c. Digital subtraction angiography
- d. Clinical examination

25. Which of the following is not a clinical test for Thoracic outlet syndrome?
- a. Allen's test
- b. Adson's test
- c. Roos test
- d. Hyperabduction maneuver

26. Dislocation of which one of the following carpal bones can present with a median nerve palsy?
- a. Scaphoid
- b. Hamate
- c. Lunate
- d. Trapezium

27. Ape thumb deformity is observed in lesions of
- a. Radial nerve injury
- b. Ulnar nerve injury
- c. Median nerve injury
- d. Circumflex humeral nerve injury

28. The "Card test" tests the function of
- a. Median nerve
- b. Ulnar nerve
- c. Axillary nerve
- d. Radial nerve

29. Disability of hands is maximum with a lesion of
- a. Median nerve at elbow
- b. Median nerve at wrist
- c. Ulnar nerve at elbow
- d. Ulnar nerve at wrist

30. Ulnar nerve transaction above elbow causes (PGI type)
- a. Complete loss of sensation in 4th and 5th finger
- b. Paralysis of all lumbricals
- c. Paralysis of all interossei
- d. Paralysis of flexor carpi ulnaris
- e. Paralysis of flexor digitorum profundus

31. A patient presents with loss of sensation of ring and little finger with wasting of hypothenar muscles. Where is the likely site of lesion?
- a. Deep branch of ulnar nerve is injured
- b. Median nerve is involved
- c. Ulnar nerve is transected prior to division into superficial and deep branches
- d. Superficial branch of ulnar nerve is injured

32. In a patient with Claw hand due to leprosy, the deformity would be classified as
- a. Grade 0
- b. Grade I
- c. Grade II
- d. Grade III

33. Damage to the radial nerve in the spinal groove spares which muscle
- a. Lateral head of triceps
- b. Long head of triceps
- c. ECRB
- d. Anconeus

34. Which of the following factor does not predispose to carpal tunnel syndrome?
- a. Hypertension
- b. Hypothyroidism
- c. Pregnancy
- d. Acromegaly

35. Phalen's test is positive in
- a. Carpal tunnel syndrome
- b. DeQuervain's disease
- c. Tennis elbow
- d. Ulnar bursitis

36. Meralgia paraesthetica involves
- a. Axillary nerve
- b. Sural nerve
- c. Median nerve
- d. Lateral cutaneous nerve of thigh

37. Which nerve has been reported to be injured during McRobert's procedure performed for delivering a child?
- a. Axillary nerve
- b. Sural nerve
- c. Median nerve
- d. Lateral cutaneous nerve of thigh

38. The most common cause of Tarsal tunnel syndrome
- a. Osteoarthritis
- b. Ankylosing spondylitis
- c. Psoriatic arthritis
- d. Rheumatoid arthritis

39. Which of the following does not involve nerve damage?
- a. Guillian-Barré syndrome
- b. Volkmann's ischemic contracture
- c. Neurotmesis
- d. Erb's paralysis

40. Schaefer's test is for assesment of
- a. Palmaris longus
- b. Flexor hallucis longus
- c. Brachioradialis
- d. Coracobrachialis

41. The most common nerve injury in a typist involved in computer-related work would be
- a. Ulnar nerve
- b. Radial nerve
- c. Median nerve
- d. Axillary nerve

42. Compression of median nerve in carpal tunnel produces
- a. Loss of adduction of thumb
- b. Loss of opposition of thumb
- c. Loss of abduction of thumb
- d. Failure of flexion of DIP joint

43. Which nerve is involved in people involved in repetitive typing work?
- a. Radial
- b. Ulnar
- c. Median
- d. Axillary

44. Axillary crutch paralyzes which nerve?
- a. Axillary
- b. Median
- c. Radial
- d. Ulnar

45. Which of the following does not involve nerve damage?
 a. Guillain-Barré syndrome b. Erb's paralysis
 c. Volkmann paralysis d. Neurotmesis

INFECTIONS

1. Spina ventosa results from
 a. Tuberculosis (TB) b. Sarcoidosis
 c. Both d. None
2. Caries sicca is seen in
 a. Hip b. Knee
 c. Shoulder d. None
3. TB of spine commonly affects all of the following parts of vertebrae except
 a. Body b. Lamina
 c. Spinous process d. Pedicle
4. TB of spine starts in
 a. Body b. Nucleosus pulposus
 c. Annulus fibrosus d. Paravertebral fascia
5. Investigation for rapid diagnosis of osteomyelitis
 a. X- ray b. CT scan
 c. MRI d. Isotope scanning
6. The most common cause of osteomyelitis in sickle cell disease is
 a. Salmonella b. Staph aureus
 c. Pseudomonas d. *Streptococcus pyogenes*
7. Hong Kong procedure is useful for treating
 a. Tuberculosis of cervical spine
 b. Gout
 c. AVN of hip
 d. Caffey's disease patients
8. Wandering acetabulum is seen in
 a. Fracture acetabulum b. CDH
 c. Dislocation of femur d. TB hip
9. Triple deformity of knee is classically seen in
 a. Fracture patella b. TB knee
 c. RA d. Rickets
10. Kanavel sign are seen in
 a. Tenosynovitis b. Trigger finger
 c. Carpal tunnel syndrome d. Dupuytren's contracture
11. Compound palmar ganglion is
 a. Pyogenic affection of ulnar bursa
 b. Tuberculosis affection of ulnar bursa
 c. Nonspecific affection of ulnar bursa
 d. Ulnar bursitis due to compound injury
12. Brodie's abcess is
 a. Acute osteomyelitis b. Subacute osteomyelitis
 c. Chronic osteomyelitis d. Septic arthritis
13. The most common organism causing infection after open fractures
 a. *Staphylococcus aureus* b. *Psudomonas*
 c. *Klebsiella* d. *Gonococcus*
14. True about HIV osteomyelitis is all except?
 a. Bilateral b. Necrosis is absent
 c. Periosteal new bone formation
 d. Most common cause is *Staph aureus*
15. Earliest change of osteomyelitis on X-Ray
 a. Lytic defects b. Loss of soft tissue planes
 c. Sequestrum d. Periosteal reaction
16. The most common joint involved in septic arthritis
 a. Knee b. Shoulder
 c. Hip d. Elbow
17. A 7-year-old boy presented with abrupt onset of pain in right hip with the hip held in abduction. Hemogram and X-ray are normal but the ESR is raised. Appropriate line of management is from here would be
 a. Hospitalize and observe b. Intravenous antibiotics
 c. Ambulatory observation d. USG-guided aspiration of hip

18. Tom Smith arthritis manifests as
 a. Hip stiffness
 b. Ankylosis
 c. Lengthening of limb
 d. Increased hip mobility and instability
19. A 30-year-old male, HIV positive, on antiretroviral therapy, has pain in right hip region. There is flexion, abduction and external rotation deformity of right hip since 2 months. Most likely diagnosis is
 a. TB Hip b. Avascular necrosis
 c. Septic arthritis d. Transient synovitis
20. The most common site of actinomycosis amongst the following is
 a. Femur b. Mandible
 c. Tibia d. Rib
21. The most common finger infected by felon is
 a. Thumb b. Index finger
 c. Middle finger d. Ring finger
22. Ring sequestrum is seen in
 a. Typhoid osteomyelitis b. Chronic osteomyelitis
 c. Amputation stump d. Tuberculosis osteomyelitis
23. The common cause of limp in a child of seven years is
 a. TB hip
 b. CDH
 c. Perthes disease
 d. Slipped capital femoral epiphysis
24. Most common cause of monoarthritis in children in India is
 a. Septic arthritis b. Osteoarthritis
 c. Tuberculous arthritis d. RA
25. The first neurological sign in a patient with TB spine is
 a. Sensory loss b. Spastic weakness
 c. Bladder involvement d. Ankle clonus
26. Poncet's disease is
 a. TB + monoarthritis b. TB+ polyarthritis
 c. RA with neutropenia d. RA with leucopenia
27. Poor prognostic factor in Pott's paraplegia are (PGI type)
 a. Acute onset paraplegia
 b. Sudden progression of paraplegia
 c. Long-standing paraplegia
 d. Motor paralysis alone
 e. Paraplegia in children
28. Apparent lengthening of the limb is seen in which stage of TB hip?
 a. Stage 1 b. Stage 2
 c. Stage 3 d. Stage 4
29. The best diagnostic modality for tuberculosis of spine is
 a. Clinical b. X-ray
 c. MRI d. CT-guided biopsy
30. Bony ankylosis may result from (PGI type)
 a. Pyogenic arthritis b. Tubercular arthritis
 c. Osteoarthritis d. Rheumatoid arthritis
31. Instillation treatment in osteomyelitis is
 a. Continuous suction and continuous drainage
 b. Intermittent suction and continuous drainage
 c. Continuous suction and intermittent drainage
 d. Intermittent suction and intermittent drainage

TUMORS

1. Classification system for bone tumors is named after
 a. Galen b. Enneking
 c. Codman d. Charnley
2. Which of the following is not true about osteoid osteoma?
 a. Generally affect diaphysis of long bones
 b. Most common bone affected—tibia
 c. Radiolucent nidus in center
 d. Premalignant

3. Sunray appearance in osteosarcoma is due to
   a. Osteonecrosis
   b. Periosteal reaction
   c. Calcification along the muscle spindles
   d. Calcification along the vessels
4. Most common malignancy that metastasizes to the spine is
   a. Lung
   b. Prostate
   c. Breast
   d. Thyroid
5. Bone to bone metastasis is most commonly seen in
   a. Osteosarcoma
   b. Ewings sarcoma
   c. Chondrosarcoma
   d. Reticulum cell carcinoma
6. Night pains are characteristically seen with
   a. Osteoid osteoma
   b. Osteosarcoma
   c. Ewing sarcoma
   d. Fibrous cortical defect
7. A 10-year-old child presents with a small lytic lesion surrounded by reactive sclerosis in the middle of shaft of tibia. The most likely diagnosis is
   a. Fibrous cortical defect
   b. Eosinophilic granuloma
   c. Osteoid osteoma
   d. Fibrous dysplasia
8. The most common site for osteochondroma is fast growing ends of long bones. Next common site is
   a. Crest of the ilium
   b. Scapula
   c. Ribs
   d. Vertebra
9. Tumor with maximum bone matrix
   a. Osteoid osteoma
   b. Chondrosarcoma
   c. Enchondroma
   d. None
10. Hyperglycemia is associated with which of the following bone tumor
    a. Multiple myeloma
    b. Ewings sarcoma
    c. Osteosarcoma
    d. Chondrosarcoma
11. The risk of malignancy in multiple osteochondromatosis is
    a. 1%
    b. 2%
    c. 5%
    d. 15%
12. Which of the following is a GCT variant?
    a. Chondroblastoma
    b. Aneurysmal bone cyst
    c. Osteosarcoma with giant cells
    d. Fibrous dysplasia
13. Increased LDH levels are a bad prognostic factor in which tumor?
    a. Osteosarcoma
    b. Osteoid osteoma
    c. Giant cell tumor
    d. Ewing's tumor
14. All of the following statements about synovial cell sarcoma are correct except
    a. Occurs more often at extra-articular sites
    b. Originates from synovial lining
    c. Usually seen in people under 50 years age
    d. Knee is the most common site
15. Most common site of Adamantinoma is
    a. Mandible near symphsis menti
    b. Mandible near the molar tooth
    c. Diaphysis of tibia
    d. Hard palate
16. A 30-year-lady presented with pain and tenderness in index finger just under the nail. She was unable to wash her hands with cold water. Patient did not reveal any history of trauma or injury. What could be probable finding noted in this case
    a. Sausage digits
    b. Ridging of nail, bluish discoloration and pin-head tenderness
    c. Stiffness of whole hand
    d. Hypersensitivity of finger
17. Generally radiotherapy should not be used for treating benign conditions, the only possible exception being
    a. Chondromyxoid fibroma
    b. Extensive pigmented vilonodular synovitis
    c. Benign fibrous histiocytoma
    d. Desmoplastic fibroma so extensive that it cannot be surgically excised
18. Vertebra plana is seen in all except
    a. Ewing's sarcoma
    b. Paget's disease
    c. Trauma disease
    d. Malignancy
19. Most common malignant tumor of hand
    a. Chondroblastoma
    b. Enchondroma
    c. Squamous cell carcinoma
    d. Melanoma
20. Chondroblastoma is a tumor of
    a. Epiphysis
    b. Metaphysis
    c. Diaphysis
    d. Flat bone
21. Most common childhood tumor metastasizing to the bones is
    a. Neuroblastoma
    b. Wilm's tumor
    c. Ewing's sarcoma
    d. Ganglioneuroma
22. All of the following tumors are benign tumors except
    a. Chondroma
    b. Osteochondroma
    c. Chordoma
    d. Enchondroma
23. According to the newer hypothesis, Ewing's sarcoma arises from
    a. Epiphysis
    b. Medullary cavity
    c. Diaphysis
    d. Cortex
24. The cell of origin in giant cell tumor is
    a. Monocyte
    b. Osteoclast
    c. Osteoblast
    d. Unknown
25. Which of the following is biphasic tumor?
    a. Rhabdomyosarcoma
    b. Osteosarcoma
    c. Synovial sarcoma
    d. Osteoblastoma
26. Fallen fragment sign is seen in
    a. Giant cell tumor
    b. Simple bone cyst
    c. Aneurysmal bone cyst
    d. Fibrous dysplasia
27. A classical expansile lytic lesion in the transverse process of the vertebra is seen in
    a. Osteosarcoma
    b. Osteoblastoma
    c. Aneurysmal bone cyst
    d. Metastasis
28. Differential diagnosis of a lesion, histologically resembling GCT in the small bones of the hands and feet includes all of the following except
    a. Aneurysmal bone cyst
    b. Osteosarcoma
    c. Fibrosarcoma
    d. Hyperparathyroidism
29. Most common radiation induced tumor is
    a. Multiple myeloma
    b. Malignant fibrous histiocytoma
    c. Chondrosarcoma
    d. Osteosarcoma
30. T-10 protocol for treatment of osteosarcoma includes all of the following except
    a. Vincristine
    b. Etoposide
    c. High dose methotrexate
    d. Bleomycin, cyclophosphamide, doxorubicin (BCD)
31. Maximum incidence of Ewing's occurs in
    a. 1st decade
    b. 2nd decade
    c. 3rd decade
    d. 4th decade
32. Most common bone tumor in the 1st decade is
    a. Multiple myeloma
    b. Ewing's sarcoma
    c. Osteosarcoma
    d. Metastasis
33. A poor prognostic sign for Ewing's sarcoma is
    a. Females
    b. Fever
    c. Grade
    d. Age <12 years
34. Pigmented villo-nodular synovitis most commonly occurs at
    a. Knee
    b. Hip
    c. Shoulder
    d. Elbow
35. True about bone metastasis (PGI type)
    a. 5% bone metastasis are symptomatic
    b. MC secondary in females is breast

c. High serum levels of alkaline phophatase
d. Prostate produces osteosclerotic lesion
e. Commonly involves hand and feet bones

36. Metastasis are least common in
a. Vertebra
b. Pelvis
c. Proximal parts of long bones of the upper limb
d. Small bones of the hand

37. Most common soft tissue tumor in a child
a. Rhabdomyosarcoma   b. Fibrosarcoma
c. Histiocytoma   d. Liposarcoma

38. Expansile lytic osseous metastases are characteristics of primary malignancy of
a. Breast   b. Prostate
c. Bronchus   d. Kidney

39. A 60-year-old male has bone pain, vertebral collapse and pathological fracture in pelvis. The most probable diagnosis is
a. Multiple myeloma   b. TB
c. Hamangioma of bone   d. Secondaries

40. A 4-year-old girl presents with history of fever and a palpable mass in thigh. X-ray shows periosteal reaction and destruction of bone. Next investigation to be done
a. Bone biopsy   b. Blood culture
c. Bone scan   d. CT scan

41. Osteosclerotic bone metastasis is seen most commonly in which carcinoma?
a. Kidney   b. Lung
c. Thyroid   d. Prostate

42. An elderly patient has back pain and urinary retention. Next investigation to be done should be
a. Alkaline phosphatase   b. Acid phosphatase
c. Serum calcium   d. Serum VMA levels

43. Most common site of osteosarcoma is
a. Upper end of femur   b. Lower end of femur
c. Lower end of humerus   d. Lower end of tibia

44. Maffucci syndrome is
a. Enchondromas with hemangioma
b. Haemangiomas and limb hyperplasia
c. Haemangiomas and precocious puberty
d. Haemangiomas and capillary malformation

45. When size of osteoclastoma exceeds the size of metaphysis (PGI type)
a. Tumor will be covered by cortex
b. Tumor will be covered by fibrous capsule
c. Tumor will be covered by a thin layer of bone
d. It is limited to metaphysis
e. It is covered by periosteum

46. The following bone tumor may cause dural deposits without causing bony changes
a. Hodgkin's lymphoma   b. Multiple myloma
c. Secondaries   d. Fibrous dysplasia

47. Which is not a feature of malignant transformation in an osteochondroma?
a. Weight loss
b. Pain
c. Rapid increase in size
d. Calcification on CT more than 2 cm

48. Shepherd crook deformity is seen in
a. Fibrous dysplasia   b. Paget's disease
c. Osteogenesis imperfecta   d. All of the above

49. The treatment of choice for Ewings sarcoma is
a. Radiotherapy   b. Chemotherapy
c. Wide surgical excision   d. Amputation

50. Intraosseous skeletal tumor is best detected by?
a. Bone scan with CT   b. X-ray
c. Bone scan   d. MRI

PEDIATRIC ORTHOPEDICS

1. A child is born with CTEV (Congenital Talipes Equinus Varus). All of the following can be the causes except
a. Poliomyelitis
b. Spina bifida
c. Idiopathic
d. Arthrogryposis multiplex congenita

2. Earliest changes in Perthe's disease are detected by
a. X-ray   b. CT
c. MRI   d. Nuclear scan

3. Which of the following is not true about development dysplasia of hip (DDH)?
a. The hourglass appearance of the joint capsule may prevent a successful closed reduction
b. It is more common in females
c. Oligohydramnios is associated with higher risk of DDH
d. When the ossification center is in the lower medial quadrant, the hip is dislocated

4. A 12-year-old obese boy was referred to emergency from endocrinology department for painful limp since 1 month. Which amongst the following will be the least helping investigation?
a. USG hip   b. CT B/L hip
c. X-ray pelvis with hip   d. MRI B/L hip

5. Congenital pseudoarthrosis of tibia is best treated by
a. Above knee POP cast
b. Below knee POP cast
c. Internal fixation
d. Internal fixation and bone grafting

6. Pollicization is
a. Thumb reconstruction
b. Thumb amputation
c. Inflammation at the base of thumb in gouty arthritis
d. A treatment method for trigger thumb

7. The characteristic triad of Klippel Fiel Syndrome includes all of the following except
a. Limited neck movements   b. Low hair line
c. Short neck   d. Elevated scapula

8. All are true for congenital torticollis except
a. It can disappear spontaneously
b. Also called as Sternomastoid tumor
c. Seen only in cases of breech vaginal delivery
d. Untreated, neglected cases can result in plagiocephaly

9. Fair banks triangle is seen in
a. SCFE (Slipped capital femoral epiphysis)
b. CTEV
c. DDH
d. Congenital coxa vara

10. An 8-year-old male presents with painless limp on examination and restricted abduction and internal rotation left hip. Most probable diagnosis is
a. CDH   b. Tuberculous arthritis of hip
c. Septic arthritis of hip   d. Perthes disease

11. Trethowan's sign is seen in
a. Perthes disease   b. CDH
c. SCFE   d. Fracture neck femur

12. Bachelor's cast is used in
a. Fracture radius   b. CTEV
c. DDH   d. Fracture calcaneum

13. Most common associated anomaly in DDH is
a. Femoral anteversion   b. Pelvic obliquity
c. Femoral retroversion   d. Shallow acetabulum

14. All of the following statements are true about DDH, except
a. More common in females
b. Twin pregnancy is a known risk factor

c. Oligohydramnios is associated with a higher risk
d. The hourglass appearance of the capsule may prevent a successful closed reduction

15. Charlie Chaplin gait is seen in
   a. Genu valgum
   b. External tibial torsion
   c. Congenital coxa vara
   d. CDH

16. Critical age of osteotomy for genu varum is
   a. 4 years
   b. 6 years
   c. 8 years
   d. 10 years

17. Rocker bottom foot is due to
   a. Malunited fracture calcaneum
   b. Neural tube defect
   c. Horizontal talus
   d. Over treatment of CTEV

18. Most common congenital anomaly of foot in India is
   a. CTEV
   b. Vertical talus
   c. Metatarsus adductus
   d. Hallux valgus

19. The ideal treatment of bilateral idiopathic clubfoot in a newborn is
   a. Manipulation by mother
   b. Manipulation and casts
   c. Manipulations and dens brown splint
   d. Surgical release

20. Triple arthrodesis involves fusion of which of the following joints?
   a. Tibiotalar, calcaneocuboid and talonavicular
   b. Calcaneocuboid, talonavicular and talocalcaneal
   c. Ankle joint, calcaneocuboid and talonavicular
   d. None of the above

21. The club foot characteristically involves
   a. Foot, ankle and leg
   b. Foot only
   c. Foot and ankle
   d. Foot, ankle, leg and knee joint

22. Most important pathology in club foot is
   a. Calcaneal fracture
   b. Tightening of tendoachilles
   c. Congenital talonavicular dislocation
   d. Lateral derangement

23. Hallux valgus is associated with all except?
   a. A bunion
   b. An exostosis on the medial side of the head of the first metatarsal
   c. Osteoarthritis of the first metatarsophalangeal joint
   d. Over riding or under riding of the second toe by the third

24. Ligament stretched in flat foot is
   a. Anterior talofibular ligament
   b. Posterior talofibular ligament
   c. Calcaneonavicular ligament
   d. Calcaneofibular ligament

25. For screening of neonatal hip instability, modality most commonly used is
   a. USG
   b. X-ray
   c. MRI
   d. CT

26. A 6-year-old boy presents to emergency department with painful limp. Clinical examination reveals tenderness in the femoral triangle and some limitation of hip movements. The X-ray is normal. What should be the next course of action?
   a. Wait and watch (Observation)
   b. USG
   c. MRI
   d. Aspiration

27. A one year old child presented with multiple fractures seen in various stages of healing. The most probable diagnosis in the case is
   a. Scurvy
   b. Rickets
   c. Battered baby syndrome
   d. Fall from height

28. Not true about B/L DDH
   a. Exaggerated lordosis
   b. B/L genu valgum
   c. Wadding gait
   d. Shenton's line broken
   e. Short stature

29. The most common presentation of congenital dislocation of knee is
   a. Varus
   b. Valgus
   c. Flexion
   d. Hyperextension

30. Most common cause of genu valgum in a child is
   a. Osteoarthritis
   b. Rickets
   c. Paget's disease
   d. Rheumatoid arthritis

31. Blount's disease is associated with all of the following except
   a. Genu varum
   b. Genu recurvatum
   c. Internal tibial torsion
   d. External tibial torsion

32. Rocker bottom foot is seen in (PGI type)
   a. Congenital vertical talus
   b. Excessive correction of Grice procedure
   c. Arthrogryposis
   d. Holding club foot in too long corrected position
   e. Force dorsiflexion against equinus

33. In correction of clubfoot by manipulation, which deformity should be corrected first?
   a. Forefoot adduction
   b. Varus
   c. Tibia torsion
   d. Equinus

34. Child 3¼ years is treated for CTEV by
   a. Triple arthrodesis
   b. Posteromedial soft tissue release
   c. Lateral wedge resection
   d. Tendo-Achilles lengthening

35. Pseudoarthrosis after triple arthrodesis is seen at the joint of
   a. Calcaneocuboid
   b. Calcaneonavicular
   c. Naviculocuboid
   d. Talonavicular

36. Sprengel's deformity is
   a. Absence of clavicle
   b. Acromioclavicular dislocation
   c. Congenital elevation of scapula
   d. Recurrent dislocation of shoulder

37. Jaw tumor is seen in
   a. Osteoporosis
   b. Osteomalacia
   c. Osteopetrosis
   d. Caffey's disease

38. Treatment of choice for Caffey's disease is
   a. Multiple drilling
   b. Penicillin
   c. Tetracycline
   d. Curettage

39. Jones operation is done for
   a. CTEV
   b. Hallus valgus correction
   c. Cavus deformity of foot
   d. Claw hallux

40. Excision arthroplasty is indicated in all of the following except
   a. Hallux valgus
   b. TB hip
   c. Lateral condyle humerus fracture
   d. Caries elbow

41. Siffert Katz sign is seen in
   a. Perthes disease
   b. Blount's disease
   c. Osteogenesis imperfecta
   d. Pulled elbow

42. Flexion deformity in hammer toe is at
   a. PIP
   b. DIP b
   c. Metatarsophalangeal
   d. Calcaneonavicular

43. All are features favouring amputation in Congenital pseudoarthrosis of tibia except
   a. Shortening more than 3 inches
   b. History of multiple failed surgical procedures
   c. Association with neurofibromatosis
   d. Marked joint stiffness

NEUROMUSCULAR DISORDERS

1. In a post-polio case, iliotibial tract contracture is likely to result in
   a. Extension at the hip and knee
   b. Extension at the hip
   c. Flexion at the hip and the knee
   d. Extension at the knee

2. Test for tight iliotibial band is
   a. Ober's test
   b. Simmond's test
   c. Osner's test
   d. Charnley's test
3. In a 3-year-old child with polio paralysis, tendon transfer operation is done at?
   a. 2 months after the disease
   b. 2 years after the disease
   c. 6–12 months after the disease
   d. After skeletal maturation
4. Tendon transfers in polio should be done after the age of
   a. 6 months
   b. 5 months–1 year
   c. 2 years
   d. 5 years
5. Post-poliomyelitis, a patient has grade II power in Gastrocnemius, grade III is Peroneus, grade IV in tibialis anterior. The resultant deformity would be
   a. Calcaneovalgus
   b. Equinovarus
   c. Calcaneovarus
   d. Genu valgus
6. Muscle most commonly affected in polio is
   a. Tensor fascia lata
   b. Tibialis posterior
   c. Tibialis anterior
   d. Quadriceps
7. Polio most commonly involves which one of the following upper limb muscles
   a. Pectoralis major
   b. Trapezium
   c. Deltoid
   d. Triceps

GENETIC AND DEVELOPMENTAL DISORDERS

1. Bone dysplasia is due to
   a. Faulty nutrition
   b. Faulty development
   c. Trauma
   d. Parathyroid tumor
2. Not seen in osteopetrosis
   a. Compression of cranial nerves
   b. Osteomyelitis of mandible
   c. Pancytopenia
   d. Delayed healing of bone
3. Musculoskeletal abnormalities seen in neurofibromatosis
   a. Pseudoarthrosis
   b. Hypertrophy of limb
   c. Scoliosis
   d. All of the above
4. The most common cause of congenital pseudoarthrosis is
   a. Fibrous dysplasia
   b. Neurofibromatosis
   c. Intrauterine fracture
   d. Unknown
5. A 3-year-old male presented with progressive anemia, hepatosplenomegaly and osteomyelitis of jaw with pathological fracture. X-ray shows chalky white deposits in bone. Probable diagnosis is
   a. Alkaptonuria
   b. Osteopetrosis
   c. Myositis ossificans progerssiva
   d. Osteopoikilosis
6. Dripping candle wax appearance on X-ray of spine is seen in
   a. Osteopetrosis
   b. Metastasis
   c. TB spine
   d. Melorheostosis
7. The following is false about achondroplasia
   a. Due to gene mutation
   b. Mental retardation
   c. AD
   d. Shortening of limbs present
8. A 9-year-old child has high arched palate with shoulders meeting in front of his chest. Diagnosis is?
   a. Cleidocranial dysostosis
   b. Erb's palsy
   c. Chondro-osteodystrophy
   d. Cortical hyperostosis
9. Phocomelia is characterized by
   a. Absence of short bones
   b. Complete absence of extremities
   c. Defects of long bones of limb
   d. Partial absence of extremities
10. Pseudoarthrosis is seen in all of the following except
    a. Idiopathic
    b. Fracture
    c. Osteomyelitis
    d. Neurofibromatosis

11. Nail patella syndrome is characterized by
    a. Iliac horn
    b. Sacral horn
    c. Knee deformity
    d. Dislocation of patella
12. "Trident hand" is seen in
    a. Achondroplasia
    b. Mucopolysaccharidosis
    c. Diphyseal achalasia
    d. Cleidocranial dystosis
13. The features of Achondroplasia include all except
    a. Defective head
    b. No mental retardation
    c. Autosomal recessive
    d. Familial
14. The characteristics of Morquio's disease include all except
    a. Spinal kyphosis
    b. Subnormal intelligence
    c. Excessive excretion of keratin-sulphate in urine
    d. Dwarfism
15. Ring shaped epiphysis is seen in
    a. Osteogenesis imperfecta
    b. Morquio syndrome
    c. Zwelleger syndrome
    d. Multiple epiphyseal dysplasia
16. Not true about osteogenesis imperfecta
    a. Deafness
    b. Laxity of joints
    c. Fragile fracture
    d. Impaired healing of fracture
17. In which of the following conditions, bilateral symmetrical fractures occur?
    a. Rickets
    b. Osteogenesis imperfecta
    c. Fluorosis
    d. Osteopetrosis
18. Wormian bones are seen in
    a. Paget's disease
    b. Osteoclastoma
    c. Scheurmann's disease
    d. Osteogenesis imperfect
19. Not true about osteogenesis imperfecta
    a. Autosomal dominant disease
    b. Blue sclera
    c. Associated with otosclerosis
    d. Defect in collagen type I

METABOLIC BONE DISEASES

1. Which of the following statement is incorrect regarding osteoporosis?
   a. i/v parathormone is useful in severe osteoporosis
   b. T-score is more than 2.5 SD below normal
   c. Bisphosphonates are the mainstay of treatment
   d. Calcitonin is useful in acute pain
2. The maximum change in bone mineral density in hemiplegic patients after 1 year is seen in
   a. Lumbar spine
   b. Proximal femur of the paretic side
   c. Distal radius of the paretic side
   d. Humerus of the paretic side
3. Blade of grass lesion is seen in
   a. Thalassemia
   b. Osteoporosis
   c. Carcinoma prostate
   d. Paget's disease
4. An elderly female is on treatment for osteoporosis with alendronate for 7 years. She now presents with complaints of hip pain. The next investigation for her should be
   a. X-ray
   b. DEXA scan
   c. Vitamin D levels
   d. ALP levels
5. Hypervitaminosis of which of the following vitamins can cause bony abnormalities? (PGI type)
   a. Vitamin A
   b. Vitamin C
   c. Vitamin D
   d. Vitamin K
   e. Vitamin E
6. As per current recommendations which vitamin is required with vitamin D for treatment of osteoporosis?
   a. Vitamin A
   b. Vitamin B
   c. Vitamin C
   d. Vitamin K

7. What is the biochemical analysis in osteoporosis?
   a. Decreased Ca and P and alkaline phosphatase
   b. Increased Ca, P and alkaline phosphatase
   c. Decreased Ca and P but increased alkaline phosphatase
   d. Normal Ca, P and alkaline phosphatase

8. All of the following statements regarding Paget's disease are correct except
   a. Females are affected more than males
   b. It can lead to osteogenic sarcoma
   c. Serum alkaline phosphate level is increased
   d. Also called as osteitis deformans

9. Which of the following is not a recognized risk factor for osteoporosis?
   a. Early menarche   b. Sedentary life style
   c. Smoking   d. Low dietary calcium intake

10. A 6-year-old child is on calcium supplementation for rickets and has genu valgum. When can the child be referred to the surgeon for a corrective surgery?
   a. When vitamin D levels return to normal
   b. When growth plate healing is seem radio-graphically
   c. When serum alkaline phosphatase levels are normal
   d. When serum calcium levels become normal

11. Which of the following is not a treatment option for osteoporosis?
   a. Denosumab   b. Alendronate
   c. Vertebroplasty   d. Corticosteroids

12. Denosumab—a monoclonal antibody against RANKL receptor is used in the treatment of?
   a. Osteoarthritis   b. RA
   c. SLE   d. Osteoporosis

13. Which is the drug of choice in Paget's disease?
   a. Alendronate   b. Steroids
   c. Allopurinol   d. Calcitonin

14. Pain in Paget's disease is best relieved by?
   a. Radiation   b. Calcitonin
   c. Simple analgesics   d. Narcotic analgesics

15. True about osteoclasts are all except
   a. Derived from monocyte   b. Stimulated by PTH
   c. Phagocytosis of foreign bodies
   d. Resorption of bone

16. Rickets in infancy is characterized by all of the following except
   a. Wide open fontanella   b. Bow legs
   c. Rachitic rosary   d. Craniotabes

17. Oncogenic rickets not seen in
   a. Osteosarcoma   b. Nonossifying fibroma
   c. Chondroblastoma   d. Angiosarcoma

18. Salt and pepper skull is a feature of
   a. Eosinophilic granuloma b. Paget's syndrome
   c. Primary hyperparathyroidism
   d. Multiple myeloma

19. Absence of lamina dura in the alveolus occurs in
   a. Rickets   b. Deficiency of vitamin
   c. Osteomalacia   d. Hyperparathyroidism

20. Looser's zones are seen in
   a. Osteomalacia   b. Renal osteodystrophy
   c. Paget's ds   d. All of the above

21. Short 4th metacarpal is a feature of?
   a. Hypoparathyroidism
   b. Hyperparathyroidism
   c. Pseudohypoparathyroidism
   d. Scleroderma

22. Milkman's fracture is?
   a. Fracture humerus
   b. Fracture 1st metacarpal
   c. Fracture of clavicle in children
   d. Pseudo-fracture in adults

23. Barton's disease is
   a. Rickets and fracture   b. Scurvy and fracture
   c. Scurvy and rickets   d. Scurvy and syphilis

24. Osteoporosis is caused by all except
   a. Fluorosis   b. Hyperthyroidism
   c. Hypogonadism   d. Hyperparathyroidism

25. Most common manifestation of osteoporosis is
   a. Loss of weight   b. Bowing of legs
   c. Compression fracture of the spine
   d. Backache

26. Diagnostic radiological finding in skeletal fluorosis
   a. Interosseous membrane ossification
   b. Osteosclerosis of vertebral body
   c. Ossification of ligaments of knee joint
   d. Sclerosis of sacroiliac joint

27. Increased density in skull vault is seen in?
   a. Fluorosis   b. Renal osteodystrophy
   c. Multiple myeloma   d. Hyperparathyroidism

28. A 67-year-old man on biochemical analysis was found to have three fold rise in level of serum alkaline phosphatase (ALP) above that of upper limit of normal value during a routine check up. However, serum calcium and phosphorous concentration and LFTs were normal. He is asymptomatic. Probable cause could be
   a. Paget's disease of bone
   b. Multiple myeloma
   c. Primary hyperparathyroidism
   d. Osteomalacia

29. Rotting fence postappearance of femur is seen in
   a. Fibrous dysplasia   b. Hyperparathyroidism
   c. Paget's disease   d. Fracture neck of femur

30. Drug induced osteomalacia is known to be associated with the use of
   a. Steroids   b. Heparin
   c. Phenytoin   d. Gentamycin

31. Alkaline phosphatase is elevated in all except
   a. Rickets   b. Osteomalacia
   c. Hypoparathyroidism   d. Hypophosphatemia

32. The characteristic finding in osteomalacia is
   a. $\downarrow$P   b. $\downarrow$Ca
   c. $\downarrow$Ca and $\uparrow$P   d. $\downarrow$Ca and $\downarrow$P

33. The most common cause of primary hyperparathyroidism is
   a. Solitary adenoma   b. Chief cell hyperplasia
   c. Multiple adenoma   d. Werner's syndrome

34. In hyperparathyroidism bone resorption is seen in all these sites except
   a. Jaws   b. Metacarpals
   c. Ribs   d. End of long bones

35. A 50-year-old man presented with multiple pathological fractures. His serum calcium was 11.5 mg/dL and phosphate was 2.5 mg/dL while alkaline phosphatase was 940 IU/dL. The most probable diagnosis is
   a. Osteoporosis   b. Osteomalacia
   c. Multiple myeloma   d. Hyperparathyroidism

36. Paget's disease of bone most commonly affects
   a. Skull   b. Vertebra
   c. Pelvis   d. Femur

37. Deafness in cases of Paget's disease is due to
   a. Thickened cranium
   b. Narrowing of foramina of skull
   c. Brain compression
   d. Otosclerosis

38. Osteoporosis is seen in all the following except
   a. Thyrotoxicosis   b. Rheumatoid arthritis
   c. Hypoparathyroidism   d. Steroid therapy

39. The most common site of fracture of bone in senile osteoporosis is
   a. Vertebra
   b. Neck of femur
   c. Radius
   d. Shaft of femur

40. Risk factors for osteoporosis (PGI type)
   a. Late menopause
   b. COPD
   c. Obesity
   d. Smoking
   e. OCPs

41. Drug of choice for senile osteoporosis is
   a. Estrogens
   b. DEXA scan
   c. Calcitonin
   d. Etidronate

42. Treatment of choice for postmenopausal osteoporosis
   a. Calcitonin
   b. Alendronate
   c. Progesterone
   d. Tamoxifen

43. Least useful anti-rachitic
   a. 1,25-hydroxycholecalciferol
   b. Cholecalciferol
   c. 25-hydroxycholecalciferol
   d. Calcium

44. Vitamin D deficiency rickets is confirmed by demonstration of
   a. Epiphyseal changes in X-ray
   b. Hypocalcemia and hypophosphatemia
   c. Raised serum alkaline phosphatase
   d. Healing with physiologic doses of vitamin D3

45. Drug of choice for bisphosphonate resistant osteoporosis
   a. Teriparatide
   b. Denosumab
   c. Anakinra
   d. Calcitonin

46. Drug not used in Paget's disease of bone
   a. Plicamycin
   b. Bisphosphonates
   c. Sodium EDTA
   d. Calcitonin

47. Which of the following drugs used in osteoporosis treatment has both antiresorptive and bone formative properties?
   a. Strontium ranelate
   b. Allendronate
   c. Calcitonin
   d. Teriperatide

ARTHRITIS AND RELATED DISORDERS

1. In articular cartilage, greatest density of active chondrocytes is seen in
   a. Zone 1
   b. Zone 2
   c. Zone 3
   d. Zone 4

2. Synovial fluid of low viscosity is seen in all except
   a. Gout
   b. Osteoarthritis
   c. Septic arthritis
   d. Rheumatoid arthritis (RA)

3. What is the polymorph percentage in tubercular arthritis knee?
   a. 20%
   b. 40%
   c. 60%
   d. 90%

4. All of the following are properties of synovial fluid except
   a. It is a pale yellow, clear and sufficiently viscous fluid that droplets expelled from a needle tip fall in a long string
   b. Normally it does not contain any crystals
   c. It does not clot since it lacks in fibrinogen
   d. Normal WBC count in synovial fluid is 350–3500/mm³

5. Bouchards nodes are present over
   a. DIP
   b. PIP
   c. MCP
   d. Wrist

6. A female presents with swelling over the base of thumb and tenderness and 1st CMC joint. What is the probable diagnosis?
   a. DeQuervain's disease
   b. Osteoarthritis
   c. Rheumatoid arthritis
   d. Ankylosing spondylitis

7. Earliest radiological sign in ankylosing spondylitis (AS)
   a. Squaring of lumbar vertebrae
   b. Widening and haziness around SI joints
   c. Bamboo spine
   d. Narrowing and sclerosis around the SI joints

8. Plantar calcaneal spur is not seen in (PGI type)
   a. Reiters syndrome
   b. Scleroderma
   c. RA
   d. Psoriatic arthropathy (PsA)
   e. AS

9. Most common cause of AVN hip is
   a. Steroids
   b. Alcohol
   c. Idiopathic
   d. Sickle cell disease

10. All of the following are done in osteoarthritis of knee except
   a. Arthroscopy
   b. Osteoclasis
   c. Arthroplasty
   d. Osteotomy

11. Osteochondritis dissecans involves
   a. Medial part of lateral femoral condyle
   b. Lateral part of medial femoral condyle
   c. Inferior pole of patella
   d. Tibial tuberosity

12. A 40-year-old man presents with acute onset pain left great toe. On investigation, punched out lesions with overhanging margins are seen on phalanx and adjacent soft tissue. Most likely diagnosis is
   a. Rheumatoid arthritis (RA)
   b. Gout
   c. Reiter's ds
   d. Psoriatic arthropathy (PsA)

13. Chondrocalcinosis is seen in
   a. Rickets
   b. Ochronosis (Alkaptonuria)
   c. Hypoparathyroidism
   d. Hypervitaminosis

14. Most common joint involved joint in pseudogout
   a. Knee
   b. Hip
   c. Elbow
   d. Great toe

15. Multiple loose bodies are seen most commonly in
   a. Synovial chondromatosis
   b. Osteochondritis dissecans
   c. Osteoarthritis
   d. Osteochondral fracture
   e. RA

16. The most common cause of loose bodies in the knee joint
   a. Osteochondral fracture
   b. Osteoarthritis
   c. Synovial chondromatosis
   d. Osteochondritis dissecans

17. Joint not involved in osteoarthritis
   a. PIP
   b. DIP
   c. MCP
   d. Knee

18. PIP, DIP and 1st carpometacarpal joint involvement and sparing of wrist and MCP joints is a characteristic feature of
   a. Psoriatic arthropathy
   b. RA
   c. Pseudogout
   d. Osteoarthritis

19. A 35-year-old male develops involvement of PIP, DIP and MCP with sparing of wrist and carpometacarpal joints. Probable diagnosis is
   a. RA
   b. Psoriatic arthropathy
   c. Osteoarthritis
   d. Pseudogout

20. A middle aged female of RA on treatment develops upper motor neuron signs in her limbs. The investigation required to evaluate her further is
   a. Open mouth view
   b. Swimmers view
   c. Brodens view
   d. Cervical spine flexion and extension lateral views

21. Earliest radiological sign in RA
   a. Decreased joint space
   b. Periarticular osteopenia
   c. Articular erosion
   d. Subchondral cyst

22. Joint mostly spared in RA is
   a. Wrist
   b. MCP
   c. PIP
   d. DIP

23. Which is the most pathognomic feature of RA?
   a. Rheumatoid factor
   b. Morning stiffness
   c. Ulnar drift of fingers
   d. Rheumatoid nodules

24. Swan neck deformity refers to
   a. Flexion at PIP and extension at DIP
   b. Flexion at MCP and extension at interphalangeal joint

c. Extension at PIP and flexion at DIP
d. Extension at MCP and flexion at interphalangeal joint
25. Wind swept deformity is seen in
 a. Scurvy
 b. RA
 c. Rickets
 d. Ankylosing spondylitis
26. Most common cause of reactive arthritis
 a. *S. aureus*
 b. *S. flexneri*
 c. *N. gonorrhoeae*
 d. *E. coli*
27. A 65-year-old man has history of back pain since 3 months. His ESR is raised. He also has dorsolumbar tenderness on examination and mild restriction of chest movements. On X-ray, syndesmophytes are present in vertebrae. Diagnosis is
 a. Degenerative osteoarthritis of spine
 b. Ankylosing spondylitis
 c. Ankylosing hyperostosis
 d. Lumbar canal stenosis
28. Pencil in cup deformity is seen in
 a. AVN
 b. RA
 c. Ankylosing spondylitis
 d. Psoriatic arthritis
29. Most common muscle for pseudotumor like growth in hemophilic arthropathy
 a. Quadriceps femoris
 b. Gastrocnemius
 c. Hamstring muscle
 d. Iliopsoas
30. Most common cause for neuropathic joints
 a. Leprosy
 b. Diabetes
 c. Tabes dorsalis
 d. Nerve injury
31. Clutton joints are feature of
 a. Congenital syphilis
 b. Primary syphilis
 c. Secondary syphilis
 d. Tertiary syphilis
32. Sausage digits are seen in
 a. Psoriatic arthritis
 b. Osteoarthritis
 c. Lyme arthritis
 d. None
33. A 60-year-old man with diabetes mellitus presents with painless, swollen right ankle joint. Radiographs of the ankle show destroyed joint with large number of loose bodies. Most probable diagnosis is?
 a. Osteoarthritis
 b. Charcot's joint
 c. Clutton's joint
 d. RA
34. In a patient suffering from tabes dorsalis, charcot's joints most commonly occurs at
 a. Knee
 b. Elbow
 c. Wrist
 d. Tarsometatarsal joint
35. Which of the following joint is least affected by neuropathy
 a. Hip
 b. Shoulder
 c. Wrist
 d. Elbow
36. Tophi in gout do not involve
 a. Muscle
 b. Cartilage
 c. Bursa
 d. Skin
37. In a patient of gouty arthritis, best investigation is
 a. Uric acid in urine
 b. Serum uric acid
 c. Detection of urate crystal in synovial fluid
 d. Serum calcium level
38. Calcification of menisci is seen in
 a. Renal osteodystrophy
 b. Hyperparathyroidism
 c. Pseudogout
 d. Acromegaly
39. A lady presents with right knee swelling, aspiration was done in which calcium pyrophosphate crystals were obtained. Next best investigation would be
 a. RF
 b. CPK
 c. ANA
 d. TSH
40. X-ray of a young man shows heterotopic calcification around bilateral knee joints. Next investigation is
 a. Serum phosphate
 b. Serum PTH
 c. Serum calcium
 d. Serum alkaline phosphatase

41. Deforming polyarthritis is associated with all of the following except
 a. Psoriatic arthritis
 b. RA
 c. Behçet's syndrome
 d. Ankylosing spondylitis
42. Erosion of the bone is seen in all except
 a. Gout
 b. Psoriasis
 c. SLE
 d. RA
43. A 85-year-old woman presented with bilateral osteoarthritis of knees with no history of any previous GI disease. The first line treatment drug for her should be
 a. Paracetamol
 b. Naproxen
 c. Celecoxib
 d. Dihydrocodeine
44. A 68-year-old man came with pain and swelling of right knee. Ahlback grade 2 osteoarthritis changes were noted on X-ray. What should be the further management?
 a. Conservative
 b. Arthroscopic washout
 c. High tibial osteotomy
 d. Total knee replacement
45. A patient of nephrotic syndrome taking steroids for 6 years presented with a limp. He had limitation of abduction and internal rotation. He most probably had
 a. Renal osteodystrophy
 b. Avascular necrosis of hip
 c. Septic arthritis
 d. Osteomyelitis of hip joint
46. Which of the following in not a variety of osteochondritis
 a. Pellegrini stieda
 b. Panner's
 c. Calve's
 d. Kohler's
47. Iselin's disease is osteochondritis of
 a. 2nd metacarpal
 b. 5th metacarpal
 c. 2nd metatarsal
 d. 5th metatarsal
48. Least common site to be involved in osteoarthritis amongst the following is
 a. Hip joint
 b. Knee joint
 c. Carpometacarpal joint of thumb
 d. Metacarpophalangeal joint
49. The most common site of primary osteoarthritis is
 a. Hip joint
 b. Knee joint
 c. Ankle joint
 d. Shoulder joint
50. Earliest radiological sign of the osteoarthritis is
 a. Narrowing of joint space
 b. osteophyte formation
 c. Cystic lesion in cancellous bone
 d. Sclerosis in subchondral bone
51. The most common arthritis that affects the wrist is
 a. Osteoarthritis
 b. Tuberculous arthritis
 c. Rheumatoid arthritis
 d. Gout
52. Boutonniere's deformity occurs due to
 a. Flexion at proximal interphalangeal joint
 b. Flexion at distal interphalangeal joint
 c. Extension at distal interphalangeal joint
 d. Extension at metacarpophalangeal joint
53. The type of anemia seen in rheumatoid arthritis is
 a. Microcytic hypochromic anemia
 b. Macrocytic hypochromic anemia
 c. Normocytic hypochromic anemia
 d. Normocytic normochromic anemia
54. Which of the following is an indication for systemic steroids in rheumatoid arthritis
 a. Mononeuritis multiplex
 b. Carpal tunnel syndrome
 c. Presence of deformities
 d. Articular cartilage involvement
55. Disease where distal interphalangeal joint is characteristically involved
 a. Psoriatic arthritis
 b. Rheumatoid
 c. SLE
 d. Gout

56. Which of the following joint is least involved in ankylosing spondylitis
    - a. Knee and ankle
    - b. Sacroiliac joint
    - c. Wrist and elbow
    - d. Spine
57. The earliest diagnosis of ankylosing spondylitis can be made on
    - a. MRI STIR sequence
    - b. Bone scan
    - c. CT scan
    - d. X-ray
58. All are features of hemophilic knee joint, except:
    - a. Juxta-articular osteosclerosis
    - b. Subchondral cyst formation
    - c. Widening of intercondylar notch
    - d. Squaring of patella
59. Arthroscopy is contraindicated in
    - a. Chronic joint disease
    - b. Loose bodies
    - c. Hemophilia
    - d. Meniscal tear
60. Painless effusions in joints in congenital syphilis are called as
    - a. Clutton's joint
    - b. Higouménakis sign
    - c. Barton's joint
    - d. Chronic osteomyelitis
61. Most common joint involved in gout
    - a. Knee
    - b. Hip
    - c. MTP joint of the big toe
    - d. MP joint of thumb
62. The most commonly involved joint in pseudo-gout
    - a. Knee
    - b. Great toe
    - c. Hip
    - d. Elbow
63. Heterotropic calcification is seen in (PGI type)
    - a. Ankylosing spondylitis
    - b. Gouty arthritis
    - c. Forestier's disease
    - d. Traumatic paraplegia
64. Snowstorm appearance of knee joint on arthroscopy is seen in
    - a. Ewing's sarcoma of knee joint
    - b. Synovial chondromatosis
    - c. Fracture involving articular surface
    - d. Chondromalacia patellae
65. Osgood Schlatters disease involves
    - a. Medial malleolus
    - b. Lateral malleolus
    - c. Femoral condyle
    - d. Tibial tuberosity
66. Arthritis mutilans is seen in
    - a. SLE
    - b. Psoriatic arthropathy
    - c. Osteoarthritis
    - d. Gout
67. Which arthritis causes no periosteal reaction?
    - a. Psoriatic arthritis
    - b. Reactive arthritis
    - c. Neuropathic arthritis
    - d. Rheumatoid arthritis
68. Investigation of choice for avascular necrosis of bone is
    - a. Bone scan
    - b. CT scan
    - c. MRI
    - d. USG
69. Avascular necrosis affects which part of femoral head?
    - a. Anteromedial
    - b. Anterolateral
    - c. Posteromedial
    - d. Posterolateral
70. A 30-year-old HIV positive male who is on antiretroviral therapy (protease inhibitor) has pain in the right hip joint since 2 months. He has difficulty in abduction and internal rotation. Most likely diagnosis is
    - a. Septic arthritis
    - b. Tubercular arthritis
    - c. AVN
    - d. Osteoarthritis
71. Rheumatoid factor is
    - a. IgG against IgM
    - b. IgM against IgG
    - c. IgA against IgE
    - d. Anti-IgE auto-antibody
72. HLAs that are specific for RA (PGI type)
    - a. HLA DR-1
    - b. HLA-DR-2
    - c. HLA-DR-3
    - d. HLA-DR-4
73. True statements about RA are (PGI type)
    - a. Associated with HLA DR4
    - b. Limited to articular cartilage
    - c. More common in females
    - d. Extra-articular manifestations are there in 20% patients
    - e. Hand, elbow and knee joints are commonly involved
74. A 45-year-old coal mine worker presents with cutaneous nodules, joint pains and occasional cough with dyspnea. His chest radiographs show multiple, small nodules in bilateral lung fields. Some of the nodules show cavitation and specks of calcification. Most likely diagnosis is
    - a. Caplan's syndrome
    - b. Sjögren's syndrome
    - c. Silicosis
    - d. Wegener's granulomatosis
75. True regarding Felty's syndrome are all except
    - a. Splenomegaly
    - b. Neutropenia
    - c. RA
    - d. Nephropathy
76. All of the following are DMARDS except
    - a. Chloroquine
    - b. Penicillamine
    - c. Gold
    - d. BAL
77. Most common cause of mononeuritis multiplex in India is
    - a. Hansen's ds
    - b. Tuberculosis
    - c. RA
    - d. PAN
78. All of the following are observed in gout except
    - a. Uric acid nephrolithiasis
    - b. Deficiency of xanthine oxidase
    - c. Increase in serum urate concentration
    - d. Renal tissue involving interstitial tissue
79. NSAID of choice in seronegative spondyloarthritis is
    - a. Phenylbutazone
    - b. Indomethacin
    - c. Aspirin
    - d. Corticosteroid
80. A young man back from leisure trip has swollen knee joints and foreign body sensations in eyes. Likely cause is
    - a. Behçet's disease
    - b. Reiter's disease
    - c. Sarcoidosis
    - d. SLE
81. Most common pattern of cardiac involvement in RA is
    - a. Pancarditis
    - b. Myocarditis
    - c. Pericarditis
    - d. Endocarditis
82. Etanercept used in RA acts by blocking
    - a. TNF-α
    - b. TGF-β
    - c. IL-2
    - d. IL -6
83. Which of the following is least likely to occur in late extra- articular seropositive rheumatoid arthritis?
    - a. Neutropenia
    - b. Leg ulcers
    - c. Dry eyes
    - d. Hepatitis
84. Which of the following is not a presentation of calcium pyrophosphate deposition disease (CPPD)?
    - a. Pseudogout
    - b. Pseudoankylosing spondylitis
    - c. Apical plate excrescences (APE)
    - d. Chondrocalcinosis
85. Which of the following is true about HIV related arthritis
    - a. Cutaneous and mucosal lesions are rare
    - b. Enthesopathy is common
    - c. Associated with HLA B 27
    - d. Hip is the most common joint involved

SOFT TISSUE DISORDERS

1. Infrapatellar bursitis is also called as
    - a. Housemaid's knee
    - b. Clergyman's knee
    - c. Tailor's knee
    - d. Tuberculous knee
2. Clergyman's knee is inflammation of
    - a. Superficial later of infrapatellar bursa
    - b. Deep layer of infrapatellar bursa
    - c. Superficial layer of prepatellar bursa
    - d. Deep layer of prepatellar bursa
3. A 60-year-old diabetic has restricted motion at right shoulder in all directions in both active and passive range. An X-ray was done but did not reveal anything. What is the best management at this stage?
    - a. Physiotherapy
    - b. MRI for evaluation
    - c. Arthroscopy for evaluation
    - d. Mantoux test
4. Movie sign/Cinema sign is seen in
    - a. Chondromalacia patella
    - b. Osteochondritis dissecans

c. Arthrogryposis multiplex congenita

d. Infantile tibia vara

5. Simmonds test helps in diagnosis in rupture of which tendon?

a. Extensor pollicis longus
b. Gastrosoleus
c. Biceps
d. Iliopsoas

6. The most common cause for neuralgic pain in foot is

a. Injury to deltoid ligament
b. Compression of communication between medial and lateral plantar nerves
c. Exaggeration of longitudinal arches
d. Shortening of plantar aponeurosis

7. Bunion is commonly seen at

a. Great toe MTP joint
b. Medial malleolus
c. Lateral malleolus
d. Shin of tibia

8. A 40-year-old man was repairing his wooden shed in the morning. By afternoon, he felt that the hammer was becoming heavier and heavier. He felt pain on the lateral side of the elbow and also found that squeezing water out of sponge hurt his elbow. Which muscles are most likely involved?

a. Flexor digitorum superficialis
b. Extensor carpi radialis brevis
c. Biceps brachii and supinator
d. Triceps brachii and anconeus

9. Which of the following is a risk factor for developing Dupuytren's contracture?

a. Eptoin
b. Diabetes
c. Alcohol
d. All of the above

10. A 50 years old diabetic patient, presented with 15° flexion deformity of the little finger. Most appropriate management at this stage is?

a. Wait and watch
b. Subtotal fasciectomy
c. Total fasciectomy
d. Percutaneous fasciotomy

11. Trigger finger occurs in?

a. RA
b. Trauma
c. Osteosarcoma
d. Osteoarthritis

12. In trigger finger, constriction in the tendon sheath is most commonly present at the level of

a. Middle phalanx
b. PIP joint
c. Proximal phalanx
d. MCP joint

13. Constriction in trigger finger is present around which pulley?

a. A1
b. A2
c. A3
d. A4

14. A teen-aged girl complains of anterior knee pain on climbing stairs and on getting up after prolonged sitting. Which of the following is the most likely diagnosis?

a. Chondromalacia patellae
b. Plica syndrome
c. Bipartite patella
d. Patellofemoral osteoarthritis

15. Muscle most commonly affected by congenital absence is

a. Pectoralis major
b. Semimembranosus
c. Teres minor
d. Gluteus maximus

16. Finkelstein test is used for the diagnosis of?

a. Thoracic outlet syndrome
b. De Quervain disease
c. Dupuytren's contracture
d. Carpal tunnel syndrome

17. Haglund deformity involves which area?

a. Wrist
b. Ankle
c. Spine
d. Knee

18. Rupture of EPL tendon occurs in all except

a. RA
b. Colles fracture
c. Drummer boy's palsy
d. De Quervain disease

AMPUTATIONS, PROSTHOTICS AND ORTHOTICS

1. Which of the following is the ideal length of bone for a below knee stump

a. 12.5 cm–17.5 cm
b. Less than 5 cm long
c. 7.5 cm–10 cm long
d. 20 cm long

2. Procedure contraindicated in diabetics?

a. Ray amputation
b. Forefoot amputation
c. Syme's amputation
d. Below knee amputation

3. Best treatment modality for postamputation neuroma is?

a. Compression bandage
b. Ultrasound
c. Infrared
d. Interferential therapy

4. Pain due to post-amputation neuroma is best treated by:

a. Infrared therapy
b. Interference therapy
c. Ultrasound therapy
d. Surgical excision

5. Pain due to post-amputation neuroma can be managed by all except

a. Infrared therapy
b. Interference therapy
c. Ultrasound therapy
d. Stump bandaging

6. An amputation through fore arm where you make a fork of the two fore arm bones is is k/a

a. Chopart's amputation
b. Krukenberg amputation
c. Pirogoff amputation
d. Syme's amputation

7. Energy consumption in an above knee amputation is approximately

a. 20%
b. 40%
c. 55%
d. 65%

8. Regarding SACH foot, all are true except?

a. Solid ankle cushion heel
b. Prosthesis
c. Squatting is easy
d. Does not look like a normal foot

9. In flap method of amputation which structure is kept shorter that the level of amputation

a. Bone
b. Muscles
c. Nerves
d. Skin
e. Vessels

10. Myodesis is employed in amputations for all of the following indications except

a. Trauma
b. Tumor
c. Children
d. Ischemia

ORTHOPEDIC SURGERIES, EVOLUTION AND LATEST TRENDS

1. Which of the following is an absolute contraindication for total joint replacement?

a. Very young patients
b. Recent or current joint sepsis
c. Osteoporotic bone
d. Limb length inequality

2. After knee replacement surgery, proprioceptors of joints are altered. Effect is

a. Loss of sensation at joint in dynamic stage
b. Complete loss of sensation at joint in resting stage
c. Normal movement
d. All sensations lost

3. Most common cause of death after total hip replacement is

a. Infection
b. Pulmonary embolism
c. Deep vein thrombosis
d. Pneumonia

4. Aseptic loosening in cemented total hip replacement, occurs as a result of hypersensitivity response to

a. High density polythene debris
b. Titanium debris
c. N,N-dimethyltryptamine
d. Free radicals

5. Metal on metal articulation should be avoided in

a. Osteonecrosis
b. Young female
c. Inflammatory arthritis
d. Revision surgery

6. Tourniquet paralysis is an unfortunate complication that often leads to

a. Neuropraxia
b. Axonotmesis
c. Neurotmesis
d. None of the above

7. Bone cement setting time is

a. 30 sec
b. 1–2 min
c. 8–10 min
d. >30 min

8. Structures difficult to see with anterolateral arthroscopy of knee are all except
    a. Posterior cruciate ligament
    b. Anterior portion of lateral meniscus
    c. Patella-femoral articulation
    d. Posterior horn of medial meniscus
9. Watson jones procedure is done for?
    a. Polio
    b. Neglected clubfoot
    c. Chronic ankle instability
    d. Muscle paralysis
10. Watson Jones approach is used for?
    a. Neglected club foot
    b. Muscle paralysis
    c. Valgus deformity
    d. Hip replacement
11. All of the following are used for giving traction except?
    a. Bohler's stirrup
    b. Steinmann's pin
    c. K-wire
    d. Rush pin
12. Action of intramedullary 'k' nail is?
    a. Compression
    b. 2 point fixation
    c. 3 point fixation
    d. Weight concentration
13. Which of the following approaches is best suited for performing triple arthodesis at the ankle?
    a. Ollier's approach
    b. Gatellier and chastang's approach
    c. Posterior approach to the ankle
    d. Colonna's approach
14. In anterolateral approach for hip surgery after retracting tensor fascia lata which structure comes before reaching to hip?
    a. Gluteus Maximus
    b. Gluteus Minimus
    c. Gluteus Medius
    d. Gemellus
15. All indicate that the intramedullary Kuntscher nail is properly seated except
    a. Slot facing posteromedially
    b. The distal end at about the level of the superior end of patella
    c. Eye faces posteromedially
    d. The proximal end about 2.5 cm proximal to the trochanter
16. Kocher-Langenbeck approach is useful in acetabular fracture in all mentioned situations except
    a. Open fractures of acetabulum
    b. Sciatic nerve injury
    c. Recurrent dislocation despite of closed reduction
    d. Morel Lavallee lesion
17. Cobra plate is used for
    a. For three part proximal humeral fracture fixation
    b. For hip arthrodesis
    c. For distal femoral fracture
    d. For unstable intertrochanteric fracture fixation

PICTURE QUIZ

1. Nerve most commonly injured in the dislocation shown below is

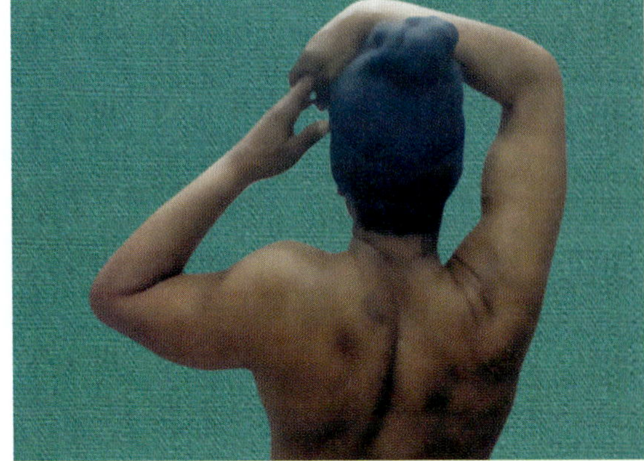

    a. Axillary nerve
    b. Ulnar nerve
    c. Median nerve
    d. Radial nerve

2. What surgery would you offer to treat the shown deformity?

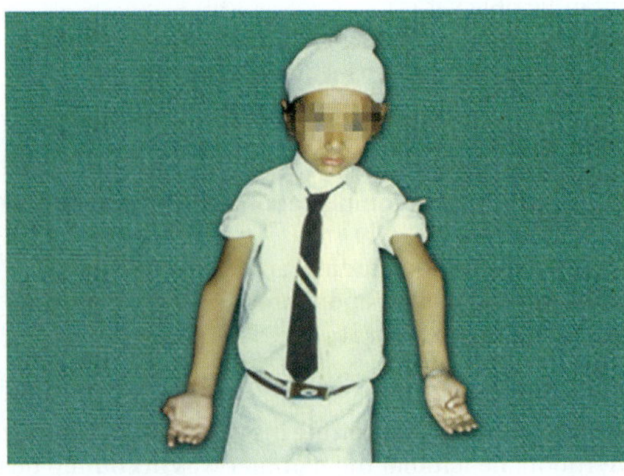

    a. Milch osteotomy
    b. Pauwel osteotomy
    c. French osteotomy
    d. McMurray osteotomy
3. Name the angle drawn in the figure

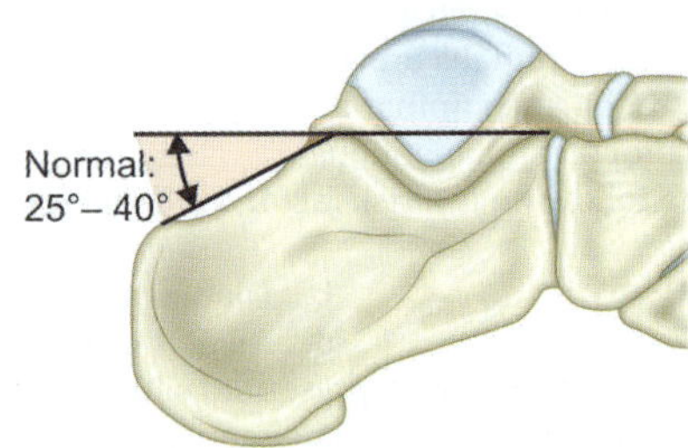

    a. Gissane's angle
    b. Neutral angle
    c. Bohler's angle
    d. Kite's angle
4. This X-ray picture of osteosarcoma is the result of

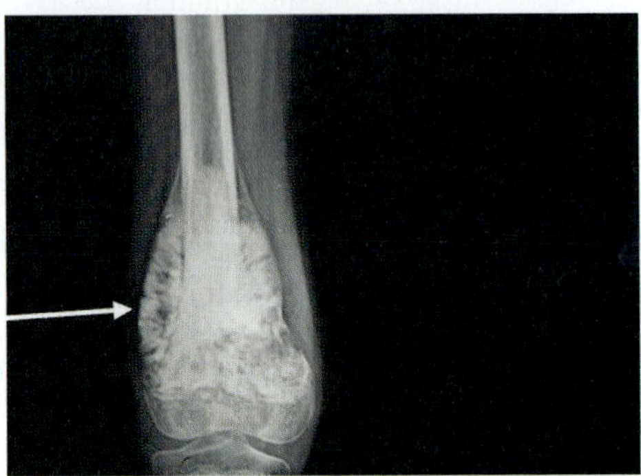

    a. Periosteal reaction
    b. Calcification along blood vessels
    c. Callus due to pathological fracture
    d. None of these
5. The X-ray below shows a patient with scoliosis. What is the angle to measure the severity of curve called as?

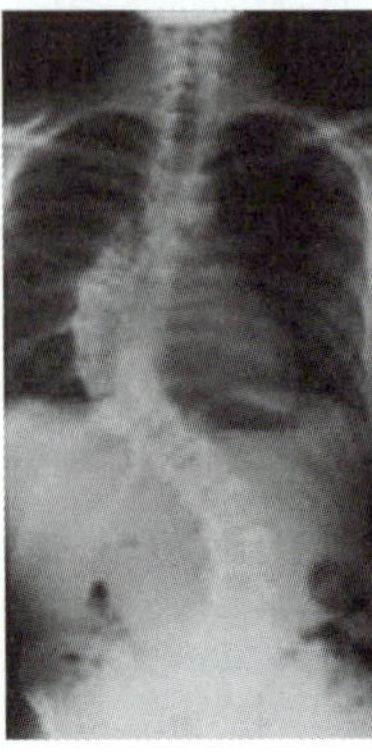
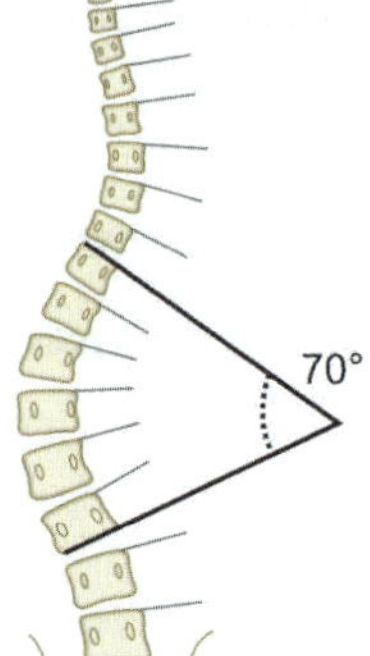

a. Reisser's angle
b. Boston's angle
c. Cobb's angle
d. Milwaukee's angle

6. Identify this X-ray sign of TB hip

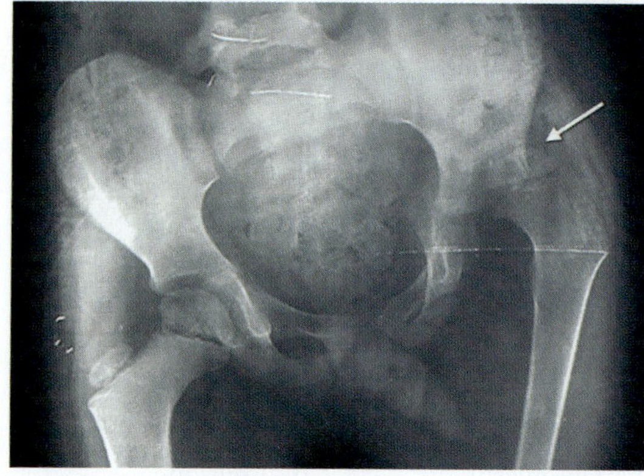

a. Wandering acetabulum
b. Pestle and mortar appearance
c. Babcock's sign
d. Ward's sign

7. Shown in the figure below is a bone cyst. The arrow in the figure is indicating

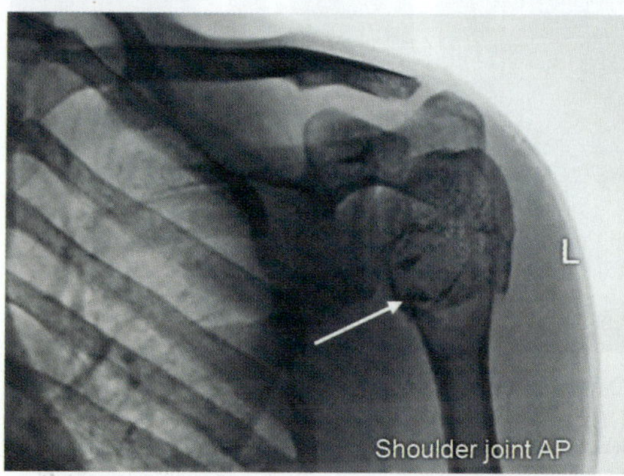

a. Fallen fragment
b. Ground glass appearance
c. Shepherd Crook fragment
d. Thurston Holland fragment

8. Figure below shows the treatment of a 3-month-child who had congenital dislocation of hip (CDH). What is the apparatus in use called as?

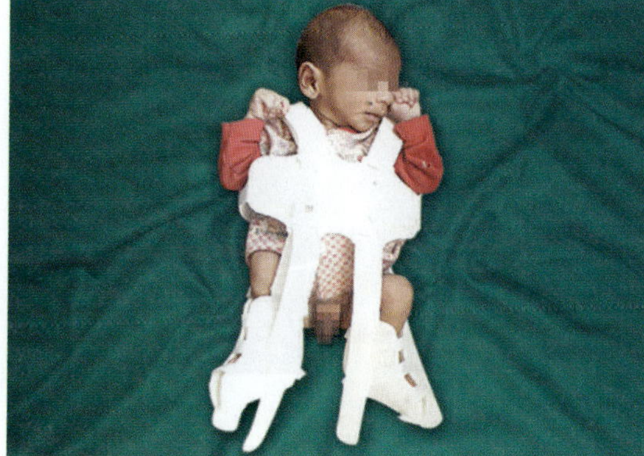

a. Von Rosen splint
b. Pavlik harness
c. Petrie's orthosis
d. Boston brace

9. What is this mode of treatment called as?

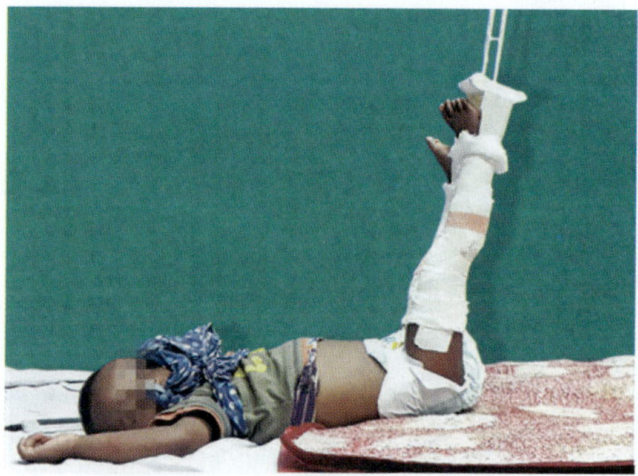

a. Russell's traction
b. 90–90 traction
c. Buck's traction
d. Gallows traction

10. What is the probable diagnosis?

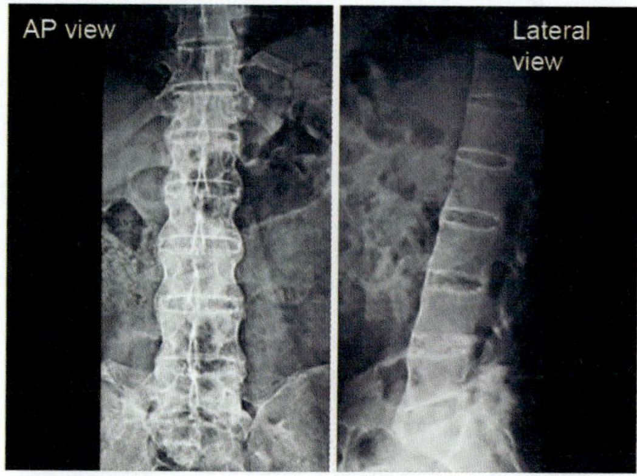

a. Ankylosing spondylitis
b. Diffuse idiopathic skeletal hyperostosis (DISH)
c. OA spine
d. Osteopetrosis

11. The child in this figure probably has

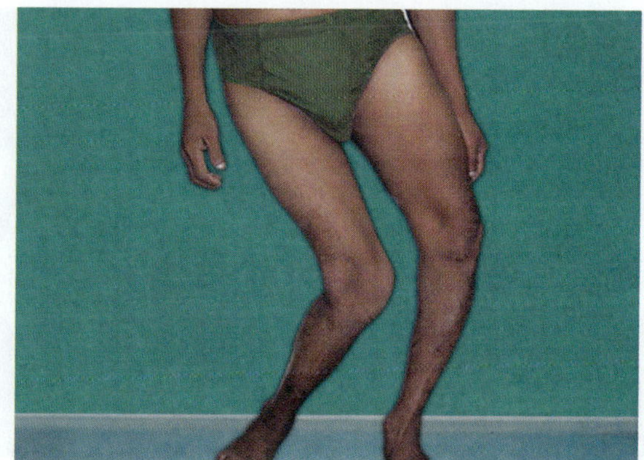

a. Juvenile chronic arthritis
b. Pseudoarthrosis of tibia
c. Hyperparathyroidism
d. Rickets

12. Identify the disease from the X-ray

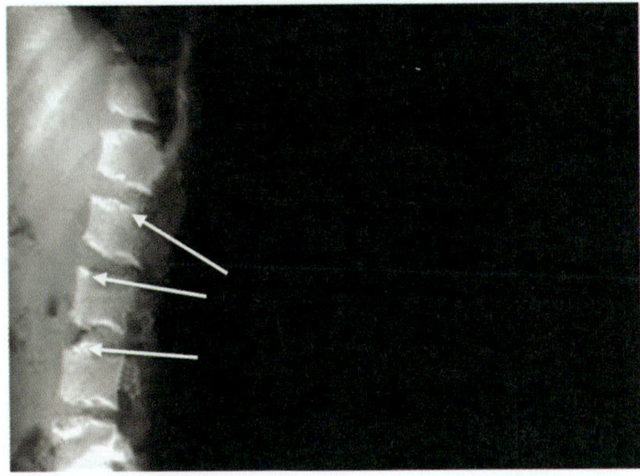

  a. Keinböck's disease
  b. Freiberg's disease
  c. Scheuermann's disease
  d. Severe disease

13. What is this child being treated for?

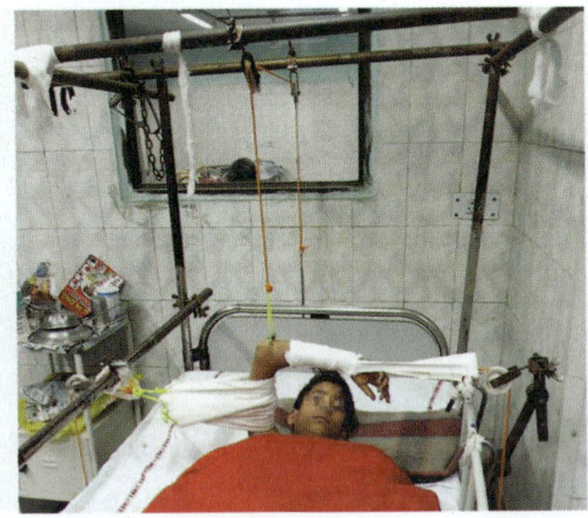

  a. Elbow flexion deformity
  b. Supracondylar humerus fracture
  c. Shaft humerus fracture
  d. Unreducible elbow dislocation

14. The line marked in the figure is

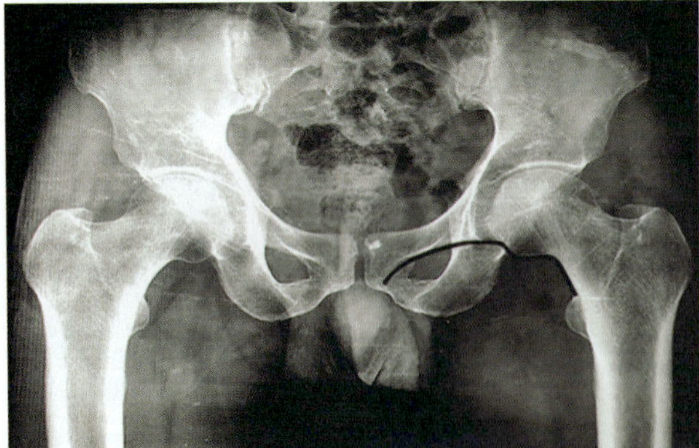

  a. Shenton's line
  b. Shoemaker's line
  c. Nelaton's line
  d. Chinese line

15. A CT cross-section of a patient is shown in the figure below. Which of the following is not a routine treatment option for this lesion?

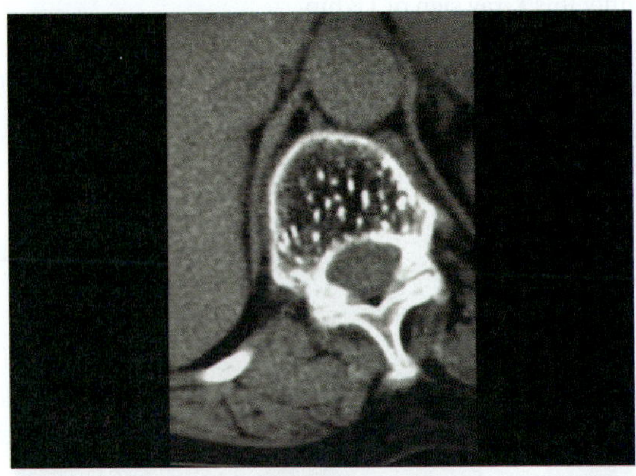

  a. Vertebroplasty   b. Excision
  c. Embolization   d. Radiotherapy

16. Identify the tumor in the X-ray

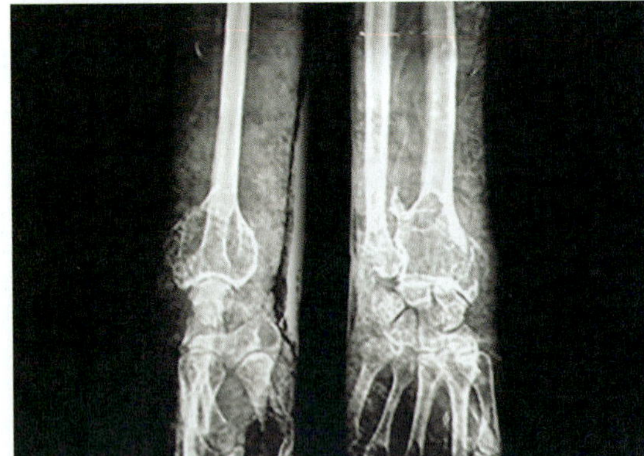

  a. Osteosarcoma
  b. GCT
  c. ABC
  d. Ewing's sarcoma

17. The shape of the femur as shown below may be seen in all of the following conditions except

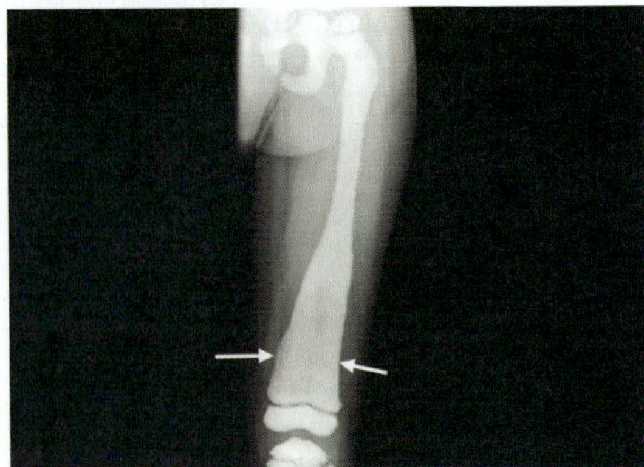

  a. Achondroplasia
  b. Osteopetrosis
  c. Pyle's disease
  d. Langerhan cell histiocytosis

18. What would be the diagnosis if the clinical test depicted in the figure is positive?

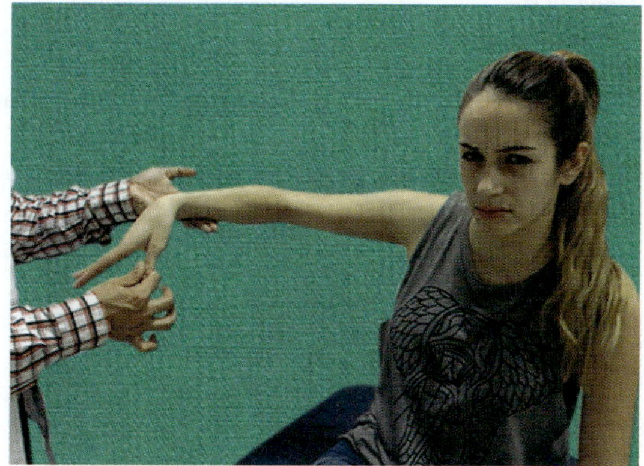

a. Trigger thumb   b. Intersection syndrome
c. De Quervain's disease   d. Tennis elbow

19. Which muscle is being tested by the examiner in the figure?

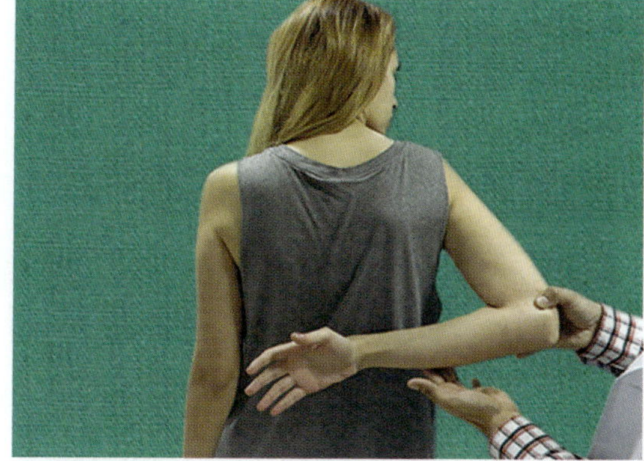

a. Supraspinatus
b. Infraspinatus
c. Teres minor
d. Subscapularis

20. This deformity of the proximal femur could be a result of all of the following conditions except

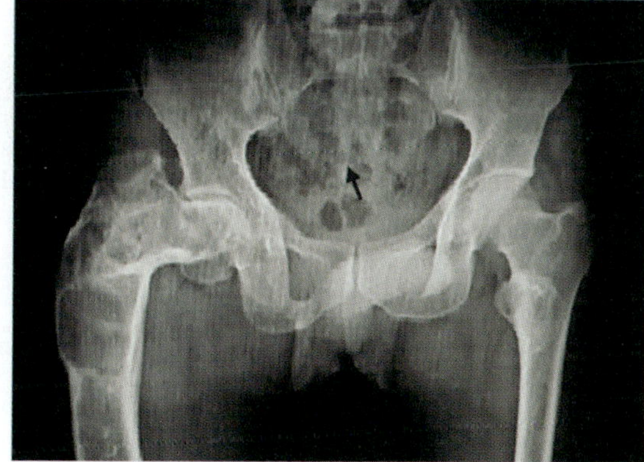

a. Fibrous dysplasia
b. Multiple myeloma
c. Paget's disease
d. Osteogenesis imperfecta

21. Based on Bado classification, the Monteggia fracture shown below will be classified into

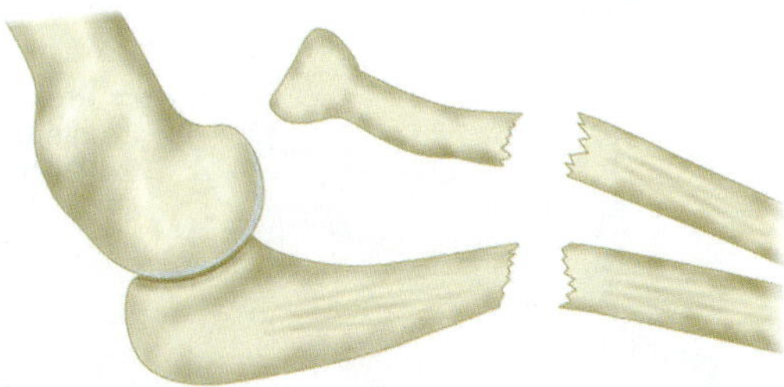

a. Type III
b. Type I
c. Type IV
d. Type II

22. Shown below is X-ray of a 45 years old male who sustained injury 4 weeks back. What would be the best treatment option for this patient?

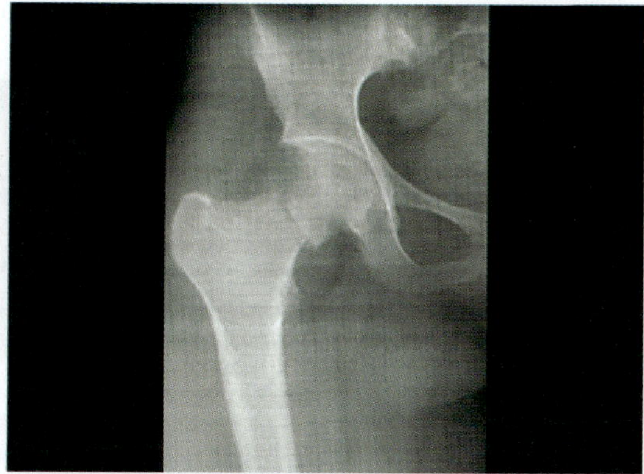

a. McMurray's osteotomy
b. Hemiarthroplasty
c. THR
d. Fixation with cannulated cancellous screws

23. If a hand X-ray of a patient has an appearance as shown below, all of the following can be differentials except

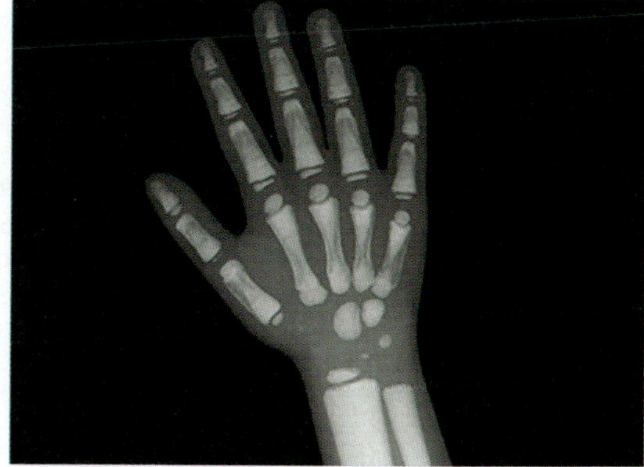

a. Marble bone disease
b. Sickle cell disease
c. Masada syndrome
d. Paget's disease

24. The deformity of the toe shown below is

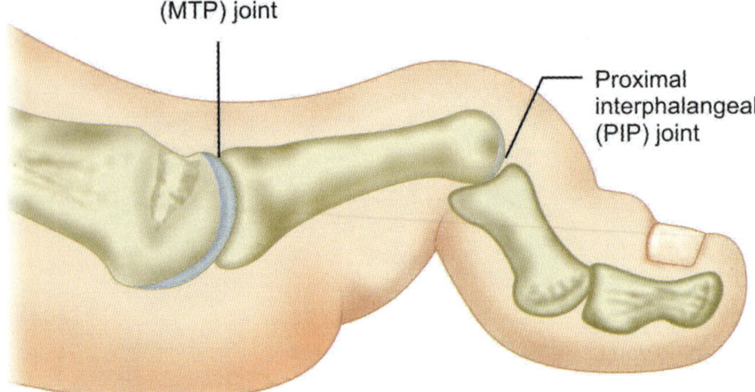

a. Claw toe
b. Hammer toe
c. Mallet toe
d. Hallux valgus

25. Shown below is an X-ray of a patient with SCFE. The radiological sign shown is called as

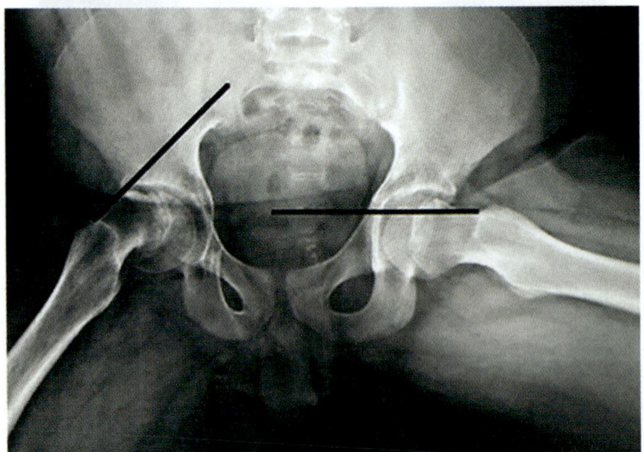

a. Metaphyseal blanch sign
b. Sagging rope sign
c. Gage sign
d. Trethowan sign

26. Procedure shown in the picture is

a. TKR
b. Unicondylar knee replacement
c. Knee resurfacing
d. None of the above

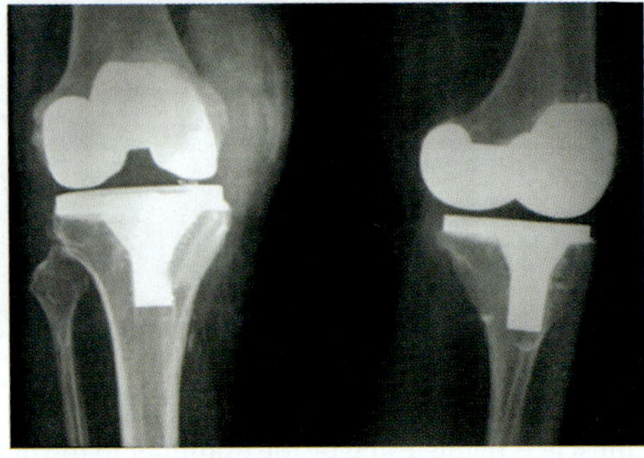

27. What is the diagnosis?

a. Congenital pseudoarthrosis of tibia
b. Fibular hemimelia
c. Tibial hemimelia
d. Ewing sarcoma

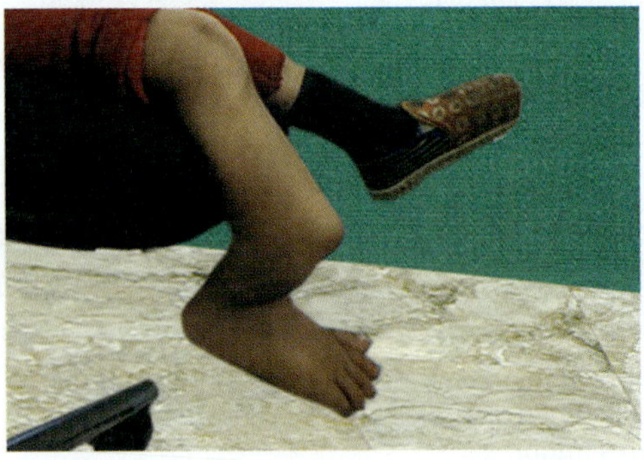

ANSWERS KEY

GENERAL ORTHOPEDICS

1. b (P-9, Col-1)
2. d (P-11, Col-1, High-yield points)
3. c (P-19, Col-2, High-yield points)
4. a (P-16, Col-1)
5. b (P-19 Col-2, High-yield points)
6. a (P-16, Col-2); Healing is generally normal in osteoporotic patients. The problem is with fixation of an osteoporotic bone that leads to increased non-union rates
7. b (P-15, Box 2.4)
8. b (P-15, Box 2.4)
9. b (P-17, Col-1)
10. a (P-19, Col-1); The best site for taking a cancellous graft is posterior superior iliac spine
11. d > c (P-13). Low impact direct blow will produce transverse fracture and if impact is high it will produce comminuted fracture. If impact of direct force (high or low) is not given then pick comminuted fracture as right choice, as transverse fracture is also produced by bending force.
12. a (P-12, Col-2); Most consistent sign of a fracture is tenderness (pain is a symptom) while the most pathognomonic sign of a fracture is abnormal mobility > crepitus

13. c (P-35, Col-1)
14. A (P-36, Col-1)
15. b
16. b, d (P-37, Col-2, High-yield points)
17. b; (P-37, Col-2) Angulation remodels better than rotation and metaphysis being cancellous active vascular bone remodels best
18. b (P-12, Box 2.2)
19. b (P-37, Box 2.12)
20. d (P-35, Col-2)
21. d (P-20, Col-2)
22. None; Thomas splint can be used in all these conditions for a temporary stabilization
23. d (P-1, Col-1)
24. c (P-27, Col-1)
25. a, b, c, d, e. All procedures are used in different situations in management of intra-articular fractures
26. c
27. a
28. b (P-17, Box 2.6)
29. c (P-41, Table 2.14)
30. b (P-41, Col-2)
31. b (P-40, Col-1)

32. b (P-39, Col-2)
33. b (P-38, Col-2)
34. d (P-38, Box 2.3)
35. d (P-46, High-yield points)
36. d > c (P-46, High-yield points, P-334, Col-2)
37. c (P-334, Col-2)
38. a (P-20, High-yield points)
39. c
40. a (P-23, Table-2.7)
41. d (P-28, Col-1). Functional cast bracing is used in fractures of limbs.
42. d.; Loose ligaments are a cause of joint instability.
43. b

POLYTRAUMA

1. b (P-58, Col-2)
2. a (P-109, Box 4.1)
3. b (P-108, Col-2)
4. d (P-53, Col-1)
5. d (P-57, Col-2)
6. c > d (P-57, Col-2)
7. b (P-57, Col-2)
8. d (P-58, Col-2)
9. c (P-109, Box 4.1)
10. b (P-53, Col-1); Airway maintenance > Pelvic fracture stabilization (immediately be a pelvic binder and earliest by external fixator)
11. b (P-56, High-yield points)
12. a (P-109, Col-1)
13. b (P-108, Col-2)
14. c; In an unconscious patient clinical examination can't be done reliably. X rays Combined with CT scan allows exclusion of cervical spine injury with >99% sensitivity in unconscious patients. There is little evidence that routine use of MRI is superior then CT scan in excluding cervical spine injury. In an unconscious patient immediate CT scan of brain is warranted to rule out head injury. Simultaneously cervical spine scan reliably rule out associated cervical spine injury.
Ref: Spinal immobilisation for unconscious patients with multiple injuries C G Morris et al. BMJ. 2004;329(7464): 495–9.

UPPER LIMB TRAUMATOLOGY

1. a (P-91, Col-2, Fig. 4.52)
2. d (P-63, Fig. 4.4a)
3. c (P-72, Col-1)
4. c (P-74, Fig. 4.2b) Velpeau bandage can be used in proximal humerus fractures, immobilizing after reducing dislocated shoulder and in acromioclavicular dislocation. The last is the most specific use.
5. d (P-75, Fig. 4.23a)
6. c (P-75, Col-1)
7. b (P-86, Col-2)
8. a (P-87, Col-1) Median nerve is commonly injured in simple elbow dislocation while Ulnar nerve is more commonly involved in complex elbow dislocation (elbow dislocation with an associated fracture);
9. a (P-87, Col-1)
10. a (P-86, Col-1); Physeal injuries are common during growth spurts as during this time the physis is relatively weaker; however elbow is an exception to the rule where physeal injuries are more common during first decade. The peak incidence of elbow dislocation is seen in adolescents and it is the commonest dislocation in children and adolescents. Supracondylar fractures of humerus occur between 3–10 years.
11. d (P-76, Col-2)
12. d (P-81, Col-1)

13. a (P-82, High-yield points)
14. b (P-80, Col-1)
15. b (P-82, Col-2) AIN > median > ulnar;
16. d (P-82, Col-1)
17. c (P-81, Col-2)
18. a (P-83, Col-2, High-yield points)
19. c (P-81,82)
20. c (P-23, Table-2.7)
21. d (P-79, Col-1)
22. c (P-85, Col-1); The patient has developed Tardy ulnar nerve palsy
23. a (P-80, Col-1)
24. c (P-80, Col-1)
25. b (P-75, Col-2); The question does not seem to be very authentic. However, authors feel that three point relationship involves olecranon process of ulna apart from the two distal epicondyles of humerus, it can be disturbed in fractures where ulna (olecranon) is involved. A weak posterior capsule may lead to posterior dislocation of elbow and thereby disturb the relationship
26. b (P-88, Col-2 High-yield points)
27. c (P-88, High-yield points)
28. c (P–89, Col-1)
29. a and c (P-88, Col-1)
30. d (P-32, Box 2.11)
31. c (P-90 High-yield points); Lateral condylar physis will be disrupted if the fragment is excised, hence excision is never an advised treatment in such patients
32. d (p-87, High-yield points)
33. b (P-94 , Col-2)
34. d. Radial impaction in Colles fracture causes positive ulnar variance.
35. d (P-99, High-yield Points); Most of the recent studies are reporting that radial length is the most important factor to be restored postsurgery and is the major determinant to functional recovery
36. d (P-97, Col-2); Term 'Causalgia' simply means burning pain. It is a symptom of Sudeck's osteodystrophy
37. b
38. d (P-99, Col-2)
39. b
40. a (P-101, High-yield points)
41. c (P-103, Col-2)
42. c (P-104, Fig. 4.69)
43. d (P-103, Col-1)
44. b (P-177, Col-1)
45. b (P-99, Fig. 4.69b)
46. c (P-107, Table 4.6)
47. b (P-84, Col-2); LCH fracture is a Salter-Harris type 4 injury. It often ends in non union that manifests as cubitus valgus deformity (followed later by tardy ulnar nerve palsy). However, most cases are surgically treated and commonest complication actually is pseudovarus due to bone spur formation on lateral condyle after surgery. So best ans to pick will be (b).
48. c > a; None of the choice is appropriate. The question has been framed inappropriately. BBFA in an adult is first given a try of CR and POP application and if CR fails ORIF with plates is opted. However, it is very difficult to reduce two bones at one time and hence most patients eventually need ORIF with plating. Still if to choose one option from the list, go with plates (C).

HIP EXAMINATION

1. c (P-119, Col-2)
2. b (P-124, Fig. 5.29)
3. a (P-121, Col-1)
4. c (P-126, Col-1)
5. b (P-124, Col-2)

PELVIS AND LOWER LIMB TRAUMA

1. d (P-117, Fig. 5.12a)
2. a (P-116, Col-2)
3. d
4. b (P-119, Col-1)
5. d (P-119, Col-1)
6. c (P-116, Col-1)
7. d (P-114, Col-2)
8. b (P-130, Table 5.9)
9. c
10. b; Patient is likely to have fracture neck of femur. Occult fractures are best diagnosed by MRI.
11. d; If age mentioned is 60–70 years prefer to mark intracapsular neck femur and if patient is more than 80 years old individual, then go with intertrochanteric fracture as the diagnosis in case there is limited information provided in the question, as in this one. If partial external rotation of lower limb and limited shortening is mentioned, then it is intracapsular fracture neck femur and if there is complete external rotation such that lateral border of the foot touches the couch then intertrochanteric fracture is the better possibility
12. b
13. b (P-125, Table 5.5)
14. c (P-126, Col-1)
15. d; Since the a mass (head) is felt in the gluteal region, it seem like a posterior dislocation of hip. When there is an associated acetabular fracture in a posteriorly dislocated hip external rotation deformity is also possible
16. a (P-125, Table 5.4); Thompson-Epstein type IV posterior dislocation of hip is associated with acetabular wall fracture (same situation as above)
17. b (P-129, Table 5.7)
18. d (P-128, Table 5.6)
19. a (P-131, Flow chart 5.2)
20. b (P-131, Flow chart 5.2)
21. c (P-131, Flow chart 5.2)
22. c (P-131, Flow chart 5.2); SP nail—An outdated implant that was used to fix neck femur fractures in the past
23. b (P-131, Flow chart 5.2)
24. b (P-131, Flow chart 5.2)
25. a, c, d
26. d (P-131, Flow chart 5.2); If on X-ray the physis is open, then Austin Moore's pins are the preferable choice. However, the option is not there in the question (rather the option is Austing Moore's prosthesis which is for hemiarthroplasty), so most appropriate choice would be (d)
27. a (P-134, High-yield points)
28. b, c, d (P-134, High-yield points)
29. d; AVN changes start in the sub-chondral area of femoral head; however the complication is most commonly seen with sub capital variety of intracapsular femoral neck fracture
30. a (P-140, *See* complications)
31. b (P-140, *See* complications)
32. a (P-138, Table 5.11)
33. c (P-142, Col-1)
34. c (P-141, Col-1)
35. c (P-141, Col-1)
36. a (P-126, Col-2)
37. b (P-142, High-yield points)
38. a (P-195, Col-2, High-yield points)
39. c (P-147, Col-1); Cylindrical cast may be given for undisplaced patellar fracture
40. d (P-147, Col-1)
41. c (P-147, Col-1)
42. d (P-145, Col-1) ABPI abnormal is 0.9 and critical limb ischemia is less than/equal to 0.4
43. b (P-154, Fig. 5.90)
44. a; Deeper muscles are more commonly involved as they travel more distally (viz FDL, FHL). Their ischemia can be tested by toe dorsiflexion which will be more specific than foot dorsiflexion (that stretches superficial muscles viz. Gastrocsoleus)
45. d (P-152, Box 5.1)
46. a (P-38, Box 2.13)
47. None. (P-160, Col-2, Fig. 5.108) Jones fracture is a fracture of the base of fifth metatarsal at junction of the metaphysis and diaphysis. It is caused by a direct blow on base of fifth metatarsal of a plantar flexed foot. Pseudo-Jones or Dancer's fracture is an avulsion fracture of the tip of the fifth metatarsal (Tuberosity avulsion fracture)
48. a (P-158, Col-2)
49. d (P-152, Box 5.1)
50. b (P-152, Box 5.1)
51. d (P-157, Col-2)
52. b (P-159, Fig. 5.102)
53. d
54. a; Recurrent dislocations are least commonly reported at ankle joint amongst the choices

SPORTS MEDICINE (LIGAMENT AND MENISCAL INJURIES OF KNEE, SHOULDER INSTABILITY AND ROTATOR CUFF TEAR)

1. b (P-183, Col-2)
2. a (P-190, Col-1 and Fig. 6.49)
3. b (P-186, Col-1)
4. b (P-183, Col-1); The posterolateral bundle of ACL is tight in extension. Laxity in extension indicates the bundle is torn.
5. b (P-193, Table 6.9)
6. a; ACL is attached to intercondylar area and a fracture in the area clearly means that the ligament is avulsed
7. b (P-195, Col-1, High-yield points)
8. d (P-187, Col-1)
9. a (P-193, Table 6.9)
10. c (P-187, Table 6.5)
11. c (P-195, High-yield points)
12. b (P-184, Table 6.4)
13. a (P-187, Col-1)
14. c
15. b.
16. c; Meniscus is injured by rotation/twisting force. Knee is locked in extension. Rotation is possible only on flexion;
17. c (P-192, Col-1)
18. d
19. b (P-192, Col-1)
20. a (P-65, Col-1)
21. b
22. b (P-65, Col-2)
23. d (P-66, Col-2)
24. d (P-164, Col-2)
25. b (P-167, Col-2)
26. c; In all varieties of shoulder dislocation, circumflex branch of axillary nerve is injured most commonly
27. d (P-164, Col-2)
28. b (P-165, Col-1)
29. d (P-178, Col-1)
30. a (P-199, Col-1)
31. a (P-172, Col-1)
32. c; No reference is there in literature. Since subscapularis tears are mostly overlooked it could be the forgotten muscle.
33. a

34. c (P-170, Fig. 6.13 b)
35. b (P-456, Col-1 and Fig. 17.14)
36. a (P-177, Col-1)
37. b (P-201, Col-1)
38. a
39. a (P-183, Col-2)
40. d (P-196, Col-2)
41. a (P-196, Col-2)
42. a (P-196, Col-2)
43. d (P-190, Col-1). This is segond fracture.
44. c (P-194, Col-2)

SPINE

1. a (P-221, Col-1, High-yield points)
2. d (P-211, Col-1); Spinal cord injury is upper motor neuron lesion so there would be hyper-reflexia below the level of lesion
3. b (P-212, Table 7.3)
4. a (P-214, Col-1)
5. b (P-215, Col-1); The complication here seems to be Neurogenic shock seen in injuries above T6 level. So site of injury is above T6. Now head injuries are most commonly associated with lower cervical spine injuries, so lower cervical spine seem to be best choice
6. c (P-216, Col-1)
7. c; Commonest level of spinal fracture is T12 vertebra
8. a (P-230 , Col-2, High-yield points)
9. b; Holdsworth classification was the earlier version of Denis three column concept
10. d (P-228, Col-1)
11. d (P-222, Col-1)
12. a (P-226, see chance fracture); More appropriate answer would be flexion distraction (Chance fracture)
13. d (P-214, Col-1)
14. a (P-243, Table 7.14)
15. d; Priapism is seen after spinal cord injury
16. c (P-242, Col-1, Fig. 7.61)
17. d (P-235, Col-2) Disk prolapse L4-L5 will compress L5 nerve root and myotome of L5 is EHL
18. a (P-249, Col-2)
19. d (P-246, Col-1)
20. b (P-211, Table 7.2, Fig. 7.6); C7 supplies the triceps reflex and middle finger.
21. b (P-228, Col-1)
22. c (P-226, Col-2)
23. c
24. b; Even in cervical spine in disk prolapse always the lower level nerve root is involved
25. c (P-237, Col-2)
26. a (P-403, Col-2)
27. b (P-389, Col-1)
28. d (P-228, Col-2)
29. c
30. d; Most dangerous is translation > flexion rotation > flexion distraction
31. a (P-221, Col-1)
32. b (P-225, Col-1)
33. a (P-222, Col-1)
34. b (P-215, Col-2, High-yield points)
35. d (see explanation of q.16)
36. a
37. a (P-251, Col-2)

PERIPHERAL NERVE INJURIES

1. c (P-255, see nerve conduction studies)
2. d (P-274, High-yield points)
3. a (P-257, Col-1, High-yield points)
4. b (P-257, Col-1 High-yield points)
5. c; Femoral nerve seems to best explain the picture. The nerve supplies the quadriceps. Although rare but if there is isolated sudden transaction of this nerve, the quadriceps will be paralyzed. This will lead to buckling of the knee as it cannot be extended and kept straight. The patient will fall onto the side of the injury and get injuries on single side of the body which has impacted the ground
6. c (P-270, Col-1)
7. b; The presentation is matching with lower plexus injury. The presence of supracondylar humerus fracture here is likely co-incidental
8. d (P-268, Col-2); Biceps and brachialis paralysis may cause some degree of elbow flexion weakness.
9. a (P-273, Table 8.2)
10. b (P-262 Col-1); Clasping sign, Pointing index and Pope sign are all synonymous terms
11. d (P-266, Col-2)
12. b (P-275, Col-1)
13. a (P-254, Col-2)
14. b
15. d (P-272, Col-2)
16. c (P-275, Col-2)
17. d (P-275, Col-2)
18. c (P-276, Table 8.3)
19. a
20. c (P-262, Fig. 8.15); Flexor pollicis longus is supplied by AIN, branch of median nerve given in proximal forearm and will cause flexion of thumb. Adductor pollicis will cause adduction as it is supplied by the ulnar nerve.
Abductor pollicis brevis (producing abduction of the thumb) and opponens pollicis (producing opposition of the thumb) are paralysed in low median nerve palsy (carpal tunnel syndrome). Abduction of the thumb is also carried out by abductor pollicis longus supplied by radial nerve so it will be maintained.
21. a (P-260, Col-2)
22. c (P-260, Fig. 8.12)
23. c
24. d (P-279, Col-2)
25. a (P-278, Col-1)
26. c (P-101, High yield points)
27. c (P-262, Col-2, see opponens pollicis)
28. b (P-260, Col-1)
29. d; Ulnar nerve supplies fine movements of the hand hence the result of injury is worse. A low lesion causes more of clawing (Ulnar paradox) and hence outcome of a low lesion is worst
30. c (P-259, Fig. 8.9)
31. d; Sensations will be carried by the superficial branch while the hypothenar muscles will be supplied by the deep branch. So, lesion is proximal to the division as both are lost
32. c (P-292, Box 9.6)
33. b (P-265, Fig. 8.23)
34. a (P-273, Col-1)
35. a (P-273, Fig. 8.37a)
36. d (P-274, Col-2)
37. d (P-274, Col-2 See Meralgia Paresthetica)
38. d (P-273, Col-2)
39. a; Guillain Barré is a demyelinating disease and a transient condition. Rest all other conditions involve permanent damage to nerves
40. a (P-272, Col-2, High-yield Points)
41. c; Carpal tunnel syndrome (Median nerve) is a common problem in patients involved in repetitive strain activities like typing etc.
42. b
43. c

44. c (P-265, Col-2)
45. a

INFECTIONS

1. a (P-310, Col-1); It is tuberculosis of phalanges (Tubercular dactylitis)
2. c (P-310, Col-1)
3. c; Facet joint > Spinous process are least involved structures in posterior TB
4. a (P-298, Col-2, see paradiskal type)
5. c
6. a (P-282, Box 9.1)
7. a (P-306, Col-1)
8. d (P-306, see stages of TB, Fig, 10.17A)
9. b (P-309, Col-1, Fig. 10.21)
10. a (P-296, Col-1)
11. b (P-296, Col-2; P-310, Col-1)
12. b (P-284, Col-1)
13. a
14. b (P-287, Col-2, High-yield Point)
15. b
16. a
17. d; Order of investigation in inflammatory joint swelling: X-Ray —> USG guided aspration of joint fluid —> MRI
18. d (P-289, Col-2)
19. a; The deformity Flexion, Abduction and External rotation points more towards TB hip. In AVN more commonly the problem would have been restricted abduction and internal rotation in early stages
20. b (P-291, Col-1, High yield points)
21. a (P-293, Col-2)
22. c (P-285, Box 9.3)
23. c; Prefer Transient synovitis over Perthes disease if it is there in the options
24. c
25. d (P-300, Col-2)
26. b (P-310, High yield points)
27. a, b, c (P-305, Table 10.3)
28. a (P-306, Col-2, stages of TB)
29. d (P-302, Col-1)
30. a, c, d; In TB arthritis ends in fibrous ankylosis while spondylitis ends in bony ankylosis. Although bony ankylosis is rare in osteoarthritis , it can occur in the joints of the fingers
31. a (P-284, Col-2)

TUMORS

1. b (P-312, Col-1)
2. d (319)
3. b (P-326, Col-1)
4. c (P-334, Box 11.5)
5. b (P-329, Col-1, High-yield Points)
6. a (P-319, Col-2)
7. c (P-319, Col-2); Both eosinophilic granuloma and osteoid osteoma can have the described picture. But since there is no mention of endosteal scalloping and considering the relative incidence, better to opt for choice (c)
8. a; Osteochondroma is common around growing end of long bones. Pelvis is although rare but next most common site.
9. a; Prefer Osteosarcoma > Osteoid Osteoma if there in choices
10. d; Some degree of hyperglycemia is associated with all malignant bone tumors. Chondrosarcoma is relatively best choice here.
11. c (P-318, Col-1)
12. b (P-323, Col-2, High-yield points); The closest variant of GCT can be taken as ABC although the authors could not find it anywhere in literature. The similarities include aggressive nature, lytic

expansile lesion, same site (GCT in young age is metaphyseal) and both have giant cells on biopsy and lack calcification that could be seen in cartilaginous lesions like Chondroblastoma
13. d (P-328, Col-2)
14. b (P-336, Col-1)
15. c (P-327, Col-2)
16. b (P-333, Col-1); This seems to be case of Glomus tumor
17. b (P-332, Col-1)
18. b (P-337, Col-2, High-yield point)
19. c
20. a (P-321, Col-1)
21. a (P-334, Box 11.5)
22. c (P-311 , Table 11.1)
23. b (P-329, Col-1, High-yield point)
24. d (P-322, Col-1)
25. c (P-336, Col-1)
26. b (P-316, Fig. 11.11)
27. c; Although osteoblastoma can occur at this site, lytic and expansile appearance goes in favor of ABC
28. b; Osteosarcoma is very rare in the small bones of hand and feet
29. d
30. b (P-327, Box 11.3)
31. b (P-328, Col-1)
32. b
33. b (P-328, Col-2)
34. a (P-332, Col-1)
35. b, c, d
36. d (P-333, Col-2)
37. a (P-336, Col-2)
38. d (P-334, Table 11.6)
39. d; It could be metastasis, more likely than multiple myeloma, considering the site, the age and the incidence.
40. a; Preference order in the case should be: X-ray > MRI > Bone biopsy
41. d (P-334, Table 11.6)
42. a; The patient can have metastasis from prostatic carcinoma or the back pain could simply be due to degenerative spine disease. Alkaline phosphatase will confirm presence of skeletal metastasis and thereafter if levels are raised, work up for prostatic carcinoma can be taken up. Going for Acid phosphatase will only detect prostatic carcinoma but not indicate whether it has metastasized or not
43. b
44. a (P-320, Col-2)
45. a, b, c, e; GCT commonly involves the epiphysis and metaphysis but rarely erodes the articular surfaces. Even while it expands it is mostly covered by a thin shell of reactive bone. So some covering will remain as the tumor will expand
46. b
47. a (P-318, Col-1)
48. d
49. b (P-328, Col-1)
50. d; Bone scans have limited ability to determine intraosseous extent of bone lesions or to demonstrate extraosseous soft tissue extensions.

PEDIATRIC ORTHOPEDICS

1. a (P-340, Col-1); Poliomyelitis is a cause of secondary (acquired CTEV)
2. c (P-371, Col-1)
3. d (P-363) Normal position of head or ossification center is lower medial quadrant.
4. a (P-374, Col-2)
5. d (P-355, Col-2)
6. a (P-378, Col-2)

7. d (P-381, Col-1)
8. c (P-380, Col-1)
9. d (P-375, Fig 12.72)
10. d; Age, limp and restricted abduction and internal rotation, all go in favor of Perthes disease
11. c (P-374, Col-1, Fig. 12.69a)
12. c (P-367, Col-2, see maintenance of reduction)
13. d
14. b (P-363)
15. b; If there is an inborn external twist in tibia (External tibial torsion), the patient will walk with feet pointing outwards (Charlie Chaplin gait)
16. a (P-360, Col-2)
17. d (P-343, Col-2); Rocker bottom foot can occur after congenital vertical talus or improper treatment in CTEV and can be associated with syndromic conditions like Arthrogryposis, Neurofibromatosis, Trisomy 13-15 and 18, Spina bifida and Prune Belly syndrome.
18. a (P-339)
19. b (P-342) Treatment should be started as soon as possible after birth.
20. b (P-345, Fig. 12.15)
21. a (P-339, Table 12.1)
22. c Talus is most deformed bone in CTEV.
23. d (P-349-50); There is overriding or under riding of first/great toe over second toe
24. c
25. a (P-365, Col-1)
26. b; Even the slightest possibility of septic arthritis needs to be ruled out in this case. So first ultrasound should be done and if it shows any collection then it should be immediately aspirated under ultrasound guidance
27. c (P-381, Col-2)
28. b Although difficult to conclude answer, Genu valgum may not be present bilaterally in these cases and is not a uniform association, so best choice to choose will be (b)
29. d (Read "Congenital dislocation of knee" from P-362, Col-1)
30. b (P-362, Box 12.4); Most common cause of genu valgum in a child is idiopathic > rickets
31. d (P-359, Col-2)
32. a, c, d, e (see explanation of Q 18 for conditions where there can be Rocker bottom foot. Choice b is not correct as Grice Green procedure is a surgical treatment option for Congenital Vertical Talus, a cause of Rocker Bottom foot)
33. a (P-343, Col-2)
34. b (P-344, Col-1)
35. d (P-354, Col-1)
36. c (P-380, Col-2)
37. d (P-382, Col-2)
38. (P-382, Col-2) None; Caffey's disease is self limiting. Steroids and Indomethacin are used during the acute flare ups
39. d (P-352, Col-1)
40. c; Lateral condyle humerus is a physeal fragment. Excision will lead to growth disturbance
41. b (P-360, Col-1)
42. a (P-353, Fig. 12.31)
43. c (P-355, Col-2)

NEUROMUSCULAR DISORDERS

1. c (P-386, Col-2)
2. a (P-386, Col-2 and Fig. 13.5)
3. b (P-387, Col-2)
4. d (P-387, Col-2); Tendon transfers in polio should be done atleast after 2 years of onset of disease as some spontaneous recovery is possible till then. However, the child must be atleast 4 years or more in age so that he can comply with the surgical rehabilitation program.
5. c; Tibialis anterior is dorsiflexor while Gastrocsoleus is plantarflexor. The former is stronger so foot will go into calcaneus. Also peronei are weak so foot will be pulled into inversion (Strong Tibialis anterior will also assist in inversion) leading finally to calcaneovarus
6. d (P-386, Col-2)
7. c (P-386, Col-2)

GENETIC AND DEVELOPMENTAL DISORDERS

1. b (P-390, Col-1, Paragraph 1)
2. d (P-392, Col-2); Here actually all options are correct, but few studies have shown fracture healing is normal and poor results are seen in fractures needing fixation. The latter is difficult due to distorted hard bone structure. So choice (d) is best to choose
3. d (P-398, Col-1); Scoliosis is the commonest of these
4. d (P-398, Col-2, see High-yield points)
5. b (P-392, Col-2)
6. d (P-394, Fig. 14.8)
7. b (P-391, Col-1)
8. a (P-393, Col-1)
9. c (P-390, Col-1, Fig. 14.1)
10. c (P-398, Col-2)
11. a (P-395, Col-1)
12. a (P-391, Col-1 and Fig. 14.2)
13. c (P-391, Col-1)
14. b (P-399, Table 14.4)
15. a; Ring shaped epiphysis is seen in Rickets, Scurvy, Osteogenesis Imperfecta, Hypothyroidism and Osteopetrosis
[*Ref.* Pediatric radiological signs textbook by Michael Grunebaum, Vol 1]
16. d (P-396) Although no choice is appropriate choice (d) seems to be best to choose. The fractures don't unite easily as the bone fixation is difficult although many studies say that the healing is normal
17. b
18. d (P-395, Col-2, High yield points)
19. c (P- 396)

METABOLIC BONE DISEASES

1. a (P-403, Col-1) Parathormone is given subcutaneously.
2. d (P-403, Col-2, see High-yield points)
3. d (P-414, Col-1, Fig. 15.11D)
4. a (P-402, Col-1). Long term use of bisphosphonate can cause atypical subtrochanteric fracture.
5. a, c
6. d (P-404, Col-1, see High-yield points)
7. d (P-400, Col-2, see investigations)
8. a (P-413, Col-2)
9. a (P-400, Table 15.1)
10. c (P-409, Col-1)
11. d; Steroids cause osteoporosis
12. d (P-403, Col-2)
13. a (P-415, Col-1)
14. b (P-415, Col-1)
15. b (P-7, Col-2)
16. b (P-405, Col-1); Long bones of legs get deformed only after the child starts weight bearing
17. d (P-410, Col-2)
18. c (P-413, Fig. 15.9 c)
19. d (P-412, Col-2)
20. d (P-410, Col-2 and see High-yield points)
21. c (See Metacarpal sign page 413, Col-1, High-yield points);
22. d (P-409, Col-2)

23. c
24. a; Bone density increases in fluorosis
25. d (P-400, Col-2)
26. a (P-415, Col-2)
27. a (P-415, Col-2)
28. a; Paget's disease can have asymptomatic presentation with high ALP, normal calcium and phosphate. Multiple myeloma will have normal ALP levels while osteomalacia and hyperparathyroidism will have abnormalities in calcium and phosphorous levels
29. b (P-409, Col-1)
30. c (P-409, Col-2)
31. c (P-409, Col-1, see High-yield points)
32. d (P-410, Col-1)
33. a (P-411, Col-2)
34. b (Bone resorption is seen in phalanges)
35. d; (P-412, Col-2) Age, raised calcium, low phosphate and markedly increased alkaline phosphatase, all suggest diagnosis of Hyperparathyroidism
36. c (P-414, Col-1)
37. d; Deafness can occur due to both cranial nerve compression and otosclerosis. The former is not consistently present and hence otosclerosis is a better choice.
38. c (P-401, Box-15.1)
39. a (P-400, Col-2)
40. d (P-400, Table 15.1)
41. d; Drug of choice for both senile and postmenopausal osteoporosis are bisphosphonates. However, where osteoporosis is resistant to bisphosphonates, Teriparatide has shown good results.
42. b (see explanation of Q.41)
43. d; Adequate vitamin D is required in the body for absorption of calcium.
44. d (P-408, Flow chart 15.3)
45. a (P-403, Col-1, see recombinant parathormone)
46. c (P-415, Col-1)
47. a

ARTHRITIS AND RELATED DISORDERS

1. c (P-417, Col-2)
2. b (P-418, Table 16.1)
3. c (P-418, Table 16.1)
4. d (P-418, Table 16.1)
5. b (P-437, Col-2, Fig. 16.26a)
6. b (P-437, Fig. 16.24) 1st CMC joint is commonly involved in OA
7. b (P-428, Col-2)
8. b; All spondyloarthropathies may be associated with calcaneal spur formation
9. c (P-446, Col-1)
10. b; Osteoclasis is surgical fracture of bone performed to correct malunion of a fractured bone
11. b (P-444, Col-2)
12. b (See Martel sign Page 434 and Fig. 16.22 B)
13. b (P-435, Col-2)
14. a (P-435, Col-2)
15. a (P-445, Col-1)
16. b; (P-445, High yield points) Commonest cause of loose body in knee in elderly and overall is osteoarthritis while in young patients it is osteochondritis dissecans.
17. c (P-437, Table 16.8)
18. d (P-437, Table 16.8)
19. b (Involvement of distal hand joints in 30–50 years age is classical of psoriatic arthropathy; P-437 Table 16.8)
20. d; RA can involve cervical spine causing instability in the C1-C2 region

21. b; (P-422, Col-1) Earliest X-ray sign of RA is soft tissue swelling > Periarticular osteopenia
22. d (P-437, Table 16.8)
23. d (P-421, Col-1) Deformities in RA are characteristic of disease but not pathognomonic
24. c (P-420, Col-1)
25. c; Wind swept deformity may be seen in both RA and Rickets; conventional use is for Rickets
26. d (P-431, Col-1); Most common cause of reactive arthritis is *Chlamydia > Shigella*
27. b (Raised ESR, restricted chest movements, syndesmophytes suggest ankylosing spondylitis although age is unfavoring. DISH is a possiblilty but see P-430, Table 16.6 to see differences between AS and DISH and reasons to rule out DISH); Ankylosing hyperostosis is same as DISH
28. d (P-432, Col-2 and Fig. 16.20)
29. a (P-441, Col-2)
30. b (P-440, Table 16.10)
31. a (P-291, Col-2)
32. a (P-432, Col-1)
33. b (P-440)
34. a (P-440, Table 16.10)
35. d; There are very few reports regarding elbow involvement by Charcot's disease
36. a (P-434, Col-1)
37. c (P-434, Col-2)
38. c (See P-435 Col-2 for causes of chondrocalcinosis)
39. d; Detection of CPPD crystals is diagnostic of CPPD arthropathy. It is often associated with hypothyroidism
40. a (See Tumoral Calcinosis on P-436, Col-1)
41. c (P-352, Col-2) In Behcet syndrome arthritis is self-limited, non-deforming, non-erosive, and mono/oligoarthritis.
42. c; Arthritis in SLE and Behçet's disease is non-erosive
43. a (The first line drug for osteoarthritis is Paracetamol/acet-aminophen)
44. d (P-439, Col-1)
45. b (A history of steroid intake, restricted abduction and internal rotation at hip is pointing towards AVN)
46. a (P-443, Col-2)
47. d (P-443, Col-2)
48. d
49. b
50. a (P-437, Col-2)
51. c (P-437, Table 16.8)
52. a (P-420, Col-1)
53. d
54. a (P-423, Col-2); Extra-articular manifestations warrant steroids in RA
55. a (P-437, Table 16.8)
56. c (P-437, Table 16.8)
57. a (P-429, Col-2)
58. a (P-442, Col-1)
59. c; Hemophilia is a relative contraindication as there is risk of uncontrolled hemorrhage
60. a (P-261, Col-2)
61. c (P-434, Col-1)
62. a (P-435, Col-2)
63. a, b, c, d
64. b (P-445, Col-2)
65. d (P-443, Col-1)

66. b (P-432, Col-1)
67. d
68. c (P-446, Col-2)
69. b (P-446, Col-2); Anterolateral part of superior weight bearing zone of head is first region to be involved
70. c (P-442, Col-1); Limitation of abduction and internal rotation is a characteristic clinical feature in AVN that occurs due to alteration in shape of femoral head. Use of protease inhibitors in HIV patients is an associated risk factor for AVN.
71. b (P-442, Col-1)
72. d, a (P-419, Col-1)
73. a, c, e; Extra-articular manifestations may be seen in up to one third patients of rheumatoid arthritis
74. a (P-425, Col-1, High-Yield points)
75. d (P-425, Col-1, High-Yield points)
76. d
77. a (P-425, Col-1)
78. b; Xanthine oxidase inhibitor (Allopurinol) is rather a treatment drug in gout
79. b (P-430, Col-2)
80. b (P-431, Col-1)
81. c (P-421, Col-2)
82. a (P-423, Table, 16.4)
83. d; (Read extra-articular manifestations of Ra from P-421)
84. b (P-435); APE are manifestation of chondrocalcinosis in monkeys
85. a (P-443, Col-1)

SOFT TISSUE DISORDERS

1. b(P-450, Col-1)
2. a (P-450, Col-1)
3. a (P-457, Col-1); The likely diagnosis is Frozen shoulder and the treatment is conservative as it is a self-limiting condition.
4. a (P-443, Col-2)
5. b (P-198, Table 6.13)
6. b
7. a (P-457, Col-2)
8. b (P-175, Col-2); The likely cause is Tennis elbow.
9. d (P-453, Col-2)
10. a (P-453, Col-2)
11. a> b (Fig. 453, Col-2)
12. d (P-453, Col-1)
13. a (P-106, Col-2) A1 pulley is present at MCP joint.
14. a;(P-443, Col-1) This is movie sign of Chondromalacia patellae (P-362)
15. a
16. b (P-452, Fig. 17.6)
17. b (P-450, Col-2, Fig. 17.2b)
18. d; RA is known to cause tendon attritions and ruptures by causing synovitis of tendon sheaths. Colles fracture has dorsal displacement of distal radius fragment that impinges and ruptures extensor tendons. Drummer's boy palsy is EPL tendon rupture due to repetitive use. Ans is Dequervain as the same does not involve EPL. It is tenosynovitis of APL and EPB.

AMPUTATIONS, PROSTHETICS AND ORTHOTICS

1. a (P-463, Col-1)
2. d; A below knee amputation is avoided in diabetics due to vascular issues
3. d (P-464, Col-1); but if TENS is a choice, it should be preferred
4. d
5. c; Least effective of the mentioned modalities is ultrasound
6. b (P-463, Fig 18.2)
7. d (P-464, Col-2, see High-Yield points)
8. c (P-466, Table 18.1)

9. c,a (P-462, Col-2)
10. d (P-462, Col-2)

ORTHOPEDIC SURGERIES, EVOLUTION AND LATEST TRENDS

1. b (P-478, 479, Box 19.6 and 7)
2. c (P-481, Col-1, see High-yield points)
3. b; Most common cause of death after THR is MI > Pulmonary embolism
4. a (P-479, Col-2)
5. b (P-478, Col-2)
6. a
7. c (P-474, Col-1)
8. c (P-476, Box 19.3)
9. c; Jones tendon transfer is for radial nerve palsy; Watson-Jones approach is for lateral exposure of hip as may be required during hip replacement surgery; modified Jones procedure is done in claw toes for deformity correction; And Watson Jones procedure is also a treatment option for chronic ankle instability.
10. d (P-493, Col-2)
11. d (P-485, Col-2); Rush pins are used for fixation of fracture shaft femur in children
12. c (P-470, Col-1)
13. a (P-494, Col-2)
14. c; (P-493, Col-2) No answer is absolutely correct but Gluteus medius seems to be most appropriate
15. a (P-470, Col-2)
16. d Morel Lavallée lesion (P-113, Col-2); is present over lateral side while Kocher Langenbeck is a posterior approach (P-493, Col-2)
17. b. Cobra plate is specially designed plate for hip arthrodesis. (P-134, Fig. 5.48)

PICTURE QUIZ

1. a; The attitude depicted in of Inferior dislocation of shoulder
2. c; The child has cubitus varus deformity secondary to malunited supracondylar humerus fracture
3. c
4. a; The X-ray is showing sun ray appearance
5. c
6. a
7. a
8. b
9. d
10. a; The X-ray is showing classical Bamboo spine appearance
11. d; The child in picture has a wind swept deformity
12. c
13. b; The patient has been put on a modified Dunlop traction
14. a
15. b; CT scan is depicting the classical polka dot pattern seen in vertebral hemangioma
16. b; The X-ray is showing soap bubble appearance classical of a Giant cell tumor. Moreover, distal end of radius is a very common site of affection
17. d; The X-ray is showing Erlenmeyer flask deformity
18. c; The examiner is performing Finkelstcin's test
19. d; The lift off test is being performed
20. b; Proximal femur has a shepherd crook deformity
21. b; Anterior angulation and anterior dislocation of head are seen in Type I
22. a; X-ray is showing intracapsular neck femur fracture
23. c; X-ray is showing the classical bone within bone appearance
24. b
25. d
26. a
27. a

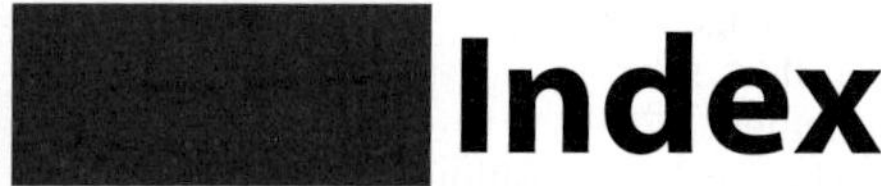# Index

Page numbers followed by *b* refer to box, *f* refer to figure, *fc* refer to flow chart, and *t* refer to table.